Psychiatric *and* Mental Health Nursing *in the* UK

Psychiatric and Mental Health Nursing in the UK

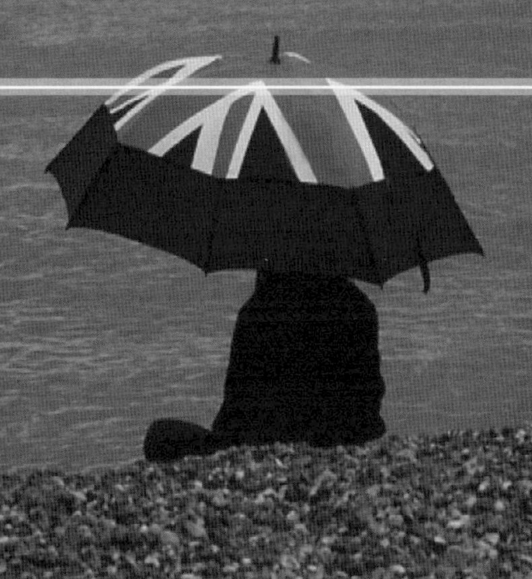

Edited by

Katie Evans RN, BA, MLitSt, PhD
Mental Health Education Consultant

Debra Nizette RN, DipAppSc (Nursing Ed), BAppSc (Nursing), MNursSt, Credentialed MHN, FACN, FACMHN
Director of Nursing, Queensland Health, Queensland, Australia

Anthony O'Brien RN, BA, MPhil (Hons), PhD, FNZMHN
Senior Lecturer in Mental Health Nursing, University of Auckland;
Nurse Specialist in Liaison Psychiatry, Auckland District Health Board, Auckland, New Zealand

UK Adapting Author

Catherine Johnson RMN, RGN
Registered General Nurse at Guy's and St. Thomas' NHS Foundation Trust;
Clinical Nurse Specialist at West London Mental Health NHS Trust, London, UK

Foreword by

Gemma Stacey MN PGCHE RN (Mental Health)
Associate Professor in the School of Health Sciences and Program Lead for Graduate Entry Nursing, University of Nottingham; Lecturer in Mental Health and Social Care, School of Nursing, Midwifery and Physiotherapy, University of Nottingham, Derby Education Centre, London Road Community Hospital, Derby, UK

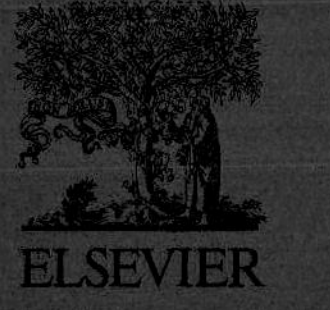

ELSEVIER

Edinburgh London New York Oxford Philadelphia St Louis Sydney 2020

ISBN: 978-0-7020-8024-1

Content Strategist: Serena Castelnovo/Poppy Garraway
Content Development Specialist: Fiona Conn
Senior Project Manager: Karthikeyan Murthy
Designer: Brian Salisbury
Marketing Manager: Samantha Page

Printed in China

Last digit is the print number: 9 8 7 6 5 4 3 2 1

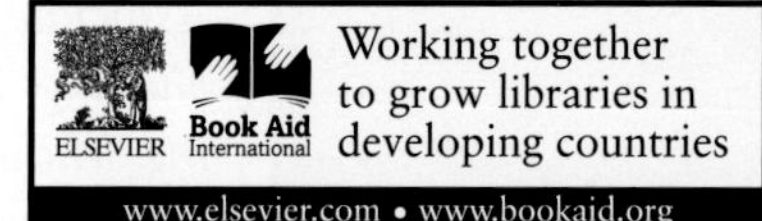

CONTENTS

FOREWORD

PSYCHIATRIC AND MENTAL HEALTH NURSING IN THE UK: FOREWORD

As student nurses embark on the field of mental health nursing or encounter people with mental health problems in their clinical placements, they are often faced with numerous questions. These can relate to the role they should adopt, how to respond to the patient in a helpful way or how to process the consequent emotions they experience. The answers to these questions are not simple as they encompass ethical dilemmas, professional issues and personal conflicts.

It is repeatedly stated that learning of this nature cannot be gained from a book as it requires a level of critical reflection underpinned by the development of self-awareness. However, *Psychiatric and Mental Health Nursing in the UK* addresses this challenge by offering the reader the opportunity to continuously consider theoretical concepts in the context of the dilemmas mental health nursing practice creates. This is a unique feature of this text as it situates theory in the authentic circumstance and encourages the reader to apply knowledge to practice in a range of complex settings.

The authenticity of the text is enabled by the variety of contributors who offer a contemporary and pragmatic account of their expertise. The reader will benefit from the accessibility of the material, which facilitates ease of understanding without over-simplifying the complexity of the skills and knowledge required to be an effective mental health nurse. The text utilises the accounts of practitioners, patients and their families throughout to illuminate key issues for the nurse. This further enhances the authenticity of the text as the stories engage the student and promote consideration of how they may feel as the professional in that scenario.

The values underpinning the text reflect a contemporary view of mental health nursing practice and reiterate the essential role of the mental health nurse in promoting person-centred care in a manner which facilitates recovery. This thread runs through the entire text to critically discuss the diversity of the populations mental health nurses work with and the social disadvantage associated with a mental health diagnosis. Consequently, the text offers a bio-psycho-social representation of mental distress and accordingly explores the range of interventions mental health nurses can implement in their practice.

The core and unique contribution of the mental health nurse is clearly articulated and advocated. This is a welcome contribution to the literature, as this is often lacking for mental health nurses due to the curriculum in the UK becoming increasingly generic in nature. Whilst an increased awareness of the needs of people with mental health problems amongst the other fields of practice is essential, the unique knowledge and skills of mental health nurses requires the level of articulation demonstrated in this text. The content of this book will speak to those who have actively selected mental health practice as their vocation and have a desire to promote effective and person-centred practice for people accessing mental health services.

Dr Gemma Stacey, PhD, MN, RN (Mental Health), PGCHE

University of Nottingham, School of Health Sciences

INTRODUCTION TO UK EDITION

I was delighted to be offered the opportunity to adapt *Psychiatric and Mental Health Nursing* for publication in the UK. Originally written for nurses training in Australia and New Zealand, the book offers a valuable resource for student nurses and newly qualified practitioners alike. It gives a global perspective on mental health nursing, and reflects on how international historical practices have shaped our services today, exploring the subject matter in an engaging and user-friendly format.

Throughout, the text has been adapted to bring it in line with UK terminology, policies, practices and service provision. Combining local, national and global perspectives in this way is intended to encourage the reader to reflect on their individual practice and examine the international body of research, literature and evidence base available, ultimately ensuring that people accessing mental health services receive the best possible evidence-based care and treatment available.

It is a very exciting time to work within the field of mental health nursing: no two days are the same and nurses are offered exceptional rewards and the privilege to make a real difference in the lives of the people that they work with. Nurses' Stories throughout the chapters, adapted in parts to increase the relevance to UK services, serve to inspire and to give insight into real-life practice.

Case Studies have been included in the text, again adapted where appropriate to the UK context. These help the reader apply theory to everyday practice, and encourage routine reflective learning; particularly beneficial when approaching the transition from being a responsible student to an accountable registered practitioner. The robust foundations built by the reader can be depended upon throughout their career, helping them to develop a toolkit of skills, approaches and knowledge.

It can be a daunting prospect making the transition to becoming a registered nurse, but every day brings new learning opportunities and chances to consolidate the skills that have been learnt and translate them into providing evidence-based services. Critical Thinking Challenges and Ethical Dilemmas explore complex issues and encourage the reader to consider and discuss them. Exercises for Class Engagement at the end of each chapter complement this learning and development, promoting the examination of nursing literature around current best practice and encouraging opportunities to learn through role play scenarios, simulating practice experiences and helping to challenge the current processes. As simulation learning is increasingly used in both practice and education settings (for example in OSCE examinations), honing these skills early will prove invaluable.

Increasingly there are opportunities for mental health nurses to work within a diverse range of settings and undertake advanced roles within specialist areas, including clinical academic pathways.

Mental health nursing offers an opportunity to connect with people, their families and broader support networks at many stages of their recovery journey and beyond, supporting people to reach their potential and live fulfilling lives, maintaining mental wellness. I hope that the readers enjoy this text as much as I do as they embark upon their mental health nursing careers.

Catherine Johnson

INTRODUCTION

We are pleased to introduce our fourth edition of *Psychiatric and Mental Health Nursing* and to inform you about the changes we have made to the content and welcome Anthony O'Brien from the University of Auckland to the editorial team. Anthony has always been a contributing author, and now he is a worthy successor to Ruth Elder who is enjoying her retirement after 35 years in the service of mental health nursing. Anthony's knowledge has been invaluable in keeping our comprehensive Australian and New Zealand focus balanced and contemporary.

Psychiatric and Mental Health Nursing was conceived in 2002 as the first comprehensive Australasian mental health nursing textbook. The book was a response to the need we as academics felt to provide Australian and New Zealand nurses with an accessible local text, designed to actively engage undergraduate nursing students with relevant examples describing the people and conditions they encountered in their learning and working environments. With the help of our contributing authors, selected for their expertise in the field of mental health, we created a local alternative to overseas productions that focussed on social, cultural, legal and legislative contexts foreign to us, our students and our mental health nursing colleagues. As the text has evolved over the past 15 years, these goals have remained our primary concern. Although we now have some local competition, our regular, stringent revisions ensure that *Psychiatric and Mental Health Nursing* will continue to be a most valuable and influential text, grounded in the realities of mental health nurses' everyday learning and working lives.

We promote the effective mental health nursing of consumers/service users who experience problems caused by mental distress and illness, while maintaining an awareness of historical influences on contemporary practice and service delivery. We have maintained our traditional focus on a broad theoretical and philosophical basis for mental health nursing while envisioning the mental health nurse as a practitioner with a recovery orientation who is highly skilled in a wide range of effective interventions.

Nurses work with people, so recovery-informed practice and person-centred care remain our primary priorities. We are privileged that the internationally known consumer, author and artist Simon Champ agreed to write the Foreword and to co-author Chapter 2. Simon was one of the first consumer advocates in Australia in the documentary *Spinning Out* (Deveson 1991) and he has been a catalyst for debate and change as an advisor on the first National Strategy for Mental Health, a board member of SANE Australia, an early member of Schizophrenia Fellowship New South Wales and an invited speaker and teacher nationally and internationally.

Our fourth edition has been revised extensively to reflect the changing views about mental health, mental health services and mental health nursing in Australia and New Zealand. We have increased the number of sections from three to five, to better focus the contents, and to address emerging issues such as the transitioning of mental health care to primary care, the development of peer- and service-user-led services, accreditation, credentialing and the MHNIP (Mental Health Nurse Incentive Program). Along with chapters on the most familiar clinical syndromes that mental health nurses and students will see in clinical practice, we have introduced new material in the areas of mental health promotion, physical healthcare and challenging behaviours.

Our aim throughout was not merely to describe the consumer's experience or diagnosis, but also to propose ways that the nurse can go beyond passive listening and offer constructive suggestions about what to say and do to help the consumer.

- Part 1 *Preparing for psychiatric and mental health nursing* explores what it means to be a nurse; the history of mental illness and mental healthcare; the consumer and recovery-focussed practice; the political, legal, ethical and professional contexts of practice; and the wide variety of settings in which mental health nurses work.
- Part 2 *Influences on mental health* aims to contextualise the influences upon both the nurse and the person with a mental disorder, examining theories about mental health and wellness across the lifespan and within societies and cultures, as well as how physical health, trauma, crisis, loss and grief can affect a person's mental wellbeing.
- Part 3 *The people with whom mental health nurses work* examines specific populations that the nurse will encounter in Australia and New Zealand: indigenous peoples; children and adolescents; older people; the families of mental health consumers; those with an intellectual disability; and people who have become involved with the criminal justice system in a forensic setting.
- Part 4 *Mental disorders that people experience* develops a better understanding of the major mental illnesses; examines DSM-5 diagnoses, interventions and effective treatments; and incorporates the client's experience of mental illness.
- Part 5 *What mental health nurses can do to help* is the active part that brings together the interventions and expertise mental health nurses can offer in clinical situations: mental health promotion; prevention; primary care; assessment and diagnosis; risk assessment; psychopharmacology; and therapeutic skill development.

Rigorous reviews were commissioned both before and after this revision. Reviewers were enormously supportive of the changes we have made. References have been updated, although we believe that the 5-year rule does not apply to seminal references. References to DSM-IV TR have been updated to DSM-5, which we chose to use because it is a consistent diagnostic system that is widely used in Australia, New Zealand and internationally, and we believe that nurses need to be aware of how diagnostic categories are used in practice and in research.

Lists of Useful Websites, Nurses' Stories and Consumer Stories have been added to every chapter, and we have included many new authors to add to the contemporary, current practice-based approach. Each chapter is structured beginning with key points, key terms and learning outcomes, and concludes with questions and exercises that will facilitate teaching and learning. Critical thinking challenges, class engagement activities, nurses' stories, case studies and research briefs encourage an active awareness of the complex issues related to mental health and illness.

One of the unique features of *Psychiatric and Mental Health Nursing* has always been the nurses' stories. Every chapter incorporates nurses' stories—short vignettes illustrating the oral, traditional knowledge possessed by practising psychiatric mental health nurses—to assist students to develop insights about the world of clinical practice. Each editor has spent a lifetime working in mental health nursing, in practical, academic and managerial roles. Our own early experiences of hospital training led us to fear that much of the concentrated practical and mentoring aspects that enlivened and enhanced our training could be lost as nurses age and leave the profession. Indeed, many of our original contributors have left the workforce in the past 8 years, and with every year that passes it seems to us to be more imperative than ever to gather, utilise and preserve the skills and knowledge of existing practitioners of mental health and psychiatric nursing.

In this new edition you will discover many new chapters and authors and other chapters that have been rigorously revised. Significant changes from the previous edition include:

- Chapter 4 *Professional, legal and ethical issues* incorporates Chapters 4 and 5 from the third edition into a new chapter that addresses aspects of the Australian and New Zealand politico-legal context, and the professional and ethical issues that guide and regulate mental health nursing practice.
- Chapter 6 *Mental health theory and influence across the lifespan* merges Chapters 8 and 9 from the third edition into a chapter that links mental health nursing theory to the lifespan approach to formulate a more holistic approach.
- Chapter 8 *Physical health* is a new chapter. It addresses the physical health of people with mental health problems and conditions that have an association with an increased risk of mental health problems.
- Chapter 10 *Working with families in mental health* is a revision of Chapter 24 from the third edition, revised and renamed to more specifically address working with the families of people with mental health problems.
- Chapter 22 *Mental health promotion, prevention and primary healthcare* is a new chapter that engages with the ways in which early intervention can either prevent or alleviate the effects of mental health problems, and how nurses are increasingly involved in different primary healthcare services.
- Chapter 24 *Challenging behaviour, risk and responses* is a new chapter. Risk assessment can be found in different contexts in many chapters, but this dedicated chapter presents a range of risk assessments specifically focussed on challenging behaviours.

We thank the students, academics and mental health professionals who have supported and accepted what we have to say. We hope that our text will continue to have a wide appeal because of its practical approach and the support it offers students and teachers as well as practitioners in any setting who work with people who have a mental health problem. In an environment where mental health nurses are moving towards greater professional autonomy and technical and professional evolution is continuous and inevitable, we want above all to stress the importance of a personal and humane approach to psychiatric mental health nursing practice.

Katie Evans
Debra Nizette
Anthony O'Brien

ABOUT THE EDITORS

Katie Evans
RN, BA, MLitSt, PhD

Katie has researched, written, taught and convened undergraduate and postgraduate mental health nursing programmes at the University of Queensland, Queensland University of Technology, Griffith University, Central Queensland University and Queensland Health. At present she designs education programmes on a freelance basis in a range of domestic and overseas contexts for nursing, mental health and forensic mental health students, as well as writing for pleasure. Her research includes a master's degree tracing the social evolution of women in the literature from Homer to Euripides, and a PhD investigating the existence of mental disorders in the ancient Greek and Roman literature, and their survival across time and culture.

Debra Nizette
RN, DipAppSc (Nursing Ed), BAppSc (Nursing), MNursSt, Credentialed MHN, FACN, FACMHN

The interpersonal nature of mental health nursing, developing practice through listening, reflection and research remain central to Deb's interest in and love of mental health nursing. Leadership, professional recognition for nurses through the development of specialisation pathways and mechanisms to support nursing practice and quality care delivery are also long-held interests. Deb has developed and convened courses in nursing and mental health nursing in health service and university settings and held practice and professional leadership roles. Deb enjoys working in partnership creating innovative and strategic projects that support nursing's contribution to health and wellbeing.

Anthony O'Brien
RN, BA, MPhil (Hons), PhD, FNZMHN

Anthony graduated as a registered male nurse in Dunedin in 1977 and as a psychiatric nurse in Auckland in 1982. Anthony is currently employed at the University of Auckland as a senior lecturer in mental health nursing and with the Auckland District Health Board as a nurse specialist in liaison psychiatry. Anthony's PhD research investigated variation in the use of mental health legislation, including the roles of social deprivation, clinical decision making and service provision. Anthony's interests are in social issues related to mental illness, and legal and ethical issues. Research areas include media reporting of suicide, advance directives and use of community treatment orders.

Catherine Johnson
RMN, RGN

Catherine initially qualified as a registered mental health nurse in Cornwall in 2005, subsequently working within inpatient services across London before moving to New Zealand to undertake a post within forensic services. On returning to the UK, Catherine worked as a community mental health nurse, during which time she became increasingly interested in holistic healthcare. This inspired her to become a dual-trained practitioner, graduating as a registered general nurse in 2014. This provided Catherine with an opportunity to work as a clinical nurse specialist addressing the physical healthcare of patients in inpatient mental health services in London.

CONTRIBUTORS

Mandy Allman, RMN, MNurs
Clinical Nurse Specialist, Te Ao Maramatanga, NZNO, New Zealand

Gail Anderson, RN, MN, Adolescent Mental Health Cert, MACN
Clinical Nurse Consultant, Adolescent Health, Westmead Hospital, Westmead, New South Wales, Australia

Peter Athanasos, RN, BA, BSc (Hons), PhD (Pharmacology)
Clinical Nurse, Emergency Department and Cramond Clinic, The Queen Elizabeth Hospital, South Australia; Adjunct Senior Lecturer, Griffith University, Queensland; Adjunct Senior Lecturer, Flinders University, South Australia, Australia

Patricia Barkway, RN, Credentialed MHN, BA, MSc (PHC), FACMHN
Senior Lecturer, Mental Health Nursing, School of Nursing and Midwifery, Flinders University, Adelaide, South Australia, Australia

Priscilla Anne Brebner, RPN, PGDip MHN
President, Te Ao Māramatanga, New Zealand College of Mental Health Nurses, New Zealand

Scott Brunero, DipApSc, BAHsc, MA (Nurs Prac)
Clinical Nurse Consultant, Prince of Wales Hospital, Sydney, New South Wales, Australia

Simon Champ, BA (Visual Arts), PostGrad Dip (Visual Arts)
Practising Artist

Michelle Cleary, RN, PhD
Professor of Mental Health Nursing, School of Health Sciences, University of Tasmania, Sydney, New South Wales, Australia

Wendy M. Cross, RN, BAppSc, MEd, PhD, FACMHN, FACN, MAICD
Associate Dean, Nursing and Allied Health, Monash University, Victoria; President, Australian College of Mental Health Nurses; Chair, Council of Deans of Nursing and Midwifery (Australia and New Zealand)

Anna Elders, PGCert Child and Adolescent MH, PGDip Cognitive Therapy, MNurs
Cognitive Behavioural Nurse Therapist, ProCare Psychological Services; Director, The CBT Clinic Ltd; Professional Teaching Fellow, The University of Auckland, Auckland, New Zealand

Kim Foster, RN, DipAppSc, BN, MA, PhD, MACN, FACMHN
Professor of Mental Health Nursing, North Western Mental Health & School of Nursing, Midwifery & Paramedicine, Australian Catholic University, Melbourne, Victoria, Australia

Charles Harmon, RN, BHS (Nursing), MN, PhD (Nursing), FACMHN
Conjoint Lecturer, School of Nursing and Midwifery, Faculty of Health, University of Newcastle, New South Wales, Australia

Kerry Hawkins, BA, GradDipEd, Graduate Boston University Global Leadership Institute Recovery Class 2013
Vice President, Helping Minds; Director, Emerging Minds; Director, Western Australian Association of Mental Health, Australia

Kristin Henderson, RN, RM, RPN, DipAppSc (Nursing Ed), BNurs, GradDip Sciences Communication, MHealthSci, MACMHN
Team Leader Inpatient & Consultation-Liaison, Child & Youth Mental Health, Royal Children's Hospital, Children's Health, Queensland, Australia

Scott Lamont, RMN, RN, MN (Hons)
Clinical Nurse Consultant, Prince of Wales Hospital, Sydney; Clinical Ethics Committee, South Eastern Sydney Area Health Service, New South Wales, Australia

Tessa Maguire, RN, MMentHlthSc
Clinical Nurse Consultant, Forensicare Melbourne, Victoria; Adjunct Lecturer, Forensic Mental Health, Swinburne University of Technology, Melbourne, Victoria, Australia

Peta Marks, RPN, BN, MHP, MCFT, Credentialed MHN, FACMHN
Professional Development Manager, Australian College of Mental Health Nurses, Australia

Trish Martin, RPN, DN
Past Director of Nursing Research, Victorian Institute of Forensic Mental Health; Adjunct Associate Professor, Monash University, Victoria, Australia

Phillip Maude, RN, PhD, MN (Res), BHSci, DipMHN, Cert Addictions, FACMHN
Associate Professor, Mental Health and Addictions Programs, Coordinator, Master of Mental Health Nursing and Graduate Diploma in Mental Health Nursing, School of Health and Biomedical Sciences (Nursing), RMIT University, Victoria; Adjunct Professoriate, School of Health Sciences, University of Tasmania, Tasmania, Australia

Brian McKenna, RN, BA, MHSc, PhD
Professor of Forensic Mental Health, School of Clinical Sciences, Auckland University of Technology; Auckland Regional Forensic Psychiatry Services, Waitemata District Health Board; Adjunct Professor, Swinburne University of Technology; Visiting Professor, Department of Psychiatry, University of Melbourne

Tom Meehan, RN, MPH, MSocSc, PhD
Associate Professor, Department of Psychiatry, University of Queensland, and Service Evaluation, West Moreton HHS, Queensland, Australia

Wendy Moyle, RN, DipAppSci, BN, MHSc, PhD
Professor and Program Director, School of Nursing and Midwifery, Menzies Health Institute Queensland, Griffith University, Queensland, Australia

Louise O'Brien, RN, BA, PhD
Conjoint Professor of Nursing (Mental Health), University of Newcastle, New South Wales, Australia

Deb O'Kane, RN, ENB 603, GradDip CN, MN, GradCert Higher Education
Lecturer, School of Nursing and Midwifery, Flinders University, Adelaide, South Australia, Australia

Michael Olasoji, RN, PhD, PGDipMHN, BNurs (Hons), BSc Biochem (Hons), MACMHN, MAPNA
Lecturer, School of Nursing and Midwifery, Monash University, Victoria, Australia

Christine J. Palmer, RN, PhD, Credentialed MHN, DipAppSc (Nursing Ed), BAppSc (Nursing), MNurs, FACMHN
Lecturer, Flinders University, Adelaide, South Australia, Australia

Tanya Park, RN, BNSc, GradDip MHN, MMid, GCTT, PhD
Assistant Professor, Faculty of Nursing, University of Alberta, Canada; Adjunct Senior Lecturer, College of Healthcare Sciences, James Cook University, Queensland, Australia

Philip B. Petrie, MEdStud, BN, RN, JP, MAICD, AMICDA, AIMM, ACMHN
Executive Director, Allevia, Bankstown, New South Wales, Australia

Toby Raeburn, RN, MN, Nurse Practitioner
Lecturer in Mental Health Nursing, University of Sydney, New South Wales, Australia

Rachel Rossiter, RN, NP, Credentialed MHN, BHlthSc, BCounselling, MCounselling, MN (NP), HScD, GradCertPTT, FACMHN
Associate Professor of Nursing (Nurse Practitioner), School of Nursing, Midwifery & Indigenous Health, Charles Sturt University, New South Wales, Australia

Kim Ryan, RN, GradCert Health Services Management
Adjunct Associate Professor, Sydney University; Registered Nurse, General, Concord Hospital; Registered Nurse, Psychiatric, Rozelle Hospital, New South Wales, Australia

Robin Scott, RN, AP, Credentialed MHN, MClinSc (MHN)
Sessional Lecturer and Clinical Research Nurse, University of Newcastle & Charles Sturt University, New South Wales, Australia

Julie Sharrock, RN, Credentialed MHN, CritCareCert, PsychNursCert, BEd, MHSc (PsychNurs), AdvDip Gestalt Therapy, FACMHN, MACN, MISPN
Mental Health Nurse Consultant, Epion, Victoria, Australia

Patrica (Tish) Siaosi, Ngati Mutunga O Wharekauri, RPN, PGDip Health (MHN), PGDip Business (MD)
Kaiwhakahaere, Te Ao Māramatanga, New Zealand College of Mental Health Nurses

Vicki Stanton, RN, Credentialed MHN, BA (SocWel), MA (SocSc), GradDipPubHlth, GradCertMgmt, FACMHN
St Vincent's Hospital, Darlinghurst; Academic, Faculty of Health, University of Technology, Sydney, New South Wales, Australia

Chris Taua, RN, BN, PGCertHS (MH), CertAdTch, MN (Dist), PhD, FNZCMHN
Director/Nurse Consultant, Pumahara Partners, Christchurch, New Zealand

Barbara Tooth, BA (Hons), PhD Clinical Psychology
General & Midwifery Nurse; Management Committee, The MHS Learning Network

Kim Usher AM, RN, A/DipNEd, DipAppSc, BA, MNST, PhD, FACN, FACMHN
Professor, Head of School, School of Health, University of New England, Armidale, New South Wales, Australia

Andrew Watkins, BN, GradCert (Child & Adol MH), GradDip (MH), MN (NP)
Clinical Nurse Consultant, South East Sydney Local Health District, New South Wales, Australia

Lina Wilson, RN, PsychNursCert, GradDip Gerontological Nurs, MaNP (Psych Nurs), MACMHN

REVIEWERS

Karen-Ann Clarke, RN, MMHN, GradDip (Psychological Studies)
Lecturer in Nursing (Mental Health), University of the Sunshine Coast, Queensland, Australia

Janette Curtis, RN, Cert tutor, Cert IV Frontline Management, BA, GradDip Public Health, PhD
Honorary Senior Fellow, School of Nursing, University of Wollongong, New South Wales, Australia

Juliana Korzon, BN, MPHIL

Elijah M. Marangu, RN, MPH, PhD candidate
Lecturer, School of Nursing and Midwifery, Faculty of Health, Deakin University, Victoria, Australia

Jonathan Mould, RN, PhD, RSCN, RMN
Lecturer, Researcher, School of Nursing, Midwifery and Paramedicine, Faculty of Health Sciences, Curtin University, Bentley, Western Australia, Australia

Brian Phillips, RN, DipAppSc, MSc, PhD, MACN
Senior Lecturer, School of Health, Charles Darwin University, Northern Territory, Australia

Rachel Rossiter, RN, NP, Credentialed MHN, BHlthSc, BCounselling, MCounselling, MN (NP), HScD, GradCertPTT, FACMHN
Associate Professor of Nursing (Nurse Practitioner), School of Nursing, Midwifery & Indigenous Health, Charles Sturt University, New South Wales, Australia

Phil Whitfield, RPN, BA, GCertProfEthics, GCertOHS, MMHNursing
Clinical Nurse Educator (Mental Health), NSW Health, New South Wales, Australia

Alasdair Williamson, RN, MSc, PGCert Health Science
Lecturer, School of Nursing, Eastern Institute of Technology, New Zealand

Stacey Wilson, RN, PhD
Senior Lecturer, School of Nursing, College of Health, Massey University, New Zealand

PART 1

Preparing for Psychiatric and Mental Health Nursing

1

The Effective Nurse

Louise O'Brien

KEY POINTS

- Mental health nursing is a challenging and stimulating area of practice that draws on knowledge from both human and biological sciences.
- The development of therapeutic relationships is the key to effective mental health nursing.
- Mental health nurses and patients together develop therapeutic relationships that promote personal connections to facilitate growth and recovery.
- Self-awareness, insight and reflexivity are fundamental skills for mental health nurses.
- Mental health nursing requires sustained and close engagement with people in highly charged situations, and this has the potential to cause occupational stress that can precede burnout syndrome.
- Burnout syndrome has three elements: emotional exhaustion; depersonalisation; and feelings of reduced personal accomplishment.
- Mental health nurses are required to develop effective therapeutic relationships while maintaining clear professional boundaries.
- Supportive collegial relationships can enhance the skills and confidence of mental health nurses at all stages of their careers.

KEY TERMS

burnout
burnout syndrome
caring
clinical supervision
compassion
empathy
ethics
healing
hope
mentoring
preceptoring
professional boundaries
recovery
reflection
reflective practices
self
self-awareness
self-disclosure
spirituality
stress
therapeutic relationships

LEARNING OUTCOMES

The material in this chapter will assist you to:

- describe the nursing skills needed to care for the spiritual needs of patients.
- describe the three components of empathy.
- define self-awareness and describe a strategy for developing self-awareness.
- discuss the three phases of reflection.
- list the factors that contribute to stress and burnout in nursing.
- explain strategies for managing stress and avoiding burnout.
- explain the importance of maintaining professional boundaries.
- describe the benefits of mentoring and preceptoring.

INTRODUCTION

Mental health nursing is one of the most interesting, challenging and rewarding areas of nursing practice. The challenges of mental health nursing can include working with people in crisis, where they can be vulnerable to doubting themselves, the environment and the people around them. The rewards include the satisfaction of using knowledge and skill to provide a place of safety and care where trust in self and others can be reestablished. Mental health nursing requires a fusion of professional knowledge, clinical and interpersonal skills, and experience. Although nurses in all settings care for the mental health and wellbeing of the patients and clients in their care, those patients and clients with acute or chronic mental illnesses have complex and perhaps long-term needs. Patients and clients with chronic mental illness often engage in frequent and regular encounters with the healthcare system. The long-term and cyclic nature of some mental illnesses means that the therapeutic relationships between mental health nurses and their patients can last for long periods. They can also vary in intensity as patients move along a continuum between periods of high dependence at one end (in acute phases when they are experiencing symptoms of their illness) and independence at the other (when their symptoms are less troublesome or their mental illness has resolved). The legal aspects of mental healthcare add a further layer of complexity to the mental health nursing role.

Skilful mental health nursing requires a sound knowledge of human physiology, health and disease, and a biopsychosocial understanding of mental illnesses and their treatments, including pharmacology. In addition, in order to practise effectively, nurses working in mental health need to be open-minded and reflective and to have developed an understanding of esoteric concepts such as spirituality and hope. They also need to understand the nature and boundaries of professional and therapeutic relationships. Personal qualities such as responsiveness, self-awareness and insight are also essential. This chapter introduces some of the concepts and issues that are fundamental to effective and safe mental health nursing practice.

NURSE'S STORY 1.1 Kate's Story of Choosing Mental Health Nursing

After finishing my A-Levels in Science, Business and Psychology I decided to take a year out while I considered which university I wanted to apply for and select the right course for me. I got what I thought would be an interim job to make some money as a care support worker within an autistic spectrum disorders charity and absolutely loved it. I was fascinated by the way in which we all view the world differently as individuals and how different people learn to manage the challenges that life can present. I had always been interested in the study of human behaviour, hence I undertook A-Level Psychology. I loved my work as a care support worker and quickly realised that I wanted to pursue a career within healthcare; nursing seemed like the natural choice.

I made enquiries with a number of universities and looked into the different branches of nursing study available: Adult, Mental Health, Learning Disability and Paediatric. Reflecting on my experiences as a support worker I was confident that I wanted to work with people experiencing mental ill health and so I applied to undertake the 3-year programme. My experiences as a care support worker was invaluable in helping to me make this decision.

My clinical practice placements over the 3-year programme were very varied and all equally interesting. My placements included older adult mental health services, male inpatient acute admissions ward, community eating disorders service, inpatient psychiatric intensive care, community forensic services and a crisis intervention team. My final placement was within a male acute ward and I was fortunate to get my first job as a newly qualified nurse there, where I undertook the Preceptorship Programme. This greatly helped me to consolidate my learning and transition from being a student to a Registered Mental Health Nurse. I was grateful for this opportunity as I was very nervous to be counted in the numbers, having been supernumerary for so long. I think it was a huge support that I had already developed key working relationships with the ward staff and so I knew who go to for advice and the right pathways for escalating any concerns within the Trust. I admit that I felt nervous at times and I was very mindful that I was both responsible and accountable for my decision making. However, the ward staff were very supportive and my preceptor ensured that we had regular one-to-one meetings to reflect on my practice and to identify any additional training opportunities that were available. I really enjoy my current role within inpatient care, but in the future I am keen to explore opportunities within psychiatric liaison services, where I can help to bridge the gap between physical and mental health services.

COMPASSION AND CARING

Compassion is a concept closely associated with and underpinning caring. Compassion is linked with sensitivity to suffering and a desire to alleviate distress (Gustin & Wagner 2013; Day 2015; Sawbridge & Hewison 2015; Straughair 2012a, 2012b). Gustin and Wagner (2013) suggest that compassion inspires 'the act of the conscious intention of being present in moments of another's despair' (p. 175). Compassion underpins concepts of acceptance, a nonjudgemental attitude, awareness, being present and listening. To be able to provide compassionate care, we need to be able to imagine what it would be like to be in the person's situation, what it would be like to experience the world as they are experiencing it and to imagine what might help.

Caring is widely considered to be central to nursing theory and practice (Schofield et al. 2013; Hogan 2013). Although the word 'caring' is simple, its use in complex healthcare situations has rendered it problematic. Following a metasynthesis of research Finfgeld-Connett (2008, p. 196) conceptualised caring as a 'context-specific interpersonal process that is characterised by expert nursing practice, interpersonal sensitivity and intimate relationships'. Finfgeld-Connett further elaborated on the concept to make explicit factors related to the roles of the patient and the nurse, and to the working environment, discussing the 'recipient's need for and openness to caring, and the nurse's professional maturity and moral foundations . . . [as well as] a working environment that is conducive to caring' (p. 196). Providing nursing care in mental health settings can, however, be even more complex as people with mental illnesses may not identify the need for care, or be open to caring interventions, especially in acute phases of illness.

Over many years, and in a great deal of contemporary literature, arguments for and against nursing adopting the concept of caring as the cornerstone of the discipline have been raised. These arguments are concerned with:

- the gendered nature of caring (Grady et al. 2008; Speedy 2006; Colby 2012)

- the care/cure debate (Jackson & Borbasi 2006)
- ethical sensitivity and caring (Weaver 2007)
- caring and culture (Wikberg & Eriksson 2008)
- the inherent conflict between the concept of caring and the economic rationalism and social privilege that controls the provision of health services (Jackson & Borbasi 2006)
- the tension between caring, coercion and legal constraints (Cashin et al. 2010; Godin 2000; Wyder et al. 2015)
- caring as resilient practice (Warelow & Edward 2007)
- the dichotomy of professional nurse caring (what nurses do) and informal caring (the caring available to people through their own social networks and personal relationships) (Jackson & Borbasi 2006).
- self-knowledge and caring (Schofield et al. 2013)
- prescriptive caring versus authentic relationships (Hogan 2013)

Nurse scholars have invested much time and energy in trying to explain what it is that makes nurse caring special or different from informal caring and from the caring provided by other professionals (i.e. medical practitioners). There have also been many attempts to find a 'fit' between caring as a construct and the biomedically dominated and economically driven healthcare sectors within which nursing is situated. From a mental health perspective, there are even more issues to consider in relation to nurse caring. For example, there are special issues associated with caring for patients who are compelled (perhaps unwillingly) to accept professional care under one of the Mental Health Acts (see Chapter 4 for mental health legislation). Historically, mental health nursing has been associated with custodial care and control. Godin (2000) captured the dilemma of mental health nurses when he raised questions about the *dis*-ease between the caring and coercive roles that mental health nurses assume. Godin positioned caring as 'clean' and constructed the coercive control elements of mental health nursing (a term he used for involuntary treatment, community orders and so on) as 'dirty' (Godin 2000, p. 1396). While Godin's argument was particularly focussed on patients and nurses in the community, many of the issues he raised (related to enforced administration of medication, seclusion and detention) are still relevant to nurses in inpatient and community settings. In addition, forensic mental health units raise further challenges (Cashin et al. 2010). From the perspective of people who have been involuntarily detained for treatment, Wyder et al. (2015) found that having staff willing to listen empathically was important and that the person's involuntary legal status should not be an impediment to nurses providing compassionate care and forming therapeutic relationships. The absolute vulnerability of patients who can be detained against their will and subjected to various treatments that they may vigorously and robustly resist means that elements of the caring role, such as patient advocacy, are critical to skilful and compassionate mental health nursing practice.

HOPE AND SPIRITUALITY

There is still much that we do not know about recovery, healing and how people manage chronic health problems. Why do some people pull through a disease, while others succumb? How is it that some people seem to cope well with even very invasive treatments, while others suffer terribly? How do some people with chronic mental illnesses function well in the community, while others are in and out of hospital in a cyclic pattern? We know that factors such as personality, resilience, social support, general health and access to acceptable (to the patient) health services all play a crucial role in patient outcomes (see Chapter 2 for more on patient recovery and rehabilitation). But the importance and value of concepts such as hope, and the role hope plays in the lives of patients and their families, are areas of increasing interest. 'Hope' is a taken-for-granted term and, although it is used widely in the literature, it is seldom clearly defined. Hope is considered essential in handling illness and has been described as 'the act by which the temptation to despair is actively overcome' (Fitzgerald Miller 2007, p. 13). We know it is a complex and multidimensional variable that has optimistic and anticipatory dimensions and involves looking ahead to the future. Hope has been linked to emotional healing and better adaptation to life stress (Carretta et al. 2014) and is a central component in recovery from mental illness (Schrank et al. 2008).

In a study of qualitative literature related to hope in older people with chronic illnesses, Carretta et al. (2014, p. 1211) identify characteristics of hope as including 'transcending possibilities' and 'positive reappraisal'. Transcending possibilities involve finding meaning through searching and connecting with others. The positive role of healthcare professionals in the maintenance of hope is described as supporting hope and the search for meaning. Positive reappraisal is dependent on the ability to seek and find positives in the illness experience and healthcare professionals also have a role in supporting patients in this search.

Hope has particular relevance to mental health nursing practice, and there is growing recognition of the concept of hope and its relationship to health, wellbeing and recovery from illness or traumatic life events (Duggleby et al. 2012). Closely linked with hope, therapeutic optimism in mental health nurses is described by Hemingway et al. (2014) as a belief that they can make a difference and a belief that their patients can recover.

The need for further research to generate knowledge and enhance understanding about suffering, hope and spirituality in relation to mental health nursing is acknowledged in the literature (Cutcliffe et al. 2015; Schrank et al. 2008). However, the emphasis on the biomedical understanding of mental illness provides barriers to such research. The biomedical model values things that can be seen, measured and quantified. Although hope and spirituality can be felt, they cannot be seen, touched or smelt and cannot always be clearly articulated, and so occupy what Crawford et al. (1998, p. 214) termed 'an embarrassed silence'. However, if we recognise that spirituality underpins the meanings that people make of illness and other life events, and that hope is a variable that has some form of healing potential, then in practice we cannot ignore the importance of spirituality and the search for meaning. Indeed, Cutcliffe et al. (2015) reinforces the importance of recognising and responding to the spiritual care needs of patients and calls for nurses to develop skills in supporting patients to understand and search for meaning in their experience. The ability to maintain hope and to make meaning of the experience of illness is central to recovery, and it is important for mental health nurses to be able to do this.

This leads us to the question: What skills do nurses need if we are to care for the spiritual needs of our patients? The short answer is that we need to develop effective interpersonal skills. Being open to the belief systems of other people; intuitiveness; active listening; being alert to the cues that tell us the things that matter to a person; self-awareness; spiritual awareness and reflective skills are considered crucial in the provision of spiritual care (Ramezani et al. 2014).

CRITICAL THINKING CHALLENGE 1.1

Margaret is a 56 year old woman who has a 2 week history of becoming increasingly disorganised, thought-disordered, agitated and distressed. She reports hearing voices and finds this very upsetting. She states that these voices are calling out to her and telling her things. While admitting Margaret to the ward you note that she is visibly distressed, appears to have difficulty concentrating and sometimes makes seemingly inappropriate responses to your questions, while at other times her responses are appropriate.

Margaret has no previous history of psychotic illness, although she does have a history of alcohol-related problems. She reports that she has not been drinking at a problem level for 4 years as she is responsible for the care of her two grandchildren. However, she has been drinking more than usual over the past month. She tells you that her mother and uncle died 2 years ago in a car accident and that her husband died of a heart attack 6 weeks ago.

- What are the main issues here?
- How might Margaret's recent family and social history be related to her current health status?
- How could you respond to Margaret's distress?

ETHICAL DILEMMA 1.1

You are caring for Tom, a 28-year-old male with bipolar disorder, who was admitted to an acute ward during a manic episode. In addition to his bipolar disorder, Tom is hepatitis B positive. He has been sectioned under the Mental Health Act and is currently being nursed with several other detained patients in a close observation area. Tom is observed to spend much of his time with two young women aged 17 and 18 whom you consider highly vulnerable. Attempts to keep Tom separate from the young women by involving them in different activities are difficult to maintain due to the close confines of the area and the lengthy periods of time of unstructured activity. There is a 'no sex' policy in the unit and Tom has been reminded of this on several occasions. He finds this amusing and says: 'I don't have to force anyone—they can make their own decisions.'

Questions

1. What could you do? List the options available.
2. Identify the potential risks and benefits of each option you have identified.
3. What ethical principles need to be considered here?

THERAPEUTIC USE OF SELF

Therapeutic relationships are key within mental health nursing. Wheeler (2011) suggested that the therapeutic relationship provides a healing connection through caring, emotional connection, narrative and anxiety management, and that this process has a powerful neurobiological impact on the mental health of the person. Therapeutic relationships are the foundation upon which all other activities are based. Mental health nursing is thus primarily an interpersonal process that uses self as the means of developing and sustaining nurse–patient relationships. Therapeutic use of self involves using aspects of the nurse's personality, background, life skills and knowledge to develop a connection with a person who has a mental health problem or illness. Nurses intentionally and consciously draw on ways of establishing human connectedness in their encounters with patients. The process is based on a genuine interest in understanding who the patient is and how they have come to be in their current situation. Lees et al. (2014, p. 310) describe therapeutic engagement as the 'establishment of rapport, active listening, empathy, boundaries, relating as equals, genuineness, compassion, unconditional positive regard, trust, time and responsiveness' and suggest that most of these elements need to be present for engagement to occur.

The purpose of using self therapeutically is to establish a therapeutic relationship with the patient. Patients in mental health services may not only be suffering from frightening symptoms or perhaps overwhelming mood changes or out-of-control thoughts and feelings; they may also be suffering from alienation and isolation. Patients may be fearful of talking to others about their symptoms or difficulties because they fear being rejected and seen as 'crazy', or they may have had experiences of rejection because of their mental illness, which make it difficult for them to form relationships. Studies of patients' experiences of mental health services provide evidence that being understood and listened to in a thoughtful, sensitive manner confirms their humanity and provides hope for their future (Shattell et al. 2006; Gunasekara et al. 2014).

In the process of using self therapeutically, the nurse develops a dialogue with the patient in order to understand the patient's predicament. Patients need to feel safe enough to disclose personal, difficult and distressing information. It is in the way in which the nurse conveys genuine interest, concern and desire to understand the patient that a therapeutic relationship can be established. How the nurse relates to, and what prior understandings they bring to, the encounter will affect this relationship (Foster et al. 2006; Wyder et al. 2015).

Studies of the experiences of both mental health nurses and of the people accessing mental health services overwhelmingly attest to the importance of therapeutic relationships. Patients have identified the need to feel compassionately cared for, to have meaningful contact with nurses, to be listened to and for nurses to know them as people and understand their predicament (Gunasekara et al. 2014; Lees et al. 2014; Stewart et al. 2015; Wyder et al. 2015). Similarly, studies of nurses' experience identify that therapeutic engagement is seen by nurses to be the hallmark of good practice in mental health settings (Cleary et al. 2012; McAndrew et al. 2014).

Empathy and Therapeutic Use of Self

The ability to empathise with patients is underpinned by caring and compassion, and is positively linked with the ability to develop therapeutic relationships and the desire to alleviate suffering. As indicated earlier, the ability to engage empathically with patients is highly valued. Empathy is not merely a feeling of understanding and compassion for the patient. Empathy, as used in the therapeutic relationship, is linked to intentional actions that are aimed at reducing the person's distress. Empathic interactions have a number of components.

First, empathy involves an attempt to understand the patient's predicament and the meanings that the patient attributes to their situation. This means that the nurse makes a conscious attempt to discuss with the patient their current and past experiences and the feelings and meanings associated with these experiences.

Second, the nurse verbalises the understanding that they have developed to the patient. The understanding that the nurse has of the patient's situation will be at best tentative; we can never really know what life is like for another. However, the process of seeking to understand, and of conveying to the patient the desire to understand, creates the opportunity for further exploration in a safe relationship. In addition, maintaining the stance of trying to understand rather than making assumptions averts the tendency to make judgements about patients and their behaviour.

The third component of empathy is the patient's validation of the nurse's understanding. One of the most important aspects of the development of the therapeutic relationship through empathic understanding is that the nurse can convey to the patient a desire to understand. This level of empathic attunement allows the patient to participate in identifying those aspects of their illness and healthcare experience that are problematic (see also Chapter 24).

The Therapeutic Relationship

The value of a therapeutic relationship, developed through therapeutic use of self, has been clearly identified from the perspective of nurses and patients in qualitative studies internationally (Geanellos 2002; Graham 2001; O'Brien 2000, 2001; Welch 2005). Forming a strong, therapeutic, continued relationship has been linked with a reduction in admission rates and an improved quality of life for patients discharged from hospital (Forchuk & Reynolds 2001), and in the enhancement of rehabilitation outcomes among people with schizophrenia (Davis & Lysaker 2007). In a review of the literature on therapeutic working relationships with people with schizophrenia, Hewitt and Coffey (2005) concluded that the therapeutic relationship was greatly valued by people with a mental illness.

Numerous studies have indicated that a therapeutic relationship can significantly impact on patient outcomes and that it is possibly one of the most important factors contributing to the effectiveness of a service (Cleary et al. 2012; Johansson & Jansson 2010; Stewart et al. 2015). People who have a positive relationship with their clinician have better outcomes (Pilgrim et al. 2009). However, a therapeutic relationship may not be sufficient to sustain health improvements, and so a combination of both therapeutic relationships and the technical skill of specific therapeutic approaches may provide the best outcomes.

SELF-AWARENESS

The process of understanding others begins with understanding the self (see also Chapter 2). 'Self' is a concept that describes the core of our personality. Welch (2005, p. 164) found that nurses described 'congruency, genuineness and authenticity' as ways of projecting 'the nurse's true self'. We use the concept of self when we want to convey our uniqueness as a human being. The self has consistent attributes that pervade the way we live in and experience the world. It is awareness of these attributes of self that can enhance the way we relate to others. A strong sense of self allows us to develop resilience in dealing with the difficulties and complexities of human communication and experience. Self-awareness is about knowing how you are going to respond to specific situations; your values, attitudes and biases towards people and situations; and knowing how your human needs might manifest in your work.

The purpose of being self-aware is to know those things in our background and our way of relating that might affect how we relate to patients. The way we view people is always subjective. The lens through which we look at the world is always our own. Although there can be no true objectivity, knowledge of the things that impinge on our subjective view of the world allows us to identify how they influence our thinking.

Nurses need to be aware of the belief systems and values that arise from their cultural, social and family backgrounds. Everyone develops biases that affect the way they view other people's behaviour. Behaviour that is understandable to one nurse might not be understandable to another. However, the self is not static but constantly evolving and sensitive to experience. We bring values, biases and beliefs to nursing and to our relationships with patients, and in turn those relationships offer the opportunity for self-development. It is through the process of self-reflection and the examination of particular experiences that nurses can learn.

Work in the mental health area requires the ability to listen to, respond to and empathise with people from a range of backgrounds. Unexamined belief systems can become obstacles to the development of a therapeutic relationship with a patient. Lack of self-awareness can cause nurses to respond to a patient's distress and behaviour in ways that may not be helpful. For example, it might cause nurses to use their power coercively in the belief that this is best for the patient. Lack of self-awareness can also lead to nurses being overly concerned, refusing to allow patients choice or overwhelming them with advice, in an attempt to protect them. Alternatively, nurses may avoid contact with particular patients or fail to respond to distress. This growing self-awareness needs to take place against a background of self-compassion; to develop the ability to empathise with others requires 'the ability to be sensitive, non-judgemental and respectful to oneself' (Gustin & Wagner 2013).

REFLECTION

The first step in developing self-awareness is the ability to reflect. Reflection is 'a process of critically reviewing experience from practice so that it may be used to inform and change future practice in a positive way' (Bulman et al. 2014, p. 1219). Reflective practice and reflective practice groups were based on the early work of Schon (1983) and Carper (1978). More detailed examinations of reflection emphasise that it is a conscious practical process of simultaneously analysing thoughts, feelings and actions in the context of beliefs, assumptions and knowledge (Kim 1999). The purpose of reflection is to increase self-awareness, as well as to develop a conscious knowledge base for practice at both macro and micro levels (Cooke & Matarasso 2005). Johns (2001, p. 241) suggests that the purpose of reflection is to 'surface contradiction between what [the nurse] intends to achieve within any situation and the way she [*sic*] actually practices'. Studies of reflective practices indicate that nurses who participate in reflective practice found that it increased self-awareness and confidence in decision making (Caldwell & Grobbel 2013).

Developing Reflective Practices

All UK registered nurses must undertake revalidation every 3 years in order to maintain their registration with the Nursing and Midwifery Council (NMC). As part of this process nurses are required to write five reflective accounts examining any of the following: an instance from undertaking continuing professional development, a piece of practice-related feedback that has been received or an event or experience from their professional practice. The template provided by the NMC aligns with the four themes from The Code: Professional Standards of Practice and Behaviour for Nurses and Midwives (NMC 2015):

- Prioritise people by actively seeking and reflecting on any direct feedback received from patients and others to ensure that you are able to fulfil their needs.
- Practise effectively by reflecting on your professional development with your colleagues, identifying areas for improvement in your practice and undertaking professional development activities.
- Preserve safety by practising within your competency for the minimum number of practice hours, reflecting on feedback and addressing any gaps in your practice through Continuing Professional Development (CPD).
- Promote professionalism and trust by providing feedback and helping other NMC colleagues reflect on their professional development and being accountable to others for your professional development and revalidation.

There are a number of structured reflective models to help guide reflection, those recommend by the Royal College of Nursing (2017) include Gibb's (1988) and Johns (2001).

Gibbs' reflective cycle has six stages:

1. Description—what happened?
2. Feelings—what were you thinking and feeling?
3. Evaluation—what was good and bad about the experience?
4. Analysis—what sense can you make of the situation?
5. Conclusion—what else could you have done?
6. Action Plan—if it arose again what would you do?

Most models of reflection involve three phases (Greenwood 1998; Johns 2001).

1. In the *descriptive phase*, the nurse creates descriptive narratives of specific clinical situations. These narratives include descriptions of actions, thoughts and feelings as well as descriptions of the situation and factors surrounding the situation. This process increases the nurse's ability to include self, and the context as well as the specific patient and health problem, in their understanding of the clinical experience. To some extent, nurses do this in verbal handovers or in discussion of specific events. In these situations, however, nurses tend to be selective about their responses and the contextual factors and colleagues tend not to probe further, although they may provide a listening ear and support.
2. The *reflective phase* involves comparison of the narrative with the nurse's beliefs, biases and knowledge. This deepens the discussion beyond the 'What happened' description. This involves the identification of the nurse's knowledge base, values and belief systems and allows the identification of gaps in knowledge, as well as previously unexamined beliefs about the patient and the

situation, or the role and intentions of the nurse. The potential for further development of knowledge, clinical skills and self-awareness is enhanced by the reflective process.

3. The *conclusion/action phase* allows the nurse to identify differences between intentions and actions, thoughts/feelings and espoused values, values and practice, patient needs and the nurse's actions. This phase allows for self-critique, learning and change. It also allows for the development of greater understanding of the influence of the context on the nurse's actions.

As discussed earlier, reflection is a process and it can be undertaken alone, with trusted peers, in formal groups or informal groups. The process can use oral or written narrative of clinical encounters. Reflective practices are closely linked with clinical supervision, which is discussed later in this chapter.

PROFESSIONAL BOUNDARIES

In nursing, professional boundaries are invisible yet powerful lines that mark the territory of the nurse (see also Chapter 24). They define a role and allow the nurse to say: 'This is what I do. This is the purpose of my presence here.' Professional boundaries are important in all areas of healthcare, but in mental health nursing they have an increased importance due to the nature of the work of mental health nurses and the vulnerability of the patient population. Over time there has been a decrease in formal divisions between staff and patients in mental health services, with the encouragement of friendliness and collaborative partnerships (Brown et al. 2000; Gardner 2010). However, a power imbalance is always present in clinician/patient encounters (Henderson 2004) and there are a number of ways that boundary violations can occur. Boundary violations can involve the exertion of power through coercion, use of force, over- or undertreatment or inappropriate intimate relationships. Maintaining professional boundaries whilst being involved in therapeutic relationships is a skill that cannot be underestimated in importance. Tariman (2010) noted that social networking provided a further challenge. This medium for relationships needs to be viewed with caution when considering professional boundaries.

Mental health nurses have to be able to maintain professional boundaries while simultaneously developing close therapeutic relationships with patients based on empathy and positive connectedness. While many of the interactions and interventions of mental health nurses may appear social in nature (e.g. playing table tennis, cards or volleyball with a patient, or going for a walk or having a coffee with a patient), it is the therapeutic intent and the conscious awareness of the purpose of the relationship that put them within the professional role. It is when interventions and interactions lose their therapeutic intent and are instead primarily for the benefit of the nurse that professional boundaries are breached. Any breach of professional boundaries has the potential to cause serious harm to patients and is a violation of professional ethics (Campbell et al. 2005).

PATIENT STORY 1.1 Sheena

You are working in Accident and Emergency as a new nurse, and you have been assigned Sheena. You are aware of the other staff's negative feelings about this patient. Some of the staff know her from previous presentations and see her problems as self-inflicted. However, you approach Sheena and, as you take the necessary observations, you ask her about what has happened to her.

Sheena tells her own story: I am 28 years old and have had lots of presentations to accident and emergency departments. I often used to cut myself or take overdoses. However, in the past 3 years I have hardly had any presentations and no admissions to hospital. I have 2 children aged 4 and 2 and I am trying to get my act together for them. I do not want to lose my children. My childhood was chaotic with lots of foster care. I spent time in refuges and took drugs for a while. I do not take drugs or drink alcohol now. I have had a community mental health nurse who has been seeing me regularly for more than 3 years. Tonight I took an overdose of antidepressants that I had been prescribed. I feel ashamed, as it was impulsive and stupid. I can see the staff talking about me and saying all the old things. They do not think I deserve care as I inflicted this on myself and everyone else here is physically ill or has had an accident. I just got to the end of my tether. I had a boyfriend who moved in and I did not like how he treated the kids so he has gone now. My community nurse is on leave. I could not contact anyone, I just felt so alone, empty and lost. I thought the kids would be better off without me.

If my community nurse were here she would ask me what happened, how I was feeling. She would treat me with respect without condoning what I did. She would help me identify how I can get out of this mess I have made. We would talk about the crisis plan that is on my fridge and how I can get through the next few days keeping myself and my children safe.

1. How are you going to respond to Sheena?
2. What interventions might be helpful to her at the moment, and in the longer term?

Professional boundaries are maintained by nurses having a clear understanding of their therapeutic role, being able to reflect on therapeutic interactions and being able to document and narrate their interventions. Maintaining professional boundaries is always the responsibility of the nurse.

Self-Disclosure

Mental health nurses use self-disclosure as a way of developing therapeutic relationships with patients. Many of the relationships that nurses have with patients are very long term, either by repeated admissions to hospital or by continued contact in community settings, so nurses and patients may come to know each other well. In a study of nurse–patient relationships between community mental health nurses and patients with long-term mental illness, nurses described the use of self-disclosure: 'The nurses used their own experiences of living a life to: be seen as ordinary people; be credible; illustrate aspects of being-in-the-world; allow the patients to identify with them; and to normalise the patient's fears and difficulties' (O'Brien 2000, p. 188). Patients described the nurse as 'a friend—but different . . . not like other friends' (O'Brien 2001, p. 180). Patients were able to identify that the therapeutic relationship was different even though they knew things about the nurse's life (O'Brien 2001, p. 180). Similarly, Geanellos (2002) noted in a study of adolescent mental health nursing that there was a close relationship between nurses and adolescent patients. Participants in her study commented that the nurse 'was more like a person than a nurse' (p. 178), and Welch (2005) also identified self-disclosure as part of the therapeutic relationship.

However, self-disclosure should be used consciously and carefully. The boundary issue is not whether disclosure of information occurs or does not occur. The issue is the nature of the disclosure and whether the nurse burdens the patient with their own personal problems. The decision about what to disclose to patients about your life needs to be made in advance. Self-disclosure does not include unburdening your personal problems. In the previously described studies, the experienced nurse clinicians were able to use their own life experiences to relate in ways that were beneficial to patients without overburdening them. These experienced clinicians also made decisions about what to share with patients according to the length of the relationship and what each patient could use productively.

ETHICAL DILEMMA 1.2

You are a newly graduated nurse working in an acute psychiatric inpatient unit. One evening you become aware of how much time a male colleague, who is team leader of the shift, is spending with a young female patient. Later you realise the patient is not on the unit and go in search of her. Concerned for her safety, you go to the staff tearoom to report her absence to the team leader who is on a break, to find the patient and the team leader in the tearoom. You say that you were concerned as the patient was not on the unit. Later, the team leader approaches you and says he is conducting individual therapy with the patient and that her psychiatrist is aware of this; however, you note that this 'therapy' is not in the treatment plan and there are no records of their conversations in the patient's notes.

Questions

1. What are the main issues here?
2. What are the ethical issues involved?
3. What could you do in this situation?

STRESS AND BURNOUT

Stress

Stress is a physiological response to any stressor or demand and a fact of life for everyone (Cohen 2000). When a person experiences a stressor, their homeostasis is disturbed and their body activates a stress response. Any foundational anatomy and physiology textbook can provide details of the stress response, but for the purposes of this chapter it is enough to understand that the response involves the release of substances into the blood that cause a range of physiological changes, including changes to heart rate, blood pressure and the gastrointestinal tract. Prolonged stress can be harmful and can have a negative effect on physical and mental health.

Stress can be experienced as negative *(distress)* or positive *(eustress)*. A stressful event can have a positive effect because it can be a catalyst for a person to make changes such as learning new skills or a stimulant to some sort of positive action (Thorpe & Barsky 2001). Individuals may respond differently to the same stressor. For example, say you and a friend need to travel in a light aircraft. You may find the thought of flying in a light aircraft stressful and anxiety provoking, while your friend may find it exhilarating and exciting. Both of you are experiencing stress reactions, but you are experiencing them very differently.

Like other professions that involve close and sustained engagement with people, nursing is innately stressful (Hill et al. 2010; Hunsaker et al. 2015). Mental health nurses frequently have to manage situations that are unpredictable and in which other people, patients and families are distressed, and these factors can increase stress levels. In addition, therapeutic relationships can last for considerable periods of time and can be incredibly challenging at times. It is important to learn to monitor and manage your own stress because unchecked stress can become chronic and result in burnout syndrome (Hill et al. 2010; Hunsaker et al. 2015).

Burnout Syndrome

The words 'burnout' and 'stress' are often seen together because stress is seen as a precursor to burnout. However, stress is a feature of life and, when managed properly, does not lead to burnout. Unlike stress, which has some positive features (e.g. it can be a catalyst for effecting positive change, such as learning a new skill), burnout has no positive aspects for the person experiencing it or for those around them. The term 'burnout' was first seen in the literature in the mid-to-late 1970s, and burnout is widely considered to be a continuing issue of concern for nursing (Meng et al. 2014).

Burnout is used to describe a pattern of feelings of emotional exhaustion, frustration with work, patients and colleagues and feelings of failure (Hunsaker et al. 2015). While the effects of emotional exhaustion will vary from person to person, feelings of depression, irritability, a sense of having nothing more to give and of being emotionally overwhelmed by work are commonly described (Barling 2001; Haddad 2002). Distancing from professional and personal relationships is a feature of burnout and this can lead to unkind, indifferent, uninterested, deprecating, belittling and/or distant responses to patients (Barling 2001; Haddad 2002). It is not difficult to imagine how distressing it would be for a patient to be nursed by someone who responded to them and their situation in a cold and unfeeling way rather than with the warmth, caring, empathy and respect we ourselves would wish for if we were sick and needing care.

It can be seen that burnout syndrome is an undesirable state, not only because of the detrimental influence it has on nurse–patient interaction, but also because of the negative effects on the affected nurse and their immediate colleagues. In addition, it has been associated with diminished work performance, increased staff turnover and misuse of drugs and alcohol (Ewers et al. 2002). From the perspective of the affected person, there is nothing worse than going to work when feeling unhappy and distressed. Furthermore, working with colleagues who are irritable, depressed and exhausted adds to everyone's stress. When people are experiencing emotional exhaustion and reduced personal accomplishment, it is difficult for them to work effectively as a team member. They may feel too lacking in creative energy to perform properly in some areas. For example, irritability might compromise a nurse's ability to mentor and support a novice or an inexperienced nurse effectively.

Nurses are considered to be particularly susceptible to burnout syndrome because of the nature of nursing work, which involves a high level of close contact with people who are often in emotionally charged situations (such as when they or a loved one are experiencing sickness, pain, anxiety or exhaustion), as well as factors such as lack of autonomy and high workload, which are common hallmarks of the nursing workplace. Moreover, mental health nursing involves long periods of working in intensely stressful situations, which may be exacerbated by the environment (e.g. secured areas), and the literature suggests that these factors make burnout an issue of particular concern to mental health nurses (Ewers et al. 2002).

Avoiding Burnout Syndrome

Burnout syndrome has been repeatedly linked to workforce supply issues in nursing and so there have been many research studies and published research reports on ways in which nurses can reduce burnout syndrome or avoid getting it. Most of these reports acknowledge two main areas that can be manipulated to avoid burnout: (1) aspects of the individual nurse; and (2) the environment in which the nurse works. It is important that we learn to know ourselves and our limitations. In nursing we are often encouraged to develop reflective skills and these are very helpful in learning to understand ourselves and our own responses to stressors. If we are aware that we are becoming moody, irritable or short-tempered, or that we are not feeling empathetic towards patients, then this can be an indication that it is time to step back and reflect on the situation (Haddad 2002). Most healthcare organisations provide a range of measures to assist staff, and these include debriefing, counselling and other measures.

It is important to extend the same care to ourselves that we offer to those in our care. Nursing is a high-stress profession and therefore it is necessary to be active in managing stress. Several factors have been identified as being protective against burnout and other negative sequelae resulting from workplace adversity. These include hardiness, optimism, nurturing relationships and networks, emotional insight and achieving life balance (Jackson et al. 2007). Although it can be difficult to fit leisure activities around shiftwork and study, it is important to maintain a balanced and healthy lifestyle and take the time to participate in enjoyable leisure activities. Continuing to learn and develop skills can also be effective.

Although individuals can do things to reduce their risk of burnout, workplace practices are strongly implicated in nurses' susceptibility to burnout syndrome, and burnout is a systemic problem at least as much as an individual one. Therefore, it is also important to ensure that organisations and managers adopt policies and practices that support nurses rather than contribute to stress and burnout (Hunsaker et al. 2015; Sawbridge & Hewison 2015). Stress and burnout need to be considered at an individual, team and organisational level (Hill et al. 2010). The provision of professional supportive relationships can ameliorate stress levels and help prevent burnout syndrome; however, organisations need to provide time and resources to ensure their continued provision.

PROFESSIONAL SUPPORTIVE RELATIONSHIPS

Clinical Supervision

Clinical supervision is a process that focuses on the clinical work of the nurse. It provides an arena in which the nurse can reflect with another experienced clinician on their clinical interactions and interventions (Buus et al. 2013; Cleary et al. 2010). The material discussed in supervision sessions is clinical care, therapeutic relationships and interactions between the nurse and patients. These discussions have the potential to provide professional support, educational and professional development and to enhance the quality of clinical practice. Clinical supervision can also provide an opportunity for nurses to reflect upon the subjective experience of their work. In order to develop the nurse's capacity for empathy, acceptance, nurturing and honest reflection, the clinical supervisor needs to be able to model these capacities in their relationship with the supervisee. Clinical supervision can occur in one-to-one sessions or in groups. In both settings the establishment of a safe, confidential nonblaming environment in which nurses feel able to share their clinical experiences is paramount (Buus et al. 2013). Besides clinical experience, clinical supervisors need to have an educational background in the process of clinical supervision and experience in being supervised.

Clinical supervision guidelines are available that provide a definition of clinical supervision, frameworks of the supervisory relationship and standards of education for the supervisor and describe processes for implementing clinical supervision programs. A list of resources is provided in Box 1.1.

BOX 1.1 Clinical Supervision Resources

Care Quality Commission 2013 Supporting information and guidance: Supporting effective clinical supervision https://www.cqc.org.uk/sites/default/files/documents/20130625_800734_v1_00_supporting_information-effective_clinical_supervision_for_publication.pdf

Nursing and Midwifery Council 2015 Standards for competence for registered nurses. London

NMC (2015) The Code: Professional standards of practice and behaviour for nurses and midwives. London

Preceptorship and Mentoring

Preceptorship and mentoring are two different models for professional relationships that can be developed between nurses (McCloughen et al. 2006). A preceptoring relationship is usually based in the clinical area. When you are new to an area, such as when you are a student taking part in clinical learning, a new graduate entering the workforce or a new employee in a clinical setting, you will often be allocated a preceptor. The preceptor will generally be a nurse with considerable experience in a particular clinical environment and will usually have completed specialised in-service training to prepare for the preceptoring role. They will understand the difficulties and challenges facing people who are new to the area, assist you to develop skills and confidence and facilitate your becoming part of the team in the particular area (Freiburger 2002). You will remain under the guidance of the preceptor for a set period of time or until you feel confident to take your place as a fully independent and functioning member of the team. Preceptors tend to be attached to wards or units, so when you go to a new area you will probably work with a different preceptor.

Mentors have many roles, but the core of mentoring is a partnership between two people that generates mutual learning as well as positive growth and development. Mentors are usually chosen because of their personal qualities and achievements (McCloughen et al. 2006). Unlike a preceptoring relationship, a mentoring relationship is not mediated through employment in a particular ward or unit. Rather, it is a long-term relationship that continues throughout a career or for as long as the parties want it to, and is sustained through changes of employment. Mentoring helps people to grow and develop and to reach their potential. Both preceptoring and mentoring provide additional avenues for debriefing and feedback that can help in dealing effectively with confusing or upsetting incidents.

As with all relationships, certain qualities are needed by both parties, including commitment, honesty, integrity and effective interpersonal skills. Mentors and preceptors need additional skills, such as problem solving; clinical currency and expertise (in the case of preceptors or clinical mentors); appropriate scholarly, administrative or research expertise; the ability to provide constructive criticism and other feedback; understanding of professional boundaries and relationships; and the ability to maintain confidentiality where appropriate.

NURSE'S STORY 1.2 Clinical Supervision

Nicola is working in an acute inpatient unit. She has 2 years' experience. She arrives at clinical supervision saying that she feels frustrated and angry about one of her patients, a young woman with a diagnosis of depression who self-harms. Nicola had spent considerable time with the patient in the preceding days and felt that she had developed a good relationship with her. Last night, after she had gone home, the patient cut her arms with a razor blade, and today she appears to Nicola to be pleased with herself that she was able to self-harm without being stopped by the staff. Nicola says that the other staff have reinforced her belief that she was ' tricked' and she is now confused about how to proceed with this patient, feeling unsure of her judgement and risk assessment skills.

The supervisor asks Nicola to tell in detail the story of what happened. She then asks Nicola to outline her feelings about, and knowledge of, the patient before and after the incident. The supervisor listens attentively and empathically, encouraging further exploration of the incident and Nicola's feelings about it. Nicola admits to feeling guilty and is concerned that she may have said or done something to provoke the incident. Together they consider how the patient might have been feeling and what possible triggers to self-harm might have existed. They then consider what Nicola saw as important in developing the relationship with the patient. The supervisor suggests some reading that Nicola can undertake to increase her understanding of self-harm-related behaviours. Together they identify what might be the goals of nursing interventions with this patient. Nicola resolves to talk to the patient about how the patient was feeling last night and what provoked the self-harm incident.

CONCLUSION

This chapter has introduced some of the core concepts and ideas that shape and inform mental health nursing practice. To be effective and therapeutic in caring for others, nurses must understand concepts such as compassion, caring, hope and spirituality. Stress and burnout are hazards for nurses and others in the caring professions and therefore nurses must learn to recognise and manage their own stress. Accessing support through mentorship, clinical supervision and ongoing educational opportunities are some of the ways to address the demanding nature of the work. Therapeutic relationships lie at the heart of mental health nursing, and a clear understanding of professional boundaries is crucial to the development and ongoing sustainability of such relationships.

Mental health nursing is an exciting and challenging area of nursing practice. Effective mental health nursing requires the culmination of all your skills, as well as your professional and life experiences, and it offers a stimulating and rewarding career path. As we strive to meet the complex needs of diverse communities and to provide care within increasingly restrictive economic environments, there are many challenges before us. Developing positive personal qualities such as self-awareness, and fostering productive and supportive collegial relationships, will help us to meet the challenges that lie ahead.

ACKNOWLEDGEMENT

This chapter has been adapted from a chapter in the previous editions of this book by Debra Jackson and Louise O'Brien.

EXERCISES FOR CLASS ENGAGEMENT

An effective way of developing self-awareness is the use of questioning. To raise your awareness of some important issues, ask yourself the following questions and then discuss your responses with other members of your group or class.

1. What kinds of values do I hold important as a framework for living? Where do these values come from? How do they inform my understanding of what it is to be a person in this world?
2. How has my family of origin influenced how I view the world? What values did my family hold as important? What do I see as important in family life?
3. What do I know about why I chose to be a nurse? Does this still hold true or have my ideas changed over time?
4. What are the pervading social attitudes towards people in mental distress or with mental illness? What are my beliefs about people in mental distress or with mental illness?
5. What experiences have I had that influence how I feel about people with mental illness?

REFERENCES

Barling, J., 2001. Drowning not waving: burnout and mental health nursing. Contemporary Nurse 11 (2/3), 247–259.

Brown, B., Crawford, P., Darongkamas, J., 2000. Blurred roles and permeable boundaries: the experience of multidisciplinary working in community mental health. Health and Social Care in the Community 8 (6), 425–435.

Bulman, C., Lathlean, J., Gobbi, M., 2014. The process of teaching and learning about reflection: research insights from professional nurse education. Studies in Higher Education 39 (7), 1219–1236. https://doi.org/10.1080/03075079.2013.777413.

Buus, N., Cassedy, P., Gonge, H., 2013. Developing a manual for strengthening mental health nurses' clinical supervision. Issues in Mental Health Nursing 34, 344–349.

Caldwell, L., Grobbel, C.C., 2013. The importance of reflective practice. International Journal of Caring Sciences 6 (3), 319–326.

Campbell, J., Yonge, O., Austin, W., 2005. Intimacy boundaries between mental health nurses and psychiatric patients. Journal of Psychosocial Nursing and Mental Health Services 43 (5), 32–39.

Carper, B.A., 1978. Fundamental patterns of knowing in nursing. In: Chaska, M.L. (Ed.), The nursing profession: views through the mist. McGraw-Hill, New York, NY, pp. 216–224.

Carretta, C.M., Ridner, S.H., Dietrich, M.S., 2014. Hope, hopelessness, and anxiety: a pilot instrument comparison study. Archives of Psychiatric Nursing 28, 230–234.

Cashin, A., Newman, C., Eason, M., Thorpe, A., O'Discoll, 2010. An ethnographic study of forensic nursing culture in an Australian prison hospital. Journal of Psychiatric and Mental Health Nursing 17, 39–45.

Cleary, M., Horsfall, J., Happell, B., 2010. Establishing clinical supervision in acute mental health inpatient units: acknowledging the challenges. Issues in Mental Health Nursing 31, 525–531.

Cleary, M., Horsfall, J., O'Hara-Aarons, M., Jackson, D., Hunt, G.E., 2012. Mental health nurses' perceptions of good work in an acute setting. International Journal of Mental Health Nursing 21 (5), 471–479.

Cohen, J., 2000. Stress and mental health: a biobehavioral perspective. Issues in Mental Health Nursing 21 (2), 285–302.

Colby, N., 2012. Caring from the male perspective: a gender neutral concept. International Journal for Human Caring 16 (4), 36–41.

Cooke, M., Matarasso, B., 2005. Promoting reflection in mental health nursing practice: a case illustration using problem-based learning. International Journal of Mental Health Nursing 14 (4), 243–248.

Crawford, P., Nolan, P., Brown, B., 1998. Ministering to madness: the narratives of people who have left religious orders to work in the caring professions. Journal of Advanced Nursing 28 (1), 212–220.

Cutcliffe, J.R., Hummelvoll, J.K., Granerud, A., Erikson, B.G., 2015. Mental health nurses responding to suffering in the 21st century occidental world: accompanying people in their search for meaning. Archives of Psychiatric Nursing 29, 19–25.

Davis, L.W., Lysaker, P.H., 2007. Therapeutic alliance and improvements in work performance over time in patients with schizophrenia. The Journal of Nervous and Mental Disease 195 (4), 353–357.

Day, H., 2015. The meaning of compassion. British Journal of Nursing 24 (6), 342–343.

Duggleby, W., Hicks, D., Nekolaichuk, C., Holtslander, L., Williams, A., Chambers, T., Eby, J., 2012. Hope, older adults, and chronic illness: a metasynthesis of qualitative research. Journal of Advanced Nursing 68 (6), 1211–1223.

Ewers, P., Bradshaw, T., McGovern, J., et al., 2002. Does training in psychosocial interventions reduce burnout rates in forensic nursing? Journal of Advanced Nursing 37 (5), 470–476.

Finfgeld-Connett, D., 2008. Meta-synthesis of caring in nursing. Journal of Clinical Nursing 17 (2), 196–204.

Fitzgerald Miller, J., 2007. Hope: a construct central to nursing. Nursing Forum 42 (1), 12–19.

Forchuk, C., Reynolds, W., 2001. Clients' reflections on relationships with nurses: comparisons from Canada and Scotland. Journal of Psychiatric and Mental Health Nursing 8, 45–51.

Foster, K., McAllister, M., O'Brien, L., 2006. Extending the boundaries: autoethnography as an emergent method in mental health nursing research. International Journal of Mental Health Nursing 15, 44–53.

Freiburger, O., 2002. Preceptor programs: increasing student self-confidence and competency. Nurse Educator 27 (2), 58–60.

Gardner, A., 2010. Therapeutic friendliness and the development of therapeutic leverage by mental health nurses in community rehabilitation settings. Contemporary Nurse 34 (2), 140–148.

Geanellos, R., 2002. Transformative change of self: the unique focus of (adolescent) mental health nursing? International Journal of Mental Health Nursing 11, 174–185.

Gibbs, G., 1988. Learning by doing: a guide to teaching and learning methods. Further Education Unit, Sheffield.

Godin, P., 2000. A dirty business: caring for people who are a nuisance or a danger. Journal of Advanced Nursing 32 (6), 1396–1402.

Grady, C.A., Stewardson, G.A., Hall, J.L., 2008. Faculty notions regarding caring in male nursing students. The Journal of Nursing Education 47 (7), 314–323.

Graham, I., 2001. Seeking clarification of meaning: a phenomenological interpretation of the craft of mental health nursing. Journal of Psychiatric and Mental Health Nursing 8, 335–345.

Greenwood, J., 1998. The role of reflection in single and double loop learning. Journal of Advanced Nursing 27, 1048–1053.

Gunasekara, I., Pentland, T., Rodgers, T., Patterson, S., 2014. What makes an excellent mental health nurse? A pragmatic inquiry initiated and conducted by people with lived experience of service use. International Journal of Mental Health Nursing 23, 101–109.

Gustin, L.W., Wagner, L., 2013. The butterfly effect of caring—clinical nurse teachers' understanding of self-compassion as a source of compassionate care. Scandinavian Journal of Caring Sciences 27, 175–183.

Haddad, A., 2002. An ethical view of burnout. RN Journal 65 (9) 25–6, 28.

Hemingway, S., Rogers, M., Elsom, S., 2014. Measuring the influence of a mental health training module on the therapeutic optimism of advanced nurse practitioner students in the United Kingdom. American Association of Nurse Practitioners 26, 155–162.

Henderson, J., 2004. The challenge of relationship boundaries in mental health. Nursing Management 11 (6), 28–31.

Hewitt, J., Coffey, M., 2005. Therapeutic working relationships with people with schizophrenia. Journal of Advanced Nursing 52 (5), 561–570.

Hill, R.G., Atnas, C.I., Ryan, P., Ashby, K., Winnington, J., 2010. Whole team training to reduce burn-out amongst staff on an in-patient alcohol ward. Journal of Substance Abuse 15 (1), 42–50.

Hogan, K., 2013. Caring as a scripted discourse versus caring as an expression of an authentic relationship between self and other. Issues in Mental Health Nursing 34, 375–379.

Hunsaker, S., Maughan, D., Heaston, S., 2015. Factors that influence the development of compassion fatigue, burnout, and compassion satisfaction in emergency department nurses. Journal of Nursing Scholarship 47 (2), 186–194.

Jackson, D., Borbasi, S.-A., 2006. Nursing care and nurse caring: issues, concerns, debates. In: Daly, J., Speedy, S., Jackson, D. (Eds.), Contexts of nursing: an introduction, second ed. Elsevier, Sydney, NSW.

Jackson, D., Firtko, A., Edenborough, M., 2007. Personal resilience as a strategy for surviving and thriving in the face of workplace adversity: a review of the literature. Journal of Advanced Nursing 60 (1), 1–9.

Johansson, H., Jansson, J.A., 2010. Therapeutic alliance and outcome in routine psychiatric outpatient treatment: patient factors and outcome. Psychology and Psychotherapy: Theory, Research and Practice 83, 193–206.

Johns, C., 2001. Reflective practice: revealing the [he]art of caring. International Journal of Nursing Practice 7 (4), 237–245.

Kim, H.S., 1999. Critical reflective inquiry for knowledge development in nursing practice. Journal of Advanced Nursing 29 (5), 1205–1212.

Lees, D., Procter, N., Fassett, D., 2014. Therapeutic engagement between consumers in suicidal crisis and mental health nurses. International Journal of Mental Health Nursing 23 (4), 306–315.

McAndrew, S., Chambers, M., Nolan, F., Thomas, B., Watts, P., 2014. Measuring the evidence: reviewing the literature of the measurement of therapeutic engagement in acute mental health inpatient wards. International Journal of Mental Health Nursing 23, 212–220.

McCloughen, A., O'Brien, L., Jackson, D., 2006. Positioning mentorship within Australian nursing contexts: a review of the local and international literature. Contemporary Nurse 23 (1), 120–134.

Meng, L., Liu, Y., Liu, H., Hu, Y., Yang, J., Liu, J., 2014. Relationships among structural empowerment, psychological empowerment, intent to stay and burnout in nursing field in mainland China—based on a cross-sectional questionnaire research. International Journal of Nursing Practice https://doi.org/10.1111/ijn.12279.

Nursing & Midwifery Council (NMC), 2015. The code: professional standards of practice and behaviour for nurses and midwives. NMC, London.

O'Brien, L., 2000. Nurse-client relationships: the experience of community psychiatric nurses. Australian and New Zealand Journal of Mental Health Nursing 9, 184–194.

O'Brien, L., 2001. The relationship between community psychiatric nurses and clients with severe and persistent mental illness: the client experience. Australian and New Zealand Journal of Mental Health Nursing 10, 176–186.

Pilgrim, D., Rogers, A., Bentall, R., 2009. The centrality of personal relationships in the creation and amelioration of mental health problems: the current interdisciplinary case. Health (London) 13, 235–254.

Ramezani, M., Ahmadi, F., Mohammadi, E., Kazemnejad, A., 2014. Spiritual care in nursing: a concept analysis. International Nursing Review 61, 211–219. https://doi.org/10.1111/inr.12099.

Royal College of Nursing, 2017. Revalidation Requirements: Reflection and Reflective Discussion [online]. Accessed 3rd September 2017. Available at: https://www.rcn.org.uk/professional-development/revalidation/reflection-and-reflective-discussion.

Sawbridge, Y., Hewison, A., 2015. Compassion costs nothing—the elephant in the room? Practice Nursing 26 (4), 194–197.

Schofield, R., Allan, M., Jewiss, T., Hunter, A., Sinclair, N., Diamond, A., Sidwell, C., 2013. Knowing self and caring through service learning. International Journal of Nursing Education Scholarship 10 (1), 267–274.

Schon, D., 1983. The reflective practitioner: how professionals think in action. Basic Books, New York, NY.

Schrank, B., Stanghellini, G., Slade, M., 2008. Hope in psychiatry: a review of the literature. Acta Psychiatrica Scandinavica 118, 421–433.

Shattell, M.M., McAllister, S., Hogan, B., et al., 2006. 'She took the time to make sure she understood': mental health patients' experiences of being understood. Archives of Psychiatric Nursing 20 (5), 234–241.

Speedy, S., 2006. The gendered culture of nursing. In: Daly, J., Speedy, S., Jackson, D. (Eds.), Contexts of Nursing: an Introduction, second ed. Elsevier, Sydney, NSW.

Stewart, D., Burrow, H., Duckworth, A., et al., 2015. Thematic analysis of psychiatric patients' perceptions of nursing staff. International Journal of Mental Health Nursing 24 (1), 82–90.

Straughair, C., 2012a. Exploring compassion: implications for contemporary nursing. Part 1. British Journal of Nursing 21 (3), 160–164.

Straughair, C., 2012b. Exploring compassion: implications for contemporary nursing. Part 2. British Journal of Nursing 21 (4), 239–244.

Tariman, J.D., 2010. Where to draw the line: professional boundaries in social networking. ONS Connect 25 (2), 10–13.

Thorpe, K., Barsky, J., 2001. Healing through self-reflection. Journal of Advanced Nursing 35 (5), 760–768.

Warelow, P., Edward, K., 2007. Caring as resilient practice in mental health nursing. International Journal of Mental Health Nursing 16, 132–135.

Weaver, K., 2007. Ethical sensitivity: a state of knowledge and needs for further research. Nursing Ethics 14 (2), 141–155.

Welch, M., 2005. Pivotal moments in the therapeutic relationship. International Journal of Mental Health Nursing 14, 161–165.

Wheeler, K., 2011. A relationship-based model for psychiatric nursing practice. Perspectives in Psychiatric Care 47 (3), 151–159.

Wikberg, A., Eriksson, K., 2008. Intercultural caring: an abductive model. Scandinavian Journal of Caring Science 22, 485–496.

Wyder, M., Bland, R., Blythe, A., Matarasso, B., Crompton, D., 2015. Therapeutic relationships and involuntary treatment orders: service users' interactions with health-care professionals on the ward. International Journal of Mental Health Nursing 24 (2), 181–189. https://doi.org/10.1111/inm.12121.

USEFUL WEBSITES

Professional Boundaries

England, Wales, Scotland and Northern Ireland: Nursing and Midwifery Council (NMC) www.nmc.org.uk

Ireland: Bord Altranais agus Cnáimhseachais na hÉireann/Nursing and Midwifery Board of Ireland (NMBI) www.nmbi.ie

Mentoring

Royal College of Nursing: Guidance for Mentors of Nursing and Midwifery Students www.rcn.org.uk/professional-development/publications/pub-006133

2

Recovery as the Context for Practice

Vicki Stanton, Barbara Tooth and Simon Champ

KEY POINTS

- The primacy of the consumer voice is central to all current mental health contexts and areas of practice.
- The ultimate goal of mental health practice is to value and facilitate the personal recovery of all individuals. This includes promoting their personal agency, connectedness and social inclusion; self-determination; and their active participation in society. It also relates to how they can negotiate the range of resources they need to remain active citizens in the community of their choice, even during periods of mental distress.
- The quality of a person's relationships is a key determinant of their quality of life.
- The recovery paradigm provides both the framework to consider what may be necessary for people to have a meaningful life and the context and guiding principles for all mental health practice.
- The context of mental health nursing practice is dynamic and ever changing, responding to new ideas about what people need in order to live a meaningful and contributing life.
- The recovery paradigm reconceptualises the roles of mental health professionals to reemphasise the therapeutic use of self, specifically how to 'be with' rather than 'do to'.
- National and international laws protecting people's basic human rights provide the legal context for recovery-informed practice within the recovery paradigm.
- Mental health policy and plans provide the sociopolitical context for practice and the implementation of services that, ideally, are based on the recovery paradigm.
- Mental health nursing practice is ultimately influenced by the attitudes, values and beliefs of the nurse and is developed through general life experiences, education and interaction with people who experience mental distress.
- The ability to think critically and develop self-awareness is central to nursing practice.

KEY TERMS

citizenship
community-managed organisations (CMOs)
connectedness
consumer voice
enabling environments
human rights
non-government organisations (NGOs)
peer support
peer support worker
personal agency
personal narratives
recovery
reflection
rehabilitation
self-determination
social inclusion
stigma
strengths
supportive environments
trauma-informed care

LEARNING OUTCOMES

The material in this chapter will assist you to:

- identify the key importance of each person's unique experiences and histories within the context of their whole life, a part of which may be in mental health service systems.
- describe the centrality of the person's lived experience to your role as a nurse and your capacity to 'be with' people on their personal journey.
- demonstrate an understanding of the role your attitudes, values and beliefs play as key factors in what you say and do when you work with people, and of the role theories and your life experiences have in this process.
- begin to appreciate the complex interaction between the current contexts that influence mental health practice.
- appreciate that human rights and the international laws that protect them are central to the mental health field in general and to people who experience mental health challenges in particular.
- identify the key differences in the way nurses conceptualise their role and their practice between the recovery and medical paradigms.
- describe the principles of recovery-informed practice and the importance of hope and optimism in recovery.

- explain the rationale for the shift in mental health to the recovery paradigm, which values the primary role of expert knowledge that comes from the lived experience of severe mental health distress.
- appreciate the value of reflective practice and continually developing self-awareness, in particular your reaction to witnessing people's distress and fears.

INTRODUCTION

It is revolutionary when you truly understand recovery (Davidson et al. 2010). In the context of this book, it must be made crystal clear that recovery is about the person living a good life in their community. In reality, mental health and community services play only a small, but important, part in people's lives. The vast majority of a person's recovery occurs outside of services. People who work within such services can get a skewed view that they are central to the person's life. They are not. They are there to support the person and not get in the way of whatever they need in their journey. It is within this context that this chapter introduces students to the richness and depth of the many facets of recovery. It explains why it is the current context for mental health policies, plans, service provision and practice in many countries worldwide (Slade et al. 2014). The chapter also addresses how recovery differs from previous approaches in mental health.

In keeping with the importance of the centrality of people's lived experience of mental health challenges, Simon Champ coauthors this chapter. Simon was one of the first consumer advocates in Australia and has been a catalyst for debate and change. He was an advisor on the first National Strategy for Mental Health, served on the board of SANE Australia and was an early member of Schizophrenia Fellowship NSW. He played a major role in the documentary *Spinning Out* (Deveson 1991), has been a speaker and teacher both nationally and internationally and is an author and artist. It is a privilege to have his contribution.

The patient movement, referred to in Australia and New Zealand as the consumer movement, has been the main driving force behind the introduction of the concept of recovery into English-speaking countries; fundamentally, it is about the protection of people's human rights. Therefore, the Universal Declaration of Human Rights (1948), the Convention on the Rights of Persons with Disabilities (1975) and the United Nations Declaration of the Rights of Indigenous People (2008) underpin the recovery paradigm. The European Union supports the declarations and convention mentioned.

The chapter starts by looking at recovery as the current context for practice, how it is defined, the tensions in defining it, how it has evolved and how it is currently understood. This section tracks the history underlying recovery, the key differences between recovery-informed and traditional practice, and how to translate the recovery approach into practice. The chapter concludes with recovery-informed service provision.

To make sense of mental health nursing practice requires an understanding of other factors that may influence it. These include social and cultural factors and the attitudes, values and beliefs that guide our thinking. People's thinking changes over time and this is determined by their own experiences and by changes in thinking about what constitutes appropriate practice. Since the 1990s, the rate of change in thinking around mental health practice has been significant and it will continue to be so. This chapter addresses some of the major shifts in thinking that influence our understanding of what mental health nursing practice entails.

It can be tempting to think that mental health nursing is a discrete area of practice of little value to the general nurse, *but this is far from the truth.* In fact, it is argued the principles underpinning recovery-based mental health practice also underpin all areas of nursing practice. The fundamental concepts and principles underlying mental health nursing are considered so important to general nursing practice that they have been incorporated into undergraduate nursing courses. The comprehensive course is intended to provide a holistic approach to nursing care and a basis for later specialist practice.

In addition, at some point in their lives one in four people in the UK will experience mental distress severe enough to be diagnosed and warrant intervention from a mental health professional (NHS England 2018). Physical illness exacerbates such distress and people cannot isolate parts of themselves in their interactions with general health professionals. Therefore, it stands to reason that general nurses frequently work with people experiencing mental distress.

For many students, this chapter will probably raise more questions than it answers. If so, it has achieved one of its objectives. It is not possible to address here all a nurse needs to know about recovery to become a competent practitioner. To do this you will need to engage in a journey of continuing professional development in recovery-informed practice and competency.

RECOVERY AS THE CONTEXT OF PRACTICE

The current context of mental health practice is one of major transformation. The focus has changed from the traditional biomedical approach towards a recovery-informed approach. Everyone working in or connected with the mental health field is being called upon to answer the question: how will what we do assist people to live a contributing and meaningful life in their chosen community, just like every other citizen? This is a key question of the recovery paradigm.

The National Framework for Recovery-Oriented Mental Health Services: Policy and Theory defines recovery as 'being able to create and live a meaningful and contributing life in a community of choice with or without the presence of mental health issues' (Commonwealth of Australia 2013a, p. 25).

While recovery is a simple concept that all people want, the implications for services and everyone within them are huge, especially when you truly understand what recovery means. How well recovery is understood and the leadership that occurs in all service and community systems impacts the rate of transformation in mental health. To guide the student and newly qualified nurse's understanding of recovery, the different context in which the term 'recovery' is being used in mental health services will be explored. It covers such contexts as a person's journey of recovery, a recovery framework, recovery-informed practice and the recovery paradigm itself. Let's look at these more closely.

Recovery as a Personal Journey

First, it is important to understand recovery is primarily and foremost a personal journey that can only be undertaken by the person. People who have or have had mental health challenges are *the experts on personal recovery through experience*. No-one can make a person recover, do it for him or her or be the expert on the person's experience. This is key to recognising how services, everyone involved in mental health and the community as a whole can support, promote and facilitate the person's self-directed recovery journey. It is paramount that each person's unique personal journey drives the care, service provision and service structures they need. Glover (2012) refers to recovery as a natural self-righting process people undertake to grow beyond any distress that interrupts the balance of daily life. Recovery starts with the person; they determine what they need and which services and supports would work best for them. Care in the context of recovery is always collaborative and driven by the person experiencing mental health challenges. Glover also emphasises the constant need to recognise and uphold the personal nature of recovery and to support the self-applied effort and learning that a person engages in. Glover cautions that mental health workers could default to seeing recovery through a clinical gaze but she advises workers to use their skills to be in relationships with people in ways that support the ongoing, progressive nature of their personal growth.

Recovery Paradigm

A paradigm is a distinct set of concepts or thought patterns, including theories, research methods, hypotheses and standards for what constitutes legitimate contributions to a field (Oxford English Reference Dictionary; The Free Dictionary). You will already be familiar with the technological paradigm that informs the biomedical model. The recovery paradigm identifies the wide range of knowledge and research that is important to inform the mental health field and the wider community, including the body of knowledge gained from personal recovery.

Maintaining hope and optimism are overarching principles in recovery (Commonwealth of Australia 2013a) as is citizenship (Rowe 2015). Key features of the recovery paradigm include the need for self-determination, personal agency, the importance of social inclusion and having choice in a range of services. Valuing the person's imperatives rather than clinical imperatives drives the recovery paradigm: it represents a change in values (Slade 2009).

Dan Fisher, a prominent psychiatrist who has identified as having been given the label of 'schizophrenia', states that the recovery paradigm views mental health issues as challenges that a person can grow beyond, through the assistance of culturally appropriate, trauma-informed services and natural supports in the process of the person building a full and gratifying life in the community of his or her choice (Fisher 2011).

Recovery framework

A framework is a subset of the recovery paradigm. Frameworks provide the structure to inform cohesive service delivery and guide principles of practice (recovery-informed practice). There are many different recovery frameworks. They can be frameworks to guide service provision, principles of practice or competencies. Often these reflect what the person proposing the framework thinks are most important. Sometimes the terms 'framework' and 'paradigm' are used interchangeably. The Tidal Model (Barker & Buchanan-Barker 2004) is one such framework specifically developed for nurses. You are encouraged to look at their website.

Terms Used to Describe People who Experience Mental Health Challenges

Before moving on in this chapter, it is important to address the terms used to describe people who experience mental health challenges. The terms most commonly used to identify people with mental distress in the UK are 'patient', 'client', 'service user', 'survivor' and 'expert by experience'. The most appropriate term to refer to a person experiencing mental ill health provokes much debate, both by the individuals with mental health problems and the professionals who care for them. Although 'service user' is commonly used throughout the UK, research has shown this term to be disliked more than any other term by professionals, and only a significant minority of people with mental health problems wish to be referred to as 'survivor' or 'user' (Simmons et al. 2010). Due to the ongoing debate, the term 'patient' will be used throughout this text. This word is not meant to cause any offense, quite the opposite in fact and is simply following a school of thought that evidence-based terminology would adopt 'patient' in preference to 'service user' (Simmons et al. 2010), the choice of which is meant with the very best of intentions. In Australia and New Zealand the terms 'consumer', 'client' '(psychiatric) survivor', 'user', 'ex-user' and 'Person with a lived experience', which is a relatively recent term, are used. This chapter has been written specifically around the concept of recovery oriented mental health in Australia and New Zealand, but has been kept in this UK edition as it offers a valuable reflection on recovery, as such the term 'consumer' will be used throughout the rest of this chapter to reflect the approach. One of the authors, Simon Champ, was one of the first consumer advocates in Australia and has been a catalyst for debate and change as an advisor on the first National Strategy for Mental Health, a board member of SANE

Australia, an early member of Schizophrenia Fellowship New South Wales and invited speaker and teacher internationally.

The Consumer Coalition first used the term 'consumer' in the United States of America in the early 1980s (Clay 2002). The term 'survivor' is also used in the United States because of its resonance with the human rights movement, highlighting the fact that treatment often does not meet people's needs and in many cases violates their basic human rights. There is much debate around the most appropriate term. Some schools of thought believe the term 'patient' is considered too bound up with illness, the medical model, deficits and the disparity in status between person and professional. It is also suggested to imply a more passive role, with the person concerned being the recipient of care. However, others believe that this is the most appropriate, relating to a person's need for care and recovery journey through ill health, regardless of the nature. The term 'client' is argued to have similar connotations to 'patient', while the authors of this chapter believe the term 'consumer' implies a more active role, with the person having rights, responsibility and a more equitable relationship with the care provider. The key mental health organisations and policy documents in Australia use the term 'consumer'. See Box 2.1 for key mental health organisations and policy documents in Australia, peak consumer and carer advisory groups and consumer participation policies and frameworks.

BOX 2.1 Key Mental Health Organisations and Policy Documents in Australia

- National Mental Health Consumer and Carer Forum, http://nmhccf.org.au
- Private Mental Health Consumer Carer Network www.pmhccn.com.au
- Mental Health Australia (an independent peak national body for mental health that has a wide range of important resources), www.mhca.org.au
- A National Framework for Recovery-Oriented Mental Health Services: Policy and Theory (2013), www.health.gov.au/internet/main/publishing.nsf/Content/mental-pubs-n-recovpol
- A National Framework for Recovery-Oriented Mental Services: Guide for Practitioners and Providers (2013), www.health.gov.au/internet/main/publishing.nsf/Content/mental-pubs-n-recovgde
- National Mental Health Commission's Strategies and Actions 2012–2015, www.mentalhealthcommission.gov.au/media/5039/strategicactions_2012%20to2015.pdf
- National Standards for Mental Health Services 2010, www.health.gov.au/internet/main/publishing.nsf/content/mental-pubs-n-servst10
- National Mental Health Commission (numerous important resources), www.mentalhealthcommission.gov.au
- Mental Health and Addiction Action Plan 2010 (Ministry of Health Wellington 2010), www.health.govt.nz/publication/mental-health-and-addiction-action-plan-2010

Since language conveys meaning, we prefer the expression 'people who have experience of mental health challenges' because it is part of the spectrum of human experience we may all have. The reality is *everyone* is susceptible to developing mental health challenges. To normalise this and to reduce stigma, there are a number of high-profile public figures in sport, politics, the arts and business coming out and talking about their own mental health challenges. These include public personalities such as Stephen Fry, Paul Merton and Ruby Wax. An extensive list can be found at http://amandagreenauthor.co.uk/300-famous-people-celebrities-who-have-suffered-with-mental-illness-or-issues-help-highlight-the-stigma-in-our-society.

Defining Personal Recovery

Only the person who has the lived experience can define personal recovery. This poses the dilemma of finding a definition that is widely accepted. There are numerous definitions of recovery in the literature. Anthony's definition continues to be prominent and informs mental health policies and plans in a number of countries around the world (Slade et al. 2014). Anthony states that recovery is:

> *a deeply personal, unique process of changing one's attitudes, values, goals, skills and/or roles. It is a way of living a satisfying, hopeful, and contributing life even within the limitations caused by the illness. Recovery involves the development of new meaning and purpose in one's life as one grows beyond the catastrophic effects of mental illness (Anthony 1993, p. 14).*

There are other definitions of recovery espoused in seminal works of prominent consumers, academics and clinicians (Borg & Kristiansen 2007; Chamberlin 1997; Curtis 1998; Deegan 1993; Davidson 2003; Fisher 2011). Key features espoused by these authors include:

- doing something worthwhile
- being involved in things not related to their own problems
- having ordinary discussions with others
- being included in and connected to communities
- being included in ordinary work roles and settings where it is recognised that everyday ups and downs of life in these settings are an intrinsic pattern to be experienced rather than pathologised
- regaining belief in oneself
- recognising losses of rights, roles, responsibilities, decisions, potential and support, then finding out what the person wants and how they want to achieve it
- making meaning out of one's experiences
- recognising that recovery is not the same as being cured, as it is a process with no endpoint or destination
- being aware recovery is an attitude, a way of approaching day-to-day challenges and being in control
- having a life outside mental illness

The aforementioned definitions demonstrate that people who have mental health challenges want to live a life like every other citizen. Recovery is not unique to people who experience mental health challenges. Every individual will have challenging life events from which they recover. This is an essential part of normal human growth and development. The difference for people with mental health challenges is the additional significant barriers they face. They often experience social disadvantage, social isolation and have difficulty getting back into mainstream society for a variety of reasons. Frequently, they have difficulty finding accommodation, obtaining meaningful work, having meaningful connection with others, achieving an adequate income and feeling safe. Simon Champ's story in Patient Story 2.1 tells of some of his experiences and the challenges of living with mental health distress.

The many descriptions of recovery demonstrate that it is a multifaceted and deeply personal experience. It is not possible to find a single definition with which everyone agrees. This was demonstrated in a large Australian study on recovery from schizophrenia (Tooth et al. 2003). One aim of the research was to identify a consumer definition of recovery. This was not achieved with the 60 participants: there were as many views as there were participants. Overwhelmingly, the participants had not actually thought in terms of recovery until they agreed to take part in the research. They stated that they were just getting on with their lives, highlighting the very personal and complex nature of people's understanding of their experiences of mental distress. The nebulous nature of recovery continues to be identified in recent research (Le Boutillier et al. 2011).

CONSUMER STORY 2.1 Simon's Story: Living With Difference and Mental Health Challenges

I have mentioned elsewhere (Champ 1998) how schizophrenia severely ruptured the relationship I enjoyed with myself prior to my mental health challenges. To have the lived experience of a mental illness/disorder even for a brief period can be distressing and discouraging not only for the person going through the experience, but also their family and friends. At best for some a mental illness/disorder can sensitise one to the world in new ways that if harnessed can be a productive force in someone's life. Yes, many people do recover and while some recover, stigma never lets them live as such. Implicit in the treatment of people affected by and living with a mental illness there were always seemingly unrealistic expectations of their 'recovery'. People's expectations of 'prognosis' were either too high or, discouragingly, too low.

The constantly changing nature of my experiences with schizophrenia over many decades changed my relationship with myself many times and in a number of different ways. For myself my diagnosis initially came with hope. I was in the euphemistically named 'nervous breakdown' category, breaking down in my final year in high school and leaving school to work and then repeat the High School Certificate (HSC). I loved studying art, biology and English. I was an English migrant who had arrived with my family trying to adjust to country schools in Australia and already falling behind. I moved many times whilst trying to study at a tertiary level with very supportive parents. I was trying to make sense and meaning in a life that was more and more chaotic. My diagnosis moved up a notch to 'paranoid schizophrenic'. On reflection this was a label I applied to myself, becoming my illness was a very disempowered position. My diagnosis moved on to 'schizoaffective disorder'. I found myself in libraries trying to understand these diagnoses. My struggle for equilibrium and meaning led to stark realities. The prognoses I came across were highly discouraging. They gave me little hope.

Always the question of being mad, bad or both challenged me. I was too young and too immature to really understand much of the 1960s civil rights and counterculture movements that questioned these labels.

When I was recently an inpatient I wanted the nurses to know how distressing I found the environment around me. No-one seemed to understand the impact of watching others and the incomprehensible interactions between people who were distressed. I wanted nurses to mirror back to people or confront them on how their behaviour affects others whilst at the same time realising this was a hard task for nurses when behaviours are those they may not have come across before. Just as people with mental health challenges have to reflect on their own issues, so too, do nurses. I want nurses to be able to keep an open mind, to keep hope alive, especially for those around the person when they are at their worst and experiencing the most challenges.

There were many professionals who provided me with hope along the way. Others could not get through to me in spite of their best efforts. I have realised how I did use denial. I now try very hard to see what I enjoy about me and around me. Time can be a healer, time can be a teacher, and bring awareness of things that have been long hidden. The nurses I most valued were those who, rather than imposing their reality on me, helped me to explore where reality and wellbeing might exist for me.

There have been many opportunities afforded to me as an activist and advocate. I have been able to travel widely and meet people including some of the best minds in mental health and art. It has opened doors for me. It has given me insights into others and myself. In the last few years I have become less concerned with the wider picture of thinking on mental health and I have tried to return in a more positive way to my practice as an artist. As hard as it is, I once again am able to find solace and new insights into many fields of endeavour, ironically including nursing. I am at my best when I'm engaged through my art and my interactions with others. Making a meaningful contribution is important to me.

What I hope for in the future is that the extraordinary amounts of new information about the world we live in and the people we are can enable far more options to be available for people, no matter what their experiences of living with a mental health disorder. These greater options must be timely and readily available to enable people to get the help they deserve. I hope nurses and more broadly everyone in the community come to see the wonder that is the human being.

Students need to be aware of how they use language and terms such as 'recovery' with the people with whom they work. Such terms may have little or no meaning to them, or their meaning may be different from your own understanding. Successive generations of people have experienced very different practices and treatments. Therefore the current terminology of recovery may not be familiar to older people. A critical point here is that it does not matter what the term is—it is the meaning people make of their own experience and the principles and values that underpin recovery that really matter.

To illustrate the above point on differences in personal meaning, in the *Spinning Out* documentary (Deveson 1991), Simon Champ came up with the quirky mnemonic for schizophrenia. For him schizophrenia means **S**pecial **C**reatively **H**eightened **I**ndividual **Z**anily **O**verly **P**erceptive **H**umorous **R**eally **E**motional **N**eeding **I**ndividual **A**ssistance.

Tensions in Defining Recovery

The recovery paradigm and recovery frameworks acknowledge the centrality of each consumer's voice in terms of care and service provision. However, there is justified concern among consumers that they are not being listened to or heard because of a lack of dialogue, collaboration and shared decision making with professionals (Kidd et al. 2015). There is a growing perception that recovery is being colonised by professionals and services as a result of consumers not being heard. Researchers (Le Boutillier et al. 2011; Cleary et al. 2013; Bird et al. 2014) found that mental health practitioners can have different meanings for recovery that are not consistent with the consumer voice on what constitutes recovery. Some practitioners considered recovery in terms of symptomology or improvement. Others emphasised certain aspects of recovery over others in their practice, depending on their own personal views. In addition, some professionals and organisations embrace the term 'recovery' but do not fully understand what it means. They continue to practise in old ways while claiming to be recovery oriented, leading to fears the promise of recovery has been hijacked by professionals (Mental Health 'Recovery' Study Working Group 2009).

Similarly, Morrow (2011) found consumer advocates argued that the recovery paradigm had been co-opted into the biomedical frame. When this happens, the biomedical frame becomes dominant and downplays the social determinants of health, structural disadvantage and social exclusion that are so critical to mental wellbeing. Here, part of the tension is between the term 'clinical recovery', which has sprung up to refer to medical management of symptoms and functioning in acute services, and the term 'personal recovery', where the concerns are significantly broader and apply no matter where the person is in services (from acute care through to the wider community). A more constructive approach is to consider the value of both views and see how they can complement one another (Glover 2012; Slade 2009).

What Recovery is Not

Recovery is not rehabilitation. It is not always easy to distinguish between the terms 'rehabilitation' and 'recovery'. The terms have been used interchangeably and also they are spoken about as if recovery has replaced rehabilitation. The concept of recovery has not replaced rehabilitation but it has changed the way it is practised. Traditionally, psychiatric rehabilitation has been provided for people who experience severe and enduring forms of mental illness, with the primary aim of reintegrating the person into the community. Professionals, including nurses, assessed the person's deficits to determine their rehabilitation needs and the person then attended a rehabilitation service where programs (often run by nurses) would address these skill deficits. This approach to rehabilitation has been criticised by Deegan (1988; 2004) and O'Hagan (2011) because it requires people to progress through predetermined skills-based training programs regardless of individual needs. In addition, such rehabilitation programs were determined by 'experts' based on what they thought was best for the person.

In 1988 Deegan made a useful distinction between recovery and rehabilitation in mental health services that is still valid today:

Disabled persons are not passive recipients of rehabilitation services. Rather, they experience themselves as recovering a new sense of self and of purpose within and beyond the limits of the disability . . . Rehabilitation refers to services and technologies that are made available to disabled persons so they may learn to adapt to their world. Recovery refers to the lived or real life experience of persons as they accept and overcome the challenge of disability (1988, p. 11).

Recovery is not cure. In his 2005 book *Recovered, not Cured*, McLean makes some very important points about the complexity of personal experience that makes this so. In medicine, recovery from illness is the absence of symptoms of the disease or disorder, and a return to the person's premorbid level of functioning after a designated period of time. For example, for some types of cancer a person is considered recovered after a period of 5 years without symptoms. None of these conditions apply to recovery from mental health challenges for the following reasons.

- People can consider themselves to be in recovery and still have the experience of mental distress.
- Mental health challenges are transformative in nature and challenge people's concepts of normality, making the return to a premorbid level of functioning meaningless.
- Recovery is also described as an ongoing process, so timeframes are likewise meaningless. The rate of recovery varies for each person. For some it may occur in small incremental steps. Indeed, the crisis or mental health challenge may arise because of the need to recover from one situation to another.

Personal Narratives

Personal narratives are essential to recovery-informed perspectives and for determining what is important for any individual in their journey of recovery. Box 2.2 about the recovery of Mary O'Hagan, a prominent international consumer educator and consultant, illustrates the tension between what people say is important to them and what

BOX 2.2 **Story of Recovery: Mary O'Hagan**

In common with so many people who experience mental distress, Mary describes her madness as the loss of self, the solid core of her being. While this core is not evident during times of madness, it returns stronger, renewed and ready to go again. Madness is a crisis of being that is a part of the full range of human experience. Mary explains: 'My self is the solid core of my being. It is like an immutable dark sun that sits at the centre of things while all my fickle feelings, thoughts and sensations orbit around it. But my self goes into hiding during madness. Sometimes it slides into the great nothingness like a setting sun. Sometimes it gets trampled in the dust by all the whizzing in my body and mind . . . Sometimes my madness strips me bare but it is also the beginning of renewal; every time I emerge from it I feel fresh and ready to start again.'

Mary had to make friends with rather than fight her madness; get to know, understand and respect it—a complex process. 'My madness was like a boarder coming to live in my house, who turned out to be a citizen from an enemy country. Knowing I might not get rid of him meant I had to make peace with him and learn to understand his language. Once I got to know the boarder, he was no longer the stereotypical enemy, but a complex character that deserved some respect.'

Mental health professionals did not find any value in helping Mary to understand the meaning in her madness. Nor did they allow her to tap into her own power, her own resourcefulness. Mary's experience of care within mental health services was one of being 'skilled in lowered expectations'; for example, repeatedly being told that things such as studying or working would be too stressful and she would not be able to do them. The way mental healthcare was provided to Mary encouraged passivity rather than autonomy. She found the capacity to tap into her own resourcefulness only by coming across the consumer/survivor literature that inspired her. She was then able to find and use her own power to get out of the cycle of madness. Mary went on to be appointed as a mental health commissioner in New Zealand and has been an international consultant on mental health since that time.

What was most difficult for Mary was not the symptoms but how people regarded her. In retrospect her madness was a place of beauty and difficulty, madness filled with soul. Mary talks about the terrible suffering and the desperate struggle of her madness, but she also talks about the richness in her experience that she could interpret as filled with purpose and meaning. She wanted acceptance of her reality. For Mary, the best thing people could have done was to be kind and accept her reality—a basic human response.

(*Source:* O'Hagan, M., undated. Making sense of madness. Accessed 31 May 2015. We encourage you to visit Mary O'Hagan's website at: www.maryohagan.com for further reading.)

professionals and the system focus on. This tension is underscored by the fact that although many people find meaning in their madness, the people they turn to for support view madness primarily as pathology and something to be managed and medicated.

BOX 2.3 **Link to Personal Stories**

- The National Mental Health Commission's *A Contributing Life: The 2013 Report Card on Mental Health and Suicide Prevention* has some interesting links to personal stories. The following link is to Grant's story. Grant was a forensic mental health inpatient: www.mentalhealthcommission.gov.au/media/94357/07_Feeling_safe_stable_and_secure.pdf
- Recommended reading: Champ, S., 1998. A most precious thread. Australian and New Zealand Journal of Mental Health Nursing 7(2):54–59.

Is Mary O'Hagan's experience an isolated one? Is it an old story that would not happen today? No. Glover (2012) presents the stories of two women and their personal experiences of mental distress managed in Australia by involuntary inpatient admissions. The women's perceptions of their care include that they were not helped to make sense of their experiences, felt stripped of their power and were not responded to as people but as 'diagnostic categories'. Their experiences were described using the language and meaning of the professional knowledge base; their own meaning and language for their experiences were not encouraged or valued. What makes Glover's work so powerful is that while both women had very similar experiences, one story took place in 1985 and the other in 2010. The latter occurred at a time when services were promoting their model of care as recovery-informed, leading Glover to ask, what has actually changed in the past 25 years? The link to personal stories in Box 2.3, and the very influential keynote address Simon Champ gave at the Congress of the Australian College of Mental Health Nurses, might help you to better understand the consumer perspective.

BRIEF HISTORY OF RECOVERY MOVEMENT AND RESEARCH

Historically, the consumer movement has championed recovery. Effective consumer groups began to emerge in the 1980s, yet people with 'mental illness' were pursuing their own goals back in the 17th century (Campbell 2009). The consumer movement grew out of the African-American civil rights movement and the rights movements for women, LGBTQI people and those with disability in the United States. At the same time in the 1960s and 1970s, hospitals in the United States were being closed. The civil rights of people who had 'mental illness' had long been denied and people became angry about a whole range of treatments they found abusive. Consumer groups banded together to advocate for significant change in mental health services and began to develop and run their own alternative models of care.

The consumer movement is at its heart a human rights movement, with a significant role in advocating for improved care and consideration of the needs of people with an experience of mental distress (Epstein & Olsen 1999). *The Roots of*

Recovery (Davidson et al. 2010) provides an excellent resource for the history of recovery and explains why current concepts of recovery have emerged.

Simon Champ observed that the civil rights and the counterculture movements of the 1960s inspired new hopes for mental health professionals in how they could relate to their 'patients' and for their hopes for the person's recovery. The impact of these changes, he states, is often ignored in the history of the consumer movement.

In addition, people who had been given a diagnosis and treated for a mental illness started to publish and speak out about their experiences and to protest about the treatment they received and how services needed to change. These include Patricia Deegan (see www.patdeegan.com/pat-deegan/lectures/conspiracy-of-hope) and Judi Chamberlin (www.youtube.com/watch?v=FGT4xJXgmoE). Others (Lovejoy 1984 and Unzicker 1989) spoke about the importance of hope, acceptance, engagement in social life, active coping and reclaiming a positive sense of self as key factors they found helpful.

At the same time the anti-psychiatry movement, initiated by psychiatrist Thomas Szasz's book *The Myth of Mental Illness* (1961), fuelled debate in the mental health field. Similarly, another psychiatrist, Franco Basaglia (Dell'Acqua 1995), was highly influential in changing Italy's mental health institutions in the 1970s. He saw institutions as inhumane and worked tirelessly to bring people back into their community so they could reconnect with life. Basaglia (Babini 2014) was instrumental in the introduction of Law 180 in Italy that led to the closure of all mental health institutions. Ever since, Trieste in Italy, where Basaglia worked, has been a role model for a significant number of countries wanting to transform their mental health services.

The concept of recovery was cemented into services in 1993 when psychologist William Anthony coined the term the 'decade of recovery' and put forward a vision of recovery for mental health services. At the same time, researchers demonstrated that the course of illnesses such as schizophrenia was much more hopeful than had been previously accepted. As a result, recovery from mental illness could be talked about in a way that was supported by empirical research (Harding 1994; Warner 1994). In contrast to the previous doom and gloom message given to people about how they would be on medication forever and live a life defined by disability, it was found that 65% of people actually recovered fully (no symptoms), lived independently and no longer needed medication. Further, many of these people had been institutionalised for up to 30 years.

CRITICAL THINKING CHALLENGE 2.1

Access the following link and listen to the webcast: http://cpr.bu.edu/resources/webcast/recovery-vision. What are the important factors that stand out for you in terms of understanding people's journeys of recovery and what this means for your practice?

Qualitative research into recovery began to appear in the late 1990s. These researchers (Tooth et al. 1997; Tooth et al. 2003; Adame & Knudson 2007; Borg 2007; May 2010; Onken et al. 2002; Ralph 2000; Ridgeway 2001; Sells et al. 2006) believed it critical that people with a lived experience of mental distress were best placed to identify those factors that are important to their recovery. They found the important factors to be the individual's personal characteristics (the most important factor in aiding recovery), supportive others, natural supports in the community and those professionals who listened to them as 'equals'. Drawing on these findings, consumers identified the following as the most important factors in their recovery:

- having self-determination
- discovering a more active sense of self (personal agency)
- valuing themselves as a person through their interactions with others
- realising the need to help themselves and to take responsibility for their distress
- seeing the potential for richer identities other than that of a person with mental illness
- reflecting on positive experiences leading to consideration of other potentials
- exploring experiences with reference to both the present and the future self
- finding ways to monitor and manage the symptoms of distress
- tapping into their own inner wisdom
- having optimism
- recognising the importance of spirituality

Please note that whilst recovery is the current context within Australian mental health services, internationally consumers, who are the driving force behind recovery, have advanced beyond recovery to focus on wellbeing (Ning 2010). Here, recovery is the process and wellbeing is the goal. This ongoing dynamic movement in conceptualisation of recovery is demonstrative of the rapidly changing focus in mental health mentioned at the beginning of this chapter.

RECOVERY-INFORMED PRACTICE

The recovery paradigm provides us with challenges in how we give priority to the person's meaning of their experiences and use our knowledge so that consumers feel understood, heard and empowered *from their perspective*. Policies require this of us, yet it is proving difficult to put into practice (Slade et al. 2014). The aim of this section is to assist the nurse to clarify and give examples of recovery-informed practice. Many of the concepts and principles of recovery are intertwined. To focus on one at the exclusion of others is meaningless: they are all necessary. So how does recovery-informed practice differ from past mental health practices that were primarily medically focussed? The following section addresses some of these issues. See Table 2.1 and Nurse's Story 2.1, which illustrate the need for recovery-informed practice in a number of areas.

TABLE 2.1 Key Differences Between Recovery-Informed and Traditional Practice

Recovery-Informed Practice	Traditional Practice
• Person is central	• Illness and symptoms are central
• Driven by human rights agenda	• Driven by the medical model
• Connecting with and maintaining meaningful roles, relationships and community is key; many things contribute to recovery	• Propensity for person's life to revolve around and be taken over by illness
• Looks for possibilities and promotes hope	• Looks for constraints and sets limits and lower expectations
• Collaborative risk management with the person	• Focuses on risk control by others
• Learns from people's narratives of recovery	• Personal narratives not a focus of care
• The person has an expertise gained from their experience of mental health challenges	• Professional is the expert on the person's experience
• Medication is a small part of management; types and doses titrated for the individual	• Treatment of symptoms, usually with medications the main form of intervention
• Person is the change agent	• The program is the change agent
• Takes a stance of 'unknowing' and curiosity to help uncover the meaning people make of their experience	• Takes a stance of 'knowing' and looks for confirmation of symptoms to make a diagnosis
• Empowering for the person to be acknowledged for their expertise	• Symptoms more important than personal meaning
• Promotes self-directed care requiring the active involvement of the person	• Promotes passivity and compliance • Recovery primarily involves the active involvement of others
• Explores what is important to the person; recognises unique experience and takes spirituality into account	• Informs people about illness and what is important to them to manage it; spirituality not taken into account
• Connects with person's strengths and draws on them to overcome challenges	• Focuses on deficits to treat and manage
• Choice and ability to connect with a broad range of services in community	• Choice of services can be limited
• Peer support or peer run services are essential	• Peer support limited or nonexistent
• Trauma-informed care—'what has happened to you'	• Not trauma informed—background issue 'what is wrong with you' more important
• Recovery is moving beyond premorbid functioning towards thriving and developing a new sense of self	• Recovery is, at best, returning to a premorbid level of functioning
• Nonlinear process	• Linear process of interventions
• Timeframes meaningless—ongoing process	• Recovery is the end point of the process
• Crisis is a time of learning how to thrive; an active recovery space	• Crisis is viewed as a relapse and failure

The most comprehensive work to identify principles of recovery-informed practice was undertaken by Le Boutillier et al. (2011). They sought to identify a conceptual framework for the key principles of recovery-informed practice from 30 documents in six countries (United States, England, Scotland, Republic of Ireland, Denmark and New Zealand). There were differences found across countries in document type and consumer involvement in their development. However, they were able to identify four practice domains.

1. *Promoting citizenship.* Citizenship is central to supporting recovery. It involves attending to the consumer's rights, social inclusion and meaningful occupation.
2. *Organisational commitment.* Ensure the work environment and service structure are conducive to promoting recovery-oriented practice. This involves ensuring the organisational culture moves from a focus on services to focusing on the needs of the person. Recovery vision, workplace support structures, quality improvement, care pathway and workforce planning are included in this practice domain.
3. *Supporting personally defined recovery.* The heart of practice is supporting people to define their own needs, goals, dreams and plans for the future to shape the content of care. Individuality, informed choice, peer support, strengths focus and holistic approach are contained in this practice domain.
4. *Working relationships.* Therapeutic relationships are essential to supporting recovery and promoting hope. There must be genuine desire to support the person and their family.

In Australia, the National Framework for Recovery-Oriented Mental Health Services: Policy and Theory (Commonwealth of Australia 2013a) identifies five practice domains and capabilities.

NURSE'S STORY 2.1 A Case for Change

When two of the authors of this chapter began mental health nursing in the 1970s, which at the time was undertaken predominantly in large psychiatric institutions, our tasks were to observe people's signs and symptoms and document them in the person's file so that the extent of the deficits could be noted and treated by the psychiatrists. The basic aim was to alleviate symptoms, primarily through medication, so that people could return to their home environment. People often stayed within the institution for many years. During this time, the meaning and impact of these symptoms for the person were considered irrelevant. In fact, conversations along such lines were actively discouraged because it was believed that this would make the person's condition much worse.

One of the authors has a very vivid recollection of working in a 'back ward' (a ward for people with supposedly chronic and disabling illnesses requiring long-term care over many years) where one patient was described as having exhibited a fixed delusion since she was admitted at the age of 17. At the time she was 24 years old and the 'delusion' was still just as distressing: she believed that her stepfather was the devil. She would become highly distressed whenever he visited with her mother and the distress continued long after he left. The staff believed it was a delusion because they perceived the stepfather to be very caring and concerned about the woman's welfare. However, a young female doctor new to the ward decided to take up this woman's case because the delusion had not responded to medication. She went through the woman's file and found that no-one had actually talked to her about the content of the delusion (what it meant for her). When the doctor finally asked, the woman told her that her stepfather from a very young age had sexually abused her and that for her he represented the devil.

Although this is a dramatic example, it illustrates the need for practice that searches for the meaning of the experience for the person rather than practice limited to the observation of signs and symptoms. It also illustrates how people can become institutionalised.

NURSE'S STORY 2.2 Moving From Deficits-Based to Strengths-Based Practice

Sarah, a 22-year-old university student, was brought in for involuntary admission after having walked in front of traffic, unable to explain what had happened or to communicate what she was thinking or feeling. Sarah had a history of having been sexually assaulted the previous year and more recently had witnessed a woman falling in front of a train. She had also recently experienced sleeplessness and poor appetite, could not study and had great fears of herself and her family members dying. She had a very close and loving relationship with her parents and her twin brother.

Using principles of recovery-informed care, the nurse took considerable time to assist Sarah in establishing a sense of safety and control in the inpatient environment. This was achieved by allowing her family members to stay with her until she went to sleep. This involved the nurse negotiating for the hospital's visiting policy to be interpreted more flexibly, as well as negotiating with other staff to spend as long with Sarah as she required to establish a sense of safety.

Sarah had difficulty talking directly with the nurse, but talking with family members in Sarah's presence about their lives, their strengths as a family and how they had supported each other through difficult times was an approach that seemed to permit Sarah to calm herself and eventually she was able to communicate what her family could do to help her feel in control. She was able to make arrangements for the next day with her family and asked for her belongings to be brought in to the hospital and for friends to be contacted. Family members were able to tell stories of times they had overcome problems and the strengths they all brought to support each other.

Sarah's admission was very brief and she reported having felt that the nurse and her family were encouraging of her in reminding her of the resources she had in her family and friends and how they were there to support her. She appreciated the time that the nurse took to patiently wait for her to be able to communicate.

1. *Promoting a culture and language of hope (overarching domain).* Communicating positive expectations, promoting hope and optimism so the person feels valued, important, welcome and safe.
2. *Person-first and holistic.* Holistic and person centred, responsive to people with Aboriginal and Torres Strait Islander, immigrant and refugee backgrounds. Responsive to age, gender, culture, spirituality, LGBTQI people, families, carers and support people.
3. *Supporting personal recovery.* Promoting autonomy and self-determination focussing on strengths and personal responsibility while engaging in collaborative relationships and reflective practice.
4. *Organisational commitment and workforce development.* Recovery vision, commitment and culture, acknowledging, valuing and learning from lived experience with recovery promoting service partnerships with workforce development and planning.
5. *Action on social inclusion and social determinants of health, mental health and wellbeing.* Supporting social inclusion, advocacy on social determinants, challenging stigmatising attitudes and discrimination and developing partnerships with communities.

Translating Recovery-Informed Practice Into Action

The transformation to recovery currently taking place in mental health services can be confusing and challenging for both experienced and beginning nurses. Recent research (Hungerford & Fox 2014) found consumers experienced mental health professionals taking a 'hands off' approach rather than working in partnership with the person. This may be due to uncertainty about what to do. Recovery's focus on the person driving their recovery can also be mistakenly interpreted as totally keeping out of the person's way.

The following section aims to address these issues by providing some basic suggestions to guide your practice. For more in-depth information you are encouraged to refer to A National Framework for Recovery-Oriented Mental Health Services: Guide for Practitioners and Providers at www.health.gov.au/internet/main/publishing.nsf/Content/mental-pubs-n-recovgde. It is important as a nurse to keep in mind the political and social contexts that, in spite of the person's, your and the service's best efforts, may work against the person exercising their right to social inclusion, personal agency and self-determination (Clifton et al. 2012).

Citizenship

Citizenship is a basic human right. Citizenship has been a feature of mental health for more than 20 years. The concept of citizenship is founded in theory and research to support the full participation of persons who experience mental health challenges (Rowe 2015). In terms of practice, it is important to be aware of the factors involved in citizenship so the person's rights are not invalidated. This is a societal issue that extends far beyond mental health services practice but must be kept in mind. Rowe makes the following points to consider in relation to citizenship.

- Citizenship is based on the five Rs of rights, responsibilities, roles, resources and relationships.
- People must have a sense of belonging and relationships, with other members recognising them as valued members in society.
- It extends the concept of social inclusion, a part of citizenship, because a person can have social inclusion but not be treated as an equal member of society.
- People need to be able to do the things they like to do, are good at and value most so they can grow and learn.
- Citizenship involves social justice so there are no undue restraints or deprivations getting in their way or blocking them.
- For citizenship to occur, the socioeconomic, health, gender and cultural barriers need to be reduced and ultimately eliminated. This is particularly so for obtaining and maintaining meaningful work.
- To achieve citizenship requires advocacy and social change.

Maintaining people in employment as much as possible mitigates against their becoming dependent on mental health services (Davidson et al. 2010). Work is a very protective factor and every effort to keep the person in employment is paramount. People employed full time reported: the least damaging psychological factors and health behaviours; lowest levels of stress and depression; most healthy and least unhealthy eating; most physical activity and lowest levels of smoking and drinking (Rosenthal et al. 2012). Those employed part time fell in the middle, and those unemployed fell on the unhealthy end of all psychological and behavioural factors. There can be a number of factors that may impede a person's return to work and for this reason supported employment programs have been established.

Social Inclusion

Social inclusion, while inherent in mental health policies and plans, remains poorly defined (Clifton et al. 2012). In their review of the international (English language) literature on social inclusion, exclusion and mental health, Wright and Stickley (2013) identify the relationship between exclusion, inequality and injustice. They note that the complexity of the concepts is tied up with significant socioeconomic and political issues. These authors suggest mental health clinicians should shift their focus from 'doing activities' to efforts that promote individual rights and access to supports that reduce health inequalities. The concept of social inclusion is also bound up with the opposite concept of social exclusion, this being the range of things that limit the capacity of individuals and includes stigma and discrimination, unemployment, low income, isolation, poor housing and lack of access to opportunities (Clifton et al. 2012).

Keeping Hope Alive

The National Framework for Recovery-Oriented Mental Health Services promotes a culture of hope and optimism, evidenced by the language used, and emphasises ensuring that people feel valued, important, welcome and safe. To stress the importance of hope, research has found hope to correlate with wellbeing, quality of life, subjective satisfaction with life, spirituality, resilience, self-esteem and self-confidence (van Gestel-Timmermans et al. 2010). In practice, this means communicating positive expectations and supporting the person in doing what they can to maintain hope.

Hope is an essential ingredient in recovery for Simon Champ, as outlined in his personal story in this chapter. He found that diagnoses, labels, being seen as an illness rather than a person and the loss of his identity all contributed to the loss of hope for some time. It was a struggle to regain it and Simon eventually found ways that worked for him to keep hope alive. Nowadays, we are much more attuned to keeping hope alive and it is imperative we keep hope alive for the person even if they have momentarily lost sight of it.

Personal agency. Davidson et al. (2010) argue that agency is the key to the transformation needed in recovery. They see an 'emphasis on activity, doing and occupation as core aspects of agency determining a person's quality of life' (p. 15). Personal agency is the fundamental freedom to fully participate in all aspects of life in the community with the full rights of all citizens. It is also being active in making meaning of one's life and being an active agent by deciding to do particular activities (e.g. returning to work) or asserting one's basic human rights (Lysaker & Leonhardt 2012).

Personal agency is internally motivated. Fundamental to personal agency is the belief in the ability to succeed. We know people are driven to act on things that are most important to them and give them pleasure. Their life evidences this in what they do and what they surround themselves with. When people experience mental health challenges, they may lose contact with these. Active involvement of the person in their care taps into and draws on their strengths, and promotes resilience, personal agency and their sense of overcoming adversities. Personal agency is a critical concept in recovery because it realises the importance of people actively contributing to their recovery to influence change.

How the nurse can promote personal agency. To ignite a person's agency, start by being curious about what is most important to the person in their life. You could begin by asking who the person wants to be involved in their care, which family members and/or significant others they want to see, or do not want to see, and whether they want contact or support from particular people to provide some constancy in their lives.

An example of the latter occurred recently when one of the authors worked in an inpatient setting and facilitated the visits of a Pilates instructor for a woman who was receiving involuntary mental healthcare and had been given a diagnosis of bipolar disorder. This person felt that the ongoing contact with her Pilates instructor gave her a sense of continuing control over a small but very important part of her life despite her situation. Some considerations for promoting personal agency follow.

- Discover what gives most meaning to the person; for example, their passions, hobbies or work.
- For Simon Champ, one of the most important areas that drives his personal agency is visual arts. He states that he needs to immerse himself in the visual arts to function as a human being. This provides great insight into where he is most likely to become active and find meaning in his life.
- If you were assisting Simon Champ, you might be curious about why visual arts are important to him.
  - What specifically does he do in relation to visual arts?
  - When he is engaged in such activities, what does he get out of it?
  - How can he reconnect with the visual arts?
  - What can he do now or in the near future to engage further in the visual arts?
  - Identify what, if any, supports Simon could utilise to further engage with the visual arts.
  - Also sharing your connection with the visual arts builds a stronger rapport and relationship.

Self-determination. Self-determination is the basic human right to be able to make and participate in decisions about your life; having a choice in determining how you live your life; and having control over your life. These are fundamental tenets in all of the human rights declarations and conventions mentioned at the beginning of this chapter. The theory of self-determination is part of the recovery paradigm because of its centrality to a person's recovery. Self-determination theory proposes the components of self-determination are autonomy, competence and relatedness (Sheldon 2012). These are required to effectively be able to participate in and make decisions and to have choice and control over one's life. All people need these to grow and thrive (Sheldon 2012). Self-determination allows people to live a good life according to their own values and beliefs. What this looks like will vary among individuals and cultures.

The consumer movement's motto 'nothing about me without me' reflects the above. This slogan had its roots in a South African disability movement (Leff et al. 1997). Maintaining and promoting a person's right to be self-determining is a fundamental principle of mental health services standards and legislation (Commonwealth of Australia 2013a, 2013b).

How the nurse can promote self-determination. Remember that when we interact with people during times of distress or challenge, we have a skewed view of their inherent capacities. Continually reflect on the assumptions you may be making about people to keep in check the capacity we all have to act 'as if' these assumptions are true. To protect and promote a person's right to self-determine, you could consider the following:

- Maximise the person's autonomy, their ability to self-regulate by taking control of, and responsibility for, what they do.
- Maximise the person's capacity to make informed choices and make sure they are involved in decisions concerning them.
- Medications or other interventions may not be the person's choice. Pat Deegan has attempted to address this by developing Common Ground. It is a tool for maximising a person's autonomy and decision making within a treatment setting. Watch the short video at www.patdeegan.com/commonground.

Relationships are critical. Chapter 1 highlighted the need for awareness of a range of factors inherent in our relationship with others if we are to be effective nurses. We know relationships are fundamentally important, from our earliest attachment experiences and throughout our life, for our emotional, social and physical wellbeing. Yet, in mental health we have not been able to delineate those aspects of our relationships with the people with whom we work that are most important and effective (Browne et al. 2012).

Research on the outcomes of psychotherapy that are relevant to relationships in nursing has consistently found that the 'non-specifics of psychotherapy' (genuineness, empathy, warmth, positive regard, flexibility and the therapeutic alliance) are the most important in determining outcome (Arnow & Steidtmann 2014; Miller et al. 2014). Other outcomes studies (Cahill et al. 2013) report 15% of outcome effect is attributed to placebo, 15% to techniques of therapy, 30% to the therapeutic relationship and 40% to client-specific factors. Such factors revolve around what the person does outside the therapeutic relationship, but also includes knowing what the person wants. When the therapeutic relationship and client factors were considered together, Cahill proposed the importance of the person's point of view of what is helpful as being more important than what the nurse believes is helpful.

What the nurse can do to develop the relationship. To make sense of the importance of the relationship you develop with the person, reflect on a time when you or a family member had a significant health challenge. What were the most helpful factors in your or your family member's experience? What was the experience of a good nurse or health professional? Do you think this was about who the nurse or health professional was as a person and/or how they were able to uncover what was most important and helpful to you or your family member? What would be important to you if you needed mental healthcare? Chances are they are very similar to the number of factors consistently reported in the mental health literature cited above.

- During times when people are facing challenges it is important to come from a place of empathy not sympathy. Watch the YouTube clip at www.youtube.com/watch?v=1Evwgu369Jw.
- Watch the first 5½ minutes of the clip by Dr Amy Banks on understanding relationships: www.wcwonline.org/Videos-by-WCW-Scholars-and-Trainers/forming-healthy-thriving-connections.

You will learn about developing your own helpful relationships as you gain experience. Continual reflection is critical to this process. Healthy relationships also require healthy environments. The internal environment of the people providing care and the culture of the health settings you work in are also important.

TRAUMA-INFORMED CARE

An essential component of a trauma-informed, recovery-oriented approach is to practise within a framework that recognises that many people experiencing mental health challenges have a background of trauma. Significant research now demonstrates the clear links between trauma and the onset of a range of mental health problems (Atkinson 2013; Kezelman & Stavropoulos 2012; Slade & Longden 2015). (See also Chapter 7.) This makes it imperative for nurses to be sensitive to the vulnerabilities and potential triggers that may give rise to retraumatisation, and be aware that this could impede recovery. Advances in neuroscience provide critical information about trauma and how to approach our work with people in general.

You will know from your clinical education that the brain consists of three parts that develop from the bottom up. The parts talk to one another via trillions of neural pathways. The 'primitive brain' (the brain stem) is responsible for the automatic functions such as breathing, heart rate and survival. The 'emotional brain' (the limbic system) is responsible for emotions and memory; it is about survival and safety. The 'thinking brain' (the neocortex) is responsible for higher order tasks such as thinking, learning, decision making, reasoning, organising, planning, meaning making and gaining control over emotions and language.

When people experience trauma and/or severe emotional stress, it can be much harder to engage the thinking brain. Instead they 'loop' in the emotional brain and this builds stronger neural pathways, making it more likely they will experience distressing emotions in the future when challenges arise. The key here is the absolute necessity for people to feel safe so they can effectively engage with others in their ongoing care.

Consider when people come into care in an inpatient setting. Personal safety is an important basis for effective nursing care. Often, people will be frightened of the inpatient environment, including acute mental health units, particularly if it is their first experience of admission to a mental healthcare setting. You need to take time to find out how the person feels and what they need to feel safe and secure. It may be listening to them, or finding strategies that the person could use; for example, locking their bedroom door or calling for help if someone enters their room. Do not assume that the person experiencing mental distress will feel safe in the healthcare setting just because you feel comfortable in the environment as a nurse. Again, imagine the situation for yourself or a loved one coming into the same setting and you should be able to get a good sense of things that may be frightening.

People can experience trauma as a result of their contact with services and certain treatments. Since the 1990s, Simon Champ has written and spoken about the traumatising effects of symptoms, hospitalisation, solitary confinement and being torn away from his environment and connections with others who really cared about him (Champ 1998). He has heard from many people who have had similar experiences.

The essentials of trauma-informed care include recognition of the following (Atkinson 2013; Kezelman & Stavropoulos 2012):

- Complex trauma and its effects have been unrecognised in mental health systems. To counteract this, it is necessary to take a universal precaution approach that assumes that all people who seek mental healthcare may have experienced trauma.
- Services need to ensure early assessment of trauma history and supervision for staff in responding sensitively and appropriately to disclosures of trauma.
- Trauma survivors often feel a lack of safety in receiving services. Reiterating the necessity for the person to feel safe, nurses can respond by helping the person to lower their distressing emotions. For example, sitting, listening or walking with the person; using basic relaxation techniques; and ensuring a calm environment can all be important. When this occurs, they will be more likely to engage their thinking brain and find ways that work for them to feel safe.
- Impacts of trauma can affect how people react to potentially helpful relationships. Building trust is essential so you can work with the person. Remember, trauma often occurs when a person's trust in people or situations has been severely violated. Nurses need to understand how trauma and abuse may have shaped difficulties in relationships and impact on therapeutic relationships.
- Coercive interventions may retraumatise people. Be mindful that nurses are often seen as figures of authority. Using the power that comes with this to exercise control

BOX 2.4 Trauma-Informed Care Resources

- Mental Health Coordinating Council (MHCC), Trauma informed Care and Practice: Towards a cultural shift in policy reform across mental health and human services in Australia, A National Strategic Direction, Position Paper and Recommendations of the National Trauma-Informed Care and Practice Advisory Working Group, 2013, http://www.mhcc.org.au/wp-content/uploads/2018/05/nticp_strategic_direction_journal_article__vf4_-_jan_2014_.pdf
- Blue Knot Foundation: empowering recovery from childhood trauma www.childabuseroyalcommission.gov.au/sites/default/files/IND.0521.001.0001.pdf
- Australian Institute of Health and Welfare, Closing the Gap: Trauma-informed services and trauma-specific care for Indigenous Australian children, 2013, www.aihw.gov.au/uploadedfiles/closingthegap/content/publications/2013/ctg-rs21.pdf
- Mental Health Coordinating Council, Trauma Informed Care and Practice, www.mhcc.org.au/project/trauma-informed-care-and-practice-ticp/

over the person to do what you think they 'should' do will most likely be counterproductive, be seen as coercive and retraumatise the person. Recognise the person's strengths and support them to develop care plans that affirm their preferences for care and how they can manage distress.

- Interventions that may be perceived as shaming and humiliating should be avoided. Nurses are responsible for maintaining the dignity and individual rights of the person at all times and providing services in ways that are flexible, individualised, culturally competent, respectful and based on best practice.
- There is a strong need to focus on what happened to the person rather than pathologising the presenting symptoms. Nurses need to develop an understanding of presenting behaviour and symptoms in the context of past experiences.
- Increasing understanding and skills in working within a framework of trauma-informed care is vital. Many resources are available as outlined in Box 2.4.

Trauma-informed care is considered so important that there are increasingly more dedicated training programs being developed for people working in healthcare and welfare settings such as the free online training from the Australian Child and Adolescent Trauma, Loss and Grief Network at http://learn.earlytraumagrief.anu.edu.au. The Australian Childhood Foundation provides significant resources for those nurses working with young people at www.childhood.org.au/blog/home/2015/april/trauma-informed-care.

Facilitating Self-Help and Personal Responsibility

Past practices in mental health focussed on the illness to the exclusion of the person experiencing the illness.

BOX 2.5 Therapeutic Questions to Promote Self-Help

Examples of questions the nurse can ask:

- Can you help me to understand what the experience of … means for you?
- What are you most concerned about at the moment?
- Have there been other times in your life when you have had similar feelings?
- How did you overcome these difficulties in the past?
- What do you think you need now to help with your current situation?
- What do you know about yourself that will help you in your current situation?

Kalyanasundaram (2007) describes the process as follows: A person would go to a health professional for help. The professional would ask about 'the problem' (usually symptoms of illness), building a bigger and bigger picture of 'the problem'. This would lead to the person focussing more and more on 'the problem'. The problem would grow bigger and bigger and be added to by the person's family or others asking about it. Soon the person's identity would be taken over and consumed by *IT*—'the problem', 'the illness'. Further contact with mental health professionals would reinforce this by almost exclusively focussing on asking questions about *IT*. This is similar to the concept of problem saturation. Clearly, this scenario is unhelpful and disempowers the person.

Asking Questions and Sharing

Asking questions about the person and their experience, their strengths and how they have overcome adversity in the past promotes understanding and a sense of agency. It puts 'the problem' in context. The person does not become the illness, and retains a more robust sense of self. There is a tension between doing something for someone and encouraging people to care for themselves. There are times when fostering dependency by doing tasks for the person appears necessary, but in many cases it is counterproductive. The list in Box 2.5 describes the therapeutic use of questioning to promote self-help.

Consumers can be key supports for many people in terms of self-help and taking responsibility. The sharing of experiences and stories of overcoming with others who have had similar experiences can be far more powerful than workers because people learn they are not alone, that there is hope and there are many different ways that may be helpful. Within Australia and New Zealand there are a considerable range of consumer organisations that provide advice, advocacy, support and service delivery. Some of the major national and state community-managed organisations (CMOs) or non-government organisations (NGOs), focussed on consumer and carer issues are listed in Box 2.6. Many other organisations providing broader supports

BOX 2.6 Consumer Organisations and Useful Websites

- Mental Health Council of Australia (MHCA) is an independent peak national body for mental health: https://mhaustralia.org
- Sane Australia is a national charity helping people seriously affected by mental illness: www.sane.org
- Mental Illness Fellowship of Australia Inc. provides counselling and support and promotes awareness and research: www.mifa.org.au
- Mental Health Carers Australia www.mentalhealthcarersaustralia.org.au
- Te Puna Web Directory is a general directory of New Zealand and Pacific websites developed by the National Library of New Zealand/Te Puna Mātauranga o Aotearoa, http://tepuna.natlib.govt.nz
- Te Puni Kōkiri provides policy advice to government and other agencies and has links to other Māori-related websites, www.tpk.govt.nz
- The following websites contain information for the NZ and Pacific Islander Mental Health Workforce.
  - Te Rau Matatini, www.teraumatatini.com
  - Le Va, www.leva.co.nz/mental-health-and-addiction
  - Public Interest Advocacy Centre, https://www.piac.asn.au
- Patricia Deegan, Recovery and the Conspiracy of Hope, www.patdeegan.com/pat-deegan/lectures/conspiracy-of-hope
- Judi Chamberlin, www.youtube.com/watch?v=FGT4xJXgmoE

operate at the local level throughout Australia and New Zealand. There are also a growing number of peer workers and peer-run services emerging. These are addressed later in the chapter.

A number of alternative support groups have been established to support those consumers who hold firmly to their experiences, such as voice-hearing groups and groups to support people to explore unusual beliefs without having to label their experiences in professional jargon. Please see Box 2.6 to explore these groups.

Focus on Personal Strengths

The importance of focussing on strengths has already been mentioned in this chapter. Here we deal with promoting people's strengths in your practice in greater depth. Nurses are well placed to endorse the strengths-based approach (Xie 2013). Working with strengths was first used in education and is not a new concept. Educationalists found that focussing on a person's deficit and trying to fix it was likely to make the person feel more anxious, blocked or even immobilised—the problem would often be exacerbated rather than alleviated. The inability of the person (and the professional) to solve the problem led to a sense of failure, and a downward spiral was not uncommon. The strengths model proposes that all people have goals, talents and confidence, and that all environments contain resources, people and opportunities (Rapp & Goscha 2012). It supports Deegan's (1988) assertion that people who have experienced mental distress are more interested in focussing on what they can do in order to move on with their lives and live as normally as possible within their community.

Focussing on strengths and personal values promotes a person's resilience, aspirations, talents and uniqueness, focussing on what the person can do and how these strengths can be mobilised, and built on to overcome current difficulties. A key therapeutic practice is reframing from a pessimistic worldview to an optimistic one that instils hope and challenges self-stigma. For example, the nurse will want to know what the person has done in the past to overcome life's difficulties and how they can use the strengths they used previously to overcome current challenges. Nurses are well placed to *gently* prompt people from taking a less positive view by asking about the exceptions; the times they do focus on what's working and so on. It is critical here not to invalidate the person. Consider: 'I appreciate that is how you feel'; 'I wonder if there are times when things work for you?' See Nurse's Story 2.2.

The nurse will also encourage the person to think of ways that will work for them. The nurse will not impose their own ideas but may offer suggestions, and will work with the person to explore and create options. The nurse will use the knowledge gained from a variety of sources to help in this exploration. The nurse works in partnership with the person—the nurse's role is to reinforce the person's plan and remind them of it if they do become unwell.

People overwhelmingly talk about the experience of mental distress as a transformative process where the old self is let go of and a new sense of self emerges (Deegan 2004). The intense struggle of dealing with mental health challenges leads to positive outcomes and a sense of personal agency that moves the person beyond where they would have been if they had not had the experience. Daniel Fisher, a psychiatrist with lived experience of psychiatric disability (his term), highlights the importance of a strengths focus: 'I no longer search for the sickness in myself or in those I grew up with as an explanation for my woes. Instead I search for the strengths in myself and those close to me which propel me through my version of the suffering we all share but seldom face' (Fisher 1994, p. 1).

The Importance of Reflection in Relation to Recovery-Informed Practice

Reflection affects nurses' individual understanding of a range of practice issues, increases awareness and clarifies aspects of themselves and their role. It involves being open to new challenges and seeking new opportunities. This very much reflects the nurse's capacity and willingness to be open to change in attitude and thinking.

Within the emerging recovery paradigm, a significant amount of learning is gained from our interactions and relationships with people who have the lived experience of mental distress. Mental health professionals have much to learn from them about the nature of mental distress and the most important factors in helping them to get on with their lives in a way that is meaningful to them. We also learn about how we help, and frequently hinder, their self-directed recovery. Reflection, critical thinking and analysis are essential skills enabling all those involved in mental healthcare to evaluate and incorporate evolving knowledge into their practice. Reflection was dealt with in more detail in Chapter 1.

On the importance of reflection in nursing practice, we want to raise an issue that has not been satisfactorily addressed in the nursing profession. Specifically, what happens when a nurse has or develops mental health challenges? In the context of practice this is of critical importance, and discussion and debate on the topic are long overdue. Refer to Nurse's Story 2.3 by Vicki Stanton.

EXTERNAL ENVIRONMENTS THAT FACILITATE RECOVERY

We have discussed what is important to personal recovery, or the internal environments of individuals. There are numerous external environments that support the person's recovery efforts including the person's immediate family, significant others and friends; relationships and supports in the person's natural community through to the wider community with its range of options for people to develop valued social roles. People spend only a fraction of their lives in contact with services; the majority of their lives is spent in the community.

The concepts of recovery, social inclusion, self-agency and citizenship stress the importance of external environments for people to live full and meaningful lives. This section looks at what is required in the external environments and, as mentioned earlier, there is ample knowledge in this area from the many consumers who have published seminal works about their stories of recovery and experiences of care (e.g. Deegan 1988; Lovejoy 1984; Unzicker 1989). These stories indicate that recovery can occur without the involvement of mental health professionals and, unfortunately, in spite of them in some cases.

Remember that mental health services play only a small but important role in the person's overall recovery journey. The community of which the person is a member provides a wealth of resources that are essential to all people, inclusive of those people experiencing mental distress. Nurses now need to be able to extend far beyond their previous traditional roles in their ability and creativity to find and use the resources available in the person's community. This section briefly discusses community-based mental health services CMOs.

Mary O'Hagan (2011) outlines alternative ways the healthcare system can respond, such as creating an optimistic culture, environment and expectations, and shifting the focus to self-determination, personal power and resourcefulness rather than focussing on symptoms and functional limitations. While individuals may have distress that interferes with their functioning at a particular point in time, this does not mean they will not benefit from engaging in activities of everyday life. As stated earlier, there is evidence that engagement in work and other meaningful pursuits leads to a diminishing of mental distress and promotion of general wellbeing.

Supportive environments are also termed enabling environments in recognition of the fact that we have been wrong in assuming that our system environments are inherently helpful. Some environments, including those of government and non-government services, do not in and of themselves enable people to move towards recovery. Johnson & Haigh (2011) outline the core elements of *enabling environments* as follows:

- The nature and quality of relationships are highly valued.
- Responsibility is shared by all participants.
- Everyone's contribution has equal value.
- There are opportunities for creativity and initiative.
- Decision making is transparent.
- Power and authority are open for discussion.
- Behaviour is seen as meaningful and a communication to be understood.

RECOVERY-INFORMED SERVICE PROVISION

The policy frameworks of the Commonwealth and State governments guide recovery-informed service provision. The Council of Australian Governments (COAG) endorsed the Commonwealth Government's Roadmap for National Mental Health Reform 2012–2022 (2012). The Roadmap highlighted the following priority areas:

- person-centred approaches
- improve the mental health and social and emotional wellbeing of all Australians
- prevent mental illness
- focus on early detection and intervention
- improve access to high-quality services and supports
- improve the social and economic participation of people with mental illness

The Roadmap focuses on the need for social inclusion for people with mental illness through a broad range of support services that will facilitate recovery, including: increased access to education, employment and training; stable and affordable housing; community resources; and the ability to influence decisions that affect them.

The New Zealand document Like Minds, Like Mine: National Plan 2014–2019 describes a program to promote the wellbeing, human rights and social inclusion for people experiencing mental disorder. Social inclusion in the NZ Like Minds, Like Mine document is outlined as follows:

> *Social inclusion means that people with mental illness are able to participate in the community as employees, students, volunteers, carers, parents, etc. They have a personal identity, aside from ill health, and have valuable contributions to make within the many communities to which they belong (Ministry of Health and Health Promotion Agency 2014, p. 4).*

NURSE'S STORY 2.3 My Experience as a Nurse With Mental Health Problems: Vicki Stanton

As a very experienced mental health nurse, I was able to recognise my own spiral into profound anxiety and depression when it started, but my senior position within the mental health service I was working in made it difficult for me to reach out to colleagues for support. I had been a highly functioning mental health worker for my entire career, never entertaining the idea that I would need to see a psychiatrist and take medication over many years. My early life experience of the traumatic loss of my child when I was very young had been firmly buried, I thought, locked in a vault, never dealt with, until events conspired to crack the vault and I unraveled. My years of strength and resilience following trauma gave way, and I couldn't self-correct and felt completely unable to talk with my colleagues about my mental health needs. The experience also raised some important issues about whether I could continue working as a nurse.

How Did my Experience of Mental Illness Impact on my Ongoing Work as a Nurse?

When I first became acutely unwell my work involved significant responsibilities in a very senior mental health management position. Commencing medication and feeling acute distress impacted on all areas of my functioning. Medication was a double-edged sword, necessary, but side effects were distressing and impacted on my ability to function. Initially, I took considerable sick leave and negotiated lighter duties. I had to search for mental healthcare that did not involve workers who I knew in my day-to-day work, to ensure confidentiality was maintained. When I did return to work, with the workload changes, I realised that I needed to resign from the high-pressure job I had been in for decades. A significant reason for resigning was the extreme hesitation I felt, and my colleagues in the mental health service also experienced, in having any discussion about my needs as a mental health worker with mental health problems. It was like dancing around an insurmountable issue, and this change in the relationship with my colleagues negatively impacted on my identity.

After resigning, I relocated back to the city to engage long term with a psychiatrist. In the city I could do this with complete confidentiality. I took some more leave, and explored options for part-time and casual work. This gave me the flexibility to adjust work depending on how I was coping.

How Did I Manage Working in an Acute Clinical Setting?

Seeing a private psychiatrist regularly was an important part of ensuring I did not compromise my nursing practice. I also engaged in ongoing supervision, including with both a peer credentialled mental health nurse and a senior psychiatrist. I routinely discussed my clinical work in the acute mental health setting and with asylum seekers to ensure my nursing practice was safe.

How Could I Discuss This With my Colleagues?

This was a great source of stress during 4 years of mental health treatment. It created anxiety that my colleagues might find out that I was regularly seeing a psychiatrist and taking medication. I feared them viewing me as less competent, less trustworthy or scrutinising me for signs that I was not functioning. While it wasn't likely that colleagues would know unless I told them, for many years the feeling of having to hide this part of myself was difficult.

There were times when I wanted to talk with colleagues based on something I'd experienced, and could recognise in people we were working with, such as discontinuation symptoms or other symptoms. In hindsight I believe both my colleagues and I could have benefited from my insights. However, I haven't talked with colleagues to date because I don't feel that nursing has yet come to terms with mental illness within the nursing profession. The fact that we don't discuss it means we don't take advantage of the richness of experience and perspectives of nurses who have recovered from mental illness and gone on to weave these experiences into our practice. Having a dialogue about this may assist nurses in the future to feel that they can engage in recovery and continue as nurses.

What was Most Helpful to Personal Recovery?

The things that were important to me in my recovery were the same things that are the theme of this chapter: connectedness, belonging, making sense of my experience and integrating this into my identity as a nurse to reclaim my strength.

The Mental Health Service

Within mental health services, there are a number of settings in which a nurse may practise (see Chapter 5). The most common of these include inpatient services in general hospitals, crisis teams, community mental health teams and recovery-focussed services. Community-based settings are where the majority of people receive services and nursing practice in these settings will include the following aims:

- assisting the person to access the services they need and want
- promoting the person's inner resources
- actively supporting the person to achieve their self-defined goals
- promoting the person's engagement in fulfilling activities of their choice
- advocating for the upholding of the person's rights
- assisting the person to advocate on their own behalf
- facilitating access to the people, places and things the person needs to survive (e.g. shelter, meals, healthcare)
- promoting a healthy lifestyle
- assisting the person to alleviate distress and identify helpful strategies
- working with the person to ensure their own safety and that of others

The focus of practice in the various settings will be determined by the person's needs, which will change over time. Nurse's Story 2.4 illustrates how community mental health nurses can provide a range of supports for people to achieve outcomes that are not possible in hospital.

NURSE'S STORY 2.4 What Nursing can Achieve in the Community

Johanna, a 26-year-old woman, had recently emigrated from Armenia with her husband Frank and 6-month-old son. Johanna was experiencing her second episode of major depression with psychotic features. Her previous psychiatric treatment prior to coming to Australia had been entirely hospital based, and when community care was suggested for this second episode of depression, Frank was reluctant to take any risks until Johanna was completely well. Frank was at work during the day, they had no family or friends in Australia, and he could not take leave to care for Johanna. Therefore, he felt she would be safer remaining in hospital. Johanna was afraid that if she stayed in hospital as long as she did on her previous admission, she would not bond with her son. Frank was persuaded to support the option of community care when reassured that resources were available to provide support during the day. Family care workers were identified who were available to provide support in their home during the day. A small network of women from Armenia who met at the local migrant resource centre also provided much-needed social support.

Within the recovery framework the important elements in responding to Johanna included identifying her strengths in her existing relationships with family and community and emphasising these. The nurse used curious questioning to help Johanna get in touch with ways she could manage her distress and work through her fears about being in control with her son and her family life. Johanna reported that this episode of depression was not as prolonged as her previous one where she was hospitalised. She felt less isolated, more in contact with her family and other people, and wanted to get better because she was encouraged by the normal day-to-day activity around her. Johanna felt confident that with the support of the people around her she could explore her distress and learn how to manage the challenges it presented her with.

Nurses must be aware that the community setting has the potential to be a site where mental healthcare is experienced as disempowering and stigmatising. Light et al. (2014) describe the experience of people subject to community treatment orders in Australia, highlighting the concerns that while receiving such care, these consumers and carers continued to experience isolation, loss and trauma, vulnerability and distress, and disempowerment. The consumers and carers in the study by Light et al. (2014) described community treatment orders as both providing access to services, but at the same time reporting that the access was to a restricted form of service dominated by medication and an involuntary process described by some as humiliating. This tells us that being in the community setting does not guarantee social inclusion in and of itself.

Community-Managed Organisations

CMOs, otherwise known as NGOs, have increasingly been playing a key role in the provision of support to consumers and carers affected by mental distress through direct service delivery. They complement existing mental health services and strengthen community supports and partnerships. The main service types of CMOs include accommodation support and outreach; employment and education; leisure and recreation; family and carer support; self-help and peer support; helpline and counselling services; and promotion, information and advocacy.

The nurse's role is to increase their knowledge of these aspects of CMOs:

- The range of community managed organisations in the community that promote social inclusion, and how to work collaboratively with all services that are necessary to meet the needs of people experiencing mental distress. There has been considerable expansion in the range and number of support programs provided through a diverse number of agencies.
- The principles of working in ways that promote self-agency. A good overview of these principles can be found in the National Framework for Recovery-Oriented Mental Health Services at www.health.gov.au/internet/publications/publishing.nsf/Content/mental-pubs-n-recovgde-toc

Further information on the range of supports provided by CMOs can be found at the website of the Mental Health Coordinating Council, one of the peak organisations in Australia (www.mhcc.org.au). The Mental Health Foundation of New Zealand is a charity dedicated to working towards 'creating a society free from discrimination, where all people enjoy positive mental health and wellbeing'. Its website provides numerous resources including the support services available and outlines of their programs (www.mentalhealth.org.nz). See also the New Zealand Mental Health Advocacy Coalition's discussion paper Future Responses to Mental Distress and Loss of Well-being at www.mentalhealth.org.nz/assets/Our-Work/Destination-Recovery-FINAL-low-res.pdf. This is an excellent resource on New Zealand's view of future mental health services.

While it is critical to work in an integrated way with CMOs and other providers, it is essential to remember that CMOs are not whole-of-life services, but rather stepping stones for those people who choose to use them. The aim is for people to develop naturally occurring supports within the community or to use other created supports that are accessed by all members of the community.

Peer Support Workers in Mental Health

Peer support refers to the provision of support to people with mental health challenges by people who have also experienced challenges with their mental health. There are many titles describing these roles, including peer support workers (PSWs), consumer workers, peer educators and peer specialists. The essence of these various roles is to provide support based on mutual respect, shared responsibility and mutual agreement about what support is needed (Repper & Carter 2011).

The value of peer support includes: the reciprocity between people who both have a lived experience that is not a part of the exchange with non-peer workers; the aspiration that comes from working with someone who has achieved personal growth; more equality in interactions; and the capacity for people using services to maintain self-agency in these more equal relationships (Austin et al. 2014). Repper and Carter (2011) found that peer workers were able to foster those aspects of recovery such as hope, empowerment and self-efficacy that are integral to self-agency. Slade (2009) writes of the benefits of PSWs as including:

- the benefits to the workers themselves of being employed and valued for their experience
- the value to non-peer mental health workers of seeing peer workers in their roles in ways that can highlight the values and raise awareness of the values inherent in their roles
- the benefits to people with mental health challenges seeing peer workers as positive role models
- the role of peer workers as culture carriers to shape change within mental health services

The National Mental Health Commission's 2013 report A Contributing Life, the 2013 report card on mental health and suicide prevention, recommends that the peer workforce is considered essential as a component to all mental health support teams, and recommends the development of a National Mental Health Peer Workforce Development Framework, as well as targets for PSWs into the future.

In addition to peer workers within mental health services, there are growing numbers of peer-provided services. One example is the voice-hearing network that runs regular groups specifically for voice hearers. They are very successful for those who attend and facilitate their recovery (de Jager et al. 2015). The voice-hearing network now runs international conferences. Information about a variety of peer services can be found in Box 2.7.

BOX 2.7 Information About Peer Workers and Peer Services

- The consumer website 'Our consumer place' is devoted to developing practice guidelines for a sustainable consumer workforce in the mental health sector through participatory research: Our Consumer Place 2009 Real lives, real jobs: www.ourconsumerplace.com.au/files/real_lives_real_jobs.pdf
- The following links provide further information on peer support:
  - PeerZone, www.peerzone.info
  - Hearing Voices Network, https://www.hearing-voices.org
  - Hearing Voices Network Aotearoa NZ, www.hearingvoices.org.nz
  - Rufus May is highly regarded in the voice-hearing network and in mental health. He has two videos on his website that are recommended viewing: www.rufusmay.com
  - Far North Queensland Partners in Recovery has a number of great resources on a range of topics: www.fnqpartnersinrecovery.com.au
  - Intentional Peer Support is an organisation established in the 1990s by Shery Mead, one of the founders of peer support in the United States: www.intentionalpeersupport.org/about-us
  - Wellness Recovery Action Plan WRAP, www.mentalhealthrecovery.com

CONCLUSION

Mental distress is a part of human existence: it varies in degree, but it may happen to all of us. The journey of healing and recovery is salient for everyone. There is a need to talk about recovery in more humane terms because it is not something that happens to 'the other': we are all vulnerable to mental distress under certain circumstances. Nurses need to be with people in this humane context rather than in a context of pathology, difference and a reductionist focus on symptoms and diagnosis.

We encourage you to reflect on how the principles of mental health practice are fundamental to all nursing practice, regardless of setting. We hope we have encouraged you to think about how you can participate more fully in your practice by developing your awareness of the complexities and realities of the context in which practice occurs. More specifically, we hope you appreciate how your attitudes, values and beliefs play a crucial role in your everyday practice.

Mental health nursing practice is also influenced by an ever-evolving knowledge base; hence, the principles informed by this knowledge base continue to change and to evolve. Practice is time and context specific, making the ability to tolerate and incorporate change vital. Consequently, your thinking about your practice will be continually influenced by your developing self-awareness, your incorporation of new ideas into your practice, and your increasing professional and personal experience.

The primary focus of mental health nursing practice is the consumer, and how nurses can help facilitate the consumer's recovery. Nurses can assist in this process by working in partnership with consumers to help them realise their potential and tap into a wide range of community resources and supports, of which mental health services are just one. Just as importantly, we hope you find the experience of mental health nursing as rewarding as we have.

EXERCISES FOR CLASS ENGAGEMENT

Imagine yourself in the scenarios below and, in groups, answer the questions that follow.

Scenario 1

You have been hospitalised with an acute medical condition. Medical advice is that you have diabetes. You are being given instructions for self-management of insulin injections and monitoring of blood sugar levels before discharge from hospital.

Scenario 2

You have been hospitalised after an acute episode of depression. Medical advice is that there is a high likelihood that you have bipolar depression. You are being given instructions on the possible side effects of the antidepressant medication you have been prescribed and are advised that you will have to continue taking some form of medication indefinitely.

Questions

In groups of four or five, discuss your thoughts and feelings about the above scenarios. Use the following questions as discussion points. Note any similarities and differences in opinion among group members as well as between the two scenarios.

- What are your immediate concerns?
- What information would you seek?
- What type of support would you wish to receive, and from whom?
- What would be the most important knowledge and skills for nurses in the different care units?
- What could your nurse do that would be helpful or unhelpful?
- What do you think will be important considerations for the rest of your life?
- Do you think you should take an active role in your present and future care? If so, how could this best be achieved?

Scenario 3

Greta is 36 years old and married to Grant, with whom she has two sons, aged five and seven. They have recently moved to a regional centre and have no family support. Greta is currently experiencing her second episode of bipolar disorder and is in the hypomanic phase of her illness. Grant is very concerned about Greta's ability to be an effective parent, but he also has longer term fears about their relationship.

Question: How could the principles of recovery-informed practice be used to assist Greta? Focus on aspects of the client's recovery rather than symptom management.

Also, as discussed early on in this chapter, the terminology used to refer to people with mental ill health is a hotly debated topic, by the people who experience mental health problems and the professionals who care for them alike. In small groups, discuss the terms you are aware of and explore your group's feelings around them? Additional Exercise: Read the Nurse's Story 2.5 below and reflect on recovery-informed practice within an indigenous setting in Australia. In small groups, discuss how cultural differences in your local populations impact care and service provision.

NURSE'S STORY 2.5 Recovery-Informed Practice Within an Indigenous Setting

Nurses working in the mental health service in Alice Springs and the surrounding region are continually challenged to provide recovery-informed mental healthcare to Indigenous people in ways that have meaning within the cultural context—a very different context to the professional backgrounds and knowledge bases of the majority of mental health workers in the area. Indigenous people comprise approximately half of all admissions to the service. Routine practices now include the encouragement of traditional Indigenous practices alongside Western medicine. Mental health nurses provide Western treatment and counselling alongside, and informed by, Indigenous traditional healers when the family indicates that this is necessary for the wellbeing of the person. The traditional healer, or Ngangkari, is considered a crucial part of the care provided to address the cultural and spiritual issues for Indigenous people receiving mental healthcare in Central Australia. The meaning of the episode of mental distress as identified by the individual, their family and the traditional healer is considered paramount.

REFERENCES

Adame, A.L., Knudson, R.M., 2007. Beyond the counter-narrative: exploring alternate narratives of recovery from the psychiatric survivor movement. Narrative Inquiry 17 (2), 157–178.

Anthony, W.A., 1993. Recovery from mental illness: the guiding vision of the mental health service system in the 1990s. Psychosocial Rehabilitation Journal 16 (4), 11–23.

Arnow, B.A., Steidtmann, D., 2014. Harnessing the potential of the therapeutic alliance. World Psychiatry 13 (3), 238–240.

Atkinson, J., 2013. Trauma-informed services and trauma-specific care for Indigenous Australian children. Resource sheet no. 21. Produced for the Closing the Gap Clearinghouse. Australian Institute of Health and Welfare, Canberra, ACT; Australian Institute of Family Studies, Melbourne.

Austin, E., Ramakrishnan, A., Hopper, K., 2014. Embodying recovery: a qualitative study of peer work in a consumer-run service setting. Community Mental Health Journal 50, 879–885.

Babini, V.P., 2014. Looking back: Italian psychiatry from its origins to Law 180 of 1978. Journal of Mental and Nervous Disease 202 (6), 428–431.

Barker, P., Buchanan-Barker, P., 2004. The Tidal Model: psychiatric colonization, recovery and the need for a paradigm shift in mental healthcare. Available at: https://onlinelibrary.wiley.com/doi/abs/10.1046/j.1440-0979.2003.00275.x.

Bird, V., Leamy, M., Tew, J., Le Boutillier, C., Williams, J., Slade, M., 2014. Fit for purpose? Validation of a conceptual framework for personal recovery with current mental health consumers. Australian and New Zealand Journal of Psychiatry 48 (7), 644–653. https://doi.org/10.1177/0004867413520046.

Borg, M., 2007. The nature of recovery as lived in everyday life: perspectives of individuals recovering from severe mental health problems (Ph.D. thesis). Norwegian University of Science and Technology, Trondheim, Norway.

Borg, M., Kristiansen, K., 2007. Working on the edge: everyday life research from Norway on the meaning of work for people recovering from severe mental health distress (Ph.D. thesis). Norwegian University of Science and Technology, Trondheim, Norway.

Browne, G., Cashin, A., Graham, I., 2012. The therapeutic relationship and mental health nursing: it is time to articulate what we do! Journal of Psychiatric and Mental Health Nursing 19, 839–843.

Cahill, J., Paley, G., Hardy, G., 2013. What do patients find helpful in psychotherapy? Implications for the therapeutic relationship in mental health nursing Journal of Psychiatric and Mental Health Nursing 20 (9), 782–791.

Campbell, P., 2009. The service user/survivor movement. In: Reynolds, J., Muston, R., Heller, T., Leach, J., McCormick, M., Wallcraft, J., Walsh, M. (Eds.), Mental health still matters. Open University/Palgrave Macmillan, Basingstoke.

Chamberlin, J., 1997. A working definition of empowerment. Psychiatric Rehabilitation Journal 20 (4), 43–46.

Champ, S., 1998. A most precious thread. Australian and New Zealand Journal of Mental Health Nursing 7 (2), 54–59.

Clay, S., 2002. A personal history of the consumer movement. https://www.mhselfhelp.org/clearinghouse-resources/2011/6/17/a-personal-history-of-the-consumer-movement.html. Accessed 22 January 2016.

Cleary, M., Horsfall, J., O'Hara-Aarons, M., Hunt, G.E., 2013. Mental health nurses' views of recovery within an acute setting. International Journal of Mental Health Nursing 22, 205–212.

Clifton, A., Repper, J., Banks, D., Remnant, J., 2012. Co-producing social inclusion: the structure/agency conundrum. Journal of Psychiatric and Mental Health Nursing 20 (6), 514–524.

Commonwealth of Australia, 2013a. National framework for recovery-oriented mental health services: policy and theory. Australian Health Ministers Advisory Council, Canberra. Available at: www.health.gov.au/internet/main/publishing.nsf/Content/mental-pubs-n-recovpol. Accessed 22 January 2016.

Commonwealth of Australia, 2013b. National framework for recovery-oriented mental health services: guide for practitioners and providers. Australian Health Ministers Advisory Council, Canberra. Available at: www.health.gov.au/internet/main/publishing.nsf/Content/mental-pubs-n-recovgde. Accessed 22 January 2016.

Convention on the Rights of Persons with Disabilities 1975. United Nations. Available at: https://www.un.org/development/desa/disabilities/convention-on-the-rights-of-persons-with-disabilities.html. Accessed 22 Jan 2016.

Curtis, L., 1998. New directions: international overview of best practices in recovery and rehabilitation services for people with serious mental illness: a discussion paper. Mental Health Commission, New Zealand.

Davidson, L., 2003. Living outside mental illness: qualitative studies in recovery in schizophrenia. New York Press, New York.

Davidson, L., Rakfeldt, J., Strauss, J., 2010. The roots of the recovery movement in psychiatry. John Wiley and Sons, West Sussex.

Deegan, P.E., 1988. Recovery: the lived experience of rehabilitation. Psychiatr. Psychosocial Rehabilitation Journal 11 (4), 11–19.

Deegan, P.E., 1993. Recovering our sense of value after being labelled mentally ill. Journal of Psychosocial Nursing 31 (4), 7–11.

Deegan, P.E., 2004. Rethinking rehabilitation: freedom. 20th world congress of rehabilitation international, Oslo, Norway.

de Jager, A., Rhodes, P., Beavan, V., Holmes, D., McCabe, K., Thomas, N., McCarthy-Jones, S., Lampshire, D., Hayward, M., 2016. Investigating the lived experience of recovery in people who hear voices. Qualitative Health Research 26 (10), 1409–1423.

Dell'Acqua, G., 1995. Trieste twenty years after: from the criticism of psychiatric institutions to institutions of mental health. Mental Health Department Trieste. Available at: www.triestesalutementale.it/english/doc/dellacqua_1995_trieste-20yearsafter.pdf. Accessed 22 January 2016.

Deveson, A., 1991. Spinning out: a documentary special on schizophrenia. Ann Deveson Productions & the Australian Film Finance Corporation, Australia.

Epstein, M., Olsen, M.A., 1999. An introduction to consumer politics. In: Clinton, M., Nelson, S. (Eds.), Advanced practice in mental health nursing. Blackwell Science, Oxford, pp. 1–16.

Fisher, D.B., 1994. Hope, humanity and voice in recovery from psychiatric disability. Journal of the California Alliance for the Mentally Ill 5(Recovery Issue), 13–15.

Fisher, D., 2011. The Evolution of the Concept of Recovery. Available at: http://d20wqiibvy9b23.cloudfront.net/resources/resources/000/000/617/original/Fisher_The_Evolution_of_Recovery.pdf?1468370245. Accessed 22 January 2016.

Glover, H., 2012. Recovery, lifelong learning, empowerment and social inclusions: is a new paradigm emerging? In: Ryan, P., Ramon, S., Greacen, T. (Eds.), Empowerment, lifelong learning and recovery in mental health: towards a new paradigm. Palgrave publishers, London.

Harding, C., 1994. Empirical correction of seven myths about schizophrenia and implications for treatment. Acta Psychiatrica Scandinavia 90 (suppl) 384, 130–146.

Hungerford, C., Fox, C., 2014. Consumer's perceptions of recovery-oriented mental health services: an Australian case-study analysis. Nursing and Health Sciences 16, 209–215.

Johnson, R., Haigh, R., 2011. Social psychiatry and social policy for the 21st century: new concepts for new needs - The 'Enabling Environments' initiative. Mental Health and Social Inclusion 15 (1), 17–23.

Kalyanasundaram, V., 2007. Facilitating recovery oriented practice. Workshop notes, NSW Institute of Psychiatry, Sydney, 22–24 August.

Kezelman, K., Stavropoulos, P., 2012. Practice guidelines for treatment of complex trauma and trauma informed care and service delivery, adults surviving child abuse. Available at: 'The Last Frontier': Practice Guidelines for Treatment of Complex Trauma and Trauma Informed Care and Service Delivery https://www.childabuseroyalcommission.gov.au/sites/default/files/IND.0521.001.0001.pdf. Accessed 22 January 2016.

Kidd, S., Kenny, A., McKinstry, C., 2015. Exploring the meaning of recovery-oriented care: an action-research study. International Journal of Mental Health Nursing 24 (1), 38–48.

Le Boutillier, C., Leamy, M., Bird, V.J., Davidson, L., Williams, J., Slade, M., 2011. What does recovery mean in practice? A qualitative analysis of international recovery-oriented practice guidelines. Psychiatric Services 62 (12), 1470–1476.

Leff, H.S., Campbell, J., Gagne, C., Woocher, L.S., 1997. Evaluating peer providers. In: Mowbray, C.T., Moxley, D.P., Jasper, C.A., Howell, L. (Eds.), Consumers as providers in psychiatric rehabilitation. IAPSRS Press, Columbia, MD, pp. 488–501.

Light, E.M., Robertson, M.D., Boyce, P., Carney, T., Cleary, M., Hunt, G.E., O'Connor, N., Ryan, C., Kerridge, I.H., 2014. The lived experience of involuntary community treatment: a quality study of mental health consumers and carers. Australasian Psychiatry 22 (4), 345–351.

Lovejoy, M., 1984. Recovery from schizophrenia: a personal odyssey. Hospital and Community Psychiatry 35 (8), 809–812.

Lysaker, P.H., Leonhardt, B.L., 2012. Agency: its nature and role in recovery from severe mental illness. World Psychiatry 11 (3), 165–166.

May, R., 2010. Facilitating recovery workshop. NSW Institute of Psychiatry, Parramatta, April.

Mental health 'recovery' study working group, 2009. Mental health 'recovery': users and refusers. Wellesley Institute, Toronto.

Miller, S.D., Hubble, M.A., Chow, D.L., Seidel, J.A., 2014. The outcome of psychotherapy: yesterday, today and tomorrow. Psychotherapy in Australia 20 (3), 64–75.

Ministry of Health and Health Promotion Agency, 2014. Like minds like mine national plan 2014–19: programme to increase social inclusion and reduce stigma and discrimination for people with experience of mental illness. Ministry of Health, Wellington, NZ.

Morrow, M., 2011. Recovery: progressive paradigm or neoliberalism. Paper presented at beyond access: from disability rights to disability justice. Society for Disability Studies, San Jose, CA.

NHS England, 2018 Mental Health. Available at: https://www.england.nhs.uk/mental-health/. Accessed 9 September 2018.

Ning, L., 2010. Building a 'user driven' mental health system. Advances in Mental Health 9 (2), 112–115.

O'Hagan, M., 2011. Recovery-based services: the four pillars. Inside Out seminar, Parramatta, 10 March.

Onken, S.J., Dumont, J.M., Ridgeway, P., Dornan, D.H., Ralph, R.O., 2002. Mental health recovery: what helps and what hinders? National Technical Assistance Center for State Mental Health Planning (NTAC). National Association for State Mental Health Program Directors (NASMHPD), Alexandria, VA.

Ralph, R.O., 2000. Review of recovery literature: a synthesis of a sample of recovery literature. National Technical Assistance Center for State Mental Health Planning (NTAC), National Association for State Mental Health Program Directors (NASMHPD), Alexandria, VA.

Rapp, C., Goscha, R., 2012. The strengths model: case management with people with psychiatric disabilities, third ed. Oxford University Press, New York.

Repper, J., Carter, T., 2011. A review of the literature on peer support in mental health services. J Mental Health 20 (4), 392–411.

Ridgeway, P., 2001. ReStorying psychiatric disability: learning from first-person recovery narratives. Psychiatric Rehabilitation Journal 24 (4), 335–343.

Rosenthal, L., Carroll-Scott, A., Earnshaw, V.A., Santilli, A., Ickovics, J.R., 2012. The importance of full-time work for urban adults' mental and physical health. Social Science and Medicine 75 (9), 1692–1696.

Rowe, M., 2015. Citizenship and Mental Health. Oxford University Press, New York.

Sells, D., Borg, M., Marin, I., Mezzina, R., Topor, A., Davidson, L., 2006. Arenas of recovery for persons with severe mental illness. American Journal of Psychiatric Rehabilitation 9, 3–16.

Sheldon, K.M., 2012. The self-determination theory perspective on positive mental health across cultures. World Psychiatry 11 (2), 101–102.

Simmons, P., Hawley, C., Gale, T., Sivakumaran, T., 2010. Service user, patient, client, user or survivor: describing recipients of mental health services. Psychiatry 34 (1), 20–23. Available at: https://www.cambridge.org/core/journals/the-psychiatrist/article/service-user-patient-client-user-or-survivor-describing-recipients-of-mental-health-services/3B896BF3D269D2D7DC9FD0F360D-E4CDA. Accessed 7 January 2019.

Slade, M., Amering, M., Farkas, M., Hamilton, B., O'Hagan, M., Panther, G., et al., 2014. Uses and abuses of recovery: implementing recovery-oriented practices in mental health systems. World Psychiatry 13 (1), 12–20.

Slade, M., 2009. 100 Ways to support recovery: a guide for mental health professionals. Rethink Recovery Series, vol. 1. Rethink, London.

Slade, M., Longden, E., 2015. The empirical evidence about mental health recovery: how likely, how long, what helps? MI Fellowship, Victoria.

National Mental Health Commission, 2013. A contributing life: the 2013 report card on mental health and suicide prevention. NMHC, Sydney.

Tooth, B., Kalyanasundaram, V., Glover, H., 1997. Recovery from schizophrenia: a consumer perspective. Report to health and human services research and development grants program, Canberra.

Tooth, B., Kalyanasundaram, V., Glover, H., Momenzadah, S., 2003. Factors consumers identify as important to recovery from schizophrenia. Australasian Psychiatry 11 (1), 70–77.

Universal Declaration of Human Rights, 1948. Available at: www.un.org/en/universal-declaration-human-rights/index.html. Accessed 22 January 2016.

United Nations Declaration of the Rights of Indigenous People, 2008. Available at: www.un.org/esa/socdev/unpfii/documents/DRIPS_en.pdf. Accessed 22 January 2016.

Unzicker, R., 1989. On my own: a personal journey through madness and re-emergence. Psychosocial Rehabilitation Journal 13 (4), 71–77.

Van Gestel-Timmermans, H., van den Bogaard, J., Brouwers, E., Herth, K., van Nieuwenhuizen, C., 2010. Hope as a determinant of mental health recovery: a psychometric evaluation of the Herth Hope Index—Dutch version. Scandinavian Journal of Caring Sciences 24, 67–74.

Warner, R., 1994. Recovery from schizophrenia: psychiatry and political economy. Routledge & Kegan Paul, New York.

Wright, N., Stickley, T., 2013. Concepts of social inclusion, exclusion and mental health: a review of the international literature. Journal of Psychiatric Mental Health Nursing 20 (1), 71–81.

Xie, H., 2013. Strengths-based approach for mental health recovery. Iran Journal of Psychiatry and Behavioural Sciences 7 (2), 5–10.

USEFUL WEBSITES

A National Framework for Recovery-Oriented Mental Health Services: Policy and Theory, 2013. www.health.gov.au/internet/main/publishing.nsf/Content/mental-pubs-n-recovpol.

A National Framework for Recovery-Oriented Mental Services: Guide for Practitioners and Providers, 2013. www.health.gov.au/internet/main/publishing.nsf/Content/mental-pubs-n-recovgde.

Adults Surviving Child Abuse. 'The Last Frontier' Practice Guidelines for Treatment of Complex Trauma and Trauma Informed Care and Service Delivery, https://www.childabuseroyalcommission.gov.au/sites/default/files/IND.0521.001.0001.pdf.

Australian Institute of Health and Welfare, Closing the Gap: Trauma-informed Services and Trauma-specific Care for Indigenous Australian Children, 2013. www.aihw.gov.au/uploadedfiles/closingthegap/content/publications/2013/ctg-rs21.pdf.

Intentional Peer Support is an organisation established in the 1990s by Shery Mead, one of the founders of peer support in the United States. www.intentionalpeersupport.org/about-us.

Judi Chamberlin, www.youtube.com/watch?v=FGT4xJXgmoE.

Mental Health and Addiction Action Plan 2010. Ministry of Health Wellington 2010. www.health.govt.nz/publication/mental-health-and-addiction-action-plan-2010.

Mental Health Australia (an independent peak national body for mental health that has a wide range of important resources), www.mhca.org.au.

Mental Health Council of Australia (MHCA) is an independent peak national body for mental health: https://mhaustralia.org/.

Mental Health Recovery Services: The Richmond Fellowship: www.rfwa.org.au.

Mental Illness Fellowship of Australia Inc. provides counselling and support and promotes awareness and research: www.mifa.org.au.

National Mental Health Commission (numerous important resources), www.mentalhealthcommission.gov.au.

National Mental Health Commission's Strategies and Actions 2012–2015, www.mentalhealthcommission.gov.au/media/5039/strategicactions_2012%20to2015.pdf.

National Mental Health Consumer and Carer Forum, http://nmhccf.org.au.

National Standards for Mental Health Services 2010, www.health.gov.au/internet/main/publishing.nsf/content/mental-pubs-n-servst10.

NZ and Pacific Islander Mental Health Workforce:

- Le Va, www.leva.co.nz/mental-health-and-addiction

Our Consumer Place 2009 Real lives, real jobs: developing practice guidelines for a sustainable consumer workforce in the mental health sector through participatory research, www.ourconsumerplace.com.au/files/real_lives_real_jobs.pdf.

Patricia Deegan, Recovery and the Conspiracy of Hope, www.patdeegan.com/pat-deegan/lectures/conspiracy-of-hope

PeerZone, www.peerzone.info.

Rethink Mental Illness: "100 Ways to Support Recovery" at: www.rethink.org/about-us/commissioning-us/100-ways-to-support-recovery.

Rufus May is highly regarded in the voice-hearing network and mental health. He has two videos on his website that are recommended viewing: www.rufusmay.com.

Sane Australia is a national charity helping people seriously affected by mental illness: www.sane.org.

Te Puna Web Directory is a general directory of New Zealand and Pacific websites developed by the National Library of New Zealand/ Te Puna Mātauranga o Aotearoa, http://tepuna.natlib.govt.nz.

Te Puni Kōkiri provides policy advice to government and other agencies and has links to other Māori-related websites, www.tpk.govt.nz.

Wellness Recovery Action Plan WRAP, www.mentalhealthrecovery.com.

3

Historical Foundations

Katie Evans

KEY POINTS

- Ancient Greek and Roman medical writers were able to recognise and differentiate between the major categories of mental illness.
- Graeco-Roman treatment methods for mental illness were generally compassionate.
- The ancient literature shows that superstition and the supernatural influenced views about and treatment of the mentally ill less than was previously believed.
- The family has traditionally cared for and nursed mentally ill members of society for most of humankind's recorded history.
- Nursing has existed as an occupation since Graeco-Roman times but there are few references to nursing as a dedicated professional activity in the ancient literature.
- Psychiatric and mental health nursing is not distinguished from general nursing for most of recorded history.
- Medical and nursing practices were less sophisticated during mediaeval times.
- Graeco-Roman medical and other knowledge was kept alive during mediaeval times in monasteries and in the East, but revived during and after the Renaissance.
- Asylums developed as a response to social conditions and the emergence of new, chronic psychiatric conditions.
- Institutional care and hospitalisation are relatively recent alternative treatment modes.
- Historical research reveals the history and development of accepted conditions such as schizophrenia and mythical ones such as 'hysteria'.

KEY TERMS

anxiety disorders
asylum
deinstitutionalisation
doctor
family
gender
Graeco-Roman
Greece
historical
history
hysteria
mediaeval
mental disorder
mental illness
mental health
midwife
mood disorder
nurse
nursing
personality disorder
psychotic disorder
research
Rome
schizophrenia
superstition
witches

LEARNING OUTCOMES

The material in this chapter will assist you to:

- discern the different ways in which mental illness has been constructed in past times.
- examine the ways in which the literature delineates and defines mental illnesses.
- understand the ways in which diverse societies adapt to their mentally ill members.
- appreciate the various approaches that have been used to treat the mentally ill in the past.
- critique the hypothesis that treatment for mental disorders has progressively improved over time.
- discriminate between compassionate and inhumane nursing processes.

INTRODUCTION

This chapter examines mental disorders, the ways in which they have been regarded and the ways in which they have been treated in the past, beginning with ancient Greek and Roman times. A timeline for major sources and events is provided in Table 3.1. It traces the transition from individual family care to the emergence of organised care for the mentally ill. The consequent professionalisation of the people who treat and care for sufferers of mental disorders is described, and it will become clear that it is difficult to distinguish between the activity of nursing the physically ill and that of nursing the mentally ill when mental illness is often seen in physiological

TABLE 3.1 Timeline of Sources and Events

Years	Medical Writers; Biographers; Letter Writers; Tragedians; Comedy Writers; Poets; Historians and Philosophers
8th century BC	Homer
500–300 BC	Herodotus (490–425 BC) Hippocratic Corpus (c. 469–399 BC) Thucydides (c. 455–400 BC) Aristophanes (c. 457–385 BC) Plato (c. 429–347 BC) Aristotle (384–322 BC) Demosthenes (384–322 BC)
300 BC–1 AD	Plautus (c. 254–184 BC) Marcus Cato (234–149 BC, 'the Censor') Terence (c. 186–159 BC) Cicero (106–43 BC)
1–200 AD	Celsus (wrote under Tiberius 14–37 AD) Martial (c. 40–104 AD) Plutarch (c. 50–120 AD) Soranus (98–138 AD) Marcus Aurelius (121–180 AD)
476 AD	Last Roman Emperor deposed: fall of the Roman Empire
660 AD	Hotel Dieu in Paris
15th, 16th and 17th centuries	The Renaissance: hospitals and universities proliferate in Europe Bethlehem Hospital in London ('Bedlam') Sisters of Charity nurse the sick
18th and 19th centuries	Industrial Revolution; upsurge of syphilis and schizophrenia; the rise of asylums 1851 Colney Hatch in London the largest lunatic asylum in Europe Littre (1801–1881) translates the Hippocratic Corpus Nightingale (1820–1910): Nightingale School for Nurses established in 1860 Freud (1856–1939) Lucy Osborn brings nurses to Sydney Hospital in 1868
20th century	Psychiatric 'talking cures' popularised ECT in the 1930s Neuroleptic drugs in the 1950s The anti-psychiatry movement in 60s and 70s: Fromm; Szaz; RD Laing; Cooper; Arieti; Foucault; Rosenhan; et al. First Congress of Australian mental health nurses in 1974 Deinstitutionalisation process Social justice movement: Ottawa Charter (1986)

ECT, Electroconvulsive therapy.

terms. The chapter establishes what constituted a mental disorder in past times and societies and how mental disorder was regarded, and considers how these perceptions about mental disorder differ from those of today.

In more recent times, we will see how the need for asylums emerged most strongly in the 19th century, as the numbers of mentally ill people appear to increase at the same time as the availability of carers, such as religious orders, community and family members, decreases. The cycle of change reverses once more in the mid-20th century, when developments in advanced psychopharmacology and electroconvulsive therapy (ECT) enabled asylums to be reduced in size or eventually dissolved, and their inpatients returned to the community. Every historical overview has a beginning and an end point, and this chapter's overview ends with deinstitutionalisation, which involved the closure of major psychiatric hospitals, the expansion of community-based care for patients, and often the relocation of inpatient psychiatric beds into general hospitals. Chapters 4 and 5 take up the story of the modern era of mental healthcare.

Each generation and society builds upon the inherited knowledge of the past, even when they are not consciously aware of the fact. Occasionally the progression falters, as it did during the Middle Ages when the vast scholarship of the Graeco-Roman period was for centuries barely kept alive by the diligence of monastic orders in the West and by Eastern scholars. Fortunately, Graeco-Roman discoveries in science and medicine, literature and the arts were recovered during the Renaissance and society has since made immense advances in these areas. Mental health nurses are very aware that research into the history of psychiatry is a source of wisdom that contextualises and adds depth to mental health nursing practice (Leishman 2005; Warelow & Edward 2007). An opportunity to reflect upon the historical precedents for prevailing mental disorders, and the ways in which they have been diagnosed and treated in the past, can enhance the ways in which contemporary clinicians view their practice.

Mental disorder cannot be discovered by archaeology or by any means other than written sources, and sometimes the terminology cannot be translated exactly. It is inevitable that in the millennia covered briefly in this chapter, attitudes towards mental disorder and the mentally ill, and even mental disorders themselves, will have changed over time. As with our own society and culture, attitudes towards mental disorder probably would have differed within any society or culture at a given time. Both ancient and modern ideas about mental disorder and 'madness' are contextual and shifting. Sometimes the ancient world seems familiar to ours, but there are moments when we realise how different a world we inhabit now; we can learn from both the differences and the similarities. The history of a discipline or profession provides a common ground from which to evaluate clinical experience. We can learn from the mistakes of the past but we can also take pride in our predecessors' achievements.

THE VALUE OF HISTORICAL ANTECEDENTS

There is an increasing tendency to discount the historical antecedents of mental disorders and their treatment as health and medical education abandons its emphasis on the teaching of history, Latin and Greek. Sigmund Freud and his colleagues received a sound classical education, which included the study of Latin and Greek, legend and mythology (Richards 1991). Just as the Greek language determined the nomenclature of most body parts and diseases, it also influenced the naming of early psychoanalytic phenomena such as *mania* and *melancholia*, *neurosis* and *psychosis*, the *ego* and the *id* and the Oedipal and Electra complexes.

Stoic philosophy held that everything is perpetually in the process of changing and that people should strive to make their thinking as clear and accurate as possible. The early practitioners of cognitive behavioural therapy (CBT) recognised a kinship with Stoic philosophy and its premise that thoughts, feelings, behaviour, biology and the environment are interrelated (Blackburn & Davidson 1990). The 2nd century AD Roman emperor Marcus Aurelius (121–180 AD) was a Stoic, and he noted in his *Meditations* countless thoughts that seem to illustrate CBT principles, for example:

> *We shrink from change, yet is there anything that can come into being without it? Could you have a hot bath unless the firewood underwent some change? Could you be nourished if the food suffered no change? Do you not see then that change in yourself is of the same order, and no less necessary to nature?*
>
> ***Meditations 7:18***

Perhaps it is the need to believe that modern medical science holds the key to a better world that leads some writers to minimise the achievements of the past, or to ignore them completely. However, in some cases medicine, culture and society have not improved dramatically. Scull (2015) says that although we like to console ourselves with visions of progress, people with a mental illness still die around 25 years earlier than the rest of the population, and their mortality rate has actually accelerated in recent decades. Sometimes the past can hold valuable lessons and precedents that have been lost and that, when rediscovered, can assist us to achieve a better outcome for ourselves as healthcare practitioners and for our patients. A surprising amount survive: Suer (1995) says that French psychiatry is directly based on ancient medicine, and traces the survival in modern psychiatric care of ancient medical terminology, psychiatric terms (e.g. mania and melancholia), theories of aetiology (airs, climates and humours) and personality types.

Nursing is a genuinely ancient career but other professions use and even invent historical precedents to assist in the glorification of their own profession. For example, psychiatry as a profession has only slowly developed in the course of the past 160 years since the American Psychiatric Association (APA) was commenced in 1844 with 13 members. Yet the influential medical historian and psychoanalyst Bennett Simon boasts that what makes the medical model 'unique' is the unbroken line that joins ancient and modern practitioners (Simon 1978).

Alexander and Selesnick, in their classic and much-reprinted psychiatry text, maintain that psychiatrists and psychiatry are the culmination of an intellectual and professional evolution that began with witch doctors and philosophers and claim that: 'the precursor of the psychiatrist was any man who tended another in pain. The story of psychiatry thus begins with the story of the first professional healer' (Alexander & Selesnick 1966, p. 3). It is clear that the possession of a lengthy historical pedigree is considered an advantage for a profession.

Some nurses try to demonstrate that their profession has existed since ancient times. For example, Doona (1992) claims as 'nurses' three women from the ancient literature—Euryclea, Cilissa and Medea's nurse—but none of these characters can be said to be 'nurses' as we understand the term today. All three are aged women who had in their youth 'nursed' or suckled children. They would not have cared for ill or wounded patients as would their modern 'nursing' counterparts. In the present climate, which emphasises tertiary education, research and professionalisation in nursing, if nurses were to investigate and to own their own true history they could lay claim to a very distinguished lineage. Nurses do not need to invent or inflate the historical achievements of their ancient colleagues.

Burnard (2007) laments the exclusive emphasis on recent research in nursing education today and recommends that more historical research be performed by nursing scholars. Holme (2015) has similar concerns that poor understanding of nursing's history undermines both nursing education and policy decision making. Nursing scholarship in fact prides itself on being present-centred in the belief that this is the same as being innovative and progressive. But Burnard (2007) claims that in the 'clamour to cite only the latest papers . . . students are often citing older ideas without appreciating their genesis. Thus well-known scholars' work is often attributed, inaccurately, to more recent workers in the field' (p. 665). If we never use older works, how do we know if what we are reading is innovative or derived from some earlier, original thinker's work?

Mental health nurses are not well served by existing mental health nursing texts if they seek to find out more about the history of mental healthcare or mental disorders. The social context in which Western nursing takes place today has altered enormously. Today's professional nursing, undertaken outside the home in hospitals removed from the family, is an exception in the historical sense compared with the millennia during which nursing was undertaken by the family and their peripheral members, neighbours, slaves and servants, or later by religious orders.

Having a mental disorder in past times was not necessarily an impediment to leading a productive and consequential life. Ancient societies did not acknowledge many of the manifold mental disorders that are assiduously identified and isolated in the *Diagnostic and Statistical Manual of Mental Disorders* (DSM-5) (APA 2013) today, and in many ways they were more compassionate and tolerant than many societies today. It seems that the aim of modern medical or psychiatric writers in propagating exaggeratedly negative notions about the past is to emphasise the belief that things have changed for the better—a belief that might be meaningful to the health profession, but does no justice to the past.

PAST IDEAS ABOUT MENTAL DISORDER

The terms 'mad' and 'insane' are not acceptable medical terms for mental illness today, but in the past these general terms were used to describe a wide range of symptoms and behaviours. The Latin word *insana* means 'not of right mind' and the equivalent Greek term is *mania*. The term 'mad' is a middle-English, pre-12th-century word that is still used today to describe a loss of reason and judgement. Metallic mercury poisoning in the felt-hat industry produced toxic effects that gave rise to the expression 'mad as a hatter'.

The idea of 'madness' in the ancient world usually implied mania or psychotic illness. Medicine recognised and treated mainly those mental disorders that disrupted a person's normal functioning in society or that threatened the social order. Violence, agitation or excitement, being overtly out of touch with reality, experiencing hallucinations or delusions, melancholia causing inertia and inability to carry out one's normal tasks, or epilepsy usually succeeded in attracting medical attention. As is the case in our own society, sometimes a person was called 'mad' because their behaviour differed from the usual societal norms.

There are some issues that we can examine to help us understand the ways in which mental illness might have been constructed in the past. The theory of the humours was a systematic hypothesis that sought to explain why some people were susceptible to certain kinds of illness, including mental illness. The humoural theory (see below) was still being applied in the 19th century and has been correctly described as the first diagnostic classification system (Mack et al. 1994). In the past, some people thought that mental illness was a punishment from the gods or God. In this chapter we examine the role of the supernatural, the perceived influence of God/gods, as well as the survival of some mental illnesses across different times and cultures, using vignettes and case studies collected from primary source literature. Finally, we assess the different meanings of 'madness' and the mental state that it implies.

The 'Humours'

Early Greek medical texts tended on the whole to view mental disorder as a physiological illness. This is generally the case in the earliest of these, the Hippocratic Corpus (c. 469–399 BC), a collection of works that were not actually written by a doctor named Hippocrates, but by a variety of authors. The humoural theory was based on the belief that the body contained within it four humours—blood, phlegm, yellow bile and black bile—which were produced in various organs of the body. Each humour intrinsically possessed a basic quality such as heat, cold, dryness and moistness. Disease developed when internal or external factors disturbed the balance of the humours, and the imbalance produced injurious effects such as madness. Black bile and phlegm in particular caused mental illness, and an individual might be predisposed to mental illness because of hereditary factors. These theories are explained more fully in the Hippocratic Corpus: *The Nature of Man, Regimen I* and *The Sacred Disease.*

Some words that are still used to describe an individual's personality derive from humoural theory. The description of a person as 'phlegmatic' (cold and sluggish) recalls the ancient meaning that the person suffered from an excess of phlegm. The 'melancholy' person was believed to have too much black bile in their system, which led to a form of depression, and the person who could be described as 'choleric' possessed excessive yellow bile, which made them passionate and easily angered. In the 'sanguine' person, blood predominated over the other humours, and in both ancient and modern times to be sanguine is to be confident and hopeful.

Mental disorder was believed to be especially prevalent in spring and at the beginning of winter when the humours were thought to be stirred up by changes in the weather. Each person was believed to have been born with a constitution in which 'dryness' and 'wetness', 'fire' and 'water' were mixed. Those with a preponderance of 'dryness' and 'fire' could be intelligent but also impetuous and inclined to more agitated forms of insanity, while those in whom 'coldness' and 'water' predominated were prone to fearfulness and depression.

Some aspects of the humoural theory are quite sophisticated and in fact the four-factor theory of temperament and body function has not only survived, it has also been revived in the areas of personality assessment and the prediction of vulnerability to physical disease (Hawkins 1982; Lester 1990; Merenda 1987). Research such as that currently being undertaken into the human genome similarly seeks to find some intrinsic yet individual factor that will explain why certain people are vulnerable to specific diseases, a continuation of the same quest that originally led to the devising of the humoural theory 2500 years ago.

Supernatural Influences

The DSM-5 (APA 2013) cautions against labelling behaviour that is based in the religious beliefs of another culture as pathological because if the clinician is unfamiliar with an individual's cultural context, they might confuse normal variations in behaviour, belief, or experience with psychopathology.

It has always been difficult in practice to differentiate religiously motivated behaviour from mental disorder. For example, Schieffelin (1996) traces the emergence of new forms of mental and behavioural disturbance that emerged in Papua New Guinea following intense Christian evangelisation. The new disorder was named 'Evil Spirit Sickness' and it was attributed to stress and religious excitement. Ng (1999) identifies a range of psychiatric sequelae associated with Qigong, in traditional Chinese medicine a method of building vitality and warding off evil. A range of other psychic disturbances that are locally recognised in specific cultures is included in the DSM-5 Glossary of cultural concepts of distress (pp. 833–838). Research indicates that the more the religious beliefs of others deviate from the mental health professional's beliefs, the more liable the professional is to judge others' beliefs as mentally unhealthy (Sanderson et al. 1999). Knowing this, mental health professionals need to recognise their potential for making incorrect judgements based on their own religious or cultural assumptions.

Greece and Rome

Herodotus (490–425 BC) wrote *The Histories*, the first prose work ever recorded. He is our primary source of information about Cleomenes the First of Sparta, who reigned between c. 519 BC and 490 BC, so Herodotus could interview people who actually knew Cleomenes. Cleomenes' story is one of the first recorded cases of a mental illness that culminated in suicide (see Case Study 3.1).

CASE STUDY 3.1 Cleomenes of Sparta—Madness and Suicide

According to Herodotus' informants, Cleomenes could have suffered from a mild form of mental illness throughout his life, but towards the end of his life he 'went quite mad' and his family had him confined to the stocks, bound and guarded. Cleomenes' subsequent suicide is reported in some detail.

> *As he was lying there, fast bound, he asked his jailer, when no one else was there, to give him a knife. At first the man, who was a serf, refused, but Cleomenes, by threats of what he would do to him when he recovered his liberty, so frightened him that he at last consented. As soon as the knife was in his hands, Cleomenes began to mutilate himself, beginning on his shins. He sliced his flesh into strips, working upward to his thighs, and from them to his hips and sides, until he reached his belly, and while he was cutting that into strips he died*
>
> ***Herodotus,* The Histories, *vi.75.***

There are many factors that influence the decision to suicide and the ways in which the act is regarded. De Leo (2002) describes the vast differences in suicide rates that are found throughout history and across nations, taking into account age, gender, socioeconomic status, ethnicity and religion. Nurses still wrestle with the moral and ethical implications of intentional suicide and for the nurse the unforeseen emotional implications of patient suicide can be devastating (Rich & Butts 2004).

Herodotus is personally unable to decide between a superstitious cause and a rational one for Cleomenes' madness and death. He includes contemporary opinions about the cause of Cleomenes' illness and suicide. Some Greeks said Cleomenes was being punished by the gods for his impiety, but his fellow Spartans believed that 'heaven had no hand in Cleomenes' madness, but by consorting with Scythians he became a drinker of strong wine, and thence the madness came' (vi.84). The Spartans were a pragmatic people, and they were better acquainted with the man, his behaviour and the events surrounding his death. Their attribution of Cleomenes' death to prosaic, organic causes, and their specific rejection of the theory that Cleomenes' madness was divinely inflicted, is proof that mental illness was not universally believed to be the result of divine punishment.

In Case Study 3.2 Plutarch (c. 50–c. 120 AD) relates that Alexander the Great acted on religious convictions and advice when he put to death a person who was mentally ill, deluded and hallucinating.

CASE STUDY 3.2 Alexander the Great: Dealing With Delusions

> *[Alexander] was playing at ball, and when it was time to dress again, the young men who were playing with him beheld a man seated on the king's throne, in silence, wearing the royal diadem and robes. When the man was asked who he was, he was speechless for a long time; but at last he came to his senses and said that his name was Dionysius . . . and for a long time had been in chains; but just now the god Serapis had come to him and loosed his chains and brought him to this spot, bidding him put on the robe and diadem and sit on the throne and hold his peace. On hearing this, Alexander put the man out of the way, as the seers directed . . .*
>
> ***Plutarch,* Life of Alexander, *LXXIII–LXXIV.***

Alexander the Great was harsh on this man because he believed that if the god Serapis had instructed the man to wear Alexander's crown and robes, this could be an omen foreshadowing his own death. Perhaps it is scenarios such as this that lead many recent authors to believe that mental illness was always punished harshly or regarded by ancient societies with superstitious dread (Blakemore 1988; Devereux 1970; Dodds 1951; Hershkowitz 1998; Parker 1983; Rosen 1968; Simon 1978; Stone 1997). This position is not wholly supported by the evidence. Perhaps there was a clear line of demarcation between the medical position on mental disorder and 'popular' attitudes and beliefs.

The Greeks seem generally to have differentiated between disease-induced madness and divinely caused madness. The Hippocratic Corpus states that the gods were more likely to purify and sanctify than to harm, and it ridicules doctors who assigned a supernatural cause to epilepsy or mental disorder, denouncing them as charlatans who were at a loss because they did not know how to treat the patient and 'sheltered themselves behind superstition' (*The Sacred Disease* II–IV).

The medical term 'melancholia' was used by both the Greek comic playwright Aristophanes (1964) (c. 457–385 BC) and the Greek politician Demosthenes (384–322 BC), demonstrating that ordinary people who watched plays or listened to politicians were familiar with medical terminology as early as the 5th century BC. In Plautus' (c. 254–184 BC) *The Menaechmi*, the doctor enquires as to whether a patient's disorder was due to possession or hallucinations, indicating that although possession was a recognised 'disorder', the medical profession clearly knew the difference between possession and hallucinations, as did popular playwrights and their audiences.

The Hippocratic Corpus' disapproval of superstition was still shared by Roman society more than five centuries later, when Soranus of Ephesus (98–138 AD) stated in his work on gynaecology that the best midwives were free from superstition and did not 'overlook salutary measures on account of a dream or omen or some customary rite or vulgar superstition' (Book I.II.4). See Nurse's Story 3.1.

NURSE'S STORY 3.1 'Who are the Best Midwives?'

It is necessary to tell what makes the best midwives, so that on the one hand the best may recognize themselves, and on the other hand beginners may look upon them as models, and the public in time of need may know whom to summon. Now generally speaking we call a midwife faultless if she merely carries out her medical task; whereas we call her the best midwife if she goes further and in addition to her management of cases is well versed in theory . . . trained in all branches of therapy (for some cases must be treated by diet, others by surgery, while still others must be cured by drugs) . . . able to prescribe hygienic regulations for her patients . . . she will be unperturbed, unafraid in danger, able to state clearly the reasons for her measures, she will bring reassurance to her patients, and be sympathetic . . . She will be well disciplined and always sober, since it is uncertain when she may be summoned to those in danger. She will have a quiet disposition, for she will have to share many secrets of life . . . she will be free from superstition so as not to overlook salutary measures on account of a dream or omen or some customary rite or vulgar superstition

Soranus*, The Gynecology, *Book I.II.4.

Perhaps two different attitudes towards mental abnormality coexisted in classical antiquity: the traditional one, which was 'superstitious and magical' and attributed abnormal behaviour to supernatural intervention; and the other, which is found in the medical literature, which rejects the supernatural or the divine as an explanation. Medical terms were adopted and used by the public, and they coexisted with superstitious and religious beliefs about possession and divine punishment. This would be a similar situation to that in which today we might believe simultaneously in both medical technology and 'the stars' or astrology.

Mental Illness and the Supernatural in the Christian Era

The spread of Christianity did not do away with the intermittent association of mental illness with supernatural influences. Instead, the belief that the old pagan gods caused mental illness was translated into a belief that the devil could cause a person to experience hallucinations or delusions. In the late 13th century, the Inquisition began to deal with isolated cases of supposed witchcraft involving heresy, but it was not until the 15th and 16th centuries that mass persecutions took place, involving accusations of night-flying, intercourse with the devil, transformation into animals and malicious spells. Both the sufferers from mental illness and those associated with them, or believed to have injured them, could be the objects of suspicion and ill treatment.

By the 1630s, the tide was beginning to turn against the persecution of witches, and influential writers such as Robert Filmer denounced witch-hunting. The American colonies were slow to react to European trends, and in 1692, 150 'witches' were tried and 19 were hung in Salem, Massachusetts. The cause of the bizarre behaviour of the adolescent girls involved has been hypothesised by modern scholars as being due to ergot poisoning or mycotoxin (Woolf 2000), but whatever the cause, when the hysteria died down, public revulsion resulted in the annulment of the convictions and the release of those of the convicted who had survived. This event marks the virtual end of witch hunting.

During a period of around two centuries a number of so-called 'witches' were put to death, but the figures on 'wise women' killed as witches because they were healers seem to be greatly exaggerated in some sources. The emergence of the women's liberation movement in the 1970s caused early nursing scholars to explore women's unrecorded and uncelebrated role as healers. The persecution of witches for practising inherited healing arts seemed to offer some explanation for the failure of women to be recognised as health professionals. However, it is difficult to locate research evidence to support assertions that 'millions' of witches or 'wise women' were killed in societies that were basically illiterate. Neither is there any indication that all of the witches who were persecuted were practising healers or that all healers were persecuted as witches.

MENTAL DISORDERS DESCRIBED IN GRAECO-ROMAN SOURCES

What follows is the result of comprehensive research into mental disorders in the ancient Greek and Roman literature (Evans 2000).

The mood disorders or *affective disorders* (see Chapter 16), consisting of mania and depression, alone or in combination, were found to exist in the ancient literature; although the term *melancholia* evolved in meaning over the centuries, it did not exactly equate with 'depression' (Evans 2007). The most convincing and earliest conclusive instance of major depression was that suffered by the prominent Roman lawyer, statesman, philosopher and author, Marcus Tullius Cicero (106–43 BC). Patient Stories 3.1 and 3.2 are both excerpts from Cicero's letters at the time, which illustrate in his own tortured words the miserable symptoms of depression he suffered: they are authentic patient stories that have survived 2000 years intact, and which are still moving in their intensity.

PATIENT STORY 3.1 Cicero's Depression

I hate crowds and shun my fellow creatures, I can hardly bear the light of day . . . Your exhortation to me to live is only partially effective. You keep me from laying violent hands upon myself, but you cannot keep me from regretting my decision and the fact that I am alive . . . No one ever suffered so crushing a blow or had greater cause to pray for death. I might have met it with honour, but the moment was let pass. From the time that remains I do not look any longer for a remedy but only for an end to my misery

Cicero,* Letters to Atticus, *52 [III.7] Brundisium, 29 April 58 BC.

PATIENT STORY 3.2 Cicero's Depression and his Exile

'. . . no man has ever lost so much or fallen into such a pit of misery. Time, far from relieving this heartache, actually increases it. Other hurts grow less acute as they grow older, this cannot but increase from day to day from the sense of present misery and the recollection of the life that is past. I mourn the loss not only of the things and persons that were mine, but of my very self. What am I now?'

Cicero,* Letters to Atticus, *60 [III.15] Thessaloniki, 17 August 58 BC

When he was despondent, his letters show that Cicero tended to withdraw from Roman society, where he was famous and much in demand, and retire to the country. Cicero wrote to his friend Atticus on most of the days they were separated, and his copious correspondence clearly documents three diagnosable episodes of major depression (Evans 2007). Cicero's published correspondence revealed that he suffered from depressed mood, markedly diminished interest and pleasure in all activities, insomnia, weight loss, anger and suspicion, excessive feelings of guilt, diminished ability to think or concentrate, indecisiveness and recurrent suicidal ideation.

Cicero seems to have discovered for himself a self-help treatment method that really works and is recommended today to alleviate depression. Writing a daily journal that addresses emotional issues over a period of months has been found by modern researchers to lighten depression, as has writing about bereavement following the death of a loved one (Range et al. 2000). Paradoxically, it is only narrative writing that helps to alleviate depression: writing poetry does not seem to help (Kaufman & Sexton 2006).

Cicero's first episode of depression seems to have occurred in 58 BC when he was exiled from Rome following a political dispute (Evans 2007). Cicero's houses in Rome and his country houses were demolished, as well as those of his brother Quintus. He had to remain further than 500 miles from Italy, people were forbidden to offer him support and he could be killed at any time before he reached this limit, so he had good reason to be miserably unhappy. He became deeply, clinically depressed as a consequence of his exile, which damaged his ambitions, importance and self-esteem.

Cicero experienced his last and most severe episode of depression after the death of his daughter Tullia. Latham and Prigerson (2004) find that bereavement complicated by depression frequently results in a very high risk of suicide. An excerpt from one of Cicero's letters written after Tullia's death is shown in Patient Story 3.3.

PATIENT STORY 3.3 Cicero's Depression: Death of Tullia

In this lonely place I do not talk to a soul. Early in the day I hide myself in a thick, thorny wood, and don't emerge till evening. Next to yourself solitude is my best friend. When I am alone all my conversation is with my books, but it is interrupted by fits of weeping, against which I struggle as best I can. But so far it is an unequal fight

Cicero,* Letters to Atticus, *Astura, 9 March 45 BC.

The *anxiety disorders* (see Chapter 18) as they were manifested in the ancient world have not previously been the subject of a great deal of critical attention in the modern secondary literature, but convincing examples of anxiety disorders are described in the classical texts. The text from the Hippocratic Corpus in Case Study 3.3 describes two ancient examples of phobic avoidance, and that which follows (Case Study 3.4) from Plutarch describes an instance of *posttraumatic stress disorder*.

CASE STUDY 3.3 Phobias

Nicanor's affection, when he went to a drinking party, was fear of the flute girl. Whenever he heard the voice of the flute begin to play at a symposium, masses of terrors rose up. He said that he could hardly bear it when it was night, but if he heard it in the daytime he was not affected. Such symptoms persisted over a long period of time. Democles, who was with him, seemed blind and powerless of body, and could not go along a cliff, nor on to a bridge to cross a ditch of the least depth, but he could go through the ditch itself. This affected him for some time

Hippocratic Corpus, Vol. VII;* Epidemics *5.81–2.

CASE STUDY 3.4 Posttraumatic Stress Disorder (PTSD)

[Cassander] had only recently come to Babylon, and when he saw some Barbarians doing obeisance to Alexander, since he had been reared as a Greek and had never seen such a sight as this before, he laughed boisterously. But Alexander was enraged, and clutching him fiercely by the hair with both hands dashed his head against the wall . . . Cassander's spirit was deeply penetrated and imbued with a dreadful fear of Alexander, so that many years afterwards, when he was now king of Macedonia and master of Greece, as he was walking about and surveying the statues at Delphi, the sight of an image of Alexander smote him suddenly with a shuddering and trembling from which he could scarcely recover, and made his head swim

Plutarch,* Life of Alexander, *LXXIV.1–4.

Both the anxiety disorders and the *personality disorders* (see Chapter 17) were acknowledged by ancient cultures to be serious, chronic mental irregularities that could influence the sufferer's life, but they were not considered to be illnesses that required treatment. A number of examples of personality disorders have been identified, but since the concept of a personality disorder is often culturally determined, particular care has been taken to ensure that the subject of the case study was considered by their peers to have differed from societal norms (Evans 2000).

There was evidence in the ancient literature that affirmed that *epilepsy* was believed to be related to mental illness. Epilepsy can exhibit psychiatric sequelae, but whereas it was considered to be a mental disorder in the ancient world, it is not so regarded today.

The *substance-related disorders* (see Chapter 20) were, conversely, not conceded to be mental disorders in ancient times, although drunkenness might lead to socially unacceptable behaviour (then and now). *Alcohol-related disorders* proved to be a complex topic; examples of these disorders were located in ancient Greek and Roman literature. Indeed, although excessive alcohol consumption seems to have caused or complicated many medical conditions, ancient medical and societal opinion seemed to indicate that conditions such as alcohol abuse, dependence and withdrawal went largely unrecognised (Evans 2000).

Some *psychotic disorders* (see Chapter 15) were documented and recognised as such in the ancient Graeco-Roman literature, but research indicates that the full gamut of criteria that would justify a modern diagnosis of *schizophrenia* (early onset, hallucinations, delusions and a degree of chronicity) was not apparent anywhere in the ancient Greek and Roman texts (Evans et al. 2003). The reportage of symptoms for all the major mental disorders in the ancient literature was often inadequate to satisfy modern diagnostic criteria with reference to the duration and range of symptoms.

MENTAL DISORDERS NOT FOUND IN THE ANCIENT LITERATURE

Schizophrenia

Herodotus' account of the mental illness and suicide of King Cleomenes of Sparta provided evidence that, although his contemporaries might have considered Cleomenes to be chronically insane and that he had a psychotic episode that was well documented, a diagnosis of schizophrenia could not be made. Indeed, although the anxiety disorders and major depression appear to have survived in the exact form in which they present nowadays, indicating that these disorders can be said to be stable across time and culture, schizophrenia appears not to have manifested in the same way, or perhaps not to have existed in classical times (Evans et al. 2003).

Evans et al. (2003) concluded that schizophrenia did not exist in its present form in ancient Graeco-Roman times and other reputable researchers have theorised that schizophrenia appeared in recent centuries. For example, H Fuller Torrey and colleagues have investigated the origins of schizophrenia and they believe that schizophrenia is the product of a genetic mutation that occurred in recent centuries (Torrey & Miller 2002). Torrey (1980, p. 27) states definitively that there was a distinct point at the beginning of the 18th century when cases of schizophrenia began to multiply, and suddenly schizophrenia's symptoms were being described everywhere.

Michel Foucault, the French philosopher considered by many to have made a significant contribution to our understanding of the social construction of madness, commenced his study with the 15th century but he did not describe schizophrenia (Foucault 1967). Foucault had no medical background and did not describe his subjects with sufficient clarity to allow clinical diagnoses to be made. To Foucault, 'madness' encompassed a bizarre collection of disorders: melancholia with delusional guilt, melancholy allied with mania, nymphomania, delirium, vertigo, hysterical convulsions, hysteria and hypochondria. Some of Foucault's subjects appear to suffer from a form of chronic, lifelong 'madness' that disabled them from undertaking productive work, so they are identified with 'the indigent'. They are represented as deluded, demented and hallucinated, reduced to an animal state in which they are inured to 'hunger, heat, cold, pain' (Foucault 1967, p. 74). Frequent references to the ability of the 'mad' to endure physiological hardship suggest a degree of neurological damage. Perhaps they were the victims of syphilis, which Grmek (1991) believes had emerged in Europe by then. Perhaps they suffered from chronic schizophrenia, if indeed this disorder had evolved by the late Middle Ages.

Research into the origins of schizophrenia has led some to conclude that not only has schizophrenia changed in its manifestation within the past 50 years, but also it might exhibit such different symptoms in different cultures as to cause one to question whether the diagnostic criteria refer to the same condition (Ellard 1987; Jeste et al. 1985). Polimeni and Reiss (2003) reviewed the data concerned with the emergence of schizophrenia, cautiously evaluating whether it is a disadvantageous by-product of normal brain evolution or whether it might have some evolutionary advantage. They come to no definitive conclusion, but evidence does exist of viral-associated sequences in the brains of individuals suffering from schizophrenia (Yolken et al. 1997). It has been hypothesised that urban birth, household crowding and/or the transmission of a virus from household cats could assist the spread of the virus (Torrey & Yolken 1995, 1998; Torrey et al. 1997).

The state of medical knowledge at present can assist in tracking the development and dissemination of new or unfamiliar diseases, but if schizophrenia had emerged in a technical and literate society, its advent would have been documented. Mental illness leaves no trace on skeletal remains; it can be traced only in the surviving literature.

CRITICAL THINKING CHALLENGE 3.1

If schizophrenia were proved to be of viral origin, how would that change the way in which the disorder is regarded by society and the medical profession?

Hysteria: a Translation Error

It is a remarkably durable belief that hysteria is a feminine mental disorder that has been recognised since the days of Hippocrates. Tasca et al. as recently as 2012 seriously discuss hysteria as a mental disorder 'discovered' by the ancient medical writers, but the term 'hysteria' is not an ancient Greek word and it does not appear in any Greek dictionary or lexicon of Greek words. It has been proven conclusively that the term 'hysteria' was invented by Emile Littre (1801–1881), the French translator of the Hippocratic Corpus in the late 19th century.

The problem resides in the translation. A number of ancient passages that have been interpreted as referring to a mental affliction arising in the womb actually refer only to physical gynaecological complaints. The evidence suggests that Littre has bestowed a modern and anachronistic meaning upon the Greek text that is not supported by the evidence (King 1993). Helen King's informative scholarship is included below because hysteria is still considered to be one of psychiatry's most celebrated apparent legacies from the ancient medical literature, and once something passes into the inherited 'knowledge' associated with a discipline, it is hard to eradicate, even if it is untrue.

Since Sigmund Freud (1856–1939) 'rediscovered' hysteria in the late 19th century, it seems that male therapists have been especially keen to reinforce the notion that women have always been prone to gender-specific ills, and that men can cure them. Bennett Simon (1978) imaginatively described Freud's psychoanalysis of a female patient's 'hysterical expression of the thwarted sexuality of the recently widowed young woman' and added that 'Greek doctors knew that virgins and widows were most susceptible to those diseases of the womb called "hysterical"' (Simon 1978, p. 25). In fact, Simon devoted an entire chapter in his book about mental illness in ancient Greece to hysteria and social issues, commencing with the statement that 'Hysteria, the disease of the "wandering uterus", was given its name by the Greeks' (Simon 1978, p. 238). The respected psychiatric textbook *Synopsis of Psychiatry* attributed Hippocrates with having 'introduced the terms "mania" and "hysteria" as forms of mental illness in the fifth century BC' (Sadock & Sadock 2007). But 'hysteria' is not a Greek word and Hippocrates did not use it.

Those who say hysteria was a mental illness typically found in women and first described in the Hippocratic Corpus are reliant on an incorrect translation of the Greek words *hysterike*, *hysterika* and *hysterikos*, words that actually translate as 'afflicted with suffering in the womb'. King (1993) found that hysteria is in reality 'but a mare's nest, a spurious entity' (Gilman et al. 1993, p. xi). In the ancient literature, *hysterikos* was not considered to have connotations of mental illness. Littre's edition of the Hippocratic Corpus (1839–1861) translates *hysterikos* as 'hysteria', in French *hysterie* (King 1993, p. 7). By examining the original Greek texts, King found that Littre's chapter headings, such as 'Hysterie', have no analogies in the Greek manuscripts; Littre freely transposed the medical categories of his own time. King concluded that Littre translated the Hippocratic Corpus in the mid-19th century, when the psychiatric condition 'hysteria' had begun to be a debated ideology. He expected to find hysteria in the text, and of course he found it, and composed his headings accordingly. The diagnosis was therefore made by the translator (King 1993, p. 8).

The Roman medical writer Celsus wrote at the time of the Emperor Tiberius (14–37 AD), but his translator Spencer perpetuated a similar error in his 1935–1938 translation of Celsus' work. Spencer noted, for example, that in *De Medicina* 5.21.6 the woman's 'fits' would have been 'hysterical fits'. Similarly, Spencer appended a footnote to indicate that the *Hippocratic Corpus: Aphorisms* V 35 was 'a description of hysteria', when it is more properly translated as 'suffering from illness in the womb'. Freud collaborated with Joseph Breuer to produce *Studies in Hysteria* in 1895. If *hysterikos*, meaning in Greek 'afflicted with suffering in the womb', is translated as 'suffering from hysteria', it is clear that the translation is influenced not by the original language of the text but by the meaning that Charcot, Freud and Breuer attached to the psychiatric diagnosis of hysteria in mainly female patients in the late 19th century (Evans 2000).

King (1993) suggests that in 'hysteria' we do not hear 'the insistent voice of a fixed entity calling across the centuries':

> *Nineteenth-century hysteria, a parasite in search of a history, grafts itself by name and lineage onto the centuries-old tradition of suffocation of the womb, thus making Hippocrates its adopted father. It is time that father disowned his hybrid child (p. 64).*

Unfortunately, the parasite hysteria remains attached to Hippocrates in the minds of many, despite being conclusively disowned, because historical research is too often ignored or disregarded.

ANCIENT MENTAL HEALTHCARE

In ancient Greek and Roman times, the Greek hero and god of healing, Asclepius (whose staff wound about with a snake inspired the present symbol of medicine) was commemorated by temple healing centres called 'Asclepions'. The main ceremonial treatment practised there was the ritual of incubation (sleep and the interpretation of dreams). In the Hippocratic Corpus it is said of dreams:

> *For when the body is awake the soul is its servant, and is never her own mistress, but divides her attention among many things . . . but the mind never enjoys independence. But when the body is at rest, the soul administers her own household*
>
> ***Regimen IV, LXXXVI.***

Recognising the importance of dreams as an expression of the unconscious is surprisingly sophisticated, and not equalled until Freud's work in the area 2500 years later. Yet the Asclepion was not an infallible remedy. In his play *The Wasps*, Aristophanes, the Greek writer of comedy, depicted a case of dementia that was treated initially by purification rites and a stay in the Temple of Asclepius, but the only treatment that was effective in preventing the demented patient from leaving the house was putting the house under guard and having every opening covered with netting. Graeco-Roman medical science and theory were highly sophisticated, but medical treatment was predominantly the concern of the individual, with perhaps a doctor's assistance if the family was prosperous.

Violent Behaviour

When Cleomenes showed signs of a violent mental disturbance, he was confined to the stocks by his family and was kept bound and guarded. The Roman medical writer Celsus wrote five centuries after the time of Cleomenes, but it is clear that the kind of treatment that was considered suitable for the person who was mad and violent in Roman society had not changed a great deal in the intervening centuries. Celsus differentiated between the several forms of insanity.

> *. . . some among insane persons are sad, others hilarious; some are more readily controlled and rave in words only, others are rebellious and act with violence; and of these latter, some only do harm by impulse, others are artful too, and show the most complete appearance of sanity whilst seizing occasion for mischief, but they are detected by the result of their acts*
>
> ***Celsus III.18.3.***

Celsus prescribed distinct interventions for the fearful, the violent, the melancholy and those who exhibited 'untimely laughter' (III.18.10). He allowed that those who 'merely rave in their talk, or who make but trifling misuse of their hands' ought not to be constrained unnecessarily, but he recommended that it was best to fetter those who were violent 'lest they should do harm, either to themselves or to others. Anyone so fettered, although he talks rationally and pitifully when he wants his fetters removed, is not to be trusted, for that is a madman's trick' (III.18.4).

This description fits perfectly the treatment accorded to Cleomenes. The mentally ill person who was violent presented a challenge in the era before the advent of the major tranquillisers in the 1950s. There was little alternative to physical restraint as a means of preventing the violently mentally ill from harming themselves or others, and physical restraint was, as it sometimes still is, the only means of preventing harm to the person or the environment.

Yet Celsus was basically humane and he respected individual differences. He recommended that the patient not be frightened and that they be kept in an environment that was reassuring, either in the light or in the dark, whichever was the most 'quieting of the spirit' for the patient. 'It is best, therefore, to make a trial of both, and to keep that patient in the light who is afraid of darkness, and him in darkness who is frightened by light' (III.18.5). Celsus forbade restraint for any longer than was required and recommended that the restraint be removed the moment it was unnecessary. Just as the prevention of harm to the patient or to others is still regarded as a legitimate reason for restraining a patient under the mental health legislation of many countries, including Australia, it also remains a legal requirement that restraint be alleviated as soon as is practically possible. Read Ethical Dilemma 3.1 and consider the question that follows.

ETHICAL DILEMMA 3.1

Now that those who merely rave in their talk, or who make but trifling misuse of their hands, should be coerced with the severer forms of constraint is superfluous; but those who conduct themselves more violently it is expedient to fetter, lest they should do harm, either to themselves or to others

Celsus, De Medicina, *III.18.4.*

The regulation that patients should be prevented from harming themselves or others is still regarded as a legitimate reason for restraining a patient under most mental health legislation. Celsus forbade restraint for any longer than was strictly necessary, saying: '[sometimes] there is nothing else to do but restrain the patient, but when circumstances permit, relief must be given with haste' (III.18.6).

Question: Is physical restraint too primitive a treatment for the mentally ill patient who is violent? Compulsory treatment with sedative medication is often seen as a more humane alternative. Is chemical restraint a more humane or less humane alternative to physical restraint?

Counselling

Celsus outlines a medley of responses that can be helpful in treating various mental disorders. The variety and sophistication of his suggested interventions can be seen as the birthplace of counselling techniques that are used in mental health nursing to this day. In the examples that follow, the patients are depressed and/or anxious. They are at home, and the simple yet effective suggestions were meant to be followed by family or friends.

> *Some need to have empty fears relieved, as was done for a wealthy man in dread of starvation, to whom pretended legacies were from time to time announced . . . in others, melancholy thoughts are to be dissipated, for which purpose music, cymbals, and noises are of use. More often, however, the patient is to be agreed with rather than opposed, and his mind slowly and imperceptibly is to be turned from the irrational talk to something better*
>
> ***Celsus, De Medicina, III.18.10–12.***

Reassurance was clearly used to good effect, and it is interesting that the invention of good news to enhance hopefulness was not considered unethical if it was effective. The patient was to be entertained, distracted and amused. Other suggestions included reading to the patient, playing games and storytelling, 'especially by those with which the patient was wont to be attracted when sane', and praising any work the patient was able to produce. People who the patient liked and esteemed were urged to eat with them to stimulate their appetite and to 'gently reprove his depression as being without cause' (Celsus, *De Medicina*, III.18.18).

Early Christian Healthcare

In 331 AD, around seven centuries after the Hippocratic Corpus was written and two and a half centuries after Celsus wrote, the Roman emperor Constantine the Great decreed that the Church should take responsibility for the care of the sick after a plague (perhaps anthrax) devastated the Roman Empire. The first public hospital in Europe was founded by a Roman woman, Fabiola, at Ostia near Rome in 390 AD. Europe has had a strong tradition of healthcare by religious orders, a tradition that has continued across the centuries since that time. After 430 AD, when the rebellious Christian sect, the Nestorians, had been exiled from Constantinople, taking Greek medical texts with them, India and Persia used the texts to make independent medical and scientific progress (Mellersh 1999).

After the fall of the Roman Empire in the 5th century, Greek and Roman medical texts survived, having been copied and kept by religious orders in the West. This knowledge was both adopted and enhanced by the Eastern scholars; by 660 AD, Indian physicians had developed sophisticated bladder and digestive tract surgery, and in the 9th century a hospital was established in Baghdad, which by the 10th century was the largest medical faculty in the world with 24 physicians. While Western medicine and healthcare stagnated, Muslim, Japanese and Chinese scholars developed extensive surgical, anatomical and pharmacological expertise (Mellersh 1999).

ANCIENT DOCTORS AND NURSES

The amount of medical knowledge that existed in ancient times could be learned by an educated person of average intelligence. The differences between doctors, nurses and knowledgeable amateurs were less defined than they are today and the amateur was not so sharply distinguished from the professional. The Roman senator Marcus Cato (234–149 BC), known as the 'Censor', was suspicious of Greek doctors, so he wrote a book of prescriptions, recipes and regimens and used it successfully to treat himself and his family. Plutarch says: 'By following such treatment and regimen he said he had good health himself, and kept his family in good health' (Plutarch, *Marcus Cato*, XXIII, 3–4). Even where roles such as 'doctor', 'nurse' or 'midwife' existed, their areas of expertise were quite different from what they are now. For example, a midwife might be employed for a birth by wealthier families, but she relied on family members for assistance and she handed the baby to a wet nurse, who took over the care and feeding of the infant.

Furthermore, it is impossible to distinguish between psychiatric mental health nurses and general nurses until relatively modern times because the distinction between disorders of the mind and disorders of the body is of relatively recent origin. In this respect, ancient nursing was more holistic than it is today, when the distinctions between the disciplines appear to be stressed more than the similarities.

There were instances noted as early as Homer (c. 8th century BC) of systematic nursing of patients. *The Iliad* (c. 800 BC), which describes the Trojan War, depicts the wounded as being removed to tents dedicated to healing and tended mainly by captured slave women under the direction of Greek surgeons, although on the battlefield the 'nurses' were more often men attached to the military force.

The Roman writer Celsus is an important source for the history of medicine, but it is doubtful that Celsus was a practising physician. The philosophers Plato and Aristotle, among others, wrote about medical subjects, although they had no formal medical training. The Greeks formalised scientific medical training at recognised medical schools such as Cos, Cnidos and later Alexandria. Early Greek doctors had no special status but, like craftsmen, travelled from town to town and most probably employed their pupils as nurses. There was no form of licensure, but pupils were bound by an agreement: the *Hippocratic Oath* is one early form of private contract (Hornblower & Spawforth 1996).

In the Hippocratic Corpus it appears that in the absence of the doctor, the patient was attended to by family members, slaves or medical students, who reported the patient's progress to the doctor. The sensitive advice in the Hippocratic Corpus (see Nurse's Story 3.2) would be useful for any person who cared for an individual who was physically or mentally ill.

NURSE'S STORY 3.2 Being Person-Centred

Kindnesses to those who are ill. For example to do in a clean way his food or drink or whatever he sees, softly what he touches. Things that do no great harm and are easily got, such as cool drink where it is needed. Entrance, conversation. Position and clothing for the sick person, hair, nails, scents

Hippocratic Corpus, Vol. VII;* Epidemics *6.4.7.

Women

In Western countries, we are used to considering nursing to be a profession suited to either gender. Indeed, psychiatric mental health nursing was predominantly the province of the male nurse, since asylums were created to confine the seriously mentally ill who could not be accommodated in society before the development of neuroleptic medication in the 1950s and males possessed an advantage in terms of strength.

In past centuries, nursing was considered to be the natural province of women, an extension of the maternal, caring role, but the absence of women in the literature has made nurses and nursing difficult to trace. The classicist who wrote an early essay entitled 'Ancient nursing' wrestled with what he saw as the absence of nurses in the ancient world:

'so little is told us of nurses and nursing. The conclusion we are tempted to draw from this silence is that the task of nursing fell to the women, whether slaves or free, of the household' (Jones 1923).

The usual attitude towards 'respectable' women in ancient male-dominated societies was conservative and patriarchal. Ancient ideas about how women should conduct themselves are encapsulated in Pericles' speech to the Athenian women in 430 BC: 'Perhaps I should say a word or two on the duties of women to those among you who are now widowed . . . the greatest glory of a woman is to be least talked about by men, whether they are praising you or criticising you' (Thucydides ii.46).

Women have traditionally been poorly educated, and little has survived of the writing that the educated few have accomplished. Most ancient authors wrote about their male, aristocratic peers, and because so much of the literary evidence from the centuries preceding the most recent two or three is limited by the writers' upper social class and male gender, much historical research cannot accurately report the incidence of any type of illness in the female gender. Where women are mentioned—whether in the medical literature, in the histories, in biographies of their menfolk, in fiction or in poetry—it is from the perspective of a male and any such account cannot be said with certainty to represent the authentic female experience.

Women usually appear in the ancient medical literature in their reproductive role, in relation to childbirth and any gynaecological disorders that might prevent or complicate childbirth. Most health problems a woman might have were attributed to the possession of a womb. The Roman poet Martial (c. 40–104 AD) records that when male doctors were called in to treat 'women's complaints' both they and their female patient's true motives were probably sexual. Note in the following quote from Martial that the modern, mistaken term 'hysteria' has been used by the translator instead of the more correct translation 'pain in the womb':

> *One day Leda announced to her aged husband, 'I'm suffering from hysteria. I'm sorry, but I'm told that nothing but intercourse will make me feel cheerier'*
>
> ***Martial, The Epigrams, 11.71.***

Leda had been attended by female nurses, but they leave when the doctors arrive, whereupon the doctors 'hoist and prise open her legs' with the exclamation: 'Ah, serious medicine!' The male doctors are depicted as eager to 'treat' this illness fabricated to procure the sexual services of younger lovers. In a society where medical practitioners were male, the ailments of women, being outside the experience of men, could be seen as counterfeit, even if the prevailing masculine ideas about the innate immorality of women did not intrude.

Leda was an upper-class woman, but in the course of their lives most women were unlikely to be treated by a male doctor. In fact, women probably received little medical attention that was unrelated to reproductive affairs, and they would have treated themselves and their dependants in the seclusion of the women's quarters.

Martial probably exaggerated in *The Epigrams* (later) when he said that the doctor who attended him had 45 students with 90 hands who examined him, but there would have been some students in any case. We may assume that a great deal of the information given in the clinical histories such as the *Epidemics* is the result of their observations and those of the family or carers. The information gathered about the patient required an awareness of what was significant and what was not, which means that responsible and intelligent laypersons would have been satisfactory sources of information. Nurse's Story 3.3 warns the reader of the sensitivity required when 'the practitioner' approaches the patient.

NURSE'S STORY 3.3 Interpersonal Skills

The bath and exercise and fear and anger and any other feeling of the mind is often apt to excite the pulse; so that when the practitioner makes his first visit, the solicitude of the patient who is in doubt as to what the practitioner may think of his state, may disturb his pulse. On this account a practitioner of experience does not seize the patient's forearm with his hand, as soon as he comes, but first sits down and with a cheerful countenance asks how the patient finds himself; and if the patient has any fear, he calms him with entertaining talk, and only after that moves his hand to touch the patient. If now the sight of the practitioner makes the pulse beat, how easily may a thousand things disturb it!

Celsus,* De Medicina, *Vol. 1, Book III, 6.6

Mistrust of doctors was apparently widespread in ancient society. Compare the reflective and idealistic image of holistic healthcare conveyed by Celsus in Nurse's Story 3.3 with his contemporary Martial's criticism below.

> *I was unwell. You hurried round, surrounded*
> *By ninety students, Doctor.*
> *Ninety chill, north-wind-chapped hands then pawed*
> *and probed and pounded.*
> *(I was unwell: now I'm extremely ill.)*
>
> ***Martial, The Epigrams, 5: IX.***

In the Roman-occupied lands—that is, most of what we know today as Europe, as well as North Africa and the Middle East—there existed a lively alternative culture that could be xenophobic about doctors, who were usually Greek and foreign. These people often applied and further developed traditional folk remedies in treating families and large households. Sometimes it was the male head of the household who nursed the sick or directed their treatment.

Midwives and Nurses

One male author who offers posterity a glimpse of those previously invisible in the literature—women, infants and a whole array of health personnel including midwives, nurses and assistants of various kinds—is Soranus of Ephesus (c. 98–138 AD), who wrote the earliest surviving text on gynaecology, building on some earlier sources that have not survived. Soranus was a renowned physician from the Greek city of Ephesus on the Mediterranean coast of what is now Turkey, who worked during the reigns of the emperors Trajan and Hadrian. Most of the good medical schools were Greek, and their graduates travelled the world plying their trade. However, Soranus wrote for the benefit of the female midwife and the wet nurse, who both fed the infant and treated childhood ills. Both appeared to be independent practitioners who were called in by the family when they were required.

The translation of *The Gynecology* in 1956 by Owsei Temkin, Professor Emeritus of the history of medicine and a former director of the Johns Hopkins Institute of the History of Medicine, is clearly a product of a time and culture in which the midwife had a role subordinate to that of the doctor, who made the command decisions as the natural leader of a 'medical team'. Culture-bound beliefs led Temkin to make unwarranted authorial comment about the text, in which he assumed that although the midwife herself was consistently addressed by Soranus, she must be 'working under the supervision of a physician'. This is incorrect.

The extract from *The Gynecology* in Nurse's Story 3.4 describes the necessary attributes of a midwife, and this passage has a timeless quality. Soranus could be describing the ideal modern nurse (or nursing student) and it is significant that many of the skills she must possess, such as sympathy, reassurance and the sharing of secrets, would encourage a therapeutic relationship that would benefit the mental health of the patient. Note that the midwife is required to be a female, while elsewhere in the work the doctor is presumed to be a male.

NURSE'S STORY 3.4 'What Persons are Fit to Become Midwives?'

She must be literate in order to be able to comprehend the art through theory too; she must have her wits about her so that she may easily follow what is said and what is happening; she must have a good memory to retain the imparted instructions (for knowledge arises from memory of what has been grasped). She must love work in order to persevere through all vicissitudes (for a woman who wishes to acquire such vast knowledge needs manly patience). She must be respectable since people will have to trust their household and the secrets of their lives to her . . . She must not be handicapped as regards her senses since there are things which she must see, answers which she must hear when questioning, and objects which she must grasp by her sense of touch. She needs sound limbs so as not to be handicapped in the performances of her work and she must be robust, for she takes a double task upon herself during the hardship of her professional visits

Soranus,* The Gynecology, *Book I.1.1–3.

The ancient Greek midwife was clearly well trained. The skills she was expected to master were numerous, and they included many that might be considered traditionally medical functions, such as independent practice, diagnosis, prescribing and case management. She also selected and supervised the wet nurse, who was also skilled in treating the ailments of childhood. The translator Temkin felt that it was 'more natural' to think that *The Gynecology* was addressed to physicians, who could then 'explain' it to the midwife, but Soranus' text is clear that the physician was only called to assist the midwife in her duties if the labour had been obstructed and surgical intervention was required to extract the fetus by hooks and embryotomy (IV; III [XIX], 9 [61]).

Temkin did nurses and nursing a disservice when he concealed the true role of the ancient Greek midwife as an independent professional practitioner. He removed her historical importance while simultaneously consolidating the dominant role of the physician. The reader is being instructed furtively: this is the way it always has been—the midwife would be breaking with an age-old tradition should she (or he) seek more autonomy. Remarkably, Temkin's interpretation has not previously been challenged by nursing scholars, perhaps because of an indifference to the importance of historical research and enquiry in nursing.

The midwife has retained her importance in the lives of birthing women. Many centuries after Soranus, Charles Dickens incorporated the character of the nurse and midwife Sairey (or Sarah) Gamp in his novel *Martin Chuzzelwit* (1844). Dickens exaggerates her fondness for tea and strong liquor and Gamp is usually cited by nurses as an example of the type of nurse who was made obsolete by the Nightingale training system (Summers 1997).

Society has always been simultaneously respectful and ribald about midwives. The Roman dramatist Terence (c. 186–159 BC) and Plautus were contemporaries, but his midwife Lesbia, summoned to attend a childbirth in *The Girl from Andros*, is a serious, sober and independent practitioner (Terence 1976). Perhaps Gamp was meant to be a caricature in the tradition of the midwives in classical Graeco-Roman writers of comedy, in much the same way as nurses are depicted in modern television dramas, films, books and advertisements in roles that run the gamut from skilful professional to scantily clad temptress.

RESURGENCE OF MEDICAL KNOWLEDGE

After the Catholic faith gained control in Europe in the Middle Ages, access to healthcare was limited to that provided by religious orders at hospices, which could care for those few in society who did not have family to provide services for them. The Christian Church was instrumental in forestalling some forms of medical research by forbidding practices such as the mutilation of the dead. This tended to hamper the training of medical personnel, the study of anatomy and eventually surgical interventions of most sorts.

The Hotel Dieu was opened in Paris in 660 AD. The Hotel Dieu was technically a hospital but was more concerned with treating patients' souls than their ailments. In the 15th and 16th centuries, the Renaissance had reawakened European scholarship and engendered advances in many fields, including healthcare: Nicholas Flamel (c. 1330–1418 AD) had established 14 new hospitals in Paris, St Thomas' Hospital had been established in London, and universities proliferated throughout Europe (Mellersh 1999).

As time progressed, society changed and the healthcare needs of the population changed too. During the 18th and 19th centuries, the Industrial Revolution caused rural societies to be disrupted due to many of their inhabitants deserting their rural homelands to seek work in the factories and manufacturing towns, thereby removing themselves from the traditional sources of societal and family healthcare. This coincided with an apparent upsurge of schizophrenia in industrialised societies. As noted previously, schizophrenia appears not to have existed in the ancient Greek or Roman worlds (Evans et al. 2003) and some researchers postulate that it evolved comparatively recently, sometime in the 17th century (Torrey 1980; Jeste et al. 1985), causing a crisis in the evolving healthcare systems and demanding the creation of new solutions.

The Asylum

Chronically ill and displaced populations required the creation of institutions that could cater for their needs. For some time little distinction was made between the mentally ill and other persons unable to exist independently in society. The dissolution of the monasteries in England in 1536 had restricted funding of hospitals by the Church, but previous to this many early hospitals and carers had been allied with the Church. The mentally ill were confined with others most in need of care and detention: lepers, criminals, the indigent, the unemployed and the ill. Perhaps a vestige of the confusion this caused between mental illness, indigence and wickedness can be found in the stigmatising view of the mentally ill that persists to this day in some societies, diminishing the patient's self-esteem and interfering with the delivery of supportive mental healthcare (Corrigan 2004; Grandbois 2005). By 1400, Bethlehem Hospital in London ('Bedlam') was devoted to the treatment, or more correctly the confinement, of the mentally ill.

Both Rosen (1968) and Porter (2002) discuss the French hospital Salpêtrière. Rosen is much more detailed, describing at length (pp. 163–164) regulations in 1690 that provided for 'wayward children', 'those who removed themselves from or transgressed the moral order considered appropriate to their social position, occupation, or family relationship'; those who 'used their parents badly', refused to work through laziness, or who were debauched or in danger of being so. Salpêtrière was the female section, and girls were confined in a separate part from prostitutes and women who ran bawdy houses. Boys were shut up in the partner-facility of Bicetre.

The initial intention was not malign; something had to be done by the state to provide for children whose parents were unable or unwilling to do so. But some time during the next century Salpêtrière evolved into an enormous asylum cum gaol. Rosen (1968) cites Tenon's 1788 *Memoires sur les Hospitaux de Paris* (p. 85), describing Salpêtrière as the largest hospital in Europe, housing other categories as well as well as young girls, pregnant or innocent, and women. It was separated into four sections for those 'not hopelessly depraved', 'dissolute girls', those held by order of the King and court-ordered inmates. Elsewhere in Salpêtrière were 'raving lunatics, imbeciles, epileptics, paralytics, blind persons, cripples' and 'incurables of all sorts' (p. 164).

The change, Rosen says, was brought about by a new view of 'reason', irrationality and madness. Deviations from what was then thought of as 'human nature' and reasonable behaviour needed to be corrected. Women in these institutions were not treated more harshly than men, although their detainers certainly acted on a now-outdated (for most of us) premise that extramarital sexual activity, for example, was symptomatic of madness. Men were accorded the same treatment if they were crippled, blind, epileptic, indigent, bankrupt or insane.

Built in London in 1851, Colney Hatch was the largest lunatic asylum in Europe. It was desperately needed. Torrey states definitively:

> *It was as if somebody rang a bell precisely at the turn of the nineteenth century to herald the official entrance of schizophrenia. Whereas up to that point there appear to have been at best a few scattered cases in the literature, classical schizophrenia was suddenly being described by different people in different places all at about the same time (1980, p. 27).*

At the time Colney Hatch was built, there were in the UK alone some 3579 'lunatics' in public asylums, 2559 in the 139 licensed houses devoted to the treatment of mental illness and 8000 more in workhouses or at home. The asylums were characterised as 'warehouses for the unwanted', the aged, destitute vagrants, alcoholics and syphilitics. Europe and the United States followed suit (Mellersh 1999).

Even when a patient was wealthy and able to employ private medical care, treatment methods for perceived mental disorder had not altered significantly in the two millennia since Hippocrates. Macalpine and Hunter (1969) investigated the alleged mental disorder of King George III (1738–1820), which they attributed to the medical condition porphyria. The king was cupped, bled and dosed with emetics and purgatives, secluded from family and friends and physically restrained for his own protection, in exactly the way that ancient Greek and Roman medical writers had described.

In Australia, although modern research has rediscovered the value of exercise in anxiety reduction and for aiding the improvement of cognitive function, depressed mood and lowered self-esteem (Callaghan 2004), the belief that 'fresh air, space and the climate of the country would preclude madness' proved not to be the case and it became essential for the maintenance of law and order to build and equip asylums modelled on similar establishments in the UK (Ash et al. 2001; Sands 2009). The first 'lunatic asylum' was opened at Castle Hill in New South Wales in 1811. All the 'lunatics' in the new colony were sent there, and by 1825 this facility was overcrowded. Gladesville Hospital in Sydney was opened in 1837 to accommodate the surplus, and each state soon developed its own psychiatric services (Sands 2009). See Chapter 5 for more information.

Although attempts were made to provide humane care, and numerous commissions and inquiries were conducted, overcrowding meant that custodial care was the usual strategy employed with the mentally ill. The medical model continued to see mental illness as an organic process. The psychoanalytic theories initiated by Freud in the latter part of the 19th century and the early 20th century were slow to be adopted in Australia.

The asylum was both a solution and a problem in itself. Custodial care was for a long time the only option if a mental disorder followed a chronic, disabling course, before the development of psychotropic medications less than 60 years ago which helped to change every aspect of how people with a mental illness were treated. The asylum took care of people who were ill-equipped to take care of themselves and it protected society from disruptive and violent behaviour, but asylums quickly became 'silted up with long-stay patients . . . a dustbin for hopeless cases' (Porter 2002, p. 119).

CRITICAL THINKING CHALLENGE 3.2

1. What would be some of the disadvantages, difficulties and changes for the patient, the patient's family and society if the mentally ill were cared for by the family?
2. What would be the advantages for the patient and for society if the patient's family were solely responsible for the care of the mentally ill?

PIONEERS AND PROFESSIONALISATION

To many nursing scholars, Charles Dickens' fictional character Sarah Gamp represents the earliest, and one must say the worst, historical role model in nursing. There is an understanding that previous to that time nursing was the exclusive province of the religious orders, both male and female, or the domestic amateur but, as this chapter has demonstrated, the roots of the nursing profession extend much further back than the 19th century, and for most of this time it is not possible to isolate mental health nursing from general nursing. The body of knowledge contained in the ancient texts delineates a competent practitioner: technically expert, systematic, professional and well respected. St Vincent de Paul formed the association later named the Sisters of Charity in 1617, and they combined general nursing with caring for the insane. The care delivered to the mentally ill ('lunatics') in asylums was harsh—indeed, if the asylum was overcrowded, as was often the case, the jail was considered an appropriate alternative.

It often happens that a number of advances in an area are made almost simultaneously. This was the case with nursing, and nursing the mentally ill in particular. Despite slower communication methods and transport, new ideas were shared and each advance fuelled further advances in key areas across the world. Each of the English-speaking countries has its own nursing pioneer who is credited with bettering the lot of the mentally ill.

Unusually, in the days when women were relatively constrained in what they could achieve, pioneering nurses were predominantly women. Florence Nightingale (1820–1910) wrote the highly influential *Notes on Nursing* (1969) and incorporated both religious and feminine attributes when she called nurses 'sister', spoke of nursing as a 'vocation' and dressed nurses in the nun-like uniform and coif (Chatterton 2000). However, the establishment of the asylum system in the middle of the 19th century provided both the impetus for the evolution of mental health nursing as a profession distinct from general nursing (Hamblet 2000) and a different gender balance from that which applied in general nursing. Asylums also ensured that mental health nursing developed along institutional lines in both the United Kingdom and its colonies.

In the asylums, more male attendants were employed initially for their strength, although photographs of asylums in the 19th century clearly show female nurses, dressed in the starched general nurse's garb of the period (Chatterton 2000). Since the introduction of neuroleptic medications in the middle of the 20th century, and with the increasing emphasis on professional qualifications, attendants became nurses, endowing this branch of the nursing profession with an enduring tradition of male practitioners.

The United States

Dorothea Lynde Dix (1802–1887) is credited with responsibility for mental healthcare reform in the United States. Dix was not a nurse, but a teacher who ran a Sunday school class for the inmates of the local asylum, who were kept in uncomfortable and unsanitary conditions. From the mid-1840s, Dix successfully lobbied in the United States and Canada for better mental healthcare and state-run hospitals. During the American Civil War (1861–1865), Dix was appointed Superintendent of Women Nurses. The United States was among the first to recognise that confining the mentally ill to protect society from their derangement was not necessarily of benefit to the patient. The first training for psychiatric nurses in the United States was organised at McLean Asylum in 1882.

The UK

In the UK, Florence Nightingale is usually credited with being the trailblazer for modern nursing, although Elizabeth Fry (1780–1845) opened the first institute for the training of Protestant nurses in London. Accounts of the originality of Nightingale's work also tend to ignore the fact that she initially spent time in the Lutheran deaconess facility at Kaiserwerth, Germany, which was itself a product of the centuries-old European tradition of religious nursing.

In 1854, Florence Nightingale collected and trained a force of nurses to tend the English troops who were involved in the Crimean War, in Turkey. English troops in Scutari died more frequently from diseases due to unsanitary conditions than from battle wounds. The Nightingale School for Nurses was established in 1860 at the historic St Thomas' Hospital in London (founded in 1215 AD) but she had already published *Notes on Nursing* in 1859, which addressed much that is also relevant to the nursing of the mentally ill. Nightingale wrote 147 works in all, and she included philosophy, sanitation, administration, health and hospitals, emigration, discipline and women's rights among her range of subjects. The nurse who writes eloquently can have an enormous influence on the profession and on others.

After the passing of the Lunacy Act of 1845, the numbers of public asylums and nursing staff or attendants who worked in them multiplied. These numbers were inflated after 1913 by the implementation of the Mental Deficiency Act, which led to the admission of women to mental institutions, sometimes on the basis of poverty, sexual lapses or unemployability (Walmsley 2000). In the asylums, both staff and patients were segregated on the basis of gender: males worked in the grounds or workshops under male attendants who were ex-army, prison warders or farmers; female patients performed domestic work indoors under female attendants or nurses (Chatterton 2000). This state of affairs continued until the shortage of suitable males during World War I led to the employment of more females, even in male wards, a trend that continued thereafter despite lower wages for women, until in 1922 at the first state registration examination more female nurses passed (n = 113) than males (n = 48) (Chatterton 2000).

DEINSTITUTIONALISATION

Aspects of deinstitutionalisation are addressed in many other chapters, so what follows is a brief summary of the issues and cross-references to relevant chapters. Addressing the process of deinstitutionalisation changes the focus from the professional development of nursing and nurses, back to patients and their care. Burnard (2007) recommends that nurses undertake more historical research, and he notes that seminal work is often, of necessity, old. This section will often cite sources that are older than the 5 years recommended for modern nursing research, but historical research always uses original sources in preference to secondary sources, which discuss what original authors have written.

Asylums were created to care for increasing numbers of chronically ill and displaced people at a time when independent religious orders struggled to cope with the numbers, and the Industrial Revolution shattered traditional family structures, employing men, women and children in crowded urban settings. This meant that in poor families who could not afford private care, family members who might have in the past cared for their chronically mentally ill relatives were no longer available. The only alternative was institutional care for people who might be deluded, violent, depressed or in other ways unable to care for themselves. But in the 20th century, a number of advances and innovations altered mental healthcare quite dramatically.

- Late in the 19th century, Freud and other psychotherapists had made the connection between a person's unconscious mind and its influence on the body, and the principles of psychotherapy became publicly known and popularised. This meant that not only were middle-class people able to afford private psychiatric treatment to access 'the talking cure', an alternative to the asylum, they were also freed from stigma. Having psychological problems was 'respectabilised', and even a little bit avant-garde and fashionable. More information about this movement can be found in Chapter 6.
- In 1938, Italian psychiatrists developed a physical treatment that they called electroconvulsive therapy (ECT). Initially, ECT was used unsuitably for most mental disorders, but it was refined to become useful in treating a number of previously unresponsive psychiatric symptoms (see Chapter 24).
- Penicillin was introduced in the 1940s, and an equally great advance in the treatment of mental illness was made in the 1950s with the discovery of new tranquillising and antipsychotic medications such as chlorpromazine ('the liquid cosh': Porter 2002, p. 205) and Imipramine for depression. Valium was the most-prescribed drug of the 1960s (Porter 2002). For the first time many troublesome, distressing and disruptive psychiatric symptoms could be controlled simply using medications, and without the use of restraint or utter seclusion from society (see Chapter 25).
- The different 'movements' that blossomed in the 1960s and 1970s sought universal liberation and confronted inequalities and differences in gender, race and sexuality. Social reformers turned their attention to reexamination of asylums or mental hospitals, which were perceived as repressing the human spirit and human potential, and in which doctors were seen as using psychiatry to control people who deviated from societal norms.

The Anti-Psychiatry Movement

In the 1960s, the movement commenced towards deinstitutionalisation. One of the factors accelerating the process was the 'anti-psychiatry movement' which advocated deinstitutionalisation (Porter 2002), claiming that institutional care was punitive and that it inevitably created dependency and disability or 'institutionalisation'. The leaders of the movement were, paradoxically, psychiatrists themselves, who had found it difficult to reconcile the milieu in which they worked with their liberated personal philosophies. The psychiatrist and writer RD Laing (1967) embraced existentialism and saw mental illness as potentially liberating. While rejecting the 'anti-psychiatry' label, he also rejected the policing and normalising role of the psychiatrist, instead establishing Kingsley Hall, a therapeutic community where residents and staff lived and worked as equals.

Szasz (1972) was an outspoken advocate of 'anti-psychiatry', being totally opposed to traditional psychiatric diagnosis. He did not deny that some people have difficult and disruptive behaviours, but he claimed that they were merely 'problems of living', and that it was ignorance of their cause that led to a diagnosis of 'mental illness', which does not exist.

Rosenhan (1973) published his celebrated research, *On Being Sane in Insane Places*, which encapsulated the anti-psychiatry movement's concerns about the frailties of a psychiatric system that had the power to drastically limit a person's freedom, should they be hospitalised. Rosenhan's work is still significant after four decades because, secretly, mental health practitioners might suspect that the events he documents could still occur in psychiatric facilities today. A number of 'pseudopatients' presented to psychiatric facilities complaining that they heard a voice saying 'empty', 'hollow' and 'thud'.

Without demonstrating any further symptoms, and giving perfectly honest histories undemonstrative of any kind of psychopathology, all but one of these people (psychologists, a psychiatrist, a paediatrician, a 'housewife') were admitted into psychiatric hospitals diagnosed as 'schizophrenic' and detained there for between 7 and 52 days. During their admissions, they were observed and reported upon, but despite acting normally and reporting no more symptoms, when they were eventually discharged they were considered to be 'in remission', not recovered. There are some valid points to be made here.

- Once having been labelled 'schizophrenic', there was nothing the pseudopatient could do to overcome the label: 'Once a person is designated abnormal, all of his other behaviors and characteristics are colored by that label' (Rosenhan, 1973, p. 23).
- Diagnostic manuals and criteria were developed to combat the very scenario that Rosenhan describes. Had the DSM-5 diagnostic criteria for schizophrenia been followed in this case, merely reporting a voice saying 'empty', 'hollow' and 'thud' would be totally insufficient to merit a diagnosis of schizophrenia (see Chapter 15). The first time that explicit diagnostic criteria were included in the DSM was in DSM III, published in 1980.

The rigid segregation of the sane from the insane, which the asylum had implemented, no longer made sense (Porter 2002). Deinstitutionalisation brought about a major reorientation of mental health services. People who would normally have been treated as inpatients in an institution were discharged, either to return to their family, or transferred to some form of community or, in the worst case scenario, to become homeless.

The Aftermath of Deinstitutionalisation

The deinstitutionalisation process continues, but meanwhile some after-effects have become plain. Deinstitutionalisation sounded good in theory and for many it was indeed liberating. Deinstitutionalisation was driven by humanitarian principles, but it was also expensive to staff and maintain large psychiatric hospitals, and there were realistic cost-savings to be made by delegating inpatient care to the community or the family. Politicians such as Margaret Thatcher and Ronald Reagan, who were hostile to 'welfarism', lent their support to 'community care' because they begrudged the cost of public hospital beds (Porter 2002). In contrast to the situation that engendered the deinstitutionalisation movement, wherein chronically mentally ill people were confined indefinitely to the asylum with little potential for discharge, nowadays the problem is that hospital stays are becoming shorter and shorter, and this is no longer driven by humanitarian principles concerned about unnecessary confinement.

A study examining factors that influence the length of psychiatric hospitalisation in the United States stated that:

> *... we confirmed with repeated observations that current efforts to limit access to inpatient hospitalization and management of duration of psychiatric hospitalization are driven heavily by economic factors. Remarkably, there is little research to test the clinical value and later consequences of brief, managed psychiatric inpatient care*
>
> **Masters et al. 2014:686.**

Case management was developed to assess, monitor and plan patient care, and to link the person to community services (see Chapter 5 for details), but despite the system's best efforts, the burden on families and carers has burgeoned, homelessness has risen (Foster et al. 2012), drug use has increased (Simning et al. 2012) and the life expectancy of people with mental illness in the community is significantly below that of their 'normal' peers (Viron & Stern 2010) (see Chapter 8). Foster et al. (2012) report that homelessness is an increasing problem worldwide and that among the homeless, untreated mental illness is a significant problem. For example, in Melbourne Australia alone, 50% of homeless men can be diagnosed with a mental illness (Foster et al. 2012).

Green and Griffiths (2014) found that secondary community services in the UK cannot meet the needs of significant numbers of mentally ill patients, and that the situation is becoming steadily worse. Although mental health hospital admissions continue to decline, it is the result of declining numbers of mental health beds (39% fewer beds in 2012 than in 1998), not a decline in numbers of patients requiring beds. Simning et al. (2012) found that community perceptions that mental illness, crime and drug use are related are true: communities are not absorbing deinstitutionalised patients, they are being overwhelmed by the untreated problems from which they suffer.

It is timely to consider the meaning of 'asylum', which is defined as 'sanctuary; protection . . . an institution offering shelter and support to distressed or destitute individuals esp. the mentally ill' (Pearsall & Trumble 2003, p. 83). For many former inpatients, deinstitutionalisation meant leaving a protected environment where they were fed, housed and nursed, for the free-for-all of normal life; and for some the transition was (and still is) harrowing. If deinstitutionalisation is to succeed, the discharged patient needs to be sensitively supervised, cared for and managed and the system meticulously administered. Deinstitutionalisation requires more than discharging the patient and closing the hospital: ongoing care still has to be organised and delivered for the course of that person's lifetime.

CONCLUSION

This chapter has provided an overview of the ways in which mental disorders have been experienced, treated and regarded in past eras. The disorders that have survived in the same form over two and a half millennia have been examined, as have those that appear to be of more recent origin. The interpersonal skills that were used to treat mental illness have proved to be at times as refined and humane as any we would use today, but there have also been regressive episodes featuring incarceration of, and brutality towards, the mentally ill.

The transition from family-based care to institutional care has been outlined, and the emergence and reemergence of mental health professionals has been described. The earliest documented role models for nursing are found in the Graeco-Roman era. These women were as professional and competent as the women and men who practise today. Ancient Greek nurses displayed a measure of independence in their practice that has not been equalled until the present era.

One of the important changes that the professionalisation of nursing wrought was that nursing became a commercial undertaking, a respectable source of employment and independence, for women as well as men, and an organised profession that displaced the traditional role of family members as carers for the ill. The mentally ill had been considered the responsibility of the asylum or state-run institutions for somewhat longer than the physically ill, but their treatment tended to be more humane and better regulated from the end of the 19th century to the beginning of the modern era.

This chapter's historical account in previous editions stopped short of documenting the changes that have occurred since the early 20th century because these have been so great and so many that they would require another chapter to describe them fully. However, deinstitutionalisation has been described briefly in this chapter as a corollary to the rise of asylums, and one of the great historical landmarks that ushered mental healthcare and psychiatric and mental health nursing into the modern age. The diverse consequences of deinstitutionalisation, some of them ongoing and as yet unresolved, show that we clearly have a long way to go before we achieve the ideal of humane, safe mental healthcare for all. In some countries the mental healthcare process is in its infancy (Terakye & Oflaz 2007). Nearly half of the people who were surveyed after having been treated in public-sector psychiatric settings in the United States reported that they had no communication from staff when they were distressed and that they would not want to return to a psychiatric facility (Grubaugh et al. 2007).

Mental health/psychiatric nursing has blossomed into a skilled profession. The challenges that concern a psychiatric mental health nurse, transformed in less than a century from ignorant attendant to university graduate, can be traced in Chapter 4, which deals with professional nursing issues. But let us end this chapter with Burnard's plea that all nurses and nurse education should embrace the 'true spirit of trying to understand the unfolding nature of ideas, theories and research', a process that has taken centuries and not just the past few years (Burnard 2007, p. 666).

EXERCISES FOR CLASS ENGAGEMENT

Discuss the following questions with your group or class members.

1. What traditional remedies for illness or stress have you seen or heard used in your own family? Are they effective?
2. Was there any alternative to the evolution of the asylum for the care of the mentally ill, given the numbers of sufferers?
3. In what sense is the term 'hysteric' or 'hysterical' used today? Would you still find that there is a relationship with 'disorders of the womb', or perhaps the possession of a womb?
4. Which aspects of mental healthcare in the past would you like to see incorporated into present mental health nursing practice? How would you go about doing this?

REFERENCES

Alexander, F.G., Selesnick, S.T., 1966. The History of Psychiatry: An Evaluation of Psychiatric Thought and Practice From Prehistoric Times to the Present. Harper & Row, New York.

American Psychiatric Association (APA), 2013. Diagnostic and Statistical Manual of Mental Disorders (DSM-5), fifth ed. American Psychiatric Association, Washington DC.

Aristophanes, 1964. The Wasps, the Poet and the Women, the Frogs,. tr. Barrett D. Penguin, Harmondsworth.

Ash, D., Benson, A., Farhall, J., et al., 2001. Mental health services in Australia. In: Meadows, G., Singh, B. (Eds.), Mental Health in Australia. Oxford University Press, Melbourne, pp. 51–66.

Blackburn, I., Davidson, K., 1990. Cognitive Therapy for Depression and Anxiety. Blackwell Scientific, New York.

Blakemore, C., 1988. The Mind Machine. BBC Books, London.

Burnard, P., Gill, P., 2007. The heresy of the 'recent' reference. Nurse Education Today 27, 665–666.

Callaghan, P., 2004. Exercise: a neglected intervention in mental health care? Journal of Psychiatric and Mental Health Nursing 11, 476–483.

Celsus, De Medicina Vol. I 1935–1938, rev. 1940 & 1948, tr. Spencer WG. Loeb Classical Library, William Heinemann, London.

Celsus, De Medicina Vol. III 1935–1938, tr. Spencer WG. Loeb Classical Library, William Heinemann, London.

Chatterton, C., 2000. Women in mental health nursing: angels or custodians? International History of Nursing Journal 5 (2), 11–19.

Cicero Letters to Atticus, 1978. tr. Shackleton Bailey DR. Penguin, Harmondsworth.

Corrigan, P., 2004. How stigma interferes with mental health care. American Psychologist 59 (7), 614–625.

De Leo, D., 2002. Struggling against suicide. Crisis 23 (1), 23–31.

Devereux, G., 1970. The psychotherapy scene in Euripides' 'Bacchae'. Journal of Hellenic Studies XC, 35–48.

Dodds, E.R., 1951. The Greeks and the Irrational. University of California Press, Berkeley.

Doona, M.E., 1992. Judgment: the nurse's key to knowledge. Journal of Professional Nursing 8 (4), 231–238.

Ellard, J., 1987. Did schizophrenia exist before the eighteenth century? Australian and New Zealand Journal of Psychiatry 21 (3), 306–314.

Evans, K., 2000. Representations of Mental Illness in the Classical Texts. Unpublished doctoral dissertation. University of Queensland, Brisbane.

Evans, K., 2007. 'Interrupted by fits of weeping': Cicero's major depressive disorder and the death of Tullia. History of Psychiatry 18 (1), 81–102.

Evans, K., McGrath, J., Milns, R., 2003. Searching for schizophrenia in ancient Greek and Roman literature: a systematic review. Acta Psychiatrica Scandinavica 107 (5), 323–330.

Foster, A., Gable, J., Buckley, J., 2012. Homelessness in schizophrenia. Psychiatric Clinics of North America 35, 717–734.

Foucault, M., 1967. (repr. 1999) Madness and Civilisation: A History of Insanity in the Age of Reason, tr. Howard R. Routledge, London.

Gilman, S., King, H., Porter, R., et al., 1993. Hysteria Beyond Freud. University of California Press, Berkeley.

Grandbois, D., 2005. Stigma of mental illness among American Indian and Alaska Native nations. Issues in Mental Health Nursing 26 (10), 1001–1024.

Green, B.H., Griffiths, E.C., 2014. Hospital admission and community treatment of mental disorders in England from 1998 to 2012. General Hospital Psychiatry 36, 442–448.

Grmek M 1991 Diseases in the Ancient Greek World, tr. Muellner M, Muellner L. Johns Hopkins University Press, Baltimore

Grubaugh, A.L., Frueh, B.C., Zinzow, H.M., et al., 2007. Patients' perceptions of care and safety within psychiatric settings. Psychological Services 4 (3), 193–201.

Hamblet, C., 2000. Obstacles to defining the role of the mental health nurse. Nursing Standard 14 (51), 34–37.
Hawkins, D.R., 1982. Specificity revisited: personality profiles and behavioral issues. Psychotherapy and Psychosomatics 38 (1), 54–63.
Herodotus The Histories vol. II: books III & IV 1921, tr. Godley AD. William Heinemann, London
Hershkowitz, D., 1998. The Madness of Epic: Reading Insanity from Homer to Statius. Clarendon Press, Oxford.
Hippocrates The Hippocratic Corpus, Vol. II 1923, tr. Jones WHS. Loeb Classical Library, William Heinemann, London
Hippocrates The Hippocratic Corpus, Vol. IV 1931, tr. Jones WHS. Loeb Classical Library, William Heinemann, London
Hippocrates The Hippocratic Corpus, Vol. VII 1923, tr. Smith WD. Loeb Classical Library, Harvard University Press, Cambridge, MA
Holme, A., 2015. Why History Matters to Nursing. Nurse Education Today 35 (5), 635–637.
Hornblower, S., Spawforth, A. (Eds.), 1996. The Oxford Classical Dictionary, third ed. Oxford University Press, New York.
Jeste, D.V., del Carmen, R., Lohr, J.B., et al., 1985. Did schizophrenia exist before the eighteenth century? Comprehensive Psychiatry 26 (6), 493–503.
Jones, W.H.S., 1923. Ancient nursing. In: Hippocrates, vol. 2, Introductory Essay IV. William Heinemann, London.
Kaufman, J.C., Sexton, J.D., 2006. Why doesn't the writing cure help poets? Review of General Psychology 10 (3), 268–282.
King, H., 1993. Once upon a text. In: Gilman, S., King, H., Porter, R., et al. (Eds.), Hysteria Beyond Freud. University of California Press, Berkeley.
Laing, R.D., 1967. The Politics of Experience and the Bird of Paradise. Penguin Books, Harmondsworth.
Latham, A.E., Prigerson, H.G., 2004. Suicidality and bereavement: complicated grief as psychiatric disorder presenting greatest risk for suicidality. Suicide and Life-Threatening Behavior 34 (4), 350–362.
Leishman, J.L., 2005. Back to the future: making a case for including the history of mental health nursing in nurse education programmes. International Journal of Psychiatric Nursing Research 10 (3), 1157–1164.
Lester, D., 1990. Galen's four temperaments and four-factor theories of personality: a comment on 'toward a four-factor theory of temperament and/or personality'. Journal of Personality Assessment 54 (1–2), 423–426.
Macalpine, I., Hunter, R., 1969. George III and the Mad-Business. Penguin, London.
Mack, A.H., Forman, L., Brown, R., et al., 1994. A brief history of psychiatric classification: from the ancients to DSM-IV. Psychiatric Clinics of North America 17 (3), 515–523.
Marcus Aurelius Meditations 1981, tr. Staniforth M. Penguin, Harmondsworth
Martial The epigrams 1972, tr. Michie J. Penguin, Harmondsworth
Masters, G.A., Baldessarini, R.J., Öngur, D., Centorrino, F., 2014. Factors associated with length of psychiatric hospitalization. Comprehensive Psychiatry 55, 681–687.
Mellersh, H.E.L., 1976. (rev. 1999) The Hutchinson Chronology of World History: The Ancient and Medieval World. Helicon, Oxford.
Merenda, P.F., 1987. Toward a four-factor theory of temperament and/or personality. J. Pers. Assess. 513 (3), 367–374.
Ng, Beng-Yeong, 1999. Qigong-induced mental disorders. Australian and New Zealand Journal of Psychiatry 33, 197–206.
Nightingale, F., 1859. (repr. 1969) Notes on Nursing: What it is and What it is not. Dover, New York.
Parker, R., 1983. Miasma: Pollution and Purification in Early Greek Religion. Clarendon, Oxford.
Pearsall, J., Trumble, B., 2003. Oxford English Reference Dictionary, Second ed. Rev. Oxford University Press, Oxford.
Plautus The Pot of Gold and Other Plays 1965, tr. Watling EF. Penguin Classics, Harmondsworth.
Plutarch Lives, Vol. II, Themistocles and Camillus, Aristides and Cato Major, Cimon and Lucullus 1914, tr. Perrin B. William Heinemann, London.
Polimeni, J., Reiss, J.P., 2003. Evolutionary perspectives on schizophrenia. Canadian Journal of Psychiatry 48 (1), 34–39.
Porter, R., 2002. Madness: a Brief History. Oxford University Press, Oxford.
Range, L.M., Kovac, S.H., Marion, M.S., 2000. Does writing about bereavement lessen grief following sudden, unintentional death? Death Studies 24 (2), 115–134.
Rich, K.L., Butts, J.B., 2004. Rational suicide: uncertain moral ground. Journal of Advanced Nursing 46 (3), 270–283.
Richards A (ed) 1991 Breuer J & Freud S, Studies on Hysteria, tr. Strachey J, Strachey A. Penguin, Harmondsworth.
Rosen, G., 1968. Madness in Society: Chapters in the Historical Sociology of Mental Illness. University of Chicago Press, Chicago.
Rosenhan, D.L., 1973. On being sane in insane places. Science, 179 250-258. In: Lilienfeld SO 1995 Seeing Both Sides: Classic Controversies in Abnormal Psychology. Brooks/Cole Publishing Company, Pacific Grove, CA.
Sadock, B.J., Sadock, V.A., 2007. Kaplan & Sadock's Synopsis of Psychiatry, tenth ed. Lippincott Williams & Wilkins, Philadelphia.
Sanderson, S., Vandenberg, B., Paese, P., 1999. Authentic religious experience or insanity? Journal of Clinical Psychology 55 (5), 607–616.
Sands, N.M., 2009. Round the bend: a brief history of mental health nursing in Victoria, Australia 1848 to 1950s. Issues in Mental Health Nursing 30 (6), 364–371.
Schieffelin, E.L., 1996. Evil spirit sickness, the Christian disease: the innovation of a new syndrome of mental derangement and redemption in Papua New Guinea. Culture, Medicine and Psychiatry 20 (1), 1–39.
Scull, A., 2015. From Madness in Civilization: A Cultural History of Insanity From the Bible to Freud, from the Madhouse to Modern Medicine. Princeton University Press & Thames & Hudson, London.
Simning, A., van Wijngaarden, E., Conwell, Y., 2012. The association of African Americans' perceptions of neighbourhood crime and drugs with mental illness. Social Psychiatry and Psychiatric Epidemiology 47 (7), 1159–1167.
Simon, B., 1978. Mind and Madness in Ancient Greece: the Classical Roots of Modern Psychiatry. Cornell University Press, London.
Soranus The Gynecology 1956, tr. Temkin O. Johns Hopkins University Press, Baltimore.
Stone, M.H., 1997. Healing the Mind. A History of Psychiatry From Antiquity to the Present. WW Norton, New York.
Suer, L., 1995. The survival of ancient medicine in modern French psychiatry. History of Psychiatry 6 (24/4), 493–501.
Summers, A., 1997. Sairey Gamp: generating fact from fiction. Nursing Enquiry 4 (1), 14–18.
Szasz, T.S., 1972. The Myth of Mental Illness. Granada Publishing, St Albans.
Tasca, C., Rapetti, M., Carta, M.G., Fadda, B., 2012. Women and hysteria in the history of mental health. Clinical Practice & Epidemiology in Mental Health 8, 110–119.
Terakye, G., Oflaz, F., 2007. A historical overview of psychiatric mental health nursing in Turkey. International Journal of Mental Health 36 (3), 73–83.
Terence The Comedies 1976, tr. Radice B. Penguin, Harmondsworth.
Thucydides History of the Pelopponesian War 1954, tr. Warner R. Penguin, Harmondsworth.
Torrey, E.F., 1980. Schizophrenia and Civilization. Jason Aronsen, New York.
Torrey, E.F., Miller, J., 2002. The Invisible Plague: the rise of Mental Illness From 1750 to the Present. Rutgers University Press, New Brunswick.

Torrey, E.F., Yolken, R.H., 1995. Could schizophrenia be a viral zoonosis transmitted from house cats? Schizophrenia Bulletin 21 (2), 167–171.

Torrey, E.F., Yolken, R.H., 1998. Is household crowding a risk factor for schizophrenia? Schizophrenia Research 29 (1/2), 12–13.

Torrey, E.F., Bowler, A.E., Clark, K., 1997. Urban birth and residence as risk factors for psychoses: an analysis of 1880 data. Schizophrenia Research 25 (3), 169–176.

Viron, M., Stern, T.A., 2010. The impact of serious mental illness on health and healthcare. Psychosomatics 51, 458–465.

Walmsley, J., 2000. Women and the Mental Deficiency Act of 1913: citizenship, sexuality and regulation. British Journal of Learning Disabilities 28, 65–70.

Warelow, P., Edward, K., 2007. Evidence-based mental health nursing in Australia: our history and future. International Journal of Mental Health Nursing 16 (1), 57–61.

Woolf, A., 2000. Witchcraft or mycotoxin? The Salem witch trials. Journal of Toxicology: Clinical Toxicology 38 (4), 457.

Yolken, R.H., Yee, F., Johnston, N., et al., 1997. Molecular analyses of brains from individuals with schizophrenia—evidence of viral infections. Schizophrenia Research 24 (1/2), 61.

USEFUL WEBSITES

This chapter is one of the best sources for the ancient history of nursing and mental illness, but there exist online timelines which provide a succinct historical overview for the history of nursing, although they are very vague for any date before the 17th century.

- Timeline of the history of nursing, https://en.wikipedia.org/wiki/Timeline_of_nursing_history

You could also conduct your own research into people and topics in ancient history. Many universities have access to ancient texts in translation; check your own library catalogue.

The Penelope site at The University of Chicago is valuable for many ancient Roman texts in translation; you could read more of Cicero's writings, completed despite recurrent depression, http://penelope.uchicago.edu/Thayer/E/Roman/home.html

The Black Dog Institute is devoted to assisting people to cope with mood disorders and is named after the British Prime Minister Winston Churchill's 'Black Dog' (which is how he described his recurrent depression), www.blackdoginstitute.org.au

See the medical writer Celsus's work De Medicina online, http://penelope.uchicago.edu/Thayer/E/Roman/Texts/Celsus/home.html

The Perseus Digital Library at Tufts University allows you to search for ancient texts in translation, www.perseus.tufts.edu

Florence Nightingale wrote prolifically on philosophy, sanitation, administration, health and hospitals, emigration, discipline and women's rights, which can be found at The Collected Works of Florence Nightingale, www.uoguelph.ca/cwfn

The Florence Nightingale Museum site is a rich source of material at www.florence-nightingale.co.uk

Internet Mental Health site is a free public site that features research and interesting discussion articles about disorders, diagnosis, medications and historical questions, www.mentalhealth.com/home

Neuroskeptic has discussions such as the stigma surrounding mental illness, http://blogs.discovermagazine.com/neuroskeptic/

Mind - For Better Mental Health. A UK Mental Health Charity www.mind.org.uk

4

Professional, Legal and Ethical Issues

Phillip Maude, Anthony O'Brien

KEY POINTS

- All nurses are required to have active registration with the regulatory body, they are called registered nurses (RNs).
- Professional and industrial bodies represent the interests of individual nurses and of the profession.
- Nurses are educationally prepared for practice in specialist nursing programmes.
- Accountability in nursing is achieved through adherence to professional standards of practice, codes of ethics and competency standards.
- Authority to continue to practise is determined by revalidation.
- Mental health nurses have developed advanced and extended roles, including nurse practitioner roles and prescribing authority.
- As the largest single group within the mental health workforce, mental health nurses provide essential services for people living with a mental illness and promote the development of services to support the mental health of communities.
- The claim to professional status requires nurses to practise within a code of ethics.
- Mental healthcare involves reflection on ethical issues and the use of principles of ethical reasoning.
- Codes of ethics guide members of the professions as to the nature of proper conduct and their obligations to the public.
- Mental health nurses are confronted with ethical issues on a daily basis.
- Nurses need to consider the ethical issues arising from their choice of intervention and from the treatments prescribed in psychiatry.
- A sound knowledge of legal issues is critical to contemporary mental health nursing.
- Mental health legislation contributes to community perceptions of people with a mental health problem.
- Mental health legislation is the legal framework that informs the involuntary treatment of individuals, defines their rights and ensures appropriate treatment.

KEY TERMS

advanced practice
autonomy
beneficence
code of ethics
community treatment orders
competencies
confidentiality
consent
duty of care
ethics
human rights
involuntary treatment
justice
least restrictive alternative
mental health legislation
negligence
nonmaleficence
nurse practitioner
nurse prescriber
profession
professional boundaries
regulation
standards of practice

LEARNING OUTCOMES

The material in this chapter will assist you to:

- outline the roles of professional and industrial organisations in mental health nursing.
- discuss the roles of advanced practitioner and nurse practitioner in mental health nursing.
- identify common ethical issues in mental health nursing.
- apply ethical principles to the analysis of ethical issues in mental health nursing.
- understand the importance of mental health legislation in mental healthcare.

INTRODUCTION

Mental health nursing is a regulated profession that occurs within a legal context and within a framework of professional standards, and ethical principles and values. This chapter outlines the professional, legal and ethical context of mental health nursing and provides guidance to assist nurses in maintaining professional practice that meets professional, legal and ethical standards. Mental health nurses are legally mandated to practise nursing in accordance with professional competencies and social expectations. As professionals, mental health nurses must be aware of local legislation and regulations that govern professional practice, including laws that are specific to the mental health context. Ethical principles and theory assist nurses to make decisions on issues of conflict and to maintain clear and safe boundaries around their practice. In addition to the ethical issues inherent in every practice setting, the mental health context presents unique issues of coercion and treatment without consent.

Since the 1990s, services have seen the development of new models of mental healthcare and mental health services. Education for clinical practice involves degree-level study, with further postgraduate study options becoming increasingly available once a nurse is registered. Mental health nursing has responded to changes in education and service delivery by developing career pathways, standards of practice, practice competencies and models of advanced practice. The scope of practice has been extended to include the nurse practitioner role and the nurse prescribing role. The profession has also developed responses to the complex ethical issues that the changing mental health context demands. The mental health context presents unique challenges to nurses because the use of compulsory treatment under mental health legislation involves significant departures from normally accepted human and healthcare rights. Mental health legislation provides a legal framework for treatment without consent and specific guidelines for procedures such as electroconvulsive treatment and seclusion. The United Nations Convention on the Rights of Persons with Disabilities is an international instrument aimed at protecting the rights of people with mental illness. This chapter explores the professional context of practice, including the roles of professional and industrial nursing organisations, mechanisms of professional regulation and the development of advanced practice and nurse practitioner roles. The chapter outlines the principles of ethical conduct and discusses some ethical issues commonly encountered in mental health nursing. It also outlines use of mental health legislation and the rights issues raised by compulsory treatment.

REGULATION OF PROFESSIONAL PRACTICE

As a professional discipline, mental health nursing is subject to regulation by the Nursing and Midwifery Council (NMC) who regulate all nurses and midwives in England, Wales, Scotland and Northern Ireland (NMC 2018a). All nurses require active registration with the NMC to be legally allowed to practice. The primary role of the NMC is to protect the public by ensuring that only nurses who meet the specific requirements are allowed to practice as a nurse, taking action if concerns are raised that a nurse is unfit to practice (NMC 2017). In addition, the NMC also sets standards and develops policies that guide nurses in their professional practice. This also applies to nurse training programmes, the NMC has a role in ensuring that nurses are consistently educated to high standards, ensuring that they are able to deliver safe and effective care at the point of entry to the register and throughout their careers. A programme of change for education is being delivered between 2016 and 2020 to modernise education standards (NMC 2018b).

Regulatory authorities set and monitor standards in the interests of the public and the professions and maintain registers of individuals licensed to practise nursing. In addition they provide disciplinary and complaints processes and produce publications on key areas of policy. Since April 2016, the NMC requires all nurses to undertake revalidation, a process that requires all nurses to demonstrate that they are practicing safely and effectively. The process aims to encourage nurses to reflect on their Code of Practice and demonstrate how they are 'living' the standards set out within it. The process requires a portfolio to be produced evidencing the following; 450 practice hours, 35 hours of CPD including 20 hours of participatory learning, five pieces of practice-related feedback, five written reflective accounts, a reflective discussion, health and character statement, proof of professional indemnity arrangements and a conformation statement from the person conducting the process—a mentor or manager, etc. Revalidation is required every 3 years and replaces the previous Prep requirements (NMC 2018c). Many nursing staff were educated outside of the UK

BOX 4.1 Nursing Regulatory Body

Nursing and Midwifery Council
England
Nursing and Midwifery Council
23 Portland Place
London
W1B 1PZ
Telephone: 020 7333 9333

Nursing and Midwifery Council
61 Aldwych
London
WC2B 4AE
Telephone: 020 7462 5800 / 5801

Nursing and Midwifery Council
6th Floor
2 Stratford Place
Montfichet Road
London
E20 1EJ
Telephone: 020 7462 5800/5801

1st Floor
1 Kemble Street
London
WC2B 4AN
Telephone: 0207 462 5800

SCOTLAND
Ground Floor
114–116 George Street
Edinburgh
EH2 4LH
Telephone: 0131 624 5000

WALES
Temple Court
13a Cathedral Road
Cardiff
CF11 9HA
(Postal only)

Available at: https://www.nmc.org.uk/contact-us/how-to-find-us

and can apply to the NMC for recognition and registration of their training. See Box 4.1 for NMC contact details.

Nurses are professionals who practice with a high degree of autonomy and so are expected, in addition to the regulatory requirements of registration bodies, to maintain their own system of professional monitoring and review.

The regulation of nursing practice is a political and professional issue. Definition of the mental health scope of practice and protection of patients by employing only practitioners prepared within that scope are issues that require an assertive approach on the part of professional nursing bodies. What is at stake is the specialist nature of mental healthcare, recognition of the skills of mental health nurses and acceptance that mental health patients have needs that cannot adequately be met without specialty preparation.

PROFESSIONAL AND INDUSTRIAL NURSING BODIES

Mental health nurses practise in a complex professional environment that requires a strong sense of professional identity and clear frameworks for practice. While broad frameworks for professional practice are provided by legislation and by nursing regulatory bodies, a wide range of professional issues is addressed through professional nursing bodies and unions. In addition, the profession has a role in monitoring the social context of practice through involvement in the development of legislation, policy and local services. A related issue is the maintenance and improvement of nurses' employment conditions. Much of this work is carried out by nurses within the various professional and industrial nursing bodies and unions.

Professional and industrial nursing bodies can be divided into those whose primary focus is professional issues, such as the Royal College of Nursing, and unions whose primary focus is providing workplace representation and bargaining over salary and conditions of employment. However, this distinction disguises the overlap between these bodies, as conditions of employment have a direct effect on nurses' ability to meet professional standards, and the realisation of the expectations of professional bodies can affect conditions of employment. Issues such as the number of beds provided by a mental health service and the number of staff allocated to different sections of the service demonstrate the overlapping functions of professional and industrial organisations. While these may be primarily industrial issues, because of their immediate impact on nurses' conditions of employment, they also have the potential to affect standards of professional practice. Both professional and industrial bodies have an interest in quality of service issues. Membership of a professional body or union is not compulsory. However, you need to reflect carefully on the advantages of membership and your responsibility as a health professional to support the organisations that maintain your conditions of employment and advocate on professional issues. Professional and industrial bodies and unions negotiate with employers and policy makers on employment and professional issues and play an important role in informing members on current issues in healthcare. They may also play an advocacy role in the case of disputes or inquiries and provide legal advice to nurses facing complaints or disciplinary proceedings. Some organisations offer indemnity insurance, which can provide valuable protection against the costs of legal advice. Some of the key professional and industrial bodies are listed in Box 4.2.

BOX 4.2 Professional and Industrial Bodies in Mental Health Nursing

Royal College of Nursing

The Royal College of Nursing (RCN) is the world's largest nursing union and professional body, representing more than 435,000 nurses, student nurses, midwives and health care assistants in the UK and internationally. The RCN is both a professional body, carrying out work on nursing standards, education and practice and a trade union. They represent the professional interests of nursing staff working in the public, private and voluntary sectors. The RCN sits on the NHS Staff Council, which negotiates pay, terms and conditions for NHS staff and is able to negotiate for pay, terms and conditions with independent sector organisations. They are also represented in social partnership arrangements in England, Scotland, Wales and Northern Ireland (RCN 2018b). https://www.rcn.org.uk

Unison: The Public Service Union

UNISON reports to be one of the UK's largest trade unions, serving more than 1.3 million members. They represent full-time and part-time staff who provide public services, although they may be employed in both the public and private sectors. UNISON https://www.unison.org.uk

STANDARDS OF PRACTICE

As with many professions, mental health nursing is governed by standards of practice. In the UK the standards are laid out by the Nursing and Midwifery Council The Code: Professional standards of practice and behaviour for nurses, midwives and nursing associates (The Code). The Code presents the professional standards of practice and behaviour that nurses and midwives must uphold in order to be registered in the UK (NMC 2015). This applies to all nurses, regardless of their branch of practice. The need for accountability in mental healthcare means that the development of standards has assumed increasing significance. The standards cover the broad scope of professional practice and include a rationale for each standard, attributes related to each standard and performance criteria. See Table 4.1 for The Code (NMC 2015). Standards of professional practice represent the commitment of mental health nurses to accountability in the professional practice of nursing and have been recognised as a benchmark in examining the quality of mental health nursing care. Continued monitoring of achievement of standards of practice is essential for any group claiming professional status, as self-regulation is recognised as a defining characteristic of professions.

COMPETENCIES

In order to ensure a framework of safety that will protect the public, professions specify sets of competencies that describe the expected skills of all practitioners within a particular

TABLE 4.1 The Code: Professional Standards of Practice and Behaviour for Nurses and Midwives

Prioritise people	You put the interests of people using or needing nursing or midwifery services first. You make their care and safety your main concern and make sure that their dignity is preserved and their needs are recognised, assessed and responded to. You make sure that those receiving care are treated with respect, that their rights are upheld and that any discriminatory attitudes and behaviours towards those receiving care are challenged.
Practise effectively	You assess need and deliver or advise on treatment, or give help (including preventative or rehabilitative care) without too much delay and to the best of your abilities, on the basis of the best evidence available and best practice. You communicate effectively, keeping clear and accurate records and sharing skills, knowledge and experience where appropriate. You reflect and act on any feedback you receive to improve your practice.
Preserve safety	You make sure that patient and public safety is protected. You work within the limits of your competence, exercising your professional 'duty of candour' and raising concerns immediately whenever you come across situations that put patients or public safety at risk. You take necessary action to deal with any concerns where appropriate.
Promote professionalism and trust	You uphold the reputation of your profession at all times. You should display a personal commitment to the standards of practice and behaviour set out in the Code. You should be a model of integrity and leadership for others to aspire to. This should lead to trust and confidence in the profession from patients, people receiving care, other healthcare professionals and the public.

The Code (NMC 2015) is available at: https://www.nmc.org.uk/globalassets/sitedocuments/nmc-publications/nmc-code.pdf

discipline. In nursing, competencies are set by regulatory bodies and by professional nursing organisations. The RCN provides competencies for registered nurses, as well as for nurse practitioners and nurse prescribers. Nurses must demonstrate continuing competence in order to renew their annual registration and for revalidation every 3 years. Regulatory authorities conduct audits of competence in which nurses are required to produce documentary evidence of continuing competence.

CAREER PATHWAYS

Postgraduate programmes for new practitioners have gained wide acceptance as the beginning of a career pathway, with service-based professional development programmes providing support for further career development. Many services now offer a range of clinical leadership roles such as nurse educator and nurse specialist, in some cases dependent on masters-level educational preparation. Nurses also pursue careers in management, research, education and private practice.

The nurse practitioner role (see later) represents a career pathway for nurses that recognises their clinical expertise and contribution to health outcomes and encourages their retention in the clinical nursing workforce. Thus the nurse practitioner pathway can be said to work on two levels: (1) maximising health gains to patients; and (2) providing a career structure that encourages the retention of the most experienced and skilled practitioners in the clinical nursing workforce.

ADVANCED PRACTICE

Increasingly, nurses are undertaking advanced practice roles that reflect contemporary clinical practice. In some cases, advanced practitioners extend that role to *nurse practitioner*, a title that requires licensing by the NMC. The growth of advanced practice roles is part of a global development in nursing aimed at maximising the nursing contribution to healthcare and improving health outcomes (Drew 2014). The concept of advanced practice recognises that nurses seeking career progression do not always wish to follow careers in management or education, but may wish to retain their clinical focus while incorporating aspects of research, education and service leadership into their roles. Advanced practice roles recognise the contribution that experienced clinicians make to patient outcomes and their importance to the development of the nursing workforce.

NURSE PRACTITIONERS

Nurse practitioners are those advanced practitioners who have extended their education within a defined scope of practice and who are licensed to practise within an extended role. Nurse practitioners work to shift health services from tertiary services with a tradition of treating diagnosed problems from presenting symptoms to services based on the local population's healthcare needs and primary healthcare. Masters preparation and an appropriate level of experience are usually the minimum criteria for accreditation as a nurse practitioner (NMC 2001, Ministry of Health 2014).

Development of the nurse practitioner role has not come without resistance and opposition from those who see this expanded role as encroaching on their professional domain (Elsom et al. 2009). One of the potential sources of conflict as the nurse practitioner role develops is in the area of boundaries between different healthcare providers (Lowe et al. 2013). The nurse practitioner is a collaborative health professional who develops collegial relationships with health colleagues and negotiates decision making with them.

As more nurse practitioners gain accreditation they will face challenges in defining models of practice that may be quite different from the models of clinical service delivery currently used. Suggested models include integrated nursing teams, consultancy, independent practice and provision of specialty services (Ministry of Health 2014). In developing these new models of service delivery, research will need to take account of the design and aims of services and the specific outcomes that have been planned. In addition, development of the nurse practitioner role requires attention to the social, legal and policy context of healthcare.

NURSE PRESCRIBERS

Nurses have long influenced the pattern of medications prescribed to patients by suggesting to doctors specific medications and medication regimens, based on their knowledge of patients' preferences and responses, assessment of patients' clinical presentation and knowledge of the actions, side-effect profile and interactions of psychotropic medications. In many areas, nurse practitioners have formalised this practice in the form of independent prescribing (Earle et al. 2011; Lim et al. 2014). Nurse independent prescribers are nurses who have successfully completed an NMC Independent Nurse Prescribing Course (also known as v200 or v300 courses). They are able to prescribe any medicine provided it is in their competency to do so. This includes medicines and products listed in the British National Formulary, unlicensed medicines and all controlled drugs in schedules two to five (RCN 2018a). As with the nurse practitioner role, the intention of extending prescriptive authority to nurse prescribers is to fully utilise the capacity of nurses to provide healthcare and to make healthcare more accessible to patients.

Like nurse practitioner development, this has not occurred without controversy. Medical practitioners have not always supported extension of prescribing authority to nurses (Elsom et al. 2009). But as more nurses are registered as nurse practitioners, it seems likely that there will be growth in the number of nurses applying for prescriptive authority.

ETHICS AND PROFESSIONAL PRACTICE

Medical sociologist Eliot Freidson (2001) described a profession as a group with clear definition of its roles and processes to ensure the quality of the work and knowledge produced by its members. Freidson's description asserts that an occupation earns the right to call itself a profession partly through the credibility and trust that are built with the people to whom it provides a service. For nursing to assert itself as a profession, ethics and identity are inseparable. This is because the identity of nursing and the self-regulatory processes that ensure continued trust within the community are inextricably interwoven. In other words, nursing and nursing practice are guided by the law, ethical principles and the public image of the nurse as an ethical practitioner. Nurses must practise in accordance with the law and adhere to a code of ethical conduct.

Internationally, professional nursing organisations have identified the need for a code of ethics to guide practice. The first international code of ethics for nurses was developed by the International Council of Nurses in 1953, with the most recent revision published in 2012 (International Council of Nurses 2012). Codes of ethics are guided by established ethical principles. The four most commonly quoted principles—autonomy, beneficence, nonmaleficence and justice—are explained in Box 4.3.

BOX 4.3 Seven Areas That Need to be Considered When Thinking About Clinical Scenarios and Applying Ethical Reasoning

1. *Rights.* Rights form the basis of most professional codes and legal judgements and consider ideas such as self-determination rights, rights and cultural relativism, the right to healthcare and rights to privacy and confidentiality.
2. *Autonomy.* Autonomy involves the right of self-determination, independence and freedom. Autonomy promotes the right of an individual to be able to make their own decisions and implies that the person will also take responsibility for decisions made. Respect for autonomy means that nurses recognise the individual's uniqueness, the right to lead a life as the person wants to, and are able to set personal goals. Nurses who follow the principle of autonomy respect a patient's right to make choices even if they are not always the best options in the opinion of the nurse.
3. *Beneficence and nonmaleficence.* Beneficence means 'doing good'. Nurses should work towards actions that support and benefit patients and their family members. However, in an increasingly technological healthcare system, doing the best by a person can also do harm by potentially putting that person at risk (e.g. intensive therapy programmes). Nonmaleficence means the duty to do no harm. Harm can be caused deliberately, or it may involve actions that put the person at risk of harm, even if this was unintentional. In nursing, intentional harm is always unacceptable. The risk for potential to cause harm is not always clear. For example, harm may be caused by a nursing intervention that is implemented to be helpful (e.g. medication administration).
4. *Justice.* Justice can also be considered as fairness. Nurses frequently face decisions in which a sense of justice should prevail. For example, a person may be detained under a Mental Health Act but justice requires this to be the case only while that person is at risk to themselves or other people and unable to self-assess and manage their own risk.
5. *Fidelity.* Fidelity means to be faithful to agreements and responsibilities one has undertaken. Nurses have responsibilities to patients, employers, government, society, the profession and themselves. Circumstances often affect which responsibilities take precedence at a particular time.
6. *Veracity.* Veracity refers to telling the truth. As a nurse, should I tell the truth when it is known that doing so will cause harm? This requires the nurse to follow through with patients when they have made commitments to spend time with them.
7. *Trust and reciprocity.* We trust that colleagues will act in ways that are mutually supportive and do no harm to each other. The principle of reciprocity is essential for nurses to build trust in working relationships between professionals as well as their patients. Patients also rely on trust and the principle of reciprocity to ensure that health practitioners do their best to do no harm and promote recovery.

ETHICAL FRAMEWORKS

A code of ethics provides a formal statement that reflects the ideals and values of a group. A framework incorporates ethical principles that should be shared by and should guide members of the group in practice and decision making. This framework may also be a statement that reflects the group's development and moral judgements over time. It can be presented as a standard for the group's professional actions. In contrast, an ethical theory offers a framework for reflection on potential or past action and can assist in the evaluation of moral judgements that have been made.

The theory of utilitarianism instructs us that an action is right if it produces the best consequences (or better consequences than other action/s). Actions are right if they maximise happiness/pleasure/utility/preferences and minimise unhappiness/pain/harm. Deontological theory guides the *duty* to perform acts that are *intrinsically* or *inherently good.* We have a duty to refrain from acts that are *intrinsically bad* or *wrong.* Ethical concepts guide us in our everyday work as health professionals. The seven areas shown in Box 4.3 need to be considered when thinking about clinical scenarios and applying ethical reasoning.

Ethical Issues in Mental Health Practice

People experiencing mental illness can be marginalised by their illness and this can cause them to be politically powerless through a lack of ability to plan and speak for themselves. Thus they can be a group that is vulnerable to human rights abuse and stigmatisation. The manifestations of mental illness often include low self-esteem, withdrawal, self-doubt and distortions in thinking. Consequently, people with mental illness may have difficulty in making autonomous decisions at various times in their life and may find it difficult to advocate for themselves. Because of this vulnerability, ethical issues are presented to mental health nurses daily and so there is a requirement for ethical decision making. This section considers some critical areas of mental health nursing practice, taking into consideration the need for ethical decision making

Psychiatric Diagnosis

Psychiatric diagnosis should be the most fundamental aspect of mental healthcare delivery under ethical examination. The effects of diagnosis on an individual may include loss of personal freedom, imposed treatment regimens and the possibility of being labelled for life as mentally ill. Diagnostic labelling and hospitalisation of people with mental illnesses often marginalise them from their community and thus jeopardise their chances of achieving or regaining social integration. Thus psychiatric diagnosis raises ethical issues in terms of autonomy and justice.

Diagnosis is a powerful tool. It has the capacity to label behaviour that is odd or objectionable and has been used to explain behaviour that is unlawful, such as acts of theft or violence. In the latter case, the law recognises that mental illness compromises a person's free will and can classify them as not legally responsible for their actions. Therefore, a diagnosis of mental illness can, in some cases, 'benefit' a person. However, the process of psychiatric diagnosis has been reported as being of poor or questionable reliability (Zachar et al. 2014). In mental health, objective signs of mental distress are not always evident, so diagnosis may be a difficult procedure. Patients may not always have sufficient trust in professionals to tell their story, and some aspects of their history may be too painful to recount in full. Also, people are influenced by processes such as denial and fantasy in describing their lives. Diagnosis plays a powerful role in some people's lives, but it has its limits. People can be left with a lifelong label, and care must be taken not to label culturally determined experiences as signs of mental illness.

A diagnosis of mental illness may label the patient as deviant from the normal population and result in predetermined clinical and social behaviours, in both the person diagnosed and the healthcare professionals caring for them. Illich (2001) first suggested in his classic 1977 text that people are transformed into patients, while individuals are transformed into clinicians by enculturation that attributes to them the power to diagnose and heal. If a patient is described to you as 'Mr Brown, the man who has been hearing voices and is afraid that others are talking about him', you will have certain expectations based on this description. However, if Mr Brown is described as 'the schizophrenic in room 4', how might your initial perceptions differ? In this case the ethical concern is one of nonmaleficence. Patients should not be harmed by the actions of health professionals, including the practice of diagnosis. There are strong messages in the words we use, especially when they become labels.

Some of the questions that need to be considered are: who has the right to decide which types of behaviour are considered to be mental illness rather than moral deviance? How do we classify people who become verbally abusive when drunk, who are addicted to psychoactive substances, are antisocial, have sexual preferences different from our own, hold unusual religious beliefs or gamble excessively? Some of these you may see as mental illness, but other people would disagree with you. We do have systems of classification that differentiate normal from abnormal behaviour—for example, the *Diagnostic and Statistical Manual of Mental Disorders* (DSM) (American Psychiatric Association 2013). But criticism has been aimed at the DSM for creating ever-expanding criteria for mental illness, resulting in more people being labelled with mental illness. Flaskeraud (2010) suggests that the DSM turns general problems or traits of personality into psychiatric disorders that are then treated with pharmaceuticals. The cultural sensitivity of these diagnostic criteria and the disempowerment that the patient feels from the confusing terminology used have also been questioned.

CRITICAL THINKING CHALLENGE 4.1

Consider the current diagnostic label of 'borderline personality disorder' (BPD) and the clinical signs and symptoms of BPD (see Chapter 17). People with BPD often present in states of high arousal with varying degrees of self-harm, and clinicians can find these presentations stressful and difficult. They provide major challenges to the healthcare service, and the label 'BPD' often invokes feelings of helplessness in clinicians, who may respond by attempting to dissuade the person from accessing the health service. If we were to take into account the fact that many people labelled with BPD have been invalidated in their lives, often as a result of sexual or physical abuse, and if this consideration persuaded us to view BPD as posttraumatic stress disorder, would this change our attitudes to working with people who are given this diagnostic label?

Psychiatric Treatment

Mental health patients are often critical of the use of coercive practices (such as overuse of pharmaceuticals, restraint and seclusion and community treatment orders [CTOs]) and can perceive their use by nurses as punishment (Mayers et al. 2010). Worldwide, length of stay in hospital has decreased, while admission rates have increased, resulting in changes to the overall milieu of inpatient units, where acute interventions and containment are the predominant care provided and less attention is paid to rehabilitation and comprehensive discharge planning.

CTOs raise several ethical issues that need to be considered concerning consent, autonomy, coercion, paternalism and beneficence. So too do confidentiality and how the country provides the most appropriate service within a responsive timeframe, as well as overall quality of services. There is concern that CTOs can be noninclusive and coercive by requiring the patient to comply with treatment plans and this raises issues concerning the human rights of a person diagnosed with a mental illness compared with members of the general public. CTOs are very powerful documents that can have an enormous impact on the privacy and autonomy interests of patients (Light et al. 2012b). Further discussion of CTOs is provided later in this chapter.

CRITICAL THINKING CHALLENGE 4.2

Using the four most commonly cited principles of ethical conduct (autonomy, beneficence, nonmaleficence and justice), consider when and if it is appropriate to administer an intramuscular injection of medication against a patient's will.

Psychopharmacology

The drugs prescribed for mental illness are potent agents, often causing major side effects, creating problems with toxicity and, in the case of major tranquillisers such as clozapine, cardiac complications and metabolic disorders (Moncrieff 2013). Psychotropic medications can also interact with other therapeutic agents and so need to be monitored closely. Side effects such as metabolic syndrome and dependence raise ethical issues of nonmaleficence, while administration of medication without consent, as frequently occurs in mental health nursing, compromises the patient's autonomy. People who have been taking psychotropic medication may find it difficult to stop their medication due to discontinuation syndrome (Harvey & Slabbert 2014; Salomon & Hamilton 2014), which carries further ethical implications. As with other psychiatric treatments, nurses may argue that their practice in this area is motivated by beneficence (Maude & Edwards 2011), but issues of nonmaleficence and compromised autonomy also need to be considered.

With respect to drug treatment, a question that needs to be considered is 'what are a person's rights when placed on psychopharmacological agents?' These rights should include access to effective professional treatment and information concerning the drug prescribed (desired effects, side effects, contraindications, complications) and the freedom to accept or refuse treatment. These rights may be limited if the person is an involuntary patient under the mental health legislation. However, all patients should have some voice and choice in the selection of drugs. If the side effects of a particular drug are difficult to live with, the person should be able to ask for a review and change of treatment, including a nonpharmacological alternative. Psychopharmacology is further discussed in Chapter 25.

Electroconvulsive Therapy

Electroconvulsive therapy (ECT) is used mainly for major depression (Daalen-Smith & Gallagher 2011). A significant ethical problem occurs when a psychiatrist prescribes ECT in order to reduce a patient's risk of self-harm or harm through neglect, but the individual does not give consent for the therapy. The thought of having ECT can be traumatic to patients and families due to the negative perceptions about this form of treatment and the potential for memory loss (Smith et al. 2009). All treatments need to be carefully negotiated with patients. For depressed people, their lowered mood and pessimistic outlook may mean that they are unable to see any solution to their depression. Some patients may say that they do not deserve help. In the case of refusal to consent, doctors in England and Wales can give ECT under the Mental Health Act (MHA). This requires agreement from two doctors and another professional, usually a social worker, who need to agree that ECT should be given. There must then be a second opinion from an independent specialist who is not directly involved in the person's care. The clinical team should also speak to family and other carers to find out what they think about ECT, along with the patient themselves (RCPsych 2018). Treatment without consent involves a significant limitation on the patient's autonomy and so needs sound ethical justification. Nurses need to ensure that these patients and their families are informed of the nature of the procedure and why consent has been provided by another source. ECT is also discussed in Chapter 16.

NURSE'S STORY 4.1 ECT and Patient Orientation to the Environment

I started working in mental health about 15 years ago. All clinical areas have their challenges and the challenges are often about the legal requirements, as well as ethical issues about practice and treatment options for patients. Nurses make a big difference in patient advocacy and are often the person who checks the legal requirements and thinks about ethical decision making. It is an essential part of reflective practice for a nurse. Thinking how the benefits of treatment outweigh the harm of treatment is often difficult in mental health. We have a Mental Health Act that governs our practice. That gives us a lot of power but it also places a greater amount of responsibility and decision making on the nurse working in mental health with people who are detained and prescribed treatment without their consent. We work in partnership when we can with patients and their carers, but often when a person is severely depressed or psychotic it is difficult to engage. That doesn't mean you don't try.

One of my main roles is electroconvulsive therapy (ECT) nurse coordinator. This means I work with the medical staff, the psychiatrist and the anaesthetist to administer ECT. I'm responsible for the patient's care once they come to the ECT suite, during the procedure and I manage and support the nurses who are escorting people and providing after treatment care in the recovery suite. We also have a lot of students come through as it is a teaching hospital.

ECT is a controversial topic. I have coordinated ECT for many years and seen good outcomes but there is a lot of stigma and misunderstanding about ECT as a treatment. The Mental Health Act provides direction for the procedure and that the person needs to have made a voluntary consent. If they are unable to do this then there are provisions to provide the prescribed ECT treatment against the patient's wishes. So this may be legal to do but it reduces the person's autonomy in decision making and you have to ensure that the benefits outweigh the potential harms. ECT is a safe treatment and it is conducted within local and national guidelines and in line with current standards.

Patients are often quite frightened by the thought of having ECT and this has been influenced by the media. Patients can also be passive in their treatment, especially if the psychiatrists have prescribed and consented for them. What we try to do here is invite the person to the ECT suite and show them around, explaining what happens when people receive ECT treatment. I think this really helps them to be more at ease and also to have a better recovery. The idea to do an orientation came from the number of events we had with people becoming distressed and disoriented in recovery. So we take them to a room and say this is where you will come and wait for the treatment, explain the procedure and that they need to fast and encourage questions. Then they go into the suite and we say this is where you will lay down and be given a short-acting anaesthetic and how they will be attached to some monitors. We then show them the recovery room and say you will wake up here and once you are ready you can go back to the ward area and have breakfast. I try to include student nurses in this orientation as well and always ask the patient if it would be OK to have students in the room during the procedure. It is very rare that they have a problem with students.

I like to have student nurses. They don't just observe, they can have supervised but hands-on experience with the care of the patient, placing on the monitoring equipment, turning them, taking vital signs and caring for them throughout their recovery. They also get to see the Mental Health Act in practice and how we check the consent and that it is the correct patient and the prescription is correct and current. The whole team takes an interest in students and we encourage them to ask questions and speak to the patient after the treatment once they have recovered.

Seclusion

Seclusion may occur in the mental health setting and is the involuntary supervised isolation of a person in a locked, non-stimulating room. This room may be spartan, containing only a mattress with a blanket and a toilet. Limiting furnishing is aimed at preventing patients from hurting themselves or others (Bowers et al. 2010). The wording in mental health legislation generally suggests that seclusion is not deemed in law to be a treatment per se but rather a management tool enabling other treatments such as medication or counselling to be given.

Seclusion is generally deemed lawful when it is necessary to protect the person with mental illness or any other person from imminent risk to their health or safety, and it has been approved by an authorised psychiatrist or senior psychiatric nurse on duty. The differences in relation to the prescription and practice of seclusion reflect the tension between the protection of patients when acutely unwell and the need to provide care within the least restrictive environment. Concerns prevail about both mental health patients and staff safety, with a perception that, without seclusion, staff may be at risk of physical harm.

The patient movement and some clinicians and researchers have been influential in raising awareness about the negative impact of seclusion on those who have experienced it. Patients have expressed dissatisfaction with seclusion, finding the experience negative, frightening, cold, drab and untherapeutic and increasing feelings of distress or agitation (Cummings et al. 2010; Larue et al. 2013; Mayers et al. 2010). While the World Health Organization has suggested that authorities should pursue the elimination of isolation rooms and prohibit the provision of new ones, such recommendations have not yet been fully implemented in UK policy or legislation.

However, changes are occurring in seclusion practices and seclusion reduction policies are in place, promoting the minimisation of restrictive practice. Sensory modulation can be seen as an alternative to seclusion, along with measures such as chill rooms, quiet rooms and comfort rooms. Sensory modulation helps patients to reduce their distress in times of heightened arousal and so lessens the need for seclusion. When mental health patients appear to be distressed, nurses engage with them and offer a range of strategies. These include, but are not limited to, listening to music, using a stress ball, having aromatherapy and using a massage chair. In some psychiatric units, patients' preferred strategies and self-soothing techniques are worked out early on in admission so that patients can have some control over what happens when they are acutely distressed. Although seclusion remains a practice of acute psychiatric wards, some progress has been made in the reduction of seclusion and in increasing mental health patient satisfaction with the hospitalisation experience. The continuing challenge for mental health nurses is to be aware of patients' previous experiences of hospitalisation, which may have involved seclusion or restraint and consequent trauma.

Suicidal Behaviour

Care of the suicidal person is possibly the most challenging clinical situation that mental health professionals face. The problem of suicide is well documented but few realise that the number of unsuccessful attempts at suicide is eight to ten times the figure for actual suicide (Hawton & James 2005). The high incidence of suicide and suicidal behaviour makes this problem a significant issue for mental health nurses. The prospect of members of our community considering whether they wish to live at all destroys the image of life as cherished and worthwhile and makes us face the reality of our own mortality. The ethical debate about suicide largely centres on the justification for intervening in a person's choice to live or die. Healthcare workers have a duty to intervene by preventing the suicidal act—a duty that arises from our need to abide by the law but also from our ethical obligation of nonmaleficence.

Involuntary Treatment

Guidelines for ethical conduct are particularly relevant to mental health nurses because involuntary status under mental health legislation places restrictions on the therapeutic nurse–patient relationship. Patients who feel that they have few rights and are restricted by legislation may be less likely to engage in a working relationship with a mental health nurse. In this situation, where the patient is subject to detention under the MHA, the nurse exercises social control over the patient. If the patient is involuntarily hospitalised, the nurse can initiate prn, a Latin term that stands for "pro re nata," which means "as the thing is needed," medication and restrain and seclude the patient under medical authority. However, mental health is not an area where the nurse can always refer the patient to doctors for the answers because the nurse is often the person delivering care and it is frequently the nurse's actions that the patient is questioning.

When a person is detained in a mental health facility, the major ethical debate centres on legal rights versus moral rights. When should a person be admitted involuntarily under the MHA? This question is usually answered by saying: 'When the person is a danger to themselves or others.' However, consider whether you would feel comfortable committing a person to a mental health facility if the person was a member of your family or a close friend.

NURSE'S STORY 4.2 Shared Environments

In the past when I undertook my nurse training, I was educated to believe that we should have shared male/female wards. At the end of the 1970s they had segregated wards, but this was before my time. After that wards had just beds and nurses would care for patients whether they were male or female. We always tried to allocate a female with a female nurse and a male with a male nurse when personal care was required, but largely we based the ward bed allocation not on gender but on patient need for safety. And when I went into the community you had to go to people's homes and give injections regardless of the patient's gender.

On reflection this has caused a lot of concern for patients coming into the ward environment and I am glad to say it has been identified as a major need by the Department of Health. Our ward has had funding to develop a female-only area. This provides a space for meeting and also a separate corridor for female-only beds and bathrooms. It was controversial at first but it is part of everyday practice now.

Women feel more comfortable having a separate space to go to and an area where they can rest and shower without the fear of males coming in. Doors on bathrooms often don't lock in mental health facilities and that can make many women feel uncomfortable and unsafe. No matter how hard we try to make this a welcoming and home-like environment it is still a public space. We don't want women coming in to the mental health facilities and feeling uncomfortable when there is no need for them to feel this way.

Our management team obtained the funding and we planned the redesign in collaboration with the patients. A great outcome! It was also an example of how you can work with patients, listen to them and develop ways to provide the least restrictive environment possible, as per the Mental Health Act. So in this case an environment where women can move freely and attend to their personal care in a safe-feeling environment. Where we aim to care but do no harm.

We also planned for transgender patients. There is a room with an en-suite bathroom so anyone who identifies as transgender can have the option to stay here if their risk assessment upon admission allows for this plan of care. If they need closer monitoring then we consider this as part of their care plan.

It is important to think about the restrictive environments we work in within mental health. There has been a lot of work done on reducing the use of seclusion but we often find that this means the person is within a high dependency area that has secure doors and a quite rigid routine. Nurses need to ensure that patients feel comfortable in this environment and monitor this. Once needing less observation and care we transfer people to the open ward as soon as we can. But sometimes the doors to these units are locked as well, as there are many people on the ward who are a danger to themselves. The locked ward resolves a lot of the problems that you would experience with patients in a general ward where you don't have this facility, but it poses human rights and ethical issues. Legally the wards can be locked if even one patient at the time poses a danger to themselves or to others. For example, if they were actively wanting to harm themselves. But the guidelines of the Mental Health Act do not take away from the ethical decision making we must do to always place the patient in the least restrictive environment, promote their self-advocacy and choice. We must ensure that the benefits of a locked ward area are clear and that the need for this is conveyed to the patient and their family. We must also provide provision for others to have leave from the ward to go about their business without restriction. This can be time consuming to do but it is very much part of the day-to-day work of a mental health nurse to ensure we provide the best care we can.

A patient voluntarily seeking treatment for a mental illness should be treated as fully competent and retains the right to give or withhold consent to treatment. An involuntary patient is admitted to hospital under mental health legislation and has limited legal capacity to refuse or consent to treatment (Finucane et al. 2005). As nurses we can be advocates for patients but we must ensure that we advocate in collaboration with them, or else we risk being paternalistic. Paternalism is when nurses believe that they know what is best for the patient, that they are most qualified to speak on the patient's behalf and that the patient is not sufficiently capable of doing so. Although the intention is good, patient autonomy is at risk. All patients should be treated with the same degree of respect that you would require and, whenever practicable, their autonomy should be maintained. This ensures that they maintain their integrity and do not feel so vulnerable and powerless.

CRITICAL THINKING CHALLENGE 4.3

Ashley is 23 years old and is admitted to an acute mental health inpatient unit as an involuntary patient. She has been diagnosed with a drug-induced relapse of psychosis and it is expected that she will have a short admission. Ashley remembers a past admission where a male patient came into her room at night and rummaged through her things. She is having problems sleeping on the ward this time as she remembers that experience. Should Ashley be prescribed prn sedatives? Considering contemporary beliefs concerning gender equality and mixed-sex wards, is allocating beds on a needs basis always appropriate? What gender issues arise from having integrated ward environments with involuntary patients, and what can we do about them?

Interpersonal Therapy

Patients place trust in their therapist, expecting that the therapist will not exploit it. The relationship between therapist and patient is therapy's strength and weakness. The therapist gains recognition as a health professional, but also power within the relationship. The ethical issue is how to use this power. Does the power remain egalitarian or become authoritarian? And to what extent does transference within the relationship hinder the therapeutic process? The therapist may become the most important person in the patient's life and runs the risk of assuming priority over all others.

In general, the ethical guidelines for one-on-one therapy and group work are threefold: (1) to protect the patient from exploitation, incompetence and pressure to perform; (2) to uphold the right of the patient to be provided with information and make informed decisions concerning their life; and (3) to foster personal growth and wellness (Holmes & Adshead 2009). The first two goals protect the patient and promote the patient's rights, while the third outlines the true goal of therapy. It is often taken for granted that therapy is beneficial to the patient. After all, looking at oneself or sharing beliefs during group or individual therapy should help patients to grow and understand why their lives have evolved as they have. This aim is compromised when the therapy is focussing on the needs of the therapist or institution, rather than on those of the patient. In extreme cases this can lead to unprofessional conduct, including sexual exploitation of the patient.

Professional Boundaries

The therapeutic relationship is a privileged relationship for both the patient and the clinician. However, responsibility for maintaining the required professional boundaries rests with the clinician, who needs to have safeguards in place that will enable issues involving professional boundaries to be identified and appropriately managed (Griffith & Tengnah 2013). Without adequate professional standards there is a risk that the patient may suffer emotional harm, which would be a breach of the ethical principle of nonmaleficence. Safeguards include reflective practice, especially use of a colleague or supervisor to discuss patient care confidentially. You may notice at times when you are working closely with a patient that you have feelings of friendship, wanting to save the patient from detrimental behaviour, a clinical fatigue with their lack of progress or a sense of knowing better than the patient what their needs are. These are all signs of potential counter-transference (see Chapter 24). You should be aware of the boundaries needed to keep nursing care therapeutic and patient-centred. When a nurse moves outside the therapeutic relationship and establishes a friendship or social relationship with a patient, the professional boundaries between the nurse and the patient become confused. When professional boundaries are blurred, the relationship can become nontherapeutic and potentially harmful to both the patient and the nurse. Ethical decision making principles are especially important to ensure that professional boundaries are not transgressed.

CRITICAL THINKING CHALLENGE 4.4

Kirsty has been employed in an inpatient ward for 3 months and has been working with her clinical supervisor on developing interpersonal skills and maintaining professional boundaries. One of the patients Kirsty is caring for is Marissa, a young woman close to Kirsty's age. In talking with Marissa, Kirsty becomes aware that they share certain life issues. These are to do with trust, forming intimate relationships and a fear of being abandoned if they let anyone get too close to them. Because they have so much in common, Kirsty feels able to help Marissa more than the other nurses on the ward. Kirsty's friends are having a party next weekend and she decides to invite Marissa so that Marissa can meet some new people and perhaps form some friendships. Kirsty decides to discuss this with her supervisor after the party, when she will be able to report on how the intervention has worked. Do you think Kirsty is at risk of breaking professional boundaries? What suggestions can you make that would help Kirsty to develop safe and positive interpersonal relationships?

Confidentiality

Patients often reveal personal information to nurses and ask that we keep that information secret. Confidentiality is a primary principle of the therapeutic relationship, but how can it be upheld

TABLE 4.2 Mental Health Legislation and Related Guidelines in the UK

Country	Legislation	Guidelines
England & Wales	Mental Health Act 1983 (amended 2007)	https://www.legislation.gov.uk/ukpga/2007/12/contents
England & Wales	Mental Capacity Act 2005, including the Deprivation of Liberty Safeguards.	https://www.legislation.gov.uk/ukpga/2005/9/contents
England	Care Act 2014	http://www.legislation.gov.uk/ukpga/2014/23/contents/enacted
Wales	Social Services and Well-Being (Wales) Act 2014	https://www.legislation.gov.uk/anaw/2014/4/contents
Scotland	Mental Health (Scotland) Act 2015	http://www.legislation.gov.uk/asp/2015/9/contents/enacted
Scotland	Adults with Incapacity (Scotland) Act 2000	https://www.legislation.gov.uk/asp/2000/4/contents
Scotland	Adult Support and Protection (Scotland) Act 2007	https://www.legislation.gov.uk/asp/2007/10/contents
Northern Ireland	The Mental Health (Northern Ireland) Order 1986	https://www.legislation.gov.uk/nisi/1986/595
Northern Ireland	Mental Capacity Act (Northern Ireland) 2016	http://www.legislation.gov.uk/nia/2016/18/contents
Ireland	Mental Health Act 2001	https://www.mhcirl.ie/File/Mental_Health_Act_2001.pdf

if the patient reveals information that must be shared with the rest of the team? Nurses should never promise to keep a secret. Secrets are appropriate within a friendship, but never within a therapeutic relationship. It is paramount that the patient is made aware that information will be shared with the team and that this information will remain within the team. So, too, when commencing a discussion during group therapy it is always important to remind patients that what they share with the group is for the group alone and not to be taken out of the room.

LAW AND MENTAL HEALTH

Mental healthcare is unique in the healthcare field because mental health is the only specialty in which a significant proportion of services are provided under a framework of legal compulsion. Compulsory treatment under mental health legislation carries significant human rights implications for patients and presents some unique clinical, ethical and professional issues for mental health nurses.

This section on mental health law provides an outline of the rationale for mental health legislation, the process of detaining a patient under the MHA, discussion of the rights of people subject to compulsory treatment, ethical issues for mental health nurses and human rights issues related to mental health legislation. Mental health legislation is provided in Table 4.2. Discussion of mental health legislation is followed by a section discussing the human rights implications of mental health legislation, with special reference to the United Nations Convention on the Rights of Persons with Disabilities. A list of key concepts related to mental health legislation is provided in Box 4.4.

CRITICAL THINKING CHALLENGE 4.5

1. How would you feel if a friend or a member of your family was admitted to hospital under mental health law?
2. What rights should patients have to have their involuntary status reviewed?
3. How can you support patients who express dissatisfaction at being treated under mental health legislation?
4. What long-term effects might compulsory admission to hospital have on a patient?

Rationale for Mental Health Legislation

Legal provision to protect individuals from the consequences of behaviour resulting from mental illness, or to protect others from such behaviour, has a long tradition in Western societies (Scull 2015).

In England and Wales, this provision is governed by the MHA 1983 (see Table 4.2 for legislation in other parts of the UK) by a process known as 'sectioning' or 'detaining' a person under the MHA 1983. These two terms are used interchangeably in the discussion that follows and the MHA 1983 is referred to as the Act. For the purposes of the Act, a mental disorder is defined as 'any disorder or disability of the mind', and 'medical treatment' includes nursing, psychological intervention, specialist rehabilitation care, medication and other forms of treatment. When considering treatment under the Act, this is the process of aiming to alleviate or to prevent worsening of the disorder, its symptoms or manifestations (Department of Health 2015a).

There are five overarching principles that should be considered when any decisions are made under the Act (Department of Health 2015b) which are as follows:

- Least restrictive option and maximising independence—where it is possible to treat a patient safely and lawfully without detaining them under the Act, the patient should not be detained. Wherever possible a patient's independence should be encouraged and supported with a focus on promoting recovery.
- Empowerment and involvement—patients should be fully involved in decisions about care, support and treatment. The views of families, carers and others, if appropriate, should be fully considered when taking decisions. Where decisions are taken which are contradictory to views expressed, professionals should explain the reasons for this.
- Respect and dignity—patients, their families and carers should be treated with respect and dignity and listened to by professionals.
- Purpose and effectiveness—decisions about care and treatment should be appropriate to the patient, with clear therapeutic aims, promote recovery and should be performed to current national guidelines and/or current, available best-practice guidelines.

BOX 4.4 **Glossary of Some Key Concepts and Terms Used in Mental Health Care and Legislation**

Appropriate adult People that are held by the police who are believed to have a mental health issue, have the right to be accompanied by an appropriate adult, such as a member of their family or a mental health worker.

Approved clinician A professional such as a doctor, psychologist, nurse, occupational therapist or social worker approved to carry out tasks for the purposes of the Mental Health Act (MHA) 1983.

Approved mental health professional (AMHP) Mental health professionals who have been approved by a local social services authority to carry out certain duties under the MHA 1983.

Assessment Assessment is a clinical assessment with the specific purpose of determining whether the patient meets the criteria for detention under mental health legislation.

CapacityThe ability of a patient to make informed decisions.

Coercion Care or treatment in which a patient's autonomous decision making is limited. Coercion may be formal or informal and is not limited to patients subject to mental health legislation.

Community treatment order (CTO) A form of compulsory treatment applying to patients living in the community.

Compulsory treatment or involuntary treatment Treatment provided under mental health legislation that does not involve informed consent.

Convention for the Rights of Persons With Disabilities (CRPD) A United Nations convention that sets out the rights of people with disabilities, including people with mental illness.

Court of Protection The Court of Protection makes decisions and appoints deputies to act on someone's behalf if they are unable to make decisions about their personal health, finance or welfare.

Detained A person is detained if they are kept in hospital under mental health legislation and they are not free to leave.

Duty of care The obligation owed by nurses to patients to take all reasonable actions to provide the standard of care necessary to avoid harm and support the patient's health. Failure to meet the standard of care can result in a case of negligence.

Formal patient Someone who is being detained in hospital under a section of the MHA 1983, and is therefore not free to leave.

Independent mental health advocate (IMHA) An advocate specially trained to help people to understand and find out their rights under the MHA 1983 and help them while they are detained.

Judicial review A review by a judge of a patient's legal status under mental health legislation.

Least restrictive practice The principle that requires clinicians to use the least restrictive measures possible in care and treatment.

Hospital managers (also known as Mental Health Act managers) An independent team of people in a hospital who make sure that the requirements of the Mental Health Act are properly applied.

Mental health legislation Legislation that is specific to mental health and provides for mental health treatment without consent.

Mental Health Tribunal (MHT) A special court that deals with cases relating to the MHA 1983—the Tribunal decides whether someone can be discharged from a section and can decide about suitable aftercare and make recommendations about matters such as hospital leave, transfer to another hospital, guardianship and CTOs.

Nearest relative (NR) A specified family member who has certain responsibilities and powers when their family member is detained in hospital under the MHA. These include the right to information and to discharge in some situations. The law sets out a list to decide who will be the nearest relative, this can sometimes be changed.

Patient The definition of a patient in the MHA 1983 is a person suffering or appearing to be suffering from mental disorder.

Place of safety A locally agreed place where the police may take a person to be assessed, usually a hospital, or a police station if no other options and in an emergency.

Responsible clinician (RC) The mental health professional in charge of a patient's care and treatment while they are sectioned under the MHA 1983.

Second opinion appointed doctor (SOAD) An independent doctor appointed by the Care Quality Commission in England or by the Healthcare Inspectorate Wales. Their approval is required for a person to be given or continue to be given certain forms of medical treatment under the MHA 1983.

Section Being 'sectioned' means that a person is kept in hospital under the MHA 1983.

Section 12 approved doctor A doctor trained and qualified in the use of the MHA 1983, usually a psychiatrist.

Voluntary patient (also known as informal patient) A person who agrees to admission to a psychiatric hospital voluntarily, they are not detained under the MHA 1983.

Voluntary treatment Treatment that involves informed consent and is not provided under mental health legislation.

- Efficiency and equity—providers, commissioners and other relevant organisations should work together to ensure that the quality of commissioning and provision of mental healthcare services are of high quality and are given equal priority to physical health and social care services. All relevant services should work together to facilitate timely, safe and supportive discharge from detention.

Where possible, patients should always be cared for informally, without detention under the Act. Having a mental disorder is not sufficient grounds for any compulsory measures to be taken, which are only to be permitted if specific criteria about the consequences of a person's mental disorder are met. It is important to remember that difference should not be confused with disorder; no one may be considered mentally disordered on the grounds of their religious, political or cultural beliefs unless there are clinical grounds to believe that these are manifestations of a disorder of the mind. This also applies to peoples involvement in illegal, immoral or antisocial behaviour. As highlighted by the Mental Capacity Act (MCA) (Department of Health 2005), a person is not to be treated as unable to make a decision merely because they make an unwise one.

In cases where informal admission is not possible, detention may be necessary, the terms of which are discussed in the next section. The consequences of detaining a person under the Act are that they are either physically removed from society by being hospitalised, or have conditions placed on their choices as a member of society. Conditions typically include accepting mental healthcare, including medication and may include living at a particular location. From an ethical perspective detention is usually based on an ethical justification of the need for care which means that the harm of restraining a patient's autonomy is justified by the benefits to the person restrained, or to others to whom they may pose a risk. Mental health legislation provides clinicians with a legal framework within which to provide involuntary treatment to individuals who meet the criteria of that legislation. It will be apparent that sectioning a person involves significant departures from the normally accepted rights of citizens, especially the right to personal freedom and the right to consent to treatment.

The Process of Detention Under the Act

The process of admission to hospital, either informally or formally, varies in different parts of the UK due to the different legislations governing the process (see Table 4.2). This section is intended as an overview of the process, giving examples from the MHA 1983 which governs care within England and Wales. In most jurisdictions legislation requires that the person concerned has a mental illness (sometimes termed 'mental disorder') and that a degree of risk is present. It is not sufficient that the person has a mental illness and in the opinion of professionals would benefit from treatment which the person refuses. Mental illness must coexist with a significant degree of risk. An example would be a person who hears voices commanding them to harm others, where it seems likely that the person will act on those voices if not prevented from doing so. Note that this example includes features of mental illness (hearing voices) *and* risk (risk of harm to others). It is important to note that hearing voices is not always associated with mental illness and that most people with mental illness are not at risk of harming others. Mental health legislation therefore applies only to a small minority of people with mental illness, and only at a time when their symptoms are sufficiently severe.

If an individual becomes acutely mentally unwell, others may feel that the person represents a significant risk to themselves or to others. A person who is unwell may agree to an informal admission to hospital for assessment and/or treatment. However, in cases where they are not in agreement and it is believed that the person is suffering from a mental disorder of a nature or degree which warrants their detention in hospital, then an application for detention under the Act can be made (Department of Health 2015b). The process of sectioning a person can be initiated in a variety of situations, including patients' homes, primary care settings, court hearings, police custody, emergency departments and community or inpatient mental health services. The initial step is usually an application, in which a concerned individual requests that the person with a mental illness is assessed with a view to detention under the act. An application for detention can be made by either an approved mental health professional (AMHP) or the patient's nearest relative, both of whom must understand the criteria for detention and their responsibilities under the Act. The application must be supported by two medical recommendations given in accordance with the Act, the object of which is to determine whether people agree that the criteria for detention has been met. When deciding whether detention is necessary, ways of providing less restrictive alternatives to detention must always be explored e.g. management in the community by crisis teams or informal admission. Usually, an application for detention is made under either section 2 or section 3 of the Act. Section 2 should only be used if: the extent or the nature and degree of the patient's condition is unclear; an initial inpatient assessment is required to formulate a treatment plan and to ascertain if the patient is willing to accept treatment on a voluntary basis following admission or to reformulate a plan. Under Section 2, a person can be detained in hospital for up to 28 days. Section 3 should only be used if: the patient is already detained under section 2 (which cannot be renewed); the nature and current degree of the patient's mental disorder, the essential elements of the treatment plan to be followed and the likelihood of the patient accepting treatment as an informal patient are already sufficiently established. Under Section 3 a person can be detained in hospital for up to 6 months.

There are a number of other Sections and holding powers that can be used under the Act. Section 4 can be used in an emergency, where there is only one doctor available at short notice, allowing an informal patient to be detained in hospital for up to 72 hours, giving the hospital time to arrange for a full assessment. Section 5 is a holding power, allowing a doctor or a nurse to prevent an informal person leaving hospital if they believe the person to be too unwell. A doctor's holding power is a Section 5(2) which lasts for up to 72 hours and a nurse's holding power is a Section 5(4) which lasts for up to 6 hours, allowing for further appropriate professionals to attend for further assessment.

Mental health legislation includes various support and appeal processes that allow the patient to question decisions and to have legal representation in the decision-making process. If an application for detention has been made, the patient will need to be informed of this, and about the possible decision for compulsory treatment to be given. Under sections 2 and 3 patients have the right to appeal against their detention and apply for a tribunal with assistance from a solicitor. They are also entitled to get help from an independent mental health advocate (IMHA) who can help them to understand their rights under the Act and is independent of hospital staff.

Assessment Under Mental Health Legislation

An assessment under mental health legislation is a clinical assessment that follows the standard process of comprehensive assessment (see Chapter 22) but with a particular focus on whether the patient meets legislative criteria for detention. It includes careful consideration of current and historical risk issues. Assessments under mental health legislation are usually conducted by psychiatrists. Nurses are also involved, and in some cases may have initiated the process by raising concerns about the patient and their safety. Although the psychiatrist will complete and sign the assessment document, nurses often contribute important observations and information to the assessment. Nurses may also be in a position to advocate for alternatives to detention; for example, by exploring additional community and home support, utilising respite care and negotiating the patient's voluntary engagement with the mental health team. These considerations are important to ensure that the care provided involves the least restrictions for the patient. Care should be voluntary whenever possible, and compulsory only if options for voluntary care cannot be used. It is important to understand that in most cases assessment under mental health legislation is not an assessment of the patient's capacity for informed decision making. Rather, assessment is one of mental state in the context of the person's social and clinical history, and level of risk. The issue of capacity assessment is addressed in a separate section later.

Compulsory Treatment

Once subject to detention, a patient can be treated without their consent. Treatment in this case involves measures such as hospitalisation, medication and supportive personal care. People made subject to detention have usually refused to consent to voluntary treatment: that is one of the reasons for seeking a section under the Act for compulsory treatment. The plan of compulsory treatment will include ensuring safety by providing a secure environment, ongoing clinical assessment, medication aimed at reducing acute symptoms, personal care for those patients unable to care for themselves (hygiene, hydration, nutrition) and supportive psychological care (being with the person, psychotherapeutic support, safe socialisation, visits or contact with friends or family members).

Although the power to treat without consent is provided by legislation, nurses should always attempt to negotiate consent rather than simply exercising the legal right to treat without consent. Compulsory treatment does not override nurses' ethical and professional obligation to work collaboratively with patients. For example, a patient may have medication prescribed, but might refuse to accept that medication when it is first offered. The nurse should then work with the patient to negotiate consent by explaining the intended benefits of the medication, validating any concerns the patient has about the medication and providing the patient with choices about how the medication is administered. An option might be to provide as much explanation as possible and give the patient time to reconsider their refusal. In these situations, nurses should always be honest in disclosing whether administering the medication by force is a possibility. In cases where medication does need to be administered by force, safety of the patient and the nurse is paramount. This includes psychological and physical safety. Every service has policies and procedures relating to the use of force and these should be followed carefully. In addition, these policies will outline the explanations to provide to patients, how to offer reassurance to patients about the nurse's actions and use of the least possible force necessary in the situation. Patients should be provided with subsequent opportunities to review their experience of forced medication, and nurses should have an opportunity to debrief with colleagues.

Protective Mechanisms in Mental Health Legislation

Because mental health legislation involves significant limitations on normally accepted health and human rights, MHAs include a range of measures aimed at counterbalancing the power of legislation to detain individuals and impose compulsory treatment. Protective mechanisms include the right to legal advocacy, processes of appeal and review, appointment of statutory officials to oversee the operation of legislation, complaints procedures and access to review tribunals. Readers should consult the legislation for their own jurisdiction, as well as the guidelines for the use of mental health legislation listed in Table 4.2.

As with other legislation, actions taken under mental health legislation may be subject to challenge in higher courts, where decisions can be tested and may be reversed. Legal challenges have the effect of creating a body of case law, legal decisions that test the actions and decision making of clinicians and of legal procedures of mental health legislation. Case law can, in turn, impact on clinical practice because clinicians are obliged to work with precedents established in the higher courts.

Working With Coercion and Compulsion

The concept of procedural justice provides a model for working with patients whose autonomy is restricted by their legal status or by limits imposed by the nurse. Procedural justice can be defined as the fairness with which decisions are made. Fairness relates to both decision-making processes and to the outcome of those processes. Procedural justice has some similarities to natural justice, and to due process, but in the mental health context it is different to both of these concepts as it is concerned with the quality of interactions between the nurse and the patient. Procedural justice requires nursing skills such as listening, treating people with respect, offering choices and validating the patient's experience. Because these skills are inherent in therapeutic relationships, nurses do not need to develop a new set of skills. Nurses are often closely involved with patients whose autonomy is limited by their legal status, whether in an inpatient or a community setting. It is therefore especially important for nurses to be aware of coercive actions and how they are experienced by patients (Galon & Wineman 2010). Even when interactions are coercive, using the principles of procedural justice can limit the coercive impact of those interactions.

An example of procedural justice is provided by Maguire et al. (2014) who studied the coercive practice of limit setting in a mental health inpatient setting. Limit setting can be important to the safety of inpatient setting, and can help patients by providing external boundaries on their behaviour at a time when internal boundaries are not effective. At the same time, limit setting can constrain patients' autonomy. In Maguire et al.'s (2014) study nurses and patients were interviewed about their experience of limit setting and reported that empathic engagement helped in maintaining therapeutic relationships. The researchers also found that treating patients in a fair, respectful, consistent and knowledgeable way enhanced positive outcomes compared with interactive styles that were controlling and indifferent. This example from an inpatient setting has application in many situations when nurses are working with patients who are subject to the restraints of mental health legislation or other forms of coercion. In community settings, where nurses are working with patients under compulsory community treatment, researchers have reported that procedural justice is associated with a reduced experience of coercion (Galon & Wineman 2011). Procedural justice is not a substitute for ensuring that patients' rights are respected and upheld, but it does help to guide interactions towards being less coercive.

Community Treatment Orders

Introduced in the United States in the 1970s, CTOs were originally developed as a response to the coercive nature of involuntary hospitalisation and therefore had a focus on protecting the civil rights of service users who might otherwise have been involuntarily admitted to hospital (Hiday 2006). CTOs were introduced in Canada in 1985 (O'Brien & Farrell 2005), Scotland in 2005 (Lawton-Smith 2006), England and Wales in 2007 (Woolley 2010) and Sweden in 2008 (Sjostrom et al. 2011). They have been recommended as an alternative to hospitalisation and as a means of providing care in the least restrictive environment. There are, however, concerns that CTOs represent part of an increasing preoccupation with risk and contribute to stigmatisation of mental health service users by reinforcing a perception of dangerousness. CTOs vary in their requirements, but generally require patients to attend for treatment or face the possibility of rehospitalisation. Typically, CTOs are ordered by a psychiatrist, but are subject to judicial review and appeal processes. Benefits claimed for CTOs are reduced hospitalisation, improved access to services, reduced rates of relapse and improved social functioning.

A person who is subject to a CTO will live at their own home, whether that is a private residence, a boarding house or some form of supported community accommodation. In some cases, the CTO will specify the address the patient must live at, and that the patient must refrain from the use of alcohol and other recreational drugs. Patients under CTOs will receive follow-up care from a community-based mental health service, which will provide a care coordinator/case manager and other components of care such as social support, psychological treatment, medication and support to navigate the health and social services they need. Models such as assertive outreach teams (Harvey et al. 2012) and intensive home treatment teams (George & Giri 2011) have been used to provide services to people under CTOs. Services are delivered at the patient's home, often by a community mental health nurse, at a community mental health centre or some combination of both. Most people subject to a CTO will be prescribed medication, usually an antipsychotic, and most often in depot (long-acting) form. The community mental health nurse will also monitor the patient's physical health and ensure that they receive primary healthcare from a GP. This last function is important to address the health disparities experienced by people with severe mental illness, particularly those who have been prescribed second-generation antipsychotic medication for long periods of time (see Chapter 8 for further discussion of physical health).

There is general agreement that a CTO by itself, even together with a policy of enforcement, is not sufficient to ensure improved outcomes for patients. In addition, interventions aimed at improving outcomes while reducing reliance on legal coercion have been found to be effective (Dawson 2015). Research into patients' perspectives on CTOs has yielded mixed results. Studies indicate that although some are opposed to the measure, others identify perceived benefits (Schwarz et al. 2010). Factors found to be associated with a positive service user perception of CTOs are a sense of fairness, involvement in decision making, the opportunity to have views heard and responded to and a sense of respect (Lawton-Smith 2006).

Rates of use of CTOs are high in many countries, which has led to debate about their human rights implications and effectiveness (Corring et al. 2017). Critics have argued that the CTO represents an unnecessary extension of coercion into community settings, and that this increased coercion is likely to lead to service users disengaging from services. As a nurse you need to be aware of your legal obligations towards people subject to CTOs and of their potential to affect therapeutic relationships with service users. As mental health legislation is revised, you need to be informed about both the human rights and the clinical issues inherent in this form of compulsory care.

Human Rights and Mental Health Legislation

People with mental illness have historically been subject to discriminatory laws, systemic loss of rights in legislation and breaches of those rights granted to them under mental health and other legislation. Much of this loss of rights stems from discrimination and stigma. In response, various international instruments have been developed to help protect the rights of individuals with mental illness. Until 2008 human rights under mental health legislation were protected mainly by three instruments: the 1966 International Covenant on Civil and Political Rights; the 1966 International Covenant on Economic, Social and Cultural Rights; and the 1991 United Nations Principles for the Protection of Persons with Mental Illness and the Improvement of Mental Health Care. The UK is a signatory to all three instruments. However, even with those instruments in place, people with mental illness continued to experience discrimination, often within the mental health services provided for them, and from a range of domestic legislation that did not always afford sufficient protection.

After a long period of development, the United Nations Convention on the Rights of Persons with Disabilities (the Convention) was adopted in 2006 and entered into force in May 2008. The Convention has been ratified by the UK and is considered to be the most authoritative document articulating the rights of people with mental illness. The Convention does not create new rights for people with disabilities, but clarifies existing rights under other instruments such as those mentioned previously. Unlike some other rights instruments, the Convention does not focus solely on one issue, in this case mental illness. Instead, it focuses on the concept of disability and provides a wide definition which includes mental illness alongside other disabilities. A foundation principle of the Convention is equality; that is, not only should people with disabilities enjoy the rights to be free from prejudice and discrimination, but also barriers to social inclusion should be removed so that people with disabilities are able to enjoy the full range of opportunities available to other members of society. The 50 articles of the Convention make this a very wide-ranging instrument, covering issues such as equal access to justice, gender issues, housing, rights of children and older people, and mobility. The full text of the Convention can be downloaded from www.un.org/development/desa/disabilities.

One of the major implications of the Convention is the Article 12 requirement for equality before the law. This requirement has been interpreted to mean that any legislation that limits rights on the basis of an individual's membership of a 'status group' (such as people with disabilities) is considered discriminatory. As noted in the discussion of mental health legislation earlier, most UK mental health legislation exclusively limits the rights of people with mental illness and is therefore considered discriminatory under the terms of Article 12 (Szmukler et al. 2014). The argument is that this legislation is discriminatory because it only applies to people with mental illness. The intent of the legislation is to provide needed treatment to people with mental illness when they are unwell and represent a significant risk to themselves or others, and would benefit from treatment. However, this argument is already applied to others who are unwell and presenting with significant risk issues; for example, people with delirium, acute confusional states as a result of low blood sugar or a reduced level of consciousness as a result of illness or injury. To end discrimination towards people with mental illness, it is suggested that a single test of decision-making capacity is applied to all health patients whose illness or health status impairs their ability to make safe decisions. An assumption is that we should respect the decision that the person would have made if they were not impaired.

Further reading around human rights and mental health legislation can be found at: UN Declaration of Human Rights 1948 https://www.un.org/en/udhrbook/pdf/udhr_booklet_en_web.pdf, European Convention on Human Rights (ECHR) https://www.echr.coe.int/Documents/Convention_ENG.pdf, Human Rights Act 1998 https://www.legislation.gov.uk/id/ukpga/1998/42, Equality Act 2010 Public Sector Equality Duty (PSED) https://www.gov.uk/equality-act-2010-guidance#public-sector-equality-duty.

CRITICAL THINKING CHALLENGE 4.6

1. How would you feel if a friend or a member of your family was discharged from hospital under a community treatment order?
2. What rights should apply to patients subject to community treatment orders?
3. Why is it important that countries commit to international treaties such as the United Nations Convention for the Rights of Persons with Disabilities?
4. What legislation is aimed at protecting the rights of mental health patients in your country?

Duty of Care and Decision-Making Capacity

In emergency situations where there is a threat to life or a serious threat to health, hospitalisation and treatment without consent is a common-law duty of clinicians. Emergency situations might arise in mental healthcare settings or general healthcare settings, such as mental health inpatient units, emergency departments and general hospital wards. In this section, we discuss emergency situations arising in general healthcare settings. In the emergency department individuals may temporarily lose capacity because of the toxic effects of recreational drugs or the high emotional arousal associated with self-harm. A common example of an emergency situation in a general healthcare setting is where a patient has developed delirium and become acutely confused. There are many causes of delirium, which is characterised by a rapid deterioration in mental state that can fluctuate rapidly. This may be secondary to medical illness, anaesthesia, high temperature or other causes. In some cases, the precise cause of delirium is not known and the diagnosis is based on the clinical history.

In people showing acute confusional states, clinicians commonly apply a test of capacity (or competence). Guidance can be found in the MCA 2005, which includes the Deprivation of Liberty Safeguards. There are five statutory principles of the MCA:

- A person must be assumed to have capacity unless it is established that they lack capacity.
- A person is not to be treated as unable to make a decision unless all practicable steps to help them to do so have been taken without success.
- A person is not to be treated as unable to make a decision merely because they make an unwise decision.
- An act done, or decision made, on behalf of a person who lacks capacity, must be done, or made, in their best interests.
- Before the act is done, or the decision is made, regard must be had to whether the purpose of the act or the decision can be as effectively achieved in a way that is less restrictive of the person's rights and freedom of action.

The MCA empowers individuals to make their own decisions where possible and protects the rights of those who lack capacity. Where an individual lacks capacity to make a specific decision at a particular time, the MCA provides a legal framework for others to act and make that decision on their behalf, in their best interests, including where the decision is about care and/or treatment (Department of Health 2015b).

Assessment of capacity is dependent on the seriousness of the situation the person faces. For example, making a decision to leave hospital while confused is clearly more serious than making a decision about whether or not to have a shower. Each situation must be assessed individually, and clinicians should consult with colleagues if they are unsure. Family members should also be consulted in order to establish what the person's normal preferences would be. Factors such as cultural and language differences, sensory impairment, pain and an unfamiliar environment need to be considered in assessing capacity. If a person's decision-making capacity is thought to be permanently impaired—for example, in dementia—clinicians should consider provisions for legal guardianship. This normally involves a court process, with a family member or lawyer being appointed by the court to make decisions on the person's behalf. For the patient, legal guardianship has the benefit that decisions made on their behalf can be legally scrutinised.

CONCLUSION

This chapter has explored contemporary professional, ethical and legal issues associated with mental health nursing practice. Mental health nursing needs a strong professional voice and organisation to support practitioners in the services of the future. The development of advanced practice and nurse practitioner roles represents a future in which mental health nurses will play an increasing role in the provision and development of clinical services.

Mental health nursing is fraught with ethical issues arising from the classification of mental illness, diagnoses, treatment and working within the constraints of mental health legislation. While there are existing codes of ethics for nurses, a code of ethical conduct specific to mental health nursing is required to guide practice in the complex challenges of mental healthcare. Growing recognition of the prevalence and burden of mental illness, together with increasing specialisation within mental health, will require similar resourcefulness and adaptability as mental health nurses work to maintain a profession that is both rewarding to practitioners and valued by patients.

The complexities of the ethical and legal issues concerning the care of vulnerable populations such as the mentally ill also require constant scrutiny. The United Nations Convention on the Rights of Persons with Disabilities provides guidelines to ensure legislation considers the human rights of individuals.

EXERCISES FOR CLASS ENGAGEMENT

1. Read the four scenarios below and consider appropriate responses to the questions that follow. You can either split into discussion groups or work individually.

Scenario 1

A 33-year-old woman under a community treatment order is refusing to have her regular antipsychotic medication, although she does agree that her symptoms were lessened when taking the medication. She is concerned about her increase in weight as a result of taking the medication and tells you that you do not understand what it is like taking medication with such side effects.

Scenario 2

A 59-year-old male widower, who has been diagnosed with liver and bowel cancer, presents with considerable pain and distress. He advises the nurse that he has always believed in euthanasia and has decided that his time is now up. He does not want to be a burden on his daughter and wishes to die with dignity. He is open about his wish to die and has planned his suicide. All his affairs are in order. He believes that he will carry this out sooner rather than later, as the pain is now too great and he just wants it to end.

Scenario 3

A 15-year-old girl arrived at the emergency department after ingesting 24 paracetamol tablets. She had been struggling with anorexia nervosa since she was 11 and felt that her life was heading nowhere. She was transferred as an involuntary patient to the local mental health hospital and prescribed nasogastric tube feeding, which was given without her consent. Three weeks later she remains suicidal and is still being tube fed. She wants to be left alone as she cannot face the pain of life any more.

Scenario 4

An 84-year-old famous actor has refused food and fluid for six days as she does not want to live any more. She has right-sided paralysis following a cerebrovascular accident. She wants to be remembered as young and beautiful. She feels that her life has been full and now wants it to end, as she feels that her future prospects are hopeless.

Questions

- In the above four scenarios, who is making a rational choice to die?
- What are our responsibilities in each case as health professionals?
- Do health professionals have the right to stop people when they wish to die?

2. Discuss contemporary developments in mental health services globally and in your country, and their impact on how people with mental illness are cared for in the community.
3. Think about some recent clinical experiences you have had with patients with a mental problem or illness and discuss your responses to the following questions with your group or class members.
   - Identify some controlling interventions you have been involved with or have observed. If you were involved, how did you feel about being involved?
   - Were there alternatives that could have been less restrictive?
   - What are your own beliefs about how and where people with mental illness should be cared for?
   - Should legislation have the power to contain or control people with a mental illness to protect them from themselves and/or other people?

REFERENCES

American Psychiatric Association (APA), 2013. Diagnostic and Procedural Manual of Mental Disorders, fifth ed. APA, Washington. text rev.

Bowers, L., Van Der Merwe, M., Nijman, H., et al., 2010. The practice of seclusion and time-out on English acute psychiatric wards: the City-128 study. Archives of Psychiatric Nursing 24 (4), 275–286.

Corring, D., O'Reilly, R., Sommerdyk, C., 2017. A systematic review of the views and experiences of subjects of community treatment orders. International Journal of Law and Psychiatry 52, 74–80.

Cummings, K., Grandfield, S., Coldwell, C., 2010. Caring with comfort rooms. Reducing seclusion and restraint in psychiatric facilities. Journal of Psychosocial Nursing and Mental Health Services 48 (6), 26–30.

Daalen-Smith, C.L., Gallagher, J., 2011. Electroshock: a discerning review of the nursing literature. Issues in Mental Health Nursing 32 (4), 203–213.

Dawson, J., 2015. A realistic approach to assessing mental health laws' compliance with the UNCRPD. International Journal of Law and Psychiatry 40, 70–79.

Department of Health, 2005. Mental Capacity Act. Available at: https://www.legislation.gov.uk/ukpga/2005/9/contents.

Department of Health, 2015a. Reference Guide to the Mental Health Act 1983. Available at: https://assets.publishing.service.gov.uk/government/uploads/system/uploads/attachment_data/file/417412/Reference_Guide.pdf. Accessed: 5th October 2018..

Department of Health, 2015b. Mental Health Act 1983: Code of Practice. Available at: https://assets.publishing.service.gov.uk/government/uploads/system/uploads/attachment_data/file/435512/MHA_Code_of_Practice.PDF. Accessed: 5th October 2018.

Drew, B.L., 2014. The evolution of the role of the psychiatric mental health advanced practice registered nurse in the United States. Archives of Psychiatric Nursing 28 (5), 298–300.

Earle, E.A., Taylor, J., Peet, M., et al., 2011. Nurse prescribing in specialist mental health (part 1): the views and experiences of practising and non-practising nurse prescribers and service users. Journal of Psychiatric and Mental Health Nursing 18 (3), 189–197.

Elsom, S., Happell, B., Manias, E., 2009. Nurse practitioners and medical practice: opposing forces or complementary contributions? Perspectives in Psychiatric Care 45 (1), 9–16.

Finucane, M., Mertz, C., Slovic, P., et al., 2005. Task complexity and older adults' decision-making competence. Psychology and Aging 20 (1), 71–84.

Flaskeraud, J., 2010. DSM proposed changes, part I. Criticisms and influences on changes. Issues in Mental Health Nursing 31 (10), 686–688.

Freidson, E., 2001. Professionalism, the Third Logic: on the Practice of Knowledge. University of Chicago Press, Chicago.

Galon, P.A., Wineman, N.M., 2010. Coercion and procedural justice in psychiatric care: State of the science and implications for nursing. Archives of Psychiatric Nursing 24 (5), 307–316.

Galon, P., Wineman, N.M., 2011. Quasi-experimental comparison of coercive interventions on client outcomes in individuals with severe and persistent mental illness. Archives of Psychiatric Nursing 25 (6), 404–418.

George, K., Giri, S., 2011. An intensive community team in aged persons mental health. Australasian Psychiatry 19 (1), 56–58.

Griffith, R., Tengnah, C., 2013. Maintaining professional boundaries: keep your distance. British Journal of Community Nursing 18 (1), 43–46.

Harvey, C., Killaspy, H., Martino, S., Johnson, S., 2012. Implementation of assertive community treatment in Australia: Model fidelity, patient characteristics and staff experiences. Community Mental Health Journal 48 (5), 652–661.

Harvey, B.H., Slabbert, F.N., 2014. New insights on the antidepressant discontinuation syndrome. Human Psychopharmacology: Clinical and Experimental 29 (6), 503–516.

Hawton, K., James, A., 2005. Suicide and deliberate self-harm in young people. British Medical Journal 330 (7496), 891–894.

Hiday, V.A., 2006. Putting community risk in perspective: a look at correlations, causes and controls. International Journal of Law and Psychiatry 29 (4), 316–331.

Holmes, J., Adshead, G., 2009. Ethical aspects of the psychotherapies. In: Bloch, S., Green, S. (Eds.), Psychiatric Ethics, fourth ed. Oxford University Press, Oxford, pp. 367–384.

Illich, I., 2001. Limits to Medicine. Medical Nemesis: the Expropriation of Health. Marian Boyers, London.

International Council of Nurses (ICN), 2012. The ICN Code of Ethics for Nurses. ICN, Geneva.

Larue, C., Dumais, A., Boyer, R., Goulet, M.H., Bonin, J.P., Baba, N., 2013. The experience of seclusion and restraint in psychiatric settings: perspectives of patients. Issues in Mental Health Nursing 34 (5), 317–324.

Lawton-Smith, S., 2006. Community-Based Compulsory Treatment Orders in Scotland. The Early Evidence. The King's Fund, London.

Light, E., Kerrige, I., Ryan, C., Robertson, M., 2012b. Out of sight, out of mind: making involuntary community treatment visible in the mental health system. Medical Journal of Australia 196 (9), 591–593. https://doi.org/10.5694/mja11.11216.

Lim, A.G., North, N., Shaw, J., 2014. Nurse prescribing: the New Zealand context. Nursing praxis in New Zealand 30 (2), 18–27.

Lowe, G., Plummer, V., Boyd, L., 2013. Nurse practitioner roles in Australian healthcare settings: Grainne Lowe and colleagues report on a study to explore how clinicians, managers and policymakers perceive nurse practitioner roles and to elicit their views on barriers to their introduction. Nursing Management 20 (2), 28–35.

Maguire, T., Daffern, M., Martin, T., 2014. Exploring nurses' and patients' perspectives of limit setting in a forensic mental health setting. International Journal of Mental Health Nursing 23 (2), 153–160.

Maude, P., Edwards, K., 2011. Psychopharmacology. In: Edwards, K., Munro, I., Robins, A., Welch, A. (Eds.), Mental Health Nursing: Dimensions of Praxis. Oxford University Press, South Melbourne.

Mayers, P., Keet, N., Winker, G., et al., 2010. Mental health service users' perceptions and experiences of sedation, seclusion and restraint. International Journal of Social Psychiatry 56 (1), 60–73.

Moncrieff, J., 2013. The Bitterest Pills: the Troubling Story of Antipsychotic Drugs. Palgrave Macmillan.

Nursing and Midwifery Council, 2001. Standards for Specialist Education and Practice. Available at: https://www.nmc.org.uk/standards/standards-for-post-registration/standards-for-specialist-education-and-practice/. Accessed: 17th September 2018.

Nursing and Midwifery Council, 2015. The Code: Professional Standards of Practice and Behaviour for Nurses and Midwives. Available at: https://www.nmc.org.uk/globalassets/sitedocuments/nmc-publications/nmc-code.pdf. Accessed: 17th September 2018.

Nursing and Midwifery Council (NMC), 2017. Our Values and Mission. Available at: https://www.nmc.org.uk/about-us/our-role/our-values-and-mission.

Nursing and Midwifery Council (NMC), 2018a. Registration. Available at: https://www.nmc.org.uk/registration/. Accessed: 17th September 2018.

Nursing and Midwifery Council (NMC), 2018b. Our role in education. Available at: https://www.nmc.org.uk/education/our-role-in-education/. Accessed: 17th September 2018.

Nursing and Midwifery Council (NMC), 2018c. Revalidation: Welcome to Revalidation. Available at: http://revalidation.nmc.org.uk/welcome-to-revalidation. Accessed: 17th September 2018..

New Zealand Nurses Organisation (NZNO) 1995 Code of ethics. NZNO, Auckland
O'Brien, A., Farrell, S.J., 2005. Community treatment orders: profile of Canadian experience. Canadian Journal of Psychiatry 50 (1), 27–30.
Royal College of Nursing, 2018a. Nurse Prescribing. Available at: https://www.rcn.org.uk/get-help/rcn-advice/nurse-prescribing. Accessed: 17th September 2018.
Royal College of Nursing (RCN), 2018b. What the RCN does. Available at: https://www.rcn.org.uk/about-us/what-the-rcn-does. Accessed: 17th September 2018.
Royal College of Psychiatry (RCPsych), 2018. Information about ECT (Electro-convulsive therapy). Available at: https://www.rcpsych.ac.uk/mentalhealthinformation/therapies/electroconvulsivetherapy,ect.aspx. Accessed: 17th September 2018.
Salomon, C., Hamilton, B., 2014. Antipsychotic discontinuation syndromes: a narrative review of the evidence and its integration into Australian mental health nursing textbooks. Int J Ment Health Nurs 23 (1), 69–78.
Schwarz, L., O'Brien, A.M., Morel, V., Armstrong, M., Fleming, C., Moore, P., 2010. Community treatment orders: the service user speaks. Exploring the lived experience of community treatment orders. International Journal of Psychosocial Rehabilitation 15 (1), 39–50.
Scull, A., 2015. Madness in Civilization. A Cultural History of Insanity From the Bible to Freud, From the Madhouse to Modern Medicine. Princeton University Press, New Jersey.
Sjostrom, S., Zetterburgh, L., Marksrom, U., 2011. Why community compulsion became the solution: reforming mental health law in Sweden. International Journal of Law in Society 34 (6), 419–428.
Smith, M., Vogler, J., Zarrouf, F., Sheaves, C., Jesse, J., 2009. Electroconvulsive therapy: the struggles in the decision-making process and the aftermath of treatment. Issues in Mental Health Nursing 30 (9), 554–559.
Szmukler, G., Daw, R., Callard, F., 2014. Mental health law and the UN Convention on the Rights of Persons with Disabilities. International Journal of Law and Psychiatry 37 (3), 245–252.
Woolley, S., 2010. Involuntary treatment in the community: role of community treatment orders. The Psychiatry 34 (10), 441–446.
Zachar, P., Stoyanov, D.S., Aragona, M., Jablensky, A. (Eds.), 2014. Alternative Perspectives on Psychiatric Validation: DSM, IDC, RDoC and Beyond. Oxford University Press.

FURTHER READING

Doyal, L., Sheather, J., 2005. Mental health legislation should respect decision making capacity. British Medical Journal 331 (7530), 1467.
Fawcett, B., 2007. Consistencies and inconsistencies: mental health, compulsory treatment and community capacity building in England, Wales and Australia. British Journal of Social Work 37 (6), 1027–1042.
Jacob, R., Clare, I., Holland, A., Watson, P., Maimaris, C., Gunn, M., 2005. Self-harm, capacity, and refusal of treatment: implications for emergency medical practice. A prospective observational study. Emergency Medicine Journal 22 (11), 799–802.
Marilyn, S., 2009. Electroconvulsive therapy: the struggles in the decision-making process and the aftermath of treatment. Issues in Mental Health Nursing 30 (9), 554–559.
Nolan, P., Bradley, E., Brimblecombe, N., 2011. Disengaging from acute inpatient psychiatric care: a description of service users' experiences and views. Journal of Psychiatric and Mental Health Nursing 18 (4), 359–367.
Royal College of Psychiatrists, 2008. Rethinking risk to others in mental health services. Final report of a scoping group. Royal College of Psychiatrists, London.
Stephens, M., 2007. Risk, security and surveillance: the care and control of people with serious mental health problems. Security Journal 20 (4), 211–221.

USEFUL WEBSITES

End Seclusion Now, tinyurl.com/l2y7vs2
MindFreedom ethics and mental health page, www.mindfreedom.org
Nursing and Midwifery Council https://www.nmc.org.uk/
Royal College of Nursing https:www.rcn.org.uk
UNISON https://www.unison.org.uk
United Nations Convention on the Rights of Persons with Disabilities, www.un.org/disabilities
Universal Human Rights Instruments, www.ohchr.org/EN/ProfessionalInterest/Pages/UniversalHumanRightsInstruments.aspx

5

Settings for Mental Health Care

Julie Sharrock, Phillip Maude, Lina Wilson and Michael Olasoji

KEY POINTS

- The quality of the environment is important to patient recovery.
- The principle underpinning mental healthcare is to aim for the provision of care in the least restrictive environment.
- The preferred setting for mental healthcare is the community.
- Contemporary practice includes short-term hospitalisation and ongoing community support.
- Environmental strategies in mental healthcare became more important in the 18th century, when it was noticed that patients were more manageable in a pleasant environment.
- Confinement of the mentally ill in large public asylums was largely an innovation of the 19th century.
- The therapeutic milieu is a consciously organised environment.
- Maxwell Jones in the United States and Thomas Main in the UK pioneered the concept of the hospital and environment as treatment tools.
- The principles on which the therapeutic milieu is based include open communication, democratisation, orientation to the milieu, privacy and respect for one another and group cohesion.
- The goals of the therapeutic milieu are containment, structure, support, involvement, validation, symptom management, safe environment and maintaining links with family and the community.
- In all settings the patient is supported as a person in interactions with others, rather than as someone suffering from a health problem or disability.
- The predominant forms of service delivery in the community are case management and care coordination, which has been found to be most effective for people with enduring mental illnesses.
- There is a range of community services depending on the needs of the patient at a particular time.
- The principles of caring in the community are collaboration, recovery and goal setting, working with patients' strengths in collaboration with non-government agencies and specialist community support services.
- There are opportunities for mental health nurses to work in a variety of settings with a range of patient groups across the lifespan.

KEY TERMS

care coordination
collaboration
community care
least restrictive environment
multidisciplinary team
partnership
recovery
therapeutic milieu

LEARNING OUTCOMES

The material in this chapter will assist you to:

- define and describe the components of a therapeutic milieu.
- discuss the historical antecedents of the therapeutic milieu.
- appraise the characteristics and goals of the therapeutic milieu.
- discuss the role of the nurse in various settings.
- describe the components and functions of the multidisciplinary team.
- gain an understanding of community accommodation for people experiencing mental illness.
- examine principles of caring in the community.

INTRODUCTION

In March 2015 the Independent Mental Health Taskforce was set up by National Health Service (NHS) England, the body responsible for the delivery of the NHS on behalf of the Government. NHS England leads the NHS in England and the following discussion is used as an example of health care delivery; however, it is important for nurses working in other parts of the UK such as Scotland, Northern Ireland and Wales to familiarise themselves with the separate arrangements in other parts of the UK. NHS England sets the priorities and direction of the NHS in England and encourages and informs debate to improve health and care. The Taskforce were asked to develop the Mental Health Five Year Forward View, which was published in February 2016. The current state of mental health service provision in England was examined and recommendations were made for the next 5 years.

This chapter begins by providing the historical context within which the development of ideas about the therapeutic potential of the environment emerged. A continuum of services of bed-based and community services provided by government (public), non-government and private organisations is described. These services can be generalist or specialist in nature and are provided to people across the lifespan from the perinatal and infant period, through childhood and adolescence to adulthood and older age. Services can be named according to the model of care delivery that a team may use, based on the characteristics of the patient group it provides service to or the setting in which care is provided (see Box 5.1). Given this, the names of mental health services across the UK and internationally may vary. The authors have attempted to describe services broadly, avoiding local idiosyncratic language with the aim of making this chapter broadly applicable. The role of the nurse in these services is included to demonstrate the opportunities available for mental health nurses to work in a variety of settings with a range of patient groups.

BOX 5.1 Service Settings

Examples of Services Based on Model of Service Delivery
- Crisis intervention teams
- Treatment and recovery teams
- Assertive outreach services
- Care coordination
- Case management
- Single point of access services
- Psychiatric liaison services
- Early intervention services

Examples of Services Based on Patient Group
- Eating disorders
- Substance use disorders
- First episode psychosis
- Learning disability and mental illness
- Personality disorder
- Dual diagnosis: substance misuse and mental illness
- Perinatal and infant, child and youth, adult, older persons
- Refugees and transcultural
- Homeless persons
- Forensic
- Comorbidities such as HIV and mental illness

Examples of Specialty Areas Based on Setting
- Community
- Inpatient unit
- Prisons
- Nursing homes
- Detention centres
- General hospitals
- Emergency departments
- General practice clinics and primary care
- Rural, remote
- Schools

HIV, Human Immunodeficiency Virus.

THE IMPORTANCE OF THE SETTING IN WHICH MENTAL HEALTHCARE IS DELIVERED

Irrespective of beliefs about the nature of mental disorders, responsibility for people with a mental illness has historically been considered a domestic concern (Porter 2002). However, for a significant period, confinement of the mentally ill in madhouses and later asylums dominated as a setting for service provision. In contrast, during the latter half of the 20th century, the preference for the community as the preferred setting for the provision of care emerged.

The Asylum

In the 17th century, when it was more generally believed that people with a mental illness were insane (that is, rather than possessed, they were believed to be without reason and akin to wild beasts), small, private and public asylums were developed, wherein they could be segregated from the sane. The asylums varied markedly in terms of the quality of care they provided, and many meted out brutal treatments. Two infamous madhouses of the time were St Mary of Bethlehem in London, from whence the word *bedlam* is derived, and the Hôpital Général in Paris. The inmates at both were chained and tortured, and at Bedlam they were put on display for the amusement and edification of Sunday visitors.

The 18th century enlightenment brought a general reforming zeal as well as new ideas about madness as a mental condition that could be best treated by mental means. Furthermore, greater experience with managing the mentally ill gave rise to the idea that the asylum could be used as a therapeutic tool as opposed to merely a means of confinement and segregation. One of the foremost advocates of this progressive thinking was Philippe Pinel (1745–1826). Pinel, who is considered the founder of modern psychiatry, freed the inmates of the Bicêtre and Salpêtrière asylums in Paris from their chains (Shorter 1997, 2008). He also provided the inmates with nourishing food, warm baths and useful activity; abolished whips and other instruments of torture; and treated them with kindness. Important outcomes of these changes were that many inmates improved dramatically, while others were less violent when allowed to move around. Pinel coined the term 'le traitement moral', which translated as 'moral treatment', a phrase later popularised by the Englishman and Quaker tea merchant, William Tuke (1732–1822) (Shorter 1997, 2008). Tuke's humanitarian philosophy, which was in stark contrast to the bleedings, purges, chains and denial of basic necessities for life that had marked other treatment approaches, was that mental illness was best treated by beautiful scenery, pleasant distractions and physical comfort. He put his policies of care and kindness into practice at the York Retreat, which he established for the care of members of the local Quaker community suffering from mental illnesses.

An important assumption on which moral treatment rested was that a closed environment was most conducive to the return of reason in the inmates (Porter 2002). Consequently, purpose-built and designed institutions for confining the mentally ill were constructed during the 19th century (Porter 2002). The meaning of 'asylum' is to provide shelter, protection and a place of refuge but unfortunately the humanitarian aspirations of the 18th century eventually collapsed under the weight of the huge numbers of people being housed within them. These large, public institutions were rarely intended to be therapeutic, but were custodial. The mentally ill were housed and fed, but little occurred in the way of treatment. By World War I they had become little more than vast warehouses (Shorter 1997).

The Therapeutic Use of the Environment

In the 20th century, changes and ideas that led to the development of modern therapeutic environments took two different courses. One led to changes within psychiatric asylums themselves, while the other led to the development of services outside the existing institutions of the time: services that were often developed in conjunction with new treatment modalities. In both cases their development was partly a reaction to the institutions developed in the 19th century and their effects on inmates.

The therapeutic community has been described as an important 20th century innovation in care delivery for people with a mental illness (Mills & Harrison 2007). Overturning earlier ideas about the nature of social control, its essence was the flattening of professional hierarchies and the institution of democratic as opposed to authoritarian processes. Two of the most important early contributors to the development of the therapeutic community during the 20th century were Thomas Main (1911–1990) in the UK during the late 1940s and Maxwell Jones (1907–1990) in the United States during the 1950s (Thomas et al. 2002). They were among the first modern psychiatrists to recognise the role of the social environment in effecting change in both staff and patients. The foundation for Main's therapeutic aims (Main 1946, 1980) was laid at Northfield Military Hospital in the UK, where two psychiatrists, John Rickman and Wilfred Bion, had experimented with group treatments (Mills & Harrison 2007).

Jones built his ideas on the observations made by him and other psychiatrists during World War II, that some army units created pathology among soldiers. Jones pioneered the idea that 'a hospital might become therapeutic as a social organisation' (Fischer 2012). He believed all human social organisation comprised a setting for social and interpersonal relations that could either enhance or limit human potential for health and wellbeing. Jones believed that patients should have a democratic voice in how the ward environments were run and in their individual courses of care and treatment. At the time it was considered revolutionary, but diminished in significance post-deinstitutionalisation until recent times with the resurgence of recovery-focussed care.

Jones (1953) used the concept of therapeutic community to describe his innovations in the wards of large asylums during the 1940s and 1950s, although the term 'therapeutic community' can be traced to an earlier lecture given by the American psychiatrist Harry Stack Sullivan in 1939 (Mills & Harrison 2007). For Jones, the essence of the concept of therapeutic community was a change to the organisational ethos of large mental institutions. He started this change in 1940 when he altered the structure of a psychiatric unit at the Maudsley Hospital in London from a punitive, authoritarian one to one where the patients—100 soldiers with 'effort syndrome' (a psychosomatic disorder marked by fatigue)—were encouraged to become actively involved in their own treatment, were educated about their symptoms and were given a work programme. The outcomes of these changes were that staff behaved less like custodians and more like facilitators and a more democratic ward culture emerged.

One of the most important tenets to be derived from Jones' work is that, in order to be therapeutic, a setting has to be recovery focused. A therapeutic milieu is a consciously organised environment demanding deliberate decision making and an experienced staff who understand inpatient psychiatry (Vatne & Hoem 2008). The concept of milieu means more than just the physical environment. It includes the social, emotional, interpersonal, professional and managerial elements that comprise a particular setting. In a therapeutic milieu these elements are not considered simply part of the usual background to treatment but are critical influences on therapy. The milieu is intended to meet not only patients' needs for psychiatric, medical and nursing care, but also their needs for recreation, occupation and social interaction.

The principles of a therapeutic milieu remain current in contemporary mental health settings (Mahoney et al. 2009), although modifications and additions have been made in order to meet modern challenges of service delivery. The concepts of therapeutic milieu and a recovery focus are of particular importance to bed-based settings where patients spend a significant proportion, if not all, of their day. However, there needs to be a whole-of-service approach to therapeutic work because, in contemporary practice, inpatient admissions are shorter and the work that is begun there needs to continue on into community settings.

The Changing Role of the Nurse

From what you have read about the history of mental health, you will be able to glean that the role of the nurse has adapted from being a 'custodian' or 'lunatic attendant' to the current roles of 'primary nurse', 'care coordinator' or 'key worker'. In looking back at the institutional era of mental health nursing, it is clear that the care provided by attendants was as humane and holistic as the environment of the time permitted. It is important to recognise that Pinel's reforms could never have been introduced without the support of the attendants at the time (Walk 1961).

Attendants/nurses were responsible for ensuring that people's needs were met, including basic nutritional requirements, adequate personal hygiene and clothing and recreational and social opportunities. Accommodation was made as homelike as possible. It is still nurses who are pivotal in establishing and maintaining the therapeutic milieu, as it is nurses who are entrusted with patient care 24 hours per day and who have the most contact with people in inpatient care.

As more humane attitudes to the mentally ill developed, education of the attendants and nurses was introduced. In the UK in the 18th and 19th century the term 'keeper' was commonly used, seeming to imply the nurse's role focussed on restriction and control. When the asylum system opened in 1845 the preferred term became 'attendant', indicating a more humanitarian approach to care. By the end of the 19th century 'nurse' was preferred and shows the shift in viewing nursing more as a developing profession. Today the term 'mental health nurse' is preferred, but 'psychiatric nurse' is also used interchangeably (RCN 2015). During this time the importance of concepts such as the therapeutic milieu and the therapeutic use of self made their way into the vocabulary of the mental health nurse.

The Multidisciplinary Team

The concept of the multidisciplinary team arose out of the advent of improved treatments for mental illness and the recognition of the need for professional discipline-specific assistance to facilitate patient transition from the hospital setting into the community. The professions that comprise the multidisciplinary team include registered mental health nurses, psychiatrists, psychologists, social workers and occupational therapists. In addition, complementary therapists such as art or music therapists can be a valuable addition to the team. Depending on local and national variations, other members might include speech and language therapists, support workers, housing support workers and activity coordinators. While every discipline has a specific role to fill, roles do overlap. This overlap can be observed most clearly in the conduct of various therapies, where any member of the team may take the lead role. In the community, the multidisciplinary team 'is a mechanism for case allocation, clinical decision making, teaching, training and supervision and the application of the necessary skill mix for the best outcomes for patients' (Renouf & Meadows 2001). It also offers the advantage of continuity of care. When a staff member goes on leave, there is always someone else who can fill in. The discipline-specific roles are set out in Box 5.2.

A significant philosophical change in care delivery that has occurred since the 2000s is the adoption within mental health services of recovery principles. (See Chapter 2 for a full discussion of recovery.) Recovery-informed practice supports the belief that people can recover from illness and learn to live with any limitations imposed by the illness to live rewarding and meaningful lives. The basis of all recovery-based practice is the formation of a collaborative relationship between the person and the clinician. This relationship is purposeful and assists the person to recognise their strengths and develop goals for the future. The clinician does not ignore aspects of the person's care that need to be addressed, but uses the relationship formed with the person to address issues such as safety and relapse prevention in a therapeutic manner.

The contribution of the multidisciplinary team is to support the person in their journey towards recovery. The best way of supporting an individual's recovery will vary from person to person as each person will have their own journey of recovery with their own individualised goals. Some of the characteristics of recovery are that it is:

- a unique and personal journey
- a normal human process
- an ongoing experience and not the same as an end point or cure
- a journey rarely taken alone
- nonlinear and frequently interspersed with both achievement and setbacks (Davidson & Roe 2007)

In keeping with recovery principles, lived experience peer workers/patient representatives are now included in the multidisciplinary team. The philosophy of including patient representatives within teams focusses on coproduction, putting people with lived experiences of mental health illness at the centre of planning and delivering mental health services. Coproduction values patients as experts through experience, offering empathy, validation and instilling hope in patients who have been recently diagnosed or who have lost hope in their ability to recover from mental illness. Peer support can be described as promoting a wellness model that focusses on strengths, recovery, the positive aspects of people and their ability to function effectively and supportively, rather than on an illness model. This approach ensures that the emphasis is on the individual rather than on problems or symptoms experienced. The peer worker can demonstrate the elements of recovery in a supportive manner, as the peer worker can relate to the patient in a truly empathetic way. The peer worker can instil hope and the possibility of recovery in a manner that cannot be achieved by clinicians alone (Delaney 2010; Repper & Martin 2011).

There are considerations that need to be addressed when working with the peer workforce in a professional setting (Delaney 2010; Doughty & Tse 2011; Repper & Martin 2011). It is important to ensure that peer workers receive enough support to deal with the issues they may face when working with others who are experiencing similar problems. Transferential challenges may arise and place stress on the therapeutic relationship between peer workers and patients. Professional accountability and professional boundaries may also seem blurred in coproduction and the peer workforce. More research is required to assess the benefit of this type of workforce, although the research to date has found a positive impact within services that have employed people with lived experience (Repper & Martin 2011).

A CONTINUUM OF MENTAL HEALTH SERVICES ACROSS THE LIFESPAN

Contemporary mental health services are based in hospital and community settings, with the predominant preference for services to be provided in the least restrictive environment (community and homes) where possible. Services are provided by government (public), non-government and private organisations. Services can be generalist or specialist in nature for patients across the lifespan from the perinatal and infant period through to childhood and adolescence (see Chapter 11) and onto adulthood and older age (see Chapter 12).

BOX 5.2 Members of the Multidisciplinary Team

Mental Health Nurse

Nurses make up the largest group of workers in the mental health system. In order to practise, nurses must be registered with the Nursing and Midwifery Council.

Registration as a nurse follows completion of a 3-year BSc (Hons) Nursing degree, or a 2-year MSc Graduate Entry Nursing post-graduate degree in Mental Health. Nursing education has a strong foundation in the biopsychosocial model of healthcare.

Mental health nurses work in a wide range of settings and practise with a variety of patients utilising different models of service delivery and frameworks for helping people. As in every nursing specialty, nurses range from novice to expert practitioners. Advanced practice nurses are expected to be prepared to masters level and possess a high degree of knowledge, skill and experience applied in the nurse–patient relationship in order to achieve optimal outcomes through critical analysis, problem solving and accurate decision making. The nurse's role is to assist patients to function when their ability to do this has been lost (temporarily or permanently) due to illness. For example, if a patient is unable to wash, the nurse helps them to wash; if they are unable to feed themselves, the nurse helps feed them; if they are unable to walk, the nurse assists them; if they have lost touch with hope, the nurse holds onto hope; or if they have lost touch with reality, the nurse provides reality orientation. At the centre of mental health nursing is the nurse's relationship with the patient. As identified in Chapter 1 the nurse utilises him- or herself therapeutically in the service of the patient.

The importance of the nurse–patient relationship was highlighted in a study of expert mental health nurses that described a relational interplay between nurses and their patients (Santangelo 2015). Interacting therapeutically during everyday tasks was considered an important part of mental health nursing. In addition, the ability and willingness of the nurse to be with patients in the here-and-now, in both the extreme and the mundane moments of the patient's existence, was considered an essential component of nursing care. The noticing and monitoring role of the mental health nurse was described as being alert to disruptions in health and from those observations being able to gauge what needs to be done and when. The findings of this study highlight the skill set that assists mental health nurses to work well with patients with complex needs when other disciplines find they have nothing to offer.

Psychiatrist

The psychiatrist is a medical specialist in the diagnosis and treatment of mental illness but, by virtue of their initial training, also understands physical illnesses. The psychiatrist initially undertakes a medical degree and then undergoes further specialty training in psychiatry. In the UK, the Royal College of Psychiatrists (RCPsych) is responsible for training, educating and representing psychiatrists (RCPsych 2018). In many teams the psychiatrist is responsible for diagnosing mental disorders, prescribing the biological aspects of treatment, and authorising admission, discharge, special leave or close observation, although increasingly advanced practice mental health nurses are taking up these practices. As with other professionals in the team, psychiatrists, depending on interest and training, might also engage in various forms of psychotherapy.

Psychologist

Psychologists complete an undergraduate degree but usually complete postgraduate studies before practising. The clinical psychologist is educated to at least Honours level and many will also have a master's degree or PhD. Psychologists are experts in human behaviour, having studied the brain, memory, learning, human development and the processes determining how people think, feel, behave and react. Psychologists apply their expertise using reliable and scientifically supported methods (British Psychological Society 2018).

Clinical psychologists are employed in community and inpatient mental health settings and have skills in:

- psychological assessment and diagnosis of major mental illnesses and psychological problems, with particular training in the selection and administration of psychological tests such as those designed to assess attributes like intelligence or mood states such as depression
- the delivery of a range of psychological techniques to people with mental health problems
- the application of psychological theory and scientific research to solve complex clinical psychological problems requiring individually tailored interventions
- conducting research on prevention, diagnosis, assessment, treatment and outcomes
- evaluation of psychological interventions and programmes in various settings (British Psychological Society 2018).

Social Worker

Social workers undertake an undergraduate degree in social work and underpinning their knowledge base are frameworks of social justice, human rights, collective responsibility and respect for diversity. The social worker is interested in how aspects of the social environment affect the experience of illness and recovery and their role is to assist the patient to identify and address these issues where possible. Social workers are particularly helpful in ensuring that patients receive their just entitlements in pensions and benefits, as well as assessing and accessing suitable accommodation (British Association of Social Workers 2018).

Occupational Therapist

Occupational therapists undertake a degree in occupational therapy and are interested in promoting health and wellbeing through occupation. Occupational therapists help patients to become independent in activities of daily living and focus on facilitating patients' occupational functioning and/or assessing and treating the barriers to their engagement in meaningful work or activity. They assess and evaluate a person's performance in the full range of their occupational functions, including their ability to budget for food and accommodation, to pursue meaningful leisure activities and to seek paid and voluntary employment. The occupational therapist considers the type of practical assistance a patient might need to function in the community (Royal College of Occupational Therapists 2018).

There are opportunities for mental health nurses to work in all of these services with new roles constantly emerging.

The following section describes hospital services such as acute inpatient mental health units, general hospitals and emergency departments. The discussion also covers the wide range of community services, including specialist community mental health services and other community health and primary care mental health services.

Hospital and Bed-Based Services

Hospital and bed-based services have dominated mental healthcare in the past but with the emergence of deinstitutionalisation and a focus on recovery, a preference for community-based services has become the norm. A range of bed-based services is provided depending on the patient's care needs, presenting risks and age. The level of observation, supervision and restriction provided varies from open to locked doors with access to intensive care areas and seclusion facilities. The philosophy of providing the least restrictive option possible guides the choice of setting. It can be useful to think of services providing a continuum of acute, subacute and extended care. At the acute end of the continuum is the inpatient mental health unit. For patients who need longer term and/or secure care, specially designed units are also provided.

General hospital wards and emergency departments also form part of bed-based services. Emergency departments are the key access point for health emergencies of all types, including psychiatric emergencies. For example, people who require attention after deliberate self-harm frequently present for care to emergency departments and may require ongoing care in a general hospital.

There is significant psychiatric comorbidity in both emergency department (Fulbrook & Lawrence 2015; Lee et al. 2008) and general hospital patients and this results in patient suffering, increases in morbidity and mortality, significant distress for families and staff and increases in resource usage (Aitken et al. 2014; Mental Health Network 2012; Slade et al. 2009; Zolnierek 2009). Patients of mental health services have higher rates of physical disorders than the general population (Collins et al. 2012; Happell et al. 2015; Hardy et al. 2013) and this population accesses general healthcare through mainstream health programmes. General hospitals are increasingly recognising their role in the mental healthcare of their patients by incorporating mental health services into hospital and emergency departments. In many hospitals, mental health clinicians are co-located in emergency departments, providing assessment, treatment and referral services for people presenting with mental health issues (McNamara et al. 2008; Sharrock et al. 2008; Wand et al. 2012, 2015).

Inpatient Settings

As mentioned earlier in this chapter, the idea that the setting in which mental healthcare is delivered needs to be recovery oriented is particularly true for bed-based settings. Given the preference for community-based care, bed-based settings make up a small component of the overall continuum of care. However, bed-based settings can be the most traumatising for people coming in for an admission. Inpatient units can be quite challenging for patients with no experience of inpatient care. Hospital stays have become shorter, acuity has increased and the environment is at times noisy, with multiple demands placed on both staff and patients. The inpatient unit environment also has a fluctuating community, with staff changing shifts over a 24-hour period and patients moving in and out of the unit as they are admitted and discharged.

Tensions exist between maintaining the order of the inpatient setting and ensuring that patients' choices, preferences and satisfaction are provided for. The rules and regulations of busy inpatient units can lead to patients feeling powerless and a power imbalance in their relationships with care providers (Chen et al. 2013). In order to provide an environment that is healing and therapeutic, staff are continually assessing the unit for situations that could affect the milieu in an adverse manner. Consideration is given to times when people are being admitted to the unit, or discharged from the unit, as well as to times when the unit is busy and staff are unable to be present in sufficient numbers and to any disruptions to the usual routine of the unit, including any staffing issues.

The important principles and goals governing the inpatient therapeutic milieu are described in the following sections and summarised in Box 5.3.

Principles

Open communication. In the therapeutic milieu, great value is placed on communication (Rapoport 1960). This communication begins at first greeting with a newly admitted patient. Emphasis should be placed on providing time for the relationship to develop through respectful and open communication. This begins with acceptance of the person and an inquiry into what has brought the person to hospital, including any goals that the person has about their treatment. Knowing the person's expectations will help ensure that these expectations can be met and anything that cannot be addressed during the hospital stay is very clearly articulated. For example, the person may want to improve their financial situation, but they are receiving a limited pension. The discussion of financial improvement might begin in the hospital setting but

BOX 5.3 The Inpatient Therapeutic Milieu

Principles
- Open communication
- Democratisation
- Orientation to the therapeutic milieu
- Privacy and respect for one another
- Group cohesion

Goals
- Containment
- Safe environment
- Structure
- Support
- Involvement
- Validation
- Symptom management
- Maintaining links with the patient's family or significant others
- Developing and maintaining links with the community

might not be realised until the person is discharged and able to explore options more thoroughly.

Staff and patients form part of the therapeutic milieu and work in collaboration in care provision, with each having a valuable contribution to make to the recovery journey. In order to be able to contribute effectively it is necessary that everyone, including the patient, has all the information necessary to make informed decisions. Effective decisions rely on everyone knowing and working towards the same goals.

Democratisation. Democratisation is a core element of the acute inpatient unit (Rapoport 1960). The aim is to create an environment in which patients feel free to express themselves without fear of judgement or reprisal; an environment where there are opportunities to participate in decision making about how care is to be provided in an individual manner. Patients can be expected to assist in decision making in relation to the therapeutic activities that are conducted on the unit. Every effort should be made to cater to the cultural needs of patients when planning therapeutic activities. Shared decision making about the rules of the unit will provide ownership and respectful adherence as people will have a greater understanding of why some rules are in operation. Patient participation in decision making communicates an expectation of healthy behaviour. This practice is therapeutic insofar as it recognises the strengths of patients and facilitates interaction and understanding. However, patients will vary in their ability to contribute to decision making depending on the acuity of their symptoms, which may change rapidly.

Orientation to the therapeutic milieu. Orientation to the therapeutic milieu is important in developing open communication and rapport with patients. All staff, patients and visitors who come into the inpatient unit need to know about expectations in relation to acceptable behaviours, the layout of the unit, timing of activities, the roles of the treating team, visiting hours, information about legal requirements (especially if someone is under mental health legislation) and any other information that is pertinent to ensure a comfortable stay on the unit. Conflict arises when people do not have a good understanding of expectations or of decisions that have been made without their knowledge.

When orientation is completed properly, all people who are part of the inpatient unit have comfort in knowing what to expect and how situations will be managed if they arise; there are no surprises. People are treated with courtesy and respect regardless of their role and, when this is not the case, the consequences of problematic behaviour are transparent (see Box 5.4). Any rules or policies are clearly articulated in

BOX 5.4 Limit Setting

Limits are part of the reality of everyday life. In terms of the therapeutic milieu, the establishment and maintenance of clear limits and boundaries provide a framework from within which patients, staff and visitors can function. People generally feel more secure when messages are clear and unambiguous, when they know what the rules are and when what is expected of them is consistent. People are able to function more productively when 'the goal posts do not keep shifting' (Sharrock & Rickard 2002). As a therapeutic strategy, limit setting provides a structure and a sense of caring and a greater sense of control for the patient. Establishing limits is an essential aspect of the therapeutic relationship.

Principles to Remember when Selecting Limits

- Limits must be consistent with policy and reflect the philosophy of the hospital and the unit.
- Staff must be aware that they are role models for the limits they set. Their behaviour must be consistent with what is expected of the patient and visitors.
- Patient information and orientation processes must reflect these limits consistently and clearly and yet be flexible enough so that individualised care planning can be provided.
- Limits should be clear and simple to minimise misinterpretation by staff and patients.
- Limits should have a clear rationale; that is, have some therapeutic and/or practical aim.
- Limits should not be unnecessary or controlling.
- Teamwork and consistency are essential. Where possible, the limits selected should be understood and supported by all staff involved in the care of the patient.
- Limits must be selected so that staff have the best chance to maintain the limits consistently on all shifts, remembering that unexpected contingencies will always arise. When these occur, discuss and/or document so that there is a consistent approach in place for the next time.

Principles to Remember when Enforcing Limits

- Limits should be clearly and simply stated in a nonpunitive/noncondemning manner. Be assertive, confident and do not present as angry. Explain clearly what behaviour is inappropriate and what is expected of the person. Include a brief rationale without entering into extensive debate or rationalisation.
- Negotiate only those limits that are negotiable.
- Explain the natural consequences of actions calmly and factually.
- If consequences are set, they should be enforced as soon as possible after the limit has been broken.
- Do not make threats or set consequences that cannot be followed through.
- Offer alternative actions/options/behaviour
- Be mindful of the feelings of loss of control people often experience in hospital.
- If you anticipate that there is likely to be testing of limits by a patient, plan your responses in advance.
- Be clear in your own mind what the limit is and why it is necessary.
- Do not give mixed messages
- Be aware of your own motivations and reactions to the person's behaviour and situation. Provide support to colleagues by giving the team an opportunity to discuss interactions with patients and visitors. This helps the team maintain clarity and cohesiveness, particularly in difficult situations.

(*Source:* Sharrock J., Rickard, N., 2002. Limit setting: a useful strategy in rehabilitation. Australian Journal of Advanced Nursing 19(4):21–26. Reprinted with permission of the Australian Nursing & Midwifery Federation.)

a language that can be understood by all, using interpreters if necessary for people whose first language is not English.

Privacy and respect for one another. Careful explanation should be provided to patients when they come into the hospital setting about what is expected concerning their own and other people's behaviour. This should be done in a manner that is respectful and maintains the privacy of all concerned. For some it may be their first contact with mental health services and they may be fearful about other patients. There is still much stigma associated with having a mental illness, and there are not many people who are happy to hear their diagnosis, let alone be admitted to hospital for treatment. When people are admitted to the unit they may be experiencing symptoms that interfere with their normal behaviour and it is at these times that nursing staff in particular must take on the role of protector. For example, if a person is exhibiting disinhibition and is removing their clothing in a public area, it is imperative that the person be shielded from others and guided away from public spaces into an area that is private. Careful explanation should be given for this intervention. Information should also be given to others in the area so that they understand that the person is safe and being treated in a more private space. Likewise, if there is aggression on the unit and restrictive interventions are used, it is important for all to have a good understanding as to why this intervention has been used and that the person is safe, without divulging more than is required for the situation to maintain the person's privacy.

Group cohesion. Group cohesion is important in order to create a climate of support and involvement (Rapoport 1960). Sharing among staff and patients of daily duties and unit resources facilitates a sense of community. Developing group cohesiveness has become increasingly difficult since the advent of very short lengths of stay (Watson 1992). Short lengths of stay mean patients may not get to know their co-patients and rarely know about their progress. An example of developing a sense of community is a ward barbecue, which brings staff and patients together to prepare and share a meal. Activity groups, meal times and communal areas are also important elements in bringing people together to provide support for each other.

Goals

Containment. Containment can be considered from both a psychological and a physical perspective.

Psychological (or emotional) containment arises from psychoanalytic theory and remains relevant to current practice (Beatson et al. 2010; Bowles et al. 2002). It is best understood as the creation of a relationship and an environment that makes space for and can tolerate the intense emotions experienced by patients. Containment puts boundaries around chaos and around the anxieties about being in the world (Grotstein 1997). The multidisciplinary team, and especially the nurse, creates space for psychic and emotional pain to be expressed without unnecessary restrictions; a space that is bounded by compassionate limits (see Box 5.4) to form a safe 'container' for emotional expression. This is the psychological equivalent to the physical act of holding another. The nurse is not overwhelmed by the distress but is able to 'sit with' the discomfort that is evoked by the patient. To achieve this, the nurse needs to maintain a stable and predictable emotional state and convey this to the patient. Within this context, anxiety is held and made more bearable, allowing therapy (or emotional growth) to occur (Holmes 1984). The aim is that through the recovery process, the patient will be more able to contain and regulate their own emotional states.

Physical containment (Bowers 2014) is achieved through restrictive practices that are minimised as far as possible. Inpatient units are expected to provide a place of safety, by managing risk or preventing behaviours that will lead to self-harm or the harm of others. Many patients admitted to acute mental health units can be acutely unwell and are legally detained against their will (see Chapter 4). Modern mental health inpatient units are often designed to restrict access to the community through devices such as locked doors and high-dependency units. Inpatient units seek to ensure the safety of patients and to compensate for their lack of internal controls. These goals are encoded in policies; for example, the precautions to be taken with patients deemed to be violent or suicidal, such as isolating them from other patients or providing constant supervision (Delaney et al. 2000). Measures taken include seclusion, special observation, detention in hospital, searching procedures, restrictions on inpatients, intensive care, physical restraint and enforced medication (Bowers et al. 2009). For many people with mental illness, the hospital is 'a refuge from self-destructiveness' and some patients experience the confinement of the unit as 'freeing' (Thomas et al. 2002). In other cases, locking the doors to units has been associated with depression (Haglund & Von Essen 2005) and higher levels of self-harm (Bowers et al. 2008).

Shorter stays, increased patient acuity in the acute setting and patients with more complex needs mean that a greater emphasis is placed on maintaining safety in the inpatient milieu. Two important nursing interventions to support and contribute to the therapeutic environment and safety are limit setting (see Box 5.4) and nursing observation (see Box 5.5). The therapeutic milieu needs sufficient experienced nursing staff to maintain a continuous watchful presence in a non-threatening, nonintrusive manner and to set reasonable limits on behaviour. Such watchfulness is not necessarily perceived by patients as intrusive, although it does need to be balanced with engagement and interaction (Mullen 2009). Nurses also monitor the level of environmental stimulation and provide patients with suitable activities and milieu treatments such as relaxation, sensory modulation, psychoeducation, medication, exercise, cooking and discussion groups.

? CRITICAL THINKING CHALLENGE 5.1

Intense observation at a 1:1 level presents a challenge for nurses. For example, how would you go about developing a therapeutic relationship with a patient under these circumstances? Do you think that there is a conflict between what can be seen as the 'surveillance' or 'custodial' aspect of observation and the 'caring' component?

PATIENT STORY 5.1 Catherine

Then suddenly I was moved to a place that I thought would be a relief, but in reality, was just as frightening. Tubes were inserted, veins were punctured, blood was taken, everything was monitored. I wasn't allowed to sleep by myself, I wasn't allowed to pee by myself. All I wanted to do was to escape the reality that I had become. I wanted to run into the fresh air and open my lungs and scream. I wanted to dive into the ocean and feel the salty, ice-cold water against my skin. And yet all I felt was grey. Numb. Silenced. There was no-one to trust, no-one to allow in. I was still on my own, fighting this.

Each day, three times a day, what felt like a game of Russian roulette was played. Which nurse would be on duty to watch my every move? Which nurse would become my shadow? Which nurse would have an influence on my behaviour for the next 8 hours? Subconsciously I would play a game at the start of each shift. The level of respect given to me by the nurse was relative to the amount of respect I would give back. Childish, yes. Dangerous also. The 'disrespect' I thought I was giving back to the nurse was in fact only harming myself. I would become furious with them if they didn't treat me as a person with an illness, rather than just an illness. Couldn't they see the real me underneath—or didn't they at least want to try to? Instead they became the master, simply there to control and ensure they completed their shift ticking all the boxes on the checklist. My aim then became to ensure those boxes were left unchecked. Suddenly, towels became sodden as my feeding tube was disconnected, feeders were switched off without knowledge and feeding tubes were pulled out when eyes were averted. How could I let this nurse finish their shift thinking they had won, when I was left there feeling like I was no-one?

Some shifts, there was relief. Relief because I didn't have to conjure up ways to disrespect the nurse. I could let go, knowing this shift would be ok. That I would have a support, rather than a controller. Someone to look after me and help protect me. Help protect me from myself. Help protect me from this horrible thing.

What a lot of people don't understand is how the smallest of things can either push one further down that hole, or shine the brightest of lights on it—revealing the ladder leading me out.

I experienced many of these moments lying in that hospital bed. Moments where I would think to myself—what is the point? Why shouldn't I walk down those stairs and risk my heart overloading? Why should I drink that milkshake that will bring so much angst with it that I will lay for the next 2 hours fighting the will to throw it up? But then, unexpectedly someone would say something that would allow me to see the reason for this fight. And the determination would reignite inside me to push through. I can still feel the emotion and hopelessness deep in my bones when a nurse would look at me and not see the real Catherine in my eyes. Who wouldn't ask me what inspired me, what I loved, who I wanted to be. They would read my history as if that was the story of who I was.

Parallel to that I can also still feel the profound respect I had for those that showed me respect, who would come and sit beside me and ask me who the photos on the wall were of, who would ask me what book I was reading. These people gave me the hope that I did exist beneath this horrible illness, that there was a chance I could come out the other side and still exist.

In Patient Story 5.1 Catherine describes her experience of being constantly observed when she was moved from the mental health inpatient unit to a general medical ward to receive urgent interventions for life-threatening malnourishment in the context of anorexia nervosa.

Safe environment. One important consideration when implementing a therapeutic environment is the need for safety. In the acute inpatient unit this includes the safety of the patients, the staff and other people who come into the unit as visitors or contracted workers. Len Bowers and his research team (Bowers et al. 2005, 2014) have developed an extensive intervention programme focussing on reducing the incidence of aggression within inpatient units which can be located at the Safewards website www.safewards.net (Bowers 2015).

The two vital components of Safewards are the model and the intervention. The Safewards conceptual model, derived from a large body of empirical studies in acute wards, explains the relationship between conflict and containment in this setting and the opportunities that exist for nurses to intervene, both to prevent conflict and to respond in least restrictive ways when conflict arises (Bowers 2014). The Safewards intervention is a set of specific prevention and intervention strategies, developed to correspond to diverse flashpoints identified in the model. The objective of the model is to identify what issues can create flashpoints on an acute mental health unit and work out ways that nurses and patients can stop flashpoints from becoming conflicts which can lead to containment or restrictive interventions.

Interventions range from staff reflecting on their own approach to people experiencing agitation and aggression to approaches that can be used to modify the environment or plan for situations that can be a trigger for aggression within the inpatient setting. One of the easiest interventions that can be implemented without any cost to the organisation is the language nurses use when addressing people in the acute inpatient setting. It does not cost anything for nurses to be polite and courteous to all people they come into contact with in the acute inpatient unit, regardless of the person's presentation. Even people in their most unwell state will recognise kindness and respond accordingly. At the Safewards website, clinicians can access information about a whole range of interventions that are evidence based. The site includes explanatory information on each intervention and how they can be incorporated into practice. The full range of interventions is included in

BOX 5.5 Nursing Observation in an Inpatient Setting

A major nursing activity in mental health units is observation. As was described earlier, the nurse's role in noticing and monitoring patients, being alert to disruptions in health and from those observations being able to gauge what needs to be done and when it needs to be done is important. The art of nursing is demonstrated when the nurse can effectively integrate the observation of patients with therapeutic engagement with the patients. However, this is a challenge. Observation can be experienced by both the nurse and the patient as surveillance or a custodial activity. Contemporary descriptions of observation attempt to reconcile this conflict and this is demonstrated in the following statement:

> *'. . . nursing observation is considered to be the purposeful gathering of information from people receiving care to inform clinical decision making. Undertaking observation requires nurses to be person centred and to engage therapeutically with those receiving care. Only through talking with people receiving care do nurses gain a comprehensive understanding of their most pressing issues. Underpinning all nursing observation should be the goal of supporting recovery. Implicit in this definition is the promotion of active engagement with people, rather than passively watching them from a distance' (Department of Health 2013).*

The intensity of observations varies depending on the clinical assessment. The patient may be sighted at regular intervals—for example, at the start and the end of the shift. Patients who are more acutely unwell may need to be sighted more frequently—for example, every 30 minutes or even every 10–15 minutes. If the patient is particularly at risk of harm to self and/or others and requires intensive nursing care, 1:1 nursing care may be instituted. This is also known as 'special observation' (Holyoake 2013), 'constant observation' (Pitula & Cardell 1996) or 'enhanced observation' (Cox et al. 2010). Several papers have explored the patient's perspective of 1:1 observation (Bowles et al. 2002; Thomas et al. 2002; Jones et al. 2000; Cardell & Pitula 1999; Moorehead et al. 1996; Pitula & Cardell 1996). The lived experience is both positive and negative and, not surprisingly, a key variable in the experiences documented was the attributes of the nurse undertaking the observation. Recurring themes within the positive experiences were that the nurses engaged in socially appropriate behaviour such as greeting the patients and introducing themselves. Nurses also had some form of conversation with the patients, showed an interest in and respect for the patients, managed proximity to the patients sensitively, assisted the patients to feel safe and conveyed hopeful and positive attitudes. 1:1 is the most intensive and intrusive level of observation and is used only when the risk warrants it.

Keeping these views in mind, the nurse undertaking 1:1 care of the patient at the most intense level:

- undertakes continuous visual observation, in the same room, including accompanying the patient to the shower and toilet and staying as close as possible to the patient taking into account any risk of harm to the staff member (for example, from hitting or kicking)
- monitors the patient's mental state including risk status
- assists the patient to comply with treatment to promote recovery through instruction and persuasion
- provides emotional support and skilled companionship balancing conversation, silence, distraction and activities
- supports the patient to work towards autonomous decision making and self-care
- manages the lack of privacy, sense of confinement and invasion of personal space by acknowledging the patient as a human being and the intrusion on his/her space in a sensitive but matter-of-fact manner, and being particularly sensitive during showering and toileting
- develops a therapeutic relationship with the patient demonstrating empathy, warmth, optimism, understanding, willingness to help and a nonjudgemental approach
- provides information and updates on progress to the patient
- supports the patient through distressing incidents
- assesses and monitors the environment for items that may increase the risk to the patient or others but ensures that the risk warrants any removal of important personal items
- documents a report in the patient's medical record
- provides a comprehensive handover to the incoming nurse.

Box 5.6. The beauty of the Safewards interventions is that they are simple to understand, have an evidence base, can be used independently or as a whole and, above all, have a strong recovery focus in their approach and the language used to implement each component.

Structure. The structure of the milieu refers to how time, people and places are organised. A predictable structure to a person's day provides order and stability; it establishes routines and schedules for patients, staff and the group as a whole. A sound structure is achieved by ensuring that patients are oriented to the unit as described earlier. The physical environment includes colours, lighting, furniture and unit design and layout chosen to create a healing environment. The architecture of a setting, through the provision of spaces for both private contemplation and social interaction, influences activities such as eating, talking, receiving visitors and using the telephone, as well as helping to ensure that patients maintain some control over their lives. Some inkling of the value patients place on structure can be gleaned from their approval of hospital cleanliness, availability of fresh fruit, choice of menu and well-stocked refrigerators and snack cabinets (Thomas et al. 2002).

Support. The aim of support is to help patients to feel safe, to calm themselves and to promote hope, a sense of wellbeing and self-esteem. Support is achieved by nurses being emotionally available to patients, allowing and helping them to express their emotions, and interacting in a respectful way. Patients can have an identified primary nurse or recovery partner who they know by name. Nurses can ensure their availability by being visible on the ward. Support can be conveyed by:

- listening to patients
- providing attention, praise and reassurance
- providing assistance in using and developing coping skills
- providing education and direction

BOX 5.6 Safewards Interventions

- *Clear Mutual Expectation*—this focusses on ensuring that people coming into the acute inpatient setting are given proper orientation so that they know what to expect during their stay.
- *Soft Words*—being mindful of the language we use during de-escalation techniques.
- *Talk Down*—a range of de-escalation phrases that can be used to defuse a situation.
- *Positive Words*—giving encouragement and reinforcement of positive behaviours.
- *Bad News Mitigation*—a mindful way in which to impart information that people do not necessarily want to hear as part of their inpatient stay; an example might be when informing people that they do not have permission to leave the unit at present, or that they are unable to smoke due to occupational health and safety legislation.
- *Know Each Other*—having information available about the treating team so that people coming into the inpatient unit have an idea about the people who are providing their care.
- *Mutual Help Meeting*—these information sharing meetings involve the whole of the inpatient unit population so that everyone is aware of what programmes are running each day, any issues that have arisen among the group since the last meeting, any complaints that have arisen and any other issues that may have been resolved since the previous meeting.
- *Calm Down Methods*—these interventions can be used by patients during their stay on the inpatient unit; for example, sensory modulation equipment, musical instruments, games, movies and other methods that can be safely utilised to assist people to contain their levels of anxiety, agitation and aggression.
- *Reassurance*—this is provided to people after an incident has occurred (much like debriefing). It is an opportunity to discuss what has happened, why it happened and most of all to discuss prevention of future occurrences: 'What could we do differently?' 'What could you do differently?'
- *Discharge Messages*—each time a person is discharged from the unit, the other people on the unit and the staff can leave positive messages for the person to give them positive encouragement about going home.

Mullen (2009) identifies the psychosocial interventions of stress management, self-coping skills, relapse prevention and psychoeducation as important nursing interventions in inpatient units. He also includes psychological therapies, such as cognitive behavioural strategies and motivational interviewing, as useful nursing skills. However, in providing support it is important that patients have the opportunity to interact with a wide social network and are not confined to a primary therapeutic relationship. In a supportive milieu, the patient learns to resocialise and find new ways of relating to others. Support also involves assessing the patient's social network and education of, and interaction with, the family (Delaney et al. 2000).

Involvement. In the therapeutic milieu all relationships are regarded as potentially therapeutic. Therapeutic outcome is considered a function of the patient's relationship with individuals and total social organisation of the unit. The goal of involvement requires patients to attend to and take responsibility for maladaptive behaviours. Everyone in the therapeutic milieu is required to provide and accept constructive feedback from others. Involvement encourages patients to be actively engaged in their treatment and counsels against patient passivity. The desires and interests of the patient in terms of their treatment are highly valued.

Validation. Validation means that treatment is individualised and that it is the nurse's responsibility to try to understand the meaning of individual behaviour. Each patient is treated as worthy and as able to openly discuss values, feelings and goals. Patients learn to view themselves, through validation of past negative experiences, not as 'sick' or 'bad' but as injured parties (Norton & Bloom 2004). Validation requires flexibility in the application of rules. Too-rigid adherence to structural issues such as ward routine or policies can undermine the goal of validation.

Symptom management. Relationships with patients in the acute inpatient setting tend to be short and symptom oriented. With shorter lengths of stay, the tasks of the inpatient unit are to keep patients safe, assess patients' problems, treat patients' mental illness, meet patients' basic care needs and provide physical healthcare. There is more focus on treating the person's mental illness (Bowers et al. 2005).

In order to achieve these goals, the emphasis is on communication that is practical and supportive. Nurses document the nature of symptoms and changes to their character. Nurses also administer medications and assess their efficacy in controlling patient symptoms, monitor side effects, provide medication education to patients and consider the patient's ability to follow the prescribed regimen (Delaney et al. 2000). Patient behaviours are described in terms of whether they are typical or suggest an escalation in symptomatology. Also recorded are the nursing actions that assist the patient to reorganise successfully and enable the patient to function. Self-management of psychiatric illness is a central tenet of patient-directed mental healthcare and many studies have shown better outcomes of symptom management if patients are able to plan for future remissions, develop new skills and build on strengths that they currently possess (Fakui et al. 2011). One method for patients to plan for future remissions is the use of advance directives which can inform future care (Campbell & Kisely 2009).

Maintaining links with the patient's family or significant others. In the contemporary short-stay environment, links with the patient's family and significant others need to be nurtured and maintained. Families might be confused, fearful, fed up, anxious or relieved when one of their members is admitted to a mental health unit. They often need education about the nature of mental illness, its treatment and prognosis, and they usually want to know how they can best help the patient on the road to recovery. However, families frequently report feeling neglected (Schröder et al. 2007). It is important to try to involve the family in the treatment process and encourage them to visit. The patient should be allowed to take leave with their family as soon as they are able. Such leave might begin with short outings with family members and extend to overnight and weekend stays at home. The family should also be involved in the discharge process.

Developing and maintaining links with the community. It is important to facilitate patients to know about and have access to appropriate community resources. Inpatient nurses can ensure this continuity of care by finding out about patients' support networks and by enquiring about how patients understand their illness and the options available to treat and manage symptoms. Community links are developed through collaboration and meetings between the staff of the mental health service and the community services that will provide post-discharge support for the patient.

The Role of the Nurse

The inpatient setting. Mental health nurses are the only members of the inpatient team responsible for meeting the needs of patients 24 hours a day, 365 days a year. The nurse observes patients with respect to 'daily psychopathology, sociability, social skill level and atypical and adaptive behaviours and the positive and negative consequences of treatment interventions' (Munich 2002). The role of the inpatient nurse is to manage the inpatient milieu, observe inpatients for changes in symptoms and behaviour, assess their risk for aggression and/or self-harm, observe for substance use/misuse, monitor their physical health and de-escalate emotionally charged situations. The nurse, alongside the psychiatrist, also takes some responsibility for monitoring the effects of biological treatments.

In addition, it is the nurse's role to coordinate interdisciplinary and nursing care planning. A number of strategies are used in the inpatient milieu: they are designed to facilitate consistent, goal-directed care and include case conferences and nursing/multidisciplinary team handovers. At these occasions there is opportunity to discuss patients and build a level of consensus about treatment in order to ensure a consistent and integrated approach to patients.

The general hospital and emergency department. Opportunities for mental health nurses within general hospitals are expanding (Sharrock et al. 2008). Healthcare professionals not specifically educated in mental healthcare often require assistance in the provision of mental healthcare. Specifically, nurses working in nonpsychiatric settings do not believe that they are adequately prepared to meet the mental health needs of patients, identifying a lack of knowledge, skills and confidence in the assessment and management of their patients (Marynowski-Traczyk & Broadbent 2011). In order to provide assistance to staff in general hospitals, mental health nurses are developing advanced practice roles with the aim of increasing the availability of mental health expertise to both patients and staff. One such role is that of the psychiatric liaison nurse, who works within the acute health setting most commonly but not exclusively in general hospital wards and emergency departments. The role is defined by the Psychiatric Liaison Accreditation Network (PLAN) on the Royal College of Psychiatrists website (RCPsych 2018):

The psychiatric liaison nurse:

- works with patients and their relatives providing expert mental health assessment and intervention
- provides guidance, education and support to generalist staff caring for the patient and collaborates with them in developing a plan of care
- acts as a positive role model to generalist staff in psychiatric–mental healthcare and practice
- works with the organisation or department as a mental health resource on mental health–related projects, education and policy development
- acts as a link between generalist and mental health services (public and private, hospital and community).

Mental health nurses working in emergency departments do not always identify themselves as psychiatric liaison nurses. They may focus primarily on the assessment and onward referral of people presenting to the emergency department for mental health reasons, relying on a crisis-oriented service provision. Some may see their role in broader terms that include facilitating people with mental health problems to access physical care, providing therapeutic interventions to patients including some form of follow up, providing mental health promotion within the emergency department and providing support and education to department staff in the mental healthcare of their patients (Wand et al. 2012).

There are many challenges that present to the mental health nurse placed in a general hospital and/or an emergency department. Working with clinicians not specifically educated in mental health and working in the nonpsychiatric acute health system can place the mental health nurse in the minority. These nurses face an environment where clinicians lack mental health knowledge, skills and confidence to attend to the mental health needs of their patients within a system of care that emphasises physical care and tasks (Broadbent et al. 2007; Reed & Fitzgerald 2005; Sharrock & Happell 2006). Despite these challenges, nurses working in these settings have a high level of job satisfaction citing that they enjoy the autonomy and broadened scope of practice; the challenging, stimulating and varying nature of the work; the opportunity to educate and collaborate with other professionals; and being able to use a range of skills. Advocacy, health promotion and stigma reduction are also important sources of satisfaction (McNamara et al. 2008).

Community-Based Services

The continuum of care extends into the community and the choice of service again depends on the patient's care needs at the time. Community services range from clinic-based outpatient services that patients attend, to community case management where mental health nurses/case managers visit patients in their own environments (see the following section). These living environments are as diverse as the patients themselves and are described in Box 5.7. Services may be available during business hours only or they may have extended hours, with crisis-oriented services often being available 24 hours a day, 7 days a week.

BOX 5.7 Patient Living Environments

Patients' living environments include the following:

- *The person's own home or private rental*—these can be standalone dwellings, units, flats, rooms in houses of multiple occupancy, bedsits, inner-city apartments, country dwellings or caravans. The person may live alone or with others. Some have self-contained rooms complete with en-suites and kitchenettes, while others have shared kitchen, laundry and bathroom facilities. Some have no kitchen or laundry facilities and tenants rely on soup kitchens and laundromats to meet their needs.
- *Public housing subsidised by the government*—this includes standalone dwellings, units, apartments and bed sits.
- *Supported accommodation*—levels of support vary, ranging from minimal to 24-hour, and are based on the needs and preference of the individual.
- *Hostel accommodation*—this can be transient and unsupported or have some support such as a hostel with a house supervisor.
- *Supported residential services*—these are similar to group homes and are usually run by community support services or specialist mental health support agencies, with many working in conjunction with recovery programmes to assist people to achieve their own goals and move onto independent living situations. Some have minimal staffing during daylight hours and no support overnight; others have caretakers who also live on site.
- *Emergency or crisis accommodation including homeless shelters*—these are usually provided by charitable organisations as a short-term option for people who have become homeless due to illness, financial issues or complex social issues. Some offer overnight accommodation; others offer longer stays. Most offer in-house support and assistance to find more long-term housing options.

Community Care: Care Coordination

Care coordination, also referred to in the literature as case management, is now the predominant form of service delivery in the community. The coordination of care can be taken up by an individual clinician or, as described later under 'Assertive community care', by a team of clinicians. The original goals of case management were to reduce length of time in hospital and to assist patients to navigate the community mental health system. The role has developed over the years and with the adoption of a recovery orientation to service delivery the terms 'care coordinator' or 'case manager' are more likely to be used.

A care coordinator assesses patients and provides a linking and coordination function with various identified community services in a collaborative manner with the patient. Staff in the community need to be able to assess risk and to respond quickly. In order to provide this care, staff must know the patient well, monitor the patient regularly and be attuned to signs of relapse. Patients place a very high value on their relationship with their caregiver (Boscarato et al. 2014; O'Brien et al. 2001) and care coordination has been refined to place emphasis on the development of a strong collaborative relationship with the patient. Some of the functions of care coordination are described in Box 5.8.

BOX 5.8 An Example of Care Coordination Functions

Collaboration

- Developing a therapeutic relationship and becoming a partner in the patient's recovery
- Assisting the patient to develop their own goals
- Providing education about illness and treatment and mental health legislation and associated rights and responsibilities

Symptom Management

- Using contemporary treatment—medications as well as complementary therapies which have an evidence base for their use
- Monitoring for side effects and adverse reactions, including metabolic monitoring

Monitoring Wellbeing and Recovery

- In collaboration with the patient and significant others, working towards the patient's discharge from the service at a mutually agreed upon time
- In this process, maintaining open communication, examination of treatment goals and progress towards recovery and discharge; this may include relapse management and plans for future care as required

Identifying and Working with Risk

- Using the therapeutic relationship, discussing risk issues and in collaboration with the patient developing strategies that can be enacted when risk presents

Collaborating with Other Agencies

- When care needs to be provided to the patient by other healthcare professionals outside of the mental health sector, liaising with these healthcare providers to ensure that the patient receives adequate, appropriate and timely care for other health or social issues (e.g. dental care, medical care, drug and alcohol interventions, access to counselling, access to social and vocational groups, sexual healthcare needs)

Assertive Community Care

In the assertive community treatment model (Wright et al. 2011) clinicians go out to the patient's place of living. Clinicians share a caseload rather than assuming individual responsibility for a patient and this can have benefits when a patient has complex needs that are best met by a variety of clinicians. Clinician-to-patient ratios tend to be lower in this model and this allows for the development of close relationships with patients, which have been found helpful in increasing patient tenure in the community (Rapp 1998).

An important feature of this model, and from where it derives its description as 'assertive', is case finding or outreach. The goal of outreach is to identify those individuals in greatest need and go out to them. These are often patients who have had multiple hospital admissions or who have actively avoided services. The objective is to try to find ways to interrupt the process that leads to hospitalisation. In some cases, this approach might involve relapse-prevention techniques, or supported accommodation could be required. Outreach involves developing and maintaining working relationships with hospitals and other community agencies that might come into contact with this group of patients.

The assertive model is often used with homeless persons. Homelessness and loneliness are common experiences for many people who have mental health problems (Chesters et al. 2005). There is a dearth of suitable housing for mentally ill people (Singh & Castle 2007), most of whom would prefer to live independently in ordinary housing (Chesters et al. 2005). However, the level of support many require and the lack of community acceptance mean that this goal cannot always be achieved. In helping patients acquire accommodation it is useful to keep in mind some of the goals of community living, such as the freedom to have visitors, to come and go as one pleases, and to have a private space to call one's own. Nurses working in homeless outreach services provide a specialist clinical and treatment response for people who do not engage readily with mental health services (Koekkoek et al. 2006).

Intensive Community Care

Intensive community care shares many of the features of the assertive model but caseloads are not always shared. The care coordinator provides more intensive care in the community and this model is designed for those patients with enduring problems who are high service users (Schaedle et al. 2002). A systematic review of case management practices suggests that the strength of the findings in favour of assertive and intensive models has weakened over time (Smith & Newton 2007), a finding that may be explained by the greater relevance of such a model in a post-deinstitutionalisation environment (King 2006). However, Smith and Newton (2007) found that it remains superior to standard case management in reducing the number of days patients spend in hospital, helping to engage patients in treatment, improving their adherence to treatment, promoting independence and increasing patient satisfaction.

Crisis Intervention

Murphy et al. (2012) describe an intervention model for mental health crisis developed during the 1970s as part of the deinstitutionalisation movement. It was recognised that patients with an established or emerging mental disorder tend to be more vulnerable when under stress, are more likely to experience acute symptoms at these times and need access to support. The model that was developed for patients with low prevalence disorders such as schizophrenia and bipolar disorder was based on models developed for healthy people in psychological crises. A 'crisis' can be defined as 'a situation where a person experiencing overwhelming stress due to a life event such as bereavement, rape or major illness finds that their usual coping mechanisms for everyday life break down' (Murphy et al. 2012). Chapter 7 provides a detailed discussion of crisis theory and crisis intervention.

Community teams that utilise a crisis intervention model are likely to have members of the multidisciplinary team being available to the patient and their family 24 hours a day over a limited period of time (Murphy et al. 2012). A key aim of this model is the early detection of symptoms with prompt responses and intensive interventions to prevent further deterioration in the patient's mental state and avoid a hospital admission where possible. If hospital admission occurs, then the length of stay may be reduced given that crisis support is available at discharge. An additional aim is to support and reduce carer stress and interventions include counselling, medication, practical assistance, problem solving and support and education.

In contemporary settings, the crisis intervention model is being adapted for current practice; for example, with a recovery focus (Shattell et al. 2014) and for working with emergency services (Skubby et al. 2013). In the latter model, mental health nurses work with specifically trained police officers to respond to mental health crises encountered by the police. These teams aim to improve coordination between the police, ambulances, mental health services and emergency departments. In conjunction with the team, the mental health nurse will undertake assessment, treatment and referral of people in the community experiencing a mental health crisis (Skubby et al. 2013). This results in improved service for the patient, in that timely assessment and support in a community-based setting are provided. It also results in a reduction in unnecessary emergency department presentations and a more efficient use of resources. Preliminary evidence is that while patients prefer someone they know (like a relative or care coordinator) to assist in a crisis, if police needed to be involved, they prefer it to be a collaborative and informed intervention in conjunction with mental health workers (Boscarato et al. 2014).

Early Intervention

Early intervention has developed largely from the work of Australian psychiatrist Patrick McGorry and an international network of researchers interested in the early detection and treatment of first episode psychosis (McGorry et al. 2008). Researchers such as McGorry have played a critical role in the development of early interventions and key initiatives in youth mental health such as the Headspace model (www.headspace.com). These services have demonstrated effectiveness in the first 2 to 5 years of diagnosis, which is a period that is seen to require early health intervention, as well as health teaching, to establish better prognosis and outcomes. Early intervention is reported to be effective for the treatment of both the positive and the negative symptoms of schizophrenia, to promote medication adherence, to reduce rates of relapse and to provide supportive interventions for substance use disorders.

The first episode of psychosis most often occurs between adolescence and early adulthood when a person is establishing their identity and making commitments to work, study and relationships. It is the time of life when a person is setting down the building blocks for their future (Lutgens et al. 2015). Mental illness may interfere with a person's social networks and interrupt educational achievements and employment goals. It is important to address the stigma of mental illness with the person, their family and the wider community as one person's mental illness can have more problematic outcomes if the person feels isolated. The benefits of early intervention compared with standard treatment services have been verified by randomised control trials (Garety et al. 2006; Grawe et al. 2006; Petersen et al. 2005). Harvey has published a useful metaanalytic review of the literature concerning early intervention and mental health treatment outcomes (Harvey et al. 2007). Mental health nurses utilise the principles of early intervention in assessment, intervention family work and health teaching and this links well with a recovery focus in care provision.

Residential Community Care

The focus of residential community care is more on the day-to-day functioning of patients through assessing and developing the skills required to lead a meaningful life and less on illness management. Patients need functional skills and activities of daily living such as being able to budget, plan meals and manage medication. They also need social competencies, such as being able to establish, maintain and utilise relationships with family and friends. The major goals of community care are to assist people towards independent living and to help them fit into the community and develop a sense of belonging. This focus is in keeping with recovery principles that are centred on patient wellbeing and quality of life, wellness and competence rather than illness, disability and keeping the person out of hospital.

Principles of Caring in the Community

Patients in the community require a wide range of support services according to their varying needs at any one time. The type of service offered should be determined by patient needs and goals. However, too often the focus is on what the mental health delivery system is able to provide. When patients are asked about the goals they seek for themselves, they indicate that these are, in order of priority: money, availability of healthcare, a decent place to live, transportation, socialisation and help if needed (Rapp 1998). These goals contrast with those of the mental health service delivery system, which seeks reduced hospital bed-days, integration, mainstreaming and continuity of care. They also contrast with those of many service providers, who often simply want the patient to adhere to their medication regimen.

Collaboration. The relationships developed with patients in the community are often formed over longer periods of time than those formed in the hospital setting and are more like partnerships. Patients are empowered by being helped to find their own solutions to problems, and hope is supported through recognition of their abilities. Patients have consistently demonstrated their desire to be informed and make decisions about their treatment. This independence can be supported by helping them to identify and pursue their own goals and take responsibility for their actions and behaviour as well as respecting their decisions about treatment and personal goals. A collaborative approach to care is the key to developing a partnership with patients because the patient's goals and aspirations become the centre of the relationship. Collaboration can best be achieved by engaging in activities such as:

- building a therapeutic relationship based on compassion, active engagement and good communication
- encouraging the patient's development as a person in interactions with others, rather than as someone suffering from a health problem or disability
- asking the patient to help plan the activities they want to engage in
- obtaining the patient's consent to involve their family or others in the treatment plan
- encouraging the patient to set their own goals
- ensuring that the patient can refuse, if they wish, to participate in activities

Recovery and goal setting. Goal setting can be achieved by collaborating with the patient to establish what it is they would like to achieve and how they would like to go about achieving their goals. Patients need to set the pace for their own goal attainment and the clinician should give honest feedback and encouragement to maintain motivation. For example, if a patient has a goal of wanting to make more friends, they might ask the clinician to identify suitable community groups where they can meet people. The clinician might then accompany them to their first group encounter as a form of introduction. Once the person feels comfortable, they may ask the clinician just to accompany them on public transport to the group meeting without attending the meeting as well.

Integration into the community can be assisted by encouraging patients to use mainstream health services such as the local GP for their medication rather than specialist mental health services. Patients may also need help developing work and leisure skills. For example, a patient may demonstrate artistic aptitude and skills, and wish to use their leisure time more meaningfully. The system response to this desire might be to provide a professional in a day hospital setting to teach the patient a craft. An alternative would be to find a group of patients with similar wants and then advertise for volunteers to teach the patients particular skills for a limited period or to utilise a local neighbourhood house community education programme. One of the great advantages of this method is that patients are using the resources found in their own community rather than those provided by mental health services—using the latter increases the marginalisation and stigma of people experiencing mental illness.

Success is gauged by the progress achieved working towards the patient's goals, not by the extent to which the patient has conformed to the expectations of the mental health system or service providers. From this recovery perspective, the emphasis is on *trying* to achieve the goal, rather than on whether or not the patient succeeds.

Working with patients' strengths. As has been highlighted earlier in Chapter 2, the strengths model focusses on the patient's strengths and talents rather than the problems and handicaps associated with mental illness. This approach is embedded in community care and case coordination.

Working with non-government agencies and specialist community support services. In the community, very little of the environment is under the control of mental health professionals. One of the major goals of working in the community setting is to modify the environment in which the patient lives, works, plays and interacts so that it is better aligned with their abilities. In collaboration with the patient, it is important to firstly identify the services that they would find helpful in their day-to-day or future life. These services can then be sourced by the clinician or by the patient within the community. Services that exist in most communities can be useful to help people in a multitude of ways by providing assistance or support:

- to find appropriate and affordable housing
- to find vocational training or suitable employment
- to attend social events and establish friendship groups
- to link with peer support programmes
- to use and negotiate public transport
- with shopping/cooking/cleaning and other daily tasks
- to maintain good physical and dental health
- to find a local GP
- to access other health services such as drug and alcohol services/gambling services
- to access local services such as libraries, schools and child care
- to utilise culturally specific groups

Recruiting community resources also means taking into account patients' families. In the community, families and significant others are often expected to shoulder a large burden of care for their mentally ill relative. It is not uncommon for families to feel they are being blamed for their relative's illness, and they are often ignored when it comes to being informed about diagnoses and treatment so they are not able to participate fully and meaningfully in treatment and recovery planning. However, carers are usually keen to be involved. They want up-to-date information and need to be confident that support will be prompt and available when required. Nurses provide families and caregivers with advice and education about mental illness and its treatment, and can offer linkages with resources in the community to assist families with day-to-day issues. Patient and family education has been found to make a significant positive impact on the health of patients (Lyman et al. 2014). Families may also require information about the government services they are entitled to, and the voluntary services that might assist them.

Alcohol and Other Drug Services

In contemporary mental health services, a distinction between mental health services and substance use services has emerged. This has not always been the case and can be unhelpful when clinicians try to compartmentalise a person's difficulties into 'mental health' or 'drug and alcohol'. It can lead to patients being bounced between mental health and drug and alcohol services or, at worst, falling between the cracks of the two sets of services. In reality, substance misuse is part of mental ill-health and mental health nurses with an understanding of substance use disorders are a valuable asset to services and patients alike.

Nurses are involved in a wide range of drug and alcohol treatment services from harm reduction to residential rehabilitation. The skill mix of nurses means that drug and alcohol nurses work predominantly with people with severe drug and/or alcohol dependence, especially those with coexisting conditions, such as mental health and physical health issues (Cleary et al. 2008). Nurses working in addiction are committed to the prevention, intervention, treatment and management of addictive disorders including alcohol and other drug dependencies such as nicotine dependencies. Nurses working in mental health are required to care for people with addictions, so skills such as assessment using motivational interviewing as well as therapy techniques are required. Alcohol and other substance use is further discussed in Chapter 20.

Non-Government Organisations

Non-government organisations (NGOs) have a long history internationally of providing mental health support services to the community. As has been previously mentioned, the medical model has significantly influenced the model of care within public mental health systems. In contrast, social models influence service delivery within the non-government sector; for example, some NGOs focus on the social and economic impact of mental illness, and culture change to counter stigma and discrimination to enhance recovery and social inclusion.

There are opportunities for mental health nurses to work within NGOs internationally, such as for Doctors without Borders – Medecins Sans Frontieres. However, a tension that can arise for some nurses working in NGOs is the limited access to senior mental health nurses for supervision and mentorship, lack of access to in-service education and a potential conflict between the biopsychosocial model of public mental health services and the social model of NGOs.

A peer-led workforce is an emerging trend in the development of mental health services (Doughty & Tse, 2011) provided by NGOs. Services can be stand-alone services, entirely peer led or a collaboration between government and non-government sectors. Examples of the latter are 'step-up, step-down' programmes, which are short-term residential services that provide a supportive environment for people who do not need or no longer require the intensity of inpatient treatment, or for people residing in the community who require extra support with their mental health.

The Role of the Nurse in the Community

Mental health nurses have traditionally worked across various settings including inpatient, hospital-based services, community mental health teams and other community-based organisations. However, their role within community mental health teams has changed over the years: they have become more autonomous and they now provide ongoing follow up for people with serious mental illness such as schizophrenia (Olasoji & Maude 2010; Wilkin 2001).

Mental health nurses play a major role in the way care is delivered to people with a mental illness. The process of deinstitutionalisation witnessed the transfer of care of many people with severe mental illness into the community where follow-up treatment was meant to occur. However, one of the drawbacks of the process was that many people were sometimes lost to follow up due to limited community mental health resources, with families often left to provide the much-needed ongoing support.

In the face of dwindling healthcare resources and budgetary constraints in most advanced economies there is pressure on the public mental health system to provide high-quality mental healthcare with limited funding or resources. Mental health nurses working as part of the multidisciplinary team providing case management to people with a severe mental illness are often confronted with a high caseload. Mental health nurses are reluctant or find it difficult to transfer the care of some of the patients on their caseloads to primary care due to the non-availability of adequate specialist follow up (Olasoji & Maude 2010).

Primary Healthcare

Primary healthcare is considered as the first level of contact for people accessing healthcare and it has the potential to bring healthcare close to where people live (WHO 2008). According to Starfield et al. (2005), primary healthcare has four important features that make it unique: provision of care coordination, comprehensive healthcare, longitudinal care and first health contact access.

The burden of psychiatric and psychological distress in the community is high and the WHO (2001) recommends that mental healthcare should be based in primary care. GPs are usually the first point of contact for people seeking assistance for mental health problems, with nine out of ten adults with mental health problems supported in primary care (Mental Health Taskforce 2016). In addition, the high prevalence of comorbid illnesses and the side effects of psychotropic medications in people receiving public mental health services makes the need for a strong and well-established link with general practice important for these people to access primary health services.

Despite the obviously important role that GPs play in care of people with mental health problems, they can lack interest or confidence in providing such care (Oakley Browne et al. 2007). The manner in which primary and mental healthcare systems deliver care differs a great deal. While there is a focus on multiple medical problems, diagnostic procedures and health maintenance in primary healthcare, in mental healthcare case management and a multidisciplinary care approach are common practices (Thielke et al. 2007). There is therefore a need to bring the better parts of these two systems of care together in order to provide adequate mental healthcare to people with a mental illness. Collaboration between mental healthcare providers and primary healthcare has been reported as the best way to provide care to people with mental illness and mental health nurses play a key role in fostering such collaboration (Thielke et al. 2007). Four main models of how mental healthcare is provided at the interface of primary–secondary care have been identified. They are:

- community mental health teams, which provide increased liaison and crisis intervention
- shifted outpatient clinics, whereby psychiatrists consult within health centres
- the consultation-liaison model, where specialist mental health services provide advice and skills to primary care teams
- the attachment model, where a mental health worker such as a mental health nurse provides mental healthcare to people presenting with mental health problems in primary care settings (Gask & Khanna 2011)

NURSE'S STORY 5.1 **A Patient in the Community**

One of the biggest difficulties I face is whether to admit someone to hospital or to care for them in the community when they relapse. John is a 36-year-old patient of mine with schizophrenia and substance abuse problems who I have been case managing for 2 years now.

About 6 weeks ago he started to become psychotic again. He believed the men who were renovating a block of flats next door to him were entering his flat at night and interfering with him sexually. His symptoms weren't helped by the fact that he was taking a variety of drugs including marijuana and possibly speed. I was having a hard time knowing what to do with him because he has always been reluctant to accept mental health services. Although he accepts a visit from me about every 6–8 weeks, he's never very forthcoming about what he has been up to. This reluctance, along with the fact that he had always had to be detained in hospital under the Mental Health Act, made me think he would be unwilling to go to hospital voluntarily if it came to that. So I had to think of some way in which I could respect his preferences, while at the same time ensuring he was taking his prescribed medication and not so much of the unprescribed stuff.

The other issues I had to keep in mind were that if his mental state continued to deteriorate, then he might pose a danger to himself or, more likely, other people. However, because he wasn't violent or abusive at this stage, I decided to continue to manage him in the community if I could get him to agree to more frequent visits, which he did. I also arranged to do a joint visit with one of my colleagues, a social worker, so as to get another person's perspective and to ensure that someone else was familiar with his current condition in case a crisis situation arose.

During my visits, which I had gradually increased to twice a week, we talked about his prescribed medication and it emerged that he was having problems with side effects. Although he hadn't stopped taking it completely, he was taking it erratically. I suggested that the psychiatrist might be able to help and he eventually agreed to visit him at the clinic.

At this stage John is still psychotic but I'm pretty sure he's taking his medication as prescribed and seeing the psychiatrist weekly for the moment, and I visit him once a week to monitor how he's going.

The advent of mental health nurses in the primary healthcare setting in nations such as the United States and the UK is an important development (O'Brien, et al. 2006). Mental health nurses play a pivotal role in the delivery of mental healthcare across various settings and by virtue of their training they have skills to provide specialist mental healthcare to people experiencing mental health problems in primary, secondary or tertiary systems. There are many benefits to people with mental illness receiving care provided by mental health nurses in the primary healthcare setting. For example, there is still stigma associated with mental illness, in spite of the best efforts at public education (Moses 2014), but mental health nurses working within primary healthcare have the potential to reduce this stigma. Another benefit is that people are able to receive comprehensive healthcare that brings together their physical and mental healthcare needs, especially in the light of evidence that suggests people with severe mental illness have poor physical health outcomes compared with the general population (Collins et al. 2012). In addition, specialist care is made more accessible for the general population.

For the mental health nursing profession, primary healthcare opens a new career pathway for clinicians to consider, one that provides a greater level of autonomy and flexibility and that would go a long way to promoting workforce development, which has faced decline in recent years. Mental health nurses have the opportunity to engage in health promotion, education and skill enhancement around mental health for other members of the primary healthcare team including GPs and practice nurses.

Primary healthcare remains an important aspect of the overall healthcare system of any nation. There is, however, a need to prepare nurses from the undergraduate through to the postgraduate level to take up the valuable role that awaits them in this setting.

Community Health Centres

Community health centres provide general health services to the community. Within these centres there are opportunities for mental health nurses to provide support and counselling to patients. If this is the case, it provides a great opportunity for skill sharing and improving patient access to physical healthcare.

Maternal and Child Health Services

Mental health nurses work closely with pregnant women, new mothers and their families and with midwives and other health professionals in maternal and child health services. Mental health nurses working in this practice specialty link closely with inpatient services for new parents and their infants such as mother–baby units. These units assist families with the physical, emotional and social challenges that come with having a baby. The services can be inpatient and weekend services and rely on community service support to continue the work done in the inpatient setting. Working with new parents provides a great opportunity for mental health nurses to support the healthy adjustment of parents to parenthood and the healthy development of infants.

Private Practice

Mental health nurses can choose to go into private practice, providing counselling and psychotherapy to individuals, families and/or groups, as well as clinical supervision and education. Nurses choosing to take this path need to consider their practice location, their patients, fees charged, indemnity insurance and leave coverage.

E-Mental Health

The internet is now one of the most common sources of information for patients about mental illnesses and mental health problems. It is increasingly being used in the treatment of various mental disorders. Patients may access these services independently or receive the assistance of a clinician. The programmes are of varying length and patients may participate in online discussion forums with other patients and/or clinicians, as well as undertaking online lessons and homework assignments. Email and video conferencing are commonly used for communication between e-patient and clinician. Panic (Wims et al. 2010), shyness and social phobia (Titov et al. 2009), posttraumatic stress disorder (Spence et al. 2011) and depression (Perini et al. 2009) can all be treated successfully via the internet. The major benefit of using the internet for treatment is that it provides greater flexibility in terms of when patients access the service, which is often a problem for those who work and who are unable to attend a mental health service. It is also believed to help overcome some of the stigma associated with attending a mental health service. However, it is actually older patients with the capacity to pay for services who are most likely to use e-mental health services (Lampe 2011).

Other Settings

Urban, Rural and Remote

Urban, rural and remote healthcare settings vary significantly, for example in the Highlands of Scotland and within rural Wales. Mental health nurses working in urban environments generally have ready access to education, peer support and resources. Specialist mental health services are often centred in major cities and working in urban areas tends to be popular.

Economic, political and social factors influence the delivery of mental healthcare services and the mental health problems seen in rural and remote areas. Rural populations experience healthcare inequities and there is particular concern about the access to healthcare within remote areas. Remote areas present particular challenges regarding the delivery of quality services: dispersed population, poor health status, geographic isolation, problematic transport, poor infrastructure, small economic base, limited political influence, extremes of climate and a high turnover of health professionals in all disciplines (NHS Education for Scotland 2013). Experiencing a sense of 'remoteness' is a complex subjective state, the causal factors of which are:

- geography and terrain limiting access and egress
- being socially and culturally isolated
- environmental and weather conditions resulting in isolation
- isolation due to distances

- isolation from professional peers and supports
- isolation as a result of infrastructure, communications and resources (Cliffe & Malone 2014)

The use of the internet, telephone counselling and self-help strategies offer important options for mental health service delivery and mental health education to rural and remote communities. They also benefit mental health nurses working in these communities in terms of education, peer support and linking with resources.

Forensic Mental Health Services

People with a mental illness are over-represented in prisons (Singh & Castle 2007). Forensic mental health nursing is addressed in more detail in Chapter 14 but it is important to recognise that within forensic services the mental health nurse can work in a number of different settings. These include custody centres (for both youth and adults), courts, custodial diversion services, prisons (both generalist health services and specialist mental health services) and the specialised forensic mental health services for sentenced prisoners and those deemed unfit for trial due to mental illness.

Schools

Nurses work in a range of school settings including primary and secondary schools, both public and private. Nurses may visit different schools or work as part of a specific school, becoming part of that school community. Their work involves providing students with the opportunity to have health assessments and consultations, as well as providing health education and promotion. Nurses specifically educated in mental health are well placed to contribute to student and family counselling services within their schools and work closely with the team who provide for the wellbeing of students. They provide information and advice about healthy behaviours and link students and families to community-based health and wellbeing services. Education and health promotion are provided not only to students but also to teachers and the school community as a whole. School nurses work with a school to develop health promotion strategies and liaise with community-based organisations.

Immigration Detention Centres, Asylum Seekers and Refugees

There are opportunities for mental health nurses to care for refugees and asylum seekers in onshore and offshore immigration detention centres as well as post-release and resettlement support services. While this type of work and working environment is no doubt challenging (Newman et al. 2013; Procter 2004a), the rewards of working with traumatised and disenfranchised people are great. Procter (2004b) points out that while trust is fundamental to the work of a mental health nurse, because of the history of trauma in this group of people, more attention to establishing trust is required. He also highlights the importance of understanding the stressors of the context the person is in, working with accredited interpreters and taking a collaborative approach with the person, their family and community, as well as utilising community resources where possible. Working in this type of setting also gives the mental health nurse the opportunity to work with other stakeholders such as welfare officers and teachers, national and international aid agencies (e.g. Red Cross and Save the Children) and local as well as community mental health services post release. Teamwork is essential to this work.

CONCLUSION

In this chapter it has been argued that the quality of the environment in which patient care takes place is important to patient recovery. Environmental strategies in the care of people with a mental illness have a long history, but their application over time has been patchy. These strategies reached their peak in the 18th century, when it was noticed that patients were more manageable in a pleasant environment. In the 20th century, Thomas Main and Maxwell Jones pioneered the concept of the hospital and environment as treatment tools.

The preferred contemporary setting for the provision of mental healthcare is the community, which accords best with the principle of caring for people in the least restrictive environment. The predominant form of service delivery in the community is care coordination (management), which has been found to be most effective for people with significant and enduring mental health problems. There are a range of bed-based and community settings in which mental health nurses can work to support patients toward recovery. The internet is also being used for treatment, especially of various anxiety disorders.

EXERCISES FOR CLASS ENGAGEMENT

Discuss the following questions with your tutorial group.

1. How can an emphasis on safety in the inpatient setting promote or detract from the development of therapeutic relationships?
2. How can nurses in an inpatient setting provide support to families?
3. Is it possible and/or desirable to maintain a nursing identity when working in a community setting?
4. What services are available in your community to assist patients with mental illness?

REFERENCES

Aitken, P., Robens, S., Emmens, T., 2014. An Evidence Base for Liaison Psychiatry: Guidance. Devon Partnership NHS Trust, Exeter, UK. Available at: http://mentalhealthpartnerships.com/resource/evidence-base-for-liaison-psychiatry-services. Accessed: 24 May 2015.

Beatson, J., Rao, S., Watson, C., 2010. Borderline Personality Disorder: Towards Effective Treatment. Australian Postgraduate Medicine, Melbourne.

Boscarato, K., Lee, S., Kroschel, J., Hollander, Y., Brennan, A., Warren, N., 2014. Consumer experience of formal crisis-response services and preferred methods of crisis intervention. International Journal of Mental Health Nursing 23 (4), 287–295.

Bowers, L., 2014. Safewards: a new model of conflict and containment on psychiatric wards. Journal of Psychiatric and Mental Health Nursing 21 (6), 499–508.

Bowers, L., 2015. Safewards Resources for Safewards Implementation. Available at: www.safewards.net. Accessed: 14 September 2015.

Bowers, L., Alexander, J., Bilgin, H., Botha, M., Dack, C., James, K., Jarrett, M., Jeffery, D., Nijman, H., Owiti, J., Papadopoulos, C., Ross, J., Wright, S., Stewart, D., 2014. Safewards: the empirical basis of the model and a critical appraisal. Journal of Psychiatric and Mental Health Nursing 21 (4), 354–364.

Bowers, L., Simpson, A., Alexander, J., Hackney, D., Nijman, H., Grange, A., Warren, J., 2005. The nature and purpose of acute psychiatric wards: the Tompkins acute ward study. Journal of Mental Health 14 (6), 625–635.

Bowers, L., Simpson, A., Jones, J., Van Der Merwe, M., Jeffery, D., 2009. Identifying key factors associated with aggression on acute inpatient psychiatric wards. Issues in Mental Health Nursing 30 (4), 260–271.

Bowers, L., Whittington, R., Nolan, P., Parkin, D., Curtis, S., Bhui, K., Hackney, D., Allan, T., Simpson, A., 2008. The relationship between service ecology, special observation and self-harm during acute in-patient care: the City-128 study. British Journal of Psychiatry 193 (5), 395–401.

Bowles, N., Dodds, P., Hackney, D., Sunderland, C., Thomas, P., 2002. Formal observations and engagement: a discussion paper. Journal of Psychiatric and Mental Health Nursing 9 (3), 255–260.

British Association of Social Workers (BASW), 2018. Available at: https://www.basw.co.uk.

British Psychological Society, 2018. Available at: https://www.bps.org.uk.

Broadbent, M., Moxham, L., Dwyer, T., 2007. The development and use of mental health triage scales in Australia. International Journal of Mental Health Nursing 16, 413–421.

Campbell, L., Kisely, S., 2009. Advance treatment directives for people with severe mental illness. Cochrane Database of Systematic Reviews CD005963. https://doi.org/10.1002/14651858.

Cardell, R., Pitula, C., 1999. Suicidal inpatients' perceptions of therapeutic and nontherapeutic aspects of constant observation. Psychiatric Services 50 (8), 1066–1070.

Chen, S., Krupa, T., Lysaght, R., McCay, E., Piat, M., 2013. The development of recovery competencies for in-patient mental health providers working with people with serious mental illness. Administration and Policy in Mental Health and Mental Health Services Research 40 (2), 96–116.

Chesters, J., Fletcher, M., Jones, R., 2005. Mental illness recovery and place. Australian e-Journal for the Advancement of Mental Health 4 (2), 1–9.

Cleary, M., Hunt, G., Matherson, S., Siegfied, N., Walter, G., 2008. Psychosocial interventions for people with both severe mental illness and substance misuse. Cochrane Database of Systematic Reviews CD001088. https://doi.org/10.1002/14651858.CD001088. pub2.

Cliffe, C., Malone, G., 2014. Framework for Remote and Isolated Professional Practice. CRANAplus Council of Remote Area Nurses of Australia Professional Services Division, Professional Practice.

Collins, E., Tranter, S., Irvine, F., 2012. The physical health of the seriously mentally ill: an overview of the literature. Journal of Psychiatric and Mental Health Nursing 19, 638–646.

Cox, A., Hayter, M., Ruane, J., 2010. Alternative approaches to 'enhanced observations' in acute inpatient mental health care: a review of the literature. Journal of Psychiatric and Mental Health Nursing 17 (2), 162–171.

Davidson, L., Roe, D., 2007. Recovery from versus recovery in serious mental illness: one strategy for lessening confusion plaguing recovery. Journal of Mental Health 16, 459–470.

Delaney, K., 2010. The peer specialist movement: an interview with Gayle Bluebird. RN. Issues in Mental Health Nursing 31, 232–234.

Delaney, K., Pitula, C., Perraud, S., 2000. Psychiatric hospitalization and process description: what will nursing add? Journal of Psychosocial Nursing and Mental Health Services 38 (3), 7–13.

Department of Health, 2013. Nursing Observation Through Engagement in Psychiatric Inpatient Care. Department of Health guideline. Mental Health, Drugs and Regions Division, Department of Health, State Government of Victoria, Melbourne.

Doughty, C., Tse, S., 2011. Can consumer-led mental health services be equally effective? An integrative review of CLMH services in high-income countries. Community Mental Health Journal 47 (3), 252–266.

Fakui, S., Starnino, V., Susanna, M., Davidson, L., Cook, K., Rapp, C., Gowdy, E., 2011. Effect of wellness recovery action plan (WRAP) participation on psychiatric symptoms, sense of hope and recovery. Psychiatric Rehabilitation Journal 34 (3), 214–222.

Fischer, M., 2012. Organisational turbulence, trouble and trauma: theorising the collapse of a mental health setting. Organisational Studies 33 (9), 1153–1173.

Fulbrook, P., Lawrence, P., 2015. Survey of an Australian general emergency department: estimated prevalence of mental health disorders. Journal of Psychiatric and Mental Health Nursing 22, 30–38.

Gask, L., Khanna, T., 2011. Ways of working at the interface between primary and specialist mental healthcare. The British Journal of Psychiatry 198 (1), 3–5.

Garety, P., Craig, T., Dunn, G., Fornells-Ambrojo, M., Colbert, S., Rahaman, N., 2006. Specialised care for early psychosis: symptoms, social functioning and patient satisfaction: Randomised controlled trial. British Journal of Psychiatry 188, 37–45.

Grawe, R., Falloon, I., Widen, J., Skogvol, E., 2006. Two years of continued early treatment for recent-onset schizophrenia: a randomised controlled study. Acta Psychiatric Scandinavia 114, 328–336.

Grotstein, J., 1997. Bion, The pariah of 'O'. British Journal of Psychotherapy 14 (1), 77–90.

Haglund, K., Von Essen, L., 2005. Locked entrance doors at psychiatric wards: advantages and disadvantages according to voluntarily admitted patients. Nordic Journal of Psychiatry 59 (6), 511–515.

Happell, B., Platania-Phung, C., Webster, S., McKenna, B., Millar, F., Stanton, R., Galletly, C., Castle, D., Furness, T., Liu, D., Scott, D., 2015. Applying the World Health Organization Mental Health Action Plan to Evaluate Policy on Addressing Co-Occurrence of Physical and Mental Illnesses in Australia. Australian Health Review: A Publication of the Australian Hospital Association.

Hardy, S., Hinks, P., Gray, R., 2013. Screening for cardiovascular risk in patients with severe mental illness in primary care: a comparison with patients with diabetes. Journal of Mental Health 22, 42–50.

Harvey, P., Lepage, M., Malla, A., 2007. Benefits of enriched intervention compared with standard care for patients with recent-onset psychosis: a meta-analytic approach. Canadian Journal of Psychiatry 52 (7), 464–472.

Holmes, P., 1984. Boundaries or chaos: an outpatient psychodrama group for adolescents. Journal of Adolescence 7 (4), 387–400.

Holyoake, D., 2013. I spy with my little eye something beginning with O: Looking at what the myth of 'doing the observations' means in mental health nursing culture. Journal of Psychiatric & Mental Health Nursing 20 (9), 840–850.

Jones, J., Ward, M., Wellman, N., Hall, J., Lowe, T., 2000. Psychiatric inpatients' experience of nursing observation: a United Kingdom perspective. Journal of Psychosocial Nursing 28 (12), 10–20.

Jones, M., 1953. The Therapeutic Community. Basic Books, New York.

King, R., 2006. Intensive case management: a critical re-appraisal of the scientific evidence for effectiveness. Administration and Policy in Mental Health 33 (5), 529–535.

Koekkoek, B., van Meijel, B., Hutschemaekers, G., 2006. 'Difficult patients' in mental health care: a review. Psychiatric Services 57 (6), 795–802.

Lampe, L., 2011. Internet-based therapy: too good to be true? Australian and New Zealand Journal of Psychiatry 45 (4), 342–343.

Lee, S., Brunero, S., Fairbrother, G., Cowan, D., 2008. Profiling police presentations of mental health consumers to an emergency department. International Journal of Mental Health Nursing 17, 311–316.

Lutgens, D., Iyer, S., Joober, R., Brown, T., Norman, R., Latimer, E., Schmitz, N., Baki, A., Abadi, S., Malla, A., 2015. A five-year randomized parallel and blinded clinical trial of an extended specialized early intervention vs regular care in the early phase of psychotic disorders. BMC Psychiatry 15, 22. https://doi.org/10.1186/s12888-015-0404-2.

Lyman, D., Braude, L., George, P., Dougherty, R., Daniels, A., Ghose, S., Delphin-Rittmon, M., 2014. Consumer and family psychoeducation: assessing the evidence. Psychiatric Services 65 (4), 416–428.

Mahoney, J., Palyo, N., Napier, G., Giordano, J., 2009. The therapeutic milieu reconceptualized for the 21st century. Archives of Psychiatric Nursing 23 (6), 423–429.

Main, T., 1946. The hospital as a therapeutic community. Bulletin of the Menninger Clinic 10, 66–70.

Main, T., 1980. Some basic concepts in therapeutic community work. In: Jansen, E. (Ed.), The Therapeutic Community: Outside the Hospital. Croom Helm, London, pp. 52–63.

Marynowski-Traczyk, D., Broadbent, M., 2011. What are the experiences of emergency department nurses in caring for clients with a mental illness in the emergency department? Australasian Emergency Nursing Journal 14, 172–179.

McGorry, P., Killackey, E., Yung, A., 2008. Early intervention in psychosis: concepts, evidence and future directions. World Psychiatry 7 (3), 148–156.

McNamara, P., Bryant, J., Forster, J., Sharrock, J., Happell, B., 2008. Exploratory study of mental health consultation-liaison nursing in Australia: Part 2. Preparation, support and role satisfaction. International Journal of Mental Health Nursing 17, 189–196.

Mental Health Network, 2012. Investing in Emotional and Psychological Wellbeing for Patients with Long-Term Conditions. NHS Confederation, London.

Mental Health Taskforce, 2016. The Five Year Forward View for Mental Health. Available at: https://www.england.nhs.uk/wp-content/uploads/2016/02/Mental-Health-Taskforce-FYFV-final.pdf. Accessed: 25 November 2018.

Mills, J., Harrison, T., 2007. John Rickman, Wilfred Ruprecht Bion, and the origins of the therapeutic community. History of Psychology 10 (1), 22–43.

Moorehead, S., Kennedy, J., Hodgson, C., Ruiz, P., Junaid, O., 1996. Observations of the observed: a study of inpatients' perception of being observed. Irish Journal of Psychological Medicine 13 (2), 59–61.

Moses, T., 2014. Determinants of mental illness stigma for adolescents discharged from psychiatric hospitalisation. Social Science and Medicine 109, 26–34.

Mullen, A., 2009. Mental health nurses establishing psychosocial interventions within acute inpatient settings. International Journal of Mental Health Nursing 18 (2), 83–90.

Munich, R., 2002. Efforts to preserve the mind in contemporary hospital treatment. Bulletin of the Menninger Clinic 67 (3), 167–186.

Murphy, S., Irving, C., Adams, C., Driver, R., 2012. Crisis intervention for people with severe mental illnesses. Cochrane Database of Systematic Reviews 16 (5), CD001087. https://doi.org/10.1002/14651858.CD001087.pub4.

National Health Service (NHS) Education for Scotland, 2013. Supporting Remote and Rural Healthcare. Available at: http://www.rrheal.scot.nhs.uk/media/185252/remote%20and%20rural%20healthcare%20updated.pdf. Accessed: 25 November 2018.

Newman, L., Proctor, N., Dudley, M., 2013. Seeking asylum in Australia: immigration detention, human rights and mental health care. Australasian Psychiatry 21 (4), 315–320.

Norton, K., Bloom, S., 2004. The art and challenges of long-term and short-term democratic therapeutic communities. Psychiatric Quarterly 75 (3), 249–261.

Oakley Browne, M., Lee, A., Prabhu, R., 2007. Self-reported confidence and skills of general practitioners in management of mental health disorders. Australian Journal of Rural Health 15 (5), 321–326.

O'Brien, A., Hughes, F., Kidd, J., 2006. Mental health nursing in New Zealand primary health care. Contemporary Nurse 21, 142–152.

O'Brien, A., Woods, M., Palmer, C., 2001. The emancipation of nursing practice: applying anti-psychiatry to the therapeutic community. Australian and New Zealand Journal of Mental Health Nursing 10 (1), 3–9.

Olasoji, M., Maude, P., 2010. The advent of mental health nurses in Australian general practice. Contemporary Nurse 36 (1–2), 106–117.

Perini, S., Titov, N., Andrews, G., 2009. Clinician-assisted internet-based treatment is effective for depression: randomized controlled trial. Australian and New Zealand Journal of Psychiatry 43 (6), 571–578.

Petersen, L., Jeppesen, P., Thorup, A., Abel, M.-B., Øhlenschlæger, J., Christensen, T.Ø., 2005. A randomised multicentre trial of integrated versus standard treatment for patients with a first episode of psychotic illness. British Medical Journal 331, 602.

Pitula, C., Cardell, R., 1996. Suicidal inpatients' experience of constant observation. Psychiatric Services 47 (6), 649–651.

Porter, R., 2002. Madness: A Brief History. Oxford University Press, Oxford.

Procter, N., 2004a. 'Paper Plates and Throwaway Cutlery': Aspects of Generating Trust During Mental Health Initiatives with Asylum Seekers Released from Immigration Detention Centres Synergy, pp. 8–9.

Procter, N., 2004b. Clinical update. Emergency mental health nursing for refugees and asylum seekers. Australian Nursing Journal 12, 21–23.

Rapp, C., 1998. The Strengths Model: Case Management With People Suffering From Severe and Persistent Mental Illness. Oxford University Press, New York.

Rapoport, R., 1960. Community as Doctor. Tavistock, London.

Reed, F., Fitzgerald, L., 2005. The mixed attitudes of nurses to caring for people with mental illness in a rural general hospital. International Journal of Mental Health Nursing 14, 249–257.

Renouf, N., Meadows, G., 2001. Teamwork. In: Meadows, G., Singh, B. (Eds.), Mental Health in Australia: Collaborative Community Practice. Oxford University Press, London.

Repper, J., Martin, T., 2011. A review of the literature on peer support in mental health services. Journal of Mental Health 20 (4), 392–411.

Royal College of Occupational Therapists, 2018. Available at: https://www.rcot.co.uk. Accessed: 8 September 2018.

Royal College of Psychiatrists (RCPsych), 2018. Available at: https://www.rcpsych.ac.uk. Accessed: 8 September 2018.

Royal College of Psychiatrists, 2018. Psychiatric Liaison Accreditation Network (PLAN). Available at: https://www.rcpsych.ac.uk/workinpsychiatry/qualityimprovement/qualitynetworks/liaisonpsychiatry/plan.aspx. Accessed: 9 September 2018.

Santangelo, P., 2015. What's Special About Mental Health Nursing? Being in the Here and Now, Side by Side, Co-Constructing care: a Substantive Grounded Theory of Recovery-Focused Mental Health Nursing. Submitted in Fulfilment of the Requirements for the Degree of Doctor of Philosophy. Faculty of Health, School of Health Sciences, Nursing and Midwifery, University of Tasmania.

Schaedle, R., McGrew, J., Bond, G., 2002. A comparison of experts' perspectives on assertive community treatment and intensive case management. Psychiatric Services 53 (2), 207–210.

Schröder, A., Larsson, B., Ahlström, G., 2007. Next of kin's conceptions of the quality of care in the psychiatric setting: A phenomenographic study. International Journal of Mental Health Nursing 16 (5), 307–317.
Sharrock, J., Bryant, J., McNamara, P., Forster, J., Happell, B., 2008. Exploratory study of mental health consultation-liaison nursing in Australia: part 1, demographics and role characteristics. International Journal of Mental Health Nursing 17, 180–188.
Sharrock, J., Happell, B., 2006. Competence in providing mental health care: a grounded theory analysis of nurses' experiences. Australian Journal of Advanced Nursing 24 (2), 9–15.
Sharrock, J., Rickard, N., 2002. Limit setting: a useful strategy in rehabilitation. Australian Journal of Advanced Nursing 19, 21–26.
Shattell, M., Harris, B., Beavers, J., Tomlinson, S., Prasek, L., Geevarghese, S., Emery, C., Heyland, M., 2014. A recovery-oriented alternative to hospital emergency departments for persons in emotional distress: 'The living room'. Issues in Mental Health Nursing 35, 4–12.
Shorter, E., 1997. A History of Psychiatry: from the Era of the Asylum to the Age of Prozac. John Wiley & Sons, New York.
Shorter, E., 2008. Before Prozac: the Troubled History of Mood Disorders in Psychiatry. Oxford University Press, New York.
Singh, B., Castle, D., 2007. Why are community psychiatry services in Australia doing it so hard? Medical Journal of Australia 187 (7), 410–412.
Skubby, D., Bonfine, N., Novisky, M., Munetz, M., Ritter, C., 2013. Crisis intervention team (CIT) programs in rural communities: a focus group study. Community Mental Health Journal 49, 756–764.
Slade, T., Johnston, A., Teesson, M., 2009. The Mental Health of Australians 2. Report on the 2007 National Survey of Mental Health and Wellbeing. Department of Health and Ageing, Canberra.
Spence, J., Titov, N., Dear, B., Johnston, L., Solley, K., Lorian, C., Wootton, B., Zou, J., Schwenke, G., 2011. Randomized controlled trial of internet-delivered cognitive behavioral therapy for posttraumatic stress disorder. Depression and Anxiety 28 (7), 541–550.
Smith, L., Newton, R., 2007. Systematic review of case management. Australian and New Zealand Journal of Psychiatry 41 (1), 2–9.
Starfield, B., Shi, L., Macinko, J., 2005. Contributions of primary care to health systems and health. The Milbank Quarterly 83 (3), 457–502.
Thielke, S., Vannoy, S., Unutzer, J., 2007. Integrating mental health and primary care. Primary Care Clinic Office Practice 34, 571–592.
Thomas, S., Shattell, S., Martin, T., 2002. What's therapeutic about the therapeutic milieu? Archives of Psychiatric Nursing 16 (3), 99–107.
Titov, N., Gibson, M., Andrews, G., McEvoy, P., 2009. Internet treatment for social phobia reduces comorbidity. Australian and New Zealand Journal of Psychiatry 43 (8), 754–759.
Vatne, S., Hoem, E., 2008. Acknowledging community: a milieu therapeutic approach in mental health care. Journal of Advanced Nursing 61 (6), 690–698.
Walk, A., 1961. The history of mental nursing. Journal of Mental Science 107, 2–7.
Wand, T., D'Abrew, N., Barnett, C., Acret, L., White, K., 2015. Evaluation of a nurse practitioner-led extended hours mental health liaison nurse service based in the emergency department. Australian Health Review 39, 1–8.
Wand, T., White, K., Patching, J., Dixon, J., Green, T., 2012. Outcomes from the evaluation of an emergency department-based mental health nurse practitioner outpatient service in Australia. Journal of the American Academy of Nurse Practitioners 24, 149–159.
Watson, J., 1992. Maintenance of therapeutic community principles in an age of biopharmacology and economic restraints. Archives of Psychiatric Nursing 6 (3), 183–188.
Wilkin, P., 2001. The primary care role of the community psychiatric nurse. International Journal of Psychiatry in Clinical Practice 7 (2), 79–84.
Wims, E., Titov, N., Andrews, G., Robinson, E., Schwencke, G., Johnston, L., Solley, K., Choi, I., 2010. Clinician-assisted internet-based treatment is effective for panic: a randomized controlled trial. Australian and New Zealand Journal of Psychiatry 44 (7), 599–607.
Wright, N., Callaghan, P., Bartlett, P., 2011. Mental health service users' and practitioners' experiences of engagement in assertive outreach: a qualitative study. Journal of Psychiatric and Mental Health Nursing 18 (9), 822–832.
World Health Organization (WHO), 2001. The World Health Report 2001 Mental Health: New Understanding and Hope. WHO, Geneva.
World Health Organization (WHO), 2008. The World Health Report 2008: Primary Health Care Now More than Ever. WHO, Geneva.
Zolnierek, C., 2009. Non-psychiatric hospitalization of people with mental illness: systematic review. Journal of Advanced Nursing 65 (8), 1570–1583.

USEFUL WEBSITES

Headspace, www.headspace.com
Doctors without borders – Medecins Sans Frontieres, www.msf.org.uk
Mind Charity, https://www.mind.org.uk
Reach Out, https://www.reachoutuk.org/
Rethink Mental Illness, https://www.rethink.org
Safewards, www.safewards.net
Samaritans, https://www.samaritans.org
SANE, www.sane.org.uk
Turning Point, www.turning-point.co.uk

PART 2

Influences on Mental Health

6

Mental Health Theory and Influence Across the Lifespan

Debra Nizette, Patricia Barkway

KEY POINTS

- Mental health and mental illness are complex, distinct concepts that are not mutually exclusive.
- Subjective factors influence whether human behaviour is perceived as normal or abnormal.
- In recovery, a person can experience mental health despite being diagnosed with a mental illness.
- Community attitudes about mental health and mental illness contribute to stigma.
- Personality and human behaviour theories provide explanations as to how individuals think, feel and behave, but no one theory has universal applicability.
- Personality and human behaviour theories underpin psychotherapeutic interventions for mental illness.
- Psychological and sociological theories have influenced the development of nursing theories.
- Personality development results from interactions between nature and nurture—not from nature or nurture.
- An understanding of human development across the lifespan enhances mental health assessment and the provision of holistic, recovery-oriented care.
- Self-awareness assists the nurse to better understand the patient's experience.
- Mental health vulnerability increases at various times across the lifespan due to a combination of individual and contextual factors.
- The lifespan is generally conceived of as a linear concept, the time from birth to death. Paradoxically, development across this span is more appropriately conceived of as nonlinear, multidimensional and contextual.
- Concepts of attachment and resilience play a part in the attainment and maintenance of mental health and recovery.
- Promotion of mental health across the lifespan requires a primary healthcare approach in order to address the social and environmental factors that create vulnerability to mental illness (also see Chapter 21).

KEY TERMS

attachment
developmental psychology
identity
lifespan
mental health and mental illness
mental health nursing theories
mental health promotion
protective factors
psychological theories
recovery
resilience
self
sociological theories

LEARNING OUTCOMES

The material in this chapter will assist you to:

- develop an understanding of mental health and illness from history, theoretical perspectives and individual accounts and experiences.
- describe and critique biomedical, psychological and sociological theories of personality and behaviour.
- reflect on the relevance of lifespan concepts to your own experience.
- understand the relationship of psychological and sociological theories and concepts to mental health problems and mental illness across the lifespan.
- apply these theories and concepts in all phases of the nurse–patient relationship.
- integrate strategies that promote mental health into clinical practice.

INTRODUCTION

This chapter provides a foundation for understanding mental health problems and psychopathology within the context of normal human development. It reviews the work of theorists who have contributed to our understanding of human behaviour and development, and presents emerging research and perspectives on mental health across the lifespan. The chapter also explores specific developmental issues at different stages of the lifespan and how they intersect with mental health, creating the potential for mental health vulnerability (potential for illness). Concepts such as attachment, identity and resilience, which inform our understanding of development, are addressed in providing a holistic perspective on mental health issues across the lifespan. Strategies based on health promotion and a primary healthcare approach, discussed in more detail in Chapter 21, are proposed as a means of increasing protective factors and mental health across the lifespan.

WHAT IS MENTAL HEALTH?

A succinct, universally applicable definition of mental health has long been elusive. Even though contemporary definitions address the breadth of factors that contribute to mental health, they are subjective and not easily measured. The critique about the vague nature of definitions of mental health is longstanding. In the 1980s, Doona suggested that the problem of defining mental health was derived from the fact that the concept of mental health is not a measurable scientific term. She concluded: 'health is probably a value judgement and more amenable to philosophical analysis' (Doona 1982). Her view about the subjective nature of defining mental health remains pertinent today. For example, the World Health Organization (WHO) defines mental health as: 'a state of wellbeing in which every individual realizes his or her own potential, can cope with the normal stresses of life, can work productively and fruitfully, and is able to make a contribution to her or his community' (WHO 2014). It is interesting to note that while the Third Australian Mental Health Plan included a definition of mental health in its glossary (Australian Health Ministers 2003, p 5), the fourth plan does not. It does, however, include definitions for 'mental health problem', 'mental health services' and 'mental illness' (Commonwealth of Australia 2009, p. 84).

Historical Definitions of Mental Health

Early attempts to understand human behaviour focussed more on psychopathology than mental wellness. Demon possession is mentioned in the early writings of the Chinese, the Egyptians, the Hebrews and the Greeks to explain unusual behaviour and it continued to be the predominant explanation for abnormal behaviour until the Middle Ages (Maud & Warelow 2011). However, in Europe, it was not until the 16th century that abnormal behaviour was considered to be an illness and asylums were built to house people considered to be insane. From the 19th century in Europe, the United States and the UK and its colonies biomedical explanations dominated and abnormal behaviour was considered to be a disease. Such views led to humanitarian reform, underpinned by the notion that people living with a mental illness are as deserving of care as the physically ill (Butcher et al. 2011).

Contemporary approaches to defining mental health were first proposed in the latter half of the 20th century alongside worldwide mental health reforms. Early definitions focussed on the individual's ability to respond to external factors. Kittleson (1989) cited four major components: (1) high self-esteem; (2) effective decision making; (3) values awareness; and (4) expressive communication skills. Kittleson's depiction of mental health as a positive construct separate from mental illness was welcome but limited. It was welcome because it enabled mental health to be viewed as more than merely the absence of the symptoms of mental illness. However, it was limited because a focus on individual factors implies individual responsibility, which may lead to victim blaming (McMurray 2014; Talbot & Verrinder 2013). Furthermore, a definition in terms of the individual failed to acknowledge the contribution of social, political and environmental factors to mental health.

In Australia in the 1990s, Raphael (1993) drew attention to contextual and social issues that affect mental health—namely, workplace factors, education, macroeconomic forces and other forces. These social forces are acknowledged as contributors to mental health, as are personal qualities such as resilience, coping, physical health and wellbeing (Raphael 1993). More recent definitions of mental health include social determinants such as social connectedness, acceptance of diversity, freedom from discrimination and economic participation (VicHealth 2006; WHO 2014). Seligman's research has identified five measurable attributes, which he calls pillars, that contribute to both physical and mental wellbeing. These are:

- *positive emotion*—to experience love, hope, joy etc.
- *engagement*—to be connected to community and society through work, family etc.
- *relationships*—to experience close emotional and supportive ties
- *meaning*—to have a purpose in life, and for one's life to have meaning
- *accomplishments*—to have achieved tangible goals (Seligman 2004, 2011)

The emergence of a definition of mental health that encompasses positive constructs, not just the absence of symptoms, is important because it enables mental health and mental illness to be viewed as distinct from each other, and not as two points at opposite ends of a continuum. Significantly, it means that the two states are not mutually exclusive—a position advocated by the personal recovery model (Slade 2009). A person can enjoy mental health regardless of whether or not they are diagnosed with a mental illness if they have a positive sense of self, personal and social support with which to respond to life's challenges, access to resources and support to achieve their goals and aspirations, meaningful relationships with others, access to employment and recreational activities, sufficient financial resources and suitable living arrangements. Personal recovery is distinct from a clinical recovery perspective, which only addresses symptom eradication or management (see Chapter 2).

Recovery: Mental Health Despite Mental Illness

In the latter part of the 20th century, mental health services in developed countries underwent major reform, with recovery models driving this change internationally (Prince et al. 2007). The recovery model emerged at this time and it is now the cornerstone of the reform. The New Zealand

and Australia recovery model emerged at this time, a person-centred approach to service delivery underpinned by the principles of social justice and equity, which challenges the biomedical approach of focussing mainly on symptom identification and treatment (see Chapter 2 for more discussion of the recovery paradigm) (Rickwood 2006; Ministry of Health New Zealand 2005; Victorian Government 2009). Facilitating mental health, minimising the impact of mental illness and managing the symptoms of mental illness are the goals of the recovery-informed approach. Patients in New Zealand have identified the following as requisites for recovery: having personal power; maintaining hope and optimism; staying connected with extended family and community; and access to supportive services (Mental Health Commission New Zealand 2004).

In the context of mental health reform, the language of recovery is now widely used in mental health policy, services and research—yet the interpretation of the concept varies, particularly between services and service users (Ramon et al. 2007). Slade (2009) suggests that this arises from confusion between *clinical* recovery, which means the relief of symptoms, and *personal* recovery, which Anthony (1993, p. 14) defines as: 'a deeply personal, unique process of changing one's attitudes, values, feelings, goals, skills and/or roles. It is a way of living a satisfying, hopeful and contributing life even within the limitations caused by illness. Recovery involves the development of new meaning and purpose in one's life as one grows beyond the catastrophic effects of mental illness.'

'Mental Health' as a Euphemism for 'Mental Illness'

Health professionals and the health literature have adopted the practice of using the terms 'mental health' and 'mental illness' interchangeably since the 1920s. In 1989, Kittleson drew attention to this phenomenon following an examination of undergraduate mental health texts. He found that 'personality development and emotional illness make up the bulk of mental health coverage in the texts' (1989, p. 40). A recent search of contemporary mental health literature found that this practice is still prevalent in texts and journals (Edwards et al. 2011; Meadows et al. 2012; Muir-Cochrane et al. 2014; and journals such as the *International Journal of Mental Health Nursing* and *Issues in Mental Health Nursing*). Although these publications include 'mental health' in their titles, in the main they contain chapters or articles concerning assessment of, and treatments for, mental illness or mental health problems.

The substitution of the term 'mental health' when referring to 'mental illness' is a 20th-century phenomenon that has been carried forward into the new millennium. The first references to 'mental health' being used as an alternative to 'psychiatry' occurred in the UK and the United States from the 1920s. Momentum was gained after World War II, when proponents such as Caplan (1964) advocated a shift from treatment of mental illness to prevention. In the United States, Szasz (1961) argued that mental illness was a societal ill and not an individual sickness. Amid this debate, legislators worldwide changed the term 'mental illness' to 'mental health' in the names of legislation. However, this change is nominal because the content of worldwide policy and legislation continues to be concerned with mental illness (Ministry of Health New Zealand 2012; New South Wales Government 2007). The South Australian *Mental Health Act 2009*, for example, identifies its purpose as 'to make provision for the treatment, care and rehabilitation of persons with serious mental illness with the goal of bringing about their recovery as far as is possible' (Government of South Australia 2009). Despite the title of the Act, it contains no reference to mental health as a positive concept, nor does it expand on what recovery might mean.

Following legislative name changes, organisations that provided treatment and rehabilitation services to individuals with mental illness also changed their names, replacing words like 'psychiatric' and 'mental illness/disorder' with 'mental health'—hence the emergence of organisations with titles like 'Southern Area Mental Health Service'. Nevertheless, despite the change of name there has been little shift in the focus of the services provided, as they continue to address the needs of people living with illness, with minimal focus on mental health. This is not to suggest that mental illness treatment services should not be provided; clearly there is a demonstrated need for them and they are not under scrutiny here. Rather, the assertion is that to call them mental health services is a misnomer.

A further consequence of using the euphemism 'mental health' when referring to mental illness is that this practice may in fact be contributing to the perpetuation of stigma. Implicit in the avoidance of the term 'mental illness' is the notion that mental illness is something to be avoided, hidden or shameful. Ironically, calling mental illness by another name has not reduced stigma; instead, it has broadened the application of stigma to now include mental health.

CRITICAL THINKING CHALLENGE 6.1

1. What words would you use to describe mental health?
2. How do you know when you are mentally healthy? Reflect on a time when you consider your mental health was good. Make a list of the factors that facilitated this good mental health for you.
3. Make a list of negative words used to describe mental illness and consider the impact of these words on people living with a mental illness. Then think of a more positive word or term to use for each negative word on your list.
4. How does mental health differ from mental illness?

THEORIES OF PERSONALITY

Personality can be defined as the unique set of cognitive, affective and behavioural characteristics that influence how an individual thinks, feels and acts. Various explanations of personality have been proposed by philosophers and psychologists as well as by biomedical and social scientists. In seeking to understand personality, theorists have been driven not only by curiosity and philosophical enquiry, but also to identify factors that influence both normal and abnormal behaviour.

This has enabled the development of theories to explain resilience, mental health and illness, and also to identify strategies to prevent or treat mental illness.

Explanations of personality can be broadly divided into three paradigms:

- biomedical or biological/physical models
- psychological models, including psychoanalytic, behavioural, cognitive and humanistic approaches
- sociological models

Within these paradigms, the following are the major viewpoints to offer a theory of personality development or an explanation of human behaviour.

- *Biomedical model* proposes that behaviour is influenced by physiology, with normal behaviour occurring when the body is in a state of equilibrium and abnormal behaviour being a consequence of physical pathology.
- *Psychoanalytic theory* asserts that behaviour is driven by unconscious processes and influenced by childhood/developmental conflicts that have either been resolved or remain unresolved.
- *Behavioural psychology* presents the view that behaviour is influenced by factors external to the individual. Behaviours are learned, depending on whether they are rewarded or not, by association with another event or by imitation.
- *Cognitive psychology* acknowledges the role of perception and thoughts about oneself, one's individual experience and the environment in influencing behaviour.
- *Humanistic psychology* focusses on the development of a concept of self and the striving of the individual to achieve personal goals.
- *Sociological theories* shift the emphasis from the individual to the broader social forces that influence people. These theories challenge the notion of individual pathology.

Each of these seemingly disparate perspectives makes a substantial contribution to the understanding of how and why humans think, feel and act as they do, and thereby identifies opportunities for the prevention and treatment of mental illness. Nevertheless, as a comprehensive theory of human behaviour, each also has major shortcomings and no one theory can explain all human behaviour in all circumstances. Let us now look at these theories in more detail.

Biomedical Model

Also known as psychobiology or the neuroscience perspective, the biomedical model asserts that normal behaviour is a consequence of equilibrium within the body and that abnormal behaviour results from pathological bodily or brain function. This is not a new notion—in the 4th century BC the Greek physician Hippocrates attributed mental disorder to brain pathology. His ideas were overshadowed, however, when throughout the Dark Ages, and later during the Renaissance, thinking and explanations shifted to witchcraft or demonic possession (Butcher et al. 2011; Kring et al. 2010). In the 19th century, a return to biophysical explanations accompanied the emergence of the public health movement.

In recent times, advances in technology have led to increased understanding of organic determinants of behaviour. Research and treatment have focussed on four main areas.

- *Nervous system disorders*, in particular neurotransmitter disturbance at the synaptic gap between neurons. More than 50 neurotransmitters have been identified, four of which are implicated in mental illness. These are acetylcholine (Alzheimer disease), dopamine (schizophrenia), noradrenaline (mood disorder) and serotonin (mood disorder).
- *Structural changes to the brain*, for example, following trauma or in degenerative disorders such as Huntington disease.
- *Endocrine or gland dysfunction*, as in hypothyroidism. This has a similar presentation to clinical depression, and hormonal changes are considered to be a contributing factor in postnatal depression.
- *Familial (genetic) transmission of mental illness*, for example, twin studies reviewed by Gottesman found the following lifetime risks of developing schizophrenia: general population 1%, 1 parent with schizophrenia 13%, sibling with schizophrenia 9%, dizygotic twin with schizophrenia 17%, 2 parents with schizophrenia 46%, monozygotic twin with schizophrenia 48% (Butcher et al. 2011; Cando & Gottesman 2000).

Although genetic studies demonstrate a correlation between having a close relative with schizophrenia and the likelihood of developing the disorder, a shared genetic history alone is not sufficient. If genetics were the only aetiological factor, the concordance rate for monozygotic twins could be expected to be 100%. Gottesman's research is important because it supports the diathesis-stress model, a widely held explanation for the development of mental disorder, which proposes that constitutional predisposition combined with environmental stress will lead to mental illness (Kring et al. 2010).

Critique of the Biomedical Model

Among treatments that emerge from the biomedical model are medications that alter the function, production and reabsorption of neurotransmitters in the synaptic gap. However, evidence that a particular intervention is an effective treatment is not proof of a causal link with the illness. Consider a person with type 1 insulin-dependent diabetes mellitus, for example. Because this person lacks insulin to metabolise glucose, the condition is managed with regular insulin injections. However, the lack of insulin is a symptom of the disease, not the cause. Whatever caused the pancreas to cease producing insulin is not known, despite the treatment being effective. Similarly, with schizophrenia the relationship between the use of antipsychotic medications, dopamine levels and symptom management is correlational, not causal. Therefore, although antipsychotic medication affects dopamine levels and can be an effective treatment to manage the symptoms of schizophrenia, this does not provide evidence that elevated dopamine levels caused the disorder.

Psychoanalytic Theory

Sigmund Freud developed the first psychological explanation of human behaviour—psychoanalytic theory—in the late 19th century. He placed strong emphasis on the role of unconscious processes in determining human behaviour. Central tenets of the theory are that intrapsychic (generally unconscious) forces, developmental factors and family relationships determine human behaviour. Mental illness is seen as a consequence of fixation at a particular developmental stage or conflict that has not been resolved.

Sigmund Freud (1856–1939)

Freud was an Austrian neurologist who, in his clinical practice, saw a number of patients with sensory or neurological problems for which he was unable to identify a physiological cause. In the main, these patients were middle-class Viennese women. It was from his work with these patients that Freud hypothesised that the cause of their problems was psychological. From this assumption he developed a personality theory, which he called psychoanalytic theory.

According to Freud, the mind is composed of three forces.

1. The *id* is a primitive biological force comprising two basic drives: sexual and aggressive. The id operates on the pleasure principle and seeks to satisfy life-sustaining needs such as food, love and creativity, in addition to sexual gratification.
2. The *ego* is the cognitive component of personality, which attempts to use realistic means (the reality principle) to achieve the desires of the id.
3. The *superego* is the internalised moral standards of the society in which one lives. It can be equated to a conscience.

Freud's theory proposes that personality development progresses through five stages throughout childhood. At each stage, the child's behaviour is driven by the need to satisfy sexual and aggressive drives via the mouth, anus or genitals. Failure of the child to satisfy these needs at any one of the stages will result in psychological difficulties that are carried into adulthood. For example, unresolved issues at the oral stage can lead to dependency issues in adulthood, and problems in the anal stage may lead to the child later developing obsessive-compulsive traits. Freud's stages of psychosexual development are:

- *oral*—from birth to about 18 months, the primary focus of the id is the mouth
- *anal*—from approximately 18 months to 3 years, libido shifts from the mouth to the anus and primary gratification is derived from expelling or retaining faeces
- *phallic*—from approximately 3 to 6 years, gratification of the id occurs through the genitals
- *latent*—from approximately 6 to 12 years, the child goes through a latency phase in which sexual urges are dormant
- *genital*—once the child passes through puberty, sexual urges reemerge, but now they are directed towards another person, not the self as they were at an earlier stage of development (Butcher et al. 2011; Kring et al. 2010)

Defence Mechanisms

An important contribution of psychoanalytic theory to the understanding of behaviour has been the identification of defence mechanisms and the role they play in mediating anxiety. Defence mechanisms were first described by Freud and later elaborated on by his daughter Anna Freud (1966). They are unconscious processes whereby anxiety experienced by the ego is reduced. Commonly used defence mechanisms include:

- *repression*—the primary defence mechanism and an unconscious process whereby unacceptable impulses/feelings/thoughts are barred from consciousness (e.g. memories of sexual abuse in childhood)
- *regression*—the avoidance of present difficulties by a reversion to an earlier, less mature way of dealing with the situation (e.g. a toilet-trained child who becomes incontinent following the birth of a sibling)
- *denial*—the blocking of painful information from consciousness (e.g. not accepting that a loss has occurred)
- *projection*—the denial of one's own unconscious impulses by attributing them to another person (e.g. when you dislike someone but believe it is the other person who does not like you)
- *sublimation*—an unconscious process whereby libido is transformed into a more socially acceptable outlet (e.g. creativity, art, sport)
- *displacement*—the transferring of emotion from the source to a substitute (e.g. you are unassertive in an interaction with a supervisor at work and 'kick the cat' on arriving home)
- *rationalisation*—a rational excuse is used to explain behaviour that may be motivated by an irrational force (e.g. cheating on your tax return, with the excuse that 'everyone does it')
- *intellectualisation/isolation*—feelings are cut off from the event in which they occur (e.g. after an unsuccessful job interview you say 'I didn't really want the job anyway')
- *reaction formation*—unacceptable emotions or impulses are expressed as the opposite of the original unconscious reaction (e.g. avoiding a friend's partner because you are attracted to that person)

Being aware of defence mechanisms and the role they play in managing anxiety can assist nurses to understand that a person's seemingly irrational behaviour may have an unconscious cause. For example, the child who regresses following a serious illness is not attention seeking, but reverting to behaviours from a time when they felt safe.

Critique of Psychoanalytic Theory

Although the notions of unconscious motivations and defence mechanisms are helpful in interpreting behaviours, Freud's version of psychoanalytic theory has not been without its critics. Fellow psychoanalyst Erik Erikson disagreed with Freud's theory of psychosexual stages of development and proposed instead a psychosocial theory in which development occurred throughout the lifespan, not just through childhood as in Freud's model (Erikson 1963; Santrock 2011).

The unconscious nature of Freud's concepts and stages renders them difficult to test and therefore there is little evidence to support Freudian theory. Feminists, too, object to Freud's interpretation of the psychological development of women, arguing that there is scant evidence to support the hypothesis that women view their bodies as inferior to men's because they do not have a penis (Kring et al. 2010). Nevertheless, despite these criticisms, psychoanalytic theory does provide plausible explanations for seemingly irrational behaviour.

Behavioural Psychology

Behaviourism is a school of psychology founded in the United States by JB Watson in the early 20th century with the purpose of objectively studying observable human behaviour, as opposed to examining the mind, which was the prevalent psychological method at the time in Europe. The model proposes a *scientific* approach to the study of observable behaviour, a feature that behaviourists argue is lacking in psychoanalytic theory (and in humanistic psychology, which developed later).

Behaviourism opposes the introspective, structuralist approach of psychoanalysis and emphasises the importance of the environment in shaping behaviour. The focus is on observable behaviour and conditions that elicit and maintain the behaviour (classical conditioning) or factors that reinforce behaviour (operant conditioning) or vicarious learning through watching and imitating the behaviour of others (modelling).

Three basic assumptions underpin behaviour theory:

1. personality is determined by prior learning
2. human behaviour is changeable throughout the lifespan
3. changes in behaviour are generally caused by changes in the environment

The following people were prominent figures in the development of behavioural psychology.

Ivan Pavlov (1849–1936)

Russian physiologist Ivan Pavlov was the first to describe the relationship between stimulus and response. Pavlov demonstrated that a dog could learn to salivate (respond) to a non-food stimulus (a bell) if the bell was simultaneously presented with the food. His discovery became known as classical conditioning.

John B Watson (1878–1958)

Watson, who is attributed with being the founder of behaviourism, changed the focus of psychology from the study of inner sensations to the study of observable behaviour. In his quest to make psychology a true science, Watson further developed Pavlov's work on stimulus–response learning and experimented by manipulating stimulus conditions. Watson believed that abnormal behaviour was the result of earlier faulty conditioning and that reconditioning could modify this.

Burrhus F Skinner (1904–1990)

Later, another American psychologist, BF Skinner, formulated the notion of instrumental or operant conditioning in which reinforcers (rewards) contribute to the probability of a response being either repeated or extinguished. Skinner's research demonstrated that the contingencies on which behaviour is based are external to the person, rather than internal. Consequently, changing contingencies could alter an individual's behaviour. This is an underlying principle in treatment using an operant conditioning approach (Skinner 1953).

Critique of Behaviourism

Behaviourism provided the first scientifically testable theories of human development as well as plausible explanations of conditions such as depression and anxiety. However, behavioural explanations are less convincing when applied to psychosis or organic disorders. Furthermore, most behavioural research has been conducted on animals under laboratory conditions, so to generalise findings from this research to humans is mechanistic and does not allow for intrinsic human qualities like creativity or the ability to love, think or solve problems. Finally, behavioural theory falls short in explaining the success of an individual brought up in an adverse environment (resilience), or how mental illness can occur in a person whose environment is apparently healthy and advantaged.

Cognitive Psychology

Since the 1950s, interest in the cognitive or thinking processes involved in behavioural responses has expanded. Cognitive theory proposes that people actively interpret their environment and cognitively construct their world. Therefore, behaviour is a result of the interplay of external and internal events. External events are the stimuli and reinforcements that regulate behaviour, and internal events are one's perceptions and thoughts about the world, as well as one's behaviour in the world. In other words, how one thinks about a situation will influence how one behaves in that situation. The following are prominent figures in the development of cognitive psychology.

Albert Bandura (b. 1925)

According to Bandura it is not intrapsychic or environmental forces alone that influence behaviour. Rather, human behaviour results from the interaction of the environment with the individual's perception and thinking. Self-efficacy, or the belief that one can achieve a certain goal, is the critical component in the achievement of that goal. Bandura also proposed that consequences do not have to be directly experienced by the individual for learning to occur—learning can occur vicariously through the process of modelling or learning by imitation (Bandura 2001).

Aaron T Beck (b. 1921)

Problem behaviour, says Beck, results from cognitive distortions or faulty thinking. For example, a depressed person will selectively choose information that maintains a gloomy perspective. Depression is experienced when one has a negative schema about oneself or one's situation. According to Beck, depression is a behavioural response to an attitude or a cognition of hopelessness, as opposed to hopelessness being a symptom of depression; and anxiety is experienced when one has a distorted anticipation of danger. Treatment within Beck's model involves changing one's views about oneself and one's life situation (Beck 1972).

Martin Seligman (b. 1942)

Seligman (1974) first proposed his theory of learned helplessness as an explanation for depression. The theory suggests that if an individual experiences adversity and attempts to alleviate the situation are unsuccessful, then depression follows. Seligman (1994) later expanded his model to include learned optimism, a process of challenging negative cognitions to change from a position of passivity to one of control. He subsequently founded the school of Positive Psychology, which focusses on studying positive emotions and individual strengths that enable people to flourish, rather than weaknesses (Seligman 2011; Seligman & Csikszentmihalyi 2000).

Jean Piaget (1896–1980)

Piaget was a Swiss biologist, psychologist and philosopher whose pioneering work in the field of child development has influenced healthcare and education. His theory of cognitive development proposes that children progress through four stages from birth to adolescence as they adapt to the world in which they live. These stages are sensorimotor, preoperational, concrete operational and formal operational. They are covered later in this chapter.

Critique of Cognitive Psychology

The therapeutic techniques derived from cognitive (and cognitive behavioural) theory are practical and effective and can be self-administered by the patient under the direction of a therapist. These therapies have an established record in changing problem behaviours such as phobias, obsessions and compulsions and in stress management (Butcher et al. 2011). They also make a contribution in the treatment of depression and schizophrenia, although whether the treatment result is more effective than other interventions is inconclusive in the literature (Lynch et al. 2010). Cognitive theory is criticised as being unscientific (as are psychoanalytic and humanistic theories) because mental processes cannot be objectively observed and subjective reports are not necessarily reliable (Kring et al. 2010). Additionally, the insight that one's thinking is the cause of one's problems will not in itself bring about behaviour change.

Finally, contrary to the proposal that thoughts → feelings → behaviour (a notion that underpins the cognitive approach), research conducted by Kearns and Gardiner (2010) into procrastination and motivation among postgraduate university students suggests that if the behaviour is changed first so that the student starts working on their study, then the student will feel more motivated and procrastination will be reduced. These findings can be explained by the relational model of Ivey et al. (2010), in which thoughts, feelings and behaviour interact with each other and with meaning, in contrast to the linear unidirectional explanation of cognitive psychology (see Fig. 6.1). The thrust of the interactive model is that a change in any one part of the system may result in a change in other parts as well (Ivey et al. 2010, p. 294). So while cognitions play an integral part in behavioural outcomes, they may not necessarily be the initiating factor as proposed by cognitive theory.

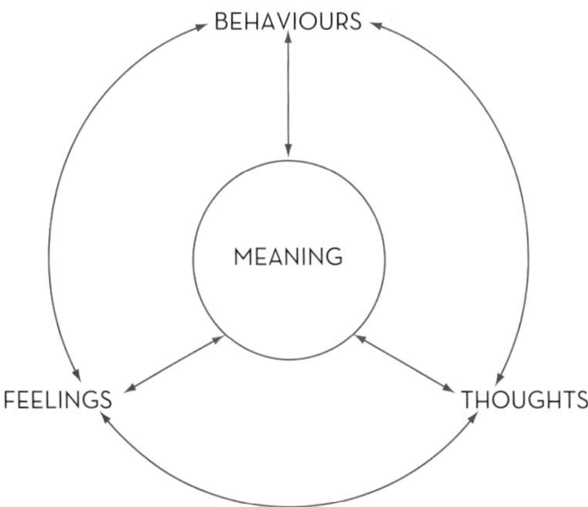

Fig. 6.1 Ivey, Ivey and Zalaquett's (2010) interactive model of cognitive psychology (*Source:* Ivey, A., Ivey, M., Zalaquett, C., 2014. Intentional Interviewing and Counselling, eighth ed. 2014 South-Western, a part of Cengage Learning, Inc. Reproduced by permission. www.cengage.com/permissions.)

Humanistic Psychology

Following disenchantment with the existing psychological theories of the time, Charlotte Bühler, Abraham Maslow, Carl Rogers and their colleagues in the United States established the Association for Humanistic Psychology in 1962. Humanistic psychology has its intellectual and social roots in philosophical humanism and existentialism, which brought psychology back to a close relationship with philosophy (Bühler & Allen 1972). This school of psychology, which became known as the Third Force, arose in response to dissatisfaction at the time with the mechanistic approach of psychoanalysis and behaviourism and the negative views that underpinned both these theoretical perspectives.

Humanistic psychologists objected to the determinism of the two prevailing theories: (1) psychoanalysis, with its emphasis on unconscious drives; and (2) behaviourism, which saw the environment as central in shaping behaviour. Humanistic psychology rejected the reductionism of explaining human behaviour, feelings, thinking and motivation merely in terms of psychological mechanisms or biological processes. It also opposed the mechanistic approach of behaviourism and psychoanalysis for the way in which they minimised human experience and qualities such as choice, creativity and spontaneity.

Humanistic psychologists focussed on the intrinsic human qualities of the individual, such as free will, altruism, freedom and self-actualisation, qualities which, they asserted, distinguished humans from other animals. Humanistic psychology therefore differed from its predecessors in its emphasis on the whole person, human emotions, experience and the meaning of experience, the creative potential of the individual, choice, self-realisation and self-actualisation. The theory also opposed dualistic (subject/object, mind/body splits), deterministic, reductionistic and mechanistic explanations of human behaviour.

The humanistic movement also reflected a historical trend in Western industrialised cultures at that time, which was to be interested in the worth of the individual and the meaning of life, and to be concerned about the rise of bureaucracy, the threat of nuclear war, the growing emphasis on scientific/positivist paradigms, alienation of the individual and consequent loss of identity in mass society. This led to humanistic psychology being aligned with existentialism as well as being associated with the human potential movements of the 1960s and 1970s, the legacy of which can be seen today in individual and group counselling approaches. Humanistic psychology also played a part in the growing interest in qualitative research methods, which seek to understand the experience of the individual and the meaning of the experience, such as phenomenology (Crotty 1996). The following people were prominent figures in the development of humanistic psychology.

Charlotte Bühler (1893–1974)

Bühler distinguished her theory from Freudian psychoanalysis with the thesis that development was lifelong, goals were personally selected and the individual was searching for meaning in life beyond one's own existence. She maintained that self-fulfilment was the key to human development and that this was achieved by living constructively, establishing a personal value system, setting goals and reviewing progress to thereby realise one's potential. Throughout the lifespan, according to Bühler, individuals strove to achieve four basic human tendencies, which were to:

- satisfy one's need for sex, love and recognition
- engage in self-limiting adaptation in order to fit in, belong and feel secure
- express oneself through creative achievements
- uphold and restore order so as to be true to one's values and conscience (Bühler & Allen 1972).

Carl Rogers (1902–1987)

Rogers proposed a more hopeful and optimistic view of humankind than that of his psychoanalytic and behaviourist contemporaries. He believed that each person contained within themselves the potential for healthy, creative growth. According to Rogers, the failure to achieve one's potential resulted from constricting and distorting influences of poor parenting, education or other social pressures. Patient-centred therapy is the counselling model that Rogers developed to assist the individual to overcome these harmful effects and take responsibility for their life (Rogers 1951, 1961).

Abraham Maslow (1908–1970)

As a frequently cited author in the nursing literature, Maslow is renowned for his theory of human needs. Maslow, like Bühler and Rogers, premised his theory on the notion that human beings are intrinsically good and that human behaviour is motivated by a drive for self-actualisation. Maslow (1968) identified three categories of human need:

1. fundamental needs
   - physiological (hunger, thirst and sex)
   - safety (security and freedom from danger)
2. psychological needs
   - belongingness and love (connection with others, to be accepted and to belong)
   - self-esteem (to achieve, be competent, gain approval and recognition)
3. self-actualisation needs
   - to achieve one's innate potential

Typically, Maslow's needs are represented in a hierarchical pyramid with fundamental needs at the base of the triangle and self-actualisation at the top, although Maslow did not describe his model in this way. Nor did he suggest that progression through the hierarchy was in one direction (i.e. ascending) as his model is often depicted. For example, one may have a positive sense of self (self-esteem needs met) but be vulnerable regarding safety needs during a natural disaster like a tsunami.

Critique of Humanistic Psychology

Intuitively, humanistic psychology appeals as a positive, optimistic view of humankind with its focus on personal growth, not disorder. However, this can also be a criticism, in that as a theory humanistic psychology is naive and incomplete. If humans are driven by a need to achieve their best and to live harmoniously with others, as Bühler, Rogers and Maslow suggest, how does this account for disturbed states like depression or antisocial behaviour like assault? Humanistic concepts can be difficult to define objectively, thereby posing a challenge for scientific investigation of the theory. Finally, there is little recognition of unconscious drives in explaining behaviour, which limits the ability of the theory to contribute to an understanding of abnormal or antisocial behaviour.

Sociological Theories

Sociological theories differ from psychological theories in that they do not seek explanations for individual behaviour; rather, they examine societal factors for their influence on the behaviour of its members. Sociologists propose that the causes of abnormal behaviour lie not in the individual's mind, but in the broader social forces of the society in which the individual lives. Demographic factors that are associated with increased incidence of mental illness include:

- age—the elderly are more likely to suffer from depression
- gender—the suicide rate for men is higher than for women, although the rate for attempted suicide is higher for women than for men
- socioeconomic status—poverty is associated with poorer physical and mental health outcomes

The following social commentators propose interpretations of mental illness that challenge the notion of individual pathology.

Emile Durkheim (1858–1917)

Durkheim's classic study of suicide led him to propose a societal rather than an individual explanation for this phenomenon. He argued that suicide was not an individual act, but that it could be understood in terms of the bonds that exist between the person and society, or the regulation of the individual by social norms. Durkheim's analysis of suicide statistics found that suicide was more prevalent in groups where the bond between the individual and the group was overly weak or excessively strong, or where the regulation of individual desires and aspirations by societal norms was either inadequate or excessive. According to Durkheim (1951) there are four types of suicide.

1. Egoistic, where the social bonds of attachment are weak and the individual is less integrated into the social group and therefore not bound by its obligations (e.g. single immigrant men).
2. Altruistic, where the social bonds of attachment are overly strong and the individual's sense of self is not distinguished from the group—the individual may be driven to suicide by a consequence of a passionate commitment to the group (e.g. suicide bombers).
3. Anomic, where regulation of the individual's desires and aspirations is not adequate. This can occur in a society undergoing rapid change, which dislocates social norms (e.g. retrenched workers).
4. Fatalistic, where there is overregulation by society which renders a sense of powerlessness in the individual and predisposes the person to suicide (e.g. deaths in custody).

Thomas Szasz (1920–2012)

Since the 1960s, prominent psychiatrist Thomas Szasz challenged the concept of mental illness, arguing that disease implies a pathology that often cannot be objectively identified (Szasz 1961, 2000). He attacked the biomedical model, claiming that its purpose is to give control over people's lives to psychiatrists, and argued that psychiatrists exercise coercive domination in the guise of protecting the public and the mad from their madness (Szasz 2000). Contrary to the illusion that psychiatry is coping well with society's vexing problems, Szasz (2000) claimed that social problems are in fact being obscured and aggravated by the disease interpretation of psychiatry.

Critique of Sociological Models

Sociological models identify social determinants of health (WHO 2008), vulnerable populations and health promotion opportunities (Navarro 2009) as well as biases that influence diagnosis and treatment. It is important to note, however, that although social determinants are associated with better or poorer mental health outcomes, the relationships are correlational and cannot be assumed to be in themselves causative. Nevertheless, the contribution of population statistics and social demographic data remains significant. By identifying social determinants that are associated with protective factors for mental health and risk factors for mental illness, potential areas for prevention and intervention are thereby identified.

Personality Theories and Explanations of Human Behaviour

Table 6.1 outlines the key features of the major biological, psychological and sociological theories which propose explanations of human behaviour. These theories inform our understanding of ourselves and others and underpin interventions for behaviour change and treatments for mental illness.

> **CRITICAL THINKING CHALLENGE 6.2**
>
> 1. Identify factors that influence whether a particular phenomenon (e.g. hearing voices) would be considered normal or a symptom of mental illness.
> 2. Compare and contrast two theories of personality development with regard to how each theory explains:
>   - mental health
>   - mental illness.
> 3. How do sociological theories differ from psychological theories of personality development and human behaviour?

A LIFESPAN APPROACH

Theories of personality development such as the biomedical, psychological (psychoanalytic, behavioural, cognitive and humanistic) and sociological assist us to understand human behaviour. Some of these theories include the concept of 'stages' to explain how changes occur across the lifespan. These 'developmental' theorists have formulated theories to assist our understanding of how growth and change affect the personality and how we become 'ourselves'. Developmental theories aim to explain normal growth and development of the personality or 'self'. A lifespan approach (lifespan developmental psychology) encompasses the sequence of events and experiences in life from birth until death. Goals of the approach are to describe development, to explain how change occurs throughout the lifespan and to optimise development through the application of theory to real life (Peterson 2013).

Contemporary lifespan theory acknowledges that individuals can learn and change at all stages throughout life. Baltes & Baltes (1990) suggest that human development does not follow a linear pathway from birth to death but that development occurs across many dimensions in a nonintegrated fashion. A nonlinear model refutes the idea that there is a definite sequential pathway for development and challenges the belief that an ideal end-state or conclusion is achieved. Baltes et al. define development as 'selective age-related change in adaptive capacity' (Baltes et al. 1999, p. 476). Baltes et al.'s view supports the idea that development consists of a series of losses and gains. Losses and gains occur throughout the lifespan as new skills are acquired, and the individual experiences certain benefits as a result; however, they may also experience a lack of continuity in other skills or abilities. For example, the older adult may not have the memory capacity of a younger person but they may develop pragmatic or problem-solving strategies (such as the use of mnemonics) that result in similar performance, thus compensating for age-related deficits (Baltes & Baltes 1990). An additional gain of development is creativity. Creativity is perceived as essential in our ability to constantly develop new strategies, such as improved problem solving, to compensate for age-related losses. Box 6.1 lists key points to an understanding of a contemporary lifespan approach.

TABLE 6.1 **Personality Theories and Explanations of Human Behaviour**

	Focus	Stage Theory	Motivation	Individual Control	Cause of Problems	Intervention
Biomedical	Physiological homeostasis/ pathology	No	Physiological homeostasis	Internal Biological	Genetics Biological/biochemical pathology	Medication Physical treatments
Psychoanalytic	Unconscious processes	Yes, e.g. Freud, Erikson	Internal drives Pleasure	Internal Psychological	Ego conflict Stage fixation	Psychoanalysis Insight therapy
Behavioural/ learning	Learning Environment	No, e.g. Pavlov, Skinner	Gain rewards Avoid punishment	External Psychological	Faulty learning	Learn new behaviours Extinguish unwanted behaviour
Cognitive	Thinking Perception	Some no, e.g. Seligman, Bandura Some developmental, e.g. Piaget	Psychological balance	Internal Psychological	Faulty perceptions Irrational beliefs	Cognitive restructuring/therapy including CBT, DBT
Humanistic	Self-concept Self-actualisation	No, e.g. Maslow, Rogers	Meet needs Goals Self-actualisation	Internal Psychological	Loss of meaning Unmet needs Incongruence Lack of unconditional positive regard	Find meaning/ understanding Patient-centred therapy
Sociological	Demographic factors Power Inequities	No, e.g. Durkheim, Szasz	Power Social equity	External Social	Society Notion of mental illness challenged	Social justice Economic and political reform

CBT, Cognitive behavioural therapy; *DBT*, dialectical behavioural therapy.

BOX 6.1 **A Lifespan Approach: Key Points**

The tenets that guide an understanding of the lifespan approach include a belief that:

- the potential for growth and development exists throughout the lifespan
- development is multidirectional, with no specific route or direction
- patterns of development vary due to social, historical, cultural and gender variables
- there are numerous dimensions to development and each may follow a different trajectory
- dimensions to development include physical–motor, cognitive–intellectual and personal–social–emotional, and each interacts with the others
- the individual and the environment influence each other
- lifespan development promotes a holistic approach to nursing practice

A Lifespan Approach to Nursing Practice

The nurse has an opportunity to provide information, resources and interventions for patients and families that will support and facilitate emotional development, cognitive growth and psychosocial wellbeing throughout the lifespan. The nurse's ability to use concepts related to development (e.g. attachment, resilience) will enhance their understanding of the patient and promote individually focussed recovery-oriented care. As well as equipping the nurse with knowledge to identify disruptions in development, developmental theories can increase the nurse's awareness of the patient, their perception of their problem and their responses to it. Moreover, knowledge of the lifespan can facilitate accurate assessment and communication, enhance empathy and promote the development of interventions that are specific and meaningful for the patient (Box 6.2 lists ways a lifespan approach informs practice). It can be useful, for example, to understand why some adolescents and young adults have difficulty relating to others and regulating their own behaviour and emotions. Additional concepts such as attachment and resilience (see Chapter 21) also need to be considered to promote person-centred care. These concepts can be protective and assist in a balanced assessment of risk at all stages of the lifespan.

BOX 6.2 **A Lifespan Approach: Role in Practice**

A lifespan approach in practice contributes to:

- communication, particularly development of rapport
- establishment of empathy
- interviewing
- identification of patient concerns and general facilitation of therapeutic communication
- risk assessment (self-harm and suicide)
- identification and implementation of appropriate interventions
- appropriate referral
- awareness of boundary issues

CRITICAL THINKING CHALLENGE 6.3

Explain what is meant by 'the lifespan' and 'a lifespan approach for nursing'. Discuss how knowledge of lifespan theories and concepts contributes to nursing practice.

MENTAL HEALTH ACROSS THE LIFESPAN

The fundamental elements of mental health are acquired throughout a person's development. Developmental theories emphasise the importance of the early months and years of life in laying a foundation for sound mental health in adulthood. Mental health, like physical health, contributes to a person's quality of life. It enhances our functioning in all aspects of life—work, relationships and social situations—and also enables us to feel that we are worthwhile and acceptable just as we are. Mental health enables us to mediate and manage distress from external events in our life, to cope with the ups and downs and to be hopeful about the future. Optimal personal development is related to and dependent on an individual's mental health.

As well as describing normal development, developmental theorists propose a set of conditions or criteria necessary for optimal development and subsequent mental health. Each theorist sets out tasks, challenges or milestones that need to be achieved for normal development. Mental health problems can result when developmental tasks and challenges are not met due to some disruption in the internal or external environment. Internal conditions include inherited characteristics and personality characteristics. External conditions include parenting, nurturing in childhood and positive or negative life events. It is important for the nurse to be aware of the tenets of the lifespan approach (outlined in Box 6.1) when considering mental health issues throughout life, as many psychological issues recur repeatedly in different forms.

CRITICAL THINKING CHALLENGE 6.4

How would your own experience affect your ability to understand the significance of events and experiences in the lives of patients? Reflect on how differences in culture may influence your understanding.

'Ideal' Development

Cognitive, perceptual, emotional and social functioning are dimensions of growth and development that are not well understood, even though they are crucial to each individual's wellbeing and mental health. Development itself is difficult to define and hints that 'improvement' is part of a developing state. The literature on ageing (Baltes & Baltes 1990; Bevan & Jeeawody 1998) explores how we can age 'successfully'. The following outcome measurements are proposed:

- length of life
- biological health
- mental health
- cognitive efficacy
- social competence and productivity
- personal control
- life satisfaction

These criteria demonstrate the multiple influences necessary for overall achievement of 'good ageing'. Multiple criteria take into account objective and subjective measures, so as to incorporate the individual's own definition of success.

'Good' outcomes of development proposed by Abraham Maslow (1968), Erik Erikson (1963) and Gordon Allport (1961) all describe criteria that are normative; that is, they assume that everyone is the same and that there is a general standard which, if achieved, can lead to an ideal end-state. As noted earlier, this assumption has been challenged. It can be useful, however, to define development as an ideal state so that factors that are barriers to achieving this state can be explored and ways of encouraging development can be addressed through health-promoting nursing interventions and a holistic approach to practice.

The ideal outcomes of development (listed in Table 6.2) highlight the characteristics of optimal wellbeing and mental health, but the course of life and significant events can disrupt this ideal. Factors that can disrupt the path of normal development are discussed further later in this chapter.

Stages and Theoretical Issues in Human Development

Stage theories were initiated by the evolutionary perspective of Charles Darwin, who believed that human development could be understood through the study of childhood. Darwin's work was significant in introducing a scientific approach to the study of development. Stage theories support the idea that individual development can be measured and monitored according to a set of expected 'norms' at average ages when certain milestones are achieved.

Stages have different meanings depending on the variable being considered. For example, biological stage theories conceive of growth being completed by adulthood, followed by a maintenance period, after which physical decline results. A sociocultural/psychosocial conception of stages describes a series of roles and age- or development-related tasks throughout life (Erikson). Cognitive–structural stages (Piaget) are conceived of as an ascending staircase along the lifeline, with later stages integrating and building upon previous cognitive functioning. Stage theories require consideration of normative variables (age or historical influences shared by most people) and nonnormative variables (events unique to individuals) that may influence growth and development across the lifespan. During assessment nurses can give consideration to normative (general) and nonnormative (unique) influences to ensure that individuals and families are assessed holistically and that the range of issues affecting development can be examined. Theories help us to understand why some people might be more vulnerable to mental health problems or at risk of developing mental illness. Freud, Erikson and Piaget were influential in contributing to a lifespan perspective of development.

TABLE 6.2 Ideal Outcomes of Development

Characteristics of the Self-actualised Person (Maslow 1968)	Dimensions of Maturity (Allport 1961)	The 'Eight Stages of Man' (Erikson 1963)
• Accurate perception of reality • Acceptance of self and others • Spontaneity • Problem centring • Detachment (emotionally self-sufficient) • Autonomy • Continued fresh appreciation • Mystic or peak experiences • Unconditional positive regard for others • Characteristic interpersonal relations • Democratic character structure • Definite moral standards • Philosophical sense of humour • Creativeness • Cultural transcendence	• Extension of the sense of self (having a life mission) • Warm relating of self to others • Emotional security • Realistic perception, skills and assignments (solves problems as required) • Self-objectification (insight or self-awareness) • Unifying philosophy on life	• Basic trust versus mistrust (0–1 year) • → Hope • Autonomy versus shame and doubt (1–3 years) • → Willpower • Initiative versus guilt (4–5 years) • → Purpose • Industry versus inferiority (6–11 years) • → Competence and accomplishment • Identity versus role confusion (12–18 years) • → Fidelity • Intimacy versus isolation (early adulthood) • → Love • Generativity versus stagnation (middle adulthood) • → Care and production • Ego integrity versus despair (older adulthood) • → Wisdom

Sigmund Freud (1856–1939)

Freud proposed three personality structures, which, if functioning in balance, help the person to resolve the conflicts of different psychosexual stages of personality development. Maturation is the desired outcome of the individual successfully moving through four psychosexual stages (from infancy to adolescence). Earlier in this chapter, the stages and characteristics of each stage were outlined and the role of defence mechanisms in managing anxiety were explained. The relevance of Freud's theory lies primarily in its ability to assist the nurse in understanding patient behaviours that appear inconsistent with age or the expected level of development, or behaviour and habits that are excessive or unexplained by other assessment frameworks.

Erik Erikson (1902–1994)

Erikson envisaged successful personality development as an outcome of conflict resolution throughout eight 'psychosocial' stages. The relevance of Erikson's psychosocial theory for nurses is that it assists the nurse with increased interpersonal understanding of the individual's biological, psychological, spiritual and social dimensions. Stages highlight the central concerns of individuals at different times in their lives and identify challenges that may contribute to vulnerability. Erikson's theory suggests that a person may be unable to achieve mastery of one of the developmental tasks due to external factors, such as a loss or injury, which may disrupt the person's development. Nurses are able to consider the tasks of each stage and integrate these understandings into appropriate assessment and planning. In addition, the nurse may convey an understanding to the patient of the importance of their concerns, increasing empathy in the nurse–patient relationship. A brief description of the conflicts and outcome of each stage is given in Table 6.2 and application of the theory to practice is outlined further in this chapter.

Evaluation of Erikson's work highlights criticisms that stage theories propose a 'normative' or standard recipe for development. Erikson has also been criticised for his optimistic view of people (Roazen, cited in Welchman 2000) that negates the complexity and flaws in human nature. Welchman (2000, p. 120) states: 'His affirmative view of human potential is a warning not to label antisocial behaviour as pathological.' Erikson used male subjects in his work, which led to criticisms that the male experience is understood as universal. Carol Gilligan, a student of Erikson, developed a critique of his work and proposed a need for a separate chart for women to account for differences in experience and challenges through life (Welchman 2000). Gilligan developed theories of women's development being associated with relationships with others; her ideas are explored later in this chapter.

Jean Piaget (1896–1980)

Piaget proposed a theory consisting of four broad stages describing the development of thinking (cognitive–developmental theory). The relevance of Piaget's theory is that it assists the nurse to understand that in the early years, infants and children require stimulation and an experience of the external world in order to learn ways of relating to their environment. Nurses can use play and simple, concrete ideas to communicate meaningfully with children in healthcare settings. An awareness by the nurse that the ability to think abstractly or conceptually is necessary for problem solving can assist the nurse with the facilitation of decision making with particular patients. For example, health-teaching

BOX 6.3 Stages of Cognitive Development

- *Sensorimotor (0–2 years).* Infants use their senses to explore and learn about the world. They are able to act on their world; for example, they can move an object (rattle) to make a noise.
- *Preoperational (2–7 years).* Preschool children are able to use symbols to represent their earlier actions, but thinking remains illogical. Children play at make-believe and acquire language.
- *Concrete operational (7–11 years).* Reasoning becomes more logical and organised. Objects can be classified according to size and other hierarchies can be established.
- *Formal operational (11 years onwards).* The ability to think in abstract terms defines this stage. Concepts and symbols can be used in advanced problem solving (advanced mathematics). A variety of options can be generated to solve problems and generate creative thought.

(Adapted from Peterson, C., 2004. Looking Forward Through the Lifespan: Developmental Psychology, fourth ed. Prentice Hall, Sydney.)

interventions with adolescents or young adults (assumed to be at the formal-operations stage) would require the nurse to be specific with information and not to assume that they are able to apply health-teaching information to a range of issues. Each issue would need to be addressed separately as some adolescents and young adults may be unable to generalise information.

There are several key concepts in Piaget's theory. Adaptation is the mechanism by which development occurs, as the structures of the mind 'adapt' to better represent the external world. According to this theory the individual develops 'schemas' or behaviour patterns. When a new item is incorporated into the existing schema, 'assimilation' occurs. 'Accommodation' occurs when the individual is unable to assimilate the new item into the existing schema. The schema is altered to accommodate the new item. An example would be when a baby reaches for and grasps an object (the baby will assimilate the action into a 'grasping schema'); the baby then accommodates as it modifies its grasp for a range of differently shaped objects. The aim of this process is to achieve equilibrium, thereby increasing the sophistication of thinking and understanding. Piaget was interested in how children think, reason and learn. He proposed the stages outlined in Box 6.3.

Moral Development

Piaget was concerned with moral as well as cognitive development. As he saw it, the maturing minds of adolescents experienced disequilibrium and conflict as a result of discussions with peers. Disequilibrium was seen as an opportunity for growth and development for the adolescent as they sought resolution of the particular dilemma (Golombok & Fivush 1994; Piaget 1977). But as with Piaget's general developmental theories, researchers have found that morality begins at a much earlier age, although not always at such a sophisticated level (Darley & Shultz 1990; Shultz & Wells 1985).

Lawrence Kohlberg (Kohlberg 1986; Kohlberg et al. 1983) developed a stage-based model in which people functioning at the higher levels were seen as being able to use a justice orientation in their moral decisions. A justice orientation emphasises the need for reason and detachment in decision making. Kohlberg saw moral development as an internal process that happens as a result of increasing cognitive maturity with little external influence. His assessment of morality was based on people's responses to hypothetical moral dilemmas. Unfortunately, many nursing authors have tended to use his theory with no recognition of the many criticisms of his work. Critics have observed that his view of justice is limited to one theoretical perspective, and that his methodology was flawed and biased as it used only young male participants and ignored family influences. Others have pointed out that moral thoughts do not always result in moral behaviours (Bailey 1986).

Carol Gilligan (Brown et al. 1991; Gilligan 1982, 1987, 1998) emphasised a care orientation, where the relatedness of individuals to each other is seen as important in moral decision making. Initially she proposed that women used a care orientation, whereas men used a justice-based approach. This aroused much controversy at the time. Her current view is that males and females use either a justice or a caring 'voice', depending on the situation and the issue, although most males and females do appear to favour the style she originally proposed for each sex. Females are therefore not seen as inferior to men in their decision making, but different. Other findings have supported this view (Donenberg & Hoffman 1988; Pratt et al. 1984).

Attachment, Parenting and Family Factors

Research has often found that a bond, or attachment, between mother and child is the most significant factor influencing development (Garmon 2000; Park & Roberts 2002). Eisenberg (2000) and Stilwell et al. (1997) carried out longitudinal research across various age groups from infancy to adolescence demonstrating how, through attachment, children and adolescents progressively develop a conscience.

Research into parenting styles has also contributed to our understanding of moral development. In the 1960s Diana Baumrind (1971) studied parents and their children. She described three parenting styles, which have since been extensively studied and are used in clinical practice.

1. *Authoritative parents* had clear expectations, but were also warm, supportive, rational and reciprocating, willing to allow an interactive level of communication. Their children tended to achieve high levels of competent and responsible independent behaviour, with mature levels of morality.
2. *Authoritarian parents* were dominant and detached, with a lower level of warmth than others, resulting in discontented, withdrawn and distrustful children. It is important to note the difference between this and the authoritative parenting style, as laypeople as well as professionals can sometimes mistakenly use the two terms interchangeably.

3. *Permissive parents* gave control to the child, were relatively warm, nondemanding and noncontrolling. Children of these parents were the least self-reliant, explorative or self-controlled, often with a poor social conscience (Baumrind 1971).

White (1996), argues that moral development is complex and cannot be fully explained by developmental stage theories. She sees family adaptability, cohesiveness and degree of family communication as critical factors. The early work of research scientist John Bowlby and Canadian psychologist Mary Ainsworth generated a model of attachment known today as secure-base phenomenon. The notion of a secure base has moved beyond the parent–child dyad to include the significance of secure attachment in all relationships. It proposes that when an individual—child or adult—has a secure attachment to a stronger, supportive other, they are then capable of responding to the needs of others (Waters et al. 1995).

Implications for Nursing Practice

Moral development theories are useful in helping nurses to understand the children and families with whom they work. Without making value judgements or blaming, one can sometimes understand, for example, that the individual who has become involved in antisocial or criminal behaviour may not have done so simply because of a 'personality problem', but possibly because of suffering deficits in childhood. The person with severe anxiety, inappropriate guilt or poor self-esteem may be so due to authoritarian parenting. We as nurses might also be helped in understanding our own moral development and its influence on our ethical behaviour as professionals. The importance of a secure base, or a reliable relationship that encourages growth and exploration of the world, is important for us all.

Bowlby had a strong conviction that relationships influence who we become and how we relate to others into adulthood. Feminist perspectives criticise the notion of attachment because of the assumption that the primary relationship is always with the mother. However, attachment theory is useful in helping us to understand the role of risk and protective factors in early development and will be further discussed later in this chapter. The concept of resilience helps explain differences in outcomes between people who have experienced similar events in their lives. It is critical for nurses to acknowledge that identity is also important and that it has multiple meanings for people. In understanding this, nurses can support each person's self-concept and self-esteem, contributing positively to their mental health. These theories reinforce the importance of families, whatever style or structure, as supportive, nurturing sources underpinning development. It is always important, when interviewing patients, to gain a thorough understanding of their families and the influence they have had and continue to have on the person's mental health.

The complex nature of human development is reflected in the diversity of theoretical approaches to its study. Each of the aforementioned theories focusses on different dimensions of human development. Theories can be used eclectically in practice and integrated into a lifespan approach to help understand human development and behaviour. Additional concepts to assist in a more comprehensive understanding of the developmental process incorporate those already mentioned, which focus on the importance of interpersonal relationships in development, and those following, which highlight the interplay between the person and their environment, which Richard Lerner (1991) popularised as 'developmental contextualism'.

CHILDHOOD

Most theorists believe that infant 'attachment' (previously discussed under moral development) and the early years of life are the most significant in building a foundation for all future development (see Chapter 11). The most important outcomes of the infant–childhood developmental phases are the acquisition of a positive sense of self, and the ability to trust others.

Development and Theoretical Issues

There is evidence that mental health in children and adults could be contingent on positive parent–child relationships (Barlow & Parsons 2002; Licence 2004). Dr John Bowlby's 1951 report, *Maternal Care and Mental Health*, commissioned by the WHO, documented his idea of the importance of 'attachment' in determining outcomes of childhood development (Bowlby 1951). Attachment has been described as 'the strong affectional tie we feel for special people in our lives that leads us to experience pleasure and joy when we interact with them and to be comforted by their nearness in times of stress' (Berk 2001, p. 190). The report noted that in the first 3 to 4 months of life, infants are observed to recognise their mother among other figures, and respond differently to her by smiling and vocalising. Attachment behaviour was also identified as occurring with others, usually fathers or family members, about a month after it was observed occurring with the mother. The behaviour of the mother (attentive or distant) and differences in the child (attractive appearance and settled behaviour or otherwise) determine how attachment behaviour occurs.

Attachment behaviour develops throughout the first 3 years of life. During this time the child protests when the mother is out of sight. However, when the child realises that the mother will return, trust increases and the child is later able to feel secure with subordinate attachment figures such as preschool teachers and relatives. Attachment to parents grows weaker throughout the lifespan, but it continues as we age and is transferred to other adults in our lives. Attachment behaviour is also directed to people outside the family and other groups and organisations. Increased need for attachment is experienced when people are under threat or stress and a need for security is felt. Secure attachments in childhood are predictive of positive sociable behaviour towards others, higher self-esteem and greater achievement throughout the lifespan.

The quality of attachment can vary and attachments have been described as 'secure' or 'anxious' (Karen 1994). Children who have a secure attachment are relaxed in the presence of their caregiver and seek to be near them when they are upset and are soothed by them. Less securely attached children are unable to be comforted by their caregiver in a consistent way and appear less relaxed when they are nearby (Wilson 2009). As they develop, these less securely attached children are more likely to experience problems with self-esteem and socialising and be more vulnerable to mental health problems and psychopathology (Arbona & Power 2003; Nakash-Eisikovits et al. 2002).

The achievement of secure attachment equates to Erikson's first stage and the ability to trust. The first four of Erikson's stages relate to infancy and childhood.

1. *Basic trust versus mistrust (0–12 months).* Resolution of the conflict at this stage requires the infant to compromise when their basic needs are not met, to develop acceptance and to cope with frustration until such time as these needs are restored. The outcome or strength the child acquires from this is 'hope'.
2. *Autonomy versus shame and doubt (1–3 years).* Resolution of this conflict is the acquisition of 'autonomy', which is experienced as a growing feeling of self-control. The child is encouraged, with appropriate limits, to be independent, to explore relationships with others and to develop curiosity about their environment. Inhibition can result if the child is overly directed or limited, whereas defiance and problems with self-regulation can result when there is no guidance or limit setting.
3. *Initiative versus guilt (4–5 years).* A sense of purpose balanced with responsibility and initiative is the desired resolution of this stage. The child has mastered the previous stages and is capable of basic social functioning and self-regulation. However, parental guidance is still required, to direct the child's initiative into constructive endeavours.
4. *Industry versus inferiority (6–11 years).* A sense of self as competent in a range of unique abilities is the desired outcome of this stage. Children are prone to suffer from comparison with others once they attend school and can acquire a sense of inferiority in certain skills that may be valued in a particular context. In this stage, children's strengths can be optimised and their weaknesses nurtured so they can work cooperatively with others and learn that they have particular contributions to make to group efforts (Erikson 1963; Welchman 2000).

Mental health is evidenced by the child entering into and maintaining relationships with others, engaging in learning and play, understanding the concepts of right and wrong, developing psychologically and exhibiting behaviour that demonstrates an ability to regulate distress (Townley 2002). All these behaviours and abilities need to be appraised in relation to the developmental level of the child as outlined in the stage theories, and the context in which the behaviour is observed.

The following behaviours occurring in a continuing pattern may be indicators of mental health problems in children: difficulties with sleep, feeding, mood and relating to others; bed wetting (enuresis) and soiling (encopresis); overly active behaviour; frequent tantrums and defiance; and somatic complaints such as 'tummy pain' without any identifiable cause (Townley 2002; see Chapter 11).

Risk Factors

A number of risk factors may predispose infants and children to mental health problems and illness in childhood or adulthood. Longitudinal research identifies numerous developmental variables and risk factors: prematurity and serious medical illness; infant temperament (behavioural inhibition); disruptions in attachment between infant and caregiver, in particular attachment involving an adolescent parent (Flaherty & Sadler 2011) or attachment to one or both parents due to acrimonious divorce or separation (Lowenstein 2010); psychopathology in parents; maternal depression; maternal substance abuse; marital quality and interactions; poverty and social class; and family violence and physical, emotional or sexual abuse and death (Salmelainen 1996; Townley 2002; Zeanah et al. 1997). Additional risk factors such as homelessness, disaster, discrimination and poverty can also affect the individual (Townley 2002).

Research on risk and protective factors also suggests a nonlinear and nonspecific transmission of risk. This suggests that the total number of risk factors is more predictive of psychopathology in later life rather than any one specific factor (Zeanah et al. 1997). However, there are examples of single factor risk in the research. For example, children who were under-controlled and impulsive at 3 years of age were identified as being more likely to meet the criteria for antisocial personality disorder as they developed; and children who exhibited inhibited behaviour were more likely to meet the diagnostic criteria for depression (Caspi et al. 1996). Several methodological issues have been identified in research into childhood mental disorders and further research using repeated observations over time and the investigation of pre- and perinatal influences on mental health disorders in children is suggested (Swanson & Wadhwa 2008). In summary, protective factors against mental health problems or mental illness in childhood are extensive and include an easy temperament, a high level of intelligence, positive relationships with a parent and early attachment to a parent, support from peers, a sense of humour, positive experiences at school, positive relationships with another adult, reflection and planning and decision-making skills.

CRITICAL THINKING CHALLENGE 6.5

Ellie is 3 years old. She lives with her parents in a block of flats in an inner-city suburb. Ellie's mother drinks a lot of alcohol and often has arguments with Sean, Ellie's stepfather. Gita, a retired woman in her 60s, lives next door. Ellie loves spending time with Gita, who has developed a close bond with Ellie.

1. Discuss the risk and protective factors in Ellie's life.
2. How could Ellie's relationship with Gita affect her future relationships?

ADOLESCENCE

Development and Theoretical Issues

The main tasks of adolescence are the successful transition to secondary schooling, learning skills for later life, psychological autonomy (self-reliance and confidence in decision making), developing close relationships within and between genders and the formation of personal identity (Masten 2001). The development of a sense of meaning and purpose in life are part of this major task of identity formation.

The ability of the adolescent to achieve these tasks will depend largely on the accomplishment of the earlier tasks of childhood. The stage of Erikson's theory that relates to adolescence is 'identity versus role confusion (12–18 years)'. During this stage, the acquisition of a relatively stable sense of self (or identity) resolves the confusion associated with this stage. The person is challenged to accommodate a range of 'self-schemas' into a comprehensive sense of self that will form a lasting identity (Welchman 2000). Schemas are various perspectives of the self, received from others. In addition, the adolescent has their own multiple perspectives of self. This stage is particularly challenging as the adolescent can experience confusion about the various roles expected of them. Adolescents have a need for ideology and occupation. This makes them vulnerable to exploitation by organisations and groups offering a particular worldview or truth. Tension is also created for the adolescent who is encouraged to select a career, but who may require an extended time between childhood and adopting an occupational identity (Erikson 1963; Welchman 2000). An absence of role modelling or poor role models makes it even more difficult to resolve this conflict, as does the complex nature of contemporary society.

Existentialism provides some guidance in understanding the conflicts faced during this stage of development as the worldview of the child makes a shift into an exploration of the meaning of life and existence, concerns of the transition to adulthood (Fitzgerald 2005). Integrative models also help to explain this complex stage of development. Research on physical changes, mood and behaviour and social and relationship variables has been explored in an integrated manner, investigating the many influences on adolescent development (Compas et al. 1995).

Identity

Erikson's theory suggests that identity develops over time and is the part of our self-concept that contributes to our overall sense of self. Formation of identity begins in infancy, as children identify with role models they perceive as attractive and important. Children aspire to become like those they admire (Phinney 2000). The concept of identity consists of both individual and group identity, and it changes over time.

Identity is most significant to the adolescent because of the risks taken as they trial their various schemas or perspectives of self. Racial, ethnic, sexual and class identities may also challenge the 'sense of self' of an individual, depending on their environment (Fitzgerald 2005; Frable 1997; Phinney 2000). The acceptability and congruence of gender identity at a personal and social level is critical for the adolescent. Nonacceptance and incongruence of identity is acknowledged as a risk factor in adolescent suicide. Family acceptance has been identified as increasing general wellbeing (self-esteem, general health and social support) in the development of identity in lesbian, gay, bisexual, transgender and intersex young people (Ryan et al. 2010).

Integrative models research the 'fit' between the individual and the environment, and suggest that the feedback adolescents receive from others contributes to either problematic or positive development (Eccles et al. 1993). The peer group is proposed as the primary influence on adolescent behaviour, and it may be that culture has more impact on behaviour than parenting (Eccles et al. 1993). Research continues, but the importance of interrelatedness between the adolescent and family, peer, school and work needs to be acknowledged, and positive relationships fostered, in order to decrease stress and confusion and to facilitate decision making and autonomy for the adolescent.

Holistic care for adolescents requires nurses to listen to the patient's personal narrative and understand that the patient may have a number of ways of seeing and expressing themselves (multiple self-schemas), depending on their environment and relationships. Family interactions that encourage adolescents to express their point of view and to disagree and participate in problem solving can contribute to the development of individuality and identity.

Risk Factors

The risks and protective factors of childhood influence adolescence, with risk increasing due to additional developmental and social challenges. Many opportunities exist to change the balance of risk and protective factors during this time because of the numerous influences the adolescent is exposed to. The risk assessment profile sheet (Fuller 1998) identifies the extensive factors that contribute to risk in this group. Among the risk factors identified are: community factors such as poverty, isolation and accommodation; school factors relating to performance and attendance; family factors including the adolescent's connectedness to family, and family violence; peer friendships and the nature of the peer association (e.g. delinquent peers); and individual characteristics such as those discussed in 'childhood', including temperament, intelligence, aggression and likeability.

Suicide is a rare event in young people under the age of 15, accounting for less than 2% of all suicides in most societies, yet there is an increased potential for suicide in young people from families where there is violence, abuse and neglect and with family histories of alcohol and drug abuse, suicide and depression (Beautrais & Mishara 2006).

CRITICAL THINKING CHALLENGE 6.6

Andrew loves sport and is on the school teams for swimming and football. He likes spending time with his friends, listening to music and going camping. Recently he has been spending increasing amounts of time with Sam, a friend who is in his swimming team. Andrew is disconcerted by feelings that he has been experiencing towards Sam and is fearful of talking to anyone about it. Discuss the factors that would support Andrew in understanding his current situation.

EARLY AND MIDDLE ADULTHOOD

Development and Theoretical Issues

Adulthood can be conceived of as a series of changes that occur after adolescence until the final stages of life. Throughout adulthood there are changes to cognitive, social, psychological and physical development, although by early adulthood many of the brain's functions have stabilised. Theories that relate to this stage of development include stages four and five of Erikson's theory, which describe early and middle adulthood. These are discussed in the following sections.

Intimacy Versus Isolation (Early Adulthood)

According to Erikson, a mutually satisfying relationship with another person in which individual identity is sustained is evidence of successful resolution of this stage. This stage also requires 'sacrifices or compromises' (Erikson, cited in Welchman 2000) as a result of a commitment to another person. The risks associated with becoming a couple can be the loss of self-identity from domination of the other, or lack of assertion of one's own desires and needs. Similarly, feelings of aloneness despite being a 'couple' can result from incomplete commitment to the relationship.

Early adulthood is a time of greater vulnerability to mental health problems than middle or late adulthood. Stresses associated with new roles at work and in relationships, accompanied by high expectations, are contributors to an increase in mental health problems and illness at this time. The person aged 20 to 30 is struggling with issues of identity and adjusting to increased responsibility as they attempt to establish a career. This period of chaos and pressure to make good decisions for the future can create vulnerability, hence the use of the term 'crisis'. Neugarten (1979) suggested that family and work roles could create conflicts for young adults as they attempt to balance responsibility with possibility and change. Chaos, confusion and change present significant challenges for young adults. Many of the risks, in particular the suicide risk for males associated with alcohol and drug abuse and depression discussed in the previous stage (adolescence), emerge in early adulthood.

Generativity Versus Self-Absorption (Middle Adulthood)

Erikson suggests the middle years are the most productive in terms of family, occupational and social contributions. This stage is characterised by the individual having altruistic tendencies and energies directed at contributing to a better world. While 'generativity' relates to guiding and supporting the next generation, it is also about contributing to the enrichment of society. Resolution of the task to achieve generativity can be achieved through a realistic appraisal of strengths, limitations and opportunity and identification of appropriate present or future achievements. Feelings of frustration and unrealised goals and potentials can create dissatisfaction with life in this stage (stagnation), which can affect the next generation if adults place their unrealised expectations on the child (Welchman 2000).

Attachment, Gender, Identity and Risk

Theories of women's development emphasise the importance of connectedness and positive relationships in maintaining women's mental health throughout the lifespan. An awareness of the work of Carol Gilligan (1982) assists nurses to understand relational issues for women. The concept that Gilligan has named 'voice' is central to this understanding. Gilligan asserts that voice is the 'core of the self' and that we use it to relate to others. Speaking and listening are ways of understanding another. She believes that women's voices need to be heard in order to enhance their personal and social development. Her book, *In a Different Voice*, asks questions about theories in which men's experiences stand for all 'human experience', excluding the experience of women (Gilligan 1982, p. xiii).

Most developmental theories support separation, detachment and autonomy as desirable outcomes of development. Gilligan (1982) proposes that 'attachment' in relationships is integral to the successful development of identity in women and that the values of interdependence, nurturing and sensitivity need to be valued as much as independence and autonomy. Unlike boys, who need to separate from their mother as they grow in order to achieve a masculine identity, girls develop their identity in the ongoing relationship they have with their mother. Self-in-relation theory was developed by Jean Baker Miller, Judith Jordan, Jan Surrey and Irene Stiver from this early work. This group, from the Stone Center at Wellesley College, espouses the importance of connection with others in developing a healthy sense of self (Jordan et al. 1991). Self-in-relation theory has been used to explain and understand the origins of mental health problems in women and also to guide appropriate interventions (Nizette & Creedy 1998).

The attachment experience of childhood is important to both sexes, as early childhood experiences of attachment can affect one's sense of self and relationships in adulthood. Research proposes that secure, avoidant or ambivalent attachment in adulthood is associated with childhood relationships and the emotional styles of parents (Hazan & Shaver, cited in Karen 1994). Hazan and Shaver found that people in a secure attachment were happy, and knew and accepted the negative as well as the positive characteristics of their partner. Avoidant people were found to suffer jealousy and fear intimacy, and ambivalent attachment led to obsessive involvement and 'ups and downs'.

CRITICAL THINKING CHALLENGE 6.7

Vivian is a 44-year-old woman who has spent the past 7 years at home being a full-time mum to her four children. Before she and her partner, Dave, had children Vivian enjoyed her work as a travel consultant in a local travel agency. She now wants to return to work but is concerned that her in-laws and other people might think she should 'just be a mum'. Vivian feels torn: she knows she can be a good mother and have a career as well. She is hesitant to express her wishes to Dave and finds herself preoccupied with the need to get back to her career, which she enjoyed so much. She finds herself losing interest in her usual daily jobs and routines.

1. What could be motivating Vivian to return to work?
2. Which 'stage' challenges is she confronting?
3. Discuss the different outcomes that may result.

OLDER ADULTHOOD

Development and Theoretical Issues

Development in older adults focusses on positive outcomes that relate to the final stages of life, such as feeling positive about one's contribution to society, having close and loving relationships with family and others, maintaining a purpose in life and having a sense of autonomy and control over one's life. Erikson's stage of 'integrity versus despair' relates to late adulthood. In this final stage, successful resolution is achieved when the person is able to transcend any feelings of guilt, self-absorption or regret for lost opportunities throughout their life. The person is able to understand and appreciate the part their life has played in society. It is a time of acceptance and reflection on the unique meaning a person may make of their life (Neugarten 1979; Welchman 2000). Despair can be identified as a fear of death. A change in time perspective occurs as the older adult's concerns relate to the time left to live rather than the years since birth (Neugarten 1979). Feelings of dissatisfaction and despair may arise with the realisation that life cannot be lived again (Welchman 2000).

The theory of gerotranscendence (Tornstam 1989, cited in Wadensten & Carlsson 2003, Tornstam 2011) focusses on the final stage of life as a period of redefining the self, one's relationships and one's view of the world. This theory on ageing differs from others in that disengagement in the older adult is explained as an increased need for reflection on the matters of life, not because of a loss of interest in life or the world. Tornstam suggests that if people believe that they only develop and mature in the first half of their life that they end up dying as half matured individuals (Tornstam 2011). Gerotranscendence provides the nurse with a different way of viewing the older person and their needs, which can lead to nursing practices in caring for the elderly that are more appropriate and holistic.

Risk Factors

The older adult may face issues of retirement, loss of functional capacity and change in family and friendship networks and supports—additional stressors that increase risk in this age group. Increased rates of depression and anxiety in the elderly can be attributed to the range of loss that is usually more commonly experienced in older age. Risk factors for these illnesses in the over-55-year age group include illness or death of a significant other or family member, premorbid personality factors, being female and self-perceived poor health (De Beurs et al. 2001). Despite the knowledge that loss is linked to risk of depression, it often goes undetected and untreated, as evidenced by high rates of suicide in this group (Bevan & Jeeawody 1998). In people aged over 75, risk for depression may increase as they have been found to be less willing to talk about mood to health professionals than younger people (Smith 2009).

For older women, poor physical health is a significant risk factor for depression because deterioration in physical health generally contributes to a person's inability to maintain relationships with others and to feel supported (Heidrich 1998). This finding is consistent with developmental theories, which propose that mental health is more likely if the individual has a positive self-perception of supportive relationships with others, autonomy, purpose and personal growth (Cantor & Sanderson 2000; Heidrich 1998). Older people from non-English-speaking backgrounds suffer more from isolation and experience particular difficulties in accessing appropriate health services (Moore, cited in Bevan & Jeeawody 1998). Isolation and loneliness can affect quality of life, as well as being significant risk factors for a range of mental health problems.

The Influence of Theories of Psychology and Sociology on Nursing

Early nursing theorists drew on the work of both psychological and social scientists to develop models of care. During the 1950s American nursing education moved into the tertiary sector, with other countries following this trend. As a consequence, teachers of nursing were required to have graduate education in addition to their nursing qualifications. Nurses undertook this study in the already established academic areas of anthropology, philosophy, education, psychology and sociology. Postgraduate study in these fields subsequently influenced the development of the thinking of many nursing theorists (King 2011; Winch et al. 2010).

The first generation of nursing theories to emerge since the 1950s was a synthesis of ideas about nursing practice and psychological/sociological theory. For instance, Madeline Leininger integrated anthropological studies with clinical nursing practice to develop her theory of transcultural nursing (Leininger 2011). In psychiatric nursing, Hildegard Peplau acknowledged the influence of the work of psychoanalyst Harry Stack Sullivan on her thinking and clinical practice (Peplau 1988; Belcher 2011),

Also evident in the writing of nurse theorists is the influence of humanistic psychology. Maslow's human needs are embraced within models of care such as those proposed by Leininger, Parse, Orem and Watson (George 2011; Reed & Crawford Shearer 2009); and existentialist and phenomenological thought are incorporated in Parse's theory of human becoming and Travelbee's human-to-human relationship model (George 2011; Parse 1992; Travelbee 1971). However, it is in the field of psychiatric nursing that the influence of psychological and sociological thought is most obvious, as seen in the theories of the following prominent psychiatric nurses.

Hildegard Peplau (1909–1999)

Peplau is acknowledged as the mother of psychiatric nursing and is known to have written the first nursing theory textbook since Nightingale (Pokorny 2010). She is also recognised as the first nursing author to use theory from other scientific fields in developing a theory of nursing and to publish without a medical co-author (Belcher 2011). Peplau's interpersonal theory of nursing is specific to practice, making it a mid-range theory, as distinct from a grand theory with broader applicability, like those of Orem and Roy, or a philosophy as espoused by earlier nursing writers such as Nightingale or Henderson (Hickman 2011).

Peplau's seminal text, Interpersonal Relations in Nursing, was first published in 1952 and outlines the therapeutic relationship between the nurse and the patient. According to Peplau, the nurse does not perform therapy on the patient, but rather, the nurse is the therapy. This heralded a shift in nursing practice from doing to a patient to being with a patient—an approach to care that today is evident in the recovery model (see Chapter 2). Further legacies of Peplau's theory are the valuing of teaching and learning about relationship skills in nursing curricula and practice, and a focus on the study of clinical phenomena as a nursing concern (Reed 2009). Peplau's theory about the nurse–patient relationship has influenced the practice and research of psychiatric nursing since the 1950s and remains applicable to nursing practice today (Belcher 2011).

In developing her theory, Peplau's thinking was influenced not only by the nursing discourse of her time, but also by several psychological clinicians, including the psychoanalyst Harry Stack Sullivan, humanistic psychologist Abraham Maslow and the social learning theorist Neal Miller. Sullivan's influence on Peplau's writing can be seen in her valuing of the individual, the intrapersonal (subjective experience) and the interpersonal (relationships). Peplau viewed utilisation of the psychological model as enabling nurses 'to move away from a disease orientation to one whereby the psychological meaning of events, feelings and behaviours could be incorporated in nursing interventions' (Peplau 1996).

Joyce Travelbee (1926–1973)

Travelbee's human-to-human relationship model is underpinned by the assumption that the purpose of nursing is achieved through the establishment of a nurse–patient relationship (Travelbee 1971). Her theory extended the work of earlier nursing theorists Peplau (1988) and Orlando (1972) on interpersonal relations in nursing and incorporated existential ideas concerning meaning from the writings of Victor Frankl (George 2011). Travelbee viewed the purpose of nursing as assisting the patient, family or community not only to prevent or cope with illness and suffering but also, if necessary, to find meaning in the experience (Travelbee 1971). Travelbee's emphasis on the emotional and psychological aspects of nursing—such as caring, empathy and rapport—is also consistent with the writings of humanistic psychologist Carl Rogers in his model of patient-centred therapy (Rogers 1951; Travelbee 1971) and is a contemporary influence in the field of palliative care nursing.

Phil Barker (b. 1946)

From his clinical research, psychiatric nurse and psychotherapist Phil Barker, in collaboration with Poppy Buchanan-Barker, developed an interdisciplinary recovery-focussed model of care, called the Tidal Model, which seeks solutions rather than solves problems (see Chapter 2). Central tenets of Barker's model include empowerment of the individual and humanistic notions of being human and helping one another. Underpinning the model are the key principles of:

- active collaboration between the mental health clinician, the individual and family in the planning and delivery of care
- the development and use of a care plan that is centred on the individual's experience, thus empowering the person
- the provision of nursing care in a multidisciplinary context
- the use of narrative-based interventions, all of which form the basis of problem resolution and mental health promotion

Barker acknowledges several influences in the development of the Tidal Model, including: his studies of philosophy and psychology in the 1960s; an initial interest in psychoanalytic, then later behavioural, cognitive and family therapies; and the work of the radical psychiatrist RD Laing. Also significant in the development of the model were the seminal writings and mentorship of Annie Altschul and Hildegard Peplau from nursing. Together, these influences contributed to Barker's development of an enduring interest in humanistic approaches and ultimately to the development of the Tidal Model, with its focus on assisting the person to find meaning in their experience (Barker & Buchanan-Barker 2005; Tidal Model 2000).

CRITICAL THINKING CHALLENGE 6.8

1. What role did psychological and other theories play in the development of psychiatric nursing theories?
2. What contribution do psychiatric nursing theories make to nursing practice?

CONCLUSION

Fluctuations in a person's mental health occur throughout the lifespan. Risk factors, both internal and external, can create vulnerability, exposing people to mental health problems and mental illness. Some of the vulnerability and risk can be mediated by health-promoting interventions. Health-promoting interventions that increase protective factors are appropriate at all times, even if risk is not apparent. Everyone is at risk or increasingly vulnerable at some stage during their life. Most importantly, nurses work within a recovery framework with patients to identify and work with their strengths to build resilience and self-efficacy.

Knowledge of theories can assist nurses to understand vulnerability and risk throughout the lifespan. Holistic assessment, including the establishment of a connection to health services through therapeutic communication, is a beginning step. During assessment, nurses can identify risk, and access and connect individuals and families to culturally appropriate resources and services. Health-promoting strategies based on an understanding of theory and applied practically can become part of nursing practice in all settings with patients and their families. Some strategies have been described in this chapter.

A greater focus on the contribution of theory to practice in curricula, professional development and policy development would support better mental health outcomes throughout the lifespan. Karen (1994), p. 420, in elaborating on the relevance of attachment in childhood, reports on studies demonstrating that 'social policy and social interventions can make a society more humane and give parents a better chance to raise secure children'. Contextual issues, environmental and social, create and maintain the internal and external factors of risk for mental health problems and illness across the lifespan. Mental health nursing practice embedded in a recovery framework and informed by theory has the potential to support the person with lived experience to build self-awareness and self-efficacy, strengths and resilience, ultimately affecting the person's quality of life throughout their lifespan.

EXERCISES FOR CLASS ENGAGEMENT

1. Go back to Critical Thinking Challenge 6.1 and answer the questions again now that you have read this chapter.
   - In small groups, compare and contrast the before and after responses.
   - If attitudes have changed, identify influences that could account for these changes.
   - Discuss how language influences how we respond to people or situations.
   - How would you feel if derogatory terms describing mental illness were used about you or a member of your family?
2. In small groups, discuss the stigma associated with mental health and mental illness.
   - Identify factors that contribute to stigma.
   - Consider how stigma might affect nursing care.
   - Devise strategies to address stigma.
   - Provide feedback to the rest of the class.
3. In small groups, discuss the following questions:
   - What contribution can theories make to mental health promotion?
   - What contribution can theories make to mental illness prevention, early intervention, treatment and recovery?
   - What contribution do theories make to nursing practice?
   - Provide feedback and debriefing to the rest of the class.
4. Prior to the tutorial, each student should interview either a registered nurse or a person with mental illness regarding the person's views on the following.
   - What contributes to the development of mental illness?
   - What enables an individual to cope with or overcome mental illness?
   - What factors might hinder an individual's recovery from mental illness?
   - What advice can the person give to nurses about caring for a person with mental illness?

   Then, in small groups, discuss the following.
   - What key issues emerged in the interview?
   - Compare and contrast professional responses with those of people who have experienced mental illness.
   - Discuss lay and professional interpretations of mental illness in the light of relevant theories.
   - What did you learn with regard to nursing a person with a mental illness?

   Provide feedback and debriefing to the rest of the class.
5. Interview a family member or friend to record their 'life history'.
   - Make notes and record events that the interviewee identifies as significant.
   - Analyse the interview and identify protective and/or risk factors from the person's story.
   - In small groups, list the protective and risk factors and categorise them as internal or external.
   - Can you identify an instance of increased vulnerability from the person's story and explain the contributing factors?
6. In small groups, identify what you consider to be the most critical time in a person's life. (Each group may identify different critical times.) Then devise a health promotion plan or strategy that includes:
   - the target group
   - examples of interventions
   - types and content of information that may be needed
   - how the plan could be implemented
7. Many of the developmental theories emerged from research undertaken on subjects who were Caucasian males.
   - Discuss and identify the issues in using these theories to understand people from different cultural backgrounds. Assign different cultural backgrounds to the people in Critical Thinking Challenges 6.5, 6.6 and 6.7 and discuss how risk and protective factors may vary.

REFERENCES

Allport, G., 1961. Pattern and Growth in Personality. Holt, Reinhart & Winston, New York.

Anthony, W.A., 1993. Recovery from mental illness: the guiding vision of the mental health service system in the 1990s. Psychosocial Rehabilitation Journal 16 (4), 11–23.

Arbona, C., Power, T., 2003. Parental attachment, self-esteem, and anti-social behaviors among African American, European American, and Mexican American adolescents. Journal of Counseling Psychology 50 (1), 40–51.

Australian Health Ministers, 2003. Third National Mental Health Plan 2003–2008. Australian Government, Canberra.

Bailey, C., 1986. Kohlberg on morality and feeling. In: Modgil, S., Modgil, C. (Eds.), Lawrence Kohlberg: Consensus and Controversy. Falmer Press, Philadelphia.

Baltes, P.B., Baltes, M.M. (Eds.), 1990. Successful Aging: Perspectives From the Behavioral Sciences. Cambridge University Press, New York.

Baltes, P.B., Staudinger, U.M., Lindenberger, U., 1999. Lifespan psychology: theory and application to intellectual functioning. Annual Review of Psychology 50, 471–507.

Bandura, A., 2001. Social cognitive theory. Annual Review of Psychology 52, 1–26.

Barker, P., Buchanan-Barker, P., 2005. The Tidal Model: A Guide for Mental Health Professionals. Brunner-Routledge, Hove.

Barlow, J., Parsons, J., 2002. Group-based training programmes for improving emotional and behavioral adjustment in 0–3-year-old children. Cochrane Database of Systematic Reviews (4).

Baumrind, D., 1971. Current patterns of parental authority. Developmental Psychology 4 (2), 1–103.

Beautrais, A.L., Mishara, B., 2006. World Suicide Prevention Day—September 10, 2007. Suicide prevention across the lifespan. Crisis 28 (2), 57–60.

Beck, A., 1972. Depression: Causes and Treatment. University of Pennsylvania Press, Philadelphia.

Belcher, J., 2011. Interpersonal relations in nursing: Hildegard E Peplau. George J Nursing Theories: the Base for Professional Nursing Practice, sixth ed. Pearson, New Jersey.

Berk, L.E., 2001. Development Through the Lifespan, second ed. Allyn & Bacon, Boston.

Bevan, C., Jeeawody, B., 1998. Successful Aging: Perspectives on Health and Social Construction. Elsevier, Sydney.

Bowlby, J., 1951. Maternal care and mental health. WHO, Geneva; HMSO, London; Columbia University Press, New York. Abridged version 1965, Child Care and the Growth of Love, second ed. Penguin, Harmondsworth.

Brown, L.M., Debold, E., Tappan, M., et al., 1991. Reading narratives of conflict and choice for self and moral voices: a relational method. In: Kurtines, W.K., Gewirtz, J.L. (Eds.), Handbook of Moral Behavior and Development Theory 2. Lawrence Erlbaum Associates, New Jersey.

Bühler, C., Allen, M., 1972. Introduction to Humanistic Psychology. Brooks/Cole, California.

Butcher, J., Mineka, S., Hooley, K., 2011. Abnormal Psychology: Care Concepts. Allyn & Bacon, Boston.

Cando, A., Gottesman, I., 2000. Twin studies of schizophrenia: from bow-and-arrow concordances to Star Wars Mx and functional genomics. American Journal of Medical Genetics 97 (1), 12–17.

Cantor, N., Sanderson, C.A., 2000. Life task participation and well-being: the importance of taking part in daily life. In: Kahneman, D., Diener, E., Schwarz, N. (Eds.), Well-being: the Foundations of Hedonic Psychology. Russell Sage Foundation, New York, pp. 230–243.

Caplan, G., 1964. Principles of Preventive Psychiatry. Basic Books, New York.

Caspi, A., Moffitt, T.E., Newman, D.L., et al., 1996. Behavioral observations at age 3 years predict adult psychiatric disorders: longitudinal evidence from a birth cohort. Archives of General Psychiatry 53 (1), 1033–1039.

Commonwealth of Australia, 2009. Fourth National Mental Health Plan: an Agenda for Collaborative Government Action in Mental Health 2009–2014. Commonwealth of Australia, Canberra.

Compas, B.E., Hinden, B.R., Gerhardt, C.A., 1995. Adolescent development: pathways and processes of risk and resilience. Annual Review of Psychology 46, 265–293.

Crotty, M., 1996. Phenomenology and Nursing Research. Churchill Livingstone, Sydney.

Darley, J.M., Schultz, T.R., 1990. Moral rules: their content and acquisition. Annual Review of Psychology 41, 525–556.

De Beurs, E., Beekman, A., Geerlings, S., et al., 2001. On becoming depressed or anxious in late life: similar vulnerability factors but different effects of stressful life events. British Journal of Psychiatry 179, 426–431.

Doona, M., 1982. Travelbee's Intervention in Psychiatric Nursing, second ed. FA Davis, Philadelphia.

Donenberg, G.R., Hoffman, L.W., 1988. Gender differences in moral development. Sex Roles 18 (11/12), 701–717.

Durkheim, E., 1951. Suicide: a Study in Sociology. Spaulding J, Simpson G tr. The Free Press, New York

Eccles, J.S., Midgley, C., Wigfield, A., et al., 1993. Development during adolescence: the impact of stage-environment fit on adolescents' experiences in schools and families. American Psychologist 48 (2), 90–101.

Edwards, K., Munro, I., Robins, A., Welsch, A., 2011. Mental Health Nursing: Dimensions of Praxis. Oxford University Press, Melbourne.

Eisenberg, N., 2000. Emotion, regulation and moral development. Annual Review of Psychology 51, 655–697.

Erikson, E.H., 1963. Childhood and Society, second ed. WW Norton, New York.

Fitzgerald, B., 2005. An existential view of adolescent development. Adolescence 40 (160), 793–799.

Flaherty, S.C., Sadler, L.S., 2011. A review of attachment theory in the context of adolescent parenting. Journal of Paediatric Health Care 25 (2), 114–120.

Frable, E.S., 1997. Gender, racial, ethic, sexual and class identities. Annual Review of Psychology 48, 139–162.

Freud, A., 1966. The Ego and the Mechanisms of Defense. International Universities Press, New York.

Fuller, A., 1998. From Surviving to Thriving: Promoting Mental Health in Young People. Australian Council for Educational Research, Melbourne.

Garmon, L.C., 2000. Relations between attachment representations and moral judgment. Doctoral thesis, Ohio State University. Dissertation Abstracts International, Section B: Sciences & Engineering DAI-B 60/11, p 5811

George, J., 2011. Nursing Theories: the Base for Professional Nursing Practice, sixth ed. Pearson, New Jersey.

Gilligan, C., 1982. In a Different Voice. Psychological Theory and Women's Development. Harvard University Press, Cambridge, MA.

Gilligan, C., 1987. Moral orientation and moral development. In: Kittay, E.F., Meyers, D.T. (Eds.), Women and Moral Theory. Rowman & Littlefield, New Jersey.

Gilligan, C., 1998. Remapping the moral domain: new images of self in relationship. In: Gilligan, C., Ward, J.V., McTaylor, L. (Eds.), Mapping the Moral Domain. Harvard University Press, Cambridge, MA.

Golombok, S., Fivush, R., 1994. Gender Development. Cambridge University Press, Cambridge.

Government of South Australia, 2009. Mental Health Act 2009. Available at: www.legislation.sa.gov.au/LZ/C/A/MENTAL%20HEALTH%20ACT%202009.aspx.

Heidrich, S.M., 1998. Older women's lives through time. Advances in Nursing Science 20 (3), 65–75.

Hickman, 2011. An introduction to nursing theory, sixth ed. George J Nursing Theories: The Base for Professional Nursing Practice, New Jersey. Pearson.

Ivey, A., Ivey, M., Zalaquett, C., 2010. Intentional Interviewing and Counselling: Facilitating Client Development in a Multicultural Society, seventh ed. Thompson Brooks/Cole, Pacific Grove, CA.

Jordan, J., Kaplan, A., Miller, J.B., et al., 1991. Women's Growth in Connection. Guilford Press, New York.

Karen, R., 1994. Becoming Attached: Unfolding the Mystery of the Infant–Mother Bond and its Impact on Later Life. Warner Books, New York.

Kearns, H., Gardiner, M., 2010. Waiting for the motivation fairy. Nature 472, 127.

King, I., 2011. Conceptual system and theory of goal attainment. George J Nursing Theories: the Base for Professional Nursing Practice, sixth ed. Pearson, New Jersey.

Kittleson, M., 1989. Mental Health vs Mental Illness: a Philosophical Discussion. Health Education 20 (2), 40–42.

Kring, A., Johnson, S., Davison, G., Neale, J., 2010. Abnormal Psychology, eleventh ed. Wiley, New York.

Kohlberg, L., 1986. A current statement on some theoretical issues. In: Modgil, S., Modgil, C. (Eds.), Lawrence Kohlberg: Consensus and Controversy. Falmer Press, Philadelphia.

Kohlberg, L., Levine, C., Hewer, H., 1983. The current formulation of the theory. In: Kohlberg, L. (Ed.), The Psychology of Moral Development. Harper & Row, New York, pp. 212–319.

Leininger, M., 2011. Theory of culture, care, diversity and universality. George J Nursing Theories: the Base for Professional Nursing practice, sixth ed. Pearson, New Jersey.

Lerner, R., 1991. Changing organism-context relations as the basic process of development: a developmental contextual perspective. Developmental Psychology 27, 27–32.

Licence, K., 2004. Promoting and protecting the health of children and young people. Child: Care, Health and Development 30, 623–635.

Lowenstein, L., 2010. Attachment theory and parental alienation. Journal of Divorce and Remarriage 51, 157–168.

Lynch, D., Laws, K., McKenna, P., 2010. Cognitive behaviour therapy for major psychiatric disorders: does it really work? A meta-analytical review of well-controlled trials. Psychological Medicine 4, 9–24.

Maslow, A.H., 1968. Toward a Psychology of Being, second ed. Van Nostrand, Princeton, NJ.

Masten, A., 2001. Ordinary magic: resilience processes in development. American Psychologist 56 (3), 227–238.

Maud, P., Warelow, P., 2011. 'Wise men, devils and fools': the history of mental illness and its treatment. In: Edwards, K., Munro, I., Robins, A., Welsch (Eds.), A 2011 Mental Health Nursing: Dimensions of Praxis. Oxford University Press, Melbourne.

McMurray, A., 2014. Community Health and Wellness: Primary Health Care in Practice, fifth ed. Elsevier, Sydney.

Meadows, G., Farhall, J., Fossey, E., Grigg, M., McDermott, F., Singh, B. (Eds.), 2012. Mental Health in Australia: Collaborative Community Practice, second ed. Oxford University Press, Australia.

Mental Health Commission New Zealand, 2004. Our Lives in 2014: a Recovery Vision from People with Experience of Mental Illness for the Second Mental Health Plan and the Development of Health and Social Sectors. Available at: www.maryohagan.com/resources/Text_Files/Our%20Lives%20in%202014.pdf.

Ministry of Health New Zealand, 2005. Te Ta¯huhu: Improving mental health 2005–2015. The Second New Zealand Mental Health and Addiction Plan. Available at: www.health.govt.nz/publication/te-tahuhu-improving-mental-health-2005-2015-second-new-zealand-mental-health-and-addiction-plan.

Ministry of Health New Zealand, 2012. Guidelines to the Mental Health (Compulsory Assessment and Treatment) Act 1992. Available at: www.health.govt.nz/publication/guidelines-mental-health-compulsory-assessment-and-treatment-act-1992.

Muir-Cochrane, E., Barkway, P., Nizette, D., 2014. Mosby's Pocket Book of Mental Health, second ed. Elsevier, Sydney.

Nakash-Eisikovits, O., Dutra, L., Westen, D., 2002. Relationship between attachment patterns and personality pathology in adolescents. Journal of the American Academy of Child and Adolescent Psychiatry 41 (9), 1111–1123.

Navarro, V., 2009. What we mean by social determinants of health. International Journal of Health Science 39 (30), 423–441.

Neugarten, B., 1979. Time, age, and the life cycle. American Journal of Psychiatry 136 (7), 887–894.

New South Wales Government, 2007. Mental Health Act 2007 No 8. Available at: www.legislation.nsw.gov.au/viewtop/inforce/act+8+2007+cd+0+N/.

Nizette, D., Creedy, D., 1998. Women and mental illness. In: Rogers Clark, C., Smith, A. (Eds.), Women's Health: A Primary Healthcare Approach. Elsevier, Sydney.

Orlando, I., 1972. The Discipline and Teaching of Nursing Process (an Evaluative Study). Putnam, New York.

Park, A., Roberts, C., 2002. The ties that bind. The 19th Report of British Social Attitudes. National Centre for Social Research, London.

Parse, R., 1992. Human becoming: Parse's theory of nursing. Nursing Science Quarterly 5, 35–42.

Peplau, H., 1988. Interpersonal Relations in Nursing. Putnam & Sons, New York.

Peplau, H., 1996. Fundamental and special—the dilemma of psychiatric and mental health nursing: commentary. Archives of Psychiatric Nursing 10 (1), 14–15.

Peterson, C., 2013. Looking Forward Through the Lifespan: Developmental Psychology, sixth ed. Pearson, Australia.

Phinney, J.S., 2000. Identity formation across cultures: the interaction of personal, societal, and historical change. History and Culture 43 (1), 27–31.

Piaget, P., 1977. Moral Judgement Development of the Child (trans. M Gabain). Penguin, Harmondsworth. Original work published 1932.

Pokorny, M., 2010. Nursing theorists of historical significance. In: Alligood, M. (Ed.), Tomey A Nursing Theorists and Their Work. Mosby Elsevier, Missouri.

Pratt, M., Golding, G., Hunter, W., 1984. Does morality have a gender? Sex, sex role and moral judgement relationships across the lifespan. Merrill-Palmer Quarterly 30 (4), 321–340.

Prince, M., Patel, V., Saxena, S., Maj, M., et al., 2007. No Health Without Mental Health. The Lancet Online 4 September. https://doi.org/10.1016/S0140-6736(07)61238-0.

Ramon, S., Healy, B., Renouf, N., 2007. Recovery from mental illness as an emergent concept and practice in Australia and the UK. International Journal of Social Psychiatry 53 (2), 108–122.

Raphael, B., 1993. Scope for prevention in mental health. National Health and Medical Research Council, Canberra.

Reed, P., 2009. Transforming practice knowledge into nursing knowledge: a revisionist analysis of Peplau. In: Reed, P. (Ed.), Crawford Shearer N Perspectives on Nursing Theory, fifth ed. Lippincott Williams & Wilkins, Philadelphia.

Reed, P., Crawford Shearer, N., 2009. Perspectives on Nursing Theory, fifth ed. Lippincott Williams & Wilkins, Philadelphia.

Rickwood, D., 2006. Pathways to Recovery: 4A's Framework for Preventing Further Episodes of Mental Illness. Commonwealth of Australia, Canberra.

Rogers, C., 1951. Client-Centered Therapy. Houghton Mifflin, Boston.

Rogers, C., 1961. On Becoming a Person: a Therapist's View of Psychotherapy. Houghton Mifflin, Boston.

Ryan, C., Russell, S., Huebner, D., Diaz, R., Sanchez, J., 2010. Family acceptance in adolescence and the health of LGBT young adults. Journal of Child and Adolescent Psychiatric Nursing 23 (4), 205–213.

Salmelainen, P., 1996. Child neglect: its causes and its role in delinquency. Contemporary Issues in Crime and Justice 33, 1–14.

Santrock, J., 2011. Life-Span Development, thirteenth ed. McGraw-Hill, New York.

Seligman, M., 1974. Depression and learned helplessness. In: Friedman, J., Katz, M. (Eds.), The Psychology of Depression: Theory and Research. Winston-Wiley, Washington.

Seligman, M., 1994. Learned Optimism. Random House, Sydney.

Seligman, M., 2004. Authentic Happiness. The Free Press, New York.

Seligman, M., 2011. Flourish: a New Understanding of Happiness and Well-Being. The Free Press, New York.

Seligman, M., Csikszentmihalyi, M., 2000. Positive psychology: an introduction. American Psychologist 55 (1), 5–14.

Shultz, T.R., Wells, D., 1985. Judging the intentionality of action-outcomes. Developmental Psychology 21 (1), 83–89.

Skinner, B., 1953. Science and Human Behaviour. Macmillan, New York.

Slade, M., 2009. 100 ways to support recovery. Available at: www.rethink.org/about-us/commissioning-us/100-ways-to-support-recovery.

Smith, P., 2009. Resilience: resistance factor for depressive symptom. Journal of Psychiatric and Mental Health Nursing 16, 829–837.

Stilwell, B.M., Galvin, M., Kopta, S.M., et al., 1997. Moralization of attachment: a fourth domain of conscious functioning. Journal of the American Academy of Child and Adolescent Psychiatry 36 (8), 1140–1147.

Swanson, J., Wadhwa, P., 2008. Developmental origins of child mental health disorders. Journal of Child Psychology and Psychiatry 49 (10), 1009–1019.

Szasz, T., 1961. The Myth of Mental Illness. Harper & Row, New York.
Szasz, T., 2000. The case against psychiatric power. In: Barker, P., Stevenson, C. (Eds.), The Construction of Power and Authority in Psychiatry. Butterworth–Heinemann, Oxford.
Talbot, L., Verrinder, G., 2013. Promoting Health: the Primary Health Care Approach, fifth ed. Elsevier, Sydney.
Tidal Model, 2000. Reclaiming Stories Recovering Lives. Available at: www.tidal-model.com.
Tornstam, L., 2011. Maturing into gerotranscendence. The Journal of Transpersonal Psychology 43 (2), 166–180.
Townley, M., 2002. Mental health needs of children and young people. Nursing Standard 16 (30), 38–47.
Travelbee, J., 1971. Interpersonal Aspects of Nursing, second ed. FA Davis, Philadelphia.
VicHealth, 2006. Evidence Based Mental Health. Vic Health Department of Human Services, Melbourne.
Victorian Government, 2009. Because mental health matters: Victorian mental health reform strategy 2009–2019. Available at: www2.health.vic.gov.au/searchresults?q=mental%20health%20reform%20strategy.
Wadensten, B., Carlsson, M., 2003. Theory-driven guidelines for practical care of older people, based on the theory of gerotranscendence. Journal of Advanced Nursing 41 (5), 462–470.
Waters, E., Vaughn, B.E., Posada, G., et al., 1995. Caregiving, Cultural, and Cognitive Perspectives on Secure-Base Behavior and Working Models: new Growing Points of Attachment Theory and Research. University of Chicago Press, Chicago.
Welchman, K., 2000. Erik Erikson: his Life, Work and Significance. Open University Press, Philadelphia.
White, F., 1996. Parent–adolescent communication and adolescent decision-making. Journal of Family Studies 2 (1), 41–56.
Wilson, S.L., 2009. Understanding and promoting attachment. Journal of Psychosocial Nursing 47 (8), 23–27.
World Health Organization (WHO), 2008. Closing the gap in a Generation: Health Equity Through Action on the Social Determinants of Health. WHO, Geneva. Available at: https://www.who.int/social_determinants/final_report/csdh_finalreport_2008.pdf.
World Health Organization (WHO), 2014. Mental health: A state of well being. Available at: www.who.int/features/factfiles/mental_health/en.
Winch, S., Henderson, A., Creedy, D., 2010. The growth of ideas and theory in nursing. In: Daly, J., Speedy, S., Jackson, D. (Eds.), Contexts of Nursing, third ed. Elsevier, Sydney.
Zeanah, C.H., Boris, N.W., Larrieu, J.A., 1997. Infant development and developmental risk: a review of the past 10 years. Journal of the American Academy of Child and Adolescent Psychiatry 36 (2), 165–178.

USEFUL WEBSITES

About.com: Psychology Theories provides an overview of the major psychological and developmental theories, http://psychology.about.com/od/psychology101/u/psychology-theories.htm

The British Psychological Society is the professional association for psychologists in the UK; the society's website contains information relevant to psychologists and health professionals and provides academic resources, publications and community information, www.bps.org.uk

7

Trauma, Crisis, Loss and Grief

Rachel Rossiter, Robin Scott

KEY POINTS

- Crises are periods of instability and chaos that arise from time to time in a person's life.
- A person's ability to negotiate the difficult periods in life depends on a range of different factors.
- Crises are frequently associated with significant loss, unexpected or unplanned-for events or with major periods of change in a person's life.
- As people pass through periods of crisis, they may build a range of additional skills that can be used to manage crises they encounter at a later stage in their lives.
- If a person is unable to get through an acute crisis effectively, they are at increased risk of future physical and mental health problems.
- In the course of their work, nurses frequently encounter individuals and families in crisis and will need to develop skills and competency in therapeutic engagement if they are to be effective helpers.
- People who have a history of early trauma and abuse are at increased risk of mental and physical illness.
- Nurses need to develop their understanding of trauma-informed care and build their competency to work sensitively and collaboratively with traumatised individuals.
- Providing assistance for people at times of crisis can be emotionally draining and stressful, and nurses need to develop a range of self-care strategies.
- Communities within the UK represent a diverse range of cultures and differing lifestyles, requiring all nurses to develop cultural awareness and sensitivity towards people whose life circumstances are different to their own.

KEY TERMS

abuse
assessment
behavioural emergency
bereavement
conflict
coping
coping strategies
crisis
culture
death
disasters
distress
emergency
emotions
feelings
grief
helping
loss
mourning
non-suicidal self-injury (NSSI)
precipitating event
psychological first aid
resilience
risk
self-harm
stress
support
suicide
trauma
traumatic events
violence
vulnerability

LEARNING OUTCOMES

The material in this chapter will assist you to:

- provide examples of the crises that people may experience across their lives.
- identify the ways in which vulnerability and resilience will impact on a person's capacity to manage crises.
- outline the impact of early trauma and loss on an individual's emotional development and psychological and physical wellbeing.
- consider the role that a trauma history or posttraumatic stress disorder (PTSD) may be contributing to a person's current presentation.
- describe therapeutic strategies that you can utilise when a person is in crisis.
- explain current perspectives on loss and bereavement.
- recognise the ways in which cultural factors may influence expressions of distress.
- explain nursing approaches to a person who is in crisis, is suicidal or has self-harmed.
- implement self-care strategies to manage the impact of working with a person who is in distress.

INTRODUCTION

Mental health nurses—in fact, nurses in general—have a pivotal role during times of trouble and difficulty in people's lives. Traumatic incidents, crisis, loss and grief often result in significant destabilisation and chaos for many people. Events such as a serious accident where there is loss of life, or serious injury, relationship breakdown, diagnosis with a life-threatening condition or sudden unemployment may well overwhelm the person. A person already living with the challenges of a physical or mental illness who then experiences events such as the death of a loved one, a break-in at their home or environmental upheavals such as flooding might need skilled support and assistance. Those that lose a loved one by a sudden, unexpected or unexplained death, such as a massive cardiac event or suicide, are profoundly affected and may well require skilled support as they negotiate the days, weeks and months that follow.

This chapter will help you to understand more about trauma, crisis, loss and grief, and the effect of these experiences on individuals and those around them. The content provides direction that will help you to develop your assessment skills, so that the information you collect and the understandings that you develop about the person and their situation will guide you towards timely, appropriate interventions. A Case Study, a Patient Story and a Parent's Story are provided to help deepen your ability to utilise the responses, treatment options and nursing actions suggested.

Your capacity to respond in an effective manner will require both well-developed assessment skills and a sound knowledge of appropriate interventions. Make sure you remember, though, that technical skills and knowledge will be effective only if you are able to approach the person with a nonjudgemental attitude, compassion and empathy. In multicultural countries such as the UK, you will care for people from many different cultures other than your own. This chapter encourages you to identify your own biases, assumptions and cultural values so that you can then approach the distressed person needing care with the level of cultural sensitivity and awareness needed to be effective and respectful.

DEFINING AND EXPLAINING CRISIS, TRAUMA, LOSS AND GRIEF

A *crisis* can be very simply described as a difficult or dangerous situation that needs attention. A crisis may be associated with aspects of a person's financial, social, environmental, political or personal life. This chapter focusses on human *crises*, defined by Belkin (1984) as 'a personal difficulty or situation that immobilises people and prevents them from controlling their lives' (p. 424). In contrast to a stressful event, such as a job interview or an exam, a specific traumatic event that the person perceives to be threatening or meaningful, such as loss of employment, the death of a loved one, assault (physical, emotional or sexual) or divorce, may trigger a state of acute crisis. In this state, usual coping strategies are overwhelmed resulting in increasing feelings of vulnerability and rising levels of anxiety and distress, along with confusion and lack of clarity in thinking. The person's usual ability to manage the demands of everyday life is disrupted, resulting in disorganisation and disequilibrium (Parad & Parad 2005, cited in Loughran 2011, p. 11). Without relief, this acute state of crisis may result in severe emotional, cognitive and behavioural dysfunction leading to a person being a risk to themselves or others (James & Gilliland 2013).

The terms 'trauma' and 'traumatic' will be used repeatedly throughout this chapter. A *trauma* or traumatic event can be described as a severe physical injury or a specific experience that triggers mental and emotional distress, and results in suffering and disruption to a person's physical and/or emotional wellbeing. While a single-incident traumatic event such as a severe car accident, an unexpected death of a close family member or natural disaster results in disruption to a person's life, it does not necessarily result in crisis. Such an event does, however, signal *a potential risk of impending crisis*. The person's reaction to and perception of the event and the nature of the trauma may lead to an acute crisis state when the person's ability to cope is overwhelmed. In contrast to popular ideas, research indicates that the majority of people exposed to a traumatic event recover after an initial period of destabilisation (Zoellner & Feeny 2014a). After a period of adjustment and recovery, some people will describe positive changes such as a renewed appreciation for life and loved ones, personal growth and enhanced coping strategies (Castelli Dransart 2013; Zoellner & Feeny 2014b).

Experiences of loss and grief are a universal part of human life. *Loss* can be described as an event where something that belongs to you and is either precious or has meaning for you has been taken away or destroyed. Loss encompasses a range of losses, from a 'minor' loss such as losing your wallet to a 'devastating loss' such as losing your home and all your belongings in a fire. *Bereavement* generally refers to being deprived of an object or a person. Bereavement is usually used in the context of losing someone you love through death. *Grief* has been defined as 'the response to the loss in all of its totality—including its physical, emotional, cognitive, behavioural and spiritual manifestations—and as a natural and normal reaction to loss' (Hall 2014).

Looking more closely at crisis, it is important to differentiate between the triggering event or trauma and the individual's response because an acute crisis state can arise from a very broad range of possible incidents. These can range from something seemingly insignificant to the outside observer, to a situation that others may view as a crisis while the person 'in crisis' does not see that there is a problem at all (Loughran 2011). You may well have experienced a time when you felt that a particular event was catastrophic and your friends or family members had difficulty understanding 'what all the fuss was about'. Perhaps failing an exam for the first time ever had shaken your confidence in your ability to complete your study programme successfully and you seriously contemplated withdrawing from your programme. You may also have found yourself feeling that your future was ruined by this failure.

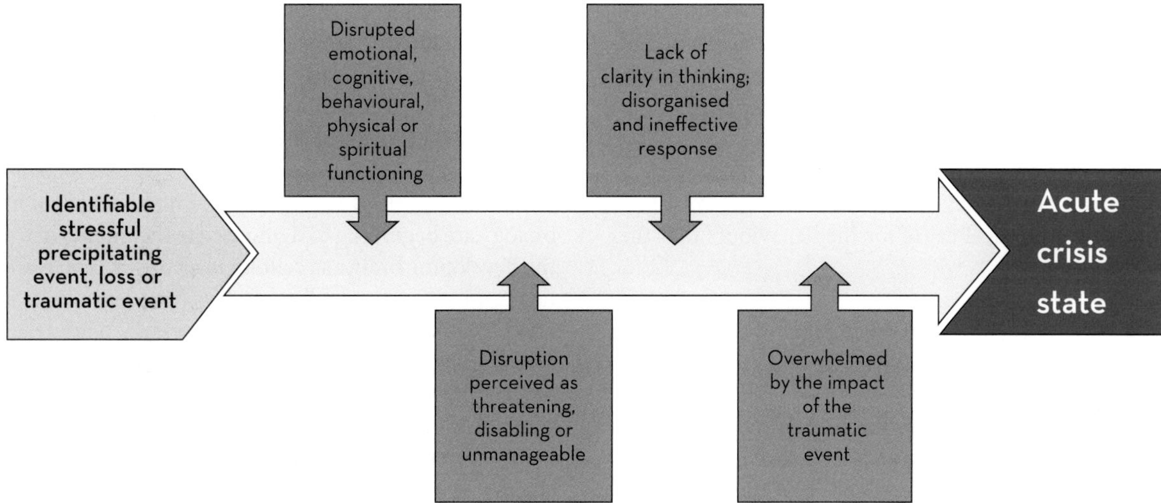

Fig. 7.1 Crisis model. (*Source:* Adapted from Glass, N., 2010. Interpersonal Relating: Health Care Perspectives on Communication, Stress and Crisis. Palgrave Macmillan, South Yarra, Victoria, p. 191.)

In contrast, you may have had a friend who from your perspective was in a crisis situation. You had had multiple discussions with your friend over a number of months about the increasing physical violence she was experiencing in her relationship. At times, you had tried to encourage her to leave the relationship and provided her with information about services for people experiencing domestic violence. Maybe your friend had come to work yet again with heavy make-up covering a black eye and you noticed bruises on her arms. While you feared for her safety, she dismissed this as 'not as bad as last time and nothing to be concerned about'. Although you saw this as a crisis situation, your friend would not access support or even acknowledge the difficulty (Loughran 2011).

The crisis model in Fig. 7.1 shows the unfolding sequence from a clearly identifiable precipitating stressor, loss or traumatic event to the acute crisis state.

Crises have been classified into different types. Table 7.1 demonstrates some of the types that are frequently used. Classifying types of crises can help to deepen understanding both of what may have triggered the crisis and what may be useful to assist the person.

TABLE 7.1 Common Types of Crisis

Types of Crisis	Description
Developmental crises	Major transitions between life stages ('rites of passage'); these can be periods of significant and at times prolonged stress, e.g. birth, adolescence, marriage, retirement, death
Situational crises or 'accidental crises'	Crises that are situation specific or culture specific, e.g. loss of employment, income or home, accidents, theft, loss of relationship, separation, divorce, domestic violence
Social crises	Arising from abuse of drugs or alcohol, criminal activities and violence
Complex crises	Not part of everyday experience or shared accumulated knowledge Severe trauma (see Box 7.1) Crises associated with: • severe mental illness • diagnosis of life-threatening physical illness • needing to seek asylum because of civil war, ethnic cleansing, religious persecution

(*Source:* Compiled from Rosen, A., 1998. Crisis management in the community. The Medical Journal of Australia 44–45; and Glass, N., 2010. Interpersonal Relating: Health Care Perspectives on Communication, Stress and Crisis. Palgrave Macmillan, South Yarra, Victoria.)

An Acute State of Crisis can Become an Emergency

The term 'emergency' is used to 'describe disruptive events that cause loss of life, property and livelihoods, injury and damage to communities' (Australian Red Cross 2013, p. 2). The term is also used within the mental health context. At times, what initially appears to be an acute state of crisis may shift rapidly to a situation requiring immediate intervention to avoid injury or death; that is, a behavioural or mental health emergency. Such emergency situations can be further classified as 'direct' behavioural emergencies or 'indirect' behavioural emergencies.

- A 'direct' behavioural emergency is a direct response to the crisis, when a person is so overwhelmed that confusion, functional decline (a marked decrease in managing everyday activities and self-care), self-injury, risk of suicide or violence towards others is an immediate threat. Suicide and/or murder as the result of relationship breakdown is an uncommon and yet typical example of such an emergency.
- 'Indirect' behavioural emergencies occur when people make bad decisions and end up placing themselves in potentially lethal situations' (James & Gilliland 2013, p. 8). For example, an indirect behavioural emergency arises when a mother who is waiting for her child to get off the school bus sees the child run directly into the path of

oncoming traffic. In her panic, she rushes forward to save the child and as a result she precipitates a car accident and she is seriously hurt. Further examples include emergency situations that arise secondary to alcohol intoxication or as a reaction to hallucinogenic drugs.

Remember that one of the major risks when assessing a person requiring emergency mental healthcare is misdiagnosis or missing a physical cause for the behaviours that the person is exhibiting.

EFFECTS OF TRAUMA, LOSS AND BEREAVEMENT ON THE INDIVIDUAL

Sadly, there are many people in our community who have experienced very significant traumas and loss during their early developmental years. It is essential that nurses build a deep understanding of the impact that trauma, abuse and neglect in the life of a child has on the development of the child's ability to regulate and manage their internal world and their emotions in adulthood.

The Effects of Early Trauma and Loss on an Individual's Development and Psychological and Physical Wellbeing

A large American study called the Adverse Childhood Events (ACE) Study was undertaken in the late 1990s. Participants were asked to report on adverse events experienced during childhood. Adverse childhood events included: experiencing psychological, physical or sexual abuse as a child; living with a mother who was being abused; or living in a household where there were people who abused substances, were suffering from mental illness, were suicidal or had ever been in prison. Researchers found that the more ACEs a child experienced, the greater the burden of physical illnesses, such as chronic obstructive pulmonary disease (COPD) and heart disease, and mental illnesses, such as depression (Felitti et al. 1998).

The researchers for this study have continued to collect data documenting the medical status from these initial participants (see the Useful Websites list at the end of this chapter for further details). These findings have been confirmed in recent research, demonstrating that adverse events occurring during the early years of life increase the risk of both physical and mental illness over the course of the person's life (Hornung & Heim 2014). Children exposed to trauma are less likely to develop resilience (De Bellis & Zisk 2014), while a recent study found a greater than 65% increased risk of depression for those experiencing early life trauma or neglect (Hanson et al. 2015).

Research has also shown evidence that changes in the developing brain as a result of early childhood abuse not only increase the risk of developing physical disorders and psychiatric illness, but also increase the risk of memory and learning processing difficulties (Trollope et al. 2012). For individuals with early trauma-related depression and anxiety, response to treatment may be less effective, thus increasing the risk of developing lifelong, treatment-resistant illness (Nanni et al. 2012; Barnhofer et al. 2014: Hornung & Heim 2014: van Loo et al. 2015). Recent evidence suggests that gene mutation resulting from early life trauma could be transgenerational; that is, passed down through the generations (Heim & Binder 2012; Provençal & Binder 2015; Lutz & Turecki 2014; Babenko et al. 2015).

This is an area of research where rapid advances in neurobiology are beginning to demonstrate the impact of trauma on the developing brain at a cellular level. Before you read further, take a moment to recall what you have learned in anatomy and physiology about DNA, mitochondria, neurotransmitters and brain structure. Advances in genetic and molecular biology are now providing some clues to the mechanisms responsible for illness in those experiencing adversity early in their lives that result in specific gene–environment interactions (Brown et al. 2013; Heim & Binder 2012; Gong & He 2015). Researchers have found that gene expression, changes in mitochondrial DNA and molecular processes involving multiple neurotransmitter systems are negatively impacted by early life trauma (Murgatroyd et al. 2015; Malki et al. 2014; Brown et al. 2013; Lutz & Turecki 2014). A study of changes to telomeres (the protective endcaps to chromosomes preventing instability in cell structure and function) which allow for multiple cell division, were shortened in depressed individuals exposed to early life trauma (Cai et al. 2015). The decreased length of the telomeres reduces the amount of cell divisions thus ultimately shortening the life of the cell. This is associated with cancer, psychiatric illness and age-related neurodegenerative disorders such as Alzheimer disease (Cai et al. 2015; Hochstrasser et al. 2012; Shammas 2011). Other brain changes include reduced hippocampal volume, hypothalamic–pituitary–adrenal axis dysfunction, structural and functional abnormalities in neuronal networks and neurotransmitter dysregulation (Appel et al. 2011; Booij et al. 2015; Provençal & Binder 2015; Gong & He 2015; Brown et al. 2013).

Early trauma increases a person's risk of physical and mental illness. Complex trauma that occurs when traumatic stressors are 'interpersonal—premeditated, planned and perpetrated by one human being on another . . . can be both violating and exploitative of another person' (Bateman et al. 2013, p. 8). The person who has a history of complex trauma may well 'present with an interrelated mix of diverse mental health and physical health issues, developmental and psychosocial problems' (Bateman et al. 2013, p. 8). Remember too that this early trauma may also place the person at increased risk of exposure to further traumatic events such as domestic violence in adulthood.

Neuroplasticity

Yet, in spite of the negative effects of psychological trauma and stress on brain structure and function, the human brain also has a remarkable ability to adapt to the changes imposed by early trauma and illness. Research (some of which dates back over 100 years) has demonstrated how individuals with significant brain damage arising from physiological disorders such as stroke (cerebral vascular accident) and traumatic brain injury can recover and regain function that seemed to have been lost as a result of the damage (Fuchs & Flugge 2014; McDonnell et al. 2015). The mechanism for this process is the brain's capacity to generate new brain cells (neurogenesis) and establish alternative neural pathways. The term 'neuroplasticity' was introduced in the 1960s as a way of understanding the reorganisation of neuronal anatomy affecting the structure and function of the brain in response to many external and internal events (Opendak & Gould 2015; Fuchs & Flugge 2014).

Given the brain's capacity to repair itself when physiological brain disease or injury occurs, it is logical to imagine that this capacity for neurogenesis and neuroplasticity could also have positive impacts on a brain affected by psychological damage associated with early trauma and mental illness. Increasingly, research is demonstrating findings that are suggestive of neuroplasticity occurring in the hippocampus and lateral ventricles of the brain, areas that influence brain changes related to psychological stress and trauma (Benninghoff et al. 2012; Wainwright & Galea 2013; Opendak & Gould 2015; Cameron & Glover 2015; Rotheneichner et al. 2014; Malykhin & Coupland 2015). Neuroplasticity has also been shown to play a key role in the development of resilience (Opendak & Gould 2015) and recent research suggests that the brain's capacity for neuroplasticity continues into late adulthood (Porto et al. 2015).

Many of the psychiatric treatments used over recent years, while effective, have relied mostly on empirical evidence (i.e. observation or experience of the benefits) rather than neurobiological evidence demonstrating the mechanism of action. Evidence is now emerging to clearly show that neuroplasticity is positively influenced by medication such as lithium and other psychotropic medications that enhance brain-derived neurotrophic factor (BDNF). Long-term, less intense and enjoyable exercise also positively influences neuroplasticity, especially in the treatment of depression. Even listening to music or playing musical instruments has a positive neuroplastic response (Reybrouck & Brattico 2015; Yang et al. 2015; Fuchs & Flugge 2014; Mandelli et al. 2014; Gray & McEwen 2013; Inoue et al. 2015; Kita 2014). Controversial treatments such as electroconvulsive therapy (ECT) and the novel treatment known as magnetic brain stimulation are also showing positive neuroplastic effects (Rajji et al. 2013; Rotheneichner et al. 2014; Schloesser et al. 2015).

Past Trauma Continues to Impact on the Present

Despite these advances in knowledge, it is essential to remember that a history of complex trauma may result in the person experiencing a range of symptoms such as 'intrusive reexperiencing of the trauma in nightmares or flashbacks, inability to recall part of the trauma and emotional numbing as well as hyper-arousal' (Bateman et al. 2013, p. 18). For some people, self-harm or non-suicidal self-injury (NSSI) becomes an 'effective, yet maladaptive strategy, to cope with trauma symptoms' (Smith et al. 2014, p. 41). NSSI has a range of functions, including reinforcing the person's painful emotions such as fear, shame, contempt for self and hostility. Conversely, NSSI may serve to stop flashbacks, distract the person from their painful memories or stop feelings of guilt. For others, NSSI may be used for self-punishment, to end states of depersonalisation or dissociation or to communicate to others the person's extreme distress (Smith et al. 2014, pp. 45–46).

Survivors of trauma are likely to make up a high percentage of the people who present to emergency departments (EDs) in crisis or who are admitted to inpatient mental health units. Unfortunately, in either setting the response from health professionals may further add to the person's trauma. It is not uncommon for health professionals to be more stigmatising towards those with mental illness than are the rest of the community.

As mental health clinicians, the authors of this chapter have at times witnessed examples of prejudice and stigma in the ED setting. In one instance, overt prejudice was expressed by the medical director of a large ED who openly stated, 'I don't want *them* in my department'. A triage nurse was overheard stating, 'I'll just triage him at a level four and hopefully he'll get sick of waiting and go home'. Statements such as, 'there's no-one here from mental health, come back tomorrow' are common in some settings, and police arriving with a person who has self-harmed are often directed to 'take them away, they are nothing but a nuisance'. Some nurses do not appear to see someone presenting with a history of mental illness or experiencing psychological and emotional distress as 'real patients'. They instead express a preference to deal with people presenting with major medical illness or trauma. ED nurses may openly admit that they 'are not specialist mental health nurses' so should not have to 'deal with them'. Such comments highlight how important it is that each nurse has a sound understanding of the impact of trauma on an individual's mental and physical wellbeing. Psychiatric liaison nurses have a key role in providing this important education within the general hospital setting.

As nurses it is imperative that you recognise the traumatising impact of 'many practices and procedures, such as ward rounds, ward rules, search procedures, locked doors, mixed-sex patient populations and the use of seclusion and restraint' (Muskett 2014, p. 58). These practices both retraumatise and disempower the person and are experienced as emotionally unsafe, and significant evidence reveals that the very services that were developed to assist people are in fact counter therapeutic (Bateman et al. 2013). When a person with a history of complex trauma suffers further traumatisation, they are likely to experience symptoms such as dissociation, a marked increase in anxiety and fear and difficulty regulating their emotional state. In this state, the person may be at increased risk of self-harm or suicidal behaviours.

Unresolved Crisis

Although the majority of people negotiate crises in their lives without long-lasting impact, some people will have difficulty bouncing back to their precrisis functioning. The *Diagnostic and Statistical Manual of Mental Disorders* (DSM-5) identifies a range of trauma- and stress-related disorders (American Psychiatric Association 2013). It is to be anticipated that individuals exposed to a situation where they face death or threatened death, serious injury or sexual violence (such as those outlined in Box 7.1) will be distressed and overwhelmed by the event.

The impact may continue beyond the initial period of being overwhelmed. For these people anxiety disorders, depressive disorders, insomnia, substance misuse, acute stress disorder (ASD) and/or PTSD may result (see Table 7.2). Trauma that results from stressors that are interpersonal and intentional (such as torture or sexual violence) increase the likelihood of longer-lasting impact (Bateman et al. 2013).

Chapter 18 will provide you with in-depth information about ASD and PTSD and nursing responses to assist people with specific aspects of these disorders.

BOX 7.1 Traumatic Events Identified as Potential Triggers for Posttraumatic Stress Disorder

The directly experienced traumatic events in Criterion A include, but are not limited to, exposure to war as a combatant or civilian, threatened or actual physical assault (e.g. physical attack, robbery, mugging, childhood physical abuse), threatened or actual sexual violence (e.g. forced sexual penetration, alcohol/drug-facilitated sexual penetration, abusive sexual contact, noncontact sexual abuse, sexual trafficking), being kidnapped, being taken hostage, terrorist attack, torture, incarceration as a prisoner of war, natural or human-made disasters and severe motor vehicle accidents.

For children, sexually violent events may include developmentally inappropriate sexual experiences without physical violence or injury.

A life-threatening illness or debilitating medical condition is not necessarily considered a traumatic event.

Medical incidents that qualify as traumatic events involve sudden, catastrophic events (e.g. waking during surgery, anaphylactic shock).

Witnessed events include, but are not limited to, observing threatened or serious injury, unnatural death, physical or sexual abuse of another person due to violent assault, domestic violence, accident, war or disaster or a medical catastrophe in one's child (e.g. a life-threatening haemorrhage).

Indirect exposure through learning about an event is limited to experiences affecting close relatives or friends and experiences that are violent or accidental (e.g. death due to natural causes does not qualify). Such events include violent personal assault, suicide, serious accident and serious injury. The disorder may be especially severe or long-lasting when the stressor is interpersonal and intentional (e.g. torture, sexual violence).

(*Source:* Reprinted with permission from the Diagnostic and Statistical Manual of Mental Disorders, Fifth Edition, (Copyright © 2013). American Psychiatric Association. All Rights Reserved.)

TABLE 7.2 Diagnostic Criteria for ASD and PTSD

Acute Stress Disorder (ASD)	Posttraumatic Stress Disorder (PTSD)
A. Exposure to actual or threatened death, serious injury or sexual violation in one (or more) of the following ways: 1. Directly experiencing the traumatic event(s). 2. Witnessing, in person, the event(s) as it occurred to others. 3. Learning that the event(s) occurred to a close family member or close friend. Note: In cases of actual or threatened death of a family member or friend, the event(s) must have been violent or accidental. 4. Experiencing repeated or extreme exposure to aversive details of the traumatic event(s) (e.g. first responders collecting human remains, police officers repeatedly exposed to details of child abuse).	A. Exposure to actual or threatened death, serious injury or sexual violence. 1. Directly experience the traumatic event. 2. Witnessing, in person, the event(s) as it occurred to others. 3. Learning that the traumatic event(s) occurred to a close family member or close friend. In cases of actual or threatened death of a family member or friend, the event(s) must have been violent or accidental. 4. Experience repeated or extreme exposure to aversive details of the traumatic event(s) (e.g. first responders collecting human remains; police officers repeatedly exposed to details of child abuse).
B. Presence of nine (or more) of the following symptoms from any of the five categories of intrusion, negative mood, dissociation, avoidance and arousal, beginning or worsening after the traumatic event(s) occurred. • ***Intrusion symptoms*** 1. Recurrent, involuntary, and intrusive distressing memories of the traumatic event(s). Note: In children, repetitive play may occur in which themes or aspects of the traumatic event(s) are expressed. 2. Recurrent distressing dreams in which the content and/or effect of the dream are related to the event(s). Note: In children, there may be frightening dreams without recognizable content. 3. Dissociative reactions (e.g. flashbacks) in which the individual feels or acts as if the traumatic event(s) were recurring. (Such reactions may occur on a continuum,	B. Presence of one (or more) of the following intrusion symptoms associated with the traumatic event(s), beginning after the traumatic event occurred. 1. Recurrent, involuntary, and intrusive distressing memories of the traumatic event(s). 2. Recurrent distressing dreams in which the content and/or effect of the dream are related to the traumatic event(s). 3. Dissociative reactions (e.g. flashbacks) in which the individual feels or acts as if the traumatic event(s) were recurring. 4. Intense or prolonged psychological distress at exposure to internal or external cues that symbolize or resemble an aspect of the traumatic event(s). 5. Marked physiological reactions to internal or external cues that symbolize or resemble an aspect of the traumatic event(s).

TABLE 7.2 **Diagnostic Criteria for ASD and PTSD—cont'd**

Acute Stress Disorder (ASD)	Posttraumatic Stress Disorder (PTSD)
with the most extreme expression being a complete loss of awareness of present surroundings.) Note: In children, trauma-specific reenactment may occur in play. 4. Intense or prolonged psychological distress or marked physiological reactions in response to internal or external cues that symbolize or resemble an aspect of the traumatic event(s). • ***Negative mood*** 5. Persistent inability to experience positive emotions (e.g. inability to experience happiness, satisfaction or loving feelings). • ***Dissociative symptoms*** 6. An altered sense of the reality of one's surroundings or oneself (e.g. seeing oneself from another's perspective, being in a daze, time slowing). 7. Inability to remember an important aspect of the traumatic event(s) (typically due to dissociative amnesia and not to other factors such as head injury, alcohol or drugs). • ***Avoidance symptoms*** 8. Efforts to avoid distressing memories, thoughts or feelings about or closely associated with the traumatic event(s). 9. Efforts to avoid external reminders (people, places, conversations, activities, objects, situations) that arouse distressing memories, thoughts, or feelings about, or closely associated with, the traumatic event(s). • ***Arousal symptoms*** 10. Sleep disturbance (e.g. difficulty falling or staying asleep, restless sleep). 11. Irritable behaviour and angry outbursts (with little or no provocation), typically expressed as verbal or physical aggression towards people or objects. 12. Hypervigilance. 13. Problems with concentration. 14. Exaggerated startle response. C. Duration of the disturbance (symptoms in Criterion B) is 3 days to 1 month after trauma exposure. • Note: Symptoms typically begin immediately after the trauma, but persistence for at least 3 days and up to a month is needed to meet disorder criteria. D. The disturbance causes clinically significant distress or impairment in social, occupational, or other important areas of functioning. E. The disturbance is not attributable to the physiological effects of a substance (e.g. medication or alcohol) or another medical condition (e.g. mild traumatic brain injury) and is not better explained by brief psychotic disorder.	C. Persistent avoidance of stimuli associated with the traumatic event(s), beginning after the traumatic event(s) occurred, as evidenced by one or both of the following. 1. Avoidance of or efforts to avoid distressing memories, thoughts or feelings about or closely associated with the traumatic event(s). 2. Avoidance of or efforts to avoid external reminders (people, places, conversations, activities, objects, situations) that arouse distressing memories, thoughts, or feelings about, or closely associated with, the traumatic event(s). D. Negative alterations in cognitions and mood associated with the traumatic event(s), beginning or worsening after the traumatic event(s) occurred, as evidenced by two (or more) of the following. 1. Inability to remember an important aspect of the traumatic event(s) (typically due to dissociative amnesia and not to other factors such as head injury, alcohol or drugs). 2. Persistent and exaggerated negative beliefs or expectations about oneself, others, or the world (e.g. 'I am bad', 'No one can be trusted', 'The world is completely dangerous', 'My whole nervous system is permanently ruined'). 3. Persistent, distorted cognitions about the cause or consequences of the traumatic event(s) that lead the individual to blame himself/herself or others. 4. Persistent negative emotional state (e.g. fear, horror, anger, guilt, or shame). 5. Markedly diminished interest or participation in significant activities. 6. Feelings of detachment or estrangement from others. 7. Persistent inability to experience positive emotions (e.g. inability to experience happiness, satisfaction, or loving feelings). E. Marked alterations in arousal and reactivity associated with the traumatic event(s), beginning or worsening after the traumatic event(s) occurred, as evidenced by two (or more) of the following. 1. Irritable behaviour and angry outbursts (with little or no provocation) typically expressed as verbal or physical aggression toward people or objects. 2. Reckless or self-destructive behaviour. 3. Hypervigilance. 4. Exaggerated startle response. 5. Problems with concentration. 6. Sleep disturbance (e.g. difficulty falling or staying asleep or restless sleep). F. Duration of the disturbance (Criteria B, C, D, and E) is more than 1 month. G. The disturbance causes clinically significant distress or impairment in social, occupational, or other important areas of functioning. H. The disturbance is not attributable to the physiological effects of a substance (e.g. medication, alcohol) or another medical condition.

(*Source:* Reprinted with permission from the Diagnostic and Statistical Manual of Mental Disorders, Fifth Edition, (Copyright © 2013). American Psychiatric Association. All Rights Reserved.)

Effects of Loss and Bereavement

Generally, the human response to loss and bereavement is to grieve. A number of theories have been developed over the past 50 years. Earlier understandings viewed grief as a series of steps through which the person needed to move in order to successfully achieve 'closure' or to 'get over' their loss. Kübler-Ross (1969) described grief as a process of five stages through which a person moves when approaching their own death: denial, anger, bargaining, depression and finally acceptance. Parkes 1998 (cited in Wright & Hogan 2008) built upon the work of Bowlby (1980) and pictured grief as the breaking of a bond with someone to whom the person was attached. While identifying four phases—shock and numbness, yearning and searching, despair and disorganisation, with grief resolving as the person reaches the fourth phase of reorganisation and recovery—the grieving process was recognised as unique to each individual.

These understandings remain popular, although extensive research has shown that the process of grieving is an individual journey and that the focus on 'closure' is unhelpful (Boss & Carnes 2012). While the intensity of grief usually diminishes with time, events such as anniversaries and many other such triggers can result in a reemergence of intense grief. Memories of loss and bereavement and the emotions associated with grieving may impact periodically throughout the person's life.

Two more recent models that are comprehensive and helpful in working with a person who is bereaved will be useful for you to explore (Hall 2014). Worden's task-based model (2009) lists a series of four key tasks that need to be completed for a person to return to a prebereavement state of stability. These are:

1. to accept the reality of the loss
2. to work through the pain of grief
3. to adjust to an environment in which the deceased is missing
4. to find an enduring connection with the deceased while embarking on a new life

In order to understand the idiosyncratic nature of each person's experience of loss, Worden (2009) identified factors that will influence the grieving process. These questions provide some prompts for you to consider as you think about a particular person's story.

- Who was the person that died?
- What was the person's relationship or attachment to the person who died?
- How did the person die?
- How were things before the person died?
- How do various aspects of the grieving person's personality impact on their grief?
- What social factors are supportive or unhelpful at this time?
- What else is happening in the person's life?

In addition to these factors, remember to make sure that you consider the cultural context and religious/spiritual framework for each person. Just as the ways in which people express distress are culturally specific, so too are practices related to dying, death and bereavement strongly influenced by cultural and religious beliefs.

The second model is shown in Fig. 7.2. The dual process model of coping with bereavement (Stroebe & Schut 1999; Stroebe et al. 2006) challenges the perception that the person must continually focus on the work of grieving to complete the tasks of grieving. Rather, this model suggests that grieving is a process of 'oscillating' back and forth between a focus on the loss or emotion-focussed coping and a focus on restoration, that is adjusting to the consequences of the loss through problem-focussed coping. Emotion-focussed coping strategies

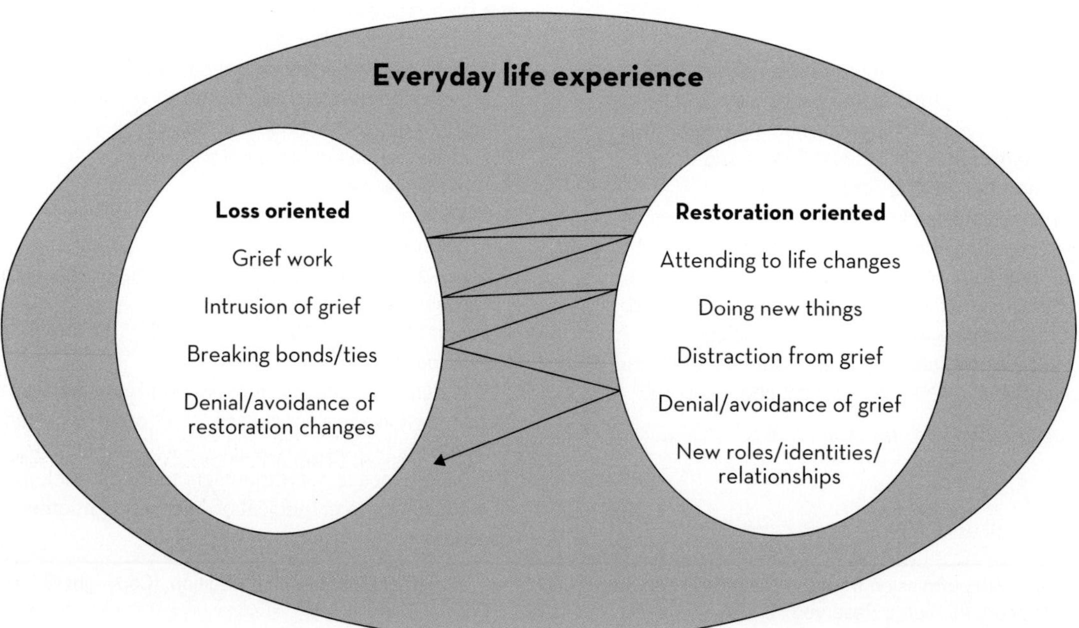

Fig. 7.2 The dual process model of coping with bereavement. (*Source:* Stroebe, H., Schut, M., 1999. The dual process model of coping with bereavement: rationale and description. Death Studies, 23[3]: 197–224, p. 213. https://doi.org/10.1080/074811899201046)

that enable a person to express and process the emotions arising from loss are essential where the situation is such that the person cannot change what has happened. Bereavement is one such situation: no matter how effective a person's capacity might be to solve problems, it is impossible for the loss to be reversed. However, bereavement will need a person to use both emotion-focussed coping and problem-solving coping. For example, the young wife with two school-age children whose husband has died will need to assume responsibility for the roles that her husband had held in the family. She may need to actively use problem-solving skills to resolve insurance issues, adjust to a reduced income and to solve the myriad other issues that are the result of her husband's death.

Remember, the impact of one person's death may be widespread. All family members will be affected, the dynamics and relationships between members of the family will be disrupted and the function of the family as a whole will be changed. 'Death ends a life but not relationships: mourning processes involve a transformation of those relationships from physical presence to continuing bonds through spiritual connections, memories, deeds and stories that are passed through kinship networks and to future generations' (Walsh & McGoldrick 2013, p. 21).

Severe and Persistent Mental Illness

For some people who live with severe and persistent mental illnesses, such as a chronic psychotic illness, severe bipolar affective disorder or severe or treatment-resistant depression, acute states of crisis may be a more frequent experience. Some of the risk factors that are likely to contribute to increased risk include poverty, limited family or social support, homelessness and comorbid physical illness (Brennaman 2012). The adverse impacts of homelessness on mental health have been clearly documented (Costello et al. 2013; Mental Health Council 2009).

OTHER FACTORS THAT INFLUENCE AN INDIVIDUAL'S RESPONSE IN TIMES OF DIFFICULTY

Factors such as an early trauma history or living with severe mental illness may indeed place a person at increased risk of experiencing an acute state of crisis. And remember that while every person's perception of and response to a stressful or traumatic event will differ, there are other factors that influence an individual's responses. Two key concepts to understand at this point are *vulnerability* and *resilience*.

Vulnerability

As humans, we are all prone to 'moments of vulnerability'; that is, we are capable of being physically or emotionally wounded or hurt. A feeling of vulnerability may arise in a social interaction or a work situation. Consider times when you have felt vulnerable, perhaps the first day in a new course of study or the first day of work, or maybe it was a time when you were ill and had just been admitted to hospital. Was your sense of vulnerability heightened by anxiety or fear or perhaps by feeling that you had no control over the situation or over what was about to happen? The term 'vulnerable' is frequently applied to specific groups in the population who are identified as a social or political problem needing a solution, for example those who are homeless or those who are seeking refuge from war and political turmoil. This term might also be used to identify a person or group of people at risk of ill health or in danger of abuse and thus needing measures to be put in place to keep them safe.

Rather than directly labelling a person as vulnerable because of factors such as their age, diagnosis or social situation (Heaslip & Ryden 2013), it is essential that vulnerability is assessed for each individual. Keep in mind that some groups, such as infants, children and those who are unable to communicate at all due to serious physical illness, frailty or extreme age, are vulnerable and need a high degree of care and support. Likewise, people arriving as refugees or seeking asylum after being exposed to war and traumatic events, such as physical and/or sexual violence and assault, being kidnapped, tortured and seeing family members killed, are extremely vulnerable and also in need of extensive care and support. However, assessing whether a person is vulnerable requires careful consideration of both personal and situational factors. Rogers' (1997) model identified vulnerability as comprising a dynamic balance between two interacting variables, personal components and environmental factors (Fig. 7.3), this model remains a useful tool to assist in assessing individual vulnerability. Also of note is the

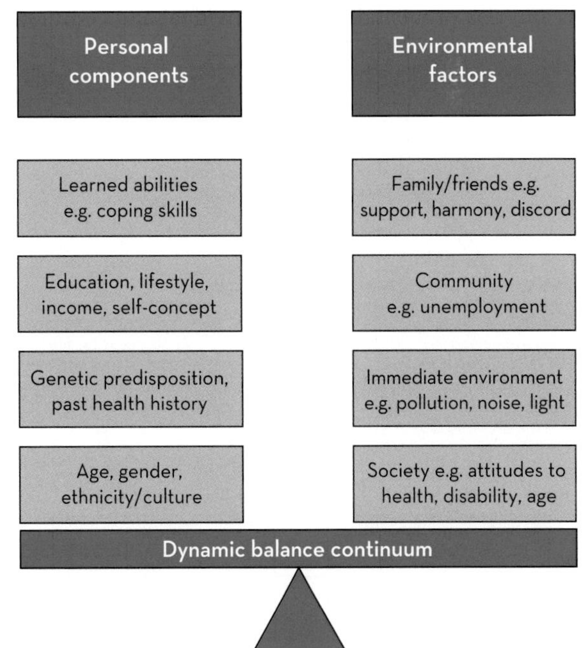

Fig. 7.3 Vulnerability: a balance-continuum model. (*Source:* Rogers model [Rogers, AC., 1997. Vulnerability, health and health care. Journal of Advanced Nursing, 26[1], 65–72. https://doi.org/10.1046/j.1365-2648.1997.1997026065.x]. Adapted by Heaslip, V., Ryden, J., [Eds.], 2013. Understanding Vulnerability: a Nursing and Healthcare Approach. John Wiley & Sons, Pondicherry, India, p. 21.)

Zubin and Spring (1997) Stress-vulnerability model, which has had considerable impact on the field of mental health. It offers hope to those who experience mental ill health as it suggests that coping mechanisms can be acquired to counter the effects of stress, hence reducing the risk of continued Illness or relapse.

Resilience

Resilience can be defined as 'a person's capacity for adapting psychologically, emotionally and physically reasonably well and without lasting detriment to self, relationships or personal development in the face of adversity, threat or challenge' (Williams 2007, quoted in Williams & Alexander 2009, p. 362). Note carefully that being resilient does not mean that there will not be occasions when a person will be 'knocked down' by a stressful or traumatic experience. Rather, being resilient gives the capacity to 'bounce back' after the event without lasting damage. A range of internal factors have been shown to influence an individual's resilience (Fig. 7.4).

Resilience fluctuates not only as individual capacity varies; multiple external factors also contribute to each person's capacity to 'bounce' back after stressful and traumatic events. Increasingly, research attention is being given to the impact of the social and cultural context on a person's resilience. Globally, large numbers of people are living under situations of extreme duress, which stretch to breaking point the resilience of even the most robust in the population (Hobfoll et al. 2011). Situations where there is heavy loss of material resources and psychosocial supports in the context of violence markedly increase psychological distress and risk of mental illness. Individual and community resilience is severely affected in regions where ongoing war and civil conflict causes loss of life and the loss of even the most basic of human needs: safe drinking water, shelter and safety.

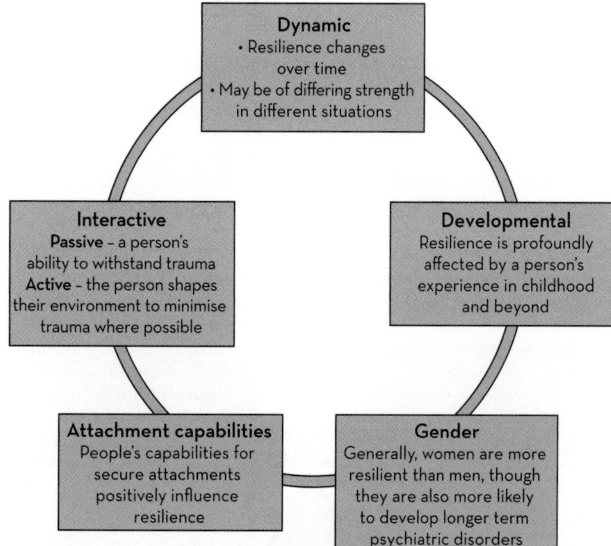

Fig. 7.4 The nature of individual resilience. (*Source:* Adapted from Williams, R., Alexander, D., 2009. Part B—Psychosocial resilience and distress in the face of adversity, conflict, terrorism, or catastrophe. In: Hopperus Buma, A.P.C.C., Burris, D.G., Hawley A., Ryan, J.M., Mahoney PF [Eds.] Conflict and Catastrophe Medicine, second ed. Springer-Verlag, London, p. 368.)

Yet, in spite of such overwhelmingly adverse circumstances and high levels of loss and psychological distress, some people retain an ability to remain active and vigorous in the face of such difficulties. For example, a person's level of education and youth appears to enable them to continue active engagement in life under difficult circumstances (Hobfoll et al. 2012). In war-affected communities in northern Uganda, researchers found that young people's resilience in the aftermath of war was positively impacted by the person's individual characteristics. Factors such as social connection with their peers, behaving respectfully and sharing with others also enable the young person to thrive. Indicators that the young person was making progress towards 'bouncing back' after the horrors of war included actively building their skills and resources and having hope for the future. The resilient young person was able to be self-reliant, look after their physical and mental health, be responsible and disciplined, but also to know how to access support from other people if needed. Spiritual health further supported resilience, with young people who described being close to God as able to 'better deal with mental distress and setbacks, and to have more strengths and hope in life' (Vindevogel et al. 2015, p. 408). The New South Wales Service for the Treatment and Rehabilitation of Torture and Trauma Survivors (STARTTS) also emphasises the amazing resilience of refugees who are able to build meaningful and productive lives when they receive support and assistance at the time when they are most vulnerable (see the Useful Websites list at the end of this chapter for examples and information).

Before reading further, go to Case Study 7.1 and read about Eilidh. As you read, consider factors that you think may have contributed to Eilidh's resilience and what factors had resulted in vulnerability at the time she rang for assistance.

People in general are remarkably resilient and many times display an enormous capacity to transcend difficulties and trauma. Remember that just as resilience is a dynamic and changeable state, levels of vulnerability likewise fluctuate over time (Heaslip & Ryden 2013). Although each person has their own unique mix of resilience and vulnerability, there are a range of factors which may impact on emotional development and psychological and physical wellbeing. Changes to environmental factors, such as sudden and unexpected unemployment in a time of high levels of unemployment, may well upset a person's balance and resilience, increasing the person's vulnerability and in some instances leading to a state of acute crisis.

Before you proceed through the next section, take time to reflect upon what you have learned so far. Each of the sections above contain essential information that you will need to keep in mind when you are working to help a person who has experienced a traumatic event, is bereaved or in crisis.

CASE STUDY 7.1

Eilidh

Eilidh was 33 years old when I first met her. She had rung the clinic where I worked as a clinical nurse consultant specialising in education and counselling for people with little-known chronic autoimmune conditions. Eilidh sounded distressed and overwhelmed, but settled once she knew that an appointment was available that day, at least until she found that the clinic was on the seventh floor of the hospital. She was scared of heights and described finding it almost impossible to get in a lift. After reassuring her that I would meet her at the lift, she agreed to come that afternoon.

Eilidh arrived as arranged and took the lift with me to the seventh floor. Although anxious, she came to my office and sat down. Eilidh had had lupus (SLE) since she was 10 years old but had not sought information or support previously. After a few moments, she started shaking and became distraught. I wondered aloud whether Eilidh would find it easier to walk up and down the corridor with me and we could talk away from the windows reminding her that she was on the seventh floor. For the next hour, I walked slowly backwards and forwards with Eilidh, as she found words to talk of the crisis that had driven her to seek assistance.

Eilidh's story revealed a remarkable level of resilience that had now faltered in the face of a marked increase in workload and relationship difficulties. Her husband James struggled to understand the fatigue and almost constant pain associated with a recent flare-up of lupus. Eilidh's father had drunk heavily and had physically and verbally abused her as a child. She had attempted to escape the abuse when she was 8 years old, writing to her grandmother asking could she go and live with her. Grandma was not able to take her, but provided love and care during school holidays. During adolescence, illness had interrupted Eilidh's schooling. In spite of this, she completed a GCSE excelling in maths and computing. Finding employment had proved difficult; no employer seemed prepared to employ someone who had a chronic relapsing illness. After more than 300 job applications, Eilidh had finally found a job and was a valued employee who had worked her way up the company, assuming more responsibility over time.

It seemed that the current workload and relationship stressors had triggered memories of Eilidh's difficult past and she was now flooded with traumatic memories and physiological responses that threatened her usual resilience. Although Eilidh had volunteered information of previous traumas, to explore those in more detail at our first meeting would likely have added further trauma and distress. As we walked, together we developed a plan and identified strategies that Eilidh could use to manage her distress. Eilidh asked if she could bring her husband James to a follow-up appointment and we planned together the focus for that meeting. Eilidh had regained her composure before leaving and felt that she would be okay until we met again later that week.

WHAT CAN YOU DO TO HELP?

This section covers information to assist you in helping people experiencing difficult times and directions on how you might develop your skills to provide effective support as a nurse.

Core Skills for 'Being With the Person in Crisis'

A wretched soul, bruised with adversity,
We bid be quiet, when we hear it cry:
But were we burdened with like weight of pain,
As much, or more, would we ourselves complain.

William Shakespeare as recorded by Heminge and Condell* (The Comedy of Errors *1623, p. 87).

Remember that a person in crisis is at a point where their usual coping strategies and resilience have been overwhelmed. As nurses, this is an opportunity to help the person at a time of increased vulnerability and need. To be effective, you need some core personal skills. An ability to remain calm and to regulate your own emotions is required. Think carefully about the ways in which you would normally settle yourself at times of distress. Have you had the experience of soothing a distressed child? Speaking gently and softly will often be effective in quietening the frightened or upset child. Likewise, bringing your attention to slowing your own breathing, speaking slowly in measured tones and appearing totally calm will not only assist the person you are helping to settle, it will also assist you to regulate and calm yourself.

Over 400 years ago, Shakespeare (recorded faithfully by John Heminge & Henry Condell 1623) suggested that when someone is troubled and 'crying', it is difficult to hear and perhaps we judge the person's behaviour as unnecessary or 'making a fuss about nothing'; but yet if we were in the same situation, we likewise would cry. If you are to be effective, it is essential that you are able to put aside your judgements and biases about both the validity of the person's distress and the 'appropriateness' of how they express their distress. Yassmin Abdel-Magied, speaking at a TEDx event in 2014 described biases 'as the filters through which we see the world around us'. (See the Useful Websites list at the end of this chapter for information about TED.) All of us have biases: this is totally normal. Our biases will be about multiple, different areas of life and against whatever is different from us (e.g. culture, sex, social class, level of education) and different from our particular social norms. Abdel-Magied (2014) described how important it is to put aside your biases. You will need to take time to identify and acknowledge these and then take care to ensure that your biases do not adversely impact on the people you are caring for. Each of you as a nurse has a responsibility to make sure that the circumstances of a person's birth do not impact on the care that you provide for a person.

The expression of crisis varies widely from person to person and is influenced by many factors including the person's culture. 'Everyone grows up with exposure to one or more cultures that teach them how to respond to crisis and grief' (Chase 2013). Each of us will have a range of idioms (phrases or expressions that mean something different to the literal definition of the actual words used) that are common to our cultural group. For example, 'got out of the wrong side of the bed' indicates that the person is in a bad mood and has been grumpy all day. In many non-Western cultures where mental distress and disorder is seen as madness, psychological distress 'is expressed through somatic complaints such as headaches, backaches, stomach aches, and general body tension . . . extreme emotions and psychological problems are expressed through somatically-oriented idioms' (Mehraby 2012, p. 55). To understand the lifeworld of the person in crisis therefore requires you to be able to put aside your judgements, to listen carefully and to 'wonder aloud' what specific idioms mean, rather than assuming that you understand (Hinton & Lewis-Fernández 2010).

Those of you who speak a second language will have some understanding of the challenges that can arise when you attempt to communicate in a language that is not your 'native tongue', unless you grew up in a bilingual household. If you have no experience of learning a second language, it is perhaps difficult to comprehend just how challenging it can be, especially as a person ages, to become even a little fluent in another language. For a person who has a basic grasp of English, this may be sufficient for the daily negotiations of everyday life; however, when difficulties arise and the person experiences a crisis, communication may become exceptionally challenging. Go back now and review the crisis model in Fig. 7.1. Key features of crisis include difficulty thinking clearly and disrupted emotional, cognitive and behavioural functioning. If the person is not extremely fluent in English, it is likely that they will have a great deal of difficulty communicating, both to express in English what is happening and to understand what is being said to them.

Think back to what you have learned about communication: do you recall what percentage of communication is nonverbal? Your ability to convey calmness and portray empathy and acceptance will be very apparent in your nonverbal communication. However, to provide effective assistance, you will also need to be able to communicate verbally. Make sure you know how to access the interpreter services in your local area. Develop your skills in using an interpreter. (See Box 7.2 for beginning instructions on how to work with an interpreter.) Links to information on providing equitable and effective care in the multicultural setting are provided in the Useful Websites list at the end of this chapter.

Now that you have calmed yourself, put aside your judgements, focussed on listening attentively (active listening) and considered how you will communicate effectively, you are well on the way to creating a safe environment and being in touch with your capacity for genuineness and empathy. These attributes, combined with self-awareness, are the essential prerequisites for therapeutic communication. They will decrease the likelihood of you jumping to conclusions about the type of help the person needs or wants. For the person in crisis, genuine concern, empathy and an awareness that you are

BOX 7.2 Working With an Interpreter

- Address the patient directly rather than speaking to the interpreter. Maintain eye contact with the patient to ensure the patient's involvement.
- Do not interrupt the patient and the interpreter. At times their interaction may take longer because of the need to clarify, and descriptions may require more time because of dialect differences or the interpreter's awareness that the patient needs more preparation before being asked a particular question.
- Ask the interpreter to give you verbatim translations so that you can assess what the patient is thinking and understanding.
- Avoid using medical jargon that the interpreter or patient may not understand.
- Avoid talking or commenting to the interpreter at length; the patient may feel left out and distrustful.
- Be aware that asking intimate or emotionally laden questions may be difficult for both the patient and the interpreter. Lead up to the questions slowly. Always ask permission to discuss these topics first, and prepare the interpreter for the content of the interview.
- When possible, allow the patient and the interpreter to meet each other ahead of time to establish some rapport. If possible, try to use the same interpreter for succeeding interviews with the patient.
- If possible, request an interpreter of the same gender as the patient and of a similar age. To make good use of the interpreter's time, decide beforehand which questions you will ask. Meet with the interpreter briefly before going to see the patient so that you can let the interpreter know what you are planning to ask. During the session, face the patient and direct your questions to the patient, not the interpreter.

(*Source:* Gorman, L.M., Sultan, D.F., 2008. Psychosocial Nursing for general patient care, third ed. Philadelphia: FA Davis. In: Townsend, M.C., 2014. Essentials of Psychiatric Mental Health Nursing: Concepts of Care in Evidence-Based Practice, sixth ed. Philadelphia: F.A. Davis.)

BOX 7.3 Mental Health First Aid Action Plan

1. Approach the person, assess and assist with any crisis.
2. Listen nonjudgmentally.
3. Give support and information.
4. Encourage the person to get appropriate professional help.
5. Encourage other supports.

(*Source:* Jorm, A.F., Kitchener, B.A., 2011. Noting a landmark achievement: mental health first aid training reaches 1% of Australian adults. Australian and New Zealand Journal of Psychiatry. 45(10), 808–813, p. 809. https://doi.org/10.3109/00048674.2011.594785.)

interested in and supportive of the person as a unique individual provide a sense of support and a glimmer of hope that it may be possible to negotiate this crisis after all (Levinson 2011; McCabe et al. 2014).

Mental Health First Aid

Mental Health First Aid (MHFA) is an initiative conceived by Professor Anthony Jorm and his wife Betty Kitchener, who was a nurse, in Australia 1997. MHFA courses are designed to improve community responses to those experiencing a mental health crisis or demonstrating signs and symptoms suggestive of a developing mental illness (Jorm 2013). The course employs a similar model to that traditionally used to deliver first aid courses and has taken off globally. The World Health Organisation (WHO 2013) published the Mental Health Action Plan 2013–2020, the first in its history, representing a formal recognition of the importance of mental health globally. The comprehensive plan is testimony to the shifts in thinking about mental health and is central to providing an effective response to mental health problems, improving mental health literacy (Saxena et al. 2013). In the UK, Public Health England launched a 3-year, £15 million campaign to train 1 million people in MHFA by 2020, aiming to improve personal resilience and help people recognise and respond effectively to the signs of mental distress in others (Department of Health 2017).

Although this is a course that enables you to deliver first aid—that is, the help provided until professional help is available or until a crisis resolves—you may find this course to be a useful addition to your studies in mental health nursing. To find out more about MHFA, see the Useful Websites list at the conclusion of this chapter.

RESPONDING AFTER DISASTERS AND TRAUMATIC EVENTS

The focus of this chapter has primarily been on what could be described as 'ordinary' crisis events affecting one individual and their immediate family. However, it is important that as nurses you are also aware of interventions developed to respond to the psychosocial needs of people impacted by large-scale emergencies. These would include events where there have been destructive natural events (e.g. floods) and man made disasters (e.g. large explosions, terrorist attacks and large plane crashes).

Psychological First Aid

Psychological First Aid (PFA) is an evidence-based response that has been developed as a Level 1 Intervention to be implemented in situations following mass disaster. It is defined as 'a humane, supportive response to a fellow human being who is suffering and who may need support' (WHO 2011). This response is designed to identify unobtrusively and quickly who is in need of immediate intervention. Rather than focussing on pathology, the emphasis is on reducing acute distress by encouraging adaptive coping. Early assistance not only reduces acute distress but may also reduce the 'development of enduring mental health problems such as PTSD and protracted grief and depression' (McCabe et al. 2014, p. 623).

PFA is part of a wider 'organised disaster response process' intended to be used as a supportive intervention in the immediate aftermath of disasters and terrorism and is designed for delivery in diverse settings including at the disaster scene, community/neighbourhood centres, schools, and other appropriate settings where there is a place of safety (Disaster Response, Resilience and Research Group, University of Western Sydney, Wooding & Raphael 2012, p. 7 & 12). Table 7.3 explains the identifying features of PFA.

To read more about PFA and obtain training to provide PFA at times of disaster, access the websites in the Useful Websites list at the end of this chapter and the References section.

CRISIS INTERVENTION MODELS

A number of different models of crisis intervention have been developed over the past 50 or more years (see Table 7.4). Each of the models is based on a different premise; however, the overall goal is to assist the person to negotiate a situation that has overwhelmed their capacity to manage at that time (James & Gilliland 2013).

Although guiding principles are important when responding to a person in an acute state of crisis, a slavish adherence to a stepwise or rigid type of model places you at risk of responding inappropriately to the needs of each person as a unique individual. The person in an acute state of crisis may be out of control, chaotic and struggling to keep their behaviour in check. As you respond to the person, you need

TABLE 7.3 Psychological First Aid (PFA)

What PFA is	What PFA is Not
It involves the following themes: • providing practical care and support, which does not intrude • assessing needs and concerns • helping people to address basic needs (e.g. food and water, information) • listening to people, but not pressuring them to talk • comforting people and helping them to feel calm • helping people connect to information, services and social supports • protecting people from further harm.	• It is not something that only professionals can do. • It is not professional counselling. • It is not 'psychological debriefing' in that PFA does not necessarily involve a detailed discussion of the event that caused the distress. • It is not asking someone to analyse what happened to them or to put time and events in order. • Although PFA involves being available to listen to people's stories, it is not about pressuring people to tell you their feelings and reactions to an event.

(*Source:* World Health Organization, War Trauma Foundation and World Vision International, 2011. Psychological First Aid: Guide For Field Workers. WHO, Geneva.)

TABLE 7.4 Crisis Intervention Models

Model	Premise	Focus	Appropriate Time to Use This Model
Equilibrium model (Caplan 1961)	People in a state of crisis are experiencing psychological or emotional disequilibrium.	To assist the person recover their precrisis equilibrium	At the point where the person is overwhelmed; when the person is in a state of emotional dysregulation and unable to make informed decisions. However, it is unhelpful to attempt to explore triggers until the person has reconnected with some of their coping strategies.
Cognitive model Based on work by Ellis (1982), Meichenbaum (1977) and Beck (1976)	The person's perception of the situation, i.e. their faulty thinking, has led to the situation becoming a crisis.	To assist the person to recognize and modify their faulty thinking and to identify their logical and rational thoughts. This will then enable the person to achieve control over their response to difficult situations.	Once the person is in a stable situation and back to their precrisis functioning.
Psychosocial transition model Theorists who have contributed to this model Adler, Ansbacher & Ansbacher (1956) Erikson (1963) and Minuchin (1974)	This is based on an assumption that the person is influenced by their genetic code and what they learned from their environments, especially the social context. Crisis may arise from the continual changes within the person and the environment.	To work closely with the person to help them identify personal and environmental factors that may have influenced the crisis. Focus then on developing additional skills and/or addressing environmental contributors to the crisis.	Once the person is in a stable situation and back to their precrisis functioning.
Developmental–ecological model Collins and Collins (2005)	This model combines understandings about developmental stages and issues occurring within the person's environment.	To be effective, the helper must identify the developmental stage at which the person is functioning and assess the environmental issues and the interaction between the two.	Depends on how the person has achieved the tasks of the developmental stage at which they are functioning.

(*Source:* Compiled from James, R.K., Gilliland, B.E., 2013. Crisis Intervention Strategies, seventh ed. Brooks/Cole Cengage Learning, Canada, pp. 17–18.)

the ability to be flexible as the person may appear to settle and then rapidly become distressed and volatile again. More recently, the Task Model of Crisis Intervention (Fig. 7.5) was developed from a review of 10 different models that each uses a series of steps to guide the clinician (Myer et al. 2013). This model demonstrates the thoughtfulness and flexibility that is needed to respond effectively to a person in crisis. The tasks required are divided into two groups, either continuous or focussed tasks.

The continuous tasks of maintaining safety for both the person and yourself, assessing the situation and the person's level of distress and providing support are the platform upon which the focussed tasks are undertaken. Each of these tasks is vital to effective crisis intervention and you will need to be able to move from one to the other throughout your work with the person. Assessment will be a task that you are undertaking continuously during your encounter with the person in crisis. Remember that the person in crisis is in a chaotic and unstable state emotionally. It is not uncommon to find that the person has settled somewhat and it seems that it is timely to move on to the next part of your intervention, only to find

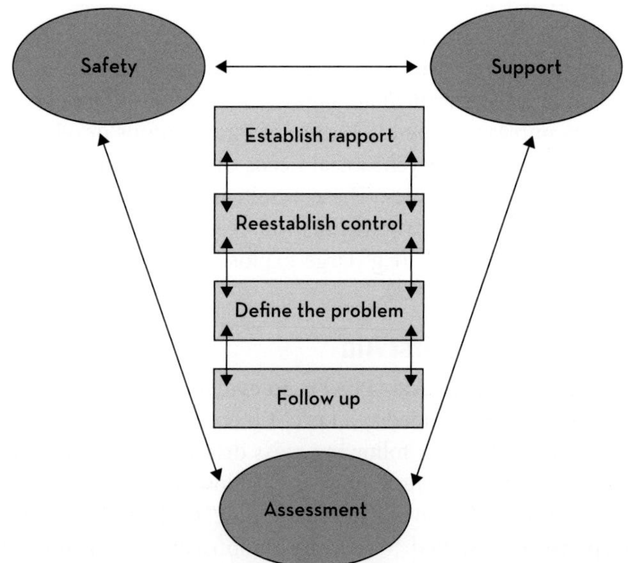

Fig. 7.5 The Task Model of Crisis Intervention. (*Source:* Adapted from Myer, R.A., Lewis, J.S, James, R.K., 2013. The introduction of a task model for crisis intervention. Journal of Mental Health Counseling 35[2], p. 99.)

that the person has slipped back into distress and despair. The process of assessment will need to continue throughout so that you can identify the capacity of the person to manage their emotions and impulses and to keep themselves safe. Chapter 22 will provide you with extensive information about developing your skills in assessment; Chapter 23 describes risk assessment, and Chapter 24 offers additional approaches to crisis intervention.

Crisis intervention also requires you to build rapport; that is, to develop a therapeutic relationship and assist the person to settle themselves. Remaining calm yourself will do much to enable the distressed person to settle. When the person has settled somewhat and you have established a connection with them, you can then proceed to finding out what has happened that triggered this crisis state. Once the person has settled and the acute distress has passed, remember that although it may seem that all is now well, your work is not yet complete. In some instances, the person may say, 'I'm fine now, I feel so embarrassed that I lost it like that. Can I please go home now?' However, it is important that you have helped them to reconnect with their coping strategies and, if possible, some external supports. While the acute state of crisis may be over, the person is likely to be shaken and still vulnerable. Before the person leaves, ensure that follow up has been arranged and that they know who they can contact should they require assistance again before the scheduled follow-up appointment.

In Nurse's Story 7.1, as you read Robin's account of working with Ryan, who had presented in crisis, compare her intervention with the Task Model of Crisis Intervention in Fig. 7.5.

If assessment reveals that the person is acutely distressed, aggressive and at risk of harming themselves or others, your skills in deescalating volatile situations will be required. This is also where your ability to empathise with the person's distress will do much to help the person settle. In many instances the person will be acutely distressed, and also anxious and frightened by their inability to cope. Again, maintaining your own emotional equilibrium and external calmness, along with reassurance that support is available, may do much to assist the person to settle. Repeatedly, research has shown that the way in which staff members respond to the person who is aggressive and potentially violent plays a very significant role in both helping the person to settle or becoming increasingly agitated and aggressive (Cutcliffe & Riahi 2013).

Nurses need to know when and how to intervene, how to engage the person and how to ensure safe conditions for deescalation. Effective deescalators (i.e. a person who is able to respond effectively to an aggressive and agitated person) are 'open, honest, supportive, self-aware, coherent, nonjudgemental, and confident, without appearing arrogant. They express genuine concern for the patient, appear nonthreatening and have a permissive, nonauthoritarian manner' (Price & Baker 2012, p. 312). Chapter 23 provides further information about effective responses where there is risk of aggression and violence.

NURSE'S STORY 7.1

Robin

Ryan, age 25, presented to the emergency department. He was distraught and overwhelmed. Several recent losses had caused him much grief and eroded his usual resilience and pragmatic coping style. He felt helpless to instigate any previously used problem-solving strategies. Ryan was very distressed and tearful as he recounted the sequence of events that had led him to think ending his life was his best course of action. My initial assessment concluded that he certainly had depressive symptoms with suicidal thoughts. Ryan had no specific plan to harm himself, but he did admit that his suicidal thoughts had scared him, as he had never previously experienced such thoughts. Given his risk of self-harm, I felt concerned about his ability to keep himself safe and my first inclination was to admit him to hospital, if necessary against his will.

Slowly, Ryan calmed a little but still felt helpless and hopeless and unable to see any way through his distress. I reassured Ryan that he was safe and he agreed that we could continue with the assessment. As I talked with him, I raised my concerns and discussed how we might work together to keep him safe through this challenging time. Admission to hospital was a possible option. Although Ryan did not refuse hospitalisation, he was clearly not keen about this suggestion. Together, we considered other options as I attempted to tap into his strengths and help him utilise his now disrupted coping strategies. I asked Ryan what he thought he needed to overcome his distress. His reply, 'I don't know'. This response was typical of a person whose thinking was affected by the emotional upset of an acute crisis state. I reframed the question, asking Ryan what his life and circumstances would look like if none of these events had happened. He described in some detail how life would be without such overwhelming grief and loss. Ryan rapidly became discouraged again when he could not think of how to live without feeling overwhelmed with grief and loss.

A shift in focus was needed again. Calming my own anxiety, I expressed my curiosity about his efforts and past success in overcoming adversities in his life. Ryan recalled several difficult events and described how he had overcome these difficulties. I reflected aloud on the strength and resilience he had demonstrated in overcoming these challenges. As Ryan acknowledged his own capacity to overcome adversity, the change in him was almost tangible. I witnessed an 'ah hah' moment. When he realised he was already working hard to recover, Ryan's level of distress dissipated markedly and he began to think of other strategies he could employ to continue his recovery. Ryan was very thankful for my help. While I accepted his thanks, at the same time I was humbled as I really hadn't worked miracles nor did I have easy answers for Ryan. Rather it had been a process of listening (really listening) while taking time to allow Ryan to reconnect with his own strength and resilience. Instead of letting my anxiety overwhelm me, I had been able to avoid reinforcing Ryan's sense of helplessness and circumvent an admission to hospital. Ryan was able to go away with renewed strength and hope for his future. Before leaving, Ryan was happy to take an appointment for follow up and phone numbers that he could call should he need to talk before we met again.

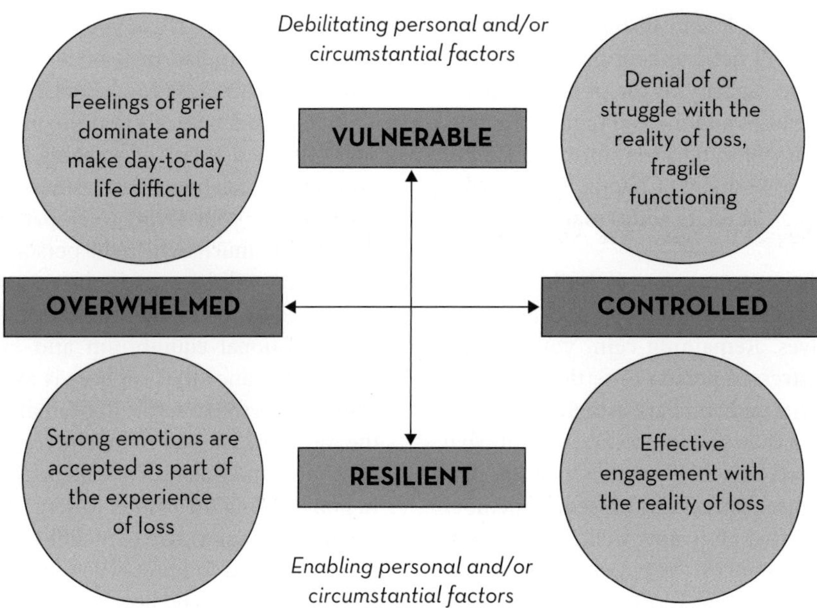

Fig. 7.6 The range of response to loss model. (*Source:* Brocklehurst, T., Hearnshaw, C., Machin, L., 2014. Bereavement needs assessment—piloting a process. Progress in Palliative Care. 22[3]:143–149. www.tandfonline.com.)

Responding to Refugees and Those Seeking Asylum

As nurses, you will also meet asylum seekers and refugees in a wide range of healthcare contexts, often at a time of great distress and need. Your response will need to be respectful, demonstrating your capacity for cultural sensitivity, and person (and family) centred. Take into account the barriers created by language difficulties and access an interpreter or health worker who speaks the person's preferred language. Remember that the person who has been greatly harmed by other humans is likely to find it very difficult to trust you and it may well take a significant period of time, patience and acceptance on your part to build a therapeutic relationship. Services such as those provided by Freedom from Torture (see Useful Websites) can be an invaluable resource. As clinicians working in a multicultural society such as the UK, ensure that you access further training to build your capacity to respond effectively to refugees and people seeking asylum.

Responding to the Person who is Bereaved or Experiencing Overwhelming Grief

When you are providing assistance to a person who has experienced a bereavement and overwhelming grief has led the person to seek assistance, remember that although these experiences are common to us all, bereaved individuals are 'at risk of developing both physical and mental health problems that may persist long after the loss has occurred' (Stroebe et al. 2006, p. 2440). The recently developed model shown in Fig. 7.6 may be useful to assist you in considering the extent to which a person is at risk of ongoing difficulties related to loss.

After you have spoken with the person and developed some understanding of their personal situation and circumstances, reference to this model can help to further consider the level of support needed. Look to identify where on the continuum between vulnerable and resilient the person is at that time and to assess the degree to which they are overwhelmed by their emotions or able to control their emotions. Take into account whether the person has debilitating contributors to their current situation or whether there are personal factors and circumstances that are supportive and enabling. Take a moment now to read Jean's story (Patient Story 7.1). See if you can identify factors that had led to Jean's feelings of distress and note what she found to be helpful and supportive.

Manner of Death Impacts Differently on the Bereaved

There are a number of additional factors that you need to be aware of when you seek to assist the person experiencing a crisis related to bereavement. Perhaps not unexpectedly, it appears that the impact of a natural or timely death in contrast with sudden and violent death or death by suicide may be markedly different. Research was undertaken to explore older people's ideas and experiences and what was helpful for them following the death of a close family member, a spouse or other person who was important to them. They spoke with 28 people aged between 71 and 90 years who had experienced a recent significant death. Rather than seeking formal support from bereavement support organisations, most people wanted to be independent and making decisions for themselves instead of relying on other people or formal support services. Death of a spouse or partner was seen to be inevitable if you live to be advanced in age

PATIENT STORY 7.1

Jean

Ten months ago, my husband, Bill, died after 5 years in a nursing home. He had Alzheimer's and no longer recognised me, but he was a gentleman to the end. He would say to the nurses, 'See that beautiful girl in the photo (our wedding photo), isn't she just the best?' We were married for almost 60 years. We couldn't have children, so we just had each other. I still miss him so much. When Bill died, my friends couldn't understand why I was so devastated. They said, 'You must be so relieved that you don't need to go to the nursing home anymore, what a blessing that he's gone.'

A few weeks after Bill's funeral, Betty and Edith invited me to go to the Rotary club. I went a few times, but it was just so difficult, I couldn't relax and they seemed to have forgotten that my beloved husband had died recently. I felt like I was spoiling their fun because I couldn't joke with them. Bill and I didn't go to clubs much, it wasn't really our thing. We enjoyed classical music concerts and art galleries much more.

Three months after Bill died, I went to see my GP. He knew Bill. I thought he would understand how devastated I was to lose Bill. He just said, 'You really wouldn't want Bill to be still suffering, he didn't know who you were anymore'. He didn't realise that Bill always smiled when I visited, even if he had forgotten who I was. When I started to sob, the doctor said, 'I'm writing a referral for you to go and see a mental health nurse who is a counsellor too, I'm concerned that you are still crying and getting so upset when we talk about Bill'. I felt so embarrassed that he thought there was something wrong with me, but I took the referral anyway.

After 2 weeks, I rang up and made an appointment for the next week. All week, I thought about cancelling, but I knew my doctor would be cross with me if I didn't go. I had never been to see a counsellor before. I worried about what I would say and whether she would also tell me to get over Bill.

You know, I am so glad that I went to that first appointment. The counsellor read the referral and smiled gently, and then she said, 'Would you like to tell me about Bill?' I went to see her every week for quite a few visits and we just talked. I was able to tell her about how I met Bill and about our life together. She was interested in all the little details that no-one else wanted to hear. Not once did she tell me that I had to get over Bill and get on with my life. It is such a relief to know that Bill can still be part of my life and my memories. I know he isn't here anymore, but it is so comforting to think about how much we loved each other. At times when I feel sad, I think about what he would have said to console me.

and was 'seen as both a "natural" and "expected" event' (Bellamy et al. 2014 p. 98). Key sources of support were seen as family and friends and contacts from organisations that the person was already associated with such as View Club, Probus Club, Rotary Club and Lions Club, while others found their membership of a church group to be helpful (Bellamy et al. 2014).

In contrast, the person who has been bereaved by suicide experiences what can be described as a life-shattering event. The work of grieving involves the person trying to make some sense of what has happened, with the first question being Why? Attempts to comprehend what has happened and why are likely to occupy the person's mind for a long time, along with efforts to understand how and what the process was that led up to suicide. Although there is growing awareness of suicide with an increasing focus on suicide prevention, levels of stigma related to death by suicide remain, and those that have been bereaved may often struggle with shame. They will also be seeking to find 'a socially acceptable interpretation of the suicide' (Castelli Dransart 2013, p. 327) such as the explanation offered by one person in Castelli Dransart's research: 'When I am asked now, I say that he was suffering a lot and that despite all the help and support we provided, he succumbed to this suffering . People don't need to know more' (2013, p. 327).

The bereaved person will also seek to make meaning of the suicide. Castelli Dransart (2013) described a continuum of ways in which people negotiated this aspect of grieving. She found that some people were able to find meaning that 'they could accept and live with' (p. 327) that then enabled them to return to actively living their lives and being involved in society in a meaningful way. At the other end of the continuum were 'people who found little meaning for the suicide and for whom the memory of the loved one still triggered mixed feelings or caused deep suffering, even years after the event' (p. 328).

Those who have lost a loved one from other forms of sudden and violent death are likewise at increased risk of mental illness. Deaths such as those outlined in Box 7.1 have been shown to have a markedly more traumatic impact than a natural and expected death. Additional stressors are linked to different types of sudden and violent death. For example, where a person has been murdered, there will be exposure to media portrayals of the death, contact with police and the legal system that are likely to continue over a lengthy period of time. War and military related losses likewise expose family members to markedly increased risk of major depressive disorder, PTSD and related conditions. Where death is as a result of a disaster, those that survive will likely have experienced horrifying scenes of destruction and may struggle with ongoing flashbacks or imagery of death and suffering. While people are remarkably resilient, it is essential that in your assessment and support of a person who presents following bereavement where the loved one died from suicide, murder or other sudden and violent cause, you are aware of the markedly increased risk of mental distress and illness (Kristensen et al. 2012).

Responding to a Person who is at Risk of Suicide

Remember that some people in an acute state of crisis may have thoughts of suicide (suicidal ideation) or have active plans to attempt suicide. A combination of factors such as bereavement, social exclusion or isolation, relationship difficulties and mental illness, rather than one specific factor, often come together to trigger a suicidal crisis. You will therefore need to build your understanding of suicidality, distress and depression. Globally, death by suicide is a serious public health issue (Bouch & Marshall 2005, Patel et al. 2014). In 2017 the Office for National Statistics reported there were 5821 suicides registered in the UK. Three-quarters of the suicides registered in 2017 were males, which has been the case since the mid-1990s. It was also reported that the male suicide rate was at the lowest it has been since the time-series began in 1981, with female rates remaining consistent with rates seen over the last 10 years (Office for National Statistics 2018). The Samaritans (2017) Suicide Statistics Report questions the figures, suggesting that the 'true' number is underestimated, with one of the main reasons for under-reporting being the misclassification of deaths, e.g. where a coroner cannot establish the intent and consequently the cause of death may be classified as 'undetermined intent' or 'accidental'. Public Health England (PHE 2018) has produced an online Suicide Prevention Atlas, which maps data on suicide, related risk factors and related service contacts for every local authority in England.

You may find that you feel uncomfortable at the prospect of asking a person directly about suicide. Many myths surround the topic of suicide, one of which is the belief that asking about thoughts of suicide is taboo and that you may put the idea into the person's head. However, the reality is that it is generally a relief for the person to have someone ask in a simple and direct way about their thoughts and plans. For example:

- You've told me a bit of what's been happening.
- Does it seem unbearable sometimes?
- Have you had thoughts of hurting yourself?
- Have you ever tried to hurt yourself?
- Do you ever have thoughts of hurting someone else?
- Have you ever had to protect yourself from others?

For the person experiencing intolerable emotional suffering and distress for which there seems to be no end, suicide is seen as a way out, a way to escape the pain permanently and to wipe out consciousness. Walsh (2012) asserts that 'the misery of the suicidal person is so profound, deep and excruciating that it is intolerable—unlivable. Moreover the pain is persistent, wearing down the person and producing profound psychic fatigue' (p. 13). When responding to the person in a suicidal crisis, the core skills identified earlier are of paramount importance. Your ability to develop a therapeutic relationship with the person in crisis will make a profound difference to the person who is distressed, isolated and feeling that they have little if any control over what is happening in their life (Lees et al. 2014).

Many initiatives have been put in place to try and improve health professionals' capacity to identify those who are at risk of suicide and to prevent these tragic deaths. A number of screening checklists designed to assess suicide risk have been developed and adopted for use in settings where people in crisis are assessed, including mental health services and EDs (NSW Health 2004). It is important to remember that assessing for suicide risk requires much more care and thought than simply completing a checklist or assessment tool.

Recent reviews of current approaches to suicide risk assessment have shown that risk factors such as previous suicide attempts or self-harm remain relevant as potential indicators of risk. Screening tools that identify static and dynamic risk factors and protective factors may be useful for research purposes, but they are not sensitive or specific enough to be reliable in clinical practice (Matheson et al. 2014). Where a tool is used to assess risk of suicide, it is still only a 'snapshot' taken at the time when the assessment is undertaken. According to 'suicidal risk is dynamic and fluctuating' (2015) even when there are significant static indicators of risk (see Table 7.5).

While the use of a screening checklist may be a component of assessment of a person's risk of suicide, assessment must include a 'detailed evaluation of suicidal behaviour and ideation, a full psychiatric assessment and determination of the psychosocial circumstances of the individual' (Matheson et al. 2014, p. 5); and where possible should include family members if available and appropriate. In all situations where there is significant risk, it is advisable to consult and work closely with colleagues rather than making decisions on your own as to the level of response required. Make sure you document clearly your decision-making process and the consultation and advice you have received when you undertake assessment and develop a management plan for the person who is at risk of suicide.

Research has found that the person who has been in a suicidal crisis and the nurses who provide the interventions described the care as having serious limitations. Attention was repeatedly drawn to the 'importance of greater therapeutic engagement between patients and nurses' and highlighted the need for nurses to access more 'effective education, training and professional development' and 'supportive clinical supervisory relationships with someone they respect' (Lees et al. 2014, p. 312). Feedback from patients who had experienced formal crisis-response services in Victoria, Australia again found that the quality of the interventions varied a great deal. People indicated their preference for an informal response with family or friends to be the ones that intervene if there is a crisis, and if that is not possible for the person's GP or case manager (if they had one), rather than formal crisis assessment and treatment team response. Where the crisis was such that there was risk of harm to self or others, people spoke of a few positive interactions where they had been treated with respect and the treatment had been humane. However, they also spoke of experiences where they felt threatened and intimidated by police or mental health staff, especially when there were two people approaching the person at once. At times where both police and mental health services were required, there were lots of difficulties with long delay times in responding, disjointed responses and difficulties with both services

TABLE 7.5 Stable, Dynamic and Protective Factors Associated With Suicide Risk

Static Risk Factors	Dynamic Risk Factors	Protective Factors
Factors that are unchangeable	Factors that are fluctuating or can change with intervention	Factors that reduce the likelihood of a negative outcome
• Age • Male gender • Marital status • History of mental disorder/illness, personality disorder, substance use disorder, previous self-harm, previous suicide attempt, previous violence, previous admission to mental health unit • Family history of suicide • Childhood adversity, neglect or abuse; early behavioural problems • Employment difficulties, history of conflict with the law	• Mental state and/or internal risk factors: > Substance abuse/dependence, especially alcohol misuse/abuse > Current diagnosis of personality disorder, especially antisocial and borderline personality disorders, impulsivity > Active symptoms of mental illness (comorbid depression or psychotic disorder and impaired rational thinking, command hallucinations) with suicidal/self-harm/harm to others ideation with plan and intent > Poor response/compliance with treatment • Situational and/or external risk factors: > Isolation (geographic and social) and poor social supports > Recent losses such as job, bereavement, separation or divorce with associated access to children issues > Recent suicide of friend, family member or public figure > Recent experience of adversity or stressful event such as admission or discharge from mental health inpatient unit > Access to means and opportunity for suicide/self-harm/harm to others > Unauthorised leave or failure to return from leave	• Previous help-seeking behaviour • Strong, dependable social supports, good relationships (friends, family, significant others) • Positive engagement with services, therapeutic alliance evident, compliance with treatment, awareness of early warning signs, concerns about effect of suicide on others • Stable employment and accommodation • Prolonged abstinence from substances

(*Source:* Compiled from: Allnutt, S., O'Driscoll, C., 2008. Statewide Clinical Risk Assessment & Management Training Program: Participant Handbook. Justice Health, Sydney; Flewett, T., 2010. Clinical Risk Management: an Introductory Text for Mental Health Clinicians. Churchill Livingstone, Chatswood; Mental Health and Drug and Alcohol Office, 2009. Mental Health for Emergency Departments—a Reference Guide. NSW Department of Health, North Sydney.)

collaborating together effectively once they were on site (Boscarato et al. 2014). Repeatedly throughout this chapter, the vital role that empathy, compassion, respect and humane treatment play in assisting the person in crisis has been emphasised. Remember, working to identify your assumptions and biases and putting those aside so that you can build rapport with the person should underpin all of your interactions with a person in crisis.

Avoid the temptation to focus solely on the person who has attempted suicide; for most people, there will be people who care about them, family or friends who too will be impacted by the crisis. If at all possible, obtain permission from the person to contact a family member, friend or colleague. Such contact is not only to assist in the assessment, but also to enable you to reconnect the person with people who can help to support them during the weeks and months to come. Review Gillian's story (see Box 7.4) and consider what the ED and mental health staff might have done differently to assist this family.

Responding to a Person who has Self-Harmed (Non-Suicidal Self-Injury)

Caring for a person who has injured themselves can be confronting and provoke a range of strong emotions in the health professional. Although you are a nurse, you are also a human being and will have the same adverse reactions as anyone else to self-inflicted bodily harm. NSSI 'violates the expectation that all people naturally seek to avoid pain and seek pleasure' and has been defined as 'intentional, self-effected, low-lethality bodily harm of a socially unacceptable nature, performed to reduce and/or communicate psychological distress' (Walsh 2012, p. 4, 273). People injure themselves in a wide range of different ways including cutting, scratching, ripping, pinching

BOX 7.4 A Parent's Story: Gillian

Although all this happened 5 years ago, it still seems like it was just yesterday. Our daughter, Jen, just 18 years old, was in her first year at university, and had been doing very well. We were so proud of her. Leroy and I had gone to the movies on a cold winter's night and Jen was out with her friends. My phone rang and when I answered, the voice on the other end said, 'This is the ED calling, your daughter has been brought here by ambulance, can you come up straight away?' The nurse told us that Jen had taken an overdose and they'd pumped her stomach and given her charcoal. When we saw her, her lips and fingers were blue and she was drowsy but recognised us. Leroy and I felt overwhelmed and frightened, what had happened to our beautiful girl? The nurse took us aside and said, 'Where have you been? Why was your daughter out by herself at night?' Her tone was so harsh, and so accusatory. We then sat and waited, no-one seemed to realise how desperately fearful we were for Jen. The message we got was they were busy and had people who were really sick to look after. There was no time to be molly-coddling parents who hadn't been responsible enough to know their daughter was trying to kill herself.

After several hours the ED registrar came, Jen was now awake, still a bit blue around the lips and drowsy. The doctor said, 'Clearly, your daughter needs a psych review, first appointment is in 1 week, here's the appointment time, you can take her home now.' Before we could ask any questions, he had gone. The nurse seemed in a hurry for us to get out of 'her ED'. I had so many questions: Would she be safe overnight? Should we let her go back to sleep? What if the drugs were still in her system? How were we to look after Jen and keep her safe for the next week?

Over the next week, Leroy and I tried to watch Jen, she got increasingly angry with our efforts to keep her safe. She said she had promised not to do it again, we just had to trust her. Finally, the appointment time came, the staff took Jen to see the psychiatrist and a psychologist talked to us. All she wanted to know was: 'What type of parents were we?' 'What had we done that led to our daughter attempting suicide?' Maybe we were both hypersensitive by then, it felt like everyone was saying this was our fault', 'we were bad parents,' 'if we had been better parents this would never have happened'. The doctor came out with Jen and said, 'She's fine, we don't need to see her again.' Because Jen was over 18, they wouldn't tell us anything further. We didn't know how to help our daughter.

The next months were agonising. My sister came to visit us. She was a mental health nurse and I still remember her saying, 'Try and remember, this was not your fault.' It was the first time anyone really listened to Leroy and me.

or tearing the skin, overdosing or poisoning, burning the skin with chemicals, hot water, cigarettes or matches, inserting objects under the skin and picking at healing wounds. It is essential that you build an understanding of how self-harm or self-injury arises. This will enable you to respond to the person with compassion and in a therapeutic manner. You will also need to further develop your ability to manage your own distress and emotional reactivity.

In contrast to the person who is planning or has attempted suicide, the majority of times when a person has self-harmed the intent is not to die, but rather to relieve the pain associated with a range of painful feeling states or with a sense of numbness or dissociation. NSSI occurs in 2% to 3% of the population and is more prevalent among adolescents; however, very few young people who harm themselves will seek assistance and those who do are more likely to talk with friends or family than to attend ED or mental health services. There have been a number of barriers to seeking help identified, including 'fear of negative reactions from others including stigmatisation, fear of confidentiality being breached and fear of being seen as "attention-seeking"' (Rowe et al. 2014, p. 1083).

Your initial response will need to focus on safety concerns. NSSI can at times accidently result in death, self-poisoning or overdose and some instances will need an emergency response; likewise for any injury that has resulted in severe bleeding and/or arterial bleeding. Attend to all other injuries with calmness and empathy, ensuring that your response is not punishing or belittling. Even if the injury is clearly not life-threatening, make sure you undertake a careful mental health assessment, including a risk assessment and ask about the intent associated with the self-injury. Suicidal ideation (thoughts) are the strongest predictor of suicide attempts; however, a history of NSSI, especially where the person uses a variety of different methods to injure themselves and is also exhibiting a sense of hopelessness, has been shown to be a moderate predictor of suicide (Victor & Klonsky 2014). Even though the person may have presented multiple times with NSSI, do not under any circumstances dismiss them as 'just another cutter'.

After completing your assessment and consulting with the mental health clinician, your focus is not on stopping the NSSI, but rather on other strategies that the person could use to alleviate the distress. Ensure that the person has the phone number of someone who they trust that they could call when they have the urge to self-harm again. Make sure that there is a follow-up appointment in place, if this is the first time that the person has presented. If the person is under the care of a therapist, or treatment programme, make sure that the treating clinician is notified.

CASE STUDY 7.2

Sayed

You are working on an acute mental health team and receive a call to see a person presenting with what is reported as a crisis. You arrive to find Sayed, a 35-year-old man sitting in the corner of the interview room with his head in his hands crying. As you introduce yourself and explain that you are from the mental health team, he becomes agitated and irritable and tells you 'there's no point me talking to you, you can't change anything'.

You ask Sayed to tell you what has been happening. As you listen, Sayed (who is still irritable) says 'It's all my wife's fault—she's the one who has caused all this.' You enquire what 'all this' is. He pauses and puts his head in his hands again and starts crying once more. He quietly says, 'She won't let me see the kids.' You give him some time to settle and he adds, 'she's doing this deliberately trying to hurt me.' You gently ask what happened that led to this situation.

Sayed slowly starts to tell you that he has been abusive and physically violent to his wife. He says, 'It's all got out of hand because of my PTSD—I can't handle it anymore, I've had enough.' You then query the circumstances that resulted in a diagnosis of PTSD. Sayed recounts an incident 5 years ago when he experienced an unprovoked serious assault. He reports an increase in his symptoms over the last 6 months. 'The flashbacks won't stop and I don't want to talk to anyone or go out—I get really snappy with my wife and the kids,' he goes onto say, 'she just doesn't get it and nags me nonstop.' He describes difficulty sleeping and no appetite and says he has lost weight over the past month. You wonder aloud how he plans to manage his stress and the relationship breakdown with his wife. Sayed declares, 'I can't see any way out of this—there's just no point anymore.'

1. Is Sayed 'in crisis' or is this an emergency?
2. Identify the specific issues in Sayed's story that you think require attention.
3. How do these issues relate to the topics covered in this chapter?
4. Identify your own assumptions and judgements that could potentially challenge your capacity to respond effectively to Sayed.
5. How would you work with Sayed to clarify and prioritise the issues confronting him and assist him at this point in his life?

Providing Trauma-Informed Care

The core features of trauma-informed care are 'safety, trustworthiness, choice, collaboration and empowerment' (Kezelman & Stavropoulos 2012, p. 88). The core skills that are required to work effectively with a person in crisis are equally important for all interactions with people who have a history of trauma. Ensure that your focus is on the person and not the disease or label; in other words, ask 'What happened to you?' rather than 'What's wrong with you?' The following points will assist you in caring for the person who has a history of trauma:

- Recognise that coercive interventions cause traumatisation/retraumatisation and are to be avoided.
- Respond empathically, be objective and use supportive language.
- Offer individually flexible plans or approaches.
- Avoid all shaming/humiliation.
- Ask questions about current abuse.
- Address the current risk and develop a safety plan for discharge.
- Presume that every person in a treatment setting may have been exposed to abuse, violence, neglect or other traumatic experiences (Bateman et al. 2013, pp. 11–12).

Nurses working in a range of settings—more specifically, those who are mental health nurses—have a key role to play in modelling trauma-informed care and reducing the likelihood that the person with whom they are working is not further traumatised. Make sure you access further information about trauma-informed care and take time to attend workshops and training that can help you to further build your skills. (See the Useful Websites list at the end of this chapter.)

The Cost of Caring

The material covered thus far has perhaps provided you with a personal challenge. When a person is experiencing an acute crisis state, is at risk of suicide or has self-harmed, they need compassionate and thoughtful assistance. As a nurse you will walk alongside people who have experienced deep pain and trauma in their lives, people who are struggling to cope with difficult experiences and people who are overwhelmed by the crisis threatening to engulf them. Many times you will be required to give assistance in the context of high levels of emotion, distress and sometimes confronting behaviours that are difficult to understand. Working with a person who is in an acute state of crisis, is self-harming or is suicidal can take a lot of emotional energy. Sometimes you too may feel overwhelmed, anxious or perhaps sad. While theoretical learning will assist you to understand current wisdom about the topics covered in this chapter, it will not be sufficient to enable you to remain calm, optimistic and able to use your technical skills effectively. You will need to make sure that you care for yourself as well.

Pearlman and Saakvitne (2013, 1995) gave advice to those working with traumatised people, reminding clinicians that it is important to follow their own prescriptions. Remember that the self-care strategies that you might prescribe for others such as yoga, exercise, mindfulness practice, healthy living, listening to music, cooking and gardening are equally important for your emotional and physical wellbeing. You are encouraged to learn and to practice self-soothing strategies such as breathing skills and to seek enhanced self-awareness. As you progress through your career, take every opportunity to reflect on your professional experiences; to confront your assumptions, biases and judgement and to develop specialist counselling skills. Take time to expand your contact with people from cultures, backgrounds and perspectives other than your own and in the process learn to enjoy the wonderful diversity and richness of the community in which you live. Such activities will enable you to be more effective as a mental health nurse and to stay healthy. Make sure that you talk about your experiences. Clinical supervision can be an excellent place to do this. Build a broad network of supportive relationships and make sure that you have a personal life outside of work. Maintaining your human connections with colleagues, friends, family and community will help you to hold 'two realities within your consciousness: humans are capable of great kindness, courage and justice and the extremes of sadism, violence and cruelty' (Everett & Gallop 2001, p. 308).

CONCLUSION

This chapter has provided a platform on which you can continue to build your capacity to work effectively with people experiencing difficult times associated with traumatic events, loss and bereavement. You now have a beginning understanding of the long-lasting impact of early trauma on a person's development and the ways in which this may influence a person's response to later difficulties. No matter where you work as a nurse, you will encounter people who will greatly benefit from the knowledge and skills you have developed from working through this chapter. The UK is a multicultural country and the populations you serve represent many different ethnic groups, a range of different religious faiths and gender diversity. As you pursue your career as a nurse, take every opportunity to build your capacity to welcome diversity and learn to appreciate the uniqueness of each individual for whom you care.

NURSE'S STORY 7.2 A Clinician's Reflection: Building Resilience

Looking back on working in a psychotherapy unit for people with borderline personality disorder and/or eating disorders and in community mental health, I realise just how much I have learned both professionally and personally during those years.

I remember vividly the first time I was introduced to a person who was regularly cutting himself severely (requiring 12-plus stitches each time). The psychiatrist introducing me to Jim (pseudonym) suggested that we meet together each week and see how we got on. We sat and looked at each other and I felt totally overwhelmed. What was I supposed to say? How could I possibly do or say anything that would be helpful? Nevertheless, Jim attended every week and we 'got on' just fine. After many struggles, things improved greatly for Jim, and I began to learn a lot more about patience and sitting with anxiety.

As part of my work, I was introduced to the practice of mindfulness. At first I found it incredibly difficult but gradually with persistence, attendance at several retreats and practice, I began to notice a difference. Being able to observe my emotions and thoughts rather than be totally caught up in my internal experience, enabled me to 'be with' people in distress. Instead of working to alleviate my anxiety or concern by giving suggestions and advice, being mindful allows me to wait for the person to find their own wisdom. Even more challenging was gradually learning to let go of my critical judgements, to let go of the frustration that arises when a person doesn't seem to be getting better, or comes back yet again and nothing seems to have changed. Over time, I realised how much time it takes for me to change my own unhelpful behaviours. I learned to remind myself that 'doing what is good for me' is not always my highest priority until I suffer the adverse effects of not doing so.

Through my years as a clinician, I have always participated in regular clinical supervision, at least second weekly and if I had a heavy load of people who were either acutely or chronically suicidal I would attend weekly. Individual clinical supervision included recording my sessions with the person's approval, and reviewing parts of the tapes with my supervisor. Totally confronting, and incredibly helpful at the same time. Working collaboratively with a team of colleagues where we had an understanding that we could contact each other for a 'second opinion' and 'coaching' any time we were concerned or overwhelmed was another key to thriving in work that is often seen as extremely difficult.

At first, I had to find ways to 'leave work at work', sometimes this involved figuratively putting the files in the filing cabinet and mentally leaving my thoughts there with the files. Other times, a brisk walk along the beach provided a way to let go of the challenges of the day. Outside of work, there are plenty of activities, such as regular exercise, gardening, fun with family and friends and reading that help to restore my energy. Often I give thanks to the many people from whom I've learned so much about resilience and courage in the face of overwhelming difficulties.

EXERCISES FOR CLASS ENGAGEMENT

1. Consider the following quote:

   The Chinese use two brush strokes to write the word 'crisis.' One brush stroke stands for danger; the other for opportunity. In a crisis, be aware of the danger—but recognise the opportunity.

   John F. Kennedy, 1959

   Think about a time when you faced a crisis in your life. Write a brief summary of the crisis that includes how you felt and how you responded to it. Think more deeply about this experience and respond to each of the following questions.
   - Can you identify the people who were most helpful to you during this time?
   - What did they say or do that helped you to get through the crisis?
   - What personal characteristics, skills and strategies did you utilise to negotiate the crisis?
   - How did this experience strengthen your capacity to cope with challenges that you have encountered since then?
2. Compile a list of strategies that you use to soothe yourself when you are upset, stressed or overwhelmed.
   - Who taught you to use these strategies?
   - Are there some that are less helpful than others?
   - For the less helpful strategies, can you identify the longer term impacts of regularly using these strategies to soothe yourself?
   - Are there times when you could use one of your strategies but don't for some reason?

   What are the barriers to self-soothing?
   What would help you to use your strategies?

3. Identify people in the class who have skills in any of the follow self-regulating strategies:
   - focussed breathing techniques
   - progressive muscle relaxation
   - gentle stretches and yoga exercises
   - mindfulness exercises

   Divide into small groups with a leader who can teach the group one of the above skills. Swap members from one group to the next so that participants have the opportunity to try several different self-regulating strategies.
4. An idiom is a phrase or expression that means something different to the literal definition of the actual words used. Pair up with a fellow student, preferably one whose culture is different to your own. Develop as long a list as possible of the idioms that each of you use when you are feeling physically unwell or emotionally distressed. Extend your list to include idioms that other members of your family use. See if you can interpret what your colleague's idioms mean.
5. Develop a brief presentation (5 minutes) to teach your colleagues how to communicate with a patient when there is no interpreter available. Include a role play to demonstrate to the class how you would communicate. *Each group member must do part of the presentation.*
   - Determine whether there is a third language that both you and the patient could use.
   - Remember that nonverbal communication is more important than verbal communication.
   - Be attentive to both your own and the patient's nonverbal messages.
   - Pantomime simple words and actions.
   - Remember, a picture is worth a thousand words. Use pen and paper and also give them to the patient.
   - Talk with your manager about the importance of using trained medical interpreters when caring for the non–English-speaking patient.
6. Develop a brief presentation (5 minutes) with instructions on how to effectively use an interpreter. *Each group member must do part of the presentation.*
   - Include a role play to demonstrate to the class how you would use an interpreter.
   - Make sure you refer to Box 7.2.
7. Choose a breathing exercise that is useful for helping a person to relax. *Each group member must do part of the presentation.*
   - Develop a brief presentation (5 minutes) with instructions on how to do the breathing exercise.
   - Include a role play to demonstrate to the class how you do the breathing exercise.
   - Then get the whole class to practise the breathing exercise with you.
8. Choose a stretching exercise that is useful for helping a person to relax. *Each group member must do part of the presentation.*
   - Develop a brief presentation (5 minutes) with instructions on how to do the stretching exercise.
   - Include a role play to demonstrate to the class how you do the stretching exercise.
   - Then get the whole class to practise the stretching exercise with you.

REFERENCES

Abdel-Magied, Y., 2014. What does my headscarf mean to you? TEDxSouthBank event, 14 December 2014, posted online 15 June 2015. Queensland, Southbank. Available at: www.ted.com/talks/yassmin_abdel_magied_what_does_my_headscarf_mean_to_you.

American Psychiatric Association, 2013. Diagnostic and Statistical Manual of Mental Disorders (DSM-5). APA, Arlington VA.

Appel, K., Schwahn, C., Mahler, J., Schulz, A., Spitzer, C., Fenske, K., Stender, J., Barnow, S., John, U., Teumer, A., Biffar, R., Nauck, M., Volzke, H., Freyberger, H.J., Grabe, H.J., 2011. Moderation of adult depression by a polymorphism in the fkbp5 gene and childhood physical abuse in the general population. Neuropsychopharmacology 36 (10), 1982–1991.

Australian Red Cross 2013 World Disasters Report 2013: Focus on technology and the future of humanitarian action. Available at: https://www.redcross.org.au/getmedia/47ab8008-d80e-4f21-9ca5-9314d689f15a/WDR-2013-Final.pdf.aspx.

Babenko, O., Kovalchuk, I., GAS, Metz, 2015. Stress-induced perinatal and transgenerational epigenetic programming of brain development and mental health. Neuroscience & Biobehavioral Reviews 48 (0), 70–91.

Barnhofer, T., Brennan, K., Crane, C., Duggan, D., Williams, J.M.G., 2014. A comparison of vulnerability factors in patients with persistent and remitting lifetime symptom course of depression. Journal of Affective Disorders 152–154 155–161.

Bateman, J., Henderson, C.M., Kezelman, C.A., 2013. Trauma-Informed Care and Practice: Towards a cultural shift in policy reform across mental health and human services in Australia, a national strategic direction. In: Position Paper and Recommendations of the National Trauma-Informed Care and Practice Advisory Working Group (Mental Health Coordinating Council (MHCC)). Mental Health Coordinating Council, Rozelle NSW, p. 116.

Belkin, G., 1984. Introduction to Counseling. William C Brown, Dubuque, IA.

Bellamy, G., Gott, M., Waterworth, S., McLean, C., Kerse, N., 2014. 'But I do believe you've got to accept that that's what life's about': older adults living in New Zealand talk about their experiences of loss and bereavement support. Health & Social Care in the Community 22 (1), 96–103. https://doi.org/10.1111/hsc.12069.

Benninghoff, J., van der Ven, A., Schloesser, R.J., Moessner, R., Möller, H.J., Rujescu, D., 2012. The complex role of the serotonin transporter in adult neurogenesis and neuroplasticity. A critical review. World Journal of Biological Psychiatry 13 (4), 240–247. https://doi.org/10.3109/15622975.2011.640941.

Booij, L., Szyf, M., Carballedo, A., Frey, E.-M., Morris, D., Dymov, S., Vaisheva, F., Ly, V., Fahey, C., Meaney, J., Gill, M., Frodl, T., 2015. DNA Methylation of the serotonin transporter gene in peripheral cells and stress-related changes in hippocampal volume: a study in depressed patients and healthy controls. PLoS ONE 10 (3), e0119061.

Boscarato, K., Lee, S., Kroschel, J., Hollander, Y., Brennan, A., Warren, N., 2014. Consumer experience of formal crisis-response services and preferred methods of crisis intervention. International Journal of Mental Health Nursing 23 (4), 287–295. https://doi.org/10.1111/inm.12059.

Boss, P., Carnes, D., 2012. The myth of closure. Family Process 51 (4), 456–469.

Bouch, J., Marshall, J.J., 2005. Suicide risk: structured professional judgement. Advances in Psychiatric Treatment 11 (2), 84–91.

Bowlby, J., 1980. Attachment and Loss: Loss, Sadness and Depression. Basic Books, New York.

Brennaman, L., 2012. Crisis emergencies for individuals with severe, persistent mental illnesses: a situation-specific theory. Archives of Psychiatric Nursing 26 (4), 251–260. https://doi.org/10.1016/j.apnu.2011.11.001.

Brown, G.W., Ban, M., Craig, T.K.J., Harris, T.O., Herbert, J., Uher, R., 2013. Serotonin transporter length polymorphism, childhood maltreatment, and chronic depression: a specific gene-environment interaction. Depression & Anxiety (1091-4269) 30 (1), 5–13.

Cai, N., Chang, S., Li, Y., Li, Q., Hu, J., Liang, J., Song, L., Kretzschmar, W., Gan, X., Nicod, J., Rivera, M., Deng, H., Du, B., Li, K., Sang, W., Gao, J., Gao, S., Ha, B., Ho, H.-Y., Hu, C., Hu, J., Hu, Z., Huang, G., Jiang, G., Jiang, T., Jin, W., Li, G., Li, K., Li, Y., Li, Y., Li, Y., Lin, Y.-T., Liu, L., Liu, T., Liu, Y., Liu, Y., Lu, Y., Lv, L., Meng, H., Qian, P., Sang, H., Shen, J., Shi, J., Sun, J., Tao, M., Wang, G., Wang, G., Wang, J., Wang, L., Wang, X., Wang, X., Yang, H., Yang, L., Yin, Y., Zhang, J., Zhang, K., Sun, N., Zhang, W., Zhang, X., Zhang, Z., Zhong, H., Breen, G., Wang, J., Marchini, J., Chen, Y., Xu, Q., Xu, X., Mott, R., Huang, G.-J., Kendler, K., Flint, J., 2015. Molecular signatures of major depression. Current Biology 25 (9), 1146–1156.

Cameron, H.A., Glover, L.R., 2015. Adult neurogenesis: beyond learning and memory. Annual Review of Psychology 66 (1), 53–81. https://doi.org/10.1146/annurev-psych-010814-015006.

Caplan, G., 1961. An Approach to Community Mental Health. Grune & Stratton, New York.

Castelli Dransart, D.A., 2013. From sense-making to meaning-making: understanding and supporting survivors of suicide. British Journal of Social Work 43 (2), 317–335.

Chase, E., 2013. Crisis intervention for nurses. Clinical Journal of Oncology Nursing 17 (3), 337–339.

Costello, L., Thomson, M., Jones, K., 2013. Mental health and homelessness. Mental Health Commission of NSW. Available at: http://nswmentalhealthcommission.com.au/sites/default/files/publication-documents/Final%20Report%20-%20AHURI%20-%20Mental%20Health%20and%20Homelessness.pdf.

Cutcliffe, J.R., Riahi, S., 2013. Systemic perspective of violence and aggression in mental health care: towards a more comprehensive understanding and conceptualization, part 1. International Journal of Mental Health Nursing 22 (6), 558–567. https://doi.org/10.1111/inm.12029.

Department of Health, 2017. Public Health England News Story: New £15 Million Programme to Help Train One Million in Mental Health First Aid. Department of Health, London.

De Bellis, M.D., Zisk, A., 2014. The biological effects of childhood trauma. Child and Adolescent Psychiatric Clinics of North America 23 (2), 185–222.

Disaster Response, Resilience and Research Group, University of Western Sydney, Wooding, S., Raphael, B., 2012. Handbook 2—Psychological First Aid (PFA): Level 1 intervention following mass disaster. Available at: www.health.nsw.gov.au/emergency_preparedness/mental/Pages/default.aspx.

Everett, B., Gallop, R., 2001. The Link Between Childhood Trauma and Mental Illness: Effective Interventions for Mental Health Professionals. Sage Publications, Thousand Oaks.

Felitti, V.J., Anda, R.F., Nordenberg, D., Williamson, D., Spitz, A., Edwards, V., Koss, M., Marks, J., 1998. Relationship of childhood abuse and household dysfunction to many of the leading causes of death in adults. American Journal of Preventive Medicine 14 (4), 245–258.

Fuchs, E., Flügge, G., 2014. Adult neuroplasticity: more than 40 years of research. Neural Plasticity 1–10. https://doi.org/10.1155/2014/541870.

Gong, Q., He, Y., 2015. Depression, neuroimaging and connectomics: a selective overview. Biological Psychiatry 77 (3), 223–235.

Gray, J.D., McEwen, B.S., 2013. Lithium's role in neural plasticity and its implications for mood disorders. Acta Psychiatrica Scandinavica 128 (5), 347–361. https://doi.org/10.1111/acps.12139.

Hall, C., 2014. Bereavement theory: recent developments in our understanding of grief and bereavement. Bereavement Care 33 (1), 7–12.

Hanson, J.L., Hariri, A.R., Williamson, D.E., 2015. Blunted ventral striatum development in adolescence reflects emotional neglect and predicts depressive symptoms. Biological Psychiatry 78 (9), 598–605.

Heaslip, V., Ryden, J. (Eds.), 2013. Understanding Vulnerability: a Nursing and Healthcare Approach. John Wiley & Sons, Pondicherry, India.

Heim, C., Binder, E.B., 2012. Current research trends in early life stress and depression: review of human studies on sensitive periods, gene–environment interactions, and epigenetics. Experimental Neurology 233 (1), 102–111.

Hinton, D.E., Lewis-Fernández, R., 2010. Idioms of distress among trauma survivors: subtypes and clinical utility. Culture, Medicine and Psychiatry 34 (2), 209–218.

Hobfoll, S.E., Johnson, R.J., Canetti, D., Palmieri, P.A., Hall, B.J., Lavi, I., Galea, S., 2012. Can people remain engaged and vigorous in the face of trauma? Palestinians in the West Bank and Gaza. Psychiatry: Interpersonal and Biological Processes 75 (1), 60–75.

Hobfoll, S.E., Mancini, A.D., Hall, B.J., Canetti, D., Bonanno, G.A., 2011. The limits of resilience: distress following chronic political violence among Palestinians. Social Science and Medicine 72 (8), 1400–1408.

Hochstrasser, T., Marksteiner, J., Humpel, C., 2012. Telomere length is age-dependent and reduced in monocytes of Alzheimer patients. Experimental Gerontology 47 (2), 160–163.

Hornung, O.P., Heim, C.M., 2014. Gene–environment interactions and intermediate phenotypes: early trauma and depression. Frontiers in Endocrinology 5, 1–12.

Inoue, K., Okamoto, M., Shibato, J., Lee, M.C., Matsui, T., Rakwai, R., Soya, H., 2015. Long-term mild, rather than intense, exercise enhances adult hippocampal neurogenesis and greatly changes the transcriptomic profile of the hippocampus. PLoS ONE 10 (7), e0133089. https://doi.org/10.1371/journal.pone.0133089.

James, R.K., Gilliland, B.E., 2013. Crisis Intervention Strategies. Brooks/Cole Cengage Learning, Canada.

Jorm, A.F., Kitchener, B.A., 2011. Noting a landmark achievement: mental health first aid training reaches 1% of Australian adults. Aust N Z J Psychiatry 45 (10), 808–813. https://doi.org/10.3109/00048674.2011.594785.

Jorm, A.F., 2013. Mental health for all. Global Health & Development. Retrieved from Project Syndicate—The World's Opinion Page. Available: www.project-syndicate.org/commentary/the-global-imperative-for-mental-health-first-aid-training-by-anthony-jorm.

Kezelman, C., Stavropoulos, P., 2012. 'The last frontier' practice guidelines for treatment of complex trauma and trauma informed care and service delivery. Blue Knot Foundation.

Kita, I., 2014. Physical exercise can induce brain plasticity and regulate mental function. Advances in Exercise & Sports Physiology 20 (1), 1–7.

Kristensen, P., Weisæth, L., Heir, T., 2012. Bereavement and mental health after sudden and violent losses: a review. Psychiatry: Interpersonal & Biological Processes 75 (1), 76–97. https://doi.org/10.1521/psyc.2012.75.1.76.

Kübler-Ross, E., 1969. On Death and Dying. Macmillan, New York.

Lees, D., Procter, N., Fassett, D., 2014. Therapeutic engagement between consumers in suicidal crisis and mental health nurses. International Journal of Mental Health Nursing 23 (4), 306–315. https://doi.org/10.1111/inm.12061.

Levinson, W., 2011. Patient-centred communication: a sophisticated procedure. BMJ Quality and Safety 20 (10), 823–825.

Loughran, H., 2011. Understanding Crisis Therapies: An Integrative Approach to Crisis Intervention and Post Traumatic Stress. Jessica Kingsley Publishers, London.

Lutz, P.E., Turecki, G., 2014. DNA methylation and childhood maltreatment: from animal models to human studies. Neuroscience 264 (0), 142–156.

Malki, K., Keers, R., Tosto, M., Lourdusamy, A., Carboni, L., Domenici, E., Uher, R., McGuffin, P., Schalkwyk, L., 2014. The endogenous and reactive depression subtypes revisited: integrative animal and human studies implicate multiple distinct molecular mechanisms underlying major depressive disorder. BMC Medicine 12 (1), 73.

Malykhin, N.V., Coupland, N.J., 2015. Hippocampal neuroplasticity in major depressive disorder. Neuroscience 309, 200–213. https://doi.org/10.1016/j.neuroscience.2015.04.047.

Mandelli, L., Emiliani, R., Porcelli, S., Fabbri, C., Albani, D., Serretti, A., 2014. Genes involved in neuroplasticity and stressful life events act on the short-term response to antidepressant treatment: a complex interplay between genetics and environment. Human Psychopharmacology: Clinical & Experimental 29 (4), 388–391. https://doi.org/10.1002/hup.2411.

Matheson, S.L., Shepherd, A.M., Carr, V.J., 2014. Management of Suicidal Behaviour—A Review of Evidence for Models of Care: An Evidence Check Rapid Review Brokered by the Sax Institute for the NSW Ministry of Health.

McCabe, O.L., Everly Jr., G.S., Brown, L.M., Wendelboe, A.M., Hamid, N.H.A., Tallchief, V.L., Links, J.M., 2014. Psychological first aid: a consensus-derived, empirically supported, competency-based training model. American Journal of Public Health 104 (4), 621–628.

McDonnell, M.N., Koblar, S., Ward, N.S., Rothwell, J.C., Hordacre, B., Ridding, M.C., 2015. An investigation of cortical neuroplasticity following stroke in adults: is there evidence for a critical window for rehabilitation? BMC Neurology 15 (1), 1–4. https://doi.org/10.1186/s12883-015-0356-7.

Mehraby, N., 2012. Lost in translation: idioms of distress. Psychotherapy in Australia 18 (3), 55–56.

Mental Health Council of Australia, 2009. Home Truths: Mental Health, Housing and Homelessness in Australia. Mental Health Australia, Canberra, Fig 1, p. 2. Ten Home Truths.

Murgatroyd, C.A., Peña, C.J., Podda, G., Nestler, E.J., Nephew, B.C., 2015. Early life social stress induced changes in depression and anxiety associated neural pathways which are correlated with impaired maternal care. Neuropeptides 52, 103–111.

Muskett, C., 2014. Trauma-informed care in inpatient mental health settings: a review of the literature. International Journal of Mental Health Nursing 23 (1), 51–59.

Myer, R.A., Lewis, J.S., James, R.K., 2013. The introduction of a task model for crisis intervention. Journal of Mental Health Counseling 35 (2), 95–107.

Nanni, V., Uher, R., Danese, A., 2012. Childhood maltreatment predicts unfavorable course of illness and treatment outcome in depression: a meta-analysis. American Journal of Psychiatry 169 (2), 141–151.

NSW Health, 2004. Framework for Suicide Risk Assessment and Management for NSW Health Staff. NSW Department of Health, North Sydney.

Office for National Statistics, 2018. Suicides in the UK: 2017 Registrations - Registered Deaths in the UK From Suicide Analysed by sex, age, Area of Usual Residence of the Deceased and Suicide Method. Available at: www.ons.gov.uk/peoplepopulationandcommunity/birthsdeathsandmarriages/deaths/bulletins/suicidesintheunitedkingdom/2017registrations.

Opendak, M., Gould, E., 2015. Adult neurogenesis: a substrate for experience-dependent change. Trends in Cognitive Sciences 19 (3), 151–161.

Parad, H., Parad, L. (Eds.), 2005. Crisis Intervention Book 2: the Practitioner's Sourcebook for Brief Therapy. Fenestra Books, Tucson, AZ.

Patel, V., Minas, H., Cohen, A., Prince, M.J. (Eds.), 2014. Global Mental Health: Principles and Practice. Oxford University Press, New York.

Pearlman, L., Saakvitne, K.W., 1995. Vicarious traumatization: how trauma therapy affects the therapist. In: Trauma and the Therapist. W. Norton & Company, New York, NY, pp. 279–294.

Pearlman, L.A., Saakvitne, K.W., 2013. Treating therapists with vicarious traumatization and secondary traumatic stress disorders. In: Figley, C.R. (Ed.), Compassion Fatigue: Coping with Secondary Traumatic Stress Disorder in Those who Treat the Traumatized. Taylor and Francis, Hoboken, pp. 150–177.

Porto, F.H., Fox, A.M., Tusch, E.S., Sorond, F., Mohammed, A.H., Daffner, K.R., 2015. Vivo evidence for neuroplasticity in older adults. Brain Research Bulletin 114, 56–61. https://doi.org/10.1016/j.brainresbull.2015.03.004.

Price, O., Baker, J., 2012. Key components of de-escalation techniques: A thematic synthesis. International Journal of Mental Health Nursing 21 (4), 310–319. https://doi.org/10.1111/j.1447-0349.2011.00793.x.

Provençal, N., Binder, E.B., 2015. The effects of early life stress on the epigenome: From the womb to adulthood and even before. Experimental Neurology 268, 10–20.

Public Health England, 2018. Suicide Prevention: Suicide Prevention Atlas. Available at: https://healthierlives.phe.org.uk/topic/suicide-prevention.

Rajji, T.K., Rogasch, N.C., Daskalakis, Z.J., Fitzgerald, P.B., 2013. Neuroplasticity-based brain stimulation interventions in the study and treatment of schizophrenia: a review. Canadian Journal of Psychiatry 58 (2), 93–98.

Recorded faithfully by John Heminge and Henry Condell (two fellow actors), 1623. The Comedy of Errors, First Folio—First Known Publication of the Collected Works of William Shakespeare. Isaac Laggard & Edward Blount, England.

Reybrouck, M., Brattico, E., 2015. Neuroplasticity beyond sounds: neural adaptations following long-term musical aesthetic experiences. Brain Sciences 5 (1), 69–91. https://doi.org/10.3390/brainsci5010069.

Rogers, A.C., 1997. Vulnerability, health and health care. Journal of Advanced Nursing 26 (1), 65–72.

Rotheneichner, P., Lange, S., O'Sullivan, A., Marschallinger, J., Zaunmair, P., Geretsegger, C., Aigner, L., Couillard-Despres, S., 2014. Hippocampal neurogenesis and antidepressive therapy: shocking relations. Neural Plasticity 1–14. https://doi.org/10.1155/2014/723915.

Rowe, S.L., French, R.S., Henderson, C., Ougrin, D., Slade, M., Moran, P., 2014. Help-seeking behaviour and adolescent self-harm: a systematic review. Australian and New Zealand Journal of Psychiatry 48 (12), 1083–1095. https://doi.org/10.1177/0004867414555718.

Samaritans, 2017. Suicide statistics report 2017. Available at: www.samaritans.org/sites/default/files/kcfinder/files/Suicide_statistics_report_2017_Final.pdf.

Saxena, S., Funk, M., Chisholm, D., 2013. Comment: World Health Assembly adopts Comprehensive Mental Health Action Plan 2013-2020. The Lancet 381 (9882), 1970–1971.

Schloesser, R.J., Orvoen, S., Jimenez, D.V., Hardy, N.F., Maynard, K.R., Sukumar, M., Manji, H.K., Gardier, A.M., David, D.J., Martinowich, K., 2015. Antidepressant-like effects of electroconvulsive seizures require adult neurogenesis in a neuroendocrine model of depression. Brain Stimulation 8 (5), 862–867.

Shammas, M.A., 2011. Telomeres, lifestyle, cancer, and aging. Current Opinion in Clinical Nutrition & Metabolic Care 14 (1), 28–34.

Smith, N.B., Kouros, C.D., Meuret, A.E., 2014. The role of trauma symptoms in nonsuicidal self-injury. Trauma, Violence, and Abuse 15 (1), 41–56. https://doi.org/10.1177/1524838013496332.

Stroebe, H., Schut, M., 1999. The dual process model of coping with bereavement: rationale and description. Death Studies 23 (3), 197–224. https://doi.org/10.1080/074811899201046.

Stroebe, M.S., Folkman, S., Hansson, R.O., Schut, H., 2006. The prediction of bereavement outcome: development of an integrative risk factor framework. Social Science and Medicine 63 (9), 2440–2451.

Trollope, A.F., Gutièrrez-Mecinas, M., Mifsud, K.R., Collins, A., Saunderson, E.A., Reul, J.M.H.M., 2012. Stress, epigenetic control of gene expression and memory formation. Experimental Neurology 233 (1), 3–11.

van Loo, H.M., Aggen, S.H., Gardner, C.O., Kendler, K.S., 2015. Multiple risk factors predict recurrence of major depressive disorder in women. Journal of Affective Disorders 180, 52–61.

Victor, S.E., Klonsky, E., 2014. Correlates of suicide attempts among self-injurers: a meta-analysis. Clinical Psychology Review 34 (4), 282–297. https://doi.org/10.1016/j.cpr.2014.03.005.

Vindevogel, S., Ager, A., Schiltz, J., Broekaert, E., Derluyn, I., 2015. Toward a culturally sensitive conceptualization of resilience: Participatory research with war-affected communities in northern Uganda. Transcultural Psychiatry 52 (3), 396–416.

Wainwright, S.R., Galea, L.A.M., 2013. The neural plasticity theory of depression: assessing the roles of adult neurogenesis and psa-ncam within the hippocampus. Neural Plasticity 1–14. https://doi.org/10.1155/2013/805497.

Walsh, B., 2012. Treating Self-Injury: A Practical Guide. The Guilford Press, New York.

Walsh, F., McGoldrick, M., 2013. Bereavement: a family life cycle perspective. Family Science 4 (1), 20–27. https://doi.org/10.1080/19424620.2013.819228.

Williams, R., Alexander, D., 2009. Part B—Psychosocial resilience and distress in the face of adversity, conflict, terrorism, or catastrophe. In: Burris, D.G., Hawley, A., Ryan, J.M., Mahoney, P.F. (Eds.), Hopperus Buma APCC. Conflict and Catastrophe Medicine. Springer Verlag, London, pp. 360–374.

Worden, J.W., 2009. Grief Counseling and Grief Therapy: A Handbook for the Mental Health Practitioner. Springer Publishing Company, New York.

World Health Organization, War Trauma Foundation & World Vision International, 2011. Psychological First Aid: Guide for field Workers. Available at: http://whqlibdoc.who.int/publications/2011/9789241548205_eng.pdf?ua=1.

World Health Organisation (WHO), 2013. Mental Health Action Plan 2013-2020. World Health Organisation, Geneva, Switzerland.

Wright, P.M., Hogan, N.S., 2008. Grief theories and models: applications to hospice nursing practice. Journal of Hospice & Palliative Nursing November/December 10 (6), 350–356.

Yang, T.-T., Lo, C.-P., Tsai, P.-S., Wu, S.-Y., Wang, T.-F., Chen, Y.-W., Jiang-Shieh, Y.-F., Kuo, Y.-M., 2015. Aging and exercise affect hippocampal neurogenesis via different mechanisms. PLoS ONE 10 (7), e0132152. https://doi.org/10.1371/journal.pone.0132152.

Zoellner, L.A., Feeny, N.C., 2014a. Conceptualizing risk and resilience following trauma exposure. In: Zoellner, L.A., Feeny, N.C. (Eds.), Facilitating Resilience and Recovery Following Trauma. The Guilford Press, New York.

Zoellner, L.A., Feeny, N.C. (Eds.), 2014b. Facilitating Resilience and Recovery Following Trauma. The Guilford Press, New York.

Zubin, J., Spring, B., 1997. Vulnerability – A new view of schizophrenia. Journal of Abnormal Psychology 86, 103–126.

USEFUL WEBSITES

Access a playlist of 13 talks that invites you to 'Check Your Assumptions', www.ted.com/playlists/292/check_your_assumptions

Anxiety UK https://www.anxietyuk.org.uk/

Emergency and Crisis Situations, www.beyondblue.org.au/the-facts/suicide-prevention/emergency-and-crisis-situations

Finding our way—inspiring personal stories of refugee and migrant people living with emotional and mental health issues, www.mhima.org.au/finding-our-way

Freedom from Torture, www.freedomfromtorture.org

Grief and Loss, www.beyondblue.org.au/the-facts/grief-and-loss

Headspace, www.headspace.com

ManKind Initiative – Helping men escape domestic abuse, https://www.mankind.org.uk

Mental Health First Aid England, https://mhfaengland.org/

MOODJUICE - Post-Traumatic Stress - Self-help Guide, http://www.moodjuice.scot.nhs.uk/posttrauma.asp

Mind: for better mental health, www.mind.org.uk.

Rethink Mental Illness, www.rethink.org

Samaritans, www.samaritans.org

SANE UK mental health charity, http://www.sane.org.uk

TED is a nonprofit organisation whose mission is to spread great ideas. The organisation describes their agenda being 'to make great ideas accessible and spark conversation'.

www.ted.com

The National Domestic Violence Helpline - run in partnership between Women's Aid & Refuge, https://www.womensaid.org.uk

The Resilience Doughnut: Combining Strengths to Thrive, www.theresiliencedoughnut.com.au/index.php.

The Resilience Doughnut is a model for building resilience that considers both the internal qualities of a resilient person as well as the factors in the person's environment which support and interact with those internal qualities. The model is based on a wide body of research (both Australian and international) examining the factors common to children and young people who have shown resilience in the face of adversity.

The Resilience Report, www.resiliencereport.com/

The Survivors Trust – no excuse for rape or sexual abuse, http://thesurvivorstrust.org

Victim Support –help after crime, https://www.victimsupport.org.uk

Women's Aid – until women and children are safe, https://www.womensaid.org.uk

8

Physical Health

Andrew Watkins, Tanya Park

KEY POINTS

- Maintaining physical health is multifaceted and is essential to wellbeing.
- Nurses play an important role in the assessment, treatment and prevention of physical health issues.
- Assessing and treating mental and physical health issues simultaneously is essential.
- Physical health issues are often overlooked when the person has a mental illness.
- Partnerships and collaboration are key to improving physical and mental health.
- The majority of premature deaths among people with mental illness are from preventable physical health issues.

KEY TERMS

cardiometabolic
cardiovascular disease
diabetes
metabolic screening
metabolic syndrome
nutrition
obesity
obstructive sleep apnoea
oral health
physical activity
premature mortality
sexual health
sexuality
sleep disturbance
sleep hygiene
tobacco

LEARNING OUTCOMES

The material in this chapter will assist you to:

- recognise the relationship between mental health and physical health.
- identify the physical health issues commonly experienced by people with a mental illness.
- develop an understanding of the experience of the person who has both physical and mental health issues.
- describe the role of the nurse in assessment of physical health.
- describe interventions for improving the physical health of people with a mental illness.
- explain the importance of assessment of physical health.
- implement nursing interventions relevant to physical health issues identified.

INTRODUCTION

People living with mental illness experience much poorer physical health outcomes compared with the general population. There is a life expectancy gap in excess of 20 years for people experiencing some types of mental illness (Brown et al. 2010). In contrast to a commonly held misconception, nearly four in every five of these premature deaths are associated with preventable physical health conditions, not suicide (Lawrence et al. 2013). There is a multitude of reasons for high levels of physical morbidity among people with mental illness. Many of the psychotropic medications prescribed to people with a serious mental illness (SMI) are associated with adverse effects on physical health, including weight gain and endocrine changes. In addition, the symptoms of many mental illnesses, such as the negative symptoms of schizophrenia, can contribute to withdrawal, isolation and increased likelihood of living a sedentary lifestyle. A survey of people living with psychosis identified that one in three people with a serious mental illness were sedentary and the large majority of the remaining two-thirds engaged in low levels of physical activity (Morgan et al. 2012). People with serious mental illness, such as schizophrenia, also have greater susceptibility to other risk factors for chronic illness, including poverty, smoking, alcohol and drug use, homelessness, unemployment, dental disease, sexually transmitted infections, sleep disorders and a poor quality diet (Steylen et al. 2013; Sweeting et al. 2013; Jones et al. 2014).

The World Health Organization (WHO) describes mental health as a state of wellbeing in which every individual realises his or her own potential, can cope with the normal stresses of life, can work productively and fruitfully and is able to make a contribution to her or his community. The WHO also acknowledges a universal right to health that includes the right to control one's health and body, to be free

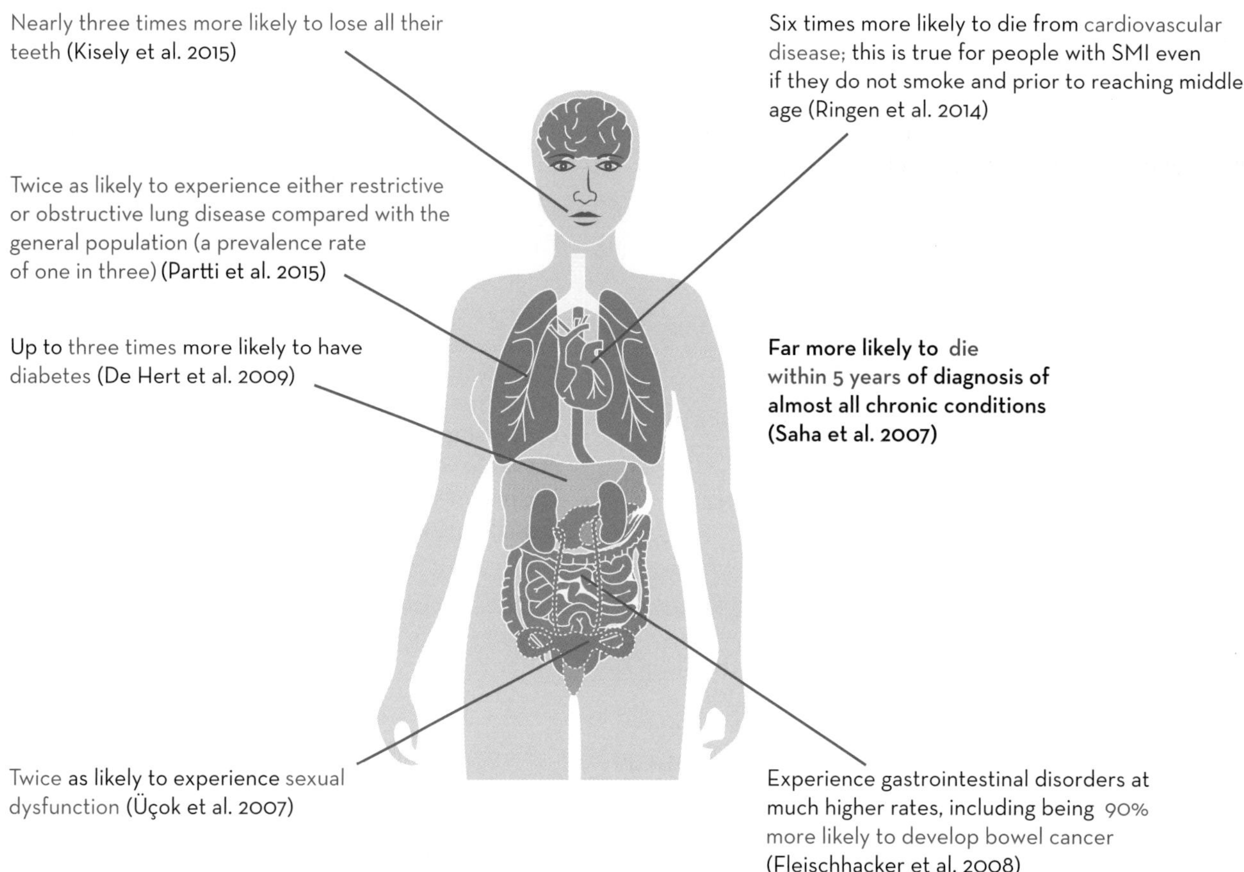

Fig. 8.1 Factors that might contribute to physical health risks in people with severe mental illness.

from interference and the right to a system of health protection that gives everyone an equal opportunity to enjoy the highest attainable level of health (WHO 2008). Historically, the physical healthcare of people with mental illness has been neglected (Thornicroft 2011). NHS England (2018) has released guidance to improve the physical health of patients with serious mental illness in primary care, calling for at least 280,000 people to have their physical health needs met from 2018/2019, thereby reducing their risks from preventable serious illnesses such as cancer, heart disease and diabetes. Nurses are well placed to take the lead in ensuring that people with a mental illness have their physical health needs considered and adequately addressed from the initial assessment right through a person's mental health journey. It is therefore vital that nurses practise in a holistic manner that incorporates physical healthcare by 'keeping the body in mind'.

It is beyond the scope of this chapter to address all the physical illnesses that are experienced by people with a mental illness. The authors have therefore chosen to focus on physical health issues that negatively impact on life expectancy, are most prevalent and most markedly affect wellbeing and quality of life. Factors contributing to physical health risks are shown in Fig. 8.1. This chapter will discuss metabolic syndrome, cardiovascular disease, diabetes, respiratory diseases, oral health, sleep and sexual health. These physical health issues require action and we believe nurses are well positioned to make a difference to the current trends.

Physical Health Neglect in Mental Health Systems

People with comorbid serious mental and physical illness frequently fall through the gaps between physical and mental healthcare systems (Lawrence et al. 2013). The healthcare system in the UK is often divided between services for physical and mental healthcare with a lack of integration. In mental healthcare systems, clinicians may focus on symptoms of mental illness often to the detriment of other health issues, a phenomenon referred to as 'diagnostic overshadowing' (Thornicroft 2011). Physical health symptoms regularly go unnoticed or are not addressed, even when people with mental illness report them to health professionals (Galletly et al. 2012). Often nurses and others working in mental health do not consider addressing physical health issues as fundamental to their duty of care or they lack the confidence to undertake a physical assessment. In the wider health system, there is often a lack of confidence in working with people who have mental illness. Commonly, many services such as medical specialists and allied health services are financially unavailable to this population. Any of these issues can form an extremely challenging obstacle to care for people with complex chronic comorbid conditions such as schizophrenia and diabetes. The upshot is that this very vulnerable population can be marginalised from health services that are a human right and essential to attaining wellbeing.

Access and availability are not the only barriers to good health faced by people with SMI. The higher rate of physical illness among people with SMI not only leads to a much shorter life expectancy but also causes a secondary effect of ongoing physical illness on top of a mental illness, such as schizophrenia and diabetes. These comorbidities increase the challenge of people being able to participate actively in the workforce and create an increased risk of poverty and welfare dependency. Despite having much higher rates of morbidity than most others in the community, people with serious mental illness actually access health services much less (Morgan et al. 2012). Reduced access has a strong disadvantageous effect on the health outcomes of this group. A comorbid physical health issue can put extra demands on family, friends and carers of people with a mental illness, by expanding their role to include physical healthcare. Chapter 10 discusses the important issue of carer roles.

METABOLIC SYNDROME

Metabolic syndrome is a cluster of abnormal clinical and metabolic findings that result in an increased risk of developing type 2 diabetes mellitus (T2DM), cardiovascular disease (CVD) and CVD mortality (Vancampfort et al. 2015a). These abnormal findings include visceral adiposity, insulin resistance, increased blood pressure, elevated triglyceride levels and low-level high-density lipoprotein (HDL) cholesterol levels (Alberti et al. 2005). The complications of metabolic syndrome involve multiple body systems including the cardiovascular, hepatic, endocrine and central nervous systems (Kaur 2014). Meeting the criteria for metabolic syndrome causes a fivefold increase in the risk of developing T2DM and twofold increase in the risk of developing CVD over the next 5 to 10 years (Kaur 2014). Thus, assertive intervention is required when metabolic syndrome risk factors are present. Fig. 8.1 highlights the risk factors of developing metabolic syndrome and Box 8.1 sets out the criteria for metabolic syndrome.

People with SMI have much higher rates of obesity and abdominal obesity in comparison with the general population (Subramaniam et al. 2014). This occurs even in the early phase of illness with or without medication. Similar to the general population, obesity in people with SMI is associated with lifestyle factors such as a poor diet and lack of physical activity (Hjorth et al. 2014). There are a number of features related to mental illness, such as sedation, amotivation and disorganisation, that exacerbate the likelihood of negative lifestyle factors that promote weight gain. There is also evidence of medication-induced effects on appetite and food intake (Cuerda et al. 2014).

Weight gain is a well-established side effect of antipsychotic medications. It is most pronounced at the beginningof treatment and generally continues with long periods of treatment. Weight gain is usually greatest with clozapine and olanzapine, while quetiapine, risperidone and paliperidone cause a more moderate gain and aripiprazole, asenapine and ziprasidone are likely to cause less weight gain (Bak et al. 2014). Without interventions, all antipsychotic medications have been found to result in significant weight gain when they are first initiated (De Hert et al. 2011). Box 8.2 specifies the physical healthcare skills that mental healthcare professionals should learn (RCPsych 2016).

BOX 8.1 International Diabetes Federation Metabolic Syndrome Criteria

Central Obesity (WC Centimetres)			Plus Any Two of:	
Ethnicity	Male	Female	TG	≥1.7 mmol/L
Europid	≥94	≥80	HDL	<1.03 (M) mmol/L <1.29 (F)
South/South-East Asian Japanese	≥90	≥80	BP	≥130/85 mmHg
Central and South American	≥90	≥80	fBSL	≥5.6 mmol/L

BP, Blood pressure; *fBSL*, fasting Blood Sugar Level; *HDL*, high-density lipoprotein; *TG*, triglycerides.

(*Source*: Alberti, K., Zimmet, P., Shaw, J., 2005. The metabolic syndrome—a new worldwide definition. Lancet. 366(9491), 1059–1062.)

Screening for Metabolic Health

To identify metabolic syndrome and to allow for early treatment, it is vital that screening be undertaken for the presence of factors that increase the risk of CVD and T2DM (Galletly et al. 2012). Screening for metabolic syndrome is well within the scope of nursing practice and should be viewed as an essential activity. Metabolic screening involves taking a person's waist circumference, blood pressure, height and weight and calculating body mass index. The best indicator of metabolic health is waist circumference and this is the most important measure to screen. Fasting lipids and glucose completes the metabolic screening process. Screening should occur every 3 months, with the exception of when someone is starting a new medication or there are concerns about a person's health, when it should occur more often. More details about how to undertake a metabolic screen are in Box 8.3.

DIABETES

T2DM is a progressive condition in which the body becomes resistant to the normal effects of insulin and/or gradually loses the capacity to produce enough insulin in the pancreas. T2DM greatly increases the risk of cardiovascular disease, renal failure, amputation and blindness and lowers life expectancy by 10 or more years (Gordon-Dseagu et al. 2015). The prevalence of T2DM in people with schizophrenia or bipolar disorder is two to three times higher than the general population (Stubbs et al. 2015). The risk of T2DM in people with depression or depressive symptoms is also elevated compared with those without depression.

PATIENT STORY 8.1

I started taking olanzapine in mid-2015, when I was 20 years old, and within 4 months I had gained over 20 kg! I was shocked—I was starting to recover from a serious episode of psychosis but I became fat so quickly, I didn't feel at all comfortable with my new body shape and started to avoid people because I was ashamed. I found myself being very hungry nearly all of the time and craving food that was fatty and sugary. No-one mentioned to me anything about the fact that I'd feel this hungry or put on this much weight.

Over the next few years, I tried to lose the weight I had put on but I couldn't seem to shift it, in fact I continued to gain weight although at a slower rate. In 3 years I put on another 15 kg. This was something that was very strange for me; I'd always been a fit and healthy person and at that point I'd hit 105 kg, a far cry from the 68 kg I was prior to starting medication. I become resigned to the fact that I was going to be fat and there was nothing I could do about it.

I then met a mental health nurse who spoke to me about what my goals in life were. I had already got back into the workforce full time, so I told her that it was my physical health I wanted to work on. She told me that she'd be very happy to help and measured my weight, took my waist measurement and blood pressure and organised for a blood test. Together we looked at areas that could be improved and she assisted me to find out information on what were the best exercises to do and how I could improve my diet.

My blood test came back and showed a higher than normal cholesterol level. This really had me concerned and I expressed this to my nurse—I was worried that this was going to kill me. She told me that sometimes medications could cause these problems in addition to weight gain. She reassured me that it was possible to make changes to my health even though things I'd tried in the past had not worked. She came with me to my next doctor's appointment and helped advocate for a change in medication. The doctor agreed and switched me to aripiprazole.

My nurse then suggested we work on some goals that were short term. We started with trying to stop my weight gain and then developed more goals that increased my fitness levels and improved my nutritional intake. I started to find that I could lose weight. I found this support and encouragement gave me a lot of motivation where I had previously given up.

Two and a half years later, I have managed to lose all of that weight and am now about the same as I was before I started seeing mental health services. I feel so much happier and have lots more energy now. My cholesterol has returned to normal and I am not feeling burdened by physical health issues like I was.

BOX 8.2 Improving the Physical Health of Adults with Severe Mental Illness: Essential Actions

A joint report by the Royal College of Psychiatrists and eight partner colleges and bodies calls for a reform of the physical healthcare received by adults with severe mental illness.

Physical healthcare activities that mental healthcare professionals should be trained in:

- Assessment of physical health: assess the physical health of patients on admission and at appropriate intervals thereafter, including assessment for the presence or absence of illness, injury or disability in addition to receiving a medical history, making a functional enquiry, undertaking a physical examination, arranging blood tests and other investigations, as necessary.
- Investigation for underlying physical causes: investigate for the presence of an underlying physical cause for the mental condition of the patient and, when appropriate, form a differential diagnosis as a basis for further investigation or referral to other health professionals.
- Monitoring physical health: monitor the physical health of the patient on the basis of clinical need and national standards of physical healthcare.
- Recognition of acute illness (the 'deteriorating patient'): this includes measuring physiological parameters, using NEWS (National Early Warning Score) system, making the 'first response' to an acute illness and using effective communication and resuscitation techniques.
- Out-of-hours medical care: where inpatient services require out-of-hours medical care to be delivered by a psychiatrist, they and certain members of the clinical team need the skills and competencies to make a diagnosis (or provisional diagnosis), to treat and/or to refer the patient to acute services, while also recognising that the patient may have comorbidities and be vulnerable for reasons relating to their mental health.
- Management of long-term conditions: monitor and provide treatment for long-term conditions in collaboration with specialists.
- Medicines: be aware of all medicines prescribed for the patient. Be able to work closely with the pharmacist to optimise the use of the medicines and be able to monitor the physical side effects of psychotropic and other medicines prescribed for physical and mental conditions.
- Referral to others: psychiatrists and other healthcare professionals should know 'when and how' to refer to other health professionals. In particular, be aware of clinical 'red flag' symptoms and signs that should prompt referral to specialists.
- Health promotion and disease prevention: be aware of health promotion and disease prevention strategies, including physical activity, diet, oral health, sexual health and smoking cessation, prevention of falls, immunisation and infection control measures. Be aware of screening tools for the assessment of physical health risks (e.g. venous thromboembolism risks, tissue viability, nutritional risk factors and cardiovascular risks).
- Specific health risks: be aware of specific risks in the patient population (e.g. homeless people and refugees).
- Rehabilitation of patients: facilitate recovery from physical illness or injury for instance by liaison with specialists who provide the services needed by the patient for physical healthcare.

(*Source*: Royal College of Psychiatrists 2016, Improving the physical health of adults with severe mental illness: essential actions. Available at: https://www.rcpsych.ac.uk/mediacentre/adultswithsmi.aspx.)

BOX 8.3 Screening for Metabolic Health

Weight
- Remove shoes, items from pockets and bulky clothing

Height
- Shoes removed, feet flat on floor and looking straight ahead

BMI
- Calculated by weight divided by height squared (normal range 18.5–25)

$$\frac{\text{weight}}{\text{height (m)}^2}$$

A useful online calculator is available at NHS BMI Healthy Weight Calculator https://www.nhs.uk/Tools/Pages/Healthy-weightcalculator.aspx.

Waist Circumference
Waist measurements should be taken after breathing out. Patients should be encouraged to relax and not contract any abdominal muscles. Align the tape measure at the level of the umbilicus (belly button) and circle the whole way around the body, back to the starting point.
- Make sure the tape is parallel to the ground and not twisted.
- The tape should be snug, without compressing the skin.
- Ask the patient to breathe in and out twice and measure on the second out breath.

Blood Pressure
- Ensure correct cuff size
- Measure when the person is relaxed
- Measure with arm resting at height of the heart

Pathology
- Ensure patient fasting
- Lipid profile (including HDL/LDL)
- Glucose
- Liver function test

BMI, body mass index; *HDL*, high-density lipoprotein; *LDL*, low-density lipoprotein.

There are a multitude of reasons for the elevated risk of T2DM for people with SMI, including lifestyle factors and genetic predisposition, as well as disease and treatment-specific effects (Stubbs et al. 2015). Antipsychotic medications carry an increased risk of developing T2DM, with olanzapine and clozapine particularly noted as carrying an increased risk (Holt & Mitchell 2014).

Despite a high prevalence of T2DM among people with SMI, screening rates remain low. This leads to prolonged periods of raised blood glucose levels, hastening the negative consequences associated with T2DM. Once diagnosed, people with SMI are more likely to be suboptimally treated and have poor glycaemic control. Even when young, after being diagnosed with T2DM, people with serious mental illness experience a rapid decline in health and premature death (Ribe et al. 2014).

CRITICAL THINKING CHALLENGE 8.1

Imagine you have gained 8 kg in the last 2 months.

1. Most of the weight gain is around your abdomen. How would you feel?
2. Consider your current lifestyle. What changes to your life would occur?
3. Imagine that you have also been diagnosed with a psychotic disorder. What changes to your life would occur? How might your psychosis and weight gain affect your self-esteem? What might that do to your ability to recover? Would you continue to take medication if you thought that it caused you significant weight gain? Why or why not?

CARDIOVASCULAR DISEASE

The term 'cardiovascular diseases' (CVD) refers to any disease that affects the heart and blood vessels. Coronary heart disease and cerebrovascular disease are the primary components of CVD. The major risk factors for CVD are smoking, obesity, hypertension, raised blood cholesterol and T2DM (Todd et al. 2014). There are many other factors that increase the risk of CVD, including genetics, an unhealthy diet, physical inactivity and low socioeconomic status.

CVD is the most common cause of death in people with SMI, with prevalence rates approximately twice that of the general population (De Hert et al. 2009). In younger people with SMI, CVD rates are three times higher when compared with matched controls (Ringen et al. 2014). People with SMI have significantly higher rates of several of the modifiable risk factors when compared with controls; they are more likely to be overweight or obese; to have T2DM, hypertension or dyslipidaemia; and to smoke (Smith et al. 2013).

Despite the high CVD mortality among people with SMI, they receive less of many specialised interventions including cardiovascular medications. Evidence suggests that people with schizophrenia are not being adequately screened and treated for dyslipidaemia and hypertension. Depression is also noted as being an independent risk factor for worsening morbidity and mortality in coronary heart disease.

People with SMI have considerably lower rates of surgical interventions, such as stenting and coronary artery bypass grafting (Mather et al. 2014). This poorer quality of medical care contributes to excess mortality for people with SMI after heart failure (Schoepf et al. 2014). An additional significant barrier is the low level of care sought by people with SMI, even during acute cardiovascular events (Reininghaus et al. 2015).

In addition to weight gain and obesity-related mechanisms, there appears to be a direct effect of antipsychotic medication that contributes to the worsening of CVD risk. T2DM antagonism can be caused by antipsychotics having a direct effect on the development of insulin resistance (Stubbs et al. 2015). Higher antipsychotic doses predict greater risk of mortality from coronary heart disease and

NURSE'S STORY 8.1

Pawel has been a nurse for 27 years and now works on an acute inpatient mental health unit. He has been leading a project to help people admitted to the mental health unit deal with smoking withdrawal and encouraging them to quit. This is his story.

When I first started working as a nurse in mental health, I was a smoker. The senior nurses I was working with at the time told me that a great way to build a relationship with the patients on the unit was to chat to them while we were all having a smoke.

Pawel ceased smoking 15 years ago after witnessing his aunt dying from lung cancer.

I saw what my aunt was going through and it was horrible, she was in so much pain and distress, I decided at that time I needed to quit for my health. So I quit. It wasn't easy at all, especially being around people smoking while I was at work. I persisted though and my health has improved significantly.

Pawel decided he wanted to support the patients he was working with to experience the same benefits that he gained after quitting smoking. When he heard about the smoking ban in mental health units, he thought it was an ideal opportunity.

I thought to myself, 'If they are not allowed to smoke while they are on the unit, they may as well use it as a launching pad to quitting smoking.' The worst part of nicotine withdrawal is the first couple of days, so it would make sense that if they could make it through that, why couldn't they quit altogether? So I learnt about withdrawal symptoms from nicotine and how to prescribe nicotine replacement therapy.

As Pawel built up the intervention, other nurses took an interest and became involved with the programme. This led to a much more comprehensive approach to addressing smoking and not just when Pawel was on shift.

The key to the intervention was giving patients who were in nicotine withdrawal support. Nicotine replacement therapy doesn't completely stop the cravings and talking to patients about how they are coping with the withdrawal was really helpful.

The programme has become quite a success, with many people successfully quitting and not taking the habit up again. Pawel and the programme have also been recognised with awards.

Just banning smoking is cruel; giving people 'smoking leave' from the unit would just restart the withdrawal process again. What's the point in making people withdraw if there is no benefit for the person in the end? What we found was that many people actually wanted to quit and had found it really hard in the past. No-one likes withdrawal symptoms, but in hindsight they were often very thankful that we supported them to actually start the quitting process properly.

cerebrovascular accident. Most antipsychotics and some antidepressants are associated with a change in the heart's electrical cycle known as QTc prolongation. A prolonged QTc puts a patient at significant risk of torsade de pointes, ventricular fibrillation and sudden cardiac death (Glassman & Bigger 2014).

MANAGEMENT OF CARDIOMETABOLIC HEALTH

While screening for metabolic health is important, it has little benefit if no action is taken after problems are identified. It is vital that nurses 'don't just screen but intervene' for metabolic health (Watkins 2014). Lifestyle interventions are at the centre of the management of cardiometabolic health. Nurses are well positioned to advise, to encourage and to implement lifestyle interventions around tobacco cessation (see Nurses Story 8.1 by Pawel), physical activity and healthy nutrition. People with SMI can benefit enormously from even small lifestyle changes. Research indicates that cardiometabolic health risks in people with mental ill health may be much greater than those reported in the general population, with antipsychotic polypharmacy and higher doses of antipsychotics as factors that may contribute towards this increased risk (Bressington et al. 2016). A positive cardiometabolic health algorithm has been developed to help guide clinicians in the management of the leading causes of mortality of people with SMI. (See Fig. 8.2.)

CRITICAL THINKING CHALLENGE 8.3

Consider the cardiometabolic algorithm in Fig. 8.2 and the screening for metabolic health information in Box 8.3 to develop a nursing care plan for a young person who has just started taking antipsychotic medications. What information do you need to tailor the plan to the individual? How will you get this information? What do you consider most important? Why?

TOBACCO-RELATED ILLNESS AND SMOKING CESSATION

Very high smoking rates are observed among people with SMI. In England, 40.5% of adults with SMI are smokers, which is more than twice the rate of the general population (16.9%) (ASH 2016a) People with a mental illness also smoke more cigarettes per day and inhale more deeply than other smokers, achieving higher blood levels of nicotine than smokers without SMI (Rüther et al. 2014).

Tobacco-related diseases make up approximately half of total deaths seen in people with SMI. Tobacco use represents the highest single factor that contributes to premature death. The high smoking rates among people with SMI

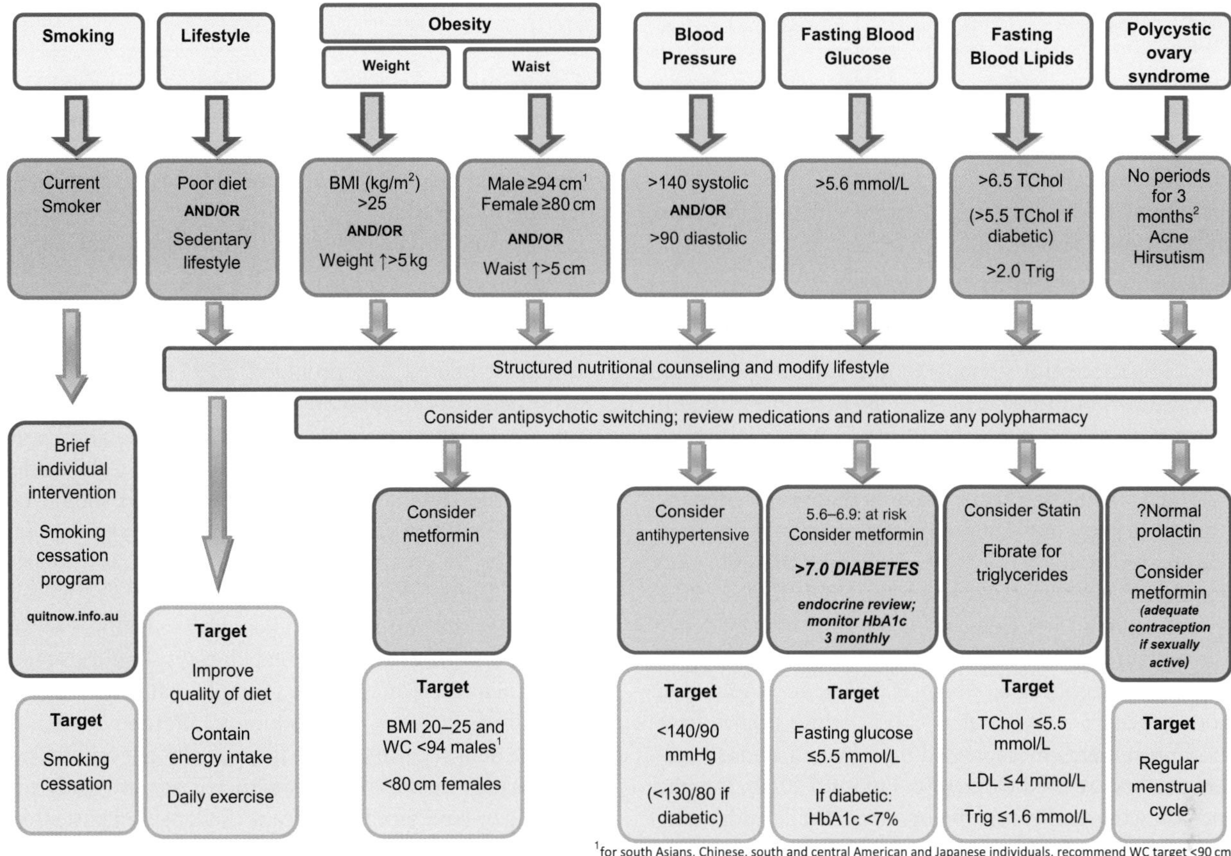

[1] for south Asians, Chinese, south and central American and Japanese individuals, recommend WC target <90 cm
[2] for premenopausal women

History: smoking, exercise, diet, FHx (diabetes, obesity, CVD), gestational diabetes, ethnicity, Polycystic ovary syndrome

Then at least 3 monthly

Examination: weight, BMI, waist circumference, BP

Investigations: Fasting blood glucose and lipids: total cholesterol (TChol); LDL, HDL, triglycerides (Trig);

Vitamin D (twice per year).

Interventions:

Nutritional counseling: reduce take away and junk food, reduce energy intake to prevent weight gain, stop soft drinks and juices, increase fibre intake.

Physical activity: structured education-lifestyle intervention. Advise daily physical activity: eg 30 minutes of walking.

If unsuccessful after 3 months in reaching targets, then consider switching and medication interventions below

Switching: Consider switching to a more weight neutral medication. Review diagnosis and ensure ongoing need for all psychotropic medications.

Don't just SCREEN →

INTERVENE

for all patients in the "red zone"

Screen cardiometabolic risk factors using screening tool (e.g. Waterreus, et al. 2009, Curtis et al. 2009 SESLHD); examine and investigate 3 monthly on all clients on psychotropic medications.

NB additional considerations for those on mood stabilizers & clozapine not included here and need to be performed (e.g. medication plasma levels, TFT's UEC's, ECHO, etc)

Always involve general practitioner, and, where appropriate and possible refer to specialist (e.g. dietitian/ physician/ diabetic clinic/ exercise physiologist).

NB: Some drugs used in metabolic disease treatment are contraindicated in pregnancy (e.g. some antihypertensives and lipid lowering drugs). If your patient on any metabolic medications is considering pregnancy, please discuss with their GP

Specific Pharmacological Interventions:

Consider metformin if:

- impaired glucose
- PCOS
- obesity or rapid weight gain

Metformin therapy: start at 500 mg x ½ tablet before breakfast and dinner for two weeks then increase to 500 mg bd. Dose can be increased to a maximum of 3 grams daily, though as this is off label treatment, no adverse effects should be tolerated. If side effects of nausea, abdominal cramping, shift to after meal.

Lipid lowering therapy: (use PBS guidelines)

Statin initiation doses for cholesterol lowering:

simvastatin 10 mg nocte — atorvastatin 10 mg nocte
pravastatin 10 mg nocte — rosuvastatin 10 mg nocte

Fibrate therapy for triglyceride lowering:

gemfibrozil 600 mg bd — fenofibrate 145 mg mane

Antihypertensive therapy: Multiple agents are available. Liaise with the GP who can monitor.

Vitamin D:

- <50 nmol/L: replenish stores: cholecalciferol 4000 IU per day for one month;
- maintenance: 1000 IU daily. Target >80 nmol/L.

References: Alberti K, Zimmet P, Shaw J. "The metabolic syndrome - a new worldwide definition". *Lancet.* 2005; 366: 1059-62. Correll, C. U., P. Manu, et al. "Cardiometabolic risk of second-generation antipsychotic medications during first-time use in children and adolescents". *JAMA.* 2009; 302: 1765-1773. De Hert M, Dekker JM, Wood D, et al. "Cardiovascular disease and diabetes in people with severe mental illness position statement from the European Psychiatric Association (EPA), supported by the European Association for the Study of Diabetes (EASD) and the European Society of Cardiology (ESC)". *European Psychiatry.* 2009; 24: 412-24. Newall H, Myles N, Ward PB, Samaras K, Shiers D, Curtis J. "Efficacy of metformin for prevention of weight gain in psychiatric populations: a review". *Int Clin Psychopharmacol.* 2012; 27: 69-75. Newcomer JW, Hennekens CH. "Severe Mental Illness and Risk of Cardiovascular Disease". *JAMA.* 2007; 298: 1794-6. Waterreus AJ, Laugharne JD. "Screening for the metabolic syndrome in patients receiving antipsychotic treatment: a proposed algorithm". *MJA.* 2009; 190:185-9. Wu, R. R., J. P. Zhao, et al. "Lifestyle intervention and metformin for treatment of antipsychotic-induced weight gain: a randomized controlled trial". *JAMA.* 2008; 299:185-193.

For online access to this fact sheet, please visit http://www.heti.nsw.gov.au/cmalgorithm

Fig. 8.2 Positive Cardiometabolic Health Algorithm An Early Intervention Framework for Patients on Psychotropic Medication. (*Source*: Curtis, J., Newall, H.D., Samaras, K., 2012. The heart of the matter: cardiometabolic care in youth with psychosis. Early Intervention in Psychiatry 6[3], 347–353.)

increases their risk of developing cancer and respiratory diseases. Tobacco smoking may be particularly problematic as it amplifies the increased risk of cardiovascular disease alongside the centralised weight gain associated with use of atypical antipsychotic medications.

The high rate of smoking among people with SMI can be attributed to a high smoking take-up rate that occurs early in life, often before a mental health diagnosis, combined with fewer and less successful attempts to quit (Myles et al. 2012; Smith et al. 2014). Addressing tobacco use in people with SMI is a major clinical and public health issue. A mental health and smoking action report by Action on Smoking and Health (ASH 2016b), The Stolen Years, suggests that people affected with mental health conditions, almost a quarter of the population, on average die 10 to 20 years younger than the general population, with smoking being the single largest cause of this difference in life expectancy. There is also evidence of positive neurocognitive effects from cigarette smoking in people with schizophrenia, which is linked to stimulation of nicotine receptors (Wing et al. 2012), while studies have shown improvements in depressed mood when transdermal nicotine patches are used (Mineur & Picciotto 2010). Despite evidence showing positive neurocognitive effects, addressing tobacco use in people with SMI is a major clinical and public health issue and there is limited clinical attention devoted to tobacco use in these groups.

There is a common misconception that people with SMI do not wish to quit smoking (Hall & Prochaska 2009). There is a strong interest in smoking cessation in people with serious mental illnesses, who are motivated for the same reasons as other smokers—to improve their health (Aschbrenner et al. 2015). An additional motivation to quit is the substantial financial cost of cigarette smoking for people who often have very low incomes, largely derived from social welfare (Ashton et al. 2013).

Another common misconception is that SMI conditions and mental illness symptoms will deteriorate by quitting smoking when the opposite it more likely. Substantial mental health benefits can be gained from quitting smoking, such as reduced symptoms of depression and anxiety. Symptoms of mental illness do not appear to deteriorate after quitting smoking.

Nurses can play a vital role in smoking cessation, influencing tobacco-related mortality. People with SMI are likely to experience more severe withdrawal symptoms compared with the general population and require extra support during cessation attempts (Rüther et al. 2014). It is important to realise that people with SMI respond to smoking cessation treatment as well as the general population in the short term, although they generally have worse long-term outcomes.

A person's current smoking status, nicotine dependency and previous attempts to quit should be assessed. Assessing nicotine dependency will help predict the level of withdrawal symptoms the patient is likely to experience upon quitting. Smoking cessation is best initiated when a person's mental state is stable. Patients should be thoroughly informed on the processes that assist quitting smoking, enabling the person to formulate their individual quit plan and to take ownership of their own attempt to quit and giving them the best chance of quitting successfully.

A person should be supported in their quit plan with cessation counselling about what to expect with withdrawal symptoms (e.g. depression and restlessness) and how to cope when these symptoms arise. Pharmacological support should be offered and provided, such as nicotine replacement therapy or bupropion when there is even mild tobacco dependence (Rüther et al. 2014). Ceasing tobacco use can affect how some medications (e.g. olanzapine, clozapine) are metabolised (Banham & Gilbody 2010). This should not be an impediment to encouraging quitting but requires careful monitoring for potential increases in side effects from psychiatric medication (Rüther et al. 2014).

Along with approaches to illicit drug use, advice on smoking to people with serious mental illnesses should also include advice on harm reduction, for example reducing frequency or strength of cigarettes or switching to alternative methods of nicotine delivery. This advice is especially relevant for people with serious mental illnesses who are not yet ready to quit smoking or have faced significant challenges in past attempts. Chapter 24 provides advice on how the nurse can use supportive therapies during this often challenging time.

Factors such as socioeconomic disadvantage and cognitive impairment are common for people with SMI. When combined with an absence of social support for abstinence from family and peers, some people will find quitting smoking much more difficult (Gartner & Hall 2015). In some people with schizophrenia, nicotine may be used as self-medication to reduce the negative symptoms of their illness, to improve their cognition or to ease the side effects caused by antipsychotic medication.

Alongside smoking cessation, exercise should be promoted among people with schizophrenia to combat weight gain and increased metabolic risk. Nurses should carefully monitor patients' medication and fluctuations in weight for a minimum of 6 months after quitting smoking (Gartner & Hall 2015). Helpful advice and support is available via NHS Smokefree https://www.nhs.uk/smokefree and ASH Action on Smoking and Health http://ash.org.uk/home/.

CRITICAL THINKING CHALLENGE 8.4

Discuss the following statement: 'People with mental illness don't have much enjoyment in life, so why would you want to take another enjoyment away and encourage them to quit cigarettes?'

RESPIRATORY DISEASES

Respiratory diseases were the leading cause of death in psychiatric institutions until 50 years ago (Brown 1997). Today, respiratory diseases are still more prevalent in people with SMI, with approximately one in three people having either restrictive or obstructive lung disease, a rate double the general population prevalence rate (Partti et al. 2015). The likelihood of developing pneumonia is also considerably raised. Not only are these conditions far more common in people experiencing SMI but they are more likely to lead to mortality (Schoepf et al. 2014). Tobacco smoking is closely associated with an increased risk of respiratory diseases and, in particular, influences chronic obstructive pulmonary disorder (COPD) in its development and progression, as well as mixed forms of asthma.

Respiratory assessment is an essential component of a physical health assessment and nurses should be vigilant and maintain regular and timely screening for respiratory conditions. Additional support and referral may be required, with consideration given to modifiable risk factors such as tobacco smoking, which is closely linked to increased cardiometabolic health risk factors. Physical activity should be promoted, since it might delay decline in lung function (Gartner and Hall 2015). Influenza is a potentially manageable public health issue that can lead to serious respiratory disease and death. Routine influenza vaccination should be encouraged among people with SMI (Partti et al. 2015). Information about influenza vaccination is readily available on the NHS website (www.nhs.uk/conditions/vaccinations/flu-influenza-vaccine). Nurses need to ensure that the patients they work with are vaccinated.

CRITICAL THINKING CHALLENGE 8.5

You are a nurse working on a busy acute mental health unit and are aware of the importance of influenza vaccination. What strategies could you develop to improve the vaccination rates of the staff and patients in the acute unit?

NUTRITION

Nutritional therapy in mental health treatment is a rapidly growing area in both the academic and clinical fields, with experts calling for nutritional medicine to be mainstream in mental health services. People experiencing SMI have poorer diets when compared with the general population. This is a significant, and importantly a modifiable, factor that contributes to severe weight gain, subsequent poor cardiometabolic health and mortality gap in this population.

People with SMI commonly have diets lower in fruit and fibre and high in saturated fat compared with the general population (Dipasquale et al. 2013). Studies that assessed caloric intake found higher intakes in those with SMI (Tsuruga et al. 2015), while evidence also demonstrated that the diets of those with SMI are lower in vegetables, legumes and dairy.

People receiving antipsychotic therapy commonly experience significantly increased hunger and an inability to sense satiety (feeling full), particularly those taking clozapine and olanzapine (Potvin et al. 2015). These medications can affect ghrelin and leptin hormones, which regulate hunger and satiety (Potvin et al. 2015). The highest increases in leptin levels are seen in patients receiving antipsychotics that produce the most weight gain.

Combining these factors with constant cravings for sugary or processed oily foods, low food preparation skills, low levels of motivation and often restricted budgets provides a potent mix for weight gain and poor metabolic health. Additionally, low mood and depression can also lead to overeating and comfort eating. Furthermore, people with SMI have a lower basal metabolic rate than the general population, contributing to rapid weight gain (Cuerda et al. 2013). Additional dietary considerations for this population include fast-eating syndrome, disordered eating habits such as only eating one main meal per day, constipation and higher levels of dental and coeliac disease (Kisely et al. 2011).

Given these dietary patterns and nutritional side effects, interventions that aim to reduce caloric intake and improve diet quality by increasing core foods and reducing discretionary foods could be seen as key factors in improving the physical health of those with SMI. Core foods reflect the five food groups: (1) vegetables; (2) fruit; (3) milk, cheese, yoghurt and alternatives; (4) lean meat, fish, poultry, eggs, seeds and nuts; and (5) grains, with some healthy oils such as olive oil. Discretionary foods reflect those that are high in energy (kilojoules/calories) and low in nutrients and are generally highly processed and refined foods (NHMRC 2013). Evidence has emerged demonstrating that people following a higher quality diet have better mental health while those whose diet quality is lower have poorer psychological functioning (Jacka et al. 2011).

An alternative dietary pattern shown to be beneficial for mental health by preventing and/or reducing depressive symptoms is the Mediterranean diet (Rienks et al. 2013). The Mediterranean diet focusses on fruits and vegetables, fish, nuts and seeds, whole grains, legumes, olive oil, feta cheese and moderate intakes of red wine, particularly with meals. In addition to improvements in mental health, this pattern of eating is protective for both diabetes and cardiovascular disease.

Key nutrients of concern in those with SMI include caffeine, omega-3 fatty acids, folate and magnesium. Caffeine overconsumption is common: people who experience schizophrenia are twice as likely to consume more than 200 mg (two cups of coffee) per day (Kim & O'Hanlon 2011). There is currently no acceptable daily intake value for caffeine; however, a review performed by Food Standards Australia New Zealand suggests increased risk of anxiety at 95 mg (one cup of coffee or two cans of cola) per day for children and 210 mg for adults (Smith et al. 2000). Low levels of omega-3 fatty acids, folate and magnesium have been linked with depression, with increased intake (oral or supplemented) proving to be an effective part of treatment (Forsyth et al. 2012).

Nutrition interventions in people with SMI to date have generally been scarce; however, studies have demonstrated that nutrition interventions in both early intervention and longer term illness have reduced health risks (Curtis et al. 2015). Although future studies need to assess the long-term impacts on anthropometric, biochemical and lifestyle (nutrition and exercise) measures, as well as quality of life, mental health symptomology and readmission rates, there is sufficient evidence to support the use of nutrition interventions in combination with exercise as core components of mental health services.

Nutritional advice and support should be integrated into routine nursing care. When providing nutrition interventions, it is crucial not only to provide both educational and practical components to ensure adequate knowledge, but also to improve shopping, label reading, food safety and culinary (food preparation) skills. With patients particularly vulnerable to increased hunger, reduced satiety and cravings for high caloric convenience foods and drinks with little nutritional value, mindfulness-based activities might also prove to be an adjunctive intervention.

PHYSICAL ACTIVITY

Physical activity can be defined as any bodily movement produced by skeletal muscle resulting in an increased energy expenditure. The term 'physical activity' encompasses both structured forms of activity, such as exercise, and unstructured forms, such as incidental activity. People experiencing mental illness are known to be less physically active than the general population and engage in prolonged periods of sedentary behaviour (Nyboe & Lund 2013). Low levels of physical activity are an established risk factor for cardiometabolic dysfunction, including diabetes and obesity. In addition to low levels of physical activity, people with mental illness have poorer cardiorespiratory fitness in comparison with the general population, which is an established risk factor for all-cause mortality and morbidity (Vancampfort, Guelinkcx et al. 2015; Vancampfort, Rosenbaum et al. 2015a). Given the high rates of premature mortality linked to preventable cardiovascular disease within this population, evidence-based physical activity interventions aimed at reducing sedentary time, increasing overall activity and increasing moderate–vigorous physical activity participation should be considered part of routine care for people living with mental illness (Vancampfort et al. 2015b).

Physical activity and exercise have been shown to have beneficial effects on psychiatric symptomatology regardless of diagnosis, while a growing body of research has reported on the benefits of exercise for improving cognition (Kimhy et al. 2014). Recent longitudinal studies have also highlighted the bidirectional relationship between activity and depressive symptoms (Pinto Pereira et al. 2014) with evidence of a protective effect of being physically active (Mammen & Faulkner 2013).

Evidence-based strategies to increase physical activity among people with mental illness include behavioural

NURSE'S STORY 8.2

The Early Intervention team works with young people between the ages of 14 and 35 years in the early stages of psychotic illness. The team operates from an interdisciplinary model within a community mental health service.

Nurses working with young people experiencing their first episode of psychosis were extremely concerned that while atypical antipsychotic medications were successful in alleviating people of many of the troubling symptoms of mental illness, they also appeared to be correlated with rapid weight gain and subsequent longer-term risks of diabetes and heart disease.

We responded to these alarms by developing an assessment tool to measure changes in weight and other metabolic abnormalities. What we found was that young people were commonly putting on 10 to 20 kg and sometimes more within their first year with the service and that alterations in a person's metabolic health deteriorated rapidly with this weight gain. These issues included elevated cholesterol and hypertension. Blood glucose levels in the body may become raised, putting these young people at much higher risk of developing diabetes.

It was also noticed by nursing staff that young people were experiencing increased rates of stigma and poor self-esteem. This in effect was like a 'double whammy' to a young person who was dealing with a new mental health diagnosis and the fact that they have to take psychiatric medication, while also trying to deal with transformations to their body image as well as disturbances to their personal life such as work, study and socialisation.

We realised that just assessing people's health was inadequate. We actually needed to make a difference and so we adopted a mantra of 'don't just screen, intervene'.

Working in conjunction with a multidisciplinary team, nursing staff established a number of lifestyle interventions and a programme called 'Keeping the Body in Mind' (KBIM). This programme aims to prevent weight gain and the accompanying deterioration in metabolic health that might in future lead to heart disease and diabetes. The programme is coordinated by a clinical nurse consultant and utilises an exercise physiologist, a dietician and a peer support worker. The lifestyle intervention programme encompasses three elements—health coaching, dietetic support and a supervised exercise programme—which are delivered with an interconnected approach. Each participant's intervention programme is tailored to suit the individual.

The programme was recently evaluated in a controlled study comparing it with another early psychosis service. The KBIM programme was compared with a similar early psychosis program with the exception of the metabolic intervention. Participants in the KBIM group (*n*=16) were provided a 12-week individualised lifestyle programme, while the comparison group (*n*=12) received standard care. The evaluation study established that the KBIM group had considerably less weight gain at 12 weeks (an average of 1.8 kg over 12 weeks) compared with standard care (an average of 7.8 kg). Only 13% of the intervention group experienced clinically significant weight gain (greater than 7% of baseline weight) compared with 75% in the non intervention group.

(*Source:* Curtis, J., Watkins, A., Rosenbaum, S., Teasdale, S., Kalucy, M., Samaras, K., Ward, P.B., 2015. Evaluating an individualized lifestyle and life skills intervention to prevent antipsychotic-induced weight gain in first-episode psychosis. Early Intervention in Psychiatry 10, 267–276. DOI:10.1111/eip.12230.)

techniques such as motivational interviewing, face-to-face and group-based exercise sessions (Rosenbaum et al. 2014, 2015b) as well as structured exercise prescriptions and interventions reflecting individual variations in mood, motivation and access to facilities and resources (Ward et al. 2015). Exercise is not a one-size-fits-all intervention and a range of individual factors should be considered when developing individualised exercise interventions. Aside from physical limitations, factors to be considered are severity of psychiatric symptomatology, previous exercise history, motivation and access to services or facilities that may affect the modality and intensity of exercise that individuals are able to undertake.

Exercise is the structured subset of physical activity and exercise prescriptions are typically described according to the FITT principle (frequency, intensity, time and type) while incorporating appropriate goal-setting strategies. The International Organization of Physical Therapists in Mental Health (IOPTMH) recommends that adults aim for 150 minutes per week of moderate intensity physical activity or 75 minutes of moderate-vigorous activity in addition to muscle-strengthening activities on at least 2 days per week (Probst 2012). Furthermore, the IOPTMH advocates that patients should avoid physical inactivity, noting that some level of physical activity regardless of intensity is better than none (Vancampfort et al. 2012). People with severe mental illness should be supported and encouraged to adhere to physical activity recommendations; however, there is growing consensus that such recommendations may be aspirational and unrealistic for many people living with severe mental illness. Positive messaging around pragmatic goals such as breaking up sitting time throughout the day and aiming to increase short duration walking should be routinely promoted (Vancampfort et al. 2015a, 2015b). Mental health nurses can provide exercise advice and physical activity counselling to mental health patients (Happell et al. 2014; Stanton et al. 2015). Examples of pragmatic interventions include using objective monitoring devices such as pedometers (or commercially available accelerometers), individualised advice on ways to accumulate greater light physical activity such as rising from a chair and moving during television commercial breaks or adding brief 5-minute walks at structured and specified points throughout the day. This may include, for example, taking less direct routes while walking to dining rooms within inpatient facilities (Vancampfort et al. 2015b). Although such limited interventions may appear trivial, encouraging small and incremental changes may assist sedentary people with severe mental illness to transition to brief bouts of moderate-intensity activity that will help them to achieve guideline-specified targets.

ORAL HEALTH

Oral health is considered integral to general health and essential for wellbeing. It influences eating, physical appearance, speech and other social and psychological factors. Oral health issues include hygiene, dental caries (cavities), periodontal disease, dental trauma and oral cancers. Oral health also plays a vital role in cardiometabolic health, with periodontal disease increasing the risk of T2DM, coronary heart disease and stroke. People with SMI experience markedly higher rates of oral health problems compared with the general population (McKibbin et al. 2015). The reasons this population has poorer oral health outcomes in comparison with the general population are multifaceted. Many psychotropic medications can reduce the amount of saliva the mouth produces leading to a dry mouth, or xerostomia, which is associated with an increase in periodontal disease. Symptoms of mental illness such as depression, amotivation and cognitive impairment can lead to apathy around dental hygiene and considerably lower rates of regular teeth brushing and flossing, which are observed in people with SMI. People with SMI are also more likely to be smokers and consume high-sugar carbonated drinks, both of which promote the likelihood of dental disease.

Nursing Management of Oral Health

People with SMI are less likely to seek dental treatment than the general population, especially for preventative dental work. Given the higher risk of dental disease in this population, it is essential that people with SMI should attend to dental care more frequently than general public recommendations. Mental health nurses have a clear role in encouraging and facilitating access to dental services. It is also important that nurses use clinical interactions as an opportunity to promote oral health as a vital part of general health. Health promotion that focusses on smoking, diet, alcohol use and dental hygiene should be routinely incorporated into mental health nursing care.

CRITICAL THINKING CHALLENGE 8.6

Consider and discuss social and economic factors that influence an individual's oral health. Consider which nursing actions/strategies you could develop to change these factors.

SLEEP

Good sleep is essential for good physical and mental health. Sleep disturbance is a symptom of almost every mental disorder, from anxiety disorders to mood disorders and psychosis (Spiegelhalder et al. 2013). Though its significance is often under-recognised, sleep disturbance can in fact be one of the more distressing and persistent symptoms of mental disorder. Sleep disturbance can present as one of the first signs of mental illness exacerbation. Poor sleep can also independently contribute to causing a mental illness and impede the recovery from a mental illness. Recognising and treating sleep disturbance can therefore be critical to the primary or secondary prevention of mental disorders and their treatment.

Sleep Disturbance

What is normal sleep? Each person has a different sleep requirement and this changes over the lifespan. On average, most adults need 7 to 8 hours per night, adolescents 9 to 10 hours and children 11 to 13 hours or more (Colten & Altebogt 2006). *Insomnia* is the most common sleep disturbance. It is a core feature of mood disorders and frequently complicates anxiety disorders and psychosis. Anxiety and severe depression are commonly associated with sleep disturbance. In schizophrenia, the sleep cycle is often disturbed, with fragmented sleep throughout the cycle or even reversal of the sleep–wake cycle so that most sleep occurs during the day. *Hypersomnia* (excessive sleep) is less common but can occur in depression and in some cases of bipolar disorder. Hypersomnia can also occur secondary to some treatments of mental illness, which have sedative side effects.

Given the high rates of obesity in people with mental disorders, the risk of obstructive sleep apnoea is high and so it is important to screen for and to treat this disorder (Kalucy et al. 2013). Obstructive sleep apnoea is the most common form of sleep disorder. Untreated, it is associated with high morbidity and mortality because of increased risks of cardio- and cerebrovascular disease, worsening of diabetes and hypertension.

CRITICAL THINKING CHALLENGE 8.7

How might poor sleep impede a person's mental health recovery? Which nursing strategies can you implement to improve sleep for someone who is experiencing insomnia?

Nursing Assessment and Intervention of Sleep Disorders

The most important primary action is to ask about a person's sleep. Depending on the clinical setting, there may be an option for nurses to take an active role in the diagnosis and management of sleep problems. There are a number of useful screening and diagnostic tools, the most simple of which is a sleep diary (freely downloadable from the internet, e.g. http://yoursleep.aasmnet.org/pdf/sleepdiary.pdf) in which the person documents times spent sleeping and influential activities such as caffeine and alcohol intake, exercise and other activities such as electronic screen time.

In established sleep disorders, nurses may play an important role in encouraging patients to manage any lifestyle issues that may be contributing to their sleep problems (see Box 8.4). The use of sedative/hypnotic medications has a place but should not necessarily be the first form of treatment offered. Benzodiazepines have a propensity for addiction and are associated with an increased risk of falls, among other serious potential side effects. (See Chapter 25 for further details regarding medications and their side effects.)

BOX 8.4 Principles of Sleep Hygiene

- Go to sleep and wake up at roughly the same time each day.
- Maintain regular meal times.
- Avoid daytime naps.
- Don't eat a big meal or exercise within 2 hours of going to bed.
- Avoid caffeinated drinks after midday.
- Minimise alcohol and cease smoking.
- Ensure the bedroom is comfortable, dark, quiet and safe and used for only sleep and sex.
- Engage in exercise (avoid this at night) and exposure to bright outside light each day, preferably in the morning.
- Do not share the bed with children or pets.
- If sleep is not achieved within 20 to 30 minutes of going to bed, get up and do something relaxing for a few minutes and then try again when feeling sleepy.
- Ensure medications are taken as directed as some can cause sedation or arousal.
- Avoid stimulating activities before bedtime (e.g. watching a violent TV programme or exposure to the blue light emitted by computer or tablet screens).

(*Source*: Malcolm, A., 2005. The nurse role in managing and treating sleep disorders. Nursing Times 101(23), 34.)

SEXUAL HEALTH

Sexuality and sexual health are important aspects of every person's health and wellbeing. Sexuality is a complex issue that encompasses not only the physical activity of sex but also gender identity, values and beliefs (Quinn & Browne 2009). Contrary to common belief, most people with SMI show an interest in sex that differs little from the general population. High-risk sexual behaviours are more likely to be observed in people with SMI, including unprotected intercourse, multiple partners, involvement in sex work and illicit drug use. The rates of blood-borne viruses, such as HIV and hepatitis C, have been found to be higher among people with SMI.

Social and interpersonal impairments commonly occur in people with SMI and limit the development of stable sexual relationships. Men with SMI in particular have poorer social outcomes, fewer (sexual) relationships and fewer offspring than the general population (de Boer et al. 2015). Women with SMI are more likely to have relatively chaotic patterns of sexual behaviours and a higher rate of non-consensual sex than their counterparts without SMI (Pandor et al. 2015). A study found that women with SMI were far less likely to use effective contraception methods and had on average three unplanned pregnancies (Hauck et al. 2014).

Another study identified that mental health nurses don't ask about sexually related topics, with the authors concluding that mental health staff need to commit to being responsive to this important aspect of a person's wellbeing and health (Davison & Huntington 2010). This is echoed in another report that found mental health nurses are reluctant to bring up the topic of sexual health (Quinn et al. 2011). To enable you to feel comfortable and confident to discuss sexual health, you will need to identify any personal issues that affect your ability to openly discuss sexual health and increase your knowledge of sexual issues. Common issues that affect a person's sexuality and sexual health include sexually transmitted infections, body image, gender identity, physiological changes, medications and stigma.

CRITICAL THINKING CHALLENGE 8.8

1. Consider and discuss social, cultural and religious beliefs that influence an individual's sexuality.
2. Consider your own personal beliefs about sexuality. Do you have any preconceived ideas about mental illness and sexuality? Do you have any concerns about conducting a sexual health assessment?

Medication and Sex

Medication-induced sexual dysfunction is a common but largely ignored side effect of most psychotropic medications (de Boer et al. 2015). Psychotropic medications are linked with sexual dysfunction such as low libido and delayed ejaculation, orgasm problems such as anorgasmia and impaired erection. Medication-induced sexual dysfunctions can lead to issues with relationships, medication adherence and quality of life (Quinn et al. 2011). Despite the fact that people with SMI consider sexual health issues to be highly relevant, it is important to remember that issues such as sexual dysfunction are unlikely to be discussed, often because of the reluctance of health professionals and mental health nurses to talk about sex. This often leads to an underestimation of their prevalence and contributes to decreased adherence to treatment. Chapter 25 discusses psychotropic medication and their side effects.

Sexual Health Screening

Health screening includes preventative testing or investigation to prevent or to ameliorate future problems. Sexual health screening includes breast, prostate, cervical and sexually transmitted infection screening. Mental health nurses can play an important role in health screening, particularly when access to services is challenging for the person with a mental illness. The mental health nurse can refer the person directly to the health screening service or they can provide the health assessment. The mental health nurse can help prevent the contraction and spread of sexually transmitted infections by providing advice and education on safe sex, for example the correct use of condoms (Pandor et al. 2015). Breast, prostate and cervical screening services are generally offered by public health services. Given the vulnerability of patients with SMI, it is essential that nurses include sexual health screening as part of holistic care. Nurses should reflect on their personal attitudes and beliefs that might be creating barriers to a thorough sexual health assessment.

WHEN PSYCHIATRIC SYMPTOMS ARE NOT A MENTAL ILLNESS

Confusion, vision problems and behaviour changes can be common symptoms for many mental illnesses but they are also common symptoms of brain tumours, infectious diseases and dehydration. Correct assessment that includes history taking and checking with relatives will lead to correct diagnosis and not missing a physical health issue (see Chapter 22 for more details of accurate assessment). One example of a disease that may be misdiagnosed as a mental illness is Lyme disease. Lyme disease is a tick-borne disease that manifests symptoms in a variety of ways. Commonly, the person presents with psychiatric symptoms such as paranoia, anxiety and depressive symptoms and because the person often does not realise they have been in contact with a tick, correct diagnosis can be difficult (Hassett et al. 2009). It is important to conduct an MRI or CT scan of the brain during a first episode of psychosis to rule out any organic causes for symptoms, such as a tumour. The symptom similarities that can occur with depression, delirium and dementia are discussed in Chapter 12.

CONCLUSION

People who experience SMI have far higher rates of morbidity and mortality across nearly all chronic health conditions. This chapter has highlighted the importance of promoting, assessing and maintaining optimum physical health for people with SMI. Specific health assessments have been highlighted in this chapter—sexual health, oral health, sleep, metabolic syndrome, cardiovascular disease, diabetes and respiratory disease. However, it is important to remember that a full physical assessment, including routine health screening, is an essential element of holistic mental healthcare. The vital role that nurses can play in improving preventable illness and disease is clear. People with SMI have physical health outcomes that are far worse than the general population. If we are to improve the unacceptable life expectancy gap that is currently experienced by those with SMI, mental health nurses need to address this important issue with primary health messages and interventions. Smoking cessation, diet and exercise advice are core interventions crucially required for the prevention of premature cardiovascular disease. Awareness and advocating the screening and intervention of other areas of physical health (especially respiratory, sexual, oral and sleep) is extremely important to improve overall quality of life. Early intervention and prevention of physical health conditions is key to improving the outcomes of people with a mental illness. Mental health nurses need to prioritise physical healthcare as one of their primary responsibilities and this involves taking the time to listen and support people's needs in a holistic way.

EXERCISES FOR CLASS ENGAGEMENT

1. Maintaining optimum physical health is multifaceted and essential to wellbeing. Nurses play an important role in the assessment, treatment and prevention of physical health issues. Working in groups, discuss the following statements:
   - Sexual health is a human right.
   - Metabolic syndrome is preventable.
   - Oral health is an important part of overall health.
   - People with schizophrenia are likely to die 20–25 years earlier than the general population.
   - SMI is as much a risk factor of cardiovascular risk as a diagnosis of diabetes.
2. Working with your group, develop nursing interventions and strategies to ensure that the issues listed in the statements are assessed, treated and not overlooked. Consider which resources you will need to implement the strategies you have identified. Are there any barriers? How can these barriers be overcome?

REFERENCES

Alberti, K., Zimmet, P., Shaw, J., 2005. The metabolic syndrome—a new worldwide definition. Lancet 366 (9491), 1059–1062.

Aschbrenner, K.A., Brunette, M.F., McElvery, R., Naslund, J.A., Scherer, E.A., Pratt, S.I., Bartels, S.J., 2015. Cigarette smoking and interest in quitting among overweight and obese adults with serious mental illness enrolled in a fitness intervention. The Journal of Nervous and Mental Disease 203 (6) 47–46.

ASH Action on Smoking and Health, 2016a. High Rates of Smoking Among People with Serious Mental Health Conditions. Available at: http://ash.org.uk/media-and-news/press-releases-media-and-news/high-rates-of-smoking-among-people-with-serious-mental-health-conditions/. Accessed: 15 September 2018.

Action on Smoking and Health (ASH), 2016b. The Stolen Years–The Mental Health and Smoking Action Report. Available at: http://ash.org.uk/download/the-stolen-years-the-mental-health-and-smoking-action-report. Accessed: 17 September 2018.

Ashton, M., Rigby, A., Galletly, C., 2013. What do 1000 smokers with mental illness say about their tobacco use? Australian and New Zealand Journal of Psychiatry 47 (7), 631–636.

Bak, M., Fransen, A., Janssen, J., van Os, J., Drukker, M., 2014. Almost all antipsychotics result in weight gain: a meta-analysis. PloS one 9 (4), e94112.

Banham, L., Gilbody, S., 2010. Smoking cessation in severe mental illness: what works? Addiction 105 (7), 1176–1189.

Bressington, D., Mui, J., Ling Tse, M., Gray, R., Cheung, E., Tong Chien, W., 2016. Cardiometabolic health, prescribed antipsychotics and health-related quality of life in people with schizophrenia-spectrum disorders: a cross-sectional study. BMC Psychiatry 16, 411.

Brown, S., 1997. Excess mortality of schizophrenia. A meta-analysis. British Journal of Psychiatry 171, 502–508.

Brown, S., Kim, M., Mitchell, C., Inskip, H., 2010. Twenty-five year mortality of a community cohort with schizophrenia. The British Journal of Psychiatry 196 (2), 116–121.

Colten, H.R., Altebogt, B.M. (Eds.), 2006. Sleep Disorders and Sleep Deprivation, an Unmet Public Health Problem. The National Academies Press, Washington, DC.

Cuerda, C., Velasco, C., Merchan-Naranjo, J., Garcia-Peris, P., Arango, C., 2014. The effects of second-generation antipsychotics on food intake, resting energy expenditure and physical activity. European Journal of Clinical Nutrition 68 (2), 146–152.

Cuerda, C., Velasco, C., Merchán-Naranjo, J., García-Peris, P., Arango, C., 2013. The effects of second-generation antipsychotics on food intake, resting energy expenditure and physical activity. European Journal of Clinical Nutrition 68, 146–152.

Curtis, J., Watkins, A., Rosenbaum, S., Teasdale, S., Kalucy, M., Samaras, K., Ward, P.B., 2015. Evaluating an individualized lifestyle and life skills intervention to prevent antipsychotic-induced weight gain in first-episode psychosis. Early Intervention in Psychiatry 10, 267–276. https://doi.org/10.1111/eip.12230.

Davison, J., Huntington, A., 2010. 'Out of sight': sexuality and women with enduring mental illness. International Journal of Mental Health Nursing 19 (4), 240–249.

de Boer, M.K., Castelein, S., Wiersma, D., Schoevers, R.A., Knegtering, H., 2015. The facts about sexual (dys) function in schizophrenia: an overview of clinically relevant findings. Schizophrenia Bulletin 41 (3), 674–686.

De Hert, M., Schreurs, V., Vancampfort, D., Van Winkel, R., 2009. Metabolic syndrome in people with schizophrenia: a review. World Psychiatry 8 (1), 15–22.

De Hert, M., Vancampfort, D., Correll, C.U., Mercken, V., Peuskens, J., Sweers, K., van Winkel, R., Mitchell, A.J., 2011. Guidelines for screening and monitoring of cardiometabolic risk in schizophrenia: systematic evaluation. The British Journal of Psychiatry 199 (2), 99–105.

Dipasquale, S., Pariante, C.M., Dazzan, P., Aguglia, E., McGuire, P., Mondelli, V., 2013. The dietary pattern of patients with schizophrenia: a systematic review. Journal of Psychiatric Research 47 (2), 197–207.

Fleischhacker, W.W., Cetkovich-Bakmas, M., De Hert, M., Hennekens, C.H., Lambert, M., Leucht, S., Maj, M., McIntyre, R.S., Naber, D., Newcomer, J.W., 2008. Comorbid somatic illnesses in patients with severe mental disorders: clinical, policy, and research challenges. Journal of Clinical Psychiatry 69 (4), 514.

Forsyth, A.K., Williams, P.G., Deane, F.P., 2012. Nutrition status of primary care patients with depression and anxiety. Australian Journal of Primary Health 18 (2), 172–176.

Galletly, C.A., Foley, D.L., Waterreus, A., Watts, G.F., Castle, D.J., McGrath, J.J., Mackinnon, A., Morgan, V.A., 2012. Cardiometabolic risk factors in people with psychotic disorders: the second Australian national survey of psychosis. Australian and New Zealand Journal of Psychiatry 46 (8), 753–761.

Gartner, C., Hall, W., 2015. Tobacco harm reduction in people with serious mental illnesses. The Lancet Psychiatry 2 (6), 485–487.

Glassman, A.H., Bigger, J.T., 2014. Antipsychotic drugs: prolonged QTc interval, torsade de pointes, and sudden death. American Journal of Psychiatry 158 (11), 1774–1782.

Gordon-Dseagu, V.L., Mindell, J.S., Steptoe, A., Moody, A., Wardle, J., Demakakos, P., Shelton, N.J., 2015. Impaired glucose metabolism among those with and without diagnosed diabetes and mortality: a cohort study using health survey for England data. PloS One 10 (3), e0119882.

Hall, S.M., Prochaska, J.J., 2009. Treatment of smokers with co-occurring disorders: emphasis on integration in mental health and addiction treatment settings. Annual Review of Clinical Psychology 5, 409.

Happell, B., Stanton, R., Hoey, W., Scott, D., 2014. Cardiometabolic health nursing to improve health and primary care access in community mental health consumers: baseline physical health outcomes from a randomised controlled trial. Issues in Mental Health Nursing 35 (2), 114–121.

Hassett, A.L., Radvanski, D.C., Buyske, S., Savage, S.V., Sigal, L.H., 2009. Psychiatric comorbidity and other psychological factors in patients with "chronic Lyme disease". The American Journal of Medicine 122 (9), 843–885.

Hauck, Y., Nguyen, T., Frayne, J., Garefalakis, M., Rock, D., 2014. Sexual and reproductive health trends among women with en-

during mental illness: a survey of Western Australian community mental health services. Health Care for Women International 36 (4), 499–510.
Hjorth, P., Davidsen, A., Kilian, R., Skrubbeltrang, C., 2014. A systematic review of controlled interventions to reduce overweight and obesity in people with schizophrenia. Acta Psychiatrica Scandinavica 130 (4), 279–289.
Holt, R.I., Mitchell, A.J., 2014. Diabetes mellitus and severe mental illness: mechanisms and clinical implications. Nature Reviews Endocrinology 11 (2), 79–89.
Jacka, F.N., Kremer, P.J., Berk, M., de Silva-Sanigorski, A.M., Moodie, M., Leslie, E.R., Pasco, J.A., Swinburn, B.A., 2011. A prospective study of diet quality and mental health in adolescents. PLoS One 6 (9), e24805.
Jones, D.R., Macias, C., Barreira, P.J., Fisher, W.H., Hargreaves, W.A., Harding, C.M., 2014. Prevalence, severity, and co-occurrence of chronic physical health problems of persons with serious mental illness. Psychiatric Services 55 (11), 1250–1257.
Kalucy, M.J., Grunstein, R., Lambert, T., Glozier, N., 2013. Obstructive sleep apnoea and schizophrenia – A research agenda. Sleep Medicine Reviews 17 (5), 357–365. https://doi:310.1016/j.smrv.2012.1010.1003.
Kaur, J., 2014. A comprehensive review on metabolic syndrome. Cardiology Research and Practice 2014. https://doi.org/10.1155/2014/943162.
Kim, A., O'Hanlon, M., 2011. Caffeine and clinical change in a patient with schizophrenia on a long-stay ward. Irish Journal of Psychological Medicine 28 (1), 42–44.
Kimhy, D., Vakhrusheva, J., Bartels, M.N., Armstrong, H.F., Ballon, J.S., Khan, S., Chang, R.W., Hansen, M.C., Ayanruoh, L., Smith, E.E., 2014. Aerobic fitness and body mass index in individuals with schizophrenia: implications for neurocognition and daily functioning. Psychiatry Research 220 (3), 784–791.
Kisely, S., Quek, L.H., Pais, J., Lalloo, R., Johnson, N.W., Lawrence, D., 2011. Advanced dental disease in people with severe mental illness: systematic review and meta-analysis. The British Journal of Psychiatry 199 (3), 187–193.
Kisely, S., Baghaie, H., Lalloo, R., Siskind, D., Johnson, N.W., 2015. A systematic review and meta-analysis of the association between poor oral health and severe mental illness. Psychosomatic Medicine 77 (1), 83–92.
Lawrence, D., Hancock, K.J., Kisely, S., 2013. The gap in life expectancy from preventable physical illness in psychiatric patients in Western Australia: retrospective analysis of population based registers. British Medical Journal 346.
Malcolm, A., 2005. The nurse role in managing and treating sleep disorders. Nursing Times 101 (23), 34.
Mammen, G., Faulkner, G., 2013. Physical activity and the prevention of depression: a systematic review of prospective studies. American Journal of Preventive Medicine 45 (5), 649–657.
Mather, B., Roche, M., Duffield, C., 2014. Disparities in treatment of people with mental disorder in non-psychiatric hospitals: a review of the literature. Archives of Psychiatric Nursing 28 (2), 80–86.
McKibbin, C.L., Kitchen-Andren, K.A., Lee, A.A., Wykes, T.L., Bourassa, K.A., 2015. Oral health in adults with serious mental illness: needs for and perspectives on care. Community Mental Health Journal 51 (2), 222–228.
Mineur, Y.S., Picciotto, M.R., 2010. Nicotine receptors and depression: revisiting and revising the cholinergic hypothesis. Trends in Pharmacological Sciences 31 (12), 580–586.
Morgan, V.A., Waterreus, A., Jablensky, A., Mackinnon, A., McGrath, J.J., Carr, V., Bush, R., Castle, D., Cohen, M., Harvey, C., 2012. People living with psychotic illness in 2010: the second Australian national survey of psychosis. Australian and New Zealand Journal of Psychiatry 46 (8), 735–752.
Myles, N., Newall, H.D., Curtis, J., Nielssen, O., Shiers, D., Large, M., 2012. Tobacco use before, at, and after first-episode psychosis: a systematic meta-analysis. Journal of Clinical Psychiatry 73 (4), 468–475.
NHMRC, 2013. Australian Dietary Guidelines. National Health and Medical Research Council, Canberra.
NHS BMI Healthy Weight Calculator. https://www.nhs.uk/Tools/Pages/Healthyweightcalculator.aspx.
NHS England, 2018. Improving The Physical Health of Patients with Serious Mental Illness. Available at: https://www.england.nhs.uk/mental-health/resources/smi/. Accessed: 15 September 2018.
Nyboe, L., Lund, H., 2013. Low levels of physical activity in patients with severe mental illness. Nordic Journal of Psychiatry 67, 43–46.
Pandor, A., Kaltenthaler, E., Higgins, A., Lorimer, K., Smith, S., Wylie, K., Wong, R., 2015. Sexual health risk reduction interventions for people with severe mental illness: a systematic review. BMC Public Health 15 (1), 138.
Partti, K., Vasankari, T., Kanervisto, M., Perälä, J., Saarni, S.I., Jousilahti, P., Lönnqvist, J., Suvisaari, J., 2015. Lung function and respiratory diseases in people with psychosis: population-based study. The British Journal of Psychiatry 1, 9.
Pinto Pereira, S.M., Geoffroy, M., Power, C., 2014. Depressive symptoms and physical activity during 3 decades in adult life: Bidirectional associations in a prospective cohort study. JAMA Psychiatry 71 (12), 1373–1380.
Potvin, S., Zhornitsky, S., Stip, E., 2015. Antipsychotic-induced changes in blood levels of leptin in schizophrenia: a meta-analysis. Canadian Journal of Psychiatry. Revue canadienne de psychiatrie 60 (3 Suppl. 2), S26.
Probst, M., 2012. The International Organization of Physical Therapists working in Mental Health (IOPTMH). Mental Health and Physical Activity 5 (1), 20–21.
Quinn, C., Browne, G., 2009. Sexuality of people living with a mental illness: a collaborative challenge for mental health nurses. International Journal of Mental Health Nursing 18 (3), 195–203.
Quinn, C., Happell, B., Browne, G., 2011. Talking or avoiding? Mental health nurses' views about discussing sexual health with consumers. International Journal of Mental Health Nursing 20 (1), 21–28.
Reininghaus, U., Dutta, R., Dazzan, P., Doody, G.A., Fearon, P., Lappin, J., Heslin, M., Onyejiaka, A., Donoghue, K., Lomas, B., 2015. Mortality in schizophrenia and other psychoses: a 10-year follow-up of the ÆSOP First-Episode Cohort. Schizophrenia bulletin 41 (3), 664–673.
Ribe, A.R., Laursen, T.M., Sandbæk, A., Charles, M., Nordentoft, M., Vestergaard, M., 2014. Long-term mortality of persons with severe mental illness and diabetes: a population-based cohort study in Denmark. Psychological Medicine 44 (14), 3097–3107.
Rienks, J., Dobson, A., Mishra, G., 2013. Mediterranean dietary pattern and prevalence and incidence of depressive symptoms in mid-aged women: results from a large community-based prospective study. European Journal of Clinical Nutrition 67 (1), 75–82.
Ringen, P.A., Engh, J.A., Birkenaes, A.B., Dieset, I., Andreassen, O.A., 2014. Increased mortality in schizophrenia due to cardiovascular disease—a non-systematic review of epidemiology, possible causes, and interventions. Frontiers in Psychiatry 5, 137.
Rosenbaum, S., Lederman, O., Stubbs, B., Vancampfort, D., Stanton, R., Ward, P.B., 2015a. How can we increase physical activity and exercise among youth experiencing first episode psychosis? A systematic review of intervention variables. Early Intervention in Psychiatry. https://doi.org/10.1111/eip.12238.
Rosenbaum, S., Tiedemann, A., Ward, P.B., Curtis, J., Sherrington, C., 2015b. Physical activity interventions: an essential component in recovery from mental illness. British Journal of Sports Medicine 49 (24), 1544–1545.

Rosenbaum, S., Tiedemann, A., Sherrington, C., Curtis, J., Ward, P.B., 2014. Physical activity interventions for people with mental illness: a systematic review and meta-analysis. Journal of Clinical Psychiatry 75 (9), 964–974.

Royal College of Psychiatrists (RCPsych), 2016. Improving The Physical Health of Adults with Severe Mental Illness: Essential Actions. Available at: https://www.rcpsych.ac.uk/mediacentre/adultswithsmi.aspx. Accessed: 15 September 2018.

Rüther, T., Bobes, J., De Hert, M., Svensson, T.H., Mann, K., Batra, A., Gorwood, P., Möller, H.J., 2014. EPA Guidance on tobacco dependence and strategies for smoking cessation in people with mental illness. European Psychiatry 29 (2), 65–82.

Saha, S., Chant, D., McGrath, J., 2007. A systematic review of mortality in schizophrenia: is the differential mortality gap worsening over time? Archives of General Psychiatry 64 (10), 1123.

Schoepf, D., Uppal, H., Potluri, R., Heun, R., 2014. Physical comorbidity and its relevance on mortality in schizophrenia: a naturalistic 12-year follow-up in general hospital admissions. European Archives of Psychiatry and Clinical Neuroscience 264 (1), 3–28.

Smith, D.J., Langan, J., McLean, G., Guthrie, B., Mercer, S.W., 2013. Schizophrenia is associated with excess multiple physical-health comorbidities but low levels of recorded cardiovascular disease in primary care: cross-sectional study. BMJ Open 3 (4).

Smith, P.F., Smith, A., Miners, J., McNeil, J., Proudfoot, A., 2000. The safety aspects of dietary caffeine. Australia. Report from the expert working group 202–223.

Smith, P.H., Mazure, C.M., McKee, S.A., 2014. Smoking and mental illness in the US population. Tobacco Control 23 (e2), e147–e153.

Spiegelhalder, K., Regen, W., Nanovska, S., Baglioni, C., Riemann, D., 2013. Comorbid sleep disorders in neuropsychiatric disorders across the life cycle. Current Psychiatry Reports 15 (6), 364.

Stanton, R., Reaburn, P., Happell, B., 2015. Barriers to exercise prescription and participation in people with mental illness: the perspectives of nurses working in mental health. Journal of Psychiatric and Mental Health Nursing 22 (6), 440–448.

Steylen, P.M., van der Heijden, F.M., Kok, H.D., Sijben, N.A., Verhoeven, W.M., 2013. Cardiometabolic comorbidity in antipsychotic treated patients: need for systematic evaluation and treatment. International Journal of Psychiatry in Clinical Practice 17 (2), 125–130.

Stubbs, B., Vancampfort, D., De Hert, M., Mitchell, A., 2015. The prevalence and predictors of type two diabetes mellitus in people with schizophrenia: a systematic review and comparative meta-analysis. Acta Psychiatrica Scandinavica 132 (2), 144–157.

Subramaniam, M., Lam, M., Guo, M.E., He, V.Y., Lee, J., Verma, S., Chong, S.A., 2014. Body mass index, obesity, and psychopathology in patients with schizophrenia. Journal of Clinical Psychopharmacology 34 (1), 40–46.

Sweeting, J., Duflou, J., Semsarian, C., 2013. Postmortem analysis of cardiovascular deaths in schizophrenia: a 10-year review. Schizophrenia Research 150 (2), 398–403.

Thornicroft, G., 2011. Physical health disparities and mental illness: the scandal of premature mortality. The British Journal of Psychiatry 199 (6), 441–442.

Todd, R.A., Lewin, A.M., Bresee, L.C., Southern, D., Rabi, D.M., Investigators, A., 2014. Coronary artery disease in adults with schizophrenia: anatomy, treatment and outcomes. IJC Heart & Vessels 4, 84–89.

Tsuruga, K., Sugawara, N., Sato, Y., Saito, M., Furukori, H., Nakagami, T., Nakamura, K., Takahashi, I., Nakaji, S., Yasui-Furukori, N., 2015. Dietary patterns and schizophrenia: a comparison with healthy controls. Neuropsychiatric Disease and Treatment 11, 1115.

Üçok, A., İncesu, C., Aker, T., Erkoç, Ş., 2007. Sexual dysfunction in patients with schizophrenia on antipsychotic medication. European Psychiatry 22 (5), 328–333.

Vancampfort, D., De Hert, M., Skjerven, L., Gyllensten, A., Parker, A., Mulders, N., Nyboe, L., Spencer, F., Probst, M., 2012. International Organization of Physical Therapy in Mental Health consensus on physical activity within multidisciplinary rehabilitation programmes for minimising cardio-metabolic risk in patients with schizophrenia. Disability and Rehabilitation 34 (1), 1–12.

Vancampfort, D., Guelinkcx, H., Probst, M., Stubbs, B., Rosenbaum, S., Ward, P.B., De Hert, M., 2015. Associations between metabolic and aerobic fitness parameters in patients with schizophrenia. The Journal of Nervous and Mental Disease 203 (1), 23–27.

Vancampfort, D., Rosenbaum, S., Probst, M., Soundy, A., Mitchell, A.J., De Hert, M., Stubbs, B., 2015. Promotion of cardiorespiratory fitness in schizophrenia: a clinical overview and meta-analysis. Acta Psychiatrica Scandinavica Aug 132 (2), 131–143.

Vancampfort, D., Stubbs, B., Ward, P., Teasdale, S., Rosenbaum, S., 2015a. Integrating physical activity as medicine in the care of people with severe mental illness. Australian and New Zealand Journal of Psychiatry 49 (8), 681–682. https://doi.org/10.1177/0004867415590831.

Vancampfort, D., Stubbs, B., Ward, P.B., Teasdale, S., Rosenbaum, S., 2015b. Why moving more should be promoted for severe mental illness. The Lancet Psychiatry 2 (4), 295.

Ward, M.C., White, D.T., Druss, B.G., 2015. A meta-review of lifestyle interventions for cardiovascular risk factors in the general medical population: lessons for individuals with serious mental illness. The Journal of Clinical Psychiatry 76 (4), e477–e486.

Watkins, A., 2014. Keeping the body in mind. Australian Nursing and Midwifery Journal 21 (11), 44–45.

World Health Organization (WHO), 2008. The Right to Health Fact Sheet No. 31. WHO, Geneva. Available at: www.who.int/hhr/activities/Right_to_Health_factsheet31.pdf. Accessed: 4 February 2016.

Wing, V.C., Wass, C.E., Soh, D.W., George, T.P., 2012. A review of neurobiological vulnerability factors and treatment implications for comorbid tobacco dependence in schizophrenia. Annals of the New York Academy of Sciences 1248 (1), 89–106.

USEFUL WEBSITES

ASH Action on Smoking and Health, http://ash.org.uk/home

Bondi Keeping the Body in Mind Program, www.youtube.com/watch?v=dFBfIq9yS_4&feature=youtu.be

British Dental Association, https://bda.org

Family Planning Advice (the sexual health charity), https://www.fpa.org.uk

International Diabetes Federation, www.idf.org

Keeping the Body in Mind in Youth with Psychosis, www.iphys.org.au

Linking the Body and Mind podcast, www.abc.net.au/radionational/programs/allinthemind/new-document/4689134

NHS Smokefree, https://www.nhs.uk/smokefree

NHS Website Vaccinations: the flu vaccine. Available at: https://www.nhs.uk/conditions/vaccinations/flu-influenza-vaccine

Oral Health Foundation: Better oral health for all, https://www.dentalhealth.org

Sleep diary, http://yoursleep.aasmnet.org/pdf/sleepdiary.pdf

World Health Organization, www.who.int/en

PART 3

The People with Whom Mental Health Nurses Work

9

Mental Health and Wellness

Wendy M. Cross, Kim Ryan, Priscilla Anne Brebner and Patrica (Tish) Siaosi

KEY POINTS

- Understanding what constitutes mental health and wellness is vital in addressing factors that contribute to mental health and wellness and how these factors may also influence mental illness.
- Social determinants of health have a significant influence on the mental health and wellbeing of individuals and communities.
- An appreciation of the prevalence of mental health problems and disorders assists mental health nurses to understand the impact of mental disorders on the health outcomes of individuals, the healthcare system and the demand for community services.
- The degree of disability associated with mental disorders influences a person's ability to function in all aspects of their life.
- The outcomes for people with mental health problems are influenced by many factors.
- Culture consists of learned behaviours and beliefs, passed on by one generation to another, through learning and tradition, which assists the individual to understand their experiences and promote social conduct including health decisions.
- Cultural awareness enhances mental health nurses' ability to offer individualised, holistic care within a therapeutic relationship and to value the contribution of cultural interventions to the therapeutic milieu.
- Openness to diversity in cultures offers mental health nurses the opportunity to reflect on their own beliefs and values about health, what it means to be healthy and what they understand as mental wellbeing.
- Culturally competent mental health nurses aim to 'enter' the patient's experience while maintaining a strongly rooted sense of their own lived experience.
- Culturally safe care is that which is deemed culturally safe by service users and their families.

KEY TERMS

comorbidity
culture
cultural awareness
cultural competence
cultural safety
cultural sensitivity
disability
diversity
ethnocentrism
incidence
mental disorder
mental health
mental illness
mortality
prevalence
service user
social determinants of health
stigma
wellness

LEARNING OUTCOMES

The material in this chapter will assist you to:

- understand the nature of mental health and wellness and the factors that influence them.
- become aware of the prevalence of mental disorders and the impact they have on the individual, communities and society.
- explain the impact of social determinants on mental health and social and emotional wellbeing.
- understand the concept of disability in relation to mental illness and how degrees of disability are determined.
- appreciate the negative influence of misconceptions and discrimination experienced by people with a mental health problem.
- describe the relevance of cultural issues to mental health outcomes for service users, their family, friends and carers.
- understand the importance of cultural diversity in negotiating healthcare strategies that achieve outcomes approved by service users.
- recognise the importance of self-reflection in the delivery of culturally safe mental health nursing care.
- appreciate how mental health nurses and others can positively influence mental health outcomes for service users, carers and communities.

INTRODUCTION

This chapter explores mental health and wellbeing, the factors that influence them and how these factors may also determine the development of a mental health problem. Social determinants of health are discussed with particular focus on implications for mental health. The chapter discusses the prevalence of mental health problems in the UK and their impact on the individual, their family, carers and health systems. The role of the media in shaping opinions and ideas is also examined. Factors such as misconceptions, stigma and stereotyping are explored and shown to have the potential to contribute to the degree of disability experienced by a person who is unwell or in the process of recovery.

This chapter also examines the impact of culture on the way in which mental health problems are perceived and managed by individuals and communities. Models of cultural sensitivity and cultural safety are introduced and the importance of self-reflection in mental health nursing practice in the delivery of culturally safe mental healthcare that takes into account the needs of the individual, their family and/or community is emphasised.

MENTAL HEALTH AND WELLNESS

Mental health is a psychological state where a person functions at a suitable level of emotional and behavioural stability and comprises the person's ability to enjoy life and balance life events and energies to achieve psychological equilibrium. The World Health Organization (WHO 2015) states that mental health includes 'subjective wellbeing, perceived self-efficacy, autonomy, competence, intergenerational dependence, and self-actualization of one's intellectual and emotional potential, among others'. The wellbeing of a person is embodied in the achievement of their abilities, coping with normal life stressors, working productively and contributing to the community (WHO 2015). Other definitions of mental health reflect cultural variances, subjective appraisals and diverse professional theories (WHO 2015). WHO emphasises that health covers a state of complete physical, mental and social wellbeing and not simply the absence of disease or illness.

Wellbeing is not the same as happiness, which can fluctuate. Wellbeing is a consistent state of being well, satisfied and content. Most of us attempt to improve our own wellbeing and quality of life, as well as the lives of those important to us (SANE 2018). According to the mental health charity Mind (2018), mental wellbeing describes a person's mental state, i.e. how they are feeling and how well they can cope with day-to-day life. Wellbeing is dynamic and can change from moment to moment, but if a person has good mental wellbeing they are able:

- to feel relatively confident in themselves and have positive self-esteem
- to feel and express a range of emotions
- to build and maintain good relationships with others
- to feel engaged with the world around them
- to live and work productively
- to cope with the stresses of daily life
- to adapt and manage in times of change and uncertainty

Therefore, a person's wellbeing is like a network, built not only on mental and physical wellness, but also on multifaceted social dynamics and perceived security.

A number of organisations across the UK work with people in all walks of life to promote mental health and wellbeing. For example, the charity Mind (2018) was initially established in 1946, called The National Association for Mental Health when three major mental health organisations were merged:

- Central Association for Mental Welfare (established 1913) led by the pioneering Dame Evelyn Fox, an organisation that worked with local groups of volunteers to help people who were mentally unwell.
- National Council for Mental Hygiene (established 1922), which had a strong educational bias and stressed the social causes of mental illness.
- Child Guidance Council (established 1927), which set up the first child guidance clinics and launched training courses for their staff.

Mind: for better mental health (2018) https://www.mind.org.uk provides advice and support to empower anyone experiencing a mental health problem; campaigning to improve services, raise awareness and promote understanding.

SANE was established in 1986 by Marjorie Wallace, who wrote a series of articles published in *The Times* entitled The Forgotten Illness, which received overwhelming public response. The articles exposed the neglect of people suffering from mental illness and the poverty of services and information for individuals and families. SANE's vision is to raise public awareness and combat stigma about mental illness; provide care and emotional support for people with mental health problems, their families and carers as well as information for other organisations and the public; excite research into the causes and treatments of serious mental illness such as schizophrenia and depression and the psychological and social impact of mental illness. SANE founded the Prince of Wales International Centre for SANE Research in Oxford in 2003, sharing this with the Oxford Mindfulness Centre, which provides mindfulness-based cognitive therapy training, integrating brain research with meditation techniques (SANE 2018). Samaritans (2018) was founded by a vicar called Chad Varah and established in London 1953. The idea for the charity came from a funeral he conducted for a 14-year-old girl; she had started her period but had no-one to talk to about this, believed that she had a sexually transmitted disease and took her own life. Chad was immensely moved by this tragic loss of life and launched Samaritans, which he called '999 for the suicidal, a man willing to listen, with a base and an emergency telephone'. Samaritans now has over 20,000 volunteers based in 201 branches across the 4 UK nations, offering 24-hour a day telephone support to people in need 7 days a week. They also work with schools, colleges and universities, workplaces, health and welfare services, homeless shelters, prisons and other charities to promote awareness of the service, including at social venues, community events and music festivals (Samaritans 2018).

Rethink Mental Illness was established in 1972 after journalist John Pringle wrote a column in *The Times* newspaper about his son's experience of schizophrenia; 400 people contacted John in response to the article and the Schizophrenia Fellowship was launched in 1972. This became the National Schizophrenia Fellowship in 1974 until 2002 when the organisation was renamed Rethink, reflecting the work done across mental health issues beyond schizophrenia. In 2011 the name was changed to its current brand, Rethink Mental Illness, calling for the public to reconsider the views they might hold about mental illness (Rethink 2018).

There are numerous organisations and charities throughout the UK (see Useful Websites) providing services and programmes to people with mental health problems and the families, friends and carers of those people. Quality support services in the community enable people to stay well for longer, remain connected with their family, friends and community and achieve a better quality of life. These organisations support people in the essential areas of their lives: home, work and relationships. They are able to signpost people to the most appropriate point of care and link with people with education and employment opportunities, to locate and to establish homes connecting them with their communities and to develop helpful relationships with families and friends. They are based on recovery models, focussing on the process that is defined and directed by the person with a mental health problem. This leads to greater independence, improved self-esteem and a meaningful quality of life in society. People are able to receive support in developing the personal resources they need in their recovery (hope, resilience, coping skills, self-acceptance and physical health) as well as accessing services that can help to empower them to achieve recovery and independence (secure accommodation, education, work etc.).

There are also specific organisations that focus on the wellbeing of children. One such initiative is the National Society for the Prevention of Cruelty to Children (NSPCC), which works across the UK, Channel Islands and Isle of Man. The NSPCC (2018) https://www.nspcc.org.uk states that 1 in 5 children in the UK has suffered abuse or neglect. Their vision is to protect children today and prevent abuse from happening tomorrow (NSPCC 2018), which includes running the Childline 24-hour telephone service https://www.nspcc.org.uk/preventing-abuse/our-services/childline/.

SOCIAL DETERMINANTS OF MENTAL HEALTH

According to the WHO, 'The social determinants of health (SDH) are the conditions in which people are born, grow, work, live, and age, and the wider set of forces and systems shaping the conditions of daily life. These forces and systems include economic policies and systems, development agendas, social norms, social policies and political systems' (www.who.int/social_determinants/en). Broadly speaking, health determinants include anything that contributes to the health of a population including the effects of behaviours on risks to health. Keleher and Murphy (2004) outline four determinants that interact in complex ways to produce overall outcomes for health: social, environmental, economic and biological.

Understanding the determinants of health leads to greater mental health promotion, prevention and early intervention. This in turn enhances social and emotional wellbeing within the community; reduces the incidence and prevalence of mental health problems and their associated effects; and augments the scope, features and suitability of approaches to improve mental health (WHO 2013). The independent Mental Health Taskforce created the Five Year Forward View for Mental Health (2016) aiming to improve access to mental health services through promotion of mental health, prevention of mental health problems, improved service quality and responsiveness and support for research, innovation and sustainability.

The Ottawa Charter (WHO 2015) sets out five principles that underpin health promotion policies:

1. Public policies must support health and policy-makers must be aware of the impact of their decisions on health.
2. Healthy living environments using a socioecological approach have positive health benefits and safeguard the natural and built environments.
3. Enabling communities offers ownership and power to people regarding their destinies.
4. The development of personal skills through provision of health information and education to promote healthy choices.
5. The obligation for promoting health is shared among individuals, groups, health professionals, service providers and governments.

The determinants of health are: housing, food, income, education, peace, social justice and equity, stable and sustainable environments and resources. With the countries of the UK being developed countries with stable political structures, established systems for addressing concerns about the environment and sustainability and sophisticated health services, they generally score well in relation to determinants of health. Nevertheless, certain groups clearly experience health outcomes lower than population norms. People with a disability, those who are socially and economically disadvantaged and prisoners are more likely than the general population to suffer from chronic illnesses or to have shorter lifespans (Morgan et al. 2014).

Housing and Food

Quality housing is affordable, secure, well maintained and not crowded. Housing insecurity can be a result of unemployment, income insecurity, low housing stock, high rents or high mortgage interest rates. Inadequate housing and homelessness are factors that affect health outcomes.

Homelessness takes many forms, but the most visible are the rough sleepers—those sleeping on the streets, in empty buildings, doorways and car parks. The Ministry of Housing, Communities and Local Government (2018) Rough Sleeping Statistics Autumn 2017 (England) reported the total number of rough sleepers counted and estimated was 4751. There is a chronic shortage of affordable housing, and while government attempt to address the issue, resources remain inadequate. Insufficient funding, combined with greater numbers of people seeking help, puts pressure on services for the homeless. Recent data from the Ministry of Housing, Communities and Local Government (2018) identified that between 1 January and 31 March 2018 local authorities accepted 13,300 households as being statutorily homeless. Homeless people come from all walks of life and include young and old, mothers and children, families and single people.

A number of charities and organisations provide support and provide advocacy for homeless people, such as Shelter, Homeless Link and Centre Point, which specifically provides services to young people (see Useful Web Sites)

Most Western populations take the local supermarket and regular nutritious meals for granted, but there are groups who cannot rely on access to sufficient nutrition on a daily basis. Food insecurity may be due to poverty, when unexpected expenses can derail a precariously balanced budget. Low prices and convenience make 'fast food' attractive to people who may be time poor or budgeting on a low income. More fast-food outlets exist in low socioeconomic areas (Inagami et al. 2009).

Remoteness can also be a factor. Where communities rely on road or sea transport to ensure regular deliveries of foodstuffs over long distances, freshness may suffer and high costs may place nutritious food out of reach for people on a restricted budget. For children, who are generally not able to secure their own food supply, food insecurity may result from parental decisions on budgetary priorities.

Where food insecurity exists, malnutrition may impact physical, social and mental health and development. Children who are malnourished or hungry do not achieve in school, compounding future disadvantage (Vinson 2009).

Activity, Employment and Income

Particularly relevant to mental health outcomes is access to employment and meaningful activity. Meaningful activity, just as much as paid employment, is part of a balanced lifestyle and gives access to social interaction and social inclusion, which are overarching social determinants (Ottawa Charter). WHO 2015 Meaningful activity includes education and training, hobbies and other leisure activities, parenting and caring, and volunteering. Meaningful activity and employment are strong factors in recovery from mental disorder and are recognised as such by people with mental illness. Mind (2015) found that over a third of people with mild to moderate mental health problems, and almost two-thirds of people with more severe mental health problems, were unemployed in 2015.

While it is known that some aspects of the work environment or unstable work can contribute to stress, work is nevertheless better for a person's mental health than unemployment (Mind 2015). Employment is strongly associated with positive mental health, including higher self-esteem and a sense of agency and purpose, whereas lack of employment erodes sense of purpose and identity (Raeburn et al. 2015). Long-term unemployment is associated with depression, low self-esteem and social isolation and contributes to the cycle of disadvantage.

Across the UK, governments make allowances and benefits available to ensure that no person need experience extreme poverty. However, within all countries there is unequal access to national wealth, and insecurity and stress that accompany a lack of income security. According to The Institute for Fiscal Studies (2018), the incomes of poorer households have been growing, but they have not grown as fast as that of middle income, with overall relative poverty figures sitting around 21% to 22%, with absolute child poverty reported to be at 26% in 2016 to 2017. People who have experienced disadvantage in early life are at greater risk of disadvantage at all critical points across their lifespan (Vinson 2009). Furthermore, disadvantages and their effects tend to accumulate throughout life and are passed across generations.

Research shows significantly increased rates of depression among low socioeconomic groups and in countries with higher levels of income inequality (Patel et al. 2010). While poverty is not the only determinant of disadvantage, unequal access to income has potentiating effects as it reduces the ability to access necessities such as secure housing, nutrition, transport and safety. In turn, these may affect the ability to access employment, education, health and community services and justice and may lead to social disconnectedness, isolation or exclusion. This is cyclical and may lead to intergenerational disadvantage (Vinson 2009).

Education

There is a strong relationship between educational attainment and health outcomes for individuals and societies. Patel et al. (2010) note a strong 'dose-relation' between education and rates of depression among populations. The UK has a diverse and multicultural population and access to mainstream education might be affected for migrant populations where English is not their first language. Cultural factors may also influence parental attitudes to the importance of education, as well as potential gender biases. Educating children not only increases their own health knowledge and empowerment, but also leads to improved health and education for their children and increased earning ability for families and communities. Empowerment and enhanced decision-making capacity increase advantage at all stages in life and in the case of women this advantage crosses generations: advantage is passed on to offspring (Sridhar 2008; UNICEF, 2015).

Peace

Every person has the right to a peaceful life, devoid of the difficulties associated with violence. Most people raised in the UK, with the exception of those in the armed forces and aid agencies working in war zones, have not experienced war or insurrection. However, some migrants are refugees from war and may also be survivors of torture (Green and Eagar 2010). Exposure to violence and trauma has serious effects on mental health and there is now ample international research indicating that the effects of trauma can present in many ways (Ball & Links 2009; Shevlin et al. 2007).

Others may experience family violence and recent exposure and public awareness have garnered support for various agencies to address this issue. Family violence, also known as domestic violence, relationship violence, spousal violence, intimate partner violence and gender-based violence, refers to acts of violence that occur within intimate relationships and take place in domestic settings. It includes physical, sexual, financial, emotional and psychological abuse. Women are more likely than men to be victims of family violence; however, the number of reports from men is rising.

Social Connectedness, Justice and Equity

Social justice and equity embody a community's aspirations and expectations of being treated fairly. Social equity is recognised as a driving principle for mental health policy and programme development. Human beings are social by nature: we need to feel valued by family and friends and that we are useful to others and contributing to society. If these needs are not met, we are prone to depression, anxiety and other mental and physical health problems (Wilkinson & Marmot 2003). A number of studies have shown that stable intimate relationships and, in particular, marriage have a protective effect for mental health (Whisman & Baucom 2011).

Mental health problems are closely associated with social exclusion and social exclusion is compounded by social inequality. Recovery model practices and resilience building capabilities as endorsed by the Nursing and Midwifery Council (NMC 2016) remind mental health nurses of their pivotal position in empowering patients, families and communities to build on strengths and social supports in institutional as well as private settings. Nurses are ideally placed to support people to remain included and valued members of society.

Gender inequality increases the risk of vulnerability to depression among women, although biological factors also contribute to the increased risk (Patel et al. 2010). Women with children face greater problems than men for transportation, economic support and childcare (Popay et al. 2008). The prevalence of depression and anxiety disorders is higher in women. However, males have a higher prevalence of attention deficit hyperactivity disorder and conduct disorder than females (ABS 2008). This can lead to problems associated with the legal system and a higher use of mental health facilities for male children and adolescents.

Females are more likely than males to report long-term mental or behavioural problems and are more likely than males to report high to very high levels of psychological distress (ABS 2008). Although women access health services, they may have concerns about taking medication for their illness if they are pregnant, are likely to become pregnant or are breastfeeding. A pregnant woman or nursing mother may well be limited in the medications she is able to take, leaving her susceptible to relapse as a result of inadequate treatment (McCauley-Elsom & Kulkarni 2007). Hormonal changes may also affect women, especially after childbirth, with some women experiencing their first episode of mental illness at this time (McCauley-Elsom & Kulkarni 2007).

Men with severe mental illnesses such as schizophrenia generally have worse outcomes than females, as measured by early onset, cognitive disabilities and social impairments. The earlier onset usually prevents males from developing personal relationships, which leads to many remaining single and childless and with reduced employment prospects (Ochoa et al. 2012).

Social exclusion also affects members of minority groups. Research shows a strong association between direct personal experiences of racism and ill health among a number of minority groups in developed countries. Ethnicity contributes to low utilisation of mental health services as well as social exclusion because fear and stigma are attached to behaviours that cannot be understood by families and communities. For many centuries and in many societies, exclusion has been the management of choice for mental illness (Cross & Singh 2012).

Of all groups in society, those incarcerated in the correctional system are socially excluded by necessity. International research consistently shows that prisoners have high rates of mental health problems. The National Audit Office (2017) reports that in 2016 there were 40,161 incidents of self-harm in prisons and 120 self-inflicted deaths; however, further work is required for the government to understand fully how many people in prison have a mental illness, how much is spent on mental health in prisons or whether it is achieving its objectives.

Imprisonment may also relate to other social factors. There is strong evidence of an association between a history of psychiatric hospitalisation and homelessness, especially after deinstitutionalisation. Homeless mentally ill people are also 40 times more likely to be arrested and 20 times more likely to be imprisoned than those with stable accommodation (Willis 2005).

For refugees, immigration detention compounds the preexisting effects of migration and trauma. Green and Eagar (2010) found that the rate of mental illness among refugees was highest for those designated 'unauthorised boat arrivals' than for other groups ('visa breach', 'visa overstay' and 'illegal foreign fisher'). Time in detention was found to have a significant additional effect: people who were detained for more than 2 years had rates of new mental illness 3.6 times higher than those who were released within 3 months. Triggs (2013) states that there have long been concerns about mental health outcomes for people in detention. She recommends the use of more humane strategies, given that 88% of asylum seekers in 2012–2013 were found to be refugees.

Stable and Sustainable Environments and Resources

'Environmental health comprises those aspects of human health, including quality of life, that are determined by physical, chemical, biological, and social and psychological problems in the environment. It also refers to the theory and practice of assessing, correcting, controlling, and preventing those factors in the environment that can potentially affect adversely the health of present and future generations' (WHO 2006, paragraph 1).

According to the Office of Disease Prevention and Health Promotion (2015), in its *Healthy People 2020*, a set of consensus-built objectives was established for public health focussing on the following six themes.

- *Outdoor air quality.* We need good-quality air to sustain life. Poor air quality is linked to premature death, cancer and long-term damage to respiratory and cardiovascular systems. Decreasing air pollution is an important step in creating a healthy environment.
- *Surface and ground water.* Surface and ground water quality applies to both drinking water and recreational waters. Contamination by infectious agents or chemicals can cause a variety of illnesses. Protecting water sources is an important component of environmental health.
- *Toxic substances and hazardous wastes.* The health effects of toxic substances and hazardous wastes are unclear. Research to appreciate fully how they may influence health is continuing, as are efforts to reduce exposure.
- *Homes and communities.* People spend most of their time at home, work or school. Some of these environments may expose people to indoor air pollution, inadequate heating and sanitation, structural problems, electrical and fire hazards and lead-based paint hazards. These threats affect health and safety.
- *Infrastructure and surveillance.* Prevention of exposure to environmental hazards depends on multiple partnerships, including between many government departments. People, data collection systems and education are important means for examining and responding to health problems, monitoring for threats and enlightening the public.
- *Global environmental health.* Water quality is an important global challenge. Diseases can be reduced by improving water quality and sanitation and increasing access to adequate water and sanitation facilities.

Healthy People 2020 has also identified several other environmental health concerns, including climate change, nanotechnologies, lead poisoning, disaster preparedness and the built environment, which appear to influence behaviours, physical activity patterns, social networks and access to resources.

Environmental health has a significant impact on the mental health of individuals and communities. Two examples of environmental contaminants that can find their way into the human body are mercury and lead. An accumulation of mercury in the brain may cause depression because mercury disturbs some neurotransmitters and this leads to lowered mood and lethargy. Similarly, lead affects the central nervous system causing neurological damage, cognitive dysfunction and behavioural problems. This is particularly noticeable in children, where high lead levels can contribute to hyperactivity, diminished play activity and difficulty learning. Infections such as meningitis, mumps and rabies may also lead to brain damage, affecting mental health.

THE INCIDENCE AND PREVALENCE OF MENTAL HEALTH PROBLEMS

Mental health problems cause considerable personal, social and financial distress to individuals and have a huge impact on healthcare funding, the implementation of service provision and community resources. In order to gauge the full extent of the problem, many countries have conducted research into the prevalence and consequent impact of mental health problems on the individual, society and healthcare funds. However, stigma can lead to considerable under-reporting of mental health problems. For example, in China and India an improved counting method showed that suicide rates are much higher than those reported in routine statistics and that self-inflicted injuries account for a quarter to half of all deaths in young women (Patel et al. 2010).

The English government has conducted extensive research to determine the prevalence of mental health problems in the community and the impact this has had on the individual, the community and government spending. A brief overview of these findings is presented below.

Five Year Forward View for Mental Health

In 2015 the independent Mental Health Taskforce was formed by NHS England, the body responsible for the delivery of the NHS on behalf of the government. The Taskforce brought together health and social care leaders, professional bodies and experts by experience; chaired by Paul Farmer (Mind CEO) and vice-chair Jacqui Dyer, an expert by experience. The Taskforce was asked to develop a 5-year strategy for mental health, resulting in the Five Year Forward View for Mental Health for the NHS in England (NHS England 2016a). Significant research was carried out and over 20,000 people gave their views to the Taskforce, including people with personal experiences of mental ill health, families, carers and professionals. The top priorities that came out of the engagement work were: improvements in access to high-quality services, choice of interventions, integrated physical and mental health care, prevention initiatives, funding and challenging stigma (NHS England 2016a). Alongside the Five Year Forward View, an implementation plan was also published (Implementing the Five Year Forward View for Mental Health, NHS England 2016b). This was to ensure cross-system working across the health delivery partners to meet the recommendations made by the Taskforce. The following is a summary of the key mental health problems identified within the population.

One in four adults is thought to experience at least one diagnosable mental health problem in any given year, with the cost to the economy estimated at £105 billion a year. Suicide rates in England have steadily increased, peaking at 4882 deaths in 2014. The rise is mostly among middle-aged men, now the leading cause of male deaths between 15 and 49 years, with men three times more likely to take their own lives than women. One in five older people in the community and 40% of people living in care homes are affected by depression.

By the age of 14 years, half of all metal health problems have been established, with 75% by the age of 24 years. One in ten children (5–16 years) have a diagnosable disorder such as conduct disorder (6%), anxiety disorder (3%), attention deficit hyperactivity disorder (2%) or depression (2%). Children from low-income families are at the highest risk. As a result, children with a conduct disorder are twice as likely to leave school without any qualifications, three times more likely to become a teenage parent, four times more likely to become dependent on drugs and 20 times more likely to end up in prison. Most young people did not access support and those who did had to wait for routine psychological therapy on average for 32 weeks (2015/16). If they required inpatient services, many were sent far from home due to inequality in service provision, with long distances from families and friends.

Maternal health problems affect one in five mothers; depression, anxiety or psychosis during pregnancy or in the first year after birth. After cardiovascular disease, suicide is the second leading cause of maternal death; however, perinatal mental health services for women with severe or complex conditions are provided at fewer than 15% of localities, with 40% offering no service at all. The mental health of mothers not only affects the women but can also have longstanding effects on the children's mental health, social and cognitive development.

Increasingly, the links between physical and mental health are being recognised, with people with severe and prolonged mental illness at risk of dying 15 to 20 years younger than the general population, which is one of the greatest health inequalities in the UK (see Chapter 8, Physical Health). Many of these deaths are avoidable, with two-thirds being from preventable illnesses, cancer and heart disease, often caused by smoking.

It is also noted that people most at risk of poor mental health are people from marginalised groups, including black, Asian and minority ethnic people (BAME), lesbian, gay, bisexual and transgender people, disabled people, homeless people and people who have had contact with the criminal justice system. It is suggested that as many as 9 out of 10 people in prison have mental health, drug or alcohol issues. People from BAME households were found to be more likely to live in poorer, over-crowded conditions, increasing their risks of developing mental ill health (NHS England 2016a).

THE COST OF MENTAL HEALTH PROBLEMS

The direct monetary cost of mental health problems is high. It is estimated that poor mental health carries an economic and social cost of £105 billion a year in England, which is approximately the cost of the entire National Health Service (NHS England 2016a). The analysis carried out by NHS England (2016a) suggests that national cost of services dedicated to mental health support across government departments in England is £34 billion each year (excluding substance abuse and dementia). Nineteen billion of this is said to be through government spending; however, there is little data available as to how 67% of this money is spent at local level. The remaining £14+ billion is spent on the support provided to unpaid carers and to voluntary and private sectors.

The Five Year Forward View (NHS England 2016a) highlights the chronic underinvestment made across mental health services and recommends that the efficiencies made through achieving better value for money should be reinvested to address the unmet needs of people with mental ill health of all ages across England. These figures do not take into account the hidden (indirect) costs of mental health problems, i.e. the health costs and loss of earnings for families and carers, the community and welfare costs, charity agencies and coronial work in the case of suicide. The actual cost of mental health problems is unknown and probably underestimated.

DISABILITY AND MENTAL HEALTH

Disability in mental health refers to an individual's impairment in one or more important areas of functioning. The worldwide burden of mental health problems and disorders is high and expected to increase.

The WHO regularly assesses disability adjusted life years (DALYs) on a global scale. DALYs are a measure of the burden of ill health obtained by calculating potential years of healthy life lost by virtue of being in a state of poor health or disability. Although mortality from mental health problems is not considered high, the impact of chronic disability on an individual's life can be measured in days out of their normal role. According to the World Health Organisation (WHO 2014), mental disorders are the largest contributor to years lived with disability (YLD) in Europe, accounting for 36.1%, which ranks neuropsychiatric disorders as the first cause of YLD. The leading chronic condition in Europe was unipolar depressive disorder making up 11% of all YDL.

Mental health problems cause considerable distress for individuals, families and friends, as well as contributing to absenteeism from work or school and to the extensive use of community support services such as crisis lines and welfare groups. Mental disorders are more prevalent in the young and therefore these people may face significant disabilities at a stage of their lives when they are completing education and establishing relationships and independence.

People with some mental health problems such as psychotic disorders or severe depression may find it a challenge to adequately attend to their personal needs, to shop and/or to prepare meals or to make sure their environment is clean and safe, thereby placing their physical wellbeing in jeopardy. Poor physical health places a greater burden on the sufferer, their family, the community and the healthcare system. A significant number of people with mental health problems live below the poverty line and require assistance from welfare groups (government and non-government). Even with assistance, some people may not have the means to provide adequate nutritious food, heating, clothing, housing, electricity, telephone or furniture for themselves and their families. Some housing and accommodation is available through a number of agencies, but the demand is greater than the resources available (Pinches 2002). A relatively small number have turbulent illnesses and often find that they are evicted from accommodation because of disruptive behaviour (Robinson 2003). Many welfare agencies run homeless shelters but have limited resources to deal with the complex needs of those with mental disorders.

MISCONCEPTIONS ABOUT MENTAL HEALTH PROBLEMS

Being diagnosed with any long-term health condition is distressing and a diagnosis of a mental health problem can be quite devastating because of people's lack of understanding of the problem. All diagnoses are socially constructed; that is, they are determined by sociological factors. Simply naming an illness allows the process and framework for treatment and care. The DSM-5 is an excellent example of the growing extent of diagnosis in mental health. Walsh and Cross (2013) note the increasing number of diagnoses in mental health and the corresponding pre-eminence of the DSM. According to Conrad and Barker (2010) three factors interact to determine the meaning of illness.

1. Culture influences how society reacts to people affected and impacts the experience of that illness.
2. As people experience illness they come to understand it, build their identity around it and live with and in spite of it, constructing their personal view over time.
3. Medical knowledge about disease is not automatically objective. It is created and established by those with vested interests, who often have a focus on outcomes. Conrad and Barker (2010) note that this does not quash scientific and medical standpoints but demonstrates that diseases and illnesses are determined socially as much as scientifically.

When negative misconceptions, stigma and discrimination accompany a diagnosis, the illness can seem insurmountable to those concerned. Misconceptions regarding mental health problems have a deleterious impact on the perception of mental health issues. Some commonly held misconceptions are:

- All people with mental health problems are unpredictable, violent and dangerous.
- People who are mentally ill have an intellectual disability or brain damage.
- People with a mental health problem will never recover.
- People with a mental health problem should be locked up and kept away from society.
- People who have schizophrenia have a split personality.

Unfortunately, misconceptions have influenced the general perception and the treatment of people with mental health problems for centuries. Ignorance and fear remain prevalent in the community, reinforcing the need for wide-ranging education as a means of increasing public awareness of mental health issues (SANE 2018; Wylie & Brown 2011).

People who develop mental disorders may have had their own preconceived ideas and prejudices with regard to mental health problems. Many believe it is the end of their life and will grieve for the life they had and for the aspirations they held for their future. While people are unwell, work or study can be interrupted, leading to financial hardship and exacerbating the feelings of frustration, low self-esteem and entrapment (LIFE 2007).

Parents and siblings also have beliefs and prejudices about their family member with mental illness. Parents may blame themselves for their child's illness or may be ashamed or embarrassed and try to hide the illness from extended family members, neighbours, friends and work colleagues (Hinshaw 2005). Siblings may feel embarrassed and stop bringing friends home. They may be fearful that they too will develop a mental illness and may become afraid of their brother or sister. Children of parents with a mental illness face unique challenges, at times taking on early parental responsibilities. The acute phase of many mental health problems, especially psychotic disorders, will cause major disruption to family life (Walton-Moss et al. 2005). Parents may need to take time out from work, which will have financial implications for the family; siblings may find it difficult to function at school or in the workplace; and children may have their schooling interrupted if they are being cared for by a relative who lives away from the family home. All family members will experience aspects similar to a grieving process as a result of the changes in their lives. Children who grow up with a parent who has a mental health problem are at higher risk of developing a mental health problem, such as depression, through either genetic susceptibility or gaps in parenting (AIHW 2009; Foster 2014).

As well as the stigma that is often experienced by people with mental health problems, immigrants with mental health problems can bear the added burden of their cultural difference and potential racial stigma. Language difficulties and culturally specific ways of expressing distress increase alienation from mainstream community groups and place this group of people at increased risk of being misdiagnosed or receiving inadequate care and support. They can be considered to have a dual vulnerability (Cross & Singh 2012).

CRITICAL THINKING CHALLENGE 9.1

1. Write a short list of what you think about people suffering from:
   - arthritis
   - depression

   How do you think these illnesses would affect people's lifestyles?
2. What would you expect to see if you walked into a psychiatric ward today? For example:
   - What would service users be doing?
   - What would the nurses be doing?
3. What influences your perceptions about people with mental illness?
4. How could you test your perceptions against reality?

NURSE'S STORY 9.1

I undertook my general nurse training at a regional base hospital in the mid-1970s. At that time, we lived in nurses' quarters. We had a month-long placement at the local psychiatric hospital and the psychiatric nurse trainees had a placement with us. I had not considered psychiatric (as it was called then) nursing at that time. During my third and final year of training I had a relationship breakup. It was very traumatic for me as the breakup was sudden. My then boyfriend was particularly nasty and made some very unkind comments about my appearance. I became quite depressed.

Living in nurses' quarters might lead you to think that everyone would have noticed me getting more and more unhappy but shared living with hundreds of student nurses also provided quite a lot of anonymity. I went about my shifts and stayed in my room most of the time. I didn't confide in my parents. My mother had suffered with depression and hypochondriasis for many years and I didn't want to burden her or my dad. I didn't want to be like her. I pretended nothing was wrong.

Over the next few months I joined a gym and started going more and more often. I also started dieting, purging and using diuretics. I lost a lot of weight. The depression lifted (I didn't have any formal treatment) but I was getting very thin. I loved it and was proud of my body. By this time we were also all gearing up for the final exams. I was able to handle the stress by working out. My weight was 45 kg and Body Mass Index (BMI) 17. This was now considered a problem, but not for me.

After a few months one of the gym instructors asked me out and I agreed. That was the turning point. He said that I was looking unwell and that he preferred it when I was fit but at a healthy weight. I was very fearful of becoming fat. He encouraged me to change to a 'lifters' high protein diet and worked with me and encouraged me. I steadily gained weight but not fat. The relationship didn't last but we have remained good friends ever since.

I moved after my graduate year and tried to get a job at a general hospital in a large regional town without success. I then considered psychiatric nursing. Although I wasn't previously interested, my personal journey created a curiosity and a greater understanding of the issues people with mental health problems face and the courtesy stigma that is attached to people who are associated with people with a mental health problem. I am so pleased I made the decision. I have never looked back. The rest is history.

The Media and Perceptions of Mental Health Problems

The media are very powerful in conveying information and influencing community attitudes and perceptions of social norms. Therefore, it follows that media coverage and reporting, be it through films, television, newspapers, magazines, posters or pamphlets, is critical when attempting to form and to influence community attitudes to mental health and mental illness and the people affected by it. Unfortunately, media coverage often reflects the widespread misunderstanding of mental health problems. This is particularly so in movies. One *Flew Over the Cuckoo's Nest* is a 1970s film that highlights the damaging portrayal of mental illness. It depicts patients in a psychiatric hospital as having few rights and being manipulated by mental health nurses. Patients who are deemed 'difficult' are subjected to medical procedures in order to make their behaviour manageable. This film is set in the mid-20th century, but there are more recent examples that also portray a negative image of people with a mental illness, including the Batman film, *The Dark Knight*. The portrayal of John Nash in A *Beautiful Mind* is a more realistic depiction of someone with schizophrenia.

To highlight the inaccurate portrayal of mental health problems in television and the media, a 1-year analysis of television drama programmes (serials, plays and films) was conducted in the US. According to the SANE website (www.sane.org), '73% of people with a mental illness were depicted as violent, while 23% of people were portrayed as homicidal maniacs'. When the same study analysed media reports about mental health problems on television and in newspapers, it found that nearly 90% of stories depicted people with mental health problems as violent and usually homicidal. This is grossly inaccurate. Newspaper reporting has a tendency to dramatise issues related to mental health problems at times, thereby perpetuating negative stereotypes and unnecessary fears in the community (Stuart 2006).

Just as the media can have a negative impact, it can also be used as an instrument to educate and to change public opinion by ensuring that accurate information is reported in a rational and sensitive manner. In order to achieve this, scriptwriters, journalists and newspaper editors need to be educated on mental health issues (www.sane.org).

Numerous organisations, both government and private, monitor and provide information to the general public, service users, teachers, nurses, universities, general practitioners and journalists in relation to mental health problems. According to Barry (2013) digital media such as the internet also have a strong influence on people's concept of mental health through a virtual presence. Mental health and wellbeing can be promoted using these media as communication instruments for information, help and support, facilitating social inclusion. The internet, and social media in particular can play a positive role in the development and maintenance of relationships and in the understanding of mental health problems (Barry 2013).

CULTURAL DIVERSITY

The UK is made up of culturally diverse communities and as such it is important that this is reflected in the care that people receive. It is important that healthcare practitioners are suitably prepared to cater for the needs of different cultural groups. However, specific guidance about how to do this is not often readily available. The NMC Code (NMC 2015) specifies under the objective 1.3 that nurses must 'avoid making assumptions and recognise diversity and individual choice'. Section 7.3 specifies nurses must 'use a range of verbal and nonverbal communication methods'. It is important that nurses consider cultural sensitivities and learn to understand and to respond better to people's personal and health needs in a holistic way that cares for people as individuals irrespective of their culture (Holland 2018). It is important to remember that the patient themselves, their family and friends can be rich sources of information.

Government figures from the 2011 Census (Office for National Statistics 2018) suggest the following facts and figures regarding regional ethnic diversity:

- The most ethnically diverse region in England and Wales was London, with 40.2% of residents identifying as Asian, Black, Mixed or Other ethnic group.
- London had the smallest percentage (44.9%) of White British people out of all regions, with the North-East having the highest (93.6%).
- People identifying in the White ethnic group were most likely to live in the South-East (16.2%).
- People identifying in Black (58.4%), Asian (35.9%), Mixed (33.1%) and Other (49.9%) ethnic groups were more likely to live in London than any other region.
- 81.5% of the general population live in urban areas, with 18.5% in rural locations.
- Ethnic groups most likely to live in urban locations were Pakistani (99.1%), Bangladeshi (98.7%) and Black African (98.2%).
- 8 out of the 10 most ethnically diverse local authorities were in London.
- Newham in London was the local authority with the lowest percentage of people identifying with the White ethnic group (29.0%).

CRITICAL THINKING CHALLENGE 9.2

1. What do you think is meant by the term 'Western culture'?
2. How helpful is this shorthand term in explaining general population health beliefs in the UK?
3. What do the advertising pages of popular magazines offer as an indication of popular 'Western' beliefs about health and wellbeing?

What is Culture?

Culture can be defined as a body of learned behaviours, passed on by role modelling, learning and tradition, common to any given human society, which is used by the individual to interpret experience and to generate social behaviour (Sadock et al. 2007). Culture shapes individual behavioural, emotional and social responses within the human environment.

Within any society there will be subgroups or subcultures, which define themselves by social norms that deviate to various extents from the given (mainstream) norm. Variations in acceptable behaviour, speech and dress may set apart social classes, religious organisations, secret societies and age groups within a society. Variations may exist between urban and rural populations within a given culture.

As noted, culture is passed on by role modelling, learning and tradition and exists in a constant state of change. Today's youth culture deviation is tomorrow's status quo. Any attempt to define a person's culture in terms of race, appearance or geography only gives rise to stereotyping, generalisation and potential inaccuracies (Flowers 2004). It is strongly recommended that mental health nurses develop relationships with cultural liaison and ethnic support workers because it is not possible to learn everything about all the cultures they will work with in their professional lives (Robinson & Harris 2006). No culture is universal or static within any given community. Although we speak of an 'Anglo-Celtic' (or more broadly a 'Western') culture as informing mainstream health beliefs, it is important to understand that this is a shorthand term that covers a multitude of cultural approaches to healthcare.

Culturally and linguistically diverse (CALD) groups frequently experience socioeconomic disadvantage and chronic stressors such as racism. Mental health nurses must also acknowledge that access to, quality of and uptake of mental healthcare varies for different ethnic groups. Furthermore, they must acknowledge that people's theories about the nature, causes and expressions of mental health and illness are shaped by ethnicity, culture, class and gender, which in turn shape help-seeking behaviour (Cross & Singh 2012). The concept of cultural self-reflection or reflexivity is as an essential component of mental health nursing practice.

Mental health nurses will work with people from many cultural and religious backgrounds who will have their own beliefs regarding mental health and illness. The terms and behaviours used to express mental distress vary among cultures. It is important that mental health nurses respect the value of other people's beliefs and understand that these beliefs shape behaviours in response to illnesses or disorders. Cultural values and beliefs also shape how people decide to access services and who is deemed an appropriate channel of communication between the service user and the health service.

In many cultures, the experience of mental illness is accompanied by stigma that prevents people from seeking help from outside the family or community. In highly patriarchal cultures, the senior male family member may decide who is to seek attention and under what circumstances (UNICEF 2006; WHO 2007). In some cultures, a senior female family member will make a decision to seek help and decide who will accompany a young patient, rather than a parent or sibling, or a group of 'aunties' may take responsibility for a baby or child on behalf of a stressed blood-mother (Parker 2011).

People from CALD groups tend to be particularly reluctant to seek assistance from mainstream services for health-related problems (Cross & Singh 2012). A number of factors contribute to low rates of help-seeking and can include: language difficulties; a lack of cultural sensitivity by service providers; inappropriate treatments, including lack of family involvement; a lack of information or misinformation; and a greater degree of stigma and shame associated with mental illnesses and related problems. The barriers most often identified relate to language, lack of information about services, cultural patterns of help-seeking, lack of cultural sensitivity by service providers, financial barriers and lack of service availability

(Hsiao et al. 2006). If services are not culturally appropriate, then data on rates of use may actually underestimate the barriers in access to service. That is, services are used but are not appropriate to the culture of a group and therefore equivalent benefits may not be derived. Hence, access should be considered to be correspondingly less.

A central tenet of cultural safety is the ability of nurses to examine their own beliefs and values and therefore mental health nurses need to be aware of their own cultural bias when seeking histories and making assessments of presenting behaviours (Gorman & Cross 2014). Flexibility in approach will ensure that due respect is accorded to the opinions and explanations of those holding cultural authority. Involving families can improve care because the knowledge and expertise of family members can be drawn upon (Cross & Bloomer 2010).

CRITICAL THINKING CHALLENGE 9.3

Consider your family unit.

1. What health beliefs do members share?
2. Do any members hold different health beliefs? If so, what has influenced their thinking?
3. Which healthcare actions are taken within the family?
4. Who makes decisions about when and how to seek healthcare outside the family?
5. Are these decisions made individually or by group negotiation?
6. How does your family's health culture influence your response to people with different health beliefs and values?

CULTURAL DIVERSITY AND MENTAL HEALTH NURSING

Models of cultural competence involve some or all of the following elements:

- respect for other people's cultural and religious beliefs and values
- respect for spiritual and religious influences on health beliefs
- awareness of variations in verbal and nonverbal communication styles
- increasing knowledge of cultural differences
- respect for the individual's explanations of their experiences
- delivering culturally sensitive care to diverse groups via negotiation and consensus
- instilling a sense of cultural safety for individuals, families and groups (Betancourt et al. 2002; Campinha-Bacote 2003)

A major criticism of the cultural competence model is that service users are not empowered to evaluate the appropriateness of service delivery or to assess health professionals' knowledge.

Cultural safety goes beyond describing the practices of other ethnic groups because merely learning about aspects of a culture does not make one fully cognisant of the complexities of that culture. Such a strategy can lead to a checklist mentality that prevents the consideration of diversity within groups and between individuals.

Culturally safe nurses are those who look at learning about themselves rather than learning about the cultures of their patients. The emphasis is on which attitudes and values nurses bring to their practice and there is an assumption that a nurse or midwife who can understand his or her own culture and the theory of power relations can be culturally safe in any context. Ramsden (2002) describes a progression towards culturally safe practice as follows:

- *Cultural awareness* is the first step and involves understanding that there is difference.
- *Cultural sensitivity* alerts students to the 'legitimacy of difference' and to self-exploration.
- *Cultural safety* is defined as 'an outcome of nursing and midwifery education that enables safe service to be defined by those that receive the service'.

A problem with cultural sensitivity relates to the underlying assumption that a group can be considered homogeneous, where all members of the group are the same. Culture is therefore seen as static, rather than something that is created by people, and does not allow for generational or other differences. Furthermore, a nurse having knowledge of a person's culture could be disempowering for someone who is disenfranchised from their own culture and could be seen as perpetuating processes that are both demeaning and disempowering (Downing et al. 2011).

Mental health nursing is about people of all cultures, socioeconomic groups and walks of life. To provide quality care nurses must acknowledge people's lived experiences, how these shape their beliefs and the acceptability of treatment. To provide quality care, nurses must acknowledge cultural diversity. Health systems that do not consider race, culture, gender or social values do not serve the people they purport to serve (Snowden 2003).

Expecting services to be accessible to all, regardless of their culture or ethnicity, is important. However, we should not underestimate the effort involved in achieving this. We need to develop practical and realistic ways of supporting those who are culturally diverse and avoid projecting our own cultural expectations of what is therapeutic. Some general principles that need to be considered in mental health nursing practice (adapted from Minas 2000) include the need:

- to acknowledge the diverse experiences of people from different religious and cultural backgrounds and the difficulties many face in getting access to effective mental health services and receiving quality acceptable and appropriate services;
- to recognise that there are vulnerable subgroups, including refugees and people who have survived trauma and torture;
- to develop an understanding of the intersection between culture and mental health, and how this influences assessment and treatment, and the need for mental health policy and service delivery to reflect the needs of the communities they serve.

Cultural respect allows mental health nurses to value the contribution that culturally appropriate interventions can make to the therapeutic environment.

PATIENT STORY 9.1

Zahra is a 30-year-old Somalian woman. She was found wandering aimlessly on a busy road by police. They were unable to engage her in conversation and were also unclear as to whether she was under the influence of drugs or alcohol. They took her to a mental health facility, where mental health clinicians were requested to assess her.

The mental health team approached Zahra and introduced themselves. At that moment, Zahra became more aware of her surroundings and became agitated. She kept repeating that she was not a prisoner and not to hurt her. Her English was limited but her meaning was clear to all. The mental health team attempted to calm her and requested that the police remain in the area but be unseen. This had a short-term calming effect.

Using an interpreter, the mental health team undertook their assessment and mental status examination. It became evident that Zahra was using multiple substances including cannabis and alcohol. She stated that she was using these substances more and more because they helped her forget the past.

Zahra had experienced terrible hardship including rape, being separated from her family and living in a detention centre for 3 years. As a result she developed posttraumatic stress disorder (PTSD).

Many refugees have experienced and witnessed appalling conditions, often perpetrated by people in authority. In Zahra's case, staff could not have predicted her response. However, when working with refugees, mental health clinicians must be mindful of the possibility of traumatic stress and the associated sequelae, including substance use.

CRITICAL THINKING CHALLENGE 9.4

You are the assigned nurse for Zahra in the patient study above. You have been asked to develop a care plan.

1. How might you go about building a therapeutic relationship with Zahra and her family?
2. Who should you involve in care planning negotiations?
3. Which cultural factors might be significant?
4. Which social factors might apply?
5. Which interventions might be of use in ensuring that Zahra receives the level of service that is her right?
6. Which treatment and management alternatives might be considered?
7. How will treatment outcomes be evaluated, and by whom?

Culture and Self-Reflection

For the mental health nurse, culture is a vital element of the therapeutic relationship. If we accept, as the basis of our human interaction, that all behaviour has meaning, then it is essential that we understand the cultural templates that shape behavioural and emotional responses. It is essential to reflect on our own beliefs and values about health, about what it means to be healthy and what we recognise as mental wellbeing.

Mental health nurses must also reflect on the assumptions of healthcare professional culture. Health education, training and practice rely strongly on an assumption that everyone involved in healthcare subscribes to 'Western' values concerning the application of scientific methods to everyday life and health behaviours. The scientific or biomedical model of healthcare also assumes a power differential between professional and patient, assigning the evaluation of healthcare services and outcomes to the professional. Mental health nurses must be aware of the power differentials inherent in social structures and service delivery models that marginalise or devalue the patient's identity, beliefs and wellbeing and actively reflect on their own professional actions in the light of this awareness (Stein-Parbury 2014).

All groups, including mental health nurses, are made up of individuals whose lived experience places them subtly apart from even their closest peers and influences their assigned and chosen behavioural styles within the peer group, with multidisciplinary colleagues and in therapeutic interactions. Nurses bring their own cultural and subcultural backgrounds, beliefs and values to all of life's interactions, including their professional healthcare beliefs and practices, as well as their position in society.

Nurses must maintain awareness of their own cultural and subcultural assumptions and of a natural tendency to ethnocentrism, i.e. the belief that one's own cultural values constitute the human norm and that differences from those values are deviant and wrong.

CRITICAL THINKING CHALLENGE 9.5

As health workers, we work within a model that is often characterised as 'Western, scientific and patriarchal'.

1. What implications might that characterisation have for:
   - the concept of care?
   - people seeking healthcare?
2. How accurate is the characterisation?

CONCLUSION

Mental health nurses have a responsibility to ensure that they are well informed regarding current statistics, trends, models and philosophies relating to all areas of mental health. They need to examine their own perceptions and belief systems in regard to mental health problems and behaviours so that they can function effectively in an unbiased manner. Reflective practice and commitment to the understanding of each individual as a person, taking into account and respecting cultural diversity, will enable mental health nurses to work with patients to establish supportive care strategies and valid outcomes.

ACKNOWLEDGEMENT

This chapter has been adapted from a chapter in the previous editions of this book by Pat Bradley and Ruth De Souza.

EXERCISES FOR CLASS ENGAGEMENT

1. Outline your ideas and thoughts about mental health and wellness. Share your ideas with other members of your group or class, and then reexamine them as you learn more about mental health and illness. Hopefully you will replace your preconceived ideas with facts and accurate information about mental health and illness.
2. How do you maintain your own mental health? What could you do to enhance it?
3. Perceptions of mental illness and people with mental health problems are socially constructed. Discuss the ways in which you developed your own views about mental health problems and how those views began and have been maintained. Use the internet to explore how the many support groups aid the community to develop positive attitudes about mental health and illness and to develop personal mental wellness plans. Make a list of useful websites.
4. How can nurses and other groups influence the social constructions of mental illness and people with mental health problems?
5. In your group, discuss the following concepts: 'stigma', 'culture', 'mental health' and 'patient/service user'.
   - What were the differences in opinions between group members? Have any group members lived experience of mental health problems or mental health services? If so, how did their views differ from other members of the group?
   - Is there any cultural variation between group members? If so, how did this influence their views?
6. Think about culture generally. (Consider the social determinants of health, ethnicity, migrant/refugee status, gender and age.) How would you describe the 'cultural mix' of your area? City? Home town? University? Year group? Discuss your answers with your group. What does your group identify as the major considerations? How do they influence healthcare utilisation and service delivery?
7. How do you define yourself culturally? How does your self-definition affect your nursing practice?
8. Cultural safety is a core value underpinning healthcare practice. Reflect upon your own cultural values and what you might need to challenge in order to provide culturally safe nursing care.

REFERENCES

Australian Institute of Health and Welfare (AIHW), 2009. A picture of Australia's children. AIHW, Canberra.

Australian Bureau of Statistics (ABS), 2008. National Survey of Mental Health and Wellbeing: summary of results. ABS, Canberra. Available at: https://www.abs.gov.au/ausstats/abs@.nsf/mf/4326.0.

Ball, J.S., Links, P.S., 2009. Borderline personality disorder and childhood trauma: evidence for a causal relationship. Current Psychiatry Reports 11 (1), 63–68.

Barry, M., 2013. Using technologies to promote mental health and wellbeing. Technology for well-being international conference. Dublin, pp. 25–26 September.

Betancourt, R., Green, A.R., Carillo, J.E., et al., 2002. Cultural competence in health care: emerging frameworks and practical approaches. Available at: https://www.commonwealthfund.org/sites/default/files/documents/media___files_publications_fund_report_2002_oct_cultural_competence_in_health_care__emerging_frameworks_and_practical_approaches_betancourt_culturalcompetence_576_pdf.pdf.

Campinha-Bacote, J., 2003. Many faces: addressing diversity in health care. Online Journal of Issues in Nursing 8 (1). Available at: http://ojin.nursingworld.org/MainMenuCategories/ANAMarketplace/ANAPeriodicals/OJIN/TableofContents/Volume82003/No1Jan2003/AddressingDiversityinHealthCare.html.

Conrad, P., Barker, K.K., 2010. The social construction of illness: key insights and policy implications. Journal of Health and Social Behavior 51 (1), S67–S79.

Cross, W.M., Bloomer, M.J., 2010. Extending boundaries: clinical communication with culturally and linguistically diverse mental health clients and carers. International Journal of Mental Health Nursing 19 (4), 268–277.

Cross, W.M., Singh, C., 2012. Dual vulnerabilities: mental illness in a culturally and linguistically diverse society. International Journal for Quality in Health Care 42 (2), 156–166.

Downing, R., Kowal, E., Paradies, A., 2011. Indigenous cultural training for healthworkers in Australia. International Journal for Quality in Health Care 23 (3), 247–257.

Flowers, D.L., 2004. Culturally competent nursing care: a challenge for the 21st century. Critical Care Nurse 24 (4), 48–52.

Foster, K., 2014. One-third of children of parents with severe mental illness are at risk of developing severe mental illness. Evidence Based Mental Health 17 (3), 73.

Gorman, D., Cross, W.M., 2014. Cultural issues in mental health. In: Mental health nursing: dimensions of praxis, second ed. Oxford University Press, Melbourne, pp. 487–504.

Green, J., Eagar, K., 2010. The health of people in Australian immigration detention centres. Medical Journal of Australia 192 (2), 65–70.

Hinshaw, S., 2005. The stigmatization of mental illness in children and parents: developmental issues, family concerns, and research needs. Journal of Child Psychology and Psychiatry 46 (7), 714–734.

Holland, K., 2018. Cultural awareness in nursing and health care: An Introductory Text, third ed. Arby Routledge, New York.

Hsiao, F.H., Klimidis, S., Minas, H., Tan, E.S., 2006. Cultural attribution of mental health suffering in Chinese societies: the views of Chinese patients with mental illness and their caregivers. Journal of Clinical Nursing 15, 998–1006.

Inagami, S., Cohen, D.A., Brown, A.F., Asch, S.M., 2009. Body mass index, neighborhood fast food and restaurant concentration, and car ownership. Journal of Urban Health 86 (5), 683–695.

Independent Mental Health Taskforce, 2016. Five Year Forward View for Mental Health. Available at: https://www.england.nhs.uk/wp-content/uploads/2016/02/Mental-Health-Taskforce-FYFV-final.pdf. Accessed: 8 October 2018.

Institute for Fiscal Studies, 2018. Living standards, poverty and inequality in the UK: 2018. Available at: https://www.ifs.org.uk/publications/13075. Accessed: 8 October 2018.

Keleher, H., Murphy, B., 2004. Understanding health: a determinants approach. Oxford University Press, Oxford, England.

LIFE, 2007. LIFE factsheet_3_web.pdf. Commonwealth of Australia. Available at: www.livingisforeveryone.com.au.

McCauley-Elsom, K., Kulkarni, J., 2007. Managing psychosis in pregnancy. ANZ Journal of Psychiatry 41 (3), 289–292.

Minas, H., 2000. Culture and psychiatric education. Australasian Psychiatry 8 (3), 204–206.

Mind, 2015. General Election 2015: briefing from Mind. Available at: https://www.mind.org.uk/media/1925604/back-bench-debate-mental-health-unemployment.pdf. Accessed: 8 October 2018.

Mind: for better mental health, 2018. Available at: https://www.mind.org.uk/information-support/tips-for-everyday-living/wellbeing/#.W7tOOGhKjIV. Accessed: 8th October 2018.

Ministry of Housing, Communities and Local Government, 2018. Rough Sleeping Statistics Autumn 2017 (England). Available at: https://assets.publishing.service.gov.uk/government/uploads/system/uploads/attachment_data/file/682001/Rough_Sleeping_Autumn_2017_Statistical_Release_-_revised.pdf. Accessed: 8 October 2018.

The Ministry of Housing, Communities and Local Government, 2018. Statutory homelessness and prevention and relief, January to March 2018: England. Available at: https://assets.publishing.service.gov.uk/government/uploads/system/uploads/attachment_data/file/721285/Statutory_Homelessness_and_Prevention_and_Relief_Statistical_Release_Jan_to_Mar_2018_-_REVISED.pdf. Accessed: 8 October 2018.

Morgan, V.A., McGrath, J.J., Jablensky, A., Badcock, J.C., Waterreus, A., Bush, R., Mackinnon, A., 2014. Psychosis prevalence and physical, metabolic and cognitive co-morbidity: data from the second Australian national survey of psychosis. Psychological Medicine 44 (10), 2163–2176.

National Audit Office, 2017. Mental health in prisons. Available at: https://www.nao.org.uk/report/mental-health-in-prisons/#. Accessed: 8 October 2018.

NHS England, 2016a. Five Year Forward View for Mental Health for the NHS in England. Available at: https://www.england.nhs.uk/wp-content/uploads/2016/02/Mental-Health-Taskforce-FYFV-final.pdf. Accessed: 8 October 2018.

NHS England, 2016b. Implementing the Five Year Forward View for Mental Health. Available at: https://www.england.nhs.uk/wp-content/uploads/2016/07/fyfv-mh.pdf. Accessed: 8 October 2018.

Nursing and Midwifery Council (NMC), 2015. The code: professional standards of practice and behaviour for nurses and midwives. Nursing and Midwifery Council, London.

Nursing and Midwifery Council (NMC), 2016. Mental Health Nursing: Field Specific Competencies. Available at: https://www.nmc.org.uk/globalassets/sitedocuments/registration/overseas/mental-health-nursing---field-specific-competencies.pdf. Accessed: 8 October 2018.

Ochoa, S., Usall, J., Cobo, J., Labad, X., Kulkarni, J., 2012. Gender differences in schizophrenia and first-episode psychosis: a comprehensive literature review. Schizophrenia Research and Treatment. https://doi.org/10.1155/2012/916198.

Office for National Statistics, 2018. Regional ethnic diversity. Available at: https://www.ethnicity-facts-figures.service.gov.uk/british-population/national-and-regional-populations/regional-ethnic-diversity/latest. Accessed: 14 October 2018.

Office of Disease Prevention and Health Promotion, 2015. Healthy People 2020. Available at: www.healthy.gov.

Parker, R., 2011. Australian Aboriginal and Torres Strait Islander mental health: an overview. In: Purdie, N., Dudgeon, P., Walker, R. (Eds.), Working together: Aboriginal and Torres Strait Islander mental health and wellbeing principles and practice. Commonwealth of Australia, Canberra. Available at: http://research.acer.edu.au/indigenous_education/24.

Patel, V., Lund, C., Hatherill, S., Plagerson, S., Corrigall, J., Funk, M., Fisher, A.J., 2010. Mental disorders: equity and social determinants. In: Blas, E., Kurup, A.S. (Eds.), Equity, social determinant s and public health programmes. World Health Organization, Geneva.

Pinches, A., 2002. Recognising not only consumers' legal rights, but also their 'community entitlements'. From an address to a mental health legal centre workshop at the National Conference of the Federation on Community Legal Centres. Melbourne.

Popay, J., Escorel, S., Hernandez, M., Johnston, H., Mathieson, J., Rispel, L., 2008. Understanding and tackling social exclusion. WHO Social Exclusion Knowledge Network, Lancaster, UK.

Raeburn, T., Schmied, V., Hungerford, C., Cleary, M., 2015. Self-determination theory: a framework for clubhouse psychosocial rehabilitation research. Issues in Mental Health Nursing 36 (2), 145–151.

Ramsden, I.M., 2002. Cultural safety and nursing education in Aotearoa and Te Waipou namu. Doctoral thesis. Victoria University, Wellington.

Rethink Mental Illness, 2018. Available at: https://www.rethink.org/about-us/people-and-history/rethink-mental-illness-timeline. Accessed: 8 October 2018.

Robinson, C., 2003. Understanding iterative homelessness: the case of people with mental disorders. Australian Housing and Urban Research Institute, UNSW-UWS Research Centre, New South Wales.

Robinson, G., Harris, A., 2006. Aboriginal mental health worker program: final evaluation report. Charles Darwin University, Darwin.

Sadock, B.J., Sadock, V.A., Kaplan, H.I., 2007. Kaplan & Sadock's synopsis of psychiatry: behavioral sciences/clinical psychiatry. Lippincott Williams & Wilkins, Philadelphia.

Samaritans, 2018. The History of Samaritans. Available at: https://www.samaritans.org/about-us/our-organisation/history-samaritans. Accessed: 8 October 2018.

SANE, 2018. About SANE. Available at: http://www.sane.org.uk/what_we_do/about_sane/. Accessed: 8 October 2018.

Shevlin, M., Dorahy, M.J., Adamson, G., 2007. Trauma and psychosis: an analysis of the national comorbidity survey. American Journal of Psychiatry 164, 166–169.

Snowden, L.R., 2003. Bias in mental health assessment and intervention: theory and evidence. American Journal of Public Health 93, 239–243.

Sridhar, D., 2008. Linkages between nutrition, ill-health and education. Background paper prepared for the Education for All Global Monitoring Report 2009, Overcoming inequality: why governance matters. Available at: www.unscn.org/layout/modules/resources/files/Linkages_between_nutrition_ill-health_and_education.pdf.

Stein-Parbury, J., 2014. Patient and person: interpersonal skills in nursing, fifth ed. Elsevier, Sydney.

Stuart, H., 2006. Media portrayal of mental illness and its treatments: what effect does it have on people with mental illness? CNS Drugs 20 (2), 99–106.

Triggs, G., 2013. Mental health and immigration detention. Medical Journal of Australia 199 (11), 721–722.

UNICEF, 2006. The state of the world's children 2007: women and children. The double dividend of gender equality. The United Nations Children's Fund, New York.

UNICEF, 2015. Girls education and gender equality. The United Nations Children's Fund, New York. Available at: www.unicef.org/education/bege_70640.html.

Vinson, T., 2009. Intergenerational disadvantage. Department of Education, Employment and Workplace Relations, Canberra.

Walsh, K., Cross, W.M., 2013. Depression, culture and the Westernisation of mental illness. In: Kocabasoglu, N. (Ed.), Mood disorders. InTech, Rijeka, Croatia.

Walton-Moss, B., Linda Gerson, L., Rose, L., 2005. Effects of mental illness on family quality of life. Issues in Mental Health Nursing 26 (6), 627–642.

Whisman, M.A., Baucom, D.H., 2011. Intimate relationships and psychopathology. Clinical Child and Family Psychology Review 15 (1), 4–13.

Wilkinson, R., Marmot, M., 2003. Social determinants of health: the solid facts, second ed. World Health Organization Europe, Copenhagen.

Willis, M., 2005. Ex-prisoners. SAAP, housing and homelessness in Australia: final report to the national SAAP coordination and development committee. Australian Institute of Criminology, Canberra.

World Health Organization (WHO), 2006. Preventing disease through healthy environments: towards an estimate of the environmental burden of disease. WHO, Geneva.

World Health Organization (WHO), 2007. Cross-cutting gender issues in women's health in the Eastern Mediterranean Region. WHO Regional Office for the Eastern Mediterranean, Cairo.
World Health Organization, 2013. (WHO) Mental Health Action Plan 2013-2020: Mental health and disorders: determinants and consequences Pg. 7. Available at: http://apps.who.int/iris/bitstream/handle/10665/89966/9789241506021_eng.pdf; jsessionid=50D30B539AC7D396407F663E0348F2F7?sequence=1. Accessed: 8 October 2018.
World Health Organization (WHO), 2014. Data and resources. Available at: http://www.euro.who.int/en/health-topics/noncommunicable-diseases/mental-health/data-and-resources. Accessed: 9 October 2018.
World Health Organization (WHO), 2015. Mental health. Available at: www.who.int/mental_health/en. Accessed December 2015.
Wyllie, A., Brown, R., 2011. Discrimination reported by users of mental health services: 2010 survey. Ministry of Health, New Zealand.

USEFUL WEBSITES

Centre Point: give homeless young people a future, www.centrepoint.org.uk
Childline, www.childline.org.uk
Depression Alliance, www.depressionalliance.org
Diversity Rx, www.DiversityRx.org
Healthy People 2020. www.healthypeople.gov
HomelessLinkwww.homeless.org.uk .
Mental Health Foundation Good mental health for all, www.mentalhealth.org.uk
National Health Service England Mental Health, www.england.nhs.uk/mental-health
PANDAS Foundation (pre [antenatal], postnatal depression or postnatal psychosis in England, Wales and Scotland), www.pandasfoundation.org.uk
Shelter, https://www.shelter.org.uk
The Centre for Mental Health, www.centreformentalhealth.org.uk
The Ottawa Charter, www.who.int/healthpromotion/conferences/previous/ottawa/en
Together: for mental wellbeing, www.together-uk.org
Transcultural Mental Health On-Line, www.priory.com/psych/trans.htm
WHO, mental health, www.who.int/mental_health/en
WHO, social determinants of health, www.who.int/topics/social_determinants/en
WHO, environmental health, www.who.int/quantifying_ehimpacts/publications/preventingdisease.pdf?ua=1
World Federation for Mental Health, www.wfmh.com

10

Working with Families in Mental Health

Kim Foster, Kim Usher and Kerry Hawkins

KEY POINTS

- An individual's mental illness and distress affects all members in their family.
- Supporting patients in their personal recovery includes recognising that their family members are also in recovery.
- Nurses play a key role in preventing intergenerational mental illness and improving wellbeing and outcomes for families through partnering with and supporting families in their recovery journey.
- Family-focussed practices in mental health include identifying the family system, providing information and support, and providing specific strategies and interventions to strengthen family capacity, build family resilience and support family recovery.

KEY TERMS

allostasis
carers
children of parents with mental illness (COPMI)
family-focussed practice (FFP)
families where a parent has mental illness (FAPMI)
family of origin
family of procreation or choice
family recovery
family resilience
intergenerational mental illness
strengths-based approach

LEARNING OUTCOMES

The material in this chapter will assist you to:

- define the key terms related to working with families in mental health.
- outline a strengths-based approach to working with families when a person has mental illness.
- describe key family assessment and family-focussed practices when working with families in mental health.
- understand the family recovery process when a family member has mental illness.
- identify how nurses can support family wellbeing, resilience and recovery through prevention and intervention strategies.

INTRODUCTION

We live within the context of our relationships with others, particularly our family and friends. When a person develops an illness such as mental illness, their experiences of the illness, recovery and treatment will inevitably affect the people with whom they are most connected. As Cowling and McGorry (2012) identify, mental illness is a family matter. Recognising the vital importance of mental health patients' relationships to their wellbeing, this chapter focusses on how nurses can provide effective care to patients that is inclusive of the needs of the whole family—the patient and their children and/or adults with whom they live and love.

DEFINING 'FAMILY'

In this chapter, the discussion focusses on family members where an individual—a child, a young person or an adult—has mental health problems such as depression, anxiety or a psychosis. The focus is not on families where the person has a neurocognitive disorder such as dementia. 'Family' can be defined in many ways. For the purposes of this chapter, the notion of 'family' and who is included in a 'family' is understood to be defined by its members (Osher & Osher 2002). That is, the family themselves determine who is 'family'. This approach acknowledges the many types of family relationships that may not be biological or necessarily resemble more traditional views of 'family' such as the nuclear family of mother, father and child(ren).

We refer to two broad types of 'family'. The first is *family of origin*. This refers to the family a person is born into, where the family includes parents and siblings of a child or an adult with mental illness. The second is *family of procreation, or choice*, where the family includes chosen relationships and partnerships. These are often not biological; for instance, when a parent is a step-parent. *Family of procreation* refers to the partner and/or children of an adult with mental illness. Both family of origin and family of procreation are inclusive of other family members such as grandparents, extended family, caregivers and others who are considered 'family' by the family members.

You will note that in mental health services, and in the literature, families of people with mental illness are also commonly referred to as family carers, carers or caregivers. The terms 'family' and 'carer' are often used interchangeably. The term 'carer' recognises the crucial role that many family members play in providing 'informal' or 'nonprofessional' unpaid care for their loved one. However, not all family members play a caregiving role and/or consider themselves caregivers or wish to be identified as carers and not all carers are family members. Therefore, throughout this chapter we mainly use the term 'family member' or family/carers and discuss the practical and emotional caregiving that many family members provide for their loved one as relevant.

WHY WORK WITH FAMILIES AND CARERS? INTRODUCING A STRENGTHS-BASED APPROACH

Over the past few decades, deinstitutionalisation has seen the care of people with mental illness shift increasingly from large mental health hospitals out into the community. This marked change to service provision has led to growing numbers of people with mental illness living with their families and carers in the community. Family members now provide vital informal caregiving; without this, there would be a greater risk of adverse outcomes and diminished quality of life for mental health patients (Jensen 2004). However, a person's illness affects not only them as an individual but also those who love them, and mental illness can be understood as existing first and foremost within the context of family and the broader community (Foster et al. 2012).

The high level of care provided by many families to their family member with mental illness means that they have an increased need for information and support in their caregiving roles. Despite their pivotal roles, family carers have consistently reported difficulty in gaining information about their loved one's mental illness (Shankar & Muthuswamy 2007). Family carers report that mental health professionals, including nurses, are often either not aware of their needs and/or are preoccupied with addressing the needs of the patient. Family carers express a need for health professionals to listen to them with nonjudgemental attitudes, respect their concerns, recognise their needs, acknowledge their strengths and include them when appropriate in decisions made about the care of their family member/loved one (Foster 2010, 2011).

In acknowledgement of the changing needs of families, there has been a paradigm shift in some areas of service provision so that the focus of care provided to families has moved to a strengths-based approach rather than the previous deficit approach. A deficit approach to healthcare focusses on what is going wrong and/or what is lacking. A strengths-based approach, however, focusses on what is working well and includes being open to recognising the positive attributes and resources of families (Darbyshire & Jackson 2005). This is also in keeping with the idea that rather than regarding families as damaged, they are viewed as challenged (Walsh 2006).

A strengths-based approach acknowledges that it is more constructive to consider the strengths that a family has and foster further positive growth and development for family members, than to continue focussing only on the difficulties they face (Usher et al. 2005). Importantly, this approach does not dismiss the patient's and family's problems, but rather focusses on the capacities and resources the family have that can be strengthened and used to support them in addressing their challenges (West et al. 2011). A strengths-based approach will be used as the framework throughout this chapter for communicating and working together with patients and their families/carers. This approach means that when we assess and work with a patient, we also recognise the need to assess their family's needs and the context within which they live. Furthermore, a family recovery lens and emphasis on developing and sustaining resilience with families will inform discussion on working with families.

A strengths-based approach includes the principles that the problems and challenges facing families with mental illness are addressed within a framework of understanding that:

- Families have strengths and limitations and the capacity to be resilient.
- The family as well as the patient experience a recovery journey.
- As mental health professionals we need to attend to the diversity of individual and family responses to the challenges of living with mental illness.

A strengths-based approach also acknowledges that while problems exist, families are the best judge of their circumstances and can be supported by healthcare professionals to find their own solutions and ways of coping. A strengths-based approach assists us as nurses to work with families with a focus on their strengths, competencies and the resources they need to deal with the particular issues they face. Using a strengths-based framework moves us away from the idea of trying to fix individual or family deficits and towards recognising their existing protective attributes and abilities and encourages the development of further skills in managing and finding solutions to their own situation. This in turn encourages nurses to view families as active agents and decision makers in their own care rather than as passive recipients of the services we provide.

CHALLENGES FOR FAMILIES WHEN A PERSON HAS MENTAL ILLNESS

Families can face a number of challenges when a family member has mental illness. For example, numerous studies have provided evidence that family members of people with mental illness provide a significant amount of care to their relatives. The Office for National Statistics (2017) reported that in the UK in 2014, it would cost an estimated £56.9 billion a year to replace the care provided by unpaid adult carers.

As a result of this caregiver role, family members experience a level of burden that places them at greater risk of poorer physical and psychological health (Bassani et al. 2009; Aguglia et al. 2004; McCann et al. 2015). The recent study of caring for an older parent with mental illness by McCann et al. (2015) reported that the caregiving experience has an unfavourable impact on the physical health of the family member, where they are more susceptible to physical illnesses and take longer to recover. The experience of caregiving in families has been loosely linked into a concept referred to as 'burden of care'—'burden' or overload as an outcome affects people in many ways including physical, emotional, social, financial and in regard to important life choices such as whether or not to continue working, career decisions and whether or not to have another child (Cummins & Hughes 2007). It is important to realise that while informal carers, who mostly care for family members, make a significant contribution to healthcare provision, this comes at a cost to the individual(s) providing the care. In fact, the impact of caregiving is experienced not only by the primary caregiver, but also by the entire family (Kenny et al. 2012).

As well as managing their relative's symptoms and dealing with the health system, Richardson et al. (2013) explain that, in common with other caregivers, family members can also be burdened by financial hardship, relationship problems, social isolation, stigmatising attitudes from others, altered daily routines, frustration and exhaustion. Caregiving can severely reduce the amount of time available for socialising with others, engaging in hobbies and self-care such as exercise (Foster 2011). Many family/carers report feeling isolated from others, often including other family members (McCann et al. 2011), leaving them without others with whom they can discuss concerns (Digiacomo et al. 2013). The study of family members' experience of caring for a parent with mental illness by McCann et al. (2015) found that the stress of caregiving can have a serious negative impact on family relationships, especially where other family members are critical of the care delivered.

Children and Families Where Parents Have Mental Illness

Children and young people in families where there is mental illness are often called on to provide care, including for their parents. Usually the person requiring care is an older adult who is cared for by their adult child. Reupert et al. (2012), however, identify that up to one in five young children under the age of 18 may live in a family where a parent has mental illness. Some children in these situations are required to provide physical and/or emotional care for their parent and/or for their siblings. Their caregiving role may continue into adulthood, where many adult children of parents with mental illness (COPMI) provide care for their ageing parents (Foster 2010).

Families where a parent has mental illness (FAPMI) face many challenges. The impact on the child may be affected by the child's age at the time of the parent's diagnosis or episodes of illness (Reupert et al. 2012), the severity of the illness and the impact of chronicity and the presence of other disorders (such as substance abuse) (Ranchandani & Psychogiou 2009). These children may be faced not only with changing parental behaviours but also a lack of other family members available to assist with the emotional needs of the child (Murphy et al. 2014). Children in families where a parent has mental illness may also be at a higher risk of developing mental and emotional problems (Maybery et al. 2009) and often experience lower levels of achievement at school (Reupert et al. 2012). These children face many challenges. For example, they are often separated from their family as a result of the parent's mental illness, especially during times when the parent requires hospitalisation (Mordoch & Hall 2008). In addition, relationship problems can occur among children of parents with mental illness where some children are reported to have 'a lack of emotional affect, distorted perceptions of others, hypervigilance of others' emotional states and a development of mistrust of others' (Murphy et al. 2011, p. 3438).

Parents Caring for a Child or Young Person with Mental Illness

Parents caring for their child or a young person with mental illness can also experience challenges. While caring for young people in these circumstances can lead to many problems for parents, such as worrying about the impact of their child's illness and symptoms on other siblings, it is also linked to a sense of loss. Parents in one study (Richardson et al. 2013) reported losses associated with their perceptions of the child's lost expectations, uncertainty for the future, loss of financial stability and loss of social and career opportunities. The parents reported experiences such as anger, disappointment, hopelessness, sadness, shock, worry and denial related to the diagnosis of mental illness and also the many challenges faced in the caregiver role. Parents caring for adult offspring often report experiencing a sense of loss for their child's potential, former ability or idealised potential (Richardson et al. 2013).

Stigma and Families

Family members of people with mental illness are not only challenged by needs of caring for the person but can also experience the stigma associated with having a relative with mental illness, which involves prejudice and/or discrimination from others. This form of stigma has been referred to as *family stigma*. It can include, for example, blaming mental illness in a child or young person on poor parenting, and/or blaming family members for not helping their relative with medications (Larson & Corrigan 2008). Stigma may make it harder for family members to accept their relative's illness (Somers 2007) and, in some cases, they may experience guilt related to the shame they feel about their relative's illness and/or behaviour (Jones 2004). This can be understood as *self-stigma*, where family members endorse negative social views of people with mental illness (Larson & Corrigan 2008).

Families of people with mental illness report being subjected to discrimination and stigma on a daily basis; this stigma may even come from extended family members (Mental Health Council of Australia 2010) and health professionals (Reed 2008). As a result, families often withdraw from social situations and connections (Murphy et al. 2014).

NURSE'S STORY 10.1

Sophie Isobel

I have been fortunate to work with children and families in adult mental health services as a family worker and coordinator of the children of parents with a mental illness (COPMI service) for almost 10 years. I fell into this role by chance when looking for something new to be involved with in mental health nursing and what started as a temporary secondment soon became my core focus and passion. Through working in the role, my understanding of mental health nursing changed dramatically as I saw the effective and meaningful work that could be done when engaging with an individual as an active part of a wider family and social context.

Everybody comes from a family and many people hold roles in families, including parenting, which forms an integral part of their self. In adult mental health services, there is an increasing push to recognise the relationship between these family roles and mental health and recovery. When a parent has a mental illness, children are often not provided with any information or support to make sense of their world and are usually not included in care planning or delivery. Advocating for family-focussed practice in mental health services is hard work, yet the opportunity to work with children and families has provided me with endless inspiration and motivation to continue.

Many mental health services have dedicated positions such as mine that exist to improve the inclusion of families in care. A big part of my role is promoting awareness of children and families at a systems level and educating clinicians about ways to work with families in the care they provide to individuals. But the role has also included running parenting programs for parents with mental illness, organising children's activity programs, running support groups and coordinating playgroups specifically for families affected by mental illness; as well as large amounts of conversations, family sessions and support provided to many children, parents and families.

My role varies on a day-to-day basis. You never quite know what might happen, which projects might be started or what a referral might entail. Most referrals come from mental health clinicians but often schools, families, early childhood services and other services also seek advice or resources. There are increasing amounts of good resources and books about mental illness for families but none of them replaces a conversation with someone exploring your experiences and questions. Conversations about mental illness can occur with parents, children, young people and family members during home visits or in hospitals or health centres. Parents can often be understandably reluctant to engage in conversations about their parenting or refuse to have a professional talk to their children about their illness, so a lot of time and thought needs to be spent building a rapport and including all family members in discussions where possible. While all parents have worries about their parenting roles and can benefit from parenting support, mental illness is an additional challenge that can be stressful for all members of a family.

No 2 days are the same in this work. One day you may find yourself walking with a teenager discussing what mental illness is, how it affects their parent and answering questions about how to tell their friends or whether they will get it too. The next you might be advocating for a parent in a family meeting on an inpatient mental health unit or navigating complex family dynamics in a home visit. Some days you might find yourself colouring with a child and talking to them about what makes them feel worried or talking with schools or other agencies about how they can support a child or family. A lot of time is spent supporting mental health clinicians to address the needs of all family members within their care planning.

Conversations with parents might focus on what their illness stops them being able to do as a parent, what they think their children may have noticed when they were unwell, how they can explain their mental illness to their child and what children need to feel safe and secure. Often parents are concerned that they are being judged as a bad parent or may find it difficult to engage in wider parenting supports. Conversations with children need to be appropriate to their age and circumstance and context. Sometimes children want lots of information and other times conversations may focus on other stressors, supports and worries. Conversations may include who the child can talk to if they need to, what understanding they have of their parent's illness and reassurance about the future. Children often think their parent's illness is their fault. It is also important to make plans for periods of separation or hospitalisation and offer truthful and simple explanations. Both children and parents are open to detailed discussions about the brain and what is known and understood about mental illness, including treatment and prognosis.

Children often notice more than we realise and their questions can be quite poignant and challenging. I generally just try to be honest and thoughtful in my answers and admit what I don't know. Children can also be very accepting so often something I am worried about talking about is not such a big deal once I start. An awkward conversation is always better than no attempt at all.

Education to other nurses about talking to children and families can be rewarding as they realise how much of it is about being willing to put aside their own fears and have a go at tricky conversations about topics such as depression, psychosis or suicide that may make us as adults feel uncomfortable. There is a privilege in stepping into the lives of families and looking at mental illness as a part of a wider structure that affects and is affected by all of its members.

A recent study of stigma experienced by family members of people diagnosed with a mental illness (McCann et al. 2011) found that being open about the situation was a strategy that helped caregivers to manage the stigma and enabled support from family and reduced social isolation. However, the study also revealed that families from a range of cultural backgrounds were likely to be secretive and hence were considered more vulnerable to the impact of stigma.

CRITICAL THINKING CHALLENGE 10.1

1. What is your understanding of self-stigma in relation to a family member having mental illness? What are some examples of self-stigma for family members?
2. How can nurses working in mental health settings help reduce family members' self-stigma?

ADDRESSING CHALLENGES AND BUILDING STRENGTHS—FAMILY RESILIENCE

While it is apparent that family members face many challenges when a relative has mental illness, there is also evidence that many families develop strengths that can enable them to address these challenges effectively. Overcoming these challenges or adversities can be understood through the lens of allostasis and resilience.

Stress and Allostasis

Living in a family where a person has mental illness, particularly if the family does not have adequate support from others, can be challenging for many family members. The concept of *allostasis* can be useful in understanding how stress in childhood or adulthood may have an impact on a person. Family members, especially children, may experience a range of stressors and/or traumatic events that can exert a negative effect on their emotional and physical health and wellbeing over time. These stressors include conflict or aggression in the family, lack of nurturing and emotional, physical and/or sexual abuse or neglect. They may also include the impact of mental illness on family members.

Allostasis refers to the adaptation process of an individual's physiological system to psychosocial, environmental or physical stressors (Logan & Barksdale 2008). The immune system and the stress response (the hypothalamic–pituitary–adrenal axis) are the two main mediators in allostasis (Repetti et al. 2011). *Allostatic load* refers to long-term outcomes of unsuccessful adaptation and the cumulative physical damage that results from repeat physical responses to stress. The impact of these stressful experiences over time negatively affects an individual's health, resulting in illness or disease (Logan & Barksdale 2008; Repetti et al. 2011).

Repetti et al. (2011) use the metaphor of meshed gears to illustrate the interrelated links between repeated short-term responses to stress or trauma and the long-term impacts of this. In a family environment, the smallest gear can be seen to represent stressful events, a child's immediate response to this as one turn of the middle gear and their long-term health outcomes as one turn of the largest gear (see Fig. 10.1).

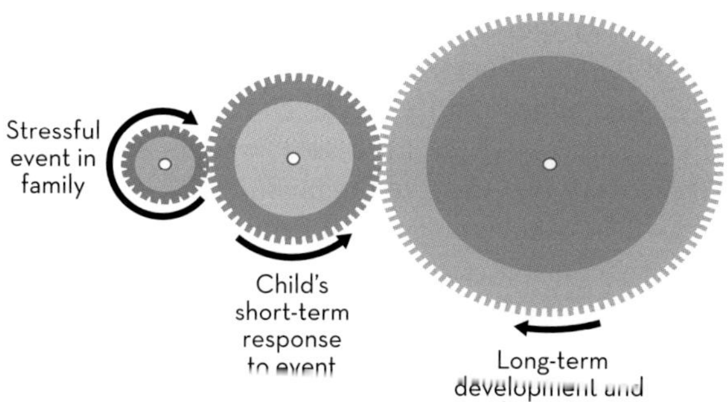

Fig. 10.1 Gears as a metaphor illustrating connections between repeated short-term reactions and their long-term outcomes. (*Source*: Repetti, R.L., Robles, T.F., Reynolds, B., 2011. Allostatic processes in the family. Development and Psychopathology, 23, 922.)

Resilience

Resilience has been variously defined, but in this context it is a process that refers specifically to risk or challenge and individual or family adaptation. Resilience is a dynamic process that involves being able to adapt positively to stress or adversity and to maintain or to restore wellbeing through the use of internal and external resources, including protective factors (Luthar et al. 2000; Foster & Robinson 2014). In this way, resilience can be understood to represent successful allostasis or adaptation. Promoting the resilience of children and families living with challenging situations such as mental illness can lead to better physical and mental health outcomes for individuals and the family as a whole (Logan & Barksdale 2008) and support the family's recovery.

Family resilience can be distinguished from that of individual resilience as it refers to the wellbeing of multiple individuals within a family system and the relationships between them, as well as the key family processes that support their resilience (Power et al. 2015). Box 10.1 outlines the key processes in family resilience. From a family resilience perspective, families are viewed as a unit with fundamental strengths and resources and potential for growth (Black & Lobo 2008; Zauszniewski et al. 2010). In families living with mental illness, resilience has been found to involve keeping a balance between stress and distress and maintaining family members' strength and optimism (Power et al. 2015).

Indicators of resilience in family members of people with mental illness include hardiness, having hope and acceptance, a sense of self-efficacy, coherence and mastery and being resourceful. Family members who have these positive characteristics seem better able to deal with the challenges they face (Zauszniewski et al. 2010). Warm and positive relationships and connections between family members are an integral resilience factor in maintaining the family's ability to withstand adversity (Walsh 2006). How the family navigates challenges such as mental illness will impact on the wellbeing of all family members (Walsh 2011).

CRITICAL THINKING CHALLENGE 10.2

Read Case Study 10.1 about Marcia.

1. Which risk factors or challenges can be identified for Marcia, Michael, the children and the family as a whole?
2. Which strengths or resources do the family have?
3. How can the family's resilience be supported by mental health clinicians?

BOX 10.1 Key Processes That Support Family Resilience

- Communication and discussion about mental illness between family members
- Maintaining rituals and routines, such as family dinners, family holidays or recreational events
- Family bonding and positive relationships between family members

(*Source*: Adapted from Power et al. 2015)

CASE STUDY 10.1

Marcia

Marcia and her husband Michael have two daughters: Nina, aged seven, and Rosie, aged three. They came to the UK from Eastern Europe 6 years ago and have no other family in the UK. Marcia's parents are divorced and Michael's father died 3 years ago. Marcia was admitted to the mental health inpatient unit after the birth of Rosie, with a diagnosis of postpartum psychosis and was recently admitted for 2 weeks for a further psychotic episode. She was then transferred to a private hospital and after discharge has been followed up by her GP.

Michael works fulltime to support the family. Nina attends a local primary school while Rosie stays home with Marcia. The children did not visit their mother in hospital and Michael had explained to them that Marcia was sick and needed a break. Marcia has not returned to work since the first episode of her illness 3 years ago. She has limited social support, with few friends and no family members in the UK.

Michael has rung the community mental health team concerned that Marcia has been keeping their eldest daughter Nina home from school. He thinks Marcia has stopped taking her antipsychotic medication but she is refusing to see the GP. Marcia has told him that she does not need help and became angry when he told her about planning to call the mental health team.

Michael describes some recent financial stress that means he has been working extra hours and they have been arguing. He describes that the children are well cared for but Nina has been teary and sleeping in their bed since Marcia was in hospital.

Planned approach to care:

- Joint home visit with the mental health team to assess the family, Marcia, the children and the environment; assessment to include family dynamics, strengths, difficulties, observation of children and parent–child interactions, state of the house, Marcia's mental state.
- Assess the impact of recent stressors on parents and children.
- Talk to both parents about their parenting concerns and the children.
- Talk about the impact of Marcia's hospitalisation on the children; explanations, support and reassurance their daughters might require; any fears the children might experience; and the impact of separation and Marcia's illness.
- Discuss Marcia's medication and its impact on her parenting (e.g. drowsiness) with her and Michael.
- Talk to Nina and Rosie about Marcia's illness and its effects, including reassurance and key messages that it isn't their fault, that she is not going to go away again unexpectedly and that she is not going to die.
- Consider making safety plans for the children and parents for managing any further episodes of separation as a result of Marcia's illness.
- Identify social and community supports for all members of the family including local playgroups or preschool groups, social groups, teachers, family support organisations, friends.
- Put Marcia in contact with parenting support, including local groups or services.
- Discuss the importance of schooling with the parents and children.
- Talk to the school and develop a plan to support the family (parents might be reluctant to talk to schools but schools can be an immense support to children; information can be provided to schools without parent consent but supporting Marcia and Michael to engage with the school and any potential supports for their daughter would be a more desirable option).
- Talk to Marcia about liaising with her GP about medication and ongoing follow up.
- Identify other family strengths and needs and develop a collaborative care plan with Marcia and Michael.

(The authors would like to acknowledge Sophie Isobel, CNC, for this case study and the genogram in Fig. 10.4).

FAMILY RECOVERY

In the context of mental illness, resilience and recovery can be understood as being interrelated (Friesen 2007). Resilience is a process that involves overcoming adversity and building strengths and recovery is a process that involves transformation in the face of challenges.

In mental health services, there has been a growing emphasis on provision of care that supports the personal recovery of patients. 'Personal recovery' has been defined as 'a deeply personal, unique process of changing one's attitudes, values, feelings, goals, skills and/or roles. It is a way of living a satisfying, hopeful and contributing life even with the limitations caused by [mental] illness' (Anthony 1993, p. 13). Implicit in this is the concept that patients define and assume responsibility for their own recovery (Wyder & Bland 2014). In personal recovery, people with mental illness can be understood as journeying through several processes. These include building *c*onnectedness with others, having *h*ope and optimism about the future, developing positive *i*dentity, finding *m*eaning in life and having *e*mpowerment (also known as CHIME) (Leamy et al. 2011).

Although there has been an increasing understanding and focus on individual patient recovery in mental health service provision, there has been minimal corresponding identification of the recovery process that families can experience as they journey alongside their family member with mental illness or distress. Yet just as the person with mental illness can experience recovery, so too can family members. These processes overlap with the personal recovery processes of the person with mental illness (Spaniol 2010) and recovery can be understood as a family process (Nicholson et al. 2014). Family recovery draws on the strengths of all members of the family, is informed by an understanding of life events and the impact of trauma and is driven by the family and their goals and needs (Nicholson et al. 2014).

Spaniol (2010) identifies four phases in the process of family recovery. Fig. 10.2 provides a visual framework of this process.

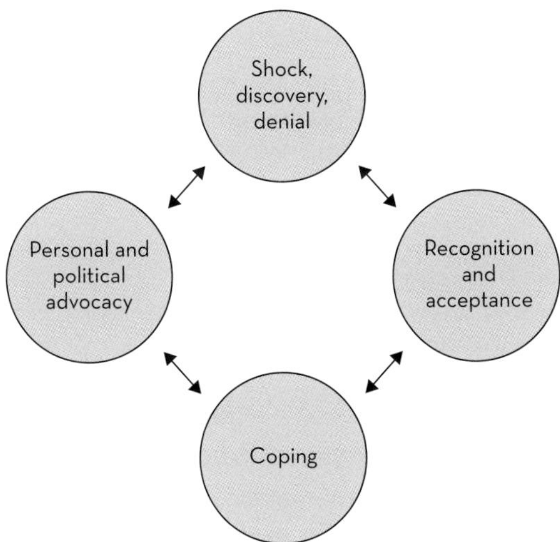

Fig. 10.2 Family recovery process. (*Source*: Spaniol, L., 2010. The pain and the possibility: the family recovery process. Community Mental Health Journal 46, 482–485.)

1. **Shock, discovery, denial:** An individual's acute mental illness can often be shocking for family members. Changes they may observe in the person can be difficult to understand. Family members may explain these away and not believe the illness is serious. Denial may persist throughout the early phase of the illness.
2. **Recognition and acceptance:** Family members may gradually gain awareness that their relative has mental illness. This can be accompanied by a sense of hope that health professionals know the answers for how to treat it, as well as feelings of guilt, embarrassment or even self-blame or responsibility for the illness. As part of the acceptance process, family members may feel a sense of loss for the life they had previously hoped for with their family member. Through grieving, over time they may come to accept this loss. Through a changing awareness of themselves, their relationships and life, family members can be transformed.
3. **Coping:** Initially, family members can struggle with the challenges of mental illness without adequate knowledge or skills. Later, family members learn to continue their lives and to identify how they can support their relative. Coping begins to replace grieving. Family members may become more assertive or angry as they question the care their relative is receiving. They may ask for additional support. Over time, the family's knowledge, confidence and coping skills may grow and they may come to view professionals as a necessary but not complete part of their ability to cope.
4. **Personal and political advocacy:** In the recovery process, family members slowly come to a new awareness of themselves. This may include a stronger sense of confidence and personal advocacy. They let go of self-blame and focus on new roles and ways of working with professionals that are more collaborative. For some family members, political advocacy and working to influence and change the system becomes more important.

TABLE 10.1 Tasks for Families in Recovery

1. Maintaining hope	Maintaining hope for themselves as individuals and their own dreams and aspirations. Holding hope is complex. Family may need to hold hope for their loved one. As they find ways to maintain hope for themselves, they are able to continue their caring responsibilities while leading their own fulfilling lives.
2. Reconnecting	Mental illness emerges within the complex network of close relationships that includes family and friends. Reconnecting includes maintaining or reestablishing relationships and support from others, being part of peer support and support groups and being part of the community.
3. Overcoming secondary trauma	Families can experience secondary traumatisation and share the trauma, isolation and stigma associated with mental illness. This can include feeling powerless to control their lives, feeling abused by the treatment system, experiencing guilt, feeling traumatised when their loved one is subjected to trauma and experiencing chronic grief and loss.
4. Journeying from carer to family	Families are often defined by their carer role. A family's journey is also an integral part of recovery. When families are able to let go of their caring role to achieve a mutually supportive role with their loved one, this ultimately enables not only their own but also their loved one's recovery.

(*Source*: Adapted from Wyder, M., Bland, R., 2014. The recovery framework as a way of understanding families' responses to mental illness: balancing different needs and recovery journeys. Australian Social Work 67(2), 179–196.)

Wyder and Bland (2014) have contributed to our emerging understanding of the interrelationship between personal and family recovery, through applying personal recovery frameworks to the family's tasks of supporting their relative and engaging in their own journey of recovery (see Table 10.1 for a summary). They conclude that the family's recovery from mental illness is an active and multidimensional process rather than limited simply to the role of caregiving.

CRITICAL THINKING CHALLENGE 10.3

1. Consider the personal recovery processes (CHIME) (Leamy et al. 2011) and the tasks for families in recovery (Wyder & Bland 2014). What are the similarities and differences between them? How can both individuals and families be supported by nurses in their recovery processes?
2. For each of the tasks for families in recovery outlined in Table 10.1, consider how nurses can support families to work through these tasks. Identify at least one strategy that nurses can use in supporting families in each family task.

WORKING WITH FAMILIES: FAMILY-FOCUSSED PRACTICE

As noted earlier, many mental health services continue to approach the care of people with mental illness through an individual lens. The focus is primarily on caring for the individual patient and managing their symptoms. If family are considered, it is often through how they can assist and support the person in their recovery, rather than from the perspective of the family's needs for information and support. Yet families/carers need to be involved in decisions about their family member's care (Foster 2010). There is need for greater recognition of family in service provision and the consequences/outcomes for family when this is not the case. An approach that focusses only on the individual and does not take into account the perspectives and needs of the people who love and care for them is an approach that fails to address the crucial family context of the lived experience of mental illness. As part of their model of care for patients, services need to provide information for families about key issues such as the patient's right to confidentiality, the patient's verbal or written consent for family/carers to have information about their illness and treatment and acknowledgment of family/carers' own needs for information about mental illness and available treatments (Rowe, 2012).

From an international perspective, best practice for working with patients and family/carers includes clinical care and communication that is empathic to family/carers (Rowe 2012), is provided in collaboration with the patient, family/carers and clinicians and where the path to recovery includes attention to financial, housing and social aspects of patients' and family/carers' lives (Wallcraft et al. 2011). Having clear standards for practice in mental health services can improve the quality of family/carer participation in mental healthcare and result in increased family/carer involvement in family care planning and improved contact between clinicians and family/carers (Lakeman 2008).

In mental health, family-focussed practice (FFP) is an approach to care that takes a 'whole of family' perspective and identifies the relationships between a mental health patient and their 'key others'. FFP involves the systematic incorporation of family member/carer health and wellbeing and the role of parenting into a family plan of care. In attending to all the family, FFP can be considered a form of preventive intervention that addresses the impact of intergenerational mental illness on family members including children and supports family recovery and resilience (Foster et al. 2015). Four key principles underpin FFP. These are a belief that:

1. Patients' (child or adult) families play a vital role in their recovery
2. Both patients and their families can be empowered to address and meet their needs
3. It is possible to support patients via their family
4. The relationships between clinician and patient, clinician and family and between patient and family members are key to enabling a 'whole of family' approach to care (Foster et al. 2015).

CRITICAL THINKING CHALLENGE 10.4

Read the paper by Goodyear et al. 2015.

1. Identify the essential and recommended practice standards for each stage of care. Which of these have you observed occurring in your clinical experience in mental health?
2. In your view, what are the barriers and enablers for clinicians engaging in these practices?
3. How could you as a student incorporate these practices into your practice on clinical placement?

Range of Family-Focussed Practice

In working with families, nurses may feel that they lack specific knowledge on the needs of children, parenting and/or the family as a whole. While there is a range of practices considered important for supporting families, it is not always feasible or necessary for nurses to provide all of them. FFP can be understood as comprising a continuum or range of intensity that moves from fundamental strategies through to more advanced or intensive approaches.

When working with families of procreation, Foster et al. (2012) recommend a minimum level of practice:

- identifying patients' parental status (as relevant) when they enter a service
- identifying the number, age, wellbeing and location of their dependent children
- supporting patients' and children's needs to maintain contact with each other
- providing relevant mental health information and resources including parenting information to patients, children and family members
- referring children and family members to family workers or services (including COPMI or FAPMI workers) as appropriate (see Fig. 10.3)

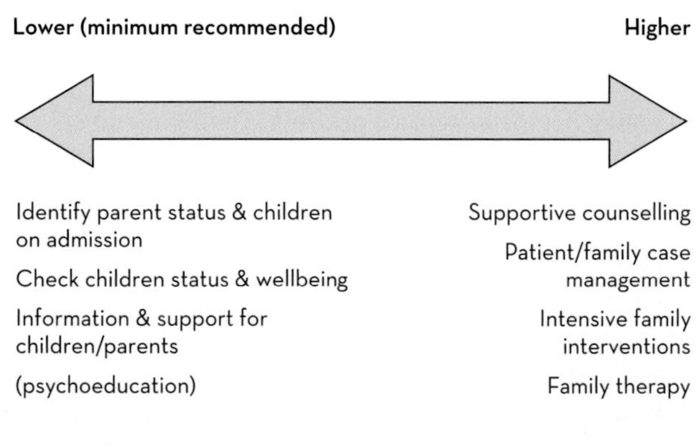

Fig. 10.3 Continuum of intensity of family-focussed practice. (*Source*: Foster, K., O'Brien, L., Korhonen, T., 2012. Developing resilient children and families where parents have mental illness: a family-focused approach. Int. J. Ment. Health Nurs. 21[1], 3–11.)

TABLE 10.2 Family-Focussed Practices

1. Assessment of family members and family functioning	Ranges from questions on family relationships at intake to service, to assessing parenting competency and/or family circumstances, impact of family member's illness on other family members and level of mental health literacy in family members.
2. Psychoeducation	Information and education on mental illness and treatment (including medication) that aims to improve family members' mental health literacy. Ranges from informal discussion and provision of written or online resources to evidence-based manualised family interventions.
3. Family care planning and goal setting	Collaborative care planning including crisis plans with family. Assisting family members to set goals in relation to patient's recovery and their own and other family members' wellbeing.
4. Liaising between the family and services	Liaising on behalf of the family between services and the family. Acting, or encouraging actions, with services to achieve better outcomes for the family.
5. Instrumental (I), emotional (E) and social (S) support	Referring family to another service and organising practical support (I). Showing empathy and compassion to family members (E). Empowering family and encouraging them to expand social connections and networks with others (S).
6. Coordinated system of care between the family and services	Coordinated system of care involving collaboration and partnership with family members, clinicians and other services. Commonly involves a wrap-around of care for the family that includes partnership between the family and service providers in a synchronised manner. Ranges from general approach involving coordinating services to defined type of service (e.g. wrap-around) with model of care.

(*Source*: Adapted from Foster, K., Maybery, D., Reupert, A., Gladstone, B., Grant, A., Ruud, T., Falkov, A., Kowalenko, N., 2015. Family focused practice in mental health care: an integrative review. Child & Youth Services, Special Edition, https://doi.org/10.1080/0145935X.2016.1104048.)

BOX 10.2 Key Areas of Family Assessment on Patient's Entry Into a Mental Health Service

- Identifying who the patient lives with and which, if any, family members or loved ones provide emotional and/or practical support for them.
- Identifying and documenting, as relevant, parent status and dependent child/children (under 18 years) status.
- If patient is a parent of dependent children, asking about child/children's care arrangements.
- Identifying family structure (family of origin and procreation/choice)[a] and the nature of key family relationships (e.g. parent/s, sibling/s, partner, children, other key family members as identified by the patient).
- Identifying recent and/or longstanding family-related stressors (e.g. illness and/or death in family, substance use, domestic violence, divorce/relationship breakdown, unemployment and financial stress, relocation, transfer of schools, lack of housing).
- Identifying patient's and family's strengths (resources including strong family relationships/supports, community support, etc.) and areas of vulnerability or need (including stressors, current illness, etc.).

[a]See Fig. 10.4 for an example of family structure in a genogram for Marcia from Case Study 10.1.

For all families, there is a range of practices that nurses and other health professionals can engage in to address the needs of all family members. A systematically conducted review of international literature on FFP identified six core practices when working with families of origin or procreation (see Table 10.2). Box 10.2 outlines assessment areas for families on intake into a service. As part of the family assessment process it is common to develop a genogram (visual display) of the family structure and key relationships. See Fig. 10.4 for an example of a genogram for Marcia from Case Study 10.1.

CONCLUSION

This chapter has focussed on the issues faced by family members when a relative has mental illness and the role nurses can play in supporting families through the recovery process and in building the family's resilience. Understanding the challenges faced by family members when their loved one has mental illness (including the need for adequate information about mental illness, its causes and treatments and the potential for negative impacts on their own physical and mental health, the risk of stigma and economic hardship, social isolation and relationship problems) can inform more relevant support provision by mental health nurses. Focussing on building family strengths and resources and on supporting family relationships has potential to help prevent intergenerational transmission of mental illness and enable families to journey through family recovery and to develop resilience and wellbeing.

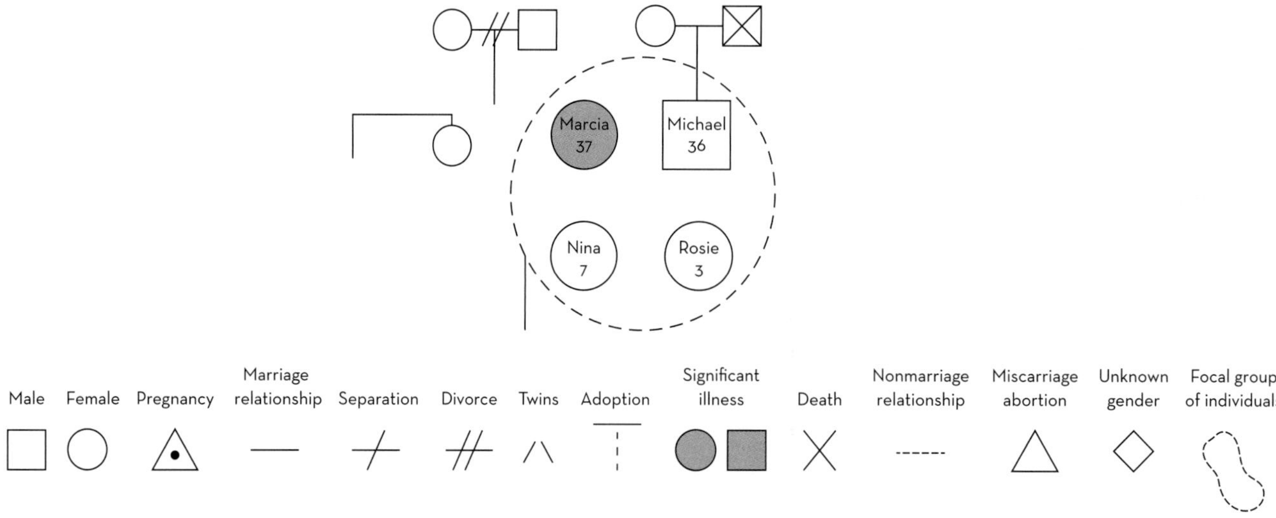

Fig. 10.4 Genogram of Marcia's family. (*Source*: Sophie Isobel, CNC.)

CASE STUDY 10.2

Stuart

Stuart is a 19-year-old man who presented to the community mental health service with suicidal ideation and a suicide plan after being referred through emergency department triage. He was accompanied by his 'adopted' father Dan. Dan was very concerned for Stuart's welfare and wanted Stuart to be seen by the mental health team. A couple of years earlier Dan befriended Stuart and became a father figure and mentor to him after meeting Stuart at a football club where they both played. Since then Dan and Stuart had developed a strong bond and connection.

Stuart had recently learnt that his biological father had died (by natural causes). Stuart did not live with his father but visited him regularly. Stuart had a history of bipolar affective disorder and had previously been a patient at a child and adolescent mental health service. Stuart's biological father had also had a history of mental illness.

On assessment at the community mental health service, the stressors in Stuart's life included the recent loss of his biological father, the related need to ensure his father had an appropriate funeral and to finalise his financial affairs and estate. Stuart's three other siblings did not have any contact with their father and wanted nothing to do with the funeral or the finalisation of the estate.

At the time of assessment, Stuart could not give any guarantee of safety and was considered a risk of harm to himself and so was admitted for further treatment and assessment to the inpatient unit. After 3 days in the unit he was prescribed antidepressant therapy and referred to the community mental health team. The community mental health service provided follow up and saw Stuart regularly in the company of Dan.

(The authors would like to acknowledge Michael Blair, RN, for this case study.)

PATIENT STORY 10.1

Kerry Hawkins (Family Carer)

Broken brain, broken hearts, shattered dreams, false starts.

My husband slowly started to become ill soon after we had our first child in 1997. By the time our third child was born in 2002, he was clearly experiencing paranoid beliefs, based on perceived interactions with people. However, he wasn't diagnosed with paranoid schizophrenia until 2008, many long and traumatic years later, with his first suicide attempt and subsequent hospitalisation.

This was not something I had planned for in my dreams around having a family. When we met, he was a solid, loving, intelligent and accomplished person. Like most people, we planned to have a family. There was no indication during our early years of marriage that he was ill. However, after our daughter was born, my husband became a little depressed and stressed and inexplicably hostile towards me. He started to change jobs regularly on the basis of increasingly paranoid beliefs. He had already become hostile towards my family and friends and actively discouraged their visits, so support from my family became limited.

By the time our third child was 6 months old, my exhaustion levels were profound. The combination of financial strain and hostility from my husband, the demands of three lovely, energetic and attention-requiring children and lack of any practical or emotional support was overwhelming. We struggled on. My husband's mental health gradually worsened. For a period of several years, our family life was characterised by despair, financial worries and fear of what lay ahead. The children were profoundly traumatised by witnessing his angry outbursts, confrontations with community members and absence from our lives.

His paranoid beliefs worsened and he was unable to keep a job for longer than several months. He hated me for not believing him, hated being a father and was full of anger. His belief that people were conspiring to remove him from the workplace degenerated into believing people were actively pursuing him with the intent to capture and harm him, believing they would eventually kill him and believing people thought he was a paedophile and were spreading rumours that followed him wherever

PATIENT STORY 10.1—cont'd

Kerry Hawkins (Family Carer)

he went. He left home periodically to escape the people he believed were seeking to destroy him. He also believed we were at risk from the same people and was shattered by the effect he was having on our family.

Finally, he became completely convinced he was about to be abducted and tortured and went on a month-long trip overseas, escaping his 'persecutors' and in fear of his life. This culminated in a suicide attempt using medication provided from a previous hospitalisation. During this period, he rang quite often and left rambling, fear-filled farewell messages on our phone, which terrified the children, who inadvertently occasionally heard them. The financial cost of the 3 years preceding this, with flights, accommodation and transport costs and gaps in employment were terrifying. With his refusal for years to apply for welfare benefits, because he did not believe he was ill, meant that for over 10 years we lived with a negative income. The distress caused by poverty is just as difficult to deal with as all the other stresses—the poverty was traumatising, disempowering, isolating and paralysing.

I made the decision to go overseas and bring my husband back to live with us, not only because I feared for his safety, but because I believed in him—believed that there had to be a way to help him recover if I could keep him safe and that he was the only person who could completely heal our children. This has been the right decision. He went straight into hospital and was diagnosed with paranoid schizophrenia. For 3 years after this, he lived in fear for his life, despite trying over 10 different neuroleptics, including combinations of clozapine and other medications. None made any difference to his paranoia or associated levels of terror, merely his sedation levels.

He has since been an inpatient several times, both in locked and open wards. These experiences have been profoundly antitherapeutic for him (his second suicide attempt was partly out of fear that I would have him hospitalised as I could see he was unwell and he said he would rather have killed himself than be readmitted) and traumatic for the children. His times in mental health units, other than stabilising him after the toxic effects of overdoses, have done him more harm than good. The facilities are also profoundly family-unfriendly, with the children torn between wanting to see their father and being reluctant to experience the hospital environment. The children were also at a very real risk of losing both parents to the effects of mental illness, as the emotional and practical strains I faced were indescribably challenging.

I gave up work in 2010 as it became clear that the mental health system was not working for him. There was no capacity within the primary care system, acute services or community mental health sector at the time to build a relationship with him, which is what he needed. I was able to encourage him to counter the effects on his body of the medication through exercise and diet, as he had gained over 30 kg, developed borderline diabetes and a life-threatening deep vein thrombosis as a consequence of his poor physical health. It was also better for the children; I could organise playtimes with their friends, take them to sports training, do community work, cook healthy meals, walk them to school and so on. It was important to protect them from the myriad of emotional, financial and social consequences of our situation as much as possible.

My time spent supporting him also enabled me to learn about recovery, something I didn't feel was mentioned enough within medical services. It really helped to hear the stories of people who had found a way through psychosis and we engaged with a number of community support groups and third-sector organisations. This led to a peer worker, also a survivor of child sexual abuse, visiting our home—and the process of enabling my husband to heal began. This process has left me wondering whether mental illness is truly a consequence of a broken brain or a broken system?

My husband is finally showing signs of recovery and I feel I have my man back. After not laughing for over 10 years, he has come alive again. He is confidently reengaging with the community. For the first time in over 10 years, he is planning our future. And the children have their father back, healing them in a way nothing else could. He is profoundly aware of the impact of his illness on all of us and the children's needs, doing everything he can to make up for the years of distress. And he's doing it brilliantly, enriching their lives every day with his presence.

Our children are robust, articulate, ebullient and kind and take delight in being a family. They have all been succeeding in their academic work, play regular sport, are well-ensconced in healthy friendship groups and are usually overtly, loudly happy. It's far from perfect, but it's perfectly normal. Different families will have different needs. But what we all need is someone to sit down with us and let us tell them what is required to help us as a family and then empower us to recover by helping us decide what we need, enabling us to access those resources with ease and dignity. For us, we had a very negative experience of the mental health system, which we found to be fractured and difficult to navigate; the array of organisations that have age, postcode and funding criteria and simply didn't deliver what we needed was just another exhausting trauma to have to deal with. It is too focussed on the individual and on the medical diagnosis.

What we needed—and found just in time—was a peer worker who didn't tell my husband what was wrong with him, but asked 'What happened to you?' But what families like us really need is a power shift where we are able to have our heads above water and get remunerated for the incredibly important work we do.

(*Source*: Adapted from ACMHN Newsletter, Spring News, pp. 16–17.)

EXERCISE FOR CLASS ENGAGEMENT

Read Patient Story 10.1 by Kerry Hawkins, 'Broken brain, broken hearts, shattered dreams, false starts'.

1. Using the framework of family recovery by Spaniol (2010), identify the relevant aspects of the family recovery process in this family's story.
2. Which elements of mental health service delivery were effective and ineffective in supporting this family's recovery?
3. How can mental health service delivery be changed or improved to provide greater support for family recovery for all family members?

REFERENCES

Aguglia, E., Onor, M.L., Trevisio, M., Negro, C., Saina, M., Maso, E., 2004. Stress in the caregivers of Alzheimer's patients: an experimental investigation in Italy. American Journal of Alzheimer's Disease and Other Dementias 19 (4), 248–252.

Anthony, W.A., 1993. Recovery from mental illness: the guiding vision of the mental health service system in the 1990s. Psychiatric Rehabilitation Journal 16 (4), 11–23.

Bassani, D.G., Padoin, C.V., Philipp, D., Veldhuizen, S., 2009. Estimating the number of children exposed to parental psychiatric disorders through a national health survey. Child and Adolescent Psychiatry and Mental Health 3, 6.

Black, K., Lobo, M., 2008. A conceptual review of family resilience factors. Journal of Family Nursing 14 (1), 33–55.

Cowling, V., McGorry, P., 2012. Parental mental illness is a family matter. Medical Journal of Australia 1 (1), 5. https://doi.org/10.5694/mjao12.10553.

Cummins, R., Hughes, J., 2007. The wellbeing of Australians: Carer health and wellbeing. Australian Unity Wellbeing Index, Survey 17.1. Deakin University, Geelong.

Darbyshire, P., Jackson, D., 2005. Using a strengths approach to understand resilience and build health capacity in families. Contemporary Nurse 18, 211–212.

Digiacomo, M., Delaney, P., Abbott, P.A., Davidson, P.M., Delaney, J., Vincent, F., 2013. 'Doing the hard yards': carer and provider focus group perspectives of accessing Aboriginal childhood disability services. BMC Health Services Research. https://doi.org/10.1186/1472-6963-13-326.

Foster, K., 2010. 'You'd think this roller coaster was never going to stop': the experience of being the adult child of a parent with serious mental illness. Journal of Clinical Nursing 19, 3143–3151.

Foster, K., 2011. 'I wanted to learn how to heal my heart': family carer experiences of receiving an emotional support service in the Well Ways program. International Journal of Mental Health Nursing 20 (1), 56–62.

Foster, K., O'Brien, L., Korhonen, T., 2012. Developing resilient children and families where parents have mental illness: a family-focused approach. International Journal of Mental Health Nursing 21 (1), 3–11.

Foster, K., Maybery, D., Reupert, A., Gladstone, B., Grant, A., Ruud, T., Falkov, A., Kowalenko, N., 2015. Family focused practice in mental health care: an integrative review. Child & Youth Services, Special Edition. https://doi.org/10.1080/0145935X.2016.1104048.

Foster, K., Robinson, T., 2014. Educating for emotional resilience in adolescence. In: Hurley, J., Linsley, P., Van der Zwan, R. (Eds.), Emotions in Education Settings. Primrose Publishing, London, pp. 56–70.

Friesen, B.J., 2007. Recovery and resilience in children's mental health: views from the field. Psychiatric Rehabilitation Journal 31 (1), 38–48.

Goodyear, M., Hill, T.-L., Allchin, B., McCormick, F., Hine, R., Cuff, R., O'Hanlon, B., 2015. Standards of practice for the adult mental health workforce: meeting the needs of families where a parent has a mental illness. International Journal of Mental Health Nursing 24 (2), 169–180.

Jensen, L.E., 2004. Mental health care experiences: listening to families. Journal of the American Psychiatric Nurses Association 10 (1), 33–41.

Jones, D.W., 2004. Families and serious mental illness: working with loss and ambivalence. British Journal of Social Work 34, 961–979.

Kenny, C., Sarma, K.M., Egan, J., 2012. An interpretive phenomenological account of the experiences of family carers of the elderly. The Irish Journal of Psychology 33, 199–214.

Lakeman, R., 2008. Practice standards to improve the quality of family and carer participation in adult mental health care: an overview and evaluation. International Journal of Mental Health Nursing 17, 44–56.

Larson, J.E., Corrigan, P., 2008. The stigma of families with mental illness. Academic Psychiatry 32, 87–91.

Leamy, M., Bird, V., Le Boutillier, C., Williams, J., Slade, M., 2011. Conceptual framework for personal recovery in mental health: systematic review and narrative synthesis. British Journal of Psychiatry 199, 445–452.

Logan, J.G., Barksdale, D.J., 2008. Allostasis and allostatic load: expanding the discourse on stress and cardiovascular disease. Journal of Clinical Nursing 17, 201–208.

Luthar, S.S., Cicchetti, D., Becker, B., 2000. The construct of resilience: a critical evaluation and guidelines for future work. Child Development 71 (3), 543–562.

Maybery, D., Reupert, A., Goodyear, M., Ritchie, R., Brann, P., 2009. Investigating the strengths and difficulties of children from families with a parental mental illness. Australian e-Journal for the Advancement of Mental Health 8 (2). Available at: www.auseinet.com/journal/vol8iss2/maybery.pdf.

McCann, T.V., Bamberg, J., McCann, F., 2015. Family carers' experience of caring for an older parent with severe and persistent mental illness. International Journal of Mental Health 24, 203–212.

McCann, T.V., Lubman, D.I., Clark, E., 2011. Responding to stigma: first time caregivers of young people with first-episode psychosis. Psychiatric Services 62, 548–550.

Mental Health Council of Australia, 2010. Mental health carers report. Available at: http://mhaustralia.org/sites/default/files/imported/component/rsfiles/publications/MHCA_CarerSurv_Layout_15-11.pdf.

Mordoch, E., Hall, W.A., 2008. Children's perceptions of living with a parent with a mental illness: finding the rhythm and maintaining the frame. Qualitative Health Research 18, 1127–1144.

Murphy, G., Peters, K., Jackson, D., Wilkes, L., 2011. A qualitative meta-synthesis of adult children of parents with a mental illness. Journal of Clinical Nursing 20, 3430–3442.

Murphy, G., Peters, K., Jackson, D., 2014. A dynamic cycle of familial mental illness. Issues in Mental Health Nursing 35, 948–953.

Nicholson, J., Wolf, T., Wilder, C., Biebel, K., 2014. Creating options for family recovery: a providers' guide to promoting parental mental health. Available at: www.employmentoptions.org.

Office for National Statistics, 2017. Unpaid carers provide social care worth £57 billion. Available at: https://www.ons.gov.uk/peoplepopulationandcommunity/healthandsocialcare/healthandlifeexpectancies/articles/unpaidcarersprovidesocialcareworth57billion/2017-07-10. Accessed: 9 October 2018.

Osher, T.W., Osher, D.M., 2002. The paradigm shift to true collaboration with families. Journal of Child & Family Studies 11, 47–60.

Power, J., Goodyear, M., Maybery, D., Reupert, A., O'Hanlon, B., Cuff, R., Perlesz, A., 2015. Family resilience in families where a parent has mental illness. Journal of Social Work. https://doi.org/10.1177/1468017314568081.

Ranchandani, P., Psychogiou, L., 2009. Paternal psychiatric disorders and children's psychosocial development. Lancet 374, 646–653.

Reed, S.I., 2008. First-episode psychosis: a literature review. International Journal of Mental Health Nursing 17 (2), 85–91.

Repetti, R.L., Robles, T.F., Reynolds, B., 2011. Allostatic processes in the family. Development and Psychopathology 23, 921–938.

Reupert, A.E., Mayberry, D.J., Kowalenko, N.M., 2012. Children whose parents have a mental illness: prevalence, need and treatment. Medical Journal of Australia Open 1 (1), 7–9.

Richardson, M., Cobham, V., McDermott, B., Murray, J., 2013. Youth mental illness and the family: parents' loss and grief. Journal of Child Family Studies 22, 719–736.

Rowe, J., 2012. Great expectations: a systematic review of the literature on the role of family carers in severe mental illness, and their relationships and engagement with professionals. Journal of Psychiatric and Mental Health Nursing 19, 70–82.
Shankar, J., Muthuswamy, S.S., 2007. Support needs of family caregivers of people who experience mental illness and the role of mental health services. Families in Society 88 (2), 302–310.
Somers, V., 2007. Schizophrenia: the impact of parental illness on children. British Journal of Social Work 37 (8), 1319–1334.
Spaniol, L., 2010. The pain and the possibility: the family recovery process. Community Mental Health Journal 46, 482–485.
Usher, K., Jackson, D., O'Brien, L., 2005. Adolescent drug abuse: helping families survive. International Journal of Mental Health Nursing 14, 209–214.
Wallcraft, J., Amering, M., Freidin, J., Davar, B., Froggatt, D., Jafri, H., Javed, A., Katontoka, S., Raja, S., et al., 2011. Partnerships for better mental health worldwide: WPA recommendations on best practices in working with service users and family carers. World Psychiatry 10, 229–236.
Walsh, F., 2006. Strengthening family resilience, second ed. Guildford Press, New York.
Walsh, F., 2011. Resilience in families with serious health challenges. In: Craft-Rosenberg, M., Pehler, S.-R. (Eds.), Sage Encyclopedia of Family Health. Sage, New York, pp. 895–899.
West, C., Usher, K., Foster, K., 2011. Family resilience: towards a new model of chronic pain management. Collegian 18 (1), 3–10.
Wyder, M., Bland, R., 2014. The recovery framework as a way of understanding families' responses to mental illness: balancing different needs and recovery journeys. Australian Social Work 67 (2), 179–196.
Zauszniewski, J.A., Bekhet, A.K., Suresky, J., 2010. Resilience in family members of persons with serious mental illness. Nursing Clinics of North America 45, 613–626.

USEFUL WEBSITES

Carers UK: Making life better for carers, www.carersuk.org
Centre for Mental Health: Supporting carers, www.centreformentalhealth.org.uk
Mind: For better mental health: How to cope when supporting someone else, www.mind.org.uk
UK Government: Advice and support for carers and the people they care for, www.gov.uk/carers-uk

11

Disorders of Childhood and Adolescence

Deb O'Kane, Kristin Henderson

KEY POINTS

- While the term 'child' generally refers to ages 0 to 13 years and the term 'adolescent' to ages 14 to 18 years, within this chapter the combined group aged 0 to18 years will at times be referred to collectively as 'children and young people'.
- The prevalence of emotional problems in the earlier years of life ranges from 20% to 26% internationally. In adolescence, anxiety and depression are among the most common mental health problems.
- More than 75% of people with serious mental illness experience their first episode before the age of 25 years. Although the highest prevalence of mental health problems occurs in the 18 to 24 age group, precursors to serious mental illness that are identified and managed during childhood and adolescence can serve to reduce this statistic.
- Mental health problems cannot be seen as operating in isolation from other aspects of young people's lives.
- Evidence of a child or an adolescent experiencing behavioural or emotional problems may be indicative of difficulties within the family.
- Working with children and adolescents can be challenging, yet very fulfilling.
- It is essential to clarify the individual's perception of the problem they are experiencing and their goals for 'treatment', as well as their parents' perceptions and desired outcomes, while working safely to protect the young person's right to confidentiality.
- 'Engagement' is the establishment of a therapeutic relationship, or rapport, in collaboration with the young person and their family to achieve desired outcomes and goals. This occurs from the initial interview. Understanding young people's language and their style of communicating is integral to effectively engaging with them.
- Children and adolescents may differ in presentation when compared with adults with similar disorders.
- Nurses involved in the care of children and adolescents may have to deal with legal issues relating to duty of care, child protection and mental health legislation.
- Child and carer participation is increasingly important when working with families.

KEY TERMS

engagement
Gillick competence
internalising and externalising problems
psychoeducation
resocialisation

LEARNING OUTCOMES

The material in this chapter will help you to:

- develop an introductory understanding of childhood and adolescent mental health problems and disorders.
- gain awareness of the extent of childhood and adolescent mental health problems in the UK and internationally.
- appreciate the range of services provided to children and adolescents.
- explore the role of the nurse in working with children and adolescents with mental health needs and supporting their families.

INTRODUCTION

Children and adolescents cannot simply be considered as 'little adults'. Within the field of mental health there are distinct differences between early life and adulthood. In recognition of the specific needs of children and young people, youth services (including mental health services) often extend their age range to include young adults up to 25 years of age.

This chapter introduces the field of child and adolescent mental health nursing. It explores the role of the nurse and, using case studies from clinical practice, provides examples of disorders experienced by children and adolescents. Furthermore, it describes interventions that nurses can implement to assist young people and their families.

Although some disorders are intergenerational, they might differ in their form of presentation during different developmental stages. For example, children suffering from depression might present as agitated or have a variety of somatic symptoms, whereas some depressed adolescents might seem antisocial, aggressive or withdrawn or become involved in substance use (Rey et al. 2015). Some problems common to adults might start in childhood or be influenced by events that occurred early in life. Some problems resolve with neurological development, emotional maturity or a stable, supportive environment. Likewise, with effective intervention and treatment there may be problems from which the young person can achieve a complete recovery.

Anxiety and depression are among the most common mental health problems experienced during adolescence. More than 75% of people with serious mental illness such as schizophrenia or bipolar disorder have their first episode before the age of 25 years and at least half of all mental health problems emerge by the age of 18 years (Layard & Hagell 2015). The highest prevalence of all mental health problems, including substance disorders, occurs in the 16 to 24 year age group, with suicide being the third highest cause of death worldwide in this age group (Gore et al. 2011). With statistics such as these, it is crucial that the mental health of children and young people should be a priority for society as a whole.

An important factor in considering the effect of any kind of illness on young people is the disruption it may bring to their development and education. In adulthood, our lives can be dramatically impacted by illness, yet we have usually completed the basic developmental tasks of life and have finished the foundations of education. For the child or adolescent, however, various problems may develop simply because of the interruption caused by illness. Similarly, a child's experiences during early development and onwards can influence subsequent developmental progress, mental health and wellbeing, giving rise to problems in adolescence and later life.

Yet despite the prevalence of child and adolescent mental health disorders, mental health issues continue to go unrecognised and untreated in children and young people, leading to poorer outcomes in areas such as health, education and occupation. This can result in a vast economic cost to society. Specialised child and adolescent mental health services are often unavailable locally in some areas of the UK, with children and families having to travel long distances to access the right support, hence many young people are unable to access the appropriate early recognition and support (Morris et al. 2011). It is with this in mind that health service policy, planning and models of care for children and young people should be targeted by strategies such as health promotion, prevention and early intervention to support tomorrow's adults and to reduce the associated financial burden (World Health Organization [WHO] 2014; Erskine et al. 2015).

DIAGNOSIS IN CHILD AND ADOLESCENT MENTAL HEALTHCARE

Unlike previous editions of the American Psychiatric Association's *Diagnostic and Statistical Manual of Mental Disorders*, the fifth edition (APA 2013) places greater emphasis on a developmental and lifespan perspective, accepting that a significant proportion of mental health problems commence in childhood and adolescence. Symptoms exhibited by young people may be transient, dynamic and changing over time and may not always fall easily into a diagnostic category. While acknowledging that these problems are not limited to a specific age group, there is a higher frequency of occurrence during periods such as early childhood, middle childhood and adolescence. Table 11.1 provides an overview of mental health issues experienced by children and young people.

The child behaviour checklist (see Box 11.1) places stronger emphasis on behaviour and problems rather than categories. Viewing problems within such a framework helps us to understand that young people have issues related to predominant personality traits, developmental factors or incidents and influences within their family and wider social environment. By contrast, static diagnostic systems can

TABLE 11.1 Overview of Mental Health Issues in Children and Young People

Neurodevelopmental Disorders	Elimination Disorders	Depressive and Bipolar Disorders	Anxiety Disorders
Autism spectrum disorder Attention deficit hyperactivity disorder Communication disorders Specific learning disorder Tic disorder	Encopresis Enuresis	Major depressive disorder Persistent depressive disorder Bipolar disorder Disruptive mood dysregulation disorder	Selective mutism Specific phobia Separation anxiety Social anxiety Panic disorder Agoraphobia Generalised anxiety
Disruptive, Impulse Control and Conduct Disorders	**Trauma and Stressor-Related Disorders**	**Schizophrenia Spectrum and Other Psychotic Disorders**	**Feeding and Eating Disorders**
Oppositional defiant disorder Intermittent explosive disorder Conduct disorder	Reactive attachment disorder Disinhibited social engagement disorder Posttraumatic stress disorder Acute stress disorder Adjustment disorder	Delusional disorder Brief psychotic disorder Schizophrenia Schizoaffective disorder	Anorexia nervosa Bulimia nervosa Binge-eating disorder Avoidant/restrictive food intake disorder Pica

(Adapted from American Psychiatric Association (APA) 2013. Diagnostic and statistical manual of mental disorders, 5th ed. APA, Washington, DC.)

BOX 11.1 Child Behaviour Checklist

General Areas

- *Internalising problems:* inhibited or over-controlled behaviours, such as anxiety or depression
- *Externalising problems:* antisocial or under-controlled behaviours, such as delinquency or aggression

Specific Areas

- *Somatic complaints:* recurring physical problems that have no known cause or cannot be medically verified; these may include headaches or a tendency to develop signs and symptoms of a medical disorder.
- *Delinquent behaviour:* behaviour where rules set by parents and/or communities are broken, such as property damage, theft of cars and other items.
- *Attention problems:* concentration difficulties and an inability to sit still, including school performance problems.
- *Aggressive behaviour:* bullying, teasing, fighting and temper tantrums.
- *Social problems:* where individuals have impairment of their relationships with peers.
- *Withdrawal:* where the individual is specifically inhibited by shyness and being socially isolated.
- *Anxious/depressed behaviour:* a range of feelings of loneliness, sadness, feeling unloved, a sense of worthlessness, anxiety and generalised fears.
- *Thought disorders:* or what might be seen as bizarre behaviour or thinking.

(Adapted from Sawyer, M.G., Miller-Lewis, L.R., Clark, J.J., 2007. The mental health of 13–17-year-olds in Australia: findings from the National Survey of Mental Health and Wellbeing. Journal of Youth Adolescence 36, 185–194.)

mask the fluid, changing and reorganising nature of young people's experience as they progress towards adulthood and may also run the risk of encouraging a focus on one 'problem' in isolation, rather than exploring a child's functioning in different settings and from different sources of information (Thompson et al. 2012; Achenbach & Ndetei 2012). For this reason, this chapter describes mental health problems in the context in which symptoms are observed, rather than in relation to categorical diagnostic criteria.

INCIDENCE

Writers in various Western countries have often expressed concern about the prevalence of emotional problems in the earlier years of life. Within countries surveyed, the incidence ranges from 10% to 20%. The World Health Organization (WHO) has predicted that these figures will double by 2020, making emotional problems one of the more common causes of illness and disability in children (WHO 2014). Figures published by Public Health England (PHE) (2016a) suggest that approximately 695,000 children (5–16 years) in England have a clinically significant, diagnosable mental health illness: conduct disorders in 68,100 children; anxiety in 39,500 children; attention deficit hyperactivity disorder (ADHD) in 18,900 children and depression in 10,800 children. This equates to approximately 1 in 10 children.

MENTAL ILLNESS IN CONTEXT

Because mental health problems can affect many aspects of young people's lives, their problems must be seen in context. It is often the case that the more significant the mental health problem, the greater the possibility of complications in other aspects of their lives. Furthermore, parents and other family members may often see these problems as affecting their own lifestyles and activities. While more needs to be understood about the long-term outlook for these young people, it is important for professionals to see the problems in the context of the child's everyday experiences. Help may be needed across a broad range of life issues—with family functioning, social skills or school problems, for example. While the mental health problem may have caused these difficulties, it is equally important to consider that a life issue may have been the cause *or* an aggravating factor in the disorder (Sawyer et al. 2007). A balanced view is required, so that causal factors are not attributed to one area without adequately observing what is happening in other aspects of the young person's life. It may be that the child or adolescent is acting as a 'barometer' for problems existing in the family—the young person may be presenting with symptoms that reflect problems in the family or between parents. This may not be recognised initially and may be revealed only after some exploration over time. This is why an important aspect of assessment of children and adolescents includes an evaluation of the family's functioning and coping skills.

ASSESSMENT

Assessing the mental health of children and young people can be very complex. Depending on the age of the child, it may not be the young person who identifies their specific problem or seeks assistance. Rather, a referral is often received from an adult (parent, teacher, health worker) presenting their view of the problem, thus providing an interpretation of what they perceive is troubling the child. It is the responsibility of the nurse to build a therapeutic relationship with all parties involved, ensuring that each person feels heard, valued and accepted.

In the process of gathering information, an assessment should include not only talking with the child or young person on their own, but also asking their consent to talk to others, such as their parents, carers, friends and teachers, in order to gain alternative perspectives. It is helpful to obtain relevant information from a number of people, given that problems may be interpreted and represented in a variety of ways by others involved in a child's life. Using a biopsychosocial assessment approach can be time consuming and is often best managed over several short sessions, rather than in one go.

Assessment will follow a similar structure to that undertaken in an adult mental health assessment; however, additional information might be required. Having a sound knowledge of normal developmental milestones enables the nurse to differentiate between the normal responses and developmental challenges of life and the significant psychological problems that may be occurring. Many mental health problems in children and young people may go undetected because signs of the problem are exhibited through their behaviour, physical manifestations or school performance. Exploring the prevalence, persistence, pervasiveness and negative impact of the problem helps appraise and conceptualise its nature and severity, so that appropriate interventions can be implemented.

Similarly, gaining an appreciation of the hopes, fears and expectations of each person present—while exploring strengths and protective factors, parenting styles and relationships between family members—can assist in placing the identified problems in context. For instance, issues such as poverty, unemployment, parental substance misuse and cultural isolation can all have a detrimental impact on a child's mental health. Therefore, it is important to collect information that allows the mental health nurse to see the problem in a wider context in order to be able to work effectively with the child and family (Layard and Hagell 2015). Observation also plays a critical role when assessing children and adolescents. The behaviour and the information provided may not always be congruent. Observing family interactions, nonverbal communication and each person's responses can highlight unrecognised family dynamics and lead to further understanding of what is happening for the child within the family or within the child's other social contexts.

Finally, assessing risk is an essential part of any child and adolescent mental health assessment (Mares & Graeff-Martins 2012). Health professionals are required by law to report any children who they believe are at risk. Thus mental health nurses have a statutory obligation to report any suspicion of risk to a child or young person with whom they are working. Significant harm or likelihood of experiencing significant harm from abuse (physical, sexual, emotional, neglect or a combination of all) must be reported. Multiagency collaboration and cohesion is essential in cases where abuse is suspected or disclosed to ensure a unified response. Risk assessment cannot be achieved through a 'tick box' exercise, since risks concerning children and adolescents are often multifactorial and complex. Risk must be assessed not only from a mental health perspective, but also within the caregiving context. Risk factors can include an immediate threat to the child's safety, as in cases of child abuse, or be cumulative, such as a child who is exposed to multiple risk factors such as adversity, neglect, parental illness or domestic violence.

Being sensitive to the prevalence of child abuse and the impact of the abuse on a child's health and psychological wellbeing is essential in any assessment. The long-term effect of abuse can have profound consequences in the developing years, leading to mental health problems, drug and alcohol dependence and associated risk taking.

As Dogra and Leighton (2009) indicate, it can be helpful for a nurse to have a framework from which all aspects of the assessment are completed (see example in Box 11.2). Ultimately, undertaking a comprehensive mental health assessment will allow the mental health nurse to gather the facts and ensure that any decisions made are in the best interests of the child and family.

BOX 11.2 Example of a Framework to Guide the Assessment Process

- Presenting concerns
- Family history
- Social history
- Developmental assessment
- Cultural issues
- Psychometric tools
- Mental state assessment
- Observation of interactions
- Risk assessment

SERVICES AVAILABLE TO CHILDREN AND YOUNG PEOPLE

In many Western countries, specialised input is most often provided by child and adolescent mental health services (CAMHS), as in the UK, or child and youth mental health services (CYMHS). These services have expanded their scope considerably, offering a range of specialist assessment and treatment options. A limitation remains that these services are often found only in main centres. However, smaller populations in rural areas in some countries, such as Australia and New Zealand, have the benefit of eCYMHS, with access to online psychiatric, nursing and allied health input via electronic media generated to smaller populations from main centres, a model that could offer significant benefits globally.

To offer a comprehensive service to meet the mental health needs of children and adolescents, the focus of service delivery requires a shift from all mental health–related issues being managed by child and adolescent mental health services to an acceptance that early-onset symptoms can effectively be managed via promotive and preventive strategies. This can be achieved through integration of and collaboration between other universal services (such as primary healthcare, education, social and community workers). These professionals, by the nature of their roles, work daily with children and adolescents and are in a prime position to recognise and to manage mental health issues early in their development. A range of broad psychosocial strategies, education and general advice can be offered and more complex mental health issues can be identified and referred to specialist services as required.

This is consistent with the pyramid framework, as advocated by the WHO (2009) (see Fig. 11.1). When planning and organising service delivery, involvement from people such as teachers, social workers, GPs and youth workers, to name but a few, would reflect the largest tier of the multilayer pyramid. This tier represents services that are frequently needed and includes interventions that can be provided at a moderately low cost. The top tier of the pyramid reflects specialist services that are often expensive and required for only a small percentage of children and young people; for instance, those with complex mental health disorders who require input from specialist

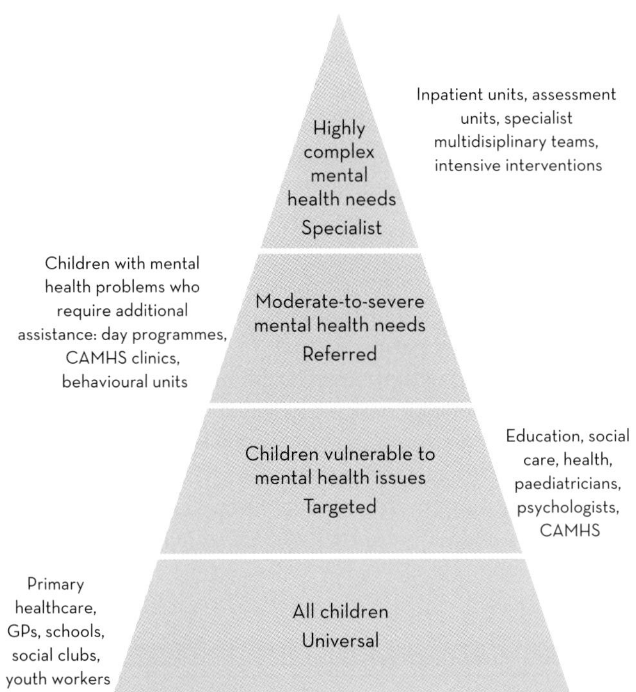

Fig. 11.1 A stepped approach to care based on a pyramid framework of healthcare delivery. (Adapted from World Health Organization [WHO], 2009. Improving health systems and services for mental health. http://apps.who.int/iris/bitstream/10665/42219/1/9789241598774_eng.pdf. © World Health Organization, 2009.)

health professionals (Servili 2012). For adolescents in particular, simply providing a traditional outpatient or inpatient service might not be enough. Many teenagers worry about what others would think if they asked for help, while others say they prefer to take care of their own problems, as they struggle with their sense of identity and relationships with adults. A variety of unhealthy or 'at-risk' behaviours may be present. An annual report (PHE 2016b) of secondary school pupils in England (11–15 years) reported similar smoking rates (3% were weekly smokers), a change in alcohol use (10% had drunk alcohol in the last week) and a rise in recreational drug use (24% had tried drugs compared with 15% in 2014, with 10% having used drugs in the last month). With prevalence rates remaining fairly high, this highlights a need for more collaboration and more funding for generalised adolescent health services and reach-out programmes that can support young people with mild-to-moderate mental health issues.

In some areas, there are adolescent health centres where no appointment is needed and teenagers can attend unaccompanied. These centres provide a wide range of services and programmes for all health and lifestyle matters. They are often based on a model of primary care promoting early intervention for a number of health needs and are delivered by a range of multidisciplinary professionals (McGorry et al. 2013). An example is the Young People's Centre run by the mental health charity Mind. This drop-in centre in Brighton offers young people aged 13 to 25 years the opportunity to access free advice, support and counselling, as well as affordable food, activities and free access to computers and the internet (see Useful Websites for details).

There is variation between regional services in the types of intervention and treatment available. As with adult services, there are usually a range of walk-in clinics and mobile crisis and support teams, backed up by separate residential units for adolescents and for children—some with programmes for families to be admitted in specific circumstances.

The treatment provided also varies from centre to centre, depending on the major problems leading young people to present locally, their age range, the treatment philosophy, theoretical models, expertise available and the living circumstances of the young person and their family. Interventions may include cognitive behavioural therapy, behaviour therapy, play therapy, psychodynamic individual or group work, socialisation and social skills programmes, systems-based family therapy, couples therapy, parenting programmes or individual therapy for a parent. Sometimes approaches are combined to achieve better outcomes. For example, a child may benefit from cognitive behavioural therapy to help them, while their parents and siblings may benefit from learning positive styles of functioning together. As with adult services, nurses have a range of roles, often developing expertise in various modes of therapy.

CRITICAL THINKING CHALLENGE 11.1

1. Why do GPs, paediatricians and schools have such a vital role to play in early detection of mental health problems in children and young people?
2. Which interventions might GPs, paediatricians and schools provide?

THE NURSING ROLE

Children and adolescents are still developing as individuals, so an intervention while they are young can often have a dramatic positive impact for the rest of their life. Early intervention is often more effective than managing difficulties that have extended into adulthood. With adequate care and a supportive environment, young people can develop resilience, emotionally, psychologically and physically. Working within a child and adolescent mental health team provides the opportunity to use a wide range of dynamic clinical treatment strategies and therapies. A multidisciplinary team approach is most frequently used. Nurses often play a significant role in various aspects of care, including that of therapist for children, adolescents and families. In the UK, nurses specialise throughout their training. There are registered children's nurses, but nurses working CAMHS services will most usually be mental health nurses, with on-the-job training and specialist courses available to help them adapt their skill set to working with children and young people. Apart from graduate nursing programmes, child and adolescent mental health nurses have options available for advanced studies in specialist areas of mental health, through postgraduate and masters programmes. In addition, nurses can take further training in counselling programmes such as family therapy, solution-focussed therapy and psychotherapy. These frameworks acknowledge the unique knowledge and skills regarded as fundamental for all professionals working in child and adolescent mental health services and focus on a number of universal key areas, each with further identified core knowledge and skills to work effectively with children and young people experiencing mental health problems.

Identifying Vulnerable Children and Young People

Parental illness, specifically mental illness, may have a significant impact on a child's life and mental health. For example, the child may have to take on extra responsibilities, may experience inconsistent parenting or may observe behaviour that is difficult to comprehend, depending on their age. As a result, children of parents who have a mental illness often have social, emotional and psychological needs different from those of children with healthy parents.

Other groups of children who may be deemed vulnerable, or at increased risk of developing mental health problems, include children in care, such as those in foster care or residential care homes, or who are adopted; young offenders; young people with a physical or learning disability; and young people from cultural and linguistically diverse groups, homeless children, refugees and asylum seekers (Dogra and Leighton 2009). As a nurse it can often be challenging because of the presenting complexity of the problem and the need to work with several agencies, each with a different agenda. It is important that the nurse remains flexible and has clear guidelines for what is expected in their role as an experienced mental health nurse.

Perinatal Mental Health Nursing

Historically, perinatal mental health included only the postpartum stage of childbirth with a focus on the mother's mental health and wellbeing. As more evidence arises, there is a better understanding that both mother and baby require sensitive assessment and the earliest possible intervention to maximise mental wellness for them both. Perinatal mental health encompasses not only the mental health of the mother and the child, but also the child–mother relationship, the emotional and psychological wellbeing of other family members and social factors that may impact the overall health of individuals within the family. Starting from preconception, perinatal mental health includes both the antenatal and the postnatal period, usually until the child is 24 months old. However, Woolhouse et al. (2015) report that a higher number of women experience symptoms related to depression *after* their child has reached 4 years old, compared with the number of women immediately after birth.

Nevertheless, whether a mother has a preexisting mental health problem or develops a mental health problem in the antenatal or postnatal stage, it can have direct and indirect consequences for the child. Research indicates that mothers experiencing mental distress may not be as sensitive or responsive to their infant's needs and can struggle to complete several activities associated with caring for an infant (Santona et al. 2015; Field 2010). With a strong evidence base demonstrating the importance of secure attachments between a child and their primary caregiver, interactions between a mother experiencing mental illness and her infant can have a detrimental impact on the bonding relationship. Evidence also suggests that the children of those mothers who suffer long-term illness, such as postnatal depression, may be prone to experiencing developmental delays in areas such as social functioning, language, cognition and behaviour (Muzik & Borovska 2010).

Recent advances in screening for perinatal mental health issues and a multitude of training courses designed to identify and to manage perinatal issues in primary care are now available. The role of the mental health nurse working in child and adolescent mental health services is to assess and to take account of any perinatal mental health issues when undertaking a psychosocial assessment. Part of planning care for the child or young person may involve referring the mother or carer to a more appropriate service to manage their own mental health.

> **CRITICAL THINKING CHALLENGE 11.2**
>
> Either individually or in a group, have a brainstorming session and list all the skills that a child and youth mental health nurse would require. Subdivide these into skills that you think might be specific to either a community mental health nurse or a mental health nurse working in an inpatient setting.

ENGAGING WITH CHILDREN AND ADOLESCENTS

Mental health nurses can become a significant resource for the child. However, to be able to intervene effectively, the nurse needs to master the art of engaging with children and young people, as individuals and with their parents or carers, in the context of *their* families.

One of the most useful skills the mental health nurse can acquire and refine is the ability to engage children and establish rapport. Engagement between nurses, young people and their families is fundamental to developing a relationship based on trust. A relationship founded on trust will foster a willingness to work together towards change. This involves communicating in a manner that is appropriate within the context of the child's development (The Werry Centre 2014). For example, the communication skills and language used when working with a 5-year-old would differ significantly from those used when working with a 16-year-old. Essentially the nurse is required to master a diverse range of communication skills that not only encourages children and teenagers to listen, but also fosters effective listening, so that the young person is more likely to communicate in response.

Mental health nurses working with children and adolescents also need to develop and to refine the skill of discreet observation of the young person's mood and behaviour and their interactions with their peers, family, friends and others. Observation of these factors, considered in the broader psychosocial context, will enable the nurse to achieve a comprehensive assessment of the factors contributing to the current difficulties experienced by the young person and their family.

Ongoing discussion with parents (carers) should clarify an understanding about which specific factors may be contributing to current problems. With a more specific diagnosis, the nurse and family may then begin the process of exploring solutions (planning). Any solutions agreed upon with the family are best implemented with the family's support and commitment, thus maximising the probability of positive change. Constant monitoring (evaluation) of behavioural interventions and responses by family members is essential to ensure that the mental health team, the young person and their family continue to share a common understanding about the management of the problem and a commitment to recovery.

The full participation of young people and their family in their mental healthcare should not be confined solely to therapeutic outcome. Organisations have much to learn from children about planning environments that are sensitive to the needs of young people. 'Family-friendly' environments also need to include processes that are responsive to the specific needs of younger people, in particular those who are experiencing significant emotional or mental health difficulties.

Engagement of young people and families across cultural contexts is key to accurate diagnosis and comprehensive treatment planning. There are implications for the way mental health professionals approach the assessment of children and their families. The nurse's understanding of specific cultural practices and beliefs held by the child and their family is imperative to developing trust. Asking for information in a way that recognises cultural norms will promote the child's confidence in the care provided. Children are more likely to provide accurate information if they believe that the nurse has an understanding of their cultural needs and a genuine respect and commitment to a recovery plan that is culturally sound.

Children

As outlined previously, a myriad of factors contribute to and affect the mental health of young people. Familial or genetic predisposition to mental illness, the presence of a coexisting medical or neurological problem, developmental problems or growing up in a chaotic or deprived environment are just a few of the considerations of which the beginning mental health nurse should be mindful during assessments of young people and their families. Furthermore, these factors will also affect the direction taken with goal planning and nursing interventions. It should be remembered that the nursing care plan is in fact a recovery plan for the young person and family; therefore, the goals must be achievable and the strategies must be practical when implemented by the child and parents (with nursing support). If the plan is based on what the nurse can achieve rather than what the family can realistically accomplish, then the medium- to long-term success for recovery may be severely impaired and continuity of care lost. Case Study 11.1 on Adam and exploration of the issues discussed thus far will illustrate some key concepts.

CASE STUDY 11.1

Adam

A mother contacts the community child and adolescent mental health service, unsure whether it is appropriate to seek help regarding her 9-year-old son, Adam, who she describes as 'becoming increasingly anxious' and who has developed 'a fixation with tidiness', so much so that it is causing disruption in the family. The family consists of two female siblings, aged 11 and 7 years, and a father who is an accomplished musician who frequently travels for extended periods performing nationally and internationally. The mental health nurse receiving the call assures the mother that her concerns warrant a further assessment by a member of the mental health team, as her child appears to be highly anxious. He is unable to relax and appears to be developing maladaptive behaviour (excessive tidying). Furthermore, his anxiety is having an adverse effect on his relationship with his siblings. The nurse gathers more specific information by phone and explains to the mother that this referral will be discussed at the next team meeting and that she will receive a call within a week regarding an appointment for her, her husband and their son, for further assessment.

Discussion of Case Study: Adam

Within the first minutes of a mother's description of her son's problem, the mental health nurse was able to predict a role for the mental health team in assisting this family. The mother was assured that her concerns were well founded. The nurse spent a little more time gathering only the information necessary to discuss the case (assessment) with the clinical team, so a plan for a further face-to-face interview could be made. Thus the mother was reassured by the prospect of another appointment (implementation). A therapeutic relationship has been initiated between the family and the mental health service.

This early process reflects the beginning of the nurse's role in engaging the family in the therapeutic relationship and emphasises how important each team member's role is in promoting a positive impression on the family (even before meeting them personally). The impression the family gains from an initial phone call can colour their perception of further interactions with the mental health team. Furthermore, the parents' feelings of confidence in the mental health nurse and other team members will possibly have an impact on the confidence that the child and siblings experience. This is important, as all family members will be involved in the child's recovery.

The foundation and building of a therapeutic relationship with the young person and the family will usually begin at the time of the initial phone call or face-to-face interview. This interview can be difficult for the young person, who may not perceive that there is a problem and therefore may not fully understand why they are attending an assessment at the mental health service. The skilled mental health nurse will use this opportunity to establish the young person's understanding of their need for an appointment. If the young person seems unsure (or unwilling to concede), they can often be encouraged to describe some difficulties that are occurring at home that they think may have led to their needing this appointment.

It is essential to clarify the child or young person's perception of the problem and their goals for treatment, as well as those of the parents. The nurse's role is to facilitate expression of the difficulties and to make explicit the goal that the child and family have regarding recovery. This is necessary so that all parties (child, family and mental health team) can agree on the treatment plan.

CRITICAL THINKING CHALLENGE 11.3

Imagine you are contacting a health service about worries and concerns you have for a family member. Which nursing attributes and skills would you find reassuring during the first phone contact?

Case Study 11.2 on Noah illustrates these key issues. While a diagnosis such as ADHD might possibly be indicated in this situation, the case illustrates that it is important to concentrate on the presenting problems and any associated difficulties, rather than giving priority to diagnostic classification. Involvement in diagnostic controversies can potentially misdirect the focus of care from the individual needs of the child and family.

CASE STUDY 11.2

Noah

Noah is a 6-year-old boy who is attending his first appointment at a community child and adolescent mental health service, accompanied by his parents. He is the oldest of three children and has a young brother and baby sister. His parents report an escalation in Noah's behaviour just before he turned 3 years: 'It's like he never grew out of the "terrible twos". He just kept on going at a hundred miles an hour', reported his mother. Noah's father concurred: 'The more limits I set, the worse he gets.' Noah's reply when asked if he knew why he was here was simply: 'I've been naughty.'

Discussion of Case Study: Noah

The skilled mental health nurse will attempt to clarify these comments using objective language and will eventually identify some very specific behaviours that the parents regard as priorities for change. The nurse will attempt to match the parents' goals with those of their son.

The nurse's response to Noah's perception that he has been 'naughty' might be: 'Naughty? What do you mean?' The aim for the nurse is to guide Noah to use specific words to tag specific behaviours, and if these match those identified by his parents, a simple goal may be developed to achieve an outcome that is satisfying to both parties. Noah's descriptions of how he sees 'the problem' may also assist the nurse to establish more accurately what the problem might be. Consider this further exchange between Noah and the nurse:

Nurse: 'Naughty'—what does that mean?

Noah: When I run away or squeal.

Nurse: So you run away?

Noah: My brother . . . he's three . . . he runs away too . . . when he runs away from Mummy, she chases him.

Nurse: And does your brother squeal?

Noah: No, but when my baby sister squeals, Daddy helps Mummy play with her.

This exchange demonstrates how, through active listening, the nurse has gathered some very specific information about the family dynamics that provides a possible explanation for some of Noah's behaviour. It could be that he is mimicking the behaviour of his younger siblings to receive the same attention from his parents that he perceives his brother and sister receive when they run away or squeal.

Encounters with children and adolescents and their families as illustrated in these case studies demonstrate how the nurse and other team members can engage young people in ongoing treatment, and how treatment will be influenced by further findings. The initiation of a sound therapeutic alliance with the child and family is an achievement, although the relationship also requires nurturing.

Generally, a therapeutic relationship is accomplished when respect is paramount in the nurse–child relationship. Like adults, young people respond most positively to being treated with genuine respect. Young people feel respected when they are listened to and given opportunities to make choices and contribute to solving problems. As Roberts et al. (2015) identify, making choices gives the child valuable practice in making decisions and opportunities for problem solving gives them courage to follow things through independently. A commitment by the mental health nurse to facilitating choice and promoting problem-solving opportunities for young people will be further enhanced by a belief in the humanistic idea that all behaviour has meaning. If we as mental health nurses explore the meaning behind the behaviours we observe, we can plan appropriate strategies to modify behaviour and to promote positive change.

Across the UK, child and adolescent mental health services work with many young people who present in acute emotional distress. Some will internalise their distress and may become withdrawn and depressed. Others may externalise their emotional pain. When this occurs, the child will demonstrate altered behaviours, which may include rigid thinking, compulsive patterns of behaviour, agitation, impulsivity and, in severe cases, aggression. If the nurse has established a therapeutic relationship with the child, the shared trust and respect will provide a foundation for choice giving and problem solving. An example from practice will best illustrate this concept.

Discussion of Case Study: Grace

Skills required. In Case Study 11.3 even though Grace is refusing to be involved in the initial assessment, her behaviour and her brief interjections are a valuable source of assessment information. The nurse will document Grace's behaviour and her comments. In context, this will reflect some family dynamics and give some indication of how Grace currently feels about her life. The challenge for the nurse will be to engage Grace initially in a shared interest of hers that is non emotional and therefore less threatening.

CASE STUDY 11.3

Grace

Grace is 12 years old and is attending the child and adolescent mental health service for the first time, accompanied by her mother, with whom she lives. Her younger brother has lived with her father since their parents separated 3 years ago. Grace's mother is extremely concerned about a gradual change in Grace's mood over the past 2 years. She has reportedly become angry and unpredictable, a dramatic change from the quiet but confident child she used to be. Her mother describes instances where Grace will impulsively run from home and engage in risky behaviour such as riding her bike recklessly on their busy street. When met by members of the mental health team, Grace is at first passive, refusing eye contact, seeming to ignore the conversation between her mother and the nurse and refusing to respond when spoken to directly. Several times during the conversation, however, Grace interrupts with a hostile comment, countering information provided by her mother.

Rather than attempting to engage Grace too early, the nurse wisely chooses to wait for an opportunity. This does not arise until the very end of the initial interview, when the nurse announces that the assessment is almost complete. 'About time', Grace grumbles, 'I just want to get in the car and listen to my new CD.' The nurse grasps this opportunity:

Nurse: Ah, a new CD ... which group?

Grace: No-one you'd know.

Nurse: Maybe not ... but try me.

To Grace's surprise, the nurse has recently bought the same CD and although Grace feigns horror that an adult would even know the band, she cannot completely disguise her admiration.

Nurse: See you in a fortnight then?

Grace: If I'm not too busy with my music.

Grace's choice of words ('if I'm not too busy ...') indicates that she is trying to sound uninterested while still leaving her options open.

Approach taken and outcome achieved. Troubled children and adolescents are not always easily engaged. Often the factors contributing to their need for mental health support have affected their ability to trust others; in many cases they have felt let down by adults. The nurse who recognises this will allow time for the young person to engage, initially on their own terms, so that the fragile therapeutic relationship can gradually strengthen. Grace's hostility was ignored; the nurse chose instead to preserve Grace's fragile sense of dignity. Respecting Grace's ability to make sound decisions, the nurse did not assume that she would be returning in a fortnight, but rather posed it as a question; this approach was aimed at reassuring Grace that she had a choice. Her choice to return in a fortnight would demonstrate her courage in recognising that a problem exists and her willingness to explore some supports.

CRITICAL THINKING CHALLENGE 11.4

1. What might the outcomes have been if the nurse had persisted in asking Grace questions early in the interview?
2. What assumptions could be made regarding Grace's need to interrupt while her mother and the nurse were speaking?

NURSE'S STORY 11.1

Kristin Henderson

As an experienced mental health nurse, I had regarded myself as a spontaneous, reflective clinician, confident that my interactions with patients were at all times respectful, helpful and kind. I was taken by surprise, then, when I began working with young people in an inpatient mental health setting—surprised that I now felt hesitant and doubtful about how to respond. What was appropriate? What would be a better response? My confidence and spontaneity had given way to feeling stilted and unsure . . . until a defining moment, when I realised that I should open my senses to cues within myself and from others, taking time to reflect upon what I was seeing in myself. This could deepen my understanding of how others see themselves. This is my story . . .

With his bath finished and his pyjamas on, 8-year-old Isaac and I stand in front of the full-length mirror looking straight at ourselves, occasionally glancing across at each other's reflection, then back to our own. As we look at our reflections, I wonder what we are *really seeing*.

I see myself: casually dressed, complete and unchanging . . . oh, and looking a wee bit tired! I suspect that Isaac, like me, sees an image of himself; but I can only speculate what self-image that might be . . .

I kneel down beside Isaac to try to observe his reflection as he might be seeing it. I note a small crack in the glass near where Isaac is standing. The mirror has been damaged, but because of the safety component of the glass, it has not shattered but simply absorbed the knock, leaving three fractures darting out from the one stress point. As I had anticipated, his image is disjointed, and the symbolic implications momentarily tug at me.

'What do you see?' I ask quietly.

No answer. He continues looking into the broken mirror. He is observing fragmented self—lots of small pieces, together, but not quite. He moves bodily up and down and sideways, all the time trying to piece together his reflection in a harmonious union. But it is not to be—whichever position he views himself from, he is in several pieces, a fragmented whole.

'I'm in pieces . . . nothing fits together properly,' he eventually says, giggling. Then for a few more minutes he moves about, trying to find where he might place himself so that the pieces of him do come together, as they should. In a short while, in frustration, he curses the mirror and leaves the room. I stand stunned. Isaac's complex and distressing childhood history symbolically laid bare before the mirror. So much about us both, reflected in this brief encounter.

Adolescents

When adolescents and their family (carers) present to a healthcare facility, there is an expectation on their part that treatment will achieve the desired outcomes, in terms of the physical, emotional and mental state of the young person. However, it is possible that these outcomes may not be achieved because of many situational factors. One such factor may be the young person's lack of willingness to be part of the referral, assessment and treatment process due to their not recognising or acknowledging that they have a significant problem. Mental health nurses providing mental healthcare for adolescents need to acknowledge that possible influencing factors such as poor insight, resistance to treatment or challenging of authority may be part of normal adolescent behaviour.

Mental health nurses should attempt to form a relationship with the young person through engagement and foster a sense of purpose with the treatment plan for the adolescent. *Engagement* is the process of forming a relationship based on person-centred interactions where there is an ongoing conversation or acknowledgement of a partnership (O'Kane 2013). Therefore, an important element of engagement is rapport building, which encompasses not only the formal aspects of mental healthcare, such as completing a diagnostic interview, but also the social interactions and nonverbal communication that occur. Geldard and Geldard (2008) state that nonverbal forms of communication may be more significant than verbal interactions when interviewing and engaging young people with mental health problems.

For mental health professionals, language is the key to open communication and creation of an environment that can augment engagement. Adolescents may use language and jargon that differs according to their age group or subculture, especially when it comes to 'street lingo'. Adolescents may have a culture that at times seems alien to their parents, caregivers and health professionals. Adolescents and their peer groups may use words and phrases that have a significantly different meaning to that which adults may be accustomed—for example, 'sick' or 'gross' may mean 'good'. Healthcare professionals who work with adolescents may need to clarify with the young person what they actually mean by their phrases or words if the professional does not understand them. This may be particularly relevant when discussing illicit drugs and the street names used for marijuana, amphetamines and hallucinogens.

Understanding language and communicating effectively is integral to engaging with young people and vital to the success of their ongoing treatment. We stated earlier that this chapter does not deal with specific classified conditions, but rather the principles of nursing care relating to groupings of disorders. The following section explores the principles of mental health nursing that promote engagement with adolescents with challenging behaviours arising from psychosis, depressive symptoms and social–emotional issues. Examples of practice situations will highlight some appropriate responses to consider.

CRITICAL THINKING CHALLENGE 11.5

As a small group exercise, discuss some strategies that nurses can use to foster engagement with an adolescent who is sullen and guarded.

Psychosis and Behaviour Issues

Psychotic symptoms can be a common reason for adolescents being admitted to child and adolescent mental health agencies. Inpatient care is often suggested to ensure safety, to stabilise the condition and to introduce appropriate medication and therapy in promoting ongoing psychological security. The symptoms associated with psychosis can be frightening for young people. It can often be a difficult time for parents, too, when their child is disturbed by hallucinations and delusions and is lacking insight into their current mental or emotional state. Nurses working with adolescents need to understand and to practise basic concepts of engagement to optimise outcomes of care provided for the adolescent and their family.

To engage the adolescent in a therapeutic relationship that will promote treatment and ultimately result in regaining wellness, nurses need to encourage and to allow the adolescent to develop trust. Trust can be difficult for a young person to develop, especially if they are attending an appointment begrudgingly or have been hospitalised against their will. To promote a therapeutic relationship that supports trust, it is essential to be honest and consistent in any approach to treatment. Adolescents can appear to be more guarded or sensitive than adults with similar disorders. For example, an adolescent may have difficulty adhering to medications. This may be for a variety of reasons, including a fear of being sedated, possible drug sensitivity, potential to develop adverse side effects from prescribed medications or, if delusional, perhaps even the suspicion of being poisoned. Adverse side effects of some antipsychotic medications may result in weight gain. Adolescents may dislike this. Young people may experience muscle spasm or rigidity as another adverse effect of antipsychotic medication. Some medications may require regular blood tests. This can be a frightening experience and some may consider it as frightening as the symptoms of the psychosis. Thus, adherence to medication can be difficult and a confusing issue for the adolescent.

Mental health nurses are pivotal in providing psychoeducation aimed at promoting wellness and in providing an opportunity for the young person to gain insight into their condition. Throughout the nurse's contact with young people, opportunities to provide psychoeducation in regard to a patient's mental health status and their treatment are vital. Early recovery can be facilitated with psychoeducation. This may include discussing issues of causation and the likely medium- to long-term outcomes of their treatment.

CASE STUDY 11.4

Jorge

A 15-year-old boy, Jorge, has been admitted to hospital. He is experiencing a psychotic episode as a result of smoking marijuana for several months. He has been having auditory hallucinations (voices telling him he is useless and a nuisance to be around). In the past 6 months there has been a decline in Jorge's academic performance and he has been isolating himself from his friends and family. Within the past 2 months he has been verbally and physically abusive towards his parents and siblings.

Discussion of Case Study: Jorge

The presentation to adolescent mental health agencies of a young person like Jorge experiencing their first episode of psychosis is not uncommon. In considering Jorge's care, the nurse's first priority is to ensure that Jorge is physically safe and that those around him also feel safe. When a person's thinking is altered by psychotic phenomena, they may act irrationally as a consequence of feeling fearful and insecure. This may include aggressive behaviour. It is important that the nurse appears confident and takes a role in calming the current situation by offering reassurance and firm guidance with statements such as, 'Jorge, what you are experiencing must be frightening. You are safe here. We will help you.' Short, clear statements made firmly but quietly and with genuine empathy will be reassuring for Jorge and his family. It is important that it is made clear that, whatever Jorge says or does, he has been heard. At this stage, the nurse should avoid disputing the patient's irrational thoughts. Rather, Jorge should be encouraged to verbalise his confusion and distress. This may assist in diffusing his agitation and may lead to him feeling calmer, thereby reducing the risk of him becoming aggressive. Aggression is often a response to feeling frightened, threatened or overwhelmed.

Another important priority is involving the family as early as possible, providing them with much-needed support, so that they can, in turn, provide support to Jorge. The family will usually be most helpful in providing an accurate history of family health. This will assist in establishing any familial predispositions to mental illness and the nature of onset. This information may help the mental health worker to establish the likely severity and prognosis for the illness and organise an individualised treatment plan that will have a higher probability of a positive outcome. Recovery from mental illness demands a high level of support from family, friends and agency staff. The best prognosis and quality of life are achieved when everyone works collaboratively.

Working with adolescents with psychosis is extremely challenging. However, if the nurse follows the aforementioned guidelines in attempting to engage them, the ability to support the child and family through the difficult times will prove ultimately rewarding. Once safety has been established and the patient and family have begun to engage with staff, the medium- to long-term relief of symptoms and psychoeducation can ensue.

Other treatment modes could include resocialisation through group therapy and individual goal setting that focusses on peer support and reestablishing a social network. Individual goal planning, peer support and group therapy can each promote socially adaptive and acceptable behaviour. Adolescence is a period of personal development involving challenging authority and pushing against the norms of society. The 'normal' adolescent behaviours should not be stifled through treatment but recognised and supported, so that Jorge can return to his peer group and family with minimal residual effects of the psychotic episode. One aspect of hospitalisation that can have negative longer-term effects is the labelling of the condition suffered by Jorge.

Depression and Suicide

Depression and risk of suicide are major problems in the community, 149 children (10–19 years old) committed suicide in England in 2014, equating to almost three children each week (PHE 2016a), with social media being a cause for concern (Jans et al. 2012). In contrast, rates of suicide in prepubertal children remain very low. This is possibly because of their lack of understanding of the concept of suicide and because they are less likely to be faced with the risk factors associated with puberty.

The psychological and physical trauma experienced by young people who have attempted suicide may be difficult for mental health nurses to come to terms with. The young person should be reassured that their safety is the treatment team's priority, while at the same time providing support to the family. Youth suicide and attempts at self-harm may challenge mental health nurses and family members to consider their own mortality and the question of why people attempt suicide. It is important that mental health nurses develop skills that enable them to feel comfortable addressing these issues directly with the child and family.

Engagement with depressed or suicidal adolescents can be extremely difficult because of their tendency towards socially withdrawn and isolative behaviour or because of cognitive impairment. Nurses are able to engage adolescents through social interactions, groups and individual therapy. It is often the nurse, who spends long hours with the young person and is present with them as their mood shifts throughout the day, who may be alerted to a subtle increase in risk to the young person's emotional or physical safety. The nurse's ability to reassure young people of their availability as needed helps young people feel free to discuss issues with the nurse when the time seems most appropriate for them.

An issue that can be confusing for nurses is that at times adolescents who are clinically depressed may present with aggressive traits or behaviours. Some adolescents are not able to communicate their emotions verbally. As a result, their only means of expressing distress may be through verbal or physical aggression, towards themselves or others. Engagement of these young people may be aided through involvement in physical activities, sport, music or art. Sharing the young person's physical space and activities may help in forging a therapeutic relationship. The use of diversional activities can enable mental health nurses to engage the young person further and to develop the therapeutic relationship. Establishing a confidante may be the turning point in the young person's treatment.

CASE STUDY 11.5

Olivia

Olivia is a 14-year-old who, over the past year, has become increasingly withdrawn from her peer group. She was previously an A-grade student in a select school, but over the past 4 months her school grades have dropped noticeably and she is not completing her homework. She is no longer interested in playing netball or attending her athletics club. Olivia's mother states that Olivia has been aggressive towards her and has been harming herself by cutting her wrists with any sharp object available. Olivia was commenced on antidepressant medication by her GP 6 weeks prior to admission but there has been minimal change in her mental state.

Discussion of Case Study: Olivia

Olivia requires intensive therapy, which may include cognitive behavioural therapy, family therapy, individual psychotherapy and a review of her medication. Psychosocial issues also need to be considered during Olivia's treatment. This may include exploring school issues, as well as whether there is any risk of Olivia having been physically, emotionally or sexually abused. Also, there may have been significant losses that have contributed to her depression.

In assisting young people like Olivia, the mental health nurse will need to establish rapport and maintain engagement. It will be important to gain the child's confidence from the initial meeting, as there will be many sensitive issues to address. Adolescents seeking help from adults will not always commit time for a therapeutic relationship to grow if they doubt in any way the sincerity of the person in whom they are confiding.

In some instances, the action of inflicting harm upon oneself can provide a sense of relief from severe emotional distress and psychic pain. It is therefore essential that the nurse recognises this possibility and, while working with the young person, makes every effort for them to feel respected and not judged on the behaviour that has led to them seeking help. Medical care, such as attention to a wound, should be addressed discreetly and professionally. The key aspect of providing care for the young person is establishing their current level of safety and working with them on how this can best be achieved. It will be helpful to ensure that the young person has adequate support networks, so that they can strengthen these connections with a view to obtaining help in more adaptive ways in the future.

CRITICAL THINKING CHALLENGE 11.6

List the potential barriers to establishing a therapeutic relationship with Olivia.

Self-Harm and Young People

Within a clinical setting, how people define self-harming behaviour may cover a wide range of actions, from being actively suicidal to causing physical pain or injury to themselves to serve other functions unassociated with suicidal intent. Historically, such a wide definition has caused considerable debate and confusion, although as we gain more understanding of self-harming behaviour it is clear there are very distinct differences in presentation, context, prevalence and treatment responsiveness between young people who self-harm with an intention of dying and those who have no intention of dying.

For the purpose of this chapter we explore self-harm in the context of non-suicidal behaviour, differentiating it by calling it non-suicidal self-injury (NSSI). While respecting that NSSI is a behaviour not a mental illness, it is important for clinicians to have a better understanding of the implications of NSSI when assessing and planning care for young people.

According to Nock (2012), NSSI can be defined as a deliberate and direct act of destruction to one's body tissue in the absence of any suicidal intent. It usually presents in the form of cutting or damaging the skin, although can involve other behaviour such as burning, scalding, hair pulling and bone breaking. There is little information regarding children younger than 10 years of age who engage in NSSI. This is because it is difficult to assess the intent and purpose of an injury in a younger child because of their developmental understanding of the implications of their own behaviour (Pointer 2013).

It has been strongly suggested that there is considerable under-reporting of NSSI. In the past and even today to an extent, studies were undertaken in hospital emergency departments where problems can arise with reporting. For instance, such data do not take into account those young people who present with their injuries as accidental or those who hurt themselves without requiring hospital treatment (Harrison and Henley 2014). In addition, many young people hide their NSSI, therefore never coming to the attention of health professionals, which makes it difficult to provide accurate information. Recently, more studies have been undertaken within schools and community-based programmes, helping us to gain a better understanding of the prevalence and factors associated with NSSI, although it still remains difficult to provide accurate data if young people choose to hide their behaviour. What we know from the research is that girls are more likely to engage in NSSI than boys and there is a definite link between NSSI and suicidal behaviour, with NSSI being one of the strongest predictors of completed suicide (Dickstein et al. 2015). It is suggested that young people who have self-harmed are 100 times more likely to die by suicide in the following year than children who have not self harmed (PHE 2016a).

Causing harm to oneself without suicidal intent and with nonfatal outcome is a sign that something is not right in the young person's life, often connected to low self-esteem and feelings of hopelessness (Greydanus 2011). Many front-line workers with adolescents mistake NSSI as a suicidal gesture or a suicide attempt. However, NSSI is something very different and must be understood in its own right. NSSI is one way that young people cope: it makes them feel better for a short period of time and allows them to manage their emotions on a day-to-day basis. It may be the only way they know to manage their feelings, with the alternative being suicide.

While for some young people NSSI may be part of their daily lives, for others there may be long periods of time when the behaviour does not occur but then escalates when they feel stressed or emotional pain. It is difficult to know precisely when self-injury will occur in young people since each person has individual reasons and purpose for engaging in NSSI. In some cases, life experiences may underlie NSSI—such as sexual, physical and/or emotional abuse; enduring chronic illness or disability; bullying; loss of a main carer; or fear and shame about their sexuality. For others, being raised in a family with high expectations or a severe lack of communication can leave the young person with feelings of unhappiness, distress and anguish. By listening to young people with experience of self-injury, it is clear that despite the shame or negativity often associated with NSSI, it serves a purpose and has multiple functions, which include:

- to relieve or regulate feelings of insufferable emotional angst or tension
- to punish oneself due to self-loathing and/or self-blame
- to cleanse in terms of symbolically removing the 'bad' feelings
- to feel in control of at least one part of one's life
- to communicate distress
- to allow time for caring for oneself in a way that is believed to be deserving
- to make the body unattractive (often associated with sexual abuse)
- to feel 'alive' when feelings of numbness or depersonalisation are present
- to distract oneself from recurring thought patterns or flashbacks of traumatic experiences
- to impact the behaviour of others (Nock 2009; Lloyd-Richardson et al. 2007)

Interventions

Reliance on such a coping mechanism can lead to repetitive and often addictive compulsive behaviour, increasing the risk of scarring, infection or accidental death. It can be frustrating for health professionals, particularly those who have no or little mental health training, to work with young people who engage in NSSI. Phrases such as 'attention seeking', 'acting out' and 'they must enjoy pain' do nothing to help young people feel safe in acknowledging their behaviour and seeking support to find alternative ways of dealing with their emotions.

It is the role of the mental health nurse to identify patterns and to help young people to recognise the triggers and receive the support they require. It is important not to focus on the injury as a measurement of distress since the type, severity or level of NSSI does not reflect the emotional distress a person is going through neither does it reflect the underlying psychopathology (Greydanus 2011).

As a clinician, it is your role to observe and to be alert for signs of NSSI since early intervention often results in improved outcomes for young people in the long term. Gently enquire about the possibility of NSSI and let the young person know that they are safe and can openly discuss their behaviour without fear of rejection or judgement. Identifying triggers, exploring reasons for the behaviour and finding alternative coping strategies help support the person through this difficult time and can reduce the frequency of NSSI (Greydanus 2011).

Undertaking a thorough risk assessment is essential to determine whether the self-harm is related to NSSI or, more seriously, a suicide attempt. Being able to discuss NSSI with the young person means the physical damage can be regularly monitored for signs of increasing frequency or gravity of wounds. The young person's safety is paramount. Undertaking a regular mental state examination identifies any related factors concerning mental illness that may require further treatment intervention such as medication. Your role may also include educating front-line professionals to gain a better understanding of NSSI and how to work effectively with the young people in their care.

FAMILY WORK

Nurses working with children and adolescents experiencing mental health issues should be aware that this group should not be seen, assessed and treated in isolation. Ideally, nurses working with this group should incorporate all members of the family who have a significant role within the household (for additional information about working with families, see Chapter 10). This ensures that the 'identified child' of child and adolescent mental health services is not perceived to be the family scapegoat. Therefore, a major component of child and adolescent mental health nursing is involvement of the family in treatment with regard to family work. Recently, there has been a shift in focus towards family-centred mental health nursing, which includes family-based assessments and treatments, spreading the attention across the whole family rather than focussing on the identified child. Family work is based on the principles of family therapy, which requires a specific way of working and requires specialist training.

Family therapy is discussed within the context of mental health therapeutic interventions in Chapter 24. However, it is important to raise the issues of family therapy within the context of child and adolescent mental health. Family therapy has been constantly evolving since its conception in the middle of the 20th century. Traditionally, it has focussed on the identified problems with the child or adolescent and how the family has dealt with these issues from a systemic perspective. Family therapy works within the following principles:

- Problems in families are best understood and treated from a circular rather than a linear perspective.
- Families experiencing problems need to discover their own problem-solving abilities.
- Family members' ability to change depends on their ability to alter their perception of the problem.
- Families' understanding of problems does not itself lead to change.
- A therapeutic context for change must be created for families.
- Problems or symptoms may serve a positive family function.
- Outcome is more positive if problems are treated from an ecosystemic perspective (Dallos & Draper 2010).

From these key aspects of family involvement, nurses can formulate their own methods of working with families that best suit their clinical environment. The skills of undertaking family work can be both challenging and rewarding. It is recommended that nurses involved in such work require ongoing clinical supervision and support in order to ensure that optimal patient/family/nurse relationships are maintained and the family achieves their desired outcomes.

CONFIDENTIALITY

An important issue for young people is being able to understand how the information shared during interactions with team members is documented and knowing who has access to these records. It is important to them that their need for confidentiality be maintained. However, when there are risk factors involved, the young person must know that nurses and their colleagues are bound to impart information that has a direct effect on their safety or the safety of others.

Interviews with adolescents should not be restricted to the formality of interview rooms. As long as safety can be assured, some adolescents may prefer to be interviewed in a more public place, such as a courtyard. Flexibility (and not a small dose of ingenuity!) is the key to providing a quality service that will encourage young people to return in crisis.

PSYCHOEDUCATION

As stated previously, having to take regular medication can be a major issue for adolescents, regardless of their condition. Many young people do not want to be different from their peer group. This may include not wanting to be seen as being different by needing to take tablets. Through psychoeducation the rationale for taking medication should be explained and adverse effects discussed, together with how to reduce the complications of medication therapy. Problem solving with the young person about ways to include taking the prescribed medication discreetly in their daily life style will be of benefit. The risk of taking nonprescribed medications should also be highlighted. This can be achieved by maximising therapeutic interventions. In adolescent mental health, engagement through developing rapport and trust are key elements to achieving change. Without these elements, minimal change might be achieved.

LEGAL ISSUES

Nurses involved in the care of young people admitted to mental health facilities often have to deal with legal issues relating to duty of care, child protection and mental health legislation. In the developed world, children and younger adolescents must have their parents' or guardians' consent to seek treatment for any form of medical intervention, including mental health assessments and treatment. Young people can give their own consent to receive medical or nursing treatment, as long as their parents are aware and the health professionals believe that the young person is competent to give consent.

The ability for young people to consent to medical treatment or seek medical consultations is referred to as 'Gillick competence' (Gillick v. West, Norfolk and Wisbech Area Health Authority 1986). Medical and nursing staff may question whether the young person is 'Gillick competent' or has the cognitive ability to make an informed judgement to give their own consent for treatment. The legal precedent is the case where a parent took the local health authority to court after one of her children received treatment from a GP without her consent. This case has had a major impact on the provision of paediatric healthcare and, consequently, health workers must assess each child's competence on a case-by-case basis, assessing both the competence and the maturity of the child (Hein et al. 2015).

In mental health, as with general healthcare, consent could be challenged by parents and doctors; however, to ensure the safety and wellbeing of young people, mental health legislation provides strong guidelines and rights of appeal. Mental health nurses who treat young people should be aware that it is unethical and legally unsafe to engage a young person in treatment without informing their parent(s). Healthcare agencies and inpatient units tend to have specific protocols and policies to address this issue.

The legal process by which young people can be admitted to mental health hospitals is similar to that for adult patients. This ensures that legal processes and due process are followed in regard to human rights, issues of liberty and the protection of the rights of others. It is always preferable that young people are admitted voluntarily. However, if the safety of an adolescent is at risk and they are unable to consent to voluntary treatment, the relevant Mental Health Act can be invoked.

The other main legal issues that need to be observed in child and adolescent mental health are child protection and statutory orders in regard to custody. The overriding principles are those of the WHO and the United Nations Convention on the Rights of the Child: all children and adolescents have legal rights to education, health and wellbeing.

CONCLUSION

This chapter has highlighted skills that a nurse requires when working for the first time with children and adolescents in the mental health field. It has focussed primarily on engagement: establishing a therapeutic relationship and forging a therapeutic bond. The authors believe that nurses must first master strategies for engaging young people and their families before more advanced skills in mental health nursing can be consolidated effectively. Engaging young people and families early and initiating a therapeutic relationship will enhance the quality of assessment information provided by children. Furthermore, a sense of trust shared between parties will promote commitment to a shared treatment plan created in partnership between the young person, their parents and the mental health team.

The case studies in this chapter have sought to reinforce the importance of engagement and working in partnerships. Demonstrating empathy and performing with absolute sincerity are important factors in caring for children and adolescents. It is important that young people feel that they are the priority for the nurse at this particular time.

EXERCISES FOR CLASS ENGAGEMENT

1. Contact your nearest child and adolescent mental health service and request information on the services available to children and young people. Share this information with your group.
   - Are these services proactive and responsive?
   - Does the service actively promote early intervention?
2. Contact a nurse working in a community setting and another from an inpatient unit and ask them to speak to your group about their roles. Note any differences between the mental health nursing of young people in the community and that of young people in an inpatient setting.
3. In small groups, nominate one person to act as a mental health nurse and another to play the role of a sullen, guarded adolescent. Remaining group members should observe and document the difficulties presented in establishing rapport.
4. Contact a child and adolescent mental health agency or community youth group and arrange to speak with a person who has experience with depressed or suicidal youth. Then clarify your responses to Critical Thinking Challenge 11.2.
5. Seek out the mental health and child protection Acts applicable in your country. Summarise key points in the application of these to establishing safety for young people. Share your findings.

REFERENCES

Achenbach, T.M., Ndetei, D.M., 2012. Clinical models for child and adolescent behavioral, emotional, and social problems. In: Rey, J.M. (Ed.), IACAPAP e-textbook of child and adolescent mental health. International Association for Child and Adolescent Psychiatry and Allied Professions, Geneva.

American Psychiatric Association (APA), 2013. Diagnostic and statistical manual of mental disorders, fifth ed. APA, Washington, DC.

Dallos, R., Draper, R., 2010. An Introduction to Family Therapy: Systemic Theory and Practice, third ed. McGraw-Hill Education, Maidenhead, UK.

Dickstein, D.P., Puzia, M.E., Cushman, G.K., Weissman, A.B., Wegbreit, E., Kim, K.L., Spirito, A., 2015. Self-injurious implicit attitudes among adolescent suicide attempters versus those engaged in nonsuicidal self-injury. Journal of Child Psychology and Psychiatry 56 (10), 1127–1136.

Dogra, N., Leighton, S., 2009. Nursing in Child and Adolescent Mental Health. McGraw-Hill/Open University Press, Maidenhead, UK.

Erskine, H.E., Moffitt, T.E., Copeland, W.E., et al., 2015. A heavy burden on young minds: the global burden of mental and substance use disorders in children and youth. Psychological Medicine 45 (7), 1551–1563.

Field, T., 2010. Postpartum depression effects on early interactions, parenting, and safety practices: a review. Infant Behaviour and Development 33 (1), 1–9.

Geldard, K., Geldard, D., 2008. Counselling Children: A Practical Introduction, third ed. Sage, London.

Gore, F.M., Bloem, P.J.N., Patton, G.C., et al., 2011. Global burden of disease in young people aged 10–24 years: a systematic analysis. Lancet 377, 2093–2102.

Greydanus, D.E., 2011. Treating self-harm in children and adolescents: a complex conundrum for the clinician. Psychiatric Times. Available at: www.psychiatrictimes.com/display/article/10168/1852801.

Harrison, J.E., Henley, G., 2014. Suicide and hospitalised self-harm in Australia: trends and analysis. Injury Research and Statistics Series No. 93. Cat. no. INJCAT 169. AIHW, Canberra.

Hein, I.M., Troost, P.W., Broersma, A., de Vries, M.C., Daams, J.G., Lindauer, R.J., 2015. Why is it hard to make progress in assessing children's decision-making competence? BMC Medical Ethics 16, 1.

Jans, T., Taneli, Y., Warnke, A., 2012. Suicide and self-harming behaviour. In: Rey, J.M. (Ed.), IACAPAP e-textbook of Child and Adolescent Mental Health. International Association for Child and Adolescent Psychiatry and Allied Professions, Geneva.

Layard, R., Hagell, A., 2015. Healthy Young Minds: Transforming the Mental Health of Children. Report of the WISH Mental Health and Wellbeing in Children Forum. World Innovation Summit in Health, Qatar.

Lloyd-Richardson, E.E., Perrine, N., Dierker, L., Kelley, M.L., 2007. Characteristics and functions of non-suicidal self-injury in a community sample of adolescents. Psychological Medicine 37, 1183–1192.

Mares, S., Graeff-Martins, A.S., 2012. The clinical assessment of infants, preschoolers and their families. In: Rey, J.M. (Ed.), IACAPAP e-textbook of Child and Adolescent Mental Health. International Association for Child and Adolescent Psychiatry and Allied Professions, Geneva.

McGorry, P., Bates, T., Birchwood, M., 2013. Designing youth mental health services for the 21st century: examples from Australia, Ireland and the UK. The British Journal of Psychiatry 202, 30–35.

Morris, J., Belfer, M., Daniels, A., et al., 2011. Treated prevalence of and mental health services received by children and adolescents in 42 low-and-middle-income countries. Journal of Child Psychology and Psychiatry 52, 1239–1246.

Muzik, M., Borovska, S., 2010. Perinatal depression: implications for child mental health. Mental Health in Family Medicine 7 (4), 239–247.

Nock, M.K., 2009. Why do people hurt themselves? New insights into the nature and functions of self-injury. Current Directions in Psychological Science 18, 78–83.

Nock, M.K., 2012. Future directions for the study of suicide and self-injury. Journal of Clinical Child and Adolescent Psychology 41 (2), 255–259.

O'Kane, D., 2013. Partnerships in health. In: Barkway, P. (Ed.), Psychology for Health Professionals, second ed. Churchill Livingston, Sydney, pp. 201–221.

Public Health England (PHE), 2016. The mental health of children and young people in England. Available at: https://assets.publishing.service.gov.uk/government/uploads/system/uploads/attachment_data/file/575632/Mental_health_of_children_in_England.pdf. Accessed: 16 October 2018.

Public Health England, 2016. Smoking, Drinking and Drug Use Among Young People in England – 2016. Available at: https://digital.nhs.uk/data-and-information/publications/statistical/smoking-drinking-and-drug-use-among-young-people-in-england/2016. Accessed: 16 October 2018.

Rey, J.M., Bella-Awusah, T.T., Jing, L., 2015. Depression in children and adolescents. In: Rey, J.M. (Ed.), IACAPAP e-textbook of Child and Adolescent Mental Health. International Association for Child and Adolescent Psychiatry and Allied Professions, Geneva.

Pointer, S., 2013. Trends in hospitalised injury, Australia, 1999–2000 to 2010–2011. Injury Research and Statistics Series No. 86. Cat. no. INJCAT 162. AIHW, Canberra.

Roberts, J., Fenton, G., Barnard, M., 2015. Developing effective therapeutic relationships with children, young people and their families. Nursing Children and Young People 27 (4), 30–35.

Santona, A., Tagini, A., Sarracino, D., De Carli, P., Pace, C.S., Parolin, L., Terrone, G., 2015. Maternal depression and attachment: the evaluation of mother–child interactions during feeding practice. Frontiers in Psychology. 6, 1235. http://doi.org/10.3389/fpsyg.2015.01235.
Sawyer, M.G., Miller-Lewis, L.R., Clark, J.J., 2007. The mental health of 13–17-year-olds in Australia: findings from the National Survey of Mental Health and Wellbeing. Journal of Youth Adolescence 36, 185–194.
Servili, C., 2012. Organizing and delivering services for child and adolescent mental health. In: Rey, J.M. (Ed.), IACAPAP e-textbook of Child and Adolescent Mental Health. International Association for Child and Adolescent Psychiatry and Allied Professions, Geneva.
The Werry Centre, 2014. Real Skills Plus ICAMH/AOD: a competency framework for the infant, child and youth mental health and alcohol and other drug workforce. The Werry Centre, Auckland.
Thompson, M., Hooper, C., Laver-Bradbury, C., Gale, C., 2012. Child and Adolescent Mental Health Theory and Practice, second ed. Hodder Arnold, UK.
Woolhouse, H., Gartland, D., Mensah, F., Brown, S.J., 2015. Maternal depression from early pregnancy to 4 years postpartum in a prospective pregnancy cohort study: implications for primary health care. BJOG: An International Journal of Obstetrics & Gynaecology 122 (3), 312–321.
World Health Organization (WHO), 2009. Improving health systems and services for mental health. Available at: http://whqlibdoc.who.int/publications/2009/9789241598774_eng.pdf.
World Health Organization (WHO), 2014. Health for the World's Adolescents: A Second Chance in the Second Decade. WHO, Geneva..

USEFUL WEBSITES

Headspace www.headspace.com
Mind: for better mental health. Young People's Centre www.mind-charity.co.uk/the-mind-directory/young-peoples-centre-ypc/
Childline www.childline.org.uk
NSPCC www.nspcc.org.uk
ADHD Foundation www.adhdfoundation.org.uk
Beat Eating Disorders www.b-eat.co.uk
Centre for Mental Health www.centreformentalhealth.org.uk
Head Meds www.headmeds.org.uk
Mind: for better mental health www.mind.org.uk
Mind Ed www.minded.org.uk
PAPYRUS: Prevention of young suicide www.papyrus-uk.org
Place2B www.place2be.org.uk
Royal College of Psychiatry www.rcpsych.ac.uk
The Mix: essential support for under 25s www.themix.org.uk
Young Minds www.youngminds.org.uk

12

Mental Disorders of Older Age

Wendy Moyle

KEY POINTS

- Populations are ageing and this increases the need for nurses to understand the mental disorders and needs of older people.
- Mental health nursing staff should not assume that deterioration in function is a normal part of ageing.
- Although the risk of mental illness increases with age, most older people are healthy and do not require health and social support.
- Staff attitudes are important in influencing the delivery of care to older people.
- Nursing management of mental illness in older people should include listening to the individual, encouraging an active and healthy lifestyle and cultivating an interactive therapeutic nurse–patient relationship.
- In assessing an older person, the nurse should avoid making ageist assumptions, such as assuming that dementia is the cause of changes in behaviour and activity.
- Mental health disorders in old age include depression, anxiety, delirium, dementia and schizophrenia. The most common disorders are depression and anxiety.

KEY TERMS

ageing
ageism
Alzheimer disease
anxiety
assessment
delirium
dementia
depression
mental disorders
nurse–patient relationship
pet therapy
schizophrenia
self-compassion
staff attitudes
substance misuse
suicide

LEARNING OUTCOMES

The material in this chapter will help you to:

- demonstrate an understanding of the common mental disorders that occur in older adults.
- explore management of the following mental disorders in older people: depression, anxiety disorders, suicide, substance misuse, delirium, dementia and schizophrenia.
- explore strategies to promote mental health in older people.
- reflect on your own and others' attitudes towards older people.

INTRODUCTION

The UK population is getting older, with 18% of the population aged 65 years and over, with 2.4% aged over 85 years. As a result of the ageing population, the old age dependency ratio (OADR) is increasing, i.e., the number of people over 65 years old for every 1000 people aged between 16 and 64 years old (traditional working age). In 2016, the OADR was 285, which is a useful measure when planning the needs of different age groups (Office for National Statistics [ONS] 2017). It is imperative that nurses understand and can work with older people, as they are likely to be the population that nurses will predominately be required to provide healthcare for in the future.

This chapter provides an overview of mental disorders that are common in the older adult population and explores the issues and principles underlying their assessment and treatment, including a number of general strategies to promote mental health. In addition, some negative attitudes towards older people are discussed, with the implications of these negative attitudes have on attempts to enhance the quality of care for older people.

DEMOGRAPHY OF AGEING IN THE UK

In 2016 the UK population was at its largest at 65.6 million, projected to increase to 74 million by 2039. With improvements in healthcare and lifestyles, the average age of the UK population is getting older. However, this is not the same across all areas of the UK. In 1996, only a small number of areas (mostly in southern England) had a local population with over 25% of people over the age of 65 years, in 2036 it is predicted that this will rise to over half of local authorities. In mid-2016 West Somerset had the highest (33.3%) and Tower Hamlets had the lowest (6.0%). The proportion is smaller for people aged over 85 years, with no local authorities having more than 3% of their population in this category in 1996. In 2016, this increased to over half and this is projected to continue rising to 4% in 2036. The highest populations are located predominantly in southern authorities, including: East Devon, Dorset, Rother, with London boroughs including Islington, Tower Hamlets and Hackney consistently having the lowest proportions (ONS 2017). Although ageing is not necessarily synonymous with illness or frailty, it does correlate with disability and impairment as chronic conditions become more common in older adults (Topinkova 2008).

Although ageing brings with it an increase in certain functional disease processes, mental illness is not a normal occurrence of ageing, although the risk of developing mental illness does increase with age. The World Health Organization (WHO 2013) reported that more than 20% of older adults have a mental or neurological disorder, with the most common disorder diagnoses in this age group being dementia and depression. The WHO (2013) also reports that anxiety disorders are found in 3.8% of the older population, as well as low levels of substance misuse (1%). In particular, risk factors for depression, such as loss and grief, social isolation, medical illness and disability and being a caregiver, are more common in older age (Fiske et al. 2009). The predicted increase in the older population is therefore expected to multiply the numbers of adults with mental illness (WHO 2013).

It is difficult to have a firm sense of how many older people have a mental illness as prevalence figures vary considerably according to the populations surveyed and the methodologies used (Volkert et al. 2013). A metaanalysis to assess the prevalence of mental disorders in older people in Europe and the United States found that the disorders with the highest prevalence were depression and alcohol-use disorders (Volkert et al. 2013). In addition, there are also a number of negative stereotypical perceptions of age and older people that may inhibit the diagnosis and treatment of physical and mental illness. In 1969, Butler coined the term 'ageism' to define the systematic stereotyping of, and discrimination against, people because they are old (cited in Butler 1975). We have come to realise that ageism can apply to any age group, not just the aged. Thus, ageism has more recently been defined as discrimination against people on the grounds of their age alone, as a consequence of which stereotypical assumptions are made about how people are viewed throughout life (Behrens 1998).

Unfortunately, health professionals are not immune to ageist attitudes (Karlin et al. 2005; Moyle 2003). Over the past decade a number of studies have investigated how healthcare professionals feel about caring for older people. Nursing students' attitudes to older people have frequently been found to be negative, inferring that older people have little value or are not seen as being exciting to care for (Henderson et al. 2008; Robinson & Cubit 2005). Furthermore, a recent study of student paramedic attitudes towards older people found that they also have negative ideas about older people (Ross et al. 2014). Ageist views may, in turn, affect the prevalence rates of mental illness in the older population through misdiagnosis or unwillingness to diagnose individuals because they are seen as 'old'. Additionally, ageism can influence treatment, in particular where tight hospital budgets can result in staff perceiving that treatment is too expensive to be given to older people (Skirbekk & Nortvedt 2014).

Although the exact numbers of older people with mental disorders in the community are not known, we do know that there are higher rates of mental illness in populations who are institutionalised in residential care settings (AIHW 2013). The most common diagnosis specified for residential care populations is schizophrenia (37.3%), followed by depression (12.1%) and schizo-affective disorder (10.8%) (AIHW 2013). Furthermore, older people living alone are more likely to be depressed and more at risk of suicide than those residing in a household with others (Purcell et al. 2012). Fewer social supports are likely to exist as people get older and this is more likely if they are living alone (O'Connor 2014).

A number of first-generation migrants to the UK are in the category of older age and some of these people speak very little English and may have a significant trauma history that predisposes them to mental health disorders. These factors impact the accessibility, assessment and care provision of this population. Nurses are in a key position to work with and to enable skilled staff to work with this population (see Chapters 6 and 7). It is important, however, not to stereotype older people as being unwell and to remember that not all older adults require hospital services and assistance.

Nurse's Story 12.1, a personal reflection by Dr Gillian Stockwell-Smith, demonstrates how ageist attitudes can negatively influence students' judgement about working with older people.

ASSESSMENT OF OLDER PEOPLE

All staff working with older people should begin by learning about healthy older people because the moment a problem appears, abnormality becomes the priority. The world is full of active, healthy older people and most older people do not require additional health and social support.

The main reasons for assessing older people are:

- to obtain a baseline assessment of function: this can assist in avoiding unrealistic goals
- to demonstrate positive changes to patients and to gather evidence for relatives, nurses and other health professionals
- for selection purposes (e.g. in research) to ensure that groups of people are of similar levels
- to evaluate a new approach, treatment programme or service
- for legal purposes (e.g. complications following a head injury)
- to assist diagnosis and prognosis

NURSE'S STORY 12.1

Dr Gillian Stockwell-Smith

As a student nurse many years ago, my compatriots and I were very concerned regarding an upcoming ward placement: 12 weeks on a long-stay older adults ward. The last thing I wanted to do at 19 was look after old people! What skill was involved in getting old people in and out of bed and dealing with incontinence?

To my surprise I found I enjoyed caring for the ladies on the ward. History came alive as they talked about their lives and the changes they had experienced, particularly during the two world wars they had lived through. Providing care for these resilient women was hard physical work, but also a privilege. I wasn't considering a career in older adult care at this point, but was merely grateful the placement hadn't been as dreadful as expected.

Later ward placements in an older adults' unit at the local mental health hospital piqued my interest in dementia. The majority of patients were in the end stages of dementia, but the distinction between different types or distinct symptoms beyond memory loss was rarely acknowledged. Care for these patients was little more than custodial; it was task orientated and frequently demeaning. In hindsight, I wince when I consider my own and others' practice during this period, but it increased my desire to improve.

Time passed and the practical and theoretical knowledge gained through general nurse training improved my skills and also my empathy with older patients. Once qualified, I went to work on a long-stay older adults ward and my love of aged care was cemented. This led to a position as Deputy Head-of-Home at an inaugural community-based long-stay older persons care unit. Once set up, the unit was considered a ground-breaking centre of excellence in residential aged care. This was mainly due to the drive and enthusiasm of the Head-of-Home. She espoused person-centred care through her innovative vision, challenging negative perceptions of older people and enhancing their participation in care at a time (early/mid-1980s) when these issues were rarely acknowledged. She greatly influenced me personally and other staff, as evidenced by the consistently high levels of care provided throughout the unit.

Postgraduate qualifications in community practice and gerontology along with workplace experience gained from a wide variety of clinical and management positions have been important in my development as an aged care practitioner. However, on reflection it is the inspirational leaders, those I have worked with and my academic supervisors, who have been critical in improving my practice and maintaining my motivation and positive outlook towards aged care. As my career progresses, I consider it is time to use my experience to mentor others. Myths and misconceptions regarding dementia continue to prevail and consequently those living with dementia often suffer from stigma.

My mission as a clinician, educator and researcher is to dispel attitudes towards older people, particularly those living with dementia, that focus on their limitations and to ensure the next generation of nurses and health professionals are aware of the essential attributes for working with older people, particularly those with dementia. Clinicians must understand the importance of good listening and communication skills, compassion and empathy in building worthwhile therapeutic relationships: to be respectful and nonjudgemental, focus on their patients' strengths and recognise their contributions, encouraging active participation in care and creating meaningful outcomes.

Most of the time nurses are involved with obtaining a baseline assessment of function and assisting with diagnosis and prognosis. However, when a patient is experiencing psychological distress there may be little time to conduct a full assessment. The use of observation skills and a brief assessment of the patient's cognitive functioning through the use of the Mini-Mental State Examination (MMSE) provide valuable baseline data on which to base subsequent observations and care (refer to Chapter 23).

When making a diagnosis of mental illness, cultural concepts related to physical and mental wellbeing must be considered. The MMSE (Folstein et al. 1975), a common cognitive screening instrument that must be purchased to use (www4.parinc.com/Products/Product.aspx?ProductID=MMSE), is available in a number of different language versions, which take into consideration an individual's educational attainment, language and culture. The consequence of using the standard MMSE in groups that differ on cultural and linguistic grounds is the potential to attribute low scores to pathological processes rather than to other factors such as education level, literacy and cultural differences in cognitive and perceptual information processing. The Rowland Universal Dementia Assessment Scale (RUDAS) is a short cognitive screening instrument designed to minimise the effects of cultural learning and language diversity (Storey et al. 2004). The RUDAS is freely available and the instrument and guide can be found at www.health.qld.gov.au/tpch/html/rudas.asp.

Furthermore, when screening older people, instruments should be used that take into account the attributes of older people as well as reporting other conditions. For example, the Cornell Scale for Depression in Dementia is useful for the identification of depression in older people with dementia (Snowdon 2010). In addition, the Mini-Cog is a short screening tool that combines the clock drawing test and the three-word recall. While some studies report the superior screening properties of the Mini-Cog compared with the MMSE (Borson et al. 2005; Milian et al. 2012), others report similar screening results (Borson et al. 2003; Dougherty et al. 2010). The Mini-Cog assessment and instructions are freely available at www.alz.org/documents_custom/minicog.pdf.

Ageism in Assessment

Although there are many safe ways to investigate the reasons behind a change in behaviour and ability in an older person, conclusions are often drawn too quickly. It is too easy to assume that if a 70-year-old person fails to recognise familiar faces and rambles and behaves strangely, a dementing condition is the cause. There could be any number of reasons for this behaviour, from acute confusion (delirium) to depression, and therefore it is important that nurses spend time with the patient and their spouse or carers, to ensure a thorough and accurate assessment and to reduce the influence of potentially ageist staff attitudes.

MENTAL HEALTH DISORDERS IN THE OLDER POPULATION

Although a number of conditions (such as anxiety disorders, depression, suicide, substance misuse, delirium, dementia and schizophrenia) fall within the context of mental illness in old age, they do not occur because of ageing. Multiple social, psychological and biological factors can determine the health of an older person. For example, many older people may lose the ability to maintain independence due to frailty or mobility problems, the challenges of physical or chronic pain, as well as a higher risk of bereavement or a drop in financial status because of retirement. All these factors can result in psychological stress that may trigger a mental health disorder. Physical and mental health are intimately tied. For example, untreated depression can lead to poor physical health and older people with heart disease have higher rates of depression (WHO 2013). Common mental health disorders are explored in the following sections in relation to older people and also in separate chapters devoted to the relevant disorder.

Anxiety Disorders

Recent research indicates that anxiety disorders may be more common than depression in older people (Byers et al. 2010). The presentation of anxiety in older people is similar to that in younger people; however, as with depression, diagnosis is complicated by the tendency of older adults to focus on physical rather than psychological illness (Zhang et al. 2015). The most common anxiety disorders in older adults are generalised anxiety disorder and phobias (Zhang et al. 2015). Prevalence rates of anxiety disorders vary and this is reported to be a result of the current anxiety criteria not adequately capturing the nature of anxiety in older adults (Jeste et al. 2006). Anxiety disorder is associated with a high number of somatic medications and a high number of chronic illnesses (Zhang et al. 2015).

There is insufficient research examining the aetiology of anxiety disorders in older adults. However, initial evidence suggests that while risk factors are similar to those for depression, social factors such as low affective support during childhood, negative parenting and experiencing negative life events are uniquely associated with anxiety (Zhang et al. 2015). Women are more likely than men to experience an anxiety disorder (AIHW 2007). Additionally, anxiety disorders and characteristics such as female gender, low education, early traumatisation, neuroticism and extraversion are common psychiatric comorbidities associated with depression in late life (van der Veen et al. 2015). The presence of anxiety symptoms decreases the efficacy of depression treatment (Andreescu et al. 2007) and although treatment for depression may reduce anxiety, this is not always the case, with anxiety symptoms persisting despite the resolution of other depressive symptoms (van der Veen et al. 2015). Comorbid anxiety disorder in patients with major depression lowers the rate of patient recovery and is also associated with a higher rate of suicide (Jeste et al. 2006).

Depression

Depression is one of the most common remediable mental disorders in older people (Laborde-Lahoz et al. 2014). Significant life changes associated with growing older can place older people at risk of depression. Depression in older adults has often been found to be associated with vascular brain changes (Lavretsky & Meeks 2009). Vascular depression is characterised by a lack of family history of depression, subcortical neurological dysfunction, cognitive impairment and psychomotor change. All of the depressive subtypes commonly recognised in younger adults are represented in older populations, along with some that are specific to older people, such as depression related to one of the neurocognitive disorders (e.g. Alzheimer disease).

> **CRITICAL THINKING CHALLENGE 12.1**
>
> There is no single cause of depression. Listen to Dr David Conn, a psychiatrist at Baycrest Hospital (Toronto, Canada), who discusses the causes and risk factors associated with depression, at: www.baycrest.org/educate/mental-health/depression/causes-and-risk-factors. As a follow up to listening to this audio recording, consider the role of the nurse in helping older people to reduce their risk of depression, in particular reducing psychological factors such as life events, illness, grief and loss.

Presentation

The presentation of depression in older age is often less obvious than in younger people, as older people often focus attention on their physical symptoms and are less likely to acknowledge feeling depressed (Hegeman et al. 2015). The criteria for a major depressive episode according to the DSM-5 (American Psychiatric Association [APA] 2013) are five or more of the symptoms outlined in Box 12.1 (see also Chapter 16) that have been present during the same 2-week period. The symptoms must result in a change in functioning and at least one of the symptoms must be either depressed mood or loss of interest or pleasure.

Although older people may exhibit the cardinal features of depression, such as lowered mood and loss of interest (APA 2013), they often attribute these feelings to their physical condition rather than to a psychological state. They also have a tendency to focus on cognitive impairments such as memory loss and concentration difficulties (Fiske et al. 2009).

It is important to interview the patient's spouse or carer to corroborate the patient's history and to substantiate a professional assessment, as well as to gather additional information to assist in the assessment. A spouse or carer will commonly

BOX 12.1 Symptoms for Major Depressive Episode (must be present nearly every day)

A. Five or more of the symptoms:
- Depressed mood most of the day
- Markedly diminished interest or pleasure
- Significant weight loss
- Insomnia or hypersomnia
- Psychomotor agitation or retardation
- Fatigue or loss of energy
- Feelings of worthlessness or excessive or inappropriate guilt
- Diminished ability to think or concentrate

B. Symptoms cause clinically significant distress or impairment in social, occupational or other important areas of functioning.

C. The symptoms are not due to the direct physiological effects of a substance.

(Adapted from American Psychiatric Association (APA) 2013. Diagnostic and statistical manual of mental disorders, 5th ed. APA, Washington, D.C.)

report changes that the individual has not recognised, such as social withdrawal, irritability, avoiding family and friends, poor hygiene and memory change. Losses such as status, income and bereavement can contribute to feelings of dejection.

Diagnosing depression in the older population is compounded by the difficulty of differentiating it clinically from dementia and delirium (explored later in this chapter). Depression and dementia may both present with psychomotor slowing, apathy, impaired memory, fatigue, sleep disturbance and poor concentration. Furthermore, distinguishing between grief and depression is not easy since they share many symptoms. Grief, however, tends to fluctuate, with the person experiencing good as well as bad days, whereas feelings of emptiness and despair are constant in the person with depression.

Prevalence

There are varying accounts of the prevalence of depression among people over the age of 65 years. However, it is believed that one in five older people in the community and 40% of people living in care homes are affected by depression (Mental Health Taskforce 2016). Variance in the rates also results from epidemiologists generally recording only cases of major depression and dysthymia; they often do not include individuals with minor depression, which is common in older age as a result of functional decline and medical symptoms. Individuals with minor depression may have significant depressive symptoms but do not fulfil all the DSM-5 criteria for major depression or dysthymia. Therefore, although people with minor depression experience at least 2 weeks of depressive symptoms, they exhibit fewer than the five diagnostic criteria required to diagnose major depression (APA 2013). Prevalence rates for depression are approximately 50% higher in women than in men (Haralambous et al. 2009).

CRITICAL THINKING CHALLENGE 12.2

Connect to the internet and download the Black Dog Institute fact sheet on depression in older people at: www.blackdoginstitute.org.au/docs/DepressioninOlderPeople.pdf. Review the signs of depression as well as the causes of depression.

Aetiology

There is a common perception that older people become depressed as a part of the normal ageing process. This is not so, but older people are vulnerable to developing a depressive illness because of age-related biochemical changes and psychological factors. Depression is frequently associated with many common medical conditions found in later life, such as stroke, cancer, myocardial infarction, diabetes, rheumatoid arthritis and Parkinson disease (Almeida et al. 2011). Psychological risk factors include bereavement, medication, a decrease in activity and losses related to physical illness, financial security, accommodation and independence (Fiske et al. 2009). Furthermore, older adults who are institutionalised face a number of changes to their normal routine as they often struggle to adjust to living in an environment where there are a lot of people, noises, rituals and habits that seem strange to them. Such factors, including limited nurse–patient interaction, may make them vulnerable to mental illness (Haugan et al. 2013).

Assessment

It is essential that nurses are involved in the assessment of older people and their psychosocial situations to assist in an early intervention nursing care plan. Assessment and management require collaboration between health professionals who are skilled and educated in the care and management of older people with mental illness (Haugan et al. 2013; Moyle & Evans 2007). It can be very difficult, especially with older patients, to distinguish between depression and dementia because both conditions share common features such as poor concentration, low mood and social isolation. To make this distinction even more difficult, depression often coexists with dementia. Furthermore, the diagnosis may be hindered if the person also has a physical illness, which leads health professionals to believe that the person's depressive symptoms are understandable given their physical status. Undiagnosed and untreated depression places the person at risk of mental suffering, poor physical health, social isolation and suicide. Screening for depression should be undertaken for people who are recently bereaved and in particular when they have unusual symptoms such as marked functional impairment, mood congruent delusions and psychomotor retardation. It is important to note that older people may use different language to describe their depressed mood. For example, rather than describing sadness they may talk about 'their nerves'.

A depression-screening instrument such as the Geriatric Depression Scale (GDS) (Yesavage et al. 1983;

see Box 12.2) may assist in making the diagnosis, referring for treatment and providing a baseline assessment against which to measure the effect of the treatment. The GDS is a well-validated screening tool for depression in older people. The GDS comes in two formats: the 30-item long form and the 15-item short form rating scale. The long form uses an 11-point cut-off and the short form uses a 7-point cut-off. The questions focus on the individual's thoughts and feelings of depression experienced over the previous week. Unlike other screening instruments, the GDS avoids asking questions about physical symptoms, as this generation of people traditionally tends to concentrate on physical symptoms and avoids discussing emotional symptoms. They may also regard the presence of depressive symptoms as a part of their ageing process and neither ask for nor expect help with such symptoms. Where a differential diagnosis cannot be made, psychiatric consultation and/or a trial of antidepressant therapy may be warranted. While cognitive deficits are common in dementia and depression in older people, they normally resolve with recovery from depression. The GDS is available in many languages (see www.stanford.edu/~yesavage/GDS.html).

The possibility of a depressive illness should be considered in older people if they develop cognitive impairment or anxiety. To assist with the diagnosis of depression, keep in mind the following when caring for older individuals:

- Check for the presence of depressive symptoms using a screening instrument for this age group, such as the GDS (see Box 12.2). Remember that individuals can suffer from depression, a physical disorder and/or dementia, all at the same time. Do not assume that symptoms can be easily related to the individual's life circumstances or their age. Approximately one in five people experiencing dementia will also experience depression (Muliyala & Varghese 2010). The reliability of the GDS is reduced when patients have cognitive impairment.
- If patients have significant cognitive impairment, the Cornell Scale for Depression in Dementia (CSDD) should be used. The CSDD is a screening tool and is not diagnostic. The nurse will interview the patient's caregiver on the 19 items of the scale. The carer reports their observations based on the previous week. The nurse then briefly interviews the patient. The tool is useful if aiming to evaluate the effect of therapy. Permission must be sought to use the CSDD. The tool and permission details can be found at: http://geropsychiatriceducation.vch.ca/docs/edu-downloads/depression/cornell_scale_depression.pdf

BOX 12.2 Geriatric Depression Scale

1. Are you basically satisfied with your life?
2. Have you dropped many of your activities and interests?
3. Do you feel that your life is empty?
4. Do you often get bored?
5. Are you hopeful about the future?
6. Are you bothered by thoughts you cannot get out of your head?
7. Are you in good spirits most of the time?
8. Are you afraid that something bad is going to happen to you?
9. Do you feel happy most of the time?
10. Do you often feel helpless?
11. Do you often get restless and fidgety?
12. Do you prefer to stay at home, rather than going out and doing new things?
13. Do you frequently worry about the future?
14. Do you feel you have more problems with memory than most?
15. Do you think it is wonderful to be alive now?
16. Do you often feel downhearted and blue?
17. Do you feel pretty worthless the way you are now?
18. Do you worry a lot about the past?
19. Do you find life very exciting?
20. Is it hard for you to get started on new projects?
21. Do you feel full of energy?
22. Do you feel that your situation is hopeless?
23. Do you think that most people are better off than you are?
24. Do you frequently get upset over little things?
25. Do you frequently feel like crying?
26. Do you have trouble concentrating?
27. Do you enjoy getting up in the morning?
28. Do you prefer to avoid social gatherings?
29. Is it easy for you to make decisions?
30. Is your mind as clear as it used to be?

Scoring for the scale

Score one point for each of the answers given below:

1. no	9. no	17. yes	25. yes
2. yes	10. yes	18. yes	26. yes
3. yes	11. yes	19. no	27. no
4. yes	12. yes	20. yes	28. yes
5. no	13. yes	21. no	29. no
6. yes	14. yes	22. yes	30. no
7. no	15. no	23. yes	
8. yes	16. yes	24. yes	

Cut-off
Normal: 0–9
Mild depressive: 10–19
Severe depressive: 20–30

(The GDS is a public domain scale developed through US government funding. Information about the scale can be found at www.stanford.edu/~yesavage/GDS.html.)

Nursing Management of Depression in Older People

Effective treatment relies on detection of depression and consideration of the factors that may have contributed to the depressive illness. Most depressive disorders in older adults respond to treatment (Fiske et al. 2009). However, in older patients with severe depression associated with dementia, the prognosis is poor.

Psychotherapeutic Support

The most effective treatment for depression is early intervention. Nurses are in a unique and important position within the healthcare team as they have more contact with patients in hospital and community settings, which makes the early recognition of depressive symptoms and early intervention possible. Nurses are invaluable in giving psychotherapeutic support to enable patients to talk about their feelings. Psychosocial therapies such as acceptance and commitment therapy (ACT), cognitive therapy (CT), cognitive behavioural therapy (CBT), mindfulness-based cognitive therapy (MBCT), compassion-focussed therapy (CFT), group therapy and counselling are useful, especially when the depressive illness is loss related. CT and CBT identify distorted or illogical thinking processes and maladaptive patterns of behaviours and then attempt to replace them with more reality-based thinking and adaptive behaviours (Wilkinson 2013). CBT may involve weekly sessions based on patient goals, the sessions guided by the therapist with the aim to highlight areas where interventions may help the person. CBT has been reported as an effective treatment for depression in older people (Jayasekara et al. 2015; Peng et al. 2009). It is also an effective treatment for anxiety disorders where the patient focus is on catastrophic thinking and where the patient uses patterns of behaviour that reinforce their anxiety (Wilkinson 2013). MBCT is a meditation-based intervention that has been reported as a promising and cost-effective treatment for older adults with depression and anxiety (Foulk et al. 2014; Smith et al. 2007). See Chapter 24 for more detail about these and other therapeutic interventions.

Pharmacotherapy and Electroconvulsive Therapy

Pharmacotherapy (e.g. antidepressants, antipsychotics) and electroconvulsive therapy (ECT) may be prescribed and used alone or in conjunction with psychosocial therapies. Although depression may be greatly improved with pharmacotherapy, it is imperative that older patients are monitored for medication side effects that can have adverse effects on their cardiac condition. For example, tricyclic antidepressants and monoamine oxidase inhibitors (MAOIs) are known to place the patient at risk of hypertensive crisis and can affect cardiac conduction (Thomas et al. 2015). Therefore, monitoring of physical functioning should be incorporated into the nurse's daily routine and results that deviate from the patient's baseline must be reported. In recent years, selective serotonin reuptake inhibitors (SSRIs) have been prescribed, as they are known to have fewer cardiac side effects. However, there is always an increased risk of drug interactions when patients are on multiple medications. It is also important to establish whether patients are on complementary and alternative medications (Hsu et al. 2009), as some of these (e.g. St John's wort) can cause potentially fatal reactions when taken with antidepressant medication. Ginseng and St John's wort, for example, may cause potentiation of MAOI activity, adverse effects and hypertensive crisis (Rahman et al. 2013).

Case Study 12.1 on Joan provides an example of how a depressive illness can affect an individual and their family. It also demonstrates the importance of an individualised nursing care plan that focusses not only on the condition but also on preparation for discharge, future rehabilitation and prevention.

> **CRITICAL THINKING CHALLENGE 12.3**
>
> Reflect on Case Study 12.1 and determine the priorities for Joan's care upon admission to hospital. How would the priorities change prior to discharge, so that recovery and the prevention of future episodes of depression could be addressed?

Suicide

Suicide rates among older people are higher than or as high as suicide rates in younger people (Lapierre et al. 2011). Effectively lethal self-harm behaviours increase with age. The most common means of suicide in men is by a violent method such as hanging and they are less likely to commit suicide by poisoning, drowning or jumping when compared with women (Sarchiapone et al. 2011). Older patients should be assessed to determine whether they are suicidal at the time of assessment for depression. The risk of suicide in the older population is very real and should never be discounted as a possibility. Suicide risk is also high in people who provide care for family members. Recent research suggests that family members who care for people with dementia, for example, are at a greater risk of suicidal behaviour. A survey of 120 family carers found that one in four (26%) had contemplated suicide more than once over the last year (O'Dwyer et al. 2013). Family members who react to the burden of the provision of care can react strongly to the behavioural signs and symptoms of dementia.

Any talk of suicide by an older individual should be taken seriously and reported to a medical practitioner or specialist services if the patient is in the community or to senior nursing staff and specialist services if the patient is hospitalised. Never assume that an older person is not capable of hoarding medications to use in a suicide attempt because they are hospitalised or in a nursing home. If the patient offers information about their intended suicide, identifying how, when and by what means will enable the level of risk to be assessed (see Chapters 7, 23, 24 for risk assessment). Personality, physical illness and recent bereavement are known contributing factors to suicide in older people not suffering from psychiatric illness at the time of death (Harwood et al. 2006).

Prevalence

Older adults tend to use more violent methods in their suicide attempts and this generally accounts for their high success rates (Conwell and Thompson 2008). Suicide rates for males show two peaks: one in younger males (aged 25–44 years) and the other in the oldest age group (80 years and over; ABS 2008). Males over 75 years have higher rates of death by suicide, which may reflect the impact of depression, social isolation, bereavement or physical illness (Department of Health 2012).

CASE STUDY 12.1

Joan

Joan is a 75-year-old married woman. Depression is prevalent in her family. Her mother suffered from depression following the birth of each of her three siblings. Joan's father found the stress of caring for his wife and children while trying to run a business too much and he divorced his wife when Joan was 10 years of age. She felt angry towards men after her father deserted his family. However, Joan met a man she learnt to trust and she got married. Following a desire to have a career she went back to high school and finished her high school certificate. She went to teachers' college to gain a teaching qualification. Life seemed to be going well for Joan until the birth of her daughter, when she experienced an episode of postnatal depression. A course of ECT helped her recover and eventually enabled her to return to teaching. She was always mindful of her history and tried to manage her life with exercise, a sensible diet and social interaction, especially through meeting with groups to play card games.

Life again seemed to be going well for Joan until her husband died suddenly around the same time that she was diagnosed with multiple sclerosis (MS) and her beloved dog Chloe also died. She was devastated and felt the same sense of abandonment as when her father left the family. She spent the next year planning her suicide, giving away her precious items such as jewellery and finalising her will. She didn't want to be a burden to her daughter, who was also troubled with depression and had a teenage family to care for. Suicide seemed the only option for Joan at the time. She spoke to no-one about her preparations but her neighbours were concerned about Joan as she slowly withdrew from their regular card game evenings.

Joan attempted suicide but was unsuccessful as a result of a neighbour finding her and calling an ambulance. Following stabilisation of her acute condition she was admitted to a large mental health unit and placed under the care of a geriatric psychiatrist. She was prescribed an antidepressant and psychotherapy.

The nursing care plan for Joan included spending time with her to establish rapport and trust and allowing Joan time to respond to her fears of her illness. Nurses used cognitive behavioural therapy (CBT) to assist Joan to talk about her feelings and helped her to identify distorted or illogical thinking processes, such as her fear that she did not want to be a burden to her family. CBT helped Joan to replace these illogical ideas with reality-based thoughts and assisted her with new coping strategies, in particular to cope with her diagnosis of multiple sclerosis. Joan responded well to the treatment and was discharged after 6 weeks into the care of a psychiatrist and a community mental health nurse. She was also referred to the MS society who visited Joan and assisted her with understanding the future requirements and planning for her disorder. The long-term plan was for Joan to stay on antidepressants and to undertake regular consultation with her healthcare team and for Joan or her family to report if she again started to feel anxious and depressed, as early intervention was important in keeping Joan well. Joan came to learn that speaking about her depression and MS were important in helping her to feel she had control again over her life.

NURSE'S STORY 12.2

As a new employee in a small private mental health hospital, I was intrigued by the number of patients admitted for depression. Janet, a 65-year-old woman, was one of those patients. She was diagnosed with major depressive disorder 6 months previously and pharmaceutical management had not improved her mood. She was admitted to the private mental health hospital and placed on suicide monitoring following family concern that she had spoken of ending her life. Janet spent the majority of her day alone in her bedroom and she was reluctant to attend any of the therapeutic groups she was prescribed. She was found with a belt around her neck, tied to the wardrobe hook, but luckily before she had caused any physical damage. She remained on suicide watch and I was assigned to be Janet's primary nurse. Although concerned that Janet was my first patient case in this institution, I was well trained in cognitive behavioural therapy (CBT) and spent each day getting to know Janet and her situation while helping her to recognise her negative patterns of thought, to evaluate their validity and to help her to replace them with healthier ways of thinking. Janet spent many months in the hospital and was eventually managed, with electroconvulsive therapy (ECT), and discharged back to community care.

While she was in the hospital, I had often felt I was not helping Janet. Seeing Janet in her very low state and constantly hearing her tell me that she would be better off dead had made me question my skills. I feared that she would commit suicide and that I would take on the blame for not being able to save Janet. Speaking with my supervisor and Janet's psychiatrist helped me to recognise that my role was valuable in Janet's recovery. I had helped her to manage her negative patterns of thought, to use classical music and deep breathing and to exercise. All of these approaches alongside ECT helped Janet to achieve a sense of self-worth and as a coordinator of Janet's care I had helped to bring together the expertise of therapists to assist Janet. I am grateful to my supervisor and Janet's psychiatrist for helping me to recognise my role as a nurse in the care of older people with depression.

Substance Misuse

Substance misuse involving illicit drugs is rare in older adults, but dependence on prescription medications such as benzodiazepines is not uncommon (Simoni-Wastila & Yang 2006), as a high proportion of older people experience sleep disturbances for which they seek medication. Older adults over the age of 60 years most commonly seek treatment for difficulties with alcohol and benzodiazepines (AIHW 2010a).

There is assumed to be a steady decline in substance abuse disorders with age; however, as substance misuse in older patients is reported to be under-recognised and undertreated the figures may actually be higher (Searby et al. 2015). One of the current concerns regarding major substance abuse relates to methamphetamine use. Given the increase in the population using methamphetamine, it is predicted that the community is likely to experience an increase in older illicit drug users as the population ages (Searby et al. 2015). As a result, the healthcare system will need to manage the significant harms of this substance on long-term cognitive deficits (Searby et al. 2015).

People who abuse alcohol are likely to suffer from major depression (Hall 2012). We also know that alcohol and drug misuse are associated with a variety of medical problems and high rates of medical treatment (Hall 2012). Furthermore, undiagnosed substance use in older patients may lead to serious withdrawal syndromes during hospitalisation (Saitz 2005). Disability is related to increased alcohol and substance use: older people with severe functional impairment have twice the rate of alcohol use than older people with no disability (AIHW 2010b).

It is imperative that nurses assess patients for substance misuse during their preliminary assessment, especially when older patients are admitted for surgery. Rather than asking whether a patient drinks alcohol, ask 'How much alcohol do you drink per day?' If they state 'not much' or 'I only drink socially', ask them to tell you exactly how much alcohol this involves. Older patients may say that they 'do not drink much' but consider that 4 pints of beer and 2 whiskies a day constitutes being a social drinker! (See also Chapter 20)

Delirium

Delirium may be defined as a transient, usually reversible, cause of cerebral dysfunction. It can occur at any age, but it occurs more commonly in older patients, especially those in hospital or a nursing home, and those with compromised mental status. Delirium is a syndrome that constitutes a characteristic pattern of signs and symptoms and can be caused by anything that rapidly damages the brain. Delirium is also associated with high rates of morbidity (APA 2013).

Differentiating between delirium and dementia can be more difficult in older people (see Table 12.1 later in the chapter). Delirium develops over a period of hours to days and tends to fluctuate during the course of a given day. Delirium is also known as acute confusion. Dementia, on the other hand, is progressive and presents as a gradual failure of brain functioning. Dementia is also referred to as chronic confusion. The exact nature of the pathophysiology of delirium is unknown. Both cortical and brainstem functions are impaired in delirium, the cortex mediating cognitive function and the brainstem wakefulness. Delirium is ruled out if a dementing syndrome accounts for the disturbance in consciousness. However, it is not unusual for delirium to coincide in people with dementia as a result of a medical condition. In this case, the person may present with additional symptoms of short duration that are above and beyond those that can be accounted for by the dementia.

There is little data on the time course of delirium in older patients, possibly because it is often missed unless family or nursing staff are in constant contact with the individual. Most patients have a prodromal stage lasting from a few hours to a day or so. This refers to a change in the person's habitual behaviour and cognitive functioning (sleep disturbance, restlessness and irritability, general malaise and anxiety).

It is important to establish early recognition of delirium because, if the disease or damage causing the delirium can be treated, the confusion will resolve. If the patient is elderly, there is a tendency for nursing staff to pass off behavioural changes as part of ageing and they may therefore avoid carrying out a thorough assessment. This may result in no treatment or inappropriate treatment being given, whereas if the delirium is related to biochemical changes caused by an infection, for example, this could be resolved by a course of antibiotics. Prevention strategies target one or more of the following risk factors.

Risk Factors

Being older places individuals at risk of delirium. There are also a number of other risk factors that predispose older people to delirium, such as:

- preexisting brain damage
- preexisting dementia
- sensory impairment

Additional risk factors are:

- infections, especially urinary tract or chest
- cardiac failure and other major heart conditions
- respiratory failure resulting in raised carbon dioxide levels
- kidney failure resulting in raised levels of protein and urea
- constipation (although the reason for this has not been established)
- medications
- drug withdrawal, including alcohol (delirium tremens, DTs)

Strategies to detect delirium earlier using cognitive assessment tools such as the Confusion Assessment Method (CAM), a tool created for clinicians to use with older people in various clinical settings, may prevent delirium in those at risk (Inouye et al. 2014). The CAM is available in both a short form (four items) for measuring delirium in hospitalised patients and a long form (ten items) for research (Inouye et al. 2014). The diagnosis of delirium is clinical because no laboratory test can diagnose delirium. In addition, individual care planning and pain management have been found to be successful in preventing delirium (Rossom et al. 2011). The goal of treatment is to determine the cause of the delirium and to stop or to reverse it.

Prior to an older person undergoing surgery, it is important that the nurse assesses the patient to ensure that any changes in behaviour following surgery can be detected and early intervention given. There are two established risk factors for older people undergoing surgery: previous alcohol or drug abuse and prolonged operating time under a general anaesthetic. Management of delirium includes supportive therapy and pharmacological management. Supportive therapy that nurses can offer includes attention to fluid and nutrition and reorientation, such as memory cues including calendars, clocks and photographs of family and pets. Delirium that may cause injury to the patient or to others may be treated by neuroleptic medication.

CRITICAL THINKING CHALLENGE 12.4

Reflect on Judy's story in Case Study 12.2. Judy understands the importance of identifying delirium early and involving family where possible to comfort the patient. Knowing the challenges that this presents, examine the situation within an acute care hospital and identify the priorities that must occur for delirium to be diagnosed early.

Neurocognitive Disorder

Prevalence

Dementia is not a normal part of life or ageing. However, the number of people with dementia is increasing because more people are living longer and the prevalence of dementia increases exponentially with age. Figures from Public Health England (2018) suggest that the recorded prevalence of dementia in the population over 65 years has shown a small but significant increase from 4.29% in 2017 to 4.33% in 2018.

People in the early stages of dementia usually live in the community, while people with higher levels of cognitive loss are usually accommodated in residential care facilities. Depression may be underdiagnosed in this population (Gaugler et al. 2014).

Aetiology

Dementia has recently been renamed in the DSM-5 as major neurocognitive disorder (NCD) (APA 2013). However, the term 'dementia' is still considered an acceptable term to use. Major NCD refers to dementia, while mild NCD refers to less severe forms of cognitive impairment and is equivalent to mild cognitive impairment. Major NCD was introduced to address the limitations of and associated stigma attached to the term 'dementia'.

Mild NCD aims to recognise the substantial clinical needs of adults living with this disorder. Mild NCD is not always a precursor of major NCD. There may be continual decline in cognition or the impairment might not progress to major NCD.

Diagnosis of major NCD requires evidence of significant cognitive decline from a previous level of performance in one or more of the cognitive domains outlined in the clinical features section. In addition, the cognitive decline must be sufficient to interfere with independence in activities of daily living. Importantly, in the DSM-5 memory, impairment was removed as a criterion for all dementias. This change takes into account that other cognitive domains such as language or attention may be impaired first, or exclusively.

Subtypes of minor and major NCD include:

- major or mild NCD due to Alzheimer disease
- major or mild frontotemporal NCD
- major or mild NCD with Lewy bodies
- major or mild vascular NCD
- major or mild NCD due to traumatic brain injury
- substance/medication-induced major or mild NCD
- major or mild NCD due to HIV infection
- major or mild NCD due to prion disease
- major or mild NCD due to Parkinson disease

CASE STUDY 12.2

Judy

Judy is a health professional who works with older people. She shares with us the challenges of delirium and how family are important in reducing a state of agitation.

Alys was 85 years old and had been admitted to the orthopaedic ward prior to undergoing emergency surgery for a fractured neck of femur. Judy admitted Alys and because she was in pain and sedated, Judy spoke with her daughter Jenny who provided information about Alys's medical history, medications and current situation. Alys lived with Jenny and her husband and until recently had been managing most of her daily care, although Jenny had noticed that Alys's short term memory had been deteriorating. The family GP told Jenny that there was nothing to worry about. He told the family to give Alys both verbal and written reminders and this would help her to manage her day. Alys spent most of her day either reading or in the garden as she loved to attend to the bonsai trees, shaping and snipping them to keep them looking good. She lost her footing one day when she walked outside and had been diagnosed with a fractured neck of femur, which was to be stabilised later that day. While waiting, Alys was given pain relief that had a sedative effect and resulted in Alys spending most of the time while she waited for surgery dozing in the hospital bed.

The surgery went to plan; however, the day following surgery Alys appeared very agitated. She lunged at the bedrails that were in place to keep her from falling and attacked the nurse who tried to comfort her. Alys told the staff to let her go, as her daughter would be waiting outside to take her home. She asked the nurse to get rid of the guards and their guns, as she was ready to go home. The staff tried to comfort Alys and informed her that she was in hospital and had surgery. They also told her that she had to rest but that they would be getting her out of bed later that day. Alys spat at the staff and accused them of holding her against her will. She didn't like the dogs or the guards who were stationed around her bed and she wanted to go home. The staff recognised that Alys probably had delirium as a result of the surgery, pain and being in a strange environment. They called the surgeon and also called Alys's daughter to ask for her help.

The staff informed Jenny that Alys appeared to have delirium and that she would benefit from having family with her during this time. Jenny arrived and was distressed to see Alys agitated and aggressive towards staff. Alys had never in the past shown aggression towards anyone. Jenny arrived as requested with family photos and she used these as prompts and reminders for Alys while telling her about her injury and surgery. Alys appeared more settled with Jenny sitting beside her and giving her comfort although she called out three more times that night and each time appeared agitated and frightened. Jenny and family took turns to sit with Alys over the next 3 days while Alys had periods of hallucinations and agitation. She soon settled and was discharged to a rehabilitation unit prior to her return to the community.

(*Source*: Webb, M., Skinner, J., Hee, L., (Eds) 2015. Stories in ageing: reflection, inquiry, action. Mosby, Sydney, p. 41.)

- major or mild NCD due to Huntington disease
- major or mild NCD due to another medical condition
- major or mild NCD due to multiple aetiologies
- unspecified NCD

Clinical Features

The following cognitive domains help to establish the presence of NCD and distinguish between mild and major NCD:

- *Complex attention*: Includes sustained attention, divided attention, selective attention and information processing speed.
- *Executive function*: Includes planning, decision making, working memory, responding to feedback, inhibition and mental flexibility.
- *Learning and memory:* Includes free recall, cued recall, recognition memory, semantic and autobiographical long-term memory, and implicit learning.
- *Language:* Includes object naming, word finding, fluency, grammar and syntax and receptive language.
- *Perceptual-motor function:* Includes visual perception, visio-constructional reasoning and perceptual-motor coordination.
- *Social cognition:* Includes recognition of emotions, theory of mind and insight.

Cognitive impairment can result in the individual displaying problems that may be identified by care staff as being challenging to manage. An increase in behavioural problems occurring in the late afternoon, evening or at night has been termed 'sundowning' (Khachiyants et al. 2011). This syndrome is often characterised by an increase in disorientation, restlessness, agitation and anxiety. Sundowning is highly prevalent among individuals with dementia. Although still up for debate, this increase in disorientation has been attributed to diurnal variations in hormones and light, as well as to fatigue and a search for familiar surroundings in which to rest. However, in some individuals this pattern is reversed and they are more disoriented in the morning. There is also an argument that this could be a socially constructed syndrome created by people around the individual.

In the mid-1980s Dr Tom Kitwood and colleagues at the Bradford Dementia Group began work on a theory of caring for people with dementia that was underpinned by the need to rebalance the 'technical framing' of dementia and complement it with a philosophy constructed from 'personhood' and 'person-centred values' (Kitwood 1988; Kitwood & Bredin 1992). Kitwood (1988) argued that dementia is not the problem, rather it is our inability to accommodate the view of the world as seen by the person with dementia. Kitwood and Bredin (1992) suggested that this created a 'them and us' dialectic tension, which is sustained by the devalued status of someone who has developed dementia. Kitwood (1988) argued that the limitations of care environments produced what he termed a 'malignant social psychology'.

This work has been advanced since the early 2000s by people such as Dawn Brooker (Brooker 2007), who promotes the following principles: the absolute *value* of all human lives regardless of age or cognitive ability; an *individualised* approach to care that recognises the individual's uniqueness; an understanding from *the perspective* of the person; and a *social environment* that supports the individual's psychological needs. Brooker called this the VIPs mode. McCormack and McCance (2010) interpret the fundamental principles of person-centred care as all individuals have dignity, autonomy, worth and a set of unique moral principles, histories and desires that need to be taken into account in the care of the person.

A person-centred approach to care aims to understand the individual and seeks to engage with, respond appropriately to their individual situation and support the individual. In such an approach, the nurse will support the individual to manage their feelings and thoughts, to deal with their stresses, to link them to their community (including a safe environment) and to support the individual and family to build resilience.

Nursing Management of the Individual with Major NCD

Although the cause of sundowning is not known, it is important to assess individuals to help guide the formulation of an individualised care plan. People with dementia are often highly responsive to the environment they find themselves in. Therefore, the environment needs to be made safe and familiar, with objects that have meaning for the individual (e.g. family photographs). Unnecessary changes to routines should be avoided. Furthermore, treatment options that have been found to help are bright light therapy, melatonin, antipsychotics and behavioural modifications (Khachiyants et al. 2011).

Verbal and physical aggression is common in major NCD and can impose a toll on care staff and families. Nurses are in a prime position to use and to advocate the use of psychosocial interventions to prevent or to reduce such behaviours. A recent review found that interventions that focus on behavioural management techniques, cognitive stimulation and physical interventions could reduce behavioural symptoms in people with NCD (Vernooij-Dassen et al. 2010). The most promising psychosocial interventions tend to be individually tailored to meet each person's needs. Therefore, one of the key features of nursing management is to understand each person's social biography and use this biography to guide inclusive care interactions (Kellett et al. 2010). Refer to Case Study 12.3 on Hilary for a story about Alzheimer disease and the impact it has on an older person and their family.

> **CRITICAL THINKING CHALLENGE 12.5**
>
> In Case Study 12.3, consider how the family might have been able to address Hilary's delusions and care provision during the early stages of her dementia.

Comparing Delirium, NCD and Depression

It is important to differentiate between delirium and NCD so that early intervention for delirium can take place and to distinguish whether features displayed by an individual are a result of NCD or depression. These conditions may present with very similar features. Table 12.1 provides an overview

CASE STUDY 12.3

Hilary

Hilary was an 83-year-old woman who had been widowed for 10 years. She lived with her daughter and son-in-law in an annex flat attached to the family house. Hilary had always been active both physically and mentally, and had contributed to the running of the household, organising meals and driving the grandchildren to school and to extracurricular activities. It came as a surprise to her friends when she voiced concern that her son-in-law wanted to take her money. She also expressed concern that as he was a psychiatrist she was convinced he was plotting against her and planned to send her to a psychiatric hospital.

Hilary's friends became concerned about her stories. They asked her to spend more time with them so that they could observe her. This created tensions in the family, as this decision meant that Hilary was not readily available to take the grandchildren to school. Her daughter talked to Hilary and she agreed that her role as the driver of the grandchildren was an important one. She recommenced driving the children again until the following week when she had a car accident. The grandchildren blamed Hilary for causing the accident and the son-in-law asked Hilary to have an older adult's assessment, as he was concerned about her poor health and behaviour. Hilary confessed to her friends that she was also concerned about her health as she recognised she had word-finding challenges. She was concerned that she might have Alzheimer disease, as her three older sisters were all diagnosed in their late 80s with Alzheimer disease. However, in spite of this confusion she also believed that her son-in-law was to blame for her ill health, as he didn't allow her to socialise with the family friends.

Hilary was referred to a geriatrician who was also a friend of the family. Hilary was angry and told the geriatrician that the only reason she was there to see him was because her son-in-law wanted to get rid of her from the family home. Following a thorough geriatric assessment, Hilary and family were informed that Hilary had Alzheimer disease. She was told she could no longer drive her car and that she needed to plan for her future care. Hilary was angry as her car gave her independence and enabled her to see her friends.

Hilary returned home with the family but continued to become more agitated. Her sleep was altered as she did not sleep for fear her son-in-law would kill her in her sleep. She also stopped eating, as she believed he was poisoning her food. Hilary carried her handbag with her worldly possessions and refused for the handbag to be out of her sight. The family maintained her care at home but became concerned when Hilary started to wander from the home and refused to shower. They worried she would be run over on the local road. A further assessment of Hilary indicated her cognition was further impaired and she was prescribed antipsychotic medication for her paranoid thoughts. As a result of this medication, Hilary sat in a chair all day dozing and was often incontinent. Although the family wanted Hilary to be cared for at home, it was becoming increasingly difficult to manage as both her daughter and son-in-law worked full-time and they were reluctant to give up their jobs to care for Hilary.

Hilary was admitted to a local nursing home where her physical and mental status continued to deteriorate. She demonstrated a poor ability to self-care, poor mobility and low motivation and cooperation. The staff were encouraged to learn about Hilary's social history and found she was a former school teacher with an interest in music. They set about decorating her room with familiar objects and music from her home. They made sure she attended music sessions each day and involved her in a resident discussion group. Hilary's mood lifted and she enjoyed the opportunity for interaction with other residents and staff and in particular attendance at music sessions. Hilary lived for 3 more years in the nursing home and her passing was felt by all staff who had cared for Hilary during her time with them.

Conclusion

The outcome for Hilary might have been different if Hilary's family had been able to spend more time with her and if she had received an earlier diagnosis, treatment and support.

TABLE 12.1 Comparison of Major Neurocognitive Disorder (Dementia), Delirium and Depression

	Major Neurocognitive Disorder (Dementia)	Delirium	Depression
Onset	Chronic	Rapid onset, usually hours or days	Often abrupt and may coincide with life events such as death of a loved one
Course	Slow, progressive cognitive failure; symptoms may be worse in evening (sundowning)	Short, diurnal fluctuations in symptoms	Diurnal fluctuations, worse in morning
Duration	Months to years	Hours to days	6 weeks to years
Signs and symptoms	Conscious	Clouding of consciousness	Conscious
	Sleep disturbance is not usually a feature but the sleep–wake cycle may be set at the wrong time frame	Sleep disturbance	Sleep–wake disturbance
	Behaviour tends to be worse in the evening	Fluctuations noted during the course of the day	Selective disorientation
	Aimless wandering or searching	Restless and uneasy	May appear to be 'slowed up'
	Hallucinations are rare	Visual hallucinations that are usually disturbing	Delusions and hallucinations are rare
	Mood may be flattened or labile	Emotional lability and distress	Sad, with feelings of hopelessness and helplessness

of the different facets of these conditions. However, patients require adequate assessment in order to establish a diagnosis.

Schizophrenia

Although schizophrenia is usually apparent before 45 years of age, it may be late onset (Desai et al. 2010). There are a greater number of women than men with late-onset schizophrenia, whereas more men than women have early-onset schizophrenia (Savla et al. 2009). Patients with psychotic disorders have been shown to have a high prevalence of aggressive behaviour (Hoptman 2015), which makes the nursing care of these patients challenging. However, the severity of day-to-day psychotic symptoms appears to be reduced in older adults who have not had recent severe psychotic episodes (Desai et al. 2010). This may be due to an ageing-related decrease in dopaminergic and other monoaminergic activities (Desai et al. 2010). Assessment of older adults with schizophrenia can be complex because this group is known to have an increased prevalence of a number of other conditions, for example obesity, diabetes and coronary artery disease (Desai et al. 2010).

Antipsychotic medications are generally effective in managing psychotic symptoms, but they are not a cure for this disorder. Some older adults with schizophrenia may no longer need antipsychotics (Ausland & Jeste 2004). However, in those who still require antipsychotics, most adverse effects are more prevalent in older adults compared with younger populations (Desai et al. 2010). In recent times, nonpharmaceutical support through therapies such as CBT, social skills training and caregiver education has proved useful to older patients with schizophrenia (Desai et al. 2010; Haddock et al. 2014). However, the most appropriate goal of such programmes may not be full recovery but a focus on improving quality of life for the patient and their family. Although further research is required, nurses may be able to assist older patients with schizophrenia using these therapeutic interventions.

The move to reduce the number of long-stay psychiatric facilities has resulted in a greater number of older patients with schizophrenia being discharged to nursing homes and into community settings. It is therefore important for nurses working in long-term and community care to understand this condition and how patients might react to the transition. Patient Story 12.1 about Jenny demonstrates the difficulties for nursing staff when they have limited mental health education and resources to assist the patient and family with the transition.

CRITICAL THINKING CHALLENGE 12.6

Read Patient Story 12.1 and address the following reflective questions:

1. In your practice have you been in contact with an older person with schizophrenia? If so, which symptoms did they exhibit? Was the diagnosis of schizophrenia a long-term or new diagnosis?
2. What role did the nurse have in the mental health team caring for Jenny?
3. What might the outcome have been for Jenny if she did not have family support?

PATIENT STORY 12.1

Jenny

Jenny is a 65-year-old married woman with a recent uncharacteristic history of paranoid thoughts and unusual behaviour. Jenny isolated herself in her house, refusing to let people into the house, including family. She feared that people entering the house were bringing in microbes that would result in an infection that would kill her. Jenny's husband tried to reason with her but when she locked him and her adult children out of the house he contacted their GP for advice.

Jenny refused to attend the GP's clinic for assessment or to allow him into the house. The GP subsequently arranged for a mental health assessment team to visit Jenny and to have the police escort Jenny to the local hospital. Jenny was uncooperative, as she feared the hospital environment placed her at a greater risk of microbes. She refused to allow the hospital staff to touch her and she required restraint to prevent her from leaving the hospital grounds. The family was distraught when they witnessed Jenny's behaviour towards the staff and her restraint. The psychiatrist who assessed Jenny made the initial diagnosis of late-onset schizophrenia. In a family conference the family confirmed that Jenny had in recent years exhibited some unusual behaviour that the family had ignored and put down to ageing and bereavement following the death of her father, to whom she was very close. She had been treated for depression in recent years and she had been isolating herself for the last 2 years.

As Jenny was uncooperative and required treatment, she was placed on a restraining order and admitted to the geriatric mental health ward. Jenny was treated with antipsychotic medication to which she responded favourably with limited side effects. After 6 weeks, Jenny was deemed to be well enough to return to her home. Prior to being discharged, the mental health team supported and educated Jenny's family about her illness and the ongoing treatment and support she would require. They also arranged to visit Jenny and her husband a week after she had returned home and provided an emergency number if Jenny's husband was concerned at any time. Jenny's husband agreed to support Jenny by monitoring her illness, supporting the taking of her medication and reducing stressors in Jenny's life. With treatment and a supportive family Jenny settled and was maintained in the community.

Nursing Management of Older People

Mental health initiatives for older people are often vague and unspecific or tend to concentrate on dementia to the exclusion of other mental disorders. There also appears to be a need for greater cohesion of services for older people so that there is a seamless integration of physical and mental health services. A number of nursing interventions have been identified as being of assistance to older people:

- It is important to listen to the individual in an active way, in particular to listen to the feelings and emotions behind the words.
- Encourage older people to participate in physical and social activities that invite them to focus on aspects of their life apart from illness.

- Assist older people to understand disease processes, how to take medications and to maintain a physically and mentally active lifestyle.
- Help them to select coping strategies to assist them with any losses such as a decline in health or financial status or bereavement.
- If bereavement is a problem, help the person to work through the pain of grief and to adjust to an environment where the deceased is no longer available.
- Identify informal supports such as whether they have social networks and/or support services.

Person-centred care approaches are useful, whereby healthcare professionals develop a collaborative and respectful partnership with the person and respect the contribution that the older adult can bring. Such an approach requires the nurse to get to know the patient—such as their needs, preferences and life history—and empower the patient by encouraging them to be involved in the decisions that affect their health and wellbeing and the provision of flexible and accessible services.

These interventions are generalised and therefore it is important to evaluate care processes regularly to ensure that the interventions are appropriate for the situation. As previously highlighted, it is also imperative that healthcare professionals consider the individual's culture because decisions about care may be affected by cultural differences. For example, some cultural groups may not be willing to seek institutional care for family members as such services may appear to be culturally inappropriate for their needs. People from non-English-speaking populations often present at later stages of mental illness because of low levels of English proficiency or unfamiliarity with mental health services. People who come to the UK as refugees or asylum seekers have frequently experienced extreme hardship in their country of origin. The effects of displacement and trauma place them at high risk of developing posttraumatic stress disorders and depression. (See Chapter 7 for further information about trauma, crisis, loss and grief.)

The Nurse–Patient Relationship

Mental health nursing promotes the importance of the therapeutic relationship and the nurse's role in the development of this relationship with the person. Hildegard Peplau promoted the nurse–patient relationship as the foundation of nursing practice (Peplau 1991). An interactive therapeutic nurse–patient relationship, where the nurse brings a positive approach and attitude to the patient and nurtures their therapeutic interaction, will assist the patient's health and wellbeing (Stenhouse 2011; Moyle 2003). This is a trusting relationship where values are respected as the nurse listens to the patient's concerns, provides information and advice, relieves the patient's distress by encouraging the expression of emotion, improves patient morale through review of their capacities or satisfaction and encourages the patient to practise self-compassion (Dossing et al. 2015, McBeth & Gumley 2012).

Self-compassion is a relatively new psychological concept. It involves accepting and having a nonjudgemental attitude towards experiences. People with low self-compassion, on the other hand, are likely to be self-judgemental and inclined to over-identify with their negative experiences. People with low self-compassion are also likely to exhibit symptoms of depression and anxiety (Macbeth & Gumley 2012). The stigma surrounding mental illness feeds the inner critic and results in feelings of shame and self-doubt. If the nurse–patient relationship develops well, it can play a large part in helping to overcome such self-doubt and sustain the patient in the face of emotional difficulties.

The nurse–patient relationship should remain professional. Identification of the nurse–patient relationship with emotion is viewed as being 'over-involved' and not therapeutic. Such an involved relationship may result in the patient being overly dependent on the nurse and losing their self-reliance. However, establishing therapeutic relationships with patients is a learned skill that does not come instinctively to nurses and nurses need to work at this skill (Moyle 2003). The reality is that nurses use a variety of therapeutic interventions to support people with mental illness. The nurse–patient relationship is the platform on which therapeutic interventions such as cognitive behavioural therapy, narrative therapy and supportive counselling can be supported.

Maintaining Health and Function

Nurses can assist older patients in maintaining function by ensuring that patients have small, frequent meals, are well hydrated and maintain bowel function through a high-fibre diet, hydration and exercise. Patients should be encouraged to mobilise and be independent and nurses should ensure that they have undisturbed rest and relaxation. Other therapies that nurses may find therapeutic for older patients are listening to music, hand and back massage and pet therapy (Moyle 2014). Massage, for example, can induce a calming sensation that may reduce anxiety (Moyle et al. 2013a). In addition, companion robots such as animal robots have also been reported to reduce agitation and to improve quality of life, in particular for older people with NCD (Moyle et al. 2013b).

Staff Attitudes

Healthcare professionals, as well as the public, often have negative images of ageing (Eymard & Douglas 2012; Robinson & Cubit 2005) and poor attitudes to and tolerance of mental illness. Stereotypical images of older people often report these individuals as being smelly, grumpy and incompetent with impaired memory (Moyle 2003). Such negative images of old age and mental health may impact on the provision of a quality mental health service for older people. It is imperative that staff counter the belief that deterioration in cognitive functioning is a normal part of ageing. This requires a refocussing of attention from disease towards education that promotes older people as skilled and valued human beings. Changing attitudes through education is challenging and it is therefore important that education programmes are constructed using research evidence (Moyle et al. 2010; Moyle 2014). Furthermore, because there are many agency and casual staff as well as care assistants working across health and social care, it is imperative that registered nurses educate these workers so that consistency in care of older people is provided.

The term 'confusion' is often used by nurses to describe any number of patient behaviours from inattention to inappropriate vocalisation and the term is used most often towards uncooperative patients. Nurses require training to be able to differentiate between acute and chronic confusion (Moyle et al. 2008).

NURSE'S STORY 12.3

Dr Marguerite Bramble

As I reflect on what a diagnosis of dementia means for me as a nurse providing care for older people with dementia, I recall a recent episode of practice in a Secure Dementia Unit (SDU) in a residential care facility. It was an afternoon shift and following handover I had been called to the SDU by Susan, an experienced personal carer, who was concerned about one resident, 77-year-old Hazel, after she had fallen in the hallway. Hazel had been diagnosed with mixed Alzheimer and vascular dementia 2 years previously after the loss of her husband and had resided in the SDU for 12 months because of her wandering and agitated behaviour.

I entered the unit to be met by Hazel attempting to walk out the door. She appeared to be unhurt from her previous fall but as I gently led her back to the main room I noted she became very distressed when a male resident, new to the unit, walked towards her. When I asked Hazel who the man was, she said: 'It's my father and he will hit me if I don't run away.' Up until the past few days Hazel had been reasonably contented in the SDU. However, despite her dizziness and unsteady gait she was now obsessed with finding a way out, away from 'her father' and could not be persuaded to stay in one place 'in case he finds me'.

My years of clinical experience in dementia care informed my assessment about the combination of psychological triggers (deluded about the man she fears is her father) together with biological changes (small infarcts causing brain damage) associated with vascular dementia, which were causing Hazel's distress and unsteadiness. As I explained my assessment to Susan we talked about immediate ways to improve Hazel's situation, such as giving her the evening meal and regular medications and settling her in her room early, calling her daughter so that she could be involved in reassuring her and additional monitoring overnight. Later, when documenting Hazel's notes, I emphasised the importance of a solution-focussed approach to Hazel's care, involving her family, general practitioner, nurses and carers to ensure her needs were met and her quality of life maintained. This approach supported my personal and professional belief that we have both a moral and an ethical duty of care as nurses to support the freedom, rights and quality of life of every individual in our care.

CONCLUSION

As people age they experience psychosocial factors such as bereavement and loss of physical and mental functioning. This may place them at risk of mental disorders and in particular depressive illness or anxiety. However, mental disorders are not a normal part of ageing and patients require adequate assessment and diagnosis to ensure that their symptoms are not related to other issues, such as adverse effects of medications.

The diagnosis and treatment of mental disorders in older adults can be difficult. Furthermore, comorbid conditions and negative stereotypical ageist assumptions make treatment and diagnosis especially difficult. However, there is a high rate of suicide in older people and therefore it is imperative that they are assessed and treated effectively.

Nurses have an important role to play in both assessment and treatment of mental disorders in older people. They have skills in establishing a therapeutic nurse–patient relationship and in using psychotherapeutic support such as CBT to assist older patients to recognise distorted or illogical thinking processes and maladaptive patterns of behaviours resulting from grief, role disputes and transitions or interpersonal deficits. These skills can, along with pharmacotherapy and, at times, ECT, improve older patients' quality of life. Although depression is a common mental disorder in older people, it is also a treatable condition. Establishing a nurse–patient relationship provides the opportunity for nursing staff to recognise the symptoms of depression and to suggest further assessment and treatment if required.

EXERCISES FOR CLASS ENGAGEMENT

Discuss the following with your group or class members.

1. Document and discuss the differences between delirium and dementia in relation to time course, cause and clinical features.
2. Identify the risk factors for delirium and discuss how you might assess for delirium.
3. Why is it important to consider the diagnosis of delirium and dementia when care planning?
4. Explore the reasons why it is difficult to differentiate depression clinically from dementia and delirium.
5. How might the symptoms of depression affect the relatives and friends of the depressed older person?

REFERENCES

Almeida, O.P., Alfonso, H., Pirkis, J., et al., 2011. A practical approach to assess depression risk and to guide risk reduction strategies in later life. International Psychogeriatrics 23, 280–291.

American Psychiatric Association (APA), 2013. Diagnostic and Statistical Manual of Mental Disorders, fifth ed. APA, Washington, DC.

Andreescu, C., Lenze, E.J., Dew, M.A., et al., 2007. Effect of comorbid anxiety on treatment response and relapse risk in late life depression: controlled study. British Journal of Psychiatry 190, 344–349.

Ausland, L.A., Jeste, D.V., 2004. Sustained remission of schizophrenia among community-dwelling older outpatients. American Journal of Psychiatry 161, 1490–1493.
Australian Bureau of Statistics (ABS), 2008. Causes of death Australia, 2008. ABS, Canberra.
Australian Institute of Health and Welfare (AIHW), 2010a. Alcohol and other Drug Treatment Services in Australia 2008–09: Report on the National Minimum Data set. Commonwealth Department of Health and Ageing, Canberra.
Australian Institute of Health and Welfare (AIHW), 2010b. Mental Health Services in Australia 2007–08. Commonwealth Department of Health and Ageing, Canberra.
Australian Institute of Health and Welfare (AIHW), 2013. Mental health services in Australia. Commonwealth Department of Health and Ageing, Canberra.
Behrens, H., 1998. Ageism: real or imagined? Elderly Care 10 (2), 10–13.
Borson, S., Scanlan, J.M., Chen, P., et al., 2003. The Mini-Cog as a screen for dementia: validation in a population-based sample. Journal of the American Geriatrics Society 51, 1451–1454.
Borson, S., Scanlan, J.M., Watanabe, J., et al., 2005. Simplifying detection of cognitive impairment: comparison of the Mini-Cog and Mini-Mental State Examination in a multiethnic sample. Journal of the American Geriatrics Society 53, 871–874.
Brooker, D., 2007. Person-Centered Dementia care: Making Services Better. Jessica Kingsley Publishers, London.
Butler, R., 1975. Why Survive? Being old in America. Harper & Row, New York.
Byers, A.L., Yaffe, K., Covinksy, K.E., et al., 2010. High occurrence of mood and anxiety disorders among older adults: the national comorbidity survey replication. Archives of General Psychiatry 67 (5), 489–496.
Conwell, Y., Thompson, C., 2008. Suicidal behaviour in elders. Psychiatric Clinics of North America 31, 333–356.
Department of Health, 2012. Preventing suicide in England: A cross-government outcomes strategy to save lives. Available at: https://assets.publishing.service.gov.uk/government/uploads/system/uploads/attachment_data/file/430720/Preventing-Suicide-.pdf. Accessed: 17 October 2018.
Desai, A.K., Seraji, M., Redden, M., Tatini, R., 2010. Schizophrenia in older adults. Current Psychiatry 9, 23–28.
Dossing, M., Nilsson, K.K., Svejstrup, S.R., Sorensen, V.V., Straarup, K.N., Hansen, T.B., 2015. Low self-compassion in patients with bipolar disorder. Comprehensive Psychiatry 60, 53–58.
Dougherty, J.H., Cannon, R., Nicholas, C.R.N., et al., 2010. The computerized self-test (CST): an interactive, internet accessible cognitive screening test for dementia. Journal of Alzheimer's Disease 20, 185–195.
Eymard, A.S., Douglas, D.H., 2012. Ageism among health care providers and interventions to improve their attitudes toward older adults: an integrative review. Journal of Gerontological Nursing 38 (5), 26–35.
Fiske, A., Loeback Wetherall, J., Gatz, M., 2009. Depression in older adults. Annual Review of Clinical Psychology 5, 363–389.
Folstein, M.F., Folstein, S.E., McHugh, P.R., 1975. Mini-Mental State: a practical method for grading the state of patients for the clinician. Journal of Psychiatric Research 12, 189–198.
Foulk, M.A., Ingersoll-Dayton, B., Kavanagh, J., et al., 2014. Mindfulness-based cognitive therapy with older adults: an exploratory study. Journal of Gerontological Social Work 57, 498–520.
Gaugler, J.E., Mittelman, M.S., Hepburn, K et al., 2014. Identifying at-risk dementia caregivers following institutionalization. Journal of Applied Gerontology 33 (5), 624–646.
Haddock, G., Eisner, E., Boone, C., et al., 2014. An investigation of the implementation of NICE-recommended CBT interventions for people with schizophrenia. Journal of Mental Health 23 (4), 162–165.
Hall, M., 2012. Alcoholism and depression. Home Healthcare Nursing 30 (9), 543–550.
Haralambous, B., Lin, X., Dow, B., et al., 2009. Depression in older age: a scoping study. Final Report. National Ageing Research Institute, Melbourne.
Harwood, D., Hawton, K., Hope, T., et al., 2006. Suicide in older people without psychiatric disorder. International Journal of Geriatric Psychiatry 21 (4), 363–367.
Haugan, G., Innstrand, S.T., Moksnes, U.K., 2013. The effect of nurse–patient interaction on anxiety and depression in cognitively intact nursing home patients. Journal of Clinical Nursing 22, 2192–2205.
Hegeman, J.M., de Waal, M.W., Comijis, H.C., Kok, R.M., van der Mast, R.C., 2015. Depression in later life: a more somatic presentation? Journal of Affective Disorders 170, 196–202.
Henderson, J., Xiao, L., Siegloff, L., et al., 2008. Older people have lived their lives: first year nursing students' attitudes towards older people. Contemporary Nurse 30 (1), 32–45.
Hoptman, M.J., 2015. Impulsivity and aggression in schizophrenia: a neural circuitry perspective with implications for treatment. CNS Spectrums 20, 280–286.
Hsu, M., Moyle, W., Creedy, D., et al., 2009. Use of antidepressants and complementary and alternative medicine among outpatients with depression in Taiwan. Archives of Psychiatric Nursing 23 (1), 75–85.
Inouye, S.K., Kosar, C.M., Tommet, D., et al., 2014. The CAM-S: development and validation of a new scoring system for delirium severity in 2 cohorts. Annals of Internal Medicine 160, 526–533.
Jayasekara, R., Procter, N., Harrison, J., Skelton, K., Hampel, S., Draper, R., Deuter, K., 2015. Cognitive behavioural therapy for older adults with depression: a review. Journal of Mental Health 24, 168–171.
Jeste, N.D., Hays, J.C., Steffens, D.C., 2006. Clinical correlates of anxious depression among elderly patients with depression. Journal of Affective Disorders 90, 37–41.
Karlin, N.J., Emick, J., Mehls, E.E., et al., 2005. Comparison of efficacy and age discrimination between psychology and nursing students. Gerontology and Geriatrics Education 26 (2), 81–96.
Kellett, U., Moyle, W., McAllister, M., King, C., Gallagher, F., 2010. Life stories and biography: a means of connecting family and staff to people with dementia. Journal of Clinical Nursing 19, 1707–1715.
Khachiyants, N., Trinkle, D., Son, S.J., Kim, K.Y., 2011. Sundown syndrome in persons with dementia: an update. Psychiatry Investigation 8, 275–287.
Kitwood, T., 1988. The technical, the personal and the framing of dementia. Social Behaviour 3, 161–180.
Kitwood, T., Bredin, M., 1992. Towards a theory of dementia care: personhood and well-being. Ageing and Society 12, 269–287.
Laborde-Lahoz, P., El-Gabalawy, R., Kinley, J., et al., 2014. Subsyndromal depression among older adults in the USA: prevalence, comorbidity, and risk for new-onset psychiatric disorders in late life. International Journal of Geriatric Psychiatry 30 (7), 677–685.
Lapierre, S., Erlangsen, A., Waern, M., et al., 2011. A systematic review of elderly suicide prevention programs. Crisis: The Journal of Crisis Intervention and Suicide Prevention 32 (2), 88–98.
Lavretsky, H., Meeks, T., 2009. Late-life depression: managing mood in patients with vascular disease. Current Psychiatry 8, 20–38.
McBeth, A., Gumley, A., 2012. Exploring compassion: a meta-analysis of the association between self-compassion and psychopathology. Clinical Psychology Review 32, 545–552.
McCormack, B., McCance, T., 2010. Person-Centred Nursing: Theory, Models and Methods. Blackwell Publishing, Oxford.
Mental Health Taskforce (MHT), 2016. The Five Year Forward View for Mental Health. Available at: https://www.england.nhs.uk/wp-content/uploads/2016/02/Mental-Health-Taskforce-FYFV-final.pdf. Accessed: 17 October 2018.

Milian, M., Leiherr, A.M., Straten, G., et al., 2012. The Mini-Cog versus the Mini-Mental State Examination and the Clock Drawing Test in daily clinical practice: screening and value in a German memory clinical. International Psychogeriatrics 24 (5), 766–774.

Moyle, W., 2003. Nurse–patient relationship: a dichotomy of expectations. International Journal of Mental Health Nursing 12 (2), 103–109.

Moyle, W., 2014. Evidence-based nursing interventions: fostering quality of life. In: Moyle, W., Parker, D., Bramble, M. (Eds.), Care of Older Adults: a Strengths Based Approach. Cambridge University Press, Sydney.

Moyle, W., Cooke, M., Beattie, E., Shum, D.H.K., O'Dwyer, S., Barrett, S., 2013a. Foot massage versus quiet presence on agitation and mood in people with dementia: a randomized controlled trial. International Journal of Nursing Studies 51, 856–864.

Moyle, W., Cooke, M., Beattie, E., Jones, C., Klein, B., Cook, G., Gray, C., 2013b. Exploring the effect of companion robots on emotional expression in older people with dementia: a pilot RCT. Journal of Gerontological Nursing 39, 46–53.

Moyle, W., Evans, K., 2007. Models of mental health care for older adults: a review of the literature. International Journal of Older People Nursing 2, 132–140.

Moyle, W., Hsu, M., Lieff, S., Vernooij-Dassen, M., 2010. Recommendations for staff education and training for older people with mental illness in long-term aged care. International Psychogeriatrics 22 (7), 1097–1106.

Moyle, W., Olorenshaw, R., Wallis, M., Borbasi, S., 2008. Best practice for the management of older people with dementia in the acute care setting: a review of the literature. International Journal of Older People Nursing 3, 121–130.

Muliyala, K.P., Varghese, M., 2010. The complex relationship between depression and dementia. Annals of Indian Academy of Neurology 13, S69–S73.

O'Dwyer, S.T., Moyle, W., Zimmer-Gembeck, M., De Leo, D., 2013. Suicidal ideation in family carers of people with dementia: a pilot study. International Journal of Geriatric Psychiatry 28, 1182–1188.

O'Connor, M., 2014. A qualitative exploration of the experiences of people living alone and receiving community based palliative care. Journal of Palliative Medicine 17, 200–203.

Office for National Statistics (ONS), 2017. Overview of the UK population: July 2017. Available at: https://www.ons.gov.uk/peoplepopulationandcommunity/populationandmigration/populationestimates/articles/overviewoftheukpopulation/july2017. Accessed: 17 October 2018.

Peng, X.D., Huang, C.Q., Chen, L.J., Lu, Z.C., 2009. Cognitive behavioural therapy and reminiscence techniques for the treatment of depression in the elderly: a systematic review. The Journal of International Medicine Research 37, 975–982.

Peplau, H.E., 1991. Interpersonal Relations in Nursing: a Conceptual Framework of Reference for Psychodynamic Nursing. Springer, New York.

Public Health England (PHE), 2018. Dementia: applying all our health. Available at: https://www.gov.uk/government/publications/dementia-applying-all-our-health/dementia-applying-all-our-health. Accessed: 7 January 2019.

Purcell, B., Heisel, M.J., Speice, J., et al., 2012. Family connectedness moderates the association between living alone and suicide ideation in a clinical sample of adults 50 years and older. American Journal of General Psychiatry 20 (8), 717–723.

Rahman, S.Z., Basilakis, J., Rahmadi, A., et al., 2013. Use of serotonergic antidepressants and St John's wort in older Australians: a population-based cohort study. Australasian Psychiatry 21 (3), 262–266.

Robinson, A., Cubit, K., 2005. Student nurses' experiences of the body in aged care. Contemporary Nurse 19 (1/2), 41–51.

Ross, L., Duigan, R., Boyle, M., Williams, B., 2014. Student paramedic attitudes towards the elderly: a cross-sectional study. Australasian Journal of Paramedicine 11 (3).

Rossom, R., Anderson, P., Greer, N., MacDonald, R., Rutks, I., Tacklind, J., 2011. Delirium: Screening, Prevention and Diagnosis. A Systematic Review of the Evidence. Department of Veterans Affairs Health Services, Research & Development Services, Washington, DC.

Saitz, R., 2005. Unhealthy alcohol use. New England Journal of Medicine 352, 596–607.

Sarchiapone, M., Mandelli, L., Iosue, M., et al., 2011. Controlling access to suicide means. International Journal of Environmental Research and Public Health 8 (12), 4550–4562.

Savla, G.N., DelaPena-Murphy, J., Sewell, D.D., et al., 2009. Schizophrenia and other psychotic disorders. In: Reichman, W., Katz, P. (Eds.), Psychiatry in Long-Term Care. Oxford University Press, New York, pp. 149–168.

Searby, A., Maude, P., McGrath, I., 2015. Dual diagnosis in older adults: a review. Issues in Mental Health Nursing 36 (2), 104–111.

Simoni-Wastila, L., Yang, H.K., 2006. Psychoactive drug abuse in older adults. The American Journal of Geriatric Pharmacotherapy 4, 380–394.

Skirbekk, H., Nortvedt, P., 2014. Inadequate treatment for elderly patients: professional norms and tight budgets could cause 'ageism' in hospitals. Health Care Analysis 22, 192–201.

Smith, A., Graham, L., Senthinathan, S., 2007. Mindfulness-based cognitive therapy for recurring depression in older people: a qualitative study. Aging and Mental Health 11, 346–357.

Snowdon, J., 2010. Depression in nursing homes. International Psychogeriatrics 22 (7), 1143–1148.

Stenhouse, R.C., 2011. 'They all said you could come and speak with us': patients' expectations and experiences of help on an acute psychiatric inpatient ward. Journal of Psychiatric and Mental Health Nursing 18 (1), 74–80.

Storey, J., Rowland, J., Basic, D., Conforti, D., Dickson, H., 2004. The Rowland Universal Dementia Assessment Scale (RUDAS): a multicultural cognitive assessment scale. International Psychogeriatrics 16 (1), 13–31.

Thomas, S.J., Shin, M., McInnis, M.G., et al., 2015. Combination therapy with monoamine oxidase inhibitors and other antidepressants or stimulants: strategies for the management of treatment-resistant depression. Pharmacotherapy 35 (4), 433–449.

Topinkova, E., 2008. Aging, disability and frailty. Annuals of Nutrition and Metabolism 52 (Suppl 1), 6–11.

van der Veen, D.C., van Zelst, W.H., Schoevers, R.A., et al., 2015. Comorbid anxiety disorders in late-life depression: results of a cohort study. International Psychogeriatrics 27, 1157–1165.

Vernooij-Dassen, M., Vasse, E., Zuidema, S., Cohen-Mansfield, J., Moyle, W., 2010. Psychosocial interventions for dementia patients in long-term care. International Psychogeriatrics 22 (7), 1121–1128.

Volkert, J., Schulz, M., Wlodarczyk, O., et al., 2013. The prevalence of mental disorders in older people in western countries: a meta-analysis. Ageing Research Reviews 12 (1), 339–353.

Wilkinson, P., 2013. Cognitive behavioural therapy with older people. Maturitas 76 (1), 5–9.

World Health Organization (WHO), 2013. Mental Health and Older Adults. Fact Sheet no. 381. WHO, Geneva.

Yesavage, J.A., Brink, T.L., Rose, T.L., 1983. Development and validation of a geriatric depression rating scale: a preliminary report. Journal of Psychiatric Research 17, 27.

Zhang, X., Norton, J., Carriere, I., et al., 2015. Generalized anxiety in community-dwelling elderly: prevalence and clinical characteristics. Journal of Affective Disorders 172, 24–29.

USEFUL WEBSITES

The following websites will help to extend your knowledge of some of the topics outlined in this chapter.

Age UK, www.ageuk.org.uk

Alzheimer's Society, www.alzheimers.org.uk

American Psychological Association, Depression and Suicide in Older Adults Resource Guide, www.apa.org/pi/aging/resources/guides/depression.aspx

Benevolent Society, Supporting Older People who are Experiencing Mental Illness of Living with a Mental Illness, file:///Users/s468521/Downloads/Olderpeoplementaldistress%20(1).pdf.

Mental Health Foundation, mental health in later life, www.mentalhealth.org.uk/help-information/mental-health-a-z/O/older-people

University of Birmingham, older people's experiences of mental health services, www.birmingham.ac.uk/research/activity/social-policy/ceimh/film-resources/older-peoples-experiences-mental-health-services.aspx

Virtual Medical Centre, delirium, www.myvmc.com/diseases/delirium-2

World Federation for Mental Health, mental health and older people, chrome-extension://oemmndcbldboiebfnladdacbdfmadadm/www.sfnsw.org.au/ArticleDocuments/921/World-Mental-Health-Day-2013-Older-People.pdf.aspx

World Health Organization, mental health and older people, www.who.int/mediacentre/factsheets/fs381/en

Assessment and Screening Tools

Cornell Scale for Depression in Dementia (CSDD), http://geropsychiatriceducation.vch.ca/docs/edu-downloads/depression/cornell_scale_depression.pdf

Geriatric Depression Scale (GDS), https://web.stanford.edu/~yesavage/GDS.html

Mini-Mental State Examination (MMSE), www4.parinc.com/Products/Product.aspx?ProductID=MMSE

Rowland Universal Dementia Assessment Scale (RUDAS), www.health.qld.gov.au/tpch/html/rudas.asp

The Mini-Cog, www.alz.org/documents_custom/minicog.pdf

13

Learning Disabilities

Charles Harmon, Philip B. Petrie and Chris Taua

KEY POINTS

- Definitions and systems of classification exist for learning disabilities.
- Mental health nurses need to liaise effectively with disability support services.
- Dual disability and dual diagnosis should be differentiated.
- People with a learning disability can fail to receive mental health services.
- Nurses are involved with the acute nursing assessment and management of individuals with a dual disability.
- Assessment and communication issues need to be considered.
- Pitfalls in the assessment process need to be negotiated.
- Continuous care for a person with dual disability needs to be facilitated.
- Discharge planning and mental health support plans are significant nursing responsibilities.

KEY TERMS

acute nursing assessment
acute nursing management
carer
challenging behaviour
continuity of care
disability services
dual disability
learning disability
mental health services
mental health support plan
normalisation
person-centred planning
social inclusion
support
support worker

LEARNING OUTCOMES

The material in this chapter will assist you to:

- analyse factors that contribute to difficulties in the diagnosis and management of people with a dual disability (i.e. people with a learning disability who also have a mental illness).
- discuss the definitions and features of learning disability according to the American Psychiatric Association (DSM-5) and the American Association on Intellectual and Developmental Disabilities.
- discuss the terminology used within the field of learning disability and how this has changed.
- discuss the factors that contribute to a thorough mental health nursing assessment for individuals with a dual disability.
- discuss the nursing management appropriate for individuals with a dual disability who have acute care requirements because of mental illness.
- discuss the nursing strategies relevant to ensuring continuity of care for people with a dual disability after their discharge from the care of a mental health service.

INTRODUCTION

This chapter provides information on the nursing care and management of people who have a dual disability, i.e. a diagnosis of a mental illness comorbid with a learning disability, in the context of mental health services. To assist readers who have little first-hand experience with people with a learning disability, a number of case studies are included.

Essentially, quality mental health nursing care for people with a learning disability is the same type of care offered to any other member of the community, with some important differences:

- It might be necessary for the mental health nurse to modify the way they communicate with the person in order to accommodate a level of understanding appropriate to the person's disability.
- A modification of the assessment process may provide the nurse with information vital to the management of the patient.
- The process of forming a therapeutic relationship with the person will be greatly enhanced by promoting a cooperative relationship between the relevant mental health professionals and the people in the person's circle of support (e.g. carers, family, advocates and/or service providers).
- The patient should be supported upon discharge from mental health services via the design and implementation of a mental health support plan (see Fig. 13.1).

THE LANGUAGE OF DISABILITY

To appreciate fully the subject of dual disability, it is necessary to learn some of the language used by disability professionals (see also the list of key terms at the beginning of this chapter). Much of the literature, particularly regarding definition of terms and the prevalence of dual disability, has been written by British or American authors, and so some guidance is provided here on interpreting the varied terminology used and applying this within a UK context.

Terminology

The term 'dual diagnosis' is most often used by mental health professionals in reference to patients who have a diagnosis of mental illness as well as a substance abuse problem. (This form of 'dual diagnosis' is addressed in Chapter 20.) There is, however, another form of 'dual diagnosis' that provides a classification for people with a mental illness who have a comorbid learning disability. To avoid confusion, the term 'dual disability' (rather than 'dual diagnosis') is used in this chapter.

Many terms have been used to describe people who in some way represent a departure from the usual. Labels such as 'feeble-minded' and 'mentally subnormal' have been used in the past to describe people with a learning disability but these terms have, thankfully, been superseded and many are now deemed highly offensive by society. Indeed, terms such as 'idiot', 'imbecile' and 'moron' were once used by the scientific community as measures of impairment but these terms are no longer in everyday professional use because of the way in which their meaning has altered over time. Internationally, the terms 'mental retardation', 'learning disability' and 'intellectual handicap' remain in use, depending on the country or jurisdiction. In the UK, the term 'learning disability' is used, although many people with learning disabilities prefer to use the term 'learning difficulty'. However, within the education services, the term 'learning difficulty' is also used to include people who have 'specific learning difficulties', e.g., dyslexia (British Institute of Learning Disabilities [BILD] 2011). In the United States, 'intellectual disability' is commonly used, which is reflected in much of the literature, therefore the terms 'learning disability' and 'intellectual disability' will be used interchangeably within this chapter.

Systems of Classification

According to the DSM-5 published by the American Psychiatric Association (APA, 2013), individuals should be assessed across a number of domains including testing for intelligence quotient (IQ), with those affected by learning

Name: Ms Sophie Jones
Date of birth: 04/07/97

Date commenced:
Written by: Isabel Greig (Clinical Nurse Consultant)

Rationale and aims

This plan is designed to give Sophie's parents and support service personnel guidance in how best to support her in managing her mental illness, including preventive strategies for minimising the occurrence of acute psychotic symptoms and reactive strategies when her symptoms are acute and difficult for her to self-manage.

Sophie has experienced an acute psychotic episode with an associated functional disability and has a moderate intellectual disability. She lives at home with her parents and works as an electronic components assembler. There is no known family history of mental illness, and Sophie's condition, while it is unclear when it began, only became a problem for her and her family about four months ago. After a period of inpatient assessment and stabilising of her condition she was discharged back into the community with community mental health services continuing to monitor her progress.

This mental health support plan has been developed through consultation with Sophie and the people in her support network and will be reviewed at least three-monthly.

The aim of the mental health support plan is to support Sophie to maintain her lifestyle in the community, including her living arrangements and her employment, through preventive treatments and strategies and through early response and intervention should her psychosis recur.

Signs and symptoms of Sophie's psychosis

When Sophie is in an acute phase of her psychosis she will be exhibiting the following signs:

- Sophie will sit and talk to herself, often looking at one place near her as she speaks (note that her speech will be conversational, as if she is talking to and listening to another person).
- Sophie will refuse to change her clothes, as she believes that her mother has been putting 'bad things' in her clothing.
- She will talk repetitively about her mother and father being 'bad'.
- She will be suspicious of other people, particularly if they are known friends of her parents.
- She will become easily distracted, often not listening to speakers or simply ignoring them, or she will need questions to be repeated several times before she answers them.
- Sophie will isolate herself in her bedroom, coming out only for meals.
- She may become aggressive towards her family or towards herself (striking the side of her head with the palm of her hand).

Triggers: things that contribute to the emergence of Sophie's symptoms

The following situations and events have been identified as having possible influence on triggering an exacerbation of her psychosis.

Fig. 13.1 An example of a mental health support plan.

These are listed to draw your attention to ensuring that they are avoided where possible:

1 **Missed medication and medication non-adherence**—Sophie has been observed spitting her medication out when she thinks no one is looking.
2 **Alcohol consumption**—while she does not seek out alcohol, it has been noticed that even light beer on a special occasion has a negative effect on her mental state.
3 **Lack of sleep**—Sophie has been more withdrawn and guarded when she has not had adequate sleep.
4 **Stress**—extra pressure at work, other people pressuring her, being 'picked on', etc.

Prevention strategies

The following strategies are to be implemented in an effort to prevent further acute episodes of psychosis in Sophie:

1 **Supervise her taking medication**—make sure she has a drink with her medication and that she takes it before a meal. Keep an eye open for discarded medication and report any incidents of medication non-adherence to her community mental health nurse.
2 The community mental health nurse is to **monitor Sophie's progress** by meeting with her weekly and responding to calls from the family or employer as required.
3 Sophie is to be seen by her psychiatrist **once every three (3) months** for a medication review. The community mental health nurse will make and attend each appointment.
4 Sophie's parents and workplace supervisors are to **report immediately any of the above signs or symptoms** of Sophie's psychosis to the community mental health nurse on the appropriate form, which can be completed and forwarded as required.

Responding to a crisis

Sophie may require more assessment and support with her psychosis than can be offered by those in her community support network. The following procedures are to be followed if the signs and symptoms of Sophie's psychosis (or any other behaviours of concern) are observed:

1 **Give her one dose of her prn medication**—Sophie has prn medication in a dosette box which she has at home and takes to work with her. She may go to sleep within 20 minutes, although when she is very ill the medication may appear to have little effect.
2 **Contact the community mental health nurse** (during business hours) **or the community mental health team** after hours (phone: 5551 9993) and inform them of Sophie's condition.
3 **Follow instructions**—a decision about how to manage the situation will be made after consultation with the psychiatrist.
4 **If she is to be taken to the local hospital for admission**, this will be done by the mental health team or the police. Make sure you pack a bag for her and send any records or notes that may assist the psychiatrist in assessing her condition and reviewing her treatment.

Note: If Sophie is admitted to the local hospital, this plan must be reviewed before discharge.

Signatures of agreement to this plan

Author's signature: ______________		Date: ______________
Name: ______________ **[Sophie Jones']**	Signature: ______________	Date: ______________
Name: ______________ **(Psychiatrist)**	Signature: ______________	Date: ______________
Name: ______________ **(Parent(s) or Guardian)**	Signature: ______________	Date: ______________
Name: ______________ **(Community mental health nurse)**	Signature: ______________	Date: ______________
Plan review date:		

Note: This sample mental health support plan has been designed to demonstrate the presentation of information for this textbook chapter. The information in this sample has been kept to a minimum and is not to be considered a clinical model for the management of any individual client who has a psychotic illness. The authors wish to acknowledge Philip Petrie (Executive Director, Allevia) for the mental health support plan format.

Fig. 13.1, cont'd

BOX 13.1 Intellectual Disability Diagnosis

Intellectual disability involves impairment of general mental abilities that impact adaptive functioning in three domains or areas. These domains determine how well an individual copes with everyday tasks:

- The conceptual domain includes skills in language, reading, writing, math, reasoning, knowledge and memory.
- The social domain refers to empathy, social judgment, interpersonal communication skills, the ability to make and retain friendships and similar capacities.
- The practical domain centres on self-management in areas such as personal care, job responsibilities, money management, recreation and organizing school and work tasks.

While intellectual disability does not have a specific age requirement, an individual's symptoms must begin during the developmental period and are diagnosed based on the severity of deficits in adaptive functioning. The disorder is considered chronic and often co-occurs with other mental conditions such as depression, attention-deficit/hyperactivity disorder and autism spectrum disorder.

(*Source*: Reprinted with permission from the Diagnostic and Statistical Manual of Mental Disorders, 2013. 5th ed. American Psychiatric Association. All Rights Reserved.)

disability having a score of 70 or below (i.e. well below the 'average' score range of 85–114). So-called functional testing must also occur, with those affected by learning disability being assessed as failing to meet developmental standards for their age across three domains (see Box 13.1).

The International Classification of Diseases (ICD-10) (World Health Organization [WHO] 1993) employed the term 'mental retardation' to describe people with a learning disability and used a system of categorisation that emphasised IQ. In the ICD-10 classification, intellectual functioning was divided into four levels of increasing severity from mild (IQ range 50–69) to moderate (IQ range 35–49), severe (IQ range 20–34) and profound (IQ below 20). In the new version of the International Classification of Diseases (ICD-11) (a version of the ICD-11 was released in June 2018, to allow Member States to prepare for implementation, with a view to reporting using ICD-11 from 1st January 2022), the term 'mental retardation' will be replaced by 'disorders of intellectual development' and the type of assessment recommended emphasises adaptive behaviour. The ICD-11 (2018) states that 'disorders of intellectual development are a group of etiologically diverse conditions originating during the developmental period characterized by significantly below average intellectual functioning and adaptive behavior that are approximately two or more standard deviations below the mean (approximately less than the 2.3rd percentile), based on appropriately normed, individually administered standardized tests'. Four levels of increasing severity remain, using the deviations below average intellectual functioning and adaptive behaviour to classify mild (2 or 3 deviations) to moderate (3 or 4 deviations), severe–profound (4+ deviations). Severe and profound classifications are differentiated exclusively on the basis of adaptive behaviour differences because standardized tests of intelligence are unable to distinguish reliably between functioning below the 0.003rd percentile (ICD-11 2018).

In a similar vein, the American Association on Intellectual and Developmental Disabilities (AAIDD) defines learning disability as '. . . a disability characterised by significant limitations both in intellectual functioning and in adaptive behavior as expressed in conceptual, social, and practical adaptive skills . . . [that] . . . originates before age 18' (Shalock et al. 2010, p. 5). This definition is similar to the DSM-5 in that it states that learning disability occurs below a threshold IQ score of around 70 and that there must be an accompanying diminishment of adaptive behaviour. According to Shalock et al. (2010, p. 109) the individual is assessed according to their support requirements and categorised according to 'the intensity of needed supports'. Intensity-of-support categories may be labelled intermittent, limited, extensive or pervasive.

Although there is no such thing as the 'typical' person with a learning disability, the following stories are nevertheless intended to give you a general idea of the characteristics of people who might fit into the intensity-of-support categories.

- Ruth has *intermittent* support needs. She is 20 years old and lives in a suburban apartment in a manner much like the rest of the community. Ruth used to attend a supported employment facility but has recently graduated to open employment in a manufacturing business, having learned the necessary vocational skills at evening class. She lives a fairly independent life with the support of her family but receives one or two visits each month from a worker from a local disability support service, who assists her in planning meals and budgeting. Ruth has limited numeracy skills but she can competently manage money transactions and perform everyday mathematical calculations. She reads slowly and hesitantly but can read an article in her local paper with few difficulties.
- Joshua is 25 years old and has *limited* support needs. He lived at home with his parents until he was 20 years old but now shares a house with two other males. Joshua works in a Social Enterprise aimed at providing employment for people with disabilities but also occasionally works on weekends as a gardener for his uncle's landscape gardening business. Although he makes friends easily and is well known at his local community football club, Joshua has difficulty budgeting and using his money wisely. He also has a history of trouble with the police because he has occasionally become involved in fights following drinking sessions. Consequently, Joshua receives 5 hours of contact per week with a disability support worker who assists him in learning financial management skills and in conducting himself responsibly when socialising.
- Emma is a 40-year-old woman who has *extensive* support needs. She has a hearing impairment and regularly takes medication for her epilepsy. After the death of her parents when she was 12 years old, Emma became institutionalised after living in a large residential facility, where she lived with 30 other individuals in a dormitory-style

unit. At the age of 25 years, she was placed in a home in the community with four other people with similar support needs. The home is staffed by support workers and the residents attend day programmes where they are provided with opportunities to participate in community activities and improve their living skills. Emma has a limited spoken vocabulary but with the assistance of a hearing aid can understand much of what is said to her. She can read important words like her own name, 'hot' and 'danger', but cannot read a newspaper or the captions in a television programme. She can perform many tasks associated with self-care and personal hygiene and assists in the preparation of meals and other domestic chores around the house.
- Petra is a 10-year-old girl who has *pervasive* support needs. Apart from her learning disability, she has cerebral palsy (a disorder that limits her ability to move and to coordinate her limbs) and epilepsy. These disabilities greatly limit her developmental opportunities and her independence. Petra lives at home with her parents and attends a school that caters for her specific needs. She has great difficulty speaking because of her cerebral palsy, but can indicate her wants and needs using sounds and gestures that her parents understand and with the aid of a 'pointer board', which she uses to point to symbols to indicate a range of things from concrete needs (such as food or drink) to emotions (such as happy). Petra also has a computer device that has a keyboard featuring the symbols on her pointer board and the capacity to 'speak' electronically for her. Petra is unable to walk independently but has a 'walker', a complex mechanical device that assists in mobilisation, and a motorised wheelchair. Petra's parents hope that she can one day lead an independent life away from her family home just like any other young adult.

Because a comprehensive description of adaptive behaviour assessment is beyond the scope of this chapter, you may wish to refer to the AAIDD text (Shalock 2010, pp. 45–55) for more information.

CAUSES OF LEARNING DISABILITIES AND ASSOCIATED DISORDERS

Learning disabilities may result from impediments to intellectual development and/or neurological damage caused by factors that include:

- heredity (e.g. genetic causes such as Down syndrome and fragile X syndrome)
- alterations in embryonic development (e.g. fetal alcohol syndrome)
- complications of pregnancy including perinatal problems (such as hypoxia or viral infections)
- environmental and teratogenic causes (including deprivation of learning/developmental opportunities resulting from an unstimulating home environment)
- general medical conditions after birth (including infections and traumas) (Regan & Willatt 2010, p. 20).

The best known are genetic causes such as Down syndrome, which occurs in approximately one in 700 live births. According to Regan and Willatt (2010, p. 20), however, about 30% to 50% of people with a learning disability have no known cause for their condition. This statistic is indicative of the problem of learning disability as an under explored field for researchers, but this situation may well change given the prominence of the human genome project and the wealth of data it has generated.

Learning disabilities may also be accompanied by other types of impacts such as hearing impairments, visual impairments and epilepsy (de Winter et al. 2011). In addition, people with a learning disability often have difficulties making healthy lifestyle choices and are especially prone to developing preventable medical disorders in adulthood (e.g. cardiovascular diseases, nutritional disorders and endocrine disorders), including mental health problems (Henderson et al. 2009; Morin et al. 2012).

SERVICE PHILOSOPHY IN DISABILITY SERVICES

Over the past four decades, the principles of normalisation, first fully articulated by Wolfensberger (1972), have been a driving force behind the creation and design of services for people with a learning disability.

O'Brien's (1987) model provided direction with respect to the normalisation of services. This model emphasises a humanist perspective in which citizens with a learning disability are given the same rights and opportunities as any other citizens, even if they need considerable support. Importantly, proponents of this model advocate the use of generic services (that is, services that any citizen would use, such as public transport, private banking services or general hospitals) rather than specialist disability-based services, in the quest for integration between those who have disabilities and those who do not.

More recently, service provision has been influenced by an extension of the O'Brien philosophy as expressed in the principles of person-centred planning (O'Brien & O'Brien 2006). *Person-centred planning* is a process whereby an individual is provided with the opportunity to take full control of setting lifestyle goals and then negotiating with others on how those goals will be achieved. It is largely based on the principle of shared responsibility, whereby the person enlists support from others (referred to as their 'circle of support') to help them to achieve their lifestyle goals (Stirk & Sanderson 2012). The person-centred model dominates social and health services, albeit in a variety of forms. The international trend to person-centredness has seen this philosophy and practice becoming fundamental to legislation across the UK. People with a disability are increasingly being educated about their rights and are campaigning for control over how they will use social and health services, including controlling personal budgets rather than selecting from government-funded services (Green & Mears 2014).

LEGISLATION AND CHANGES TO SERVICES FOR PEOPLE WITH A LEARNING DISABILITY

In the UK, most people with a learning disability live at home, either with their family or in single or shared accommodation in the general community. A smaller proportion of people with higher support needs live in supported accommodation in shared homes. Historically, there was a practice of placing people with a learning disabilities in large government-funded residential establishments (commonly referred to as 'institutions') but the proportion of individuals living in institutions has gradually diminished since the 1990s in response to pressure on governments to cease a model of support that severely restricts the human rights of people with a disability. The deinstitutionalisation of services has seen the movement of residents into community homes and other services more appropriate for their needs (Young & Ashman 2004).

The government published Building the Right Support (National Health Service [NHS] 2015), which provided commissioners with a framework around how to plan and to develop future community services for people with learning disabilities, including those with mental health conditions. This included developing 48 Transforming Care Partnerships (TCPs) (NHS 2017) to meet the needs of local populations, the ultimate aim being to reduce inpatient beds by up to 50% when the community services are in place. TCPs aim is to ensure that people are able to access care services that enable them to live in the community, close to home and near to their support networks: 'Homes not hospitals'.

The National Institute for Health and Care Excellence (NICE 2016) has produced guidelines (NG54) for the prevention, assessment and management of mental health problems in people with learning disabilities, which takes into account:

- differences in the presentation of mental health issues
- people's communications needs
- people's decision-making capacity
- the degree of a person's learning disability
- the treatment setting (e.g. primary or secondary mental health or learning disability–centred services)
- interventions designed specifically for people with learning disabilities

The aim of the guidance is to improve the assessment and support for mental health conditions experienced by people with learning disabilities, their families and carers (NICE 2016). In addition, further NICE guidance has recently been published around the care and support of people growing older with learning disabilities (NG96, NICE 2018). Because people with learning disabilities now live significantly longer, it suggested that the population of older people with a learning disability will increase four times faster than the overall population of people with learning disabilities (Emerson & Hatton 2008) and it is vital that services are ready to meet this demand. Many people with learning disabilities, especially milder disabilities, are not always in contact with disability services. As assessment improves, higher numbers of people may be identified, with subsequent increases in demand for services, which has not yet been fully quantified (NICE 2018). Many of the guidelines are available in easy read formats for people with learning disabilities and the EasyHealth website offers additional resources on a range of health issues (see Useful Websites).

Alongside mental health, physical health is equally in the spotlight, with health inequalities deemed to be 'unjust and unfair' by Public Health England (PHE) PHE (2018b) because many are avoidable. People with learning disabilities:

- have more health care needs than the general population, with 50% of people with a learning disability having at least one significant health problem
- are more likely to be obese or underweight (less than 10% of people living in supported accommodation eat a balanced diet and are less likely to engage in physical activity)
- are 20 times more likely to have epilepsy than the general population
- have a higher prevalence of psychiatric illness in childhood
- have higher rates of dementia (22%) than the general population (6%)
- are likely to have eating, drinking and swallowing difficulties, with 40% of people with dysphagia experiencing recurrent respiratory tract infections
- are more likely to have a visual impairment, and 40% report having a hearing impairment
- have a shorter life expectancy and increased risk of early death when compared with the general population (risk factors include dependence on others for mobility and feeding, environmental factors such as the family or paid carers not being listened to when concerns were raised about a person's health and factors regarding the provision of care, such as problems in advance health and care planning)

A toolkit has been produced by the Royal College of General Practitioners (RCGP 2018), described as 'health checks for people with learning disabilities toolkit', which offers healthcare workers in GP practices a step-by-step guide to performing annual health checks, seeking to reduce health inequalities. Nurses are also offered guidance from the Royal College of Nursing (RCN) (2014) on the provision of mental health care for adults who have a learning disability (RCN 2014).

Public Health England has produced 'All Our Health' (PHE 2018a), which is a resource aimed at helping healthcare professionals in England to maximise the impact they can have on improving health outcomes and reducing health inequalities. All Our Health guidance offers recommendations as to how this should apply to people with learning disabilities (PHE 2018b). This guidance highlights some of the catalysts for addressing the imbalance that has been seen in past events, such as the 'Death by indifference' report (Mencap 2007), which laid out findings of institutional discrimination within the NHS, raising concerns regarding the disparity between care received by people with a learning disability and nondisabled people.

Further health data can be found on the Learning Disabilities Observatory (PHE 2016), which was previously known as Improving Health and Lives. The Learning Disabilities Observatory is a collaboration between The Centre for Disability Research at Lancaster University and the National Development Team for Inclusion. Data are provided on the health and healthcare of people with learning disabilities and helps commissioners understand future service needs.

The financial assistance offered by governments is far too complex to cover in this chapter, with ongoing changes often made to the systems of assessment. In England and Wales, the Disability Living Allowance (DLA) for people aged between 16 and 64 years has been replaced by Personal Independence Payments (PIP), with eligibility based on a points system. People acquire a certain number of points depending on whether they meet certain descriptors for specified activities (further information can be found at: www.gov.uk/pip).

PREVALENCE OF DUAL DISABILITY

According to the DSM-5 (APA 2013, p. 38) 'intellectual disability has an overall population prevalence of 1% and prevalence rates vary by age. Prevalence for severe intellectual disability is approximately 6 per 1000.' Prevalence studies have consistently indicated higher rates of mental illness among people with a learning disability compared with the general population (Buckles et al. 2013; Cooper et al. 2007; Hatton & Taylor 2008; Taylor et al. 2004). Some authors have theorised that people with a learning disability have a higher probability of developing a mental illness than the general population because of limitations affecting communication abilities, processing skills, cognitive functioning and social skills, which cause them to be more vulnerable to stress (Deb et al. 2001; Longo & Scior 2004; Reiss 1994; Sovner 1996; Taylor et al. 2004). Gilbert et al. (1998) and Emerson et al. (2012) contend that learning disability may be accompanied by other types of impairment that have been associated with mental health problems in the general population, such as hearing impairments, visual impairments and epilepsy. Others have noted that socioeconomic factors, such as unemployment, poverty and restricted social roles may also contribute to higher rates of mental disorders in this group (Deb et al. 2001a; Hardy & Bouras 2002; Lougheed & Farrell 2013; Ouellette-Kuntz et al. 2005).

A study of people with a learning disability living in community settings in Wales (Deb et al. 2001a) found that some 4.4% of the sample (n= 90) met ICD-10 criteria for schizophrenia, 2.2% for depressive disorder, 2.2% for generalised anxiety disorder, 4.4% for phobic disorder and 1% for delusional disorder. According to Deb and coworkers (2001b, p. 495):

> *The overall rate of functional psychiatric illness (point prevalence) was similar to that found in the general community (16%). However, rates of schizophrenic illness and phobic disorder were significantly higher in the study cohort compared with those in the general population (0.4% and 1.1%, respectively).*

FALLING THROUGH THE CRACKS

CASE STUDY 13.1

Roy

Roy had his first admission to a psychiatric hospital at the age of 15 years and by the age of 20 years he was a permanent inpatient with a diagnosis of a learning disability and bipolar disorder. After considerable trial and error, his mental illness was successfully treated with the assistance of the mood stabiliser lithium carbonate and the 'typical' antipsychotic medication, thioridazine (Mellaril). By the age of 20 years, Roy was living in Cedar Lodge, a large private hostel run by a charitable organisation, where he was seen initially by a community mental health nurse and a GP.

At the age of 50 years, Roy moved from the hostel to a group-supported living home run by a different charitable organisation. He appeared to settle in well and was regarded as a bit of a joker, always attempting to cuddle the female staff. However, very little documentation accompanied him to the new service and there was a minimum of information regarding the history and management of his mental illness. Without records, there was nothing to indicate when he had commenced antipsychotic medication or why the treatment was started. The staff presumed that his medication had been initiated to manage challenging behaviours that were no longer in evidence. There were also concerns that Roy's shuffling gait and sleep difficulties were medication related. As thioridazine was about to be withdrawn worldwide in 2005, because of links with severe cardiac arrhythmias, it would no longer be available and combined with a belief that Roy no longer required medication to manage his behaviour, the new GP ceased the thioridazine with no replacement medication.

Roy's sleep pattern deteriorated rapidly, his speech and movements became accelerated, he became more insistent on cuddling both male and female staff and these physical contacts became more overtly sexual. Preexisting behaviour management techniques (such as identifying and avoiding triggers for Roy's behaviour, ignoring Roy's inappropriate behaviour, redirecting him to more appropriate tasks and asking him to spend time in the garden when he was otherwise unmanageable) became ineffective and Roy began to initiate low-level physical assaults upon staff. Additional staff were needed to support Roy at night and the overall support structure started to fracture. After 6 weeks, nurses from the local community mental health team arranged for Roy's admission to a psychiatric inpatient unit where he spent 8 weeks being stabilised on a regimen of lithium carbonate and the 'atypical' antipsychotic medication, quetiapine. Nursing management consisted of the standard practices for a person with bipolar disorder.

Following this bout of acute illness, Roy was able to return to the group home, where he managed to achieve a reasonable lifestyle, albeit after a very long turbulent period of gradual progress over the next 2 years.

CASE STUDY 13.2

Jared

Jared is a 20-year-old man who has limited support needs. He uses little verbal language but understands much of what is said to him and augments his limited speech with gestures and hand signs similar to those used by some people with severe hearing impairments. He can perform most self-care activities but is unable to read and write, except for a few words including his own name.

Jared was 17 years old when his mother died and this event marked the occurrence of challenging behaviours including sudden displays of aggression directed towards others as well as himself. Because his father could not cope with these behaviours, Jared was subsequently moved from his family home to a respite house for people with learning disabilities. Jared displayed a range of problem behaviours including high-level verbal and physical assaults, theft from staff and other residents, not telling the truth, monopolisation of staff time and self-abusive behaviours such as pulling his own hair out and picking the scabs off cuts and abrasions. The house manager sought a full physical examination because blood had been noted in the toilet bowl after Jared had used it. Jared became angry and abusive when he was asked about it, but investigations found no physiological cause for the blood in the toilet.

In his assessment, the psychologist identified a grief reaction to the loss of Jared's mother and 'a need for attention' as the primary cause of his difficult behaviours. A range of behaviour support strategies were subsequently designed and implemented by nurses, including educative programmes designed to provide him with more independence in leisure skills, and outings and other activities that Jared enjoyed. Enjoyable activities were approved on the proviso that he had not taken property that was not his or displayed aggression towards others and Jared was distracted and redirected to other activities if he engaged in inappropriate behaviours (see Chapter 24 for behaviour therapy and other therapeutic nursing interventions).

Nevertheless, over the next 6 months, the behavioural programmes appeared to be having little impact and Jared's behaviour continued to deteriorate. At the request of the house staff, Jared was seen by the mental health team but was uncommunicative and, although staff provided written and verbal information to the assessing psychiatrist describing Jared's behaviours and their possible motivation, it was determined that Jared did not have a mental illness.

Jared's behaviours continued to be highly problematic and 10 months after his placement at the respite house, he was taken by ambulance to the local hospital for the emergency surgical removal of a length of fencing wire that was lodged in his urethra. The surgeon noted that there was evidence of repeated trauma to the urethra and the neck of the bladder and that it was probable that these were self-inflicted injuries that had been sustained over a number of months (see Chapter 7 for self-harm, grief and bereavement). Concerns about the extent and apparent duration of the self-injurious behaviours resulted in a request by the surgeon for an assessment of Jared by the local hospital mental health liaison nurse. Further assessment by a psychiatrist resulted in Jared receiving a provisional diagnosis of major depression. Community mental health staff were subsequently engaged to assist disability staff with his ongoing management.

McIntyre et al. (2002) reported on the negative impact of mental illness upon individuals with a learning disability and their families. Because of a range of complexities, however, many people with an intellectual disability who also have a mental illness remain undiagnosed or do not have equitable access to mental health services (Lunsky et al. 2008; Werges 2007). Equally, however, health professionals lack skills in dealing with this population (Chaplin et al. 2009; Taua & Farrow 2009) and so much can go wrong in the care of people with dual disabilities, as the case studies of Roy (Case Study 13.1) and Jared (Case Study 13.2) illustrate.

It is clear that the outcomes in both of these case studies could have been catastrophic, particularly if either Roy or Jared had sustained a permanent injury. In Roy's case, ceasing his antipsychotic medication (thioridazine) had serious consequences that could have been avoided if adequate documentation had accompanied him in his move from one service to the next. Such documentation would have advised the new service of Roy's long-term mental health diagnosis and alerted personnel to the need to consult a specialist psychiatrist rather than generalist medical services when seeking a review of his medication. Similarly, the management of his behaviour immediately after the ceasing of his thioridazine was not informed by standard mental health management practices and, indeed, mental health professionals were not engaged until his behaviour had reached crisis point.

In Jared's case the mental health personnel were consulted at an appropriate time, but he did not receive appropriate management until his depression was severe and he had engaged in potentially serious self-harm activities. What was required in both instances was effective communication between disability and mental health services, accompanied by a thorough mental health assessment of the individuals and the creation of a management plan understood and implemented not only by mental health services but also carers in the individual's home settings (see acute assessment and management on the following pages).

CRITICAL THINKING CHALLENGE 13.1

Refer to Case Study 13.1.

1. How might the mental health nurse obtain an adequate history regarding Roy's mental illness?
2. What information should mental health nurses obtain from Roy's usual disability service carers in order to ensure a thorough assessment of his mental status?
3. How likely is it that Roy had had previous episodes of mental illness during his stay at Cedar Lodge?

CRITICAL THINKING CHALLENGE 13.2

Refer to Case Study 13.2.

1. Analyse possible factors that may have contributed to the delays in treatment for Jared's mental illness.
2. How might the mental health nurse establish communication with Jared, given his limited vocabulary?

ACUTE ASSESSMENT OF PEOPLE WITH A DUAL DIAGNOSIS

While people with learning disabilities experience the same mental health issues as other people in the community, there are sometimes differences in the way symptoms are manifested (Department for Communities and Social Inclusion 2013). Reasons for these differences could include: difficulties understanding or expressing feelings or emotions; difficulty in explaining symptoms; and different presentations or patterns to particular symptoms. For example, a person with a learning disability may cycle more rapidly between the manic and depressive phases of bipolar disorder. It is also possible that symptoms of mental illness may be 'masked' by medications that have been previously prescribed to manage other medical conditions or behavioural issues.

Just like the rest of the community, people with a learning disability can display a range of unusual or disturbed behaviours in response to adversity. However, people with a learning disability often have significant difficulty communicating with others and expressing their emotions verbally. What is often seen as a substitute for conventional communication is a wide range of behaviours, which, while serving a purpose for the individual, may not make sense to an observer. Common behaviours displayed by people with a learning disability include stereotypical or repetitive behaviours such as hand flapping or body rocking, 'acting out' behaviours such as displays of yelling and violent body movements, self-injurious behaviours such as scratching at their skin or old wounds or aggression towards others.

Sovner (1996) proposed that people with a learning disability develop unusual behaviours because they have had limited developmental opportunities and/or inappropriate learning situations when they were young. Equally, however, certain changes in behaviour may result from the pain and discomfort of general medical conditions, emotional upset, frustration, reactions to external stimuli or the distress associated with mental illness. The mental health assessment of patients with a learning disability can thus become something of an art when faced with the task of sorting out the origins of behaviour and its meaning in relation to the patient's mental illness (Ailey 2003; Devine & Taggart 2008; Slevin et al. 2008). As Sovner (1996) also pointed out, the key is working out which behaviours are purposeful (intentional) and which are signs or symptoms of a condition (unintentional) such as a mental illness.

Assessment and Communication Issues

A further difficulty for the mental health nurse is that patients with a learning disability often have limited capacity for conversation because of their primary disability or because of concurrent disabilities such as hearing impairment. In addition, patients with higher support needs may experience problems in generalising (or transferring) communication skills from familiar environments, such as their home, to less familiar environments, such as psychiatric emergency centres. Another common problem is that the patient may become shy or confused and, as a consequence, use regressed or echolalic speech (repeating what has been said), as in this example:

Nurse: How are you today, Robyn? You look a bit sad.

Robyn: A bit sad.

Acquiescence or assent is also a common issue when nursing people with learning disabilities. This is where the patient tends to answer 'Yes' to questions in order to please the interviewer or because they have interpreted questions literally:

Nurse: Do you hear voices, Robyn?

Robyn: Yes, I hear voices all the time *(Is she actually referring to hearing the nurse's voice?)*

Employing the assistance of carers, family members and significant others to help with the communication process is most advisable, particularly if the patient has a significant communication impairment (for example, is semi- or nonverbal) and uses augmentative forms of communication such as sign language (signing), pointer boards (also known as communications or symbol boards) or computer devices.

Further information on augmentative and alternative communication is beyond the scope of this chapter but is available in the literature (for example, Cascella 2005; Loncke 2014). In addition, useful websites can be found at the end of this chapter.

Note that sign languages may vary from one country to the next, just as with spoken languages. British and US hand signs are often quite different. A useful and highly recommended resource in regard to managing communication and making reasonable adjustments with people with intellectual disability is the 'five good communication standards' developed by the Royal College of Speech and Language Therapists. The five good standards are summarised as follows:

- Standard 1: There is a detailed description of how best to communicate with individuals.
- Standard 2: Services demonstrate how they support individuals with communication needs to be involved with decisions about their care and their services.
- Standard 3: Staff value and use competently the best approaches to communication with each individual they support.
- Standard 4: Services create opportunities, relationships and environments that make individuals want to communicate.
- Standard 5: Individuals are supported to understand and to express their needs in relation to their health and wellbeing (Royal College of Speech and Language Therapists 2013, p. 4).

Coombs and Martin (2002) have shown that mental health clinicians typically obtain information during the assessment and review processes either directly from the patient or from their own observations of the individual, rather than using other sources of information such as the patient's family or usual carers. However, in the case of patients with a learning disability, it is necessary to gather information from all possible sources to obtain a full clinical picture, especially if the patient has significant communications deficits and cannot participate in an assessment process that relies on their ability to respond verbally to questions (Spiller & Hardy 2004; Mansell & Beadle-Brown 2012). It could be argued that nurses working in a complex area such as this need to be highly knowledgeable and skilful (Pridding et al. 2007; Slevin et al. 2008; Taua et al. 2011).

NURSE'S STORY 13.1 Communicating

Using augmentative forms of communication can be a difficult task for the novice, but basic communication can be achieved quite quickly with the aid of motivation and some basic education. I had the pleasure of supervising a group of nursing students at a clinical placement that was both a residential facility and a school for children and adolescents with cerebral palsy. Very few of the children had speech that could be understood by the nursing students and so we commenced the process of teaching the students to communicate via pointer board, which displays symbols that can be used to indicate meaning. Needless to say, the students were daunted by the task ahead of them, particularly when they entered the classrooms and were confronted by children seated at desks decorated with symbols and enthusiastically gesturing to them to come over and 'have a chat'.

I'd tried to plan for this experience by giving the students some prior reading and a brief demonstration of the use of pointer boards. Essentially, however, the classroom teachers and I had contrived the learning environment so that the children would teach the students how to communicate via this medium. This was very exciting for me as I watched the students struggle with the new information and the pressure exerted on them by their eager 'teachers'. Within about 10 minutes, however, you could see progress being made. One nursing student yelled: 'She went to the movies with her mum, in her mum's car, and saw a movie with a handsome actor—Tom Cruise!' The child smiled proudly. When the nursing student guessed the title of the movie, the young child was absolutely delighted. The two had struck up a rapport and communication flowed much more quickly from this point.

In all instances the approach to obtaining information about a patient should be calm and nonthreatening using concrete, open-ended questions, avoiding jargon, complex technical terms or abstract questions (Devine & Taggart 2008; Hamer 1998). For patients with a learning disability, the mental health nurse will need to use skills in both observation and communication, verbal and nonverbal, in carrying out the assessment. If people in the patient's circle of support are willing to participate in this process, it is helpful to interview them to obtain information about the patient's usual behaviour patterns (O'Hara 2008) (see Chapter 10 for information on working with families). It is also important to ask how the patient's presenting behaviour is a departure from the usual. This information may help to identify the 'typical' signs that indicate mental illness as well as 'atypical' signs, which are behaviours peculiar to the patient following the onset of the mental illness, including stereotypical (or repetitive) behaviours, 'acting out' behaviours and self-abusive behaviours (Ross & Oliver 2002).

Other data pertinent to the assessment process should include information that may assist in developing the patient's history, including information from other service providers such as their GP, medical specialists and behavioural specialists. In particular, a medication history should be established.

One of the first questions asked during the initial assessment should be whether the patient has recently undergone a full medical examination. A deterioration in skills or behaviour or a change in an emotional presentation can be due to an undiagnosed physical complaint or exacerbation of an existing one. Several authors have asserted that physical illness in this group of people is often not detected and that many conditions are diagnosed too late, making treatment less effective (Bouras 2008; Deb et al. 2001; Robertson et al. 2014).

Enhancing the Assessment Process

Where possible, standard assessment formats such as the mental status examination and self-harm and/or risk assessment should be used in the assessment of all mental health patients (see Chapter 22 for the mental status examination and Chapter 23 for risk assessment and self-harm). However, in considering their usefulness in dual disability nursing it is important to keep in mind that these assessment tools are most applicable to the processes of gathering subjective data in an interview-type setting. Such an assessment can lead to the nurse gaining a diagnostic picture of the person but not necessarily a complete picture of the issues behind any behaviour that may be occurring. Nurses often state that they are constantly observing patients and recording their observations (Delaney 2006). While this might be true, Delaney stresses that 'watching and learning . . . demands that staff *pattern* and *organise* [author's italics] what they see' (2006, p. 170). Although Delaney was talking about nurses working with children in a psychiatric setting, similar issues are evident when considering the needs of people with a learning disability from a developmental perspective. Therefore, there are times when conventional assessment formats are inadequate for nursing people with a learning disability because of the numerous complex issues that they may present with.

Another common concern in the assessment process is 'diagnostic overshadowing'. This term refers to a phenomenon where the symptoms normally indicative of mental illness are erroneously attributed to a person's learning disability, with the consequence that the person's mental illness may be ignored (Devine & Taggart 2008; Johnstone et al. 2010; Reiss et al. 1982). It is vital that the assessment process is conducted professionally and that nurses and other healthcare professionals have an understanding of issues relevant to the person with a dual disability (Taua & Farrow 2009). Higgins (2004, p. 1346) discussed the need for assessments that are 'multimodal'. This ensures effective implementation and evaluation of a comprehensive plan of care, effective care management skills and ongoing review and modification. Dosen (2007) further explored a multidimensional approach that incorporates not only the biopsychosocial aspects of care but also a consideration of an individual's developmental needs. This aspect is critical in dual disability nursing given the impact of the learning disability on an individual's development. Consider the case of Jared (Case Study 13.2) and the impact of his mother's death when he was 17 years old. Nurse's Story 13.2 about Stephen also demonstrates the importance of developmental considerations.

NURSE'S STORY 13.2

Stephen

Understanding the person's experience from a developmental perspective

Stephen, aged 39 years, was first admitted to the psychiatric hospital when he was 17 years old, with a diagnosis of bipolar disorder—manic phase. He had been putting his arm around young women at his work and touching their breasts. Stephen was assessed as having a mild learning disability and therefore was admitted to a dual disability facility for compulsory treatment. Over the years, his mental state fluctuated and when his mood was elevated he would stand very close to people, becoming rather demanding and irritable when told to move back. Young female nurses and nursing students were constantly warned that Stephen was potentially 'dangerous' and told not to get too close to him. A common term used to describe his behaviour was 'predatory' and because of this he had very little physical human contact, did not get to visit the local swimming pool or go on many community outings unless there was a male staff member present.

My work with Stephen and the team involved a full case review of his history of care during his time in hospital. What came to light was that although Stephen was constantly told his behaviour was inappropriate there did not appear to have been any behaviour modification work with him to help him to understand what 'being inappropriate' meant.

The focus of his treatment from that point on was exploring Stephen's interpretation of his world, understanding it from a developmental perspective in that Stephen had not really advanced past 'adolescent type' behaviour (which is the stage he was at on admission) in always admiring young women and wanting to get close to them. When his mood elevated he was unable to place any restrictions on this behaviour. My work with him was to teach about personal space and about what is acceptable and unacceptable social behaviour (i.e. shaking hands, not hugging or touching others unless they gave him permission to). Although this took a long time, Stephen eventually came to understand the concept of personal boundaries and became very proud of himself, enjoying the positive responses he got from people (rather than the distancing and ignoring he used to get). Stephen now lives in supported residential accommodation and catches a bus to work every day. I often see him in the shopping mall buying CDs on his payday. He always shakes my hand.

There are several tools available to assist with the assessment of patients with learning disabilities when the standard tools are considered ineffective. Four such instruments are described as follows:

- The Psychiatric Assessment Schedule for Adults with Developmental Disabilities (PAS-ADD) is a diagnostic tool suitable for the mental health nurse or other mental health professional adept at clinical interviewing (Moss et al. 1993).
- The Mini Psychiatric Assessment Schedule for Adults with Developmental Disabilities (Mini PAS-ADD) is a relatively more accessible tool for most nursing staff, although specific training is required for its effective use. Essentially, the Mini PAS-ADD consists of a life events checklist as well as a four-point scale on which clinicians may 'rate' the patient's symptoms of depression, anxiety, expansive mood, obsessive compulsive disorder, psychosis and autism (Prosser et al. 1998).
- In addition to the aforementioned, Hamer (1998) recommends the use of the JOMAAC assessment tool (see Box 13.2), in which the adult patient is assessed according to observations of their Judgement, Orientation, Memory, Affect, Attitude and Cognition. The main advantage of this form of ongoing assessment is that the nurse can draw some conclusions about the patient's current mental status based on direct observation, with minimal reliance on the patient providing dialogue.
- For the assessment of children and adolescents with a learning disability, the Developmental Behaviour Checklist (DBC) (Einfeld & Tonge 1995) is a comprehensive 96-item carer-completed screening checklist that allows carers (including nurses) to rate the severity of a child's behavioural and emotional problems. This checklist has been modified to produce a version known as the Developmental Behaviour Checklist for Adults (DBC-A) (Mohr et al. 2005). Both versions of the DBC facilitate a cut-off score that indicates the level of disturbance, which may be further investigated by an expert mental health clinician.

ACUTE NURSING MANAGEMENT

Nursing people with a dual disability is complex. Nurses may be required to respond effectively to multiple medical conditions and various cognitive and developmental complexities that may be evident, as well as negotiating the individual's particular communication style. The key to nursing patients who have a mental illness comorbid with a learning disability lies in establishing effective communication with them and their supporters, combined with a thorough assessment and an ability to adapt familiar assessment and management techniques (Wallace & Beange 2008).

There is ample evidence that patients with a dual disability can benefit from a range of physical interventions, such as pharmacological treatments (Eady et al. 2013; Davis et al. 2008; Dosen 2007) and electroconvulsive therapy (Ligas et al. 2009; MacKay & Wilson 2007), in much the same way as other members of the community who experience mental illness (see Chapter 24 for a range of therapeutic interventions).

BOX 13.2 JOMAAC Assessment at a Glance

Judgement
- Perception of events or stimuli
- Appropriateness of appearance, such as grooming, touching and language
- Interpretation of vulnerable situations (observations such as hitting a bigger, stronger patient)
- Aggression towards self
- Aggression towards others
- Aggression towards property
- Suicidal gestures
- Responses to recent significant life events
- No behavioural improvement despite consistent, high-quality behavioural programming

Orientation
- Awareness of surroundings
- Awareness of internal stimuli
- Awareness of name, location and reason for hospitalisation
- Impaired level of consciousness

Memory
- Recent memory tests (What did you have for breakfast? What activity did you just do?)
- Ability to repeat what was said
- Remote memory tests (the name of community caregiver)

Affect
- Acting-out behaviour
- Emotional status (laughing, crying, flat, constricted)
- Verbalisation of fear
- Withdrawal behaviour
- Reluctance to perform a learned skill
- Reluctance to be with familiar people
- Multiple complaints, somatisation
- Reluctance to be in familiar surroundings
- Response to known upcoming event
- Response to current or near-current event
- Temper tantrum
- Change in activity level
- Facial expression, tone
- Aggression
- Hand or body gestures
- Appropriateness of emotional state
- Range of emotional state
- Sleep disturbance
- Changes in eating patterns
- Decreased concentration
- Loss of interest
- Statements regarding self-worth, suicide, hurting self or others
- Changes in person's behaviour or mood that occur in all settings, versus just some settings
- Hypersexuality

Attitude
- Uncooperative
- Sarcastic
- Perplexed
- Hostile
- Apprehensive
- Unfeeling

Cognition
- Ability to keep thoughts focussed
- Speech patterns (echolalic, mutism, intonation, pressure, rate, deterioration)
- Displays beliefs that are obviously false
- Gestured hallucinations
- Voiced hallucinations
- Poor interpersonal relationships
- Decreased ability to perform activities of daily living (feeding, dressing, toileting)
- Poor eye contact
- Bizarre rituals
- Emotional dissociation (including mood variability and impulsiveness)
- Catatonia
- Paranoid behaviour

Judgement, Orientation, Memory, Affect, Attitude, Cognition (JOMAAC) Assessment (*Source*: Hamer, B.A., 1988. Assessing mental status in persons with mental retardation. Journal of Psychosocial Nursing and Mental Health Services 36(5), 27–31)

Collins (1999) pointed out that psychotherapy for patients with a dual disability was often not used, based on the belief that the person's intellectual capacity and limited communications repertoire rendered them ineligible. There is now evidence that a range of 'talk therapies' such as behavioural and cognitive therapies are effective for those with functional language skills, albeit in an abridged form (Brown & Marshall 2006; Lindsay et al. 2015; Vereenooghe & Langdon, 2013). Similarly, Mason (2007) has commented on the reported efficacy of various relaxation techniques used to manage anxiety states for patients with a dual disability, while Yildiran and Holt (2014) have explored the efficacy of mindfulness-based interventions. The nursing interventions described in Chapter 24 can be employed in much the same way as they are for the remainder of the population, with the addition of more comprehensive discharge planning.

The case study of Erika (Case Study 13.3) provides an example of the acute nursing care that would be provided for a patient with a dual disability following their admission to an inpatient unit. In recalling our earlier discussion around diagnostic overshadowing, you can see how this played out in Erika's case in that staff did not initially recognise how her behaviour might have been indicative of a mental health issue.

Erika's Subsequent Nursing Care

In Erika's case, nursing and medical staff found that she was uncommunicative upon admission to the mental health unit and that she sat gently rocking and averting her gaze from staff. Fortunately, the staff were able to engage Erika's mother Jean in the process of taking a history and for some of the assessment process. After medical staff had performed a physical examination of Erika, it was decided to take her to

CASE STUDY 13.3

Erika

Erika is a 35-year-old woman who normally lives with her mother and has limited support needs. Erika has a small vocabulary but is able to understand much of what is said to her. She can perform self-help tasks and has developed competencies in occupational, leisure and social skills. Diagnostic overshadowing played a large part in the delay between the onset of severe symptoms and a diagnosis for Erika.

The police brought Erika into the emergency department late one Sunday after local residents reported that she had been lying on the road outside a shopping centre. Erika was very distressed and crying and when asked why she lay on the road replied: 'You will get run over lying on the road and go to heaven, sorry Mr Policeman.' She was able to give her name, phone number and address to the attending mental health nurse and a subsequent phone call found that Erika lived at home with her mother and had gone to the local shops for bread. The mental health nurse and the duty psychiatrist decided that Erika could go home to the care of her mother as there was no history of mental illness and she was able to say where she lived. Lying on the road was dismissed as 'behaviour' due to her intellectual learning disability. This proved to be diagnostic overshadowing.

Two days later, Erika's mother Jean telephoned the mental health service staff to say that a local shopkeeper had brought Erika home after he had found her lying on the road. Jean was told that someone from the mental health team would visit in the next couple of days, but this was not regarded as high priority because the behaviour was seen as part of Erika's intellectual learning disability. The following afternoon, community mental health nurses visited and questioned Erika, who became tearful and repeated: 'I'll get run over and go to heaven.' Jean told the staff that she had heard Erika crying at night and that she had been awake early in the morning and needed to be told to shower. This was unlike Erika, but Jean said that she had been sad since her grandmother died 3 months ago and seemed to lack motivation.

On their way back to the community mental health centre the nurses called in to the local shops and discovered that Erika had been lying on the road intermittently for the past 4 weeks. At first she would get up as soon as someone called out to her but over the past 2 weeks she would cry: 'No, I'll get run over and go to heaven.' The staff, recognising her behaviour as suicidal, arranged for Erika to be admitted to the mental health unit as an involuntary patient (i.e. she was deprived of her right to discharge herself from hospital on the grounds that there was a reasonable risk that she would harm herself). Erika's subsequent nursing care is described later.

her bedroom and to continue the assessment process once she had familiarised herself with her new environment. In the interim, a nurse was able to commence brief conversations with Erika using gentle open-ended questions. Erika was subsequently asked to unpack her suitcase and engage in self-care activities independently.

Erika lived at home and in such cases it is important to work with the family to gain their trust, to ensure the optimal outcome for the patient and to obtain a reliable history of the patient's mental and physical status. Over the course of the next hour, the nurse was able to ascertain from Jean that Erika was uncharacteristically withdrawn and that her movements were much slower than usual. Jean also revealed that Erika's concentration had deteriorated in recent weeks and Erika was able to add that she felt terrible and that she didn't 'want to live anymore'. Apart from these typical signs of clinical depression (see the diagnostic criteria in Chapter 16), staff noted that Erika's rocking had continued and that she made low, barely audible noises. Jean confirmed that rocking and moaning were atypical signs of Erika's depression as they were not normally part of her behavioural repertoire.

Having gained her confidence, the nurse was able to interview Erika alone and, after some encouragement, found that she had retained her plan to kill herself by lying down in the middle of a road and being run over by a car. She did not have any other plans for her own death but repeated that what she really wanted was to die and go to heaven to see her grandmother. Eventually the nurse was able to complete the initial assessments for Erika, including (but not limited to) a physical assessment, mental status assessment, risk assessment, assessment of strengths and assessment of Erika's risk of vulnerability to exploitation and abuse (see information on assessment in Chapter 22), and was able to write admission notes that described her signs and symptoms including the atypical signs of depression.

Erika was subsequently placed on half-hourly general observations with fourth-hourly observations using the JOMAAC tool as a format for further assessment of her mental status. Although primary nursing was not a part of the unit's policy on patient care, Erika was allocated a single nurse for each subsequent morning and afternoon 'shift' on the first 2 days of her admission in order to facilitate communications and to assist in the process of ongoing assessment. Despite these arrangements, Erika remained largely uncommunicative and chose to speak only with a few of the staff.

Apart from the interventions outlined previously, the management of Erika's depression was much like that afforded to other patients (see Chapter 16). While she was being stabilised on an antidepressant (in this case, venlafaxine), Erika was offered grief counselling (see Chapter 7 and 24) to help her to cope with the loss of her grandmother. Although Erika was quick to understand that she needed to take her medication with her morning and evening meals until her doctor said to stop, she was unable to grasp education given to her by staff about the physiology of her depressive illness and the need to be vigilant regarding the symptoms of relapse. She also had a very limited understanding of the way in which her medication was helping her.

At the suggestion of Erika's mother, and with Erika's permission, it was decided to devise a mental health support plan (similar to that in Fig. 13.1) in order to disseminate information about Erika's management strategies to the people in her circle of support when she had been discharged. The plan featured possible relapse signs (such as social withdrawal and 'rocking') and management strategies should Erika again decide to harm herself (such as removing Erika from harmful circumstances, clarifying Erika's intentions and contacting the community mental health team if Jean required assistance).

CRITICAL THINKING CHALLENGE 13.3

Refer to Case Study 13.3. List the ethical considerations that should be taken into account when nursing Erika in an acute-care setting. Discuss how each of these problems might be addressed.

LONG-TERM CARE

The achievement of lasting positive outcomes for patients with a dual disability and the avoidance of unnecessary hospitalisations due to acute relapse of illness is highly dependent on the discharge planning process. The following discussion about the long-term ongoing care of patients with a dual disability recognises that these patients typically access a range of services for their ongoing or continuous care and support (Alexander et al. 2011; Yohanna 2013). It is also important to recognise that those individuals living with their family or in their own home typically have contact with some form (or many different types) of support service and that those patients who live in supported accommodation services frequently maintain a high level of contact with and support from their family members. In addition, the role of the family, apart from providing typical family relationships, is often to fulfil the role of substitute decision maker or advocate.

NICE (2017) has produced quality standards (QS142) to ensure appropriate long-term care when identifying and managing mental health problems for people with learning disabilities. The quality statements are:

- Statement 1: Young people and adults with learning disabilities have an annual health check that includes a review of mental health problems.
- Statement 2: People with learning disabilities who need a mental health assessment are referred to a professional with expertise in mental health problems in people with learning disabilities.
- Statement 3: People with learning disabilities and a serious mental illness have a key worker to coordinate their care.
- Statement 4: People with learning and mental health problems who are receiving psychological interventions have them tailored to their preferences, level of understanding and strengths and needs.
- Statement 5: People with learning disabilities who are taking antipsychotic drugs that are not reduced or stopped have annual documentation on reasons for continuing this prescription.

UNDERSTANDING DISABILITY SUPPORT SERVICES

Although it is difficult to outline all of the salient features of disability support services, one common component of these services that is vital to this discussion is the process of person-centred planning. Person-centred plans, also known by a variety of other names such as lifestyle plans (O'Brien & O'Brien 2006), are considered the core documents that guide disability service providers in planning for and delivering a service that endeavours to meet the individual needs and aspirations of each person using the service. The plan is usually developed on initial entry to the service and is monitored regularly and reviewed at least annually.

In the UK, governments have moved to promote individual planning using a person-centred model. Person-centred planning focusses on what is important to the individual and is a process for continual readjustment according to the person's changing circumstances as well as their circle of support (e.g. family and friends) (Stirk & Sanderson 2012). According to Kormann and Petronko (2003, p. 434), 'person-centred practice is accepted as good practice in many countries throughout the world. It is most often used for life planning with people with a learning disability, though recently it has been advocated as a method of planning personalised support with many other sections of society who find themselves disempowered by traditional methods of service delivery, including children, people with physical disabilities, people with mental health issues and older people'. The development of the plan typically involves using a range of tools that empower the individual to recognise what is important to them and then negotiate with others to find ways to meet their needs and achieve their personal goals. In essence, the process is about personal control over choosing a lifestyle that is wanted, not what others believe is in their best interest.

Person-centred plans are based on the needs and aspirations of the individual and are a key tool in guiding the individual's circle of support in assisting them to attain a preferred lifestyle and living environment, focussed on social inclusion through inclusive means. The plans can include an array of subcomponents that encompass aspects of lifestyle support including behavioural support, health and wellbeing, accommodation and therapy, depending on what the person wants and needs (Stirk & Sanderson 2012).

Another feature of many disability support services that should be discussed is the professional background of the people they employ. There is often a misconception among mental health professionals that all disability support services, particularly those providing primary support through accommodation and case management services, are equipped to manage people with a mental illness. This is often far from reality. Many disability support organisations do not specifically employ staff with mental health nursing backgrounds but traditionally draw their staff from the fields of social welfare, disability nursing, aged care nursing or any number of unrelated and various employment backgrounds (Devine & Taggart 2008). Where a person requires a specialist service for addressing their specific needs (e.g. health needs), the role of disability service personnel is to assist the person to access appropriate generic community services (that is, the services used by any member of the community).

When a person with a dual disability is discharged back into the care of a disability accommodation support service, the mental health nurse needs to have a clear understanding of the service, its service features, the skills of the staff and the function it is funded to provide within the disability support network. This understanding should minimise confusion or misunderstandings in the implementation of management programmes and ensure that the person does not get caught in any voids created by interagency disputes over roles and responsibilities. Of course this level of understanding must be afforded to the family and carers of the person living at home because they may or may not have the skills, knowledge and experience required to effectively support the individual through the treatment process (Pridding et al. 2007; Spiller & Hardy 2004).

Discharge Planning

The purpose of discharge planning is, ideally, for the person to return to their prior environment or other suitable community-based setting. Effective discharge planning should commence at the time of the person's initial presentation to the mental health service and should include elements such as a schedule for outpatient follow up and the provision of any other additional services as required (Shepperd et al. 2010).

In facilitating the discharge planning process, the mental health nurse should first identify the people in the patient's support network and establish effective communication with them. Longo and Scior (2004) highlight the importance of primary carer involvement in the admission, treatment and discharge processes as they provide a key to achieving better health outcomes for the patient postdischarge. Involving key people from the patient's circle of support ensures that the discharge plan becomes an integral part of their support arrangements, including clarifying the goals of the patient and the roles and responsibilities of each support person in realising those goals. The plan should be documented (including monitoring and review phases) in a functional format that each person, including the patient, can follow and implement.

Shepperd et al. (2010) recommended that, before discharge, a case conference be held between all members of the patient's support network to ensure that the relevant responsibilities and processes of support are articulated, negotiated, agreed to, understood and documented, including steps to be taken that may avoid future inpatient stays, further tests or assessments and any appropriate additional referrals for further support and criteria for and processes of responding to critical incidents.

Heller and Schindler (2011) suggest that the ability of patients, family members, carers and others to respond quickly and early to an episode of acute illness is diminished if they have little insight into or knowledge about mental illness and how it affects the patient. Family members, carers and disability support workers who are educated in the issues of dual disability or who are supported in identifying and accessing information resources are more likely to provide effective support to the patient and work more effectively with (other) service professionals. With this in mind, the mental health nurse should consider including in the patient's treatment plan relevant psychoeducational strategies such as noting poor sleep patterns or agitation, which may indicate that the person is going to become acutely ill, or the effects, side effects and protocols for the administration of neuroleptic medications. Including these strategies in treatment and discharge plans has been demonstrated to have positive results in treatment compliance and the overall wellbeing of the patient (Douds et al. 2013).

The Mental Health Support Plan

Many disability support services, as part of the person-centred planning process, use a broad array of specific healthcare plans to ensure that the medical and health needs of the patient are planned, implemented and monitored by appropriate health professionals. Examples include meal-time support plans, epilepsy management plans and diabetes management plans. Specific to the discussion here is the emergence of the mental health support plan (MHSP), also known as the mental health plan or mental healthcare plan. An example of an MHSP that relates to the case study of Sophie (Case Study 13.4) is shown in Fig. 13.1. Often developed by nurses and others with specific mental health training and experience who work within the disability service network, the MHSP is increasingly being implemented by disability services and welcomed by families.

CASE STUDY 13.4

Sophie

Sophie is a 19-year-old woman with a learning disability and extensive support needs who normally lives at home with her family. She was admitted as an involuntary patient to a mental health acute ward after she was provisionally diagnosed with a first-episode psychotic illness.

Mental health personnel had obtained a history of Sophie's recent mental status changes from Sophie's parents and initially communicated with her with the assistance of her brother, whom she trusted. During her initial assessment, Sophie explained that she was afraid of her parents and that she believed them to be evil. She indicated that she had 'voices' in her head but was unable to communicate what these voices were telling her. Her parents added that, in the months before her admission, Sophie had been reluctant to shower, spent a lot of time in her room and could be heard talking to herself. When asked if anything was wrong, she became evasive, stating that she was just singing to herself. Sophie became more withdrawn and disorganised in her behaviour, eventually becoming aggressive when approached by her parents. Her personal hygiene deteriorated, she refused to change her clothes and remained in her room, coming out only for meals. Staff noted that, apart from her aggression, Sophie displayed 'atypical' signs such as making strange noises and hitting the side of her head when she became stressed.

In the weeks after her admission, staff used the JOMAAC tool to assess Sophie's progress until some of the nursing staff managed to build up a rapport with her. She continued to take her prescribed antipsychotic medication (risperidone) and otherwise received the nursing care afforded to a person with a psychotic illness (see Chapter 15). As Sophie's condition stabilised in the protective environment of the admission unit, mental health staff commenced discharge planning including the preparation of an MHSP. An example of an MHSP designed for Sophie is provided in Fig. 13.1.

The MHSP provides staff, carers, families and individuals with clearly documented guidelines that can be used for a number of purposes, including:

- providing a forum for the inclusion of significant others in the development, implementation and review of the patient's treatment
- ensuring that prescribed treatments are provided as directed by the psychiatrist and/or other related health professionals
- providing clear documentation of strategies, routines and programmes
- ensuring that early intervention strategies are identified (including understanding the early signs of acute illness and the appropriate use of medications), thus minimising the need for acute admissions

To ensure that an effective MHSP is devised, it is the responsibility of mental health nurses to make themselves available to provide input during the planning process, either through attending planning meetings held by the disability service personnel supporting the patient or by providing information as required to the author of the plan. It should also be recognised that the MHSP is an appropriate clinical tool for families and other nonprofessional or unpaid carers to ensure that treatment goals are achievable in the less formal environment of the family home and also to assist carers in their preparation for crises that may arise from exacerbation of their family member's mental illness.

NURSE'S STORY 13.3

Byron

Living with a relative with dual disability

As a community nurse working within learning disability services, I often meet people who were distressed because they lived with a relative with a dual disability. Byron's family was just one example. Byron was 26 years old and had a learning disability, along with some challenging behaviours (including screaming, punching walls and sometimes destroying furniture), which had developed since the onset of his psychotic illness 4 years previously. His parents, both aged in their mid-60s, were the only people who could engage with Byron as he was very slow to accept and trust any new people in his life. At the time of my professional involvement with them, however, they were deeply upset with their son's behaviour and confused about what they could do to take control of their lives.

It can be very difficult to maintain the required professional focus when confronted with a crisis such as this. While empathic understanding is important, it is equally important to stay objective. I have learned that, in order to help, it is important for me in my role as a nurse to recognise that the problem at hand is not my personal problem but that I have much to offer in empowering families to take control of their situation. I left that first visit filled with a deep sense of sadness for these people, but also with a tinge of excitement because I could see a future of hope. I wanted to get back to this family quickly, to understand what was happening and to assist in making things right.

The main focus of my involvement with the family was not just about addressing the more obvious problems. My role was more about helping the family to cope and stay engaged with their son. Working in partnership with Byron's parents, I was able to help them devise some strategies that would enable them to take turns in caring for their son and, when they were not, to participate in relaxation and other therapies aimed at minimising the amount of stress in their lives. I also assured Byron's parents that there were others in their situation and was able to encourage their communication with a support group for families living with mental illness. In addition, I was able to bring mental health professionals to the table who could offer interventions that enabled more effective management of Byron's symptoms and his eventual reintegration back into a community-based activities programme.

While Byron came to accept me as one of his carers, this initial engagement with his parents was the key to facilitating care. I maintained contact with Byron's family for some months after this initial contact and was delighted that his parents achieved a happy medium between caring for their son and meeting their own needs. I still see Byron and his family from time to time and take great pride in the fact that I played a small part in helping them to reestablish control of their lives. As a nurse it is tempting to try and take control of other people's problems but, for me, the biggest reward is seeing people develop to a point where I am no longer needed.

PATIENT STORY 13.1

William

My name is William. People call me Billy. I am 23.

I have a disability—I have trouble thinking and learning. But I can do lots of things for myself, except I need help with money and cooking.

I live with my mum who helps me. She is my best friend.

I was living with my mum and dad but my dad left. My mum stayed home with me because I couldn't look after myself and my dad went to work. I never saw my dad much. One day he didn't come home. My mum cried a lot and I was really scared. I thought I had done something wrong.

I had some friends who lived in my street. We would do things together, but they would make fun of me. They were my friends and we would smoke cigarettes and pot. I liked the pot, but it made me hear people talking to me but I couldn't see them. Those people told me I was bad and that my dad hated me and it was my fault he left. They talked to me a lot and made me feel very sad and sometimes angry.

My mum cried so much that I got very angry with her and when she wouldn't stop one night I hit her. I was taken away by the police and put into a hospital. There were lots of people there and some of them were sad and some of them made me scared because they yelled a lot and tried to take my things.

The nurses and doctors at the hospital told me I had a psychotic episode. I don't really know what that is, but they helped me understand that I have a problem with my brain and I did things which I could not stop, that's why I hit my mum but I would never hit my mum. Psychosis is very hard to know, but the nurses and mum know what it is and that's good for me. They gave me a needle and they told me I slept for a long time and when I woke up I was really tired but I was better.

Now I have to take tablets every morning and when I go to bed. The tablets make me tired and I am fat but I have to take them so I don't hurt anyone. The nurses told me that the people don't talk to me anymore about my dad because the medicine keeps them quiet. We had a meeting at the hospital and my mum came. The nurses told my mum what was wrong with me and how I could be fixed. My mum didn't want to let me go home because she said she was scared I might hurt her. This made me very upset.

The nurses said that if I went home then I would need a plan and some help. They told my mum and me that they would get a nurse to come and see us and see how we were going and that if we needed help, like if I was feeling bad or the people started talking again or mum was feeling scared, then we could call the nurse who would help us.

They asked me if I would like to see a special doctor who could help me and I said I would. My doctor is a psychiatrist and he asks lots of questions and lets me take my mum to see him. He asks her lots of questions too.

It has been 2 years since I hurt my mum. The doctor and the nurse have helped me and my mum and I have not hurt her again. She says that I don't scare her, but she says to me all the time that I have to keep taking my medicine and I have to keep seeing the doctor and the nurse.

I started a new job last week and I am very happy.

CONCLUSION

Providing nursing management for people with a dual disability is a challenging task that requires mental health nurses to alter their practice to accommodate the specific needs of the patient and also to liaise actively with carers and disability service personnel as a matter of priority throughout all stages of the support/intervention process. The nurse must also anticipate that not all health professionals can work effectively with this patient group, sometimes because of a lack of specific skills and knowledge and sometimes because of personal prejudices. With the improvement of support services and the greater availability of information, however, it is anticipated that future mental health nurses will be better informed about this important issue and that they may be better prepared and motivated to address the specific needs of patients with a dual disability.

EXERCISES FOR CLASS ENGAGEMENT

1. Prepare a list of derogatory terms you have heard used to describe people with a learning disability. Prepare a list of nondiscriminatory terms used to describe people with this form of disability. Compare your lists with those of your group members. Which is the longest list? What are the reasons for this discrepancy?
2. How do individual group members feel about working with people who have a learning disability? Identify the challenges to providing care for these people.
3. Which factors might interfere with the achievement of a positive outcome for the person with dual disability within mental health services and within disability services? Outline strategies to overcome these barriers.

REFERENCES

Ailey, S.H., 2003. Beyond the disability: recognising mental health issues among persons with intellectual and developmental disabilities. Nursing Clinics of North America 38 (2), 313–319.

Alexander, R.T., Hiremath, A., Chester, V., Green, F.N., Hoare, S.G., 2011. Evaluation of treatment outcomes from medium secure service for people with intellectual disability. Advances in Mental Health and Learning Disabilities 5 (1), 22–32.

American Psychiatric Association (APA), 2013. Diagnostic and Statistical Manual of Mental Disorders, fifth ed. APA, Washington, DC.

Bouras, N., 2008. Mental health of people with intellectual disabilities. Current Opinion in Psychiatry 21 (5), 439–440.

British Institute of Learning Disabilities (BILD), 2011. Factsheet: Learning Disabilities. Available at: file:///C:/Users/Catherine%20Johnson/Downloads/Learning_Disabilities_11.pdf. Accessed 14 October 2018.

Brown, M., Marshall, K., 2006. Cognitive behaviour therapy and people with learning disabilities: implications for developing nursing practice. Journal of Psychiatric and Mental Health Nursing 13 (2), 234–241.

Buckles, J., Luckasson, R., Keefe, E., 2013. A systematic review of the prevalence of psychiatric disorders in adults with intellectual disability, 2003–2010. Journal of Mental Health Research in Intellectual Disabilities 6 (3), 181–207.

Cascella, P.W., 2005. Expressive communication strengths of adults with severe to profound intellectual disabilities as reported by group home staff. Communication Disorders Quarterly 26 (3), 156–163.

Chaplin, E., O'Hara, J., Holt, G., Bouras, N., 2009. Mental health services for people with intellectual disability: challenges to care delivery. British Journal of Learning Disabilities 37 (2), 157–164.

Collins, S., 1999. Treatment and other therapeutic interventions: psychological approaches. Tizzard Learning Disability Review 4 (2), 20–27.

Coombs, T., Martin, C., 2002. Information and Risk Assessment: What do Nurses Think is Important? Paper presented to the Conference of the Australian and New Zealand College of Mental Health Nurses, Sydney, 15 -18 October.

Cooper, S.A., Smiley, E., Morrison, J., Williamson, A., Allan, L., 2007. Mental ill health in adults with intellectual disabilities: prevalence and associated factors. British Journal of Psychiatry 190 (Jan), 27–35.

Davis, E., Barnhill, L.J., Saeed, S.A., 2008. Treatment models for treating patients with combined mental illness and developmental disability. Psychiatric Quarterly 79 (3), 205–223.

Deb, S., Matthews, T., Holt, G., Bouras, N., 2001a. Practice Guidelines for the Assessment and Diagnosis of Mental Health Problems in Adults with Intellectual Disability. Pavilion, Brighton, UK.

Deb, S., Thomas, M., Bright, C., 2001b. Mental disorder in adults with intellectual disability. 1: prevalence of functional psychiatric illness among a community-based population aged between 16 and 64 years. Journal of Intellectual Disability Research 45 (6), 495–505.

Delaney, K.R., 2006. Learning to observe in context: child and adolescent inpatient mental health assessment. Journal of Child and Adolescent Psychiatric Services 19 (4), 170.

Department for Communities and Social Inclusion, 2013. Disability information. Available at: www.sa.gov.au/disability.

Devine, M., Taggart, L., 2008. Addressing the mental health needs of people with learning disabilities. Nursing Standard 22 (45), 40.

de Winter, C.F., Jansen, A.A., Evenhuis, H.M., 2011. Physical conditions and challenging behaviour in people with intellectual disabilities. Journal of Intellectual Disability Research 55 (7), 675–698.

Dosen, A., 2007. Integrative treatment in persons with intellectual disability and mental health problems. Journal of Intellectual Disability Research 51 (1), 66–74.

Douds, F., McKechanie, S., Simpson, Y., Murphy, L., 2013. 'Staying well': a psychoeducational group for people with an intellectual disability, co-morbid mental illness and offending behaviour. Journal of Intellectual Disabilities 5 (1), 54–59.

Eady, N., Courtnay, K., Strydom, A., 2013. Pharmacological management of behavioural and psychiatric symptoms in older adults with intellectual disability. Drugs & Aging 32 (2), 95–102.

Einfeld, S.L., Tonge, B.J., 1995. The developmental behaviour checklist: the development and validation of an instrument to assess behavioural and emotional disturbance in children and adolescents with mental retardation. 1: rationale and methods. Journal of Autism and Developmental Disorders 25 (2), 81–104.

Emerson, E., Glover, G., Turner, S., et al., 2012. Improving health and lives: the learning disabilities public health observatory. Advances in Mental Health and Intellectual Disabilities 6 (1), 26–32.

Emerson, E., Hatton, C., 2008. Estimating Future Need for Adult Social Care Services for People with Learning Disabilities in England. Centre for Disability Research. Available at: http://eprints.lancs.ac.uk/21049/1/CeDR_2008-6_Estimating_Future_Needs_for_Adult_Social_Care_Services_for_People_with_Learning_Disabilities_in_England.pdf. Accessed 14 October 2018.

Gilbert, T., Todd, M., Jackson, N., 1998. People with learning disabilities who also have mental health problems: practice issues and directions for learning disability nursing. Journal of Advanced Nursing 27 (6), 1151–1157.

Green, J., Mears, J., 2014. The implementation of the NDIS: who wins, who loses? Cosmopolitan Civil Societies Journal 6 (2), 3915.

Hamer, B.A., 1998. Assessing mental status in persons with mental retardation. Journal of Psychosocial Nursing 36 (5), 27–31.

Hardy, S., Bouras, N., 2002. The presentation and assessment of mental health problems in people with learning disabilities. Learning Disability Practice 5 (3), 33–38.

Hatton, C., Taylor, J.L., 2008. Factor structure of the PAS-ADD Checklist with adults with intellectual disabilities. Journal of Intellectual & Developmental Disability 33 (4), 330–336.

Heller, T., Schindler, A., 2011. Family support interventions for families of adults with intellectual and developmental disabilities. International Review of Research in Mental Retardation 37, 299–332.

Henderson, C.M., Rosasco, M., Robinson, L.M., et al., 2009. Functional impairment severity and health status amongst older adults with intellectual disability. Journal of Intellectual Disability Research 53 (11), 887–897.

Higgins, S., 2004. The mental health needs of people with severe learning disabilities. British Journal of Nursing 13 (22), 1342–1346.

Johnstone, E.C., Cunningham Owens, D., Lawrie, S.M., et al., 2010. Companion to Psychiatric Studies, eighth ed. Elsevier, China.

ICD-11 for Mortality and Morbidity Statistics (ICD-11 MMS), 2018. Available at: https://icd.who.int/browse11/l-m/en#/http%3a%2f%2fid.who.int%2ficd%2fentity%2f605267007. Accessed 14 October 2018.

Kormann, R.J., Petronko, M.R., 2003. Crisis and revolution in developmental disabilities: the dilemma of community based services. The Behavior Analyst Today 3 (4), 434–443.

Learning Disabilities Observatory 2016. People with Learning Disabilities in England 2015: Main report. Available at: https://assets.publishing.service.gov.uk/government/uploads/system/uploads/attachment_data/file/613182/PWLDIE_2015_main_report_NB090517.pdf. Accessed: 14 October 2018.

Ligas, A., Petrides, G., Istafanous, R., Kellner, C.H., 2009. Successful electroconvulsive therapy in a patient with intellectual disability and bipolar disorder, with catatonic features misdiagnosed as encephalopathy. Journal of ECT 25 (3), 202–204.

Lindsay, W.R., Tinsley, S., Beail, N., et al., 2015. A preliminary controlled trial of a trans-diagnostic programme for cognitive-behavioural therapy with adults with intellectual disability. Journal of Intellectual Disability Research 59 (4), 360–369.

Loncke, F., 2014. Augmentative and Alternative Communication: Models and Applications for Educators, Speech-Language Pathologists, Caregivers, and Users. Plural Publishing, San Diego.

Longo, S., Scior, K., 2004. Inpatient psychiatric care for individuals with intellectual disabilities: service users' and carers' perspectives. Journal of Mental Health 13 (2), 211–221.

Lougheed, D.C., Farrell, S., 2013. The challenge of a triple diagnosis: identifying and serving homeless Canadian adults with a dual diagnosis. Journal of Policy and Practice in Intellectual Disabilities 10 (3), 230–235.

Lunsky, Y., Bradley, E., Durbin, J., Koegl, C., 2008. A comparison of patients with intellectual disability receiving specialised and general services in Ontario's psychiatric hospitals. Journal of Intellectual Disability Research 52 (11), 1003–1012

MacKay, F., Wilson, C., 2007. Successful multidisciplinary and multi-treatment working for a person with learning disability who experienced major depressive disorder. Learning Disability Review 12 (3), 39–47.

Mansell, J., Beadle-Brown, J., 2012. Active Support Enabling and Empowering People with Intellectual Disabilities. Jessica Kingsley, London.

Mason, J., 2007. The provision of psychological therapy to people with intellectual disabilities: an investigation into some of the relevant factors. Journal of Intellectual Disability Research 51 (3), 244–249.

McIntyre, L.L., Blacher, J., Baker, B.L., 2002. Behaviour/mental health problems in young adults with intellectual disability: The impact on families. Journal of Intellectual Disability Research 46 (3), 239–249.

Mencap, 2007. Death by Indifference. Available at: https://www.mencap.org.uk/sites/default/files/2016-06/DBIreport.pdf. Accessed 14 October 2018.

Mohr, C., Tonge, B.J., Einfeld, S.L., 2005. The development of a new measure for the assessment of psychopathology in adults with intellectual disability. Journal of Intellectual Disability Research 49 (7), 469–480.

Morin, D., Merineau-Cote, J., Oullette-Kuntz, H., Tasse, M., Kerr, M., 2012. A comparison of the prevalence of chronic disease among people with and without intellectual disability. American Journal of Intellectual and Developmental Disabilities 117 (6), 455–463.

Moss, S.C., Patel, P., Prosser, H., et al., 1993. Psychiatric morbidity in older people with moderate and severe learning disability (mental retardation). Part 1: development and reliability of the patient interview (the PAS-ADD). British Journal of Psychiatry 163, 471–480.

National Health Service, 2015. Building the Right Support. Available at: www.england.nhs.uk/learning-disabilities/natplan. Accessed 14 October 2018.

National Health Service, 2017. Transforming Care Partnerships (TCPs). Available at: https://www.england.nhs.uk/learning-disabilities/tcp/. Accessed 14 October 2018.

National Institute for Health and Care Excellence (NICE), 2016. NG54 Mental Health Problems in People with Learning Disabilities: Prevention, Assessment and Management. Available at: https://www.nice.org.uk/guidance/ng54. Accessed 14 October 2018.

National Institute for Health and Care Excellence (NICE), 2017. QS142 Learning Disabilities: Identifying and Managing Mental Health Problems. Available at: www.nice.org.uk/guidance/qs142/chapter/Quality-statements. Accessed 14 October 2018.

National Institute for Health and Care Excellence (NICE), 2018. NG96 Care and Support of People Growing Older with Learning Disabilities. Available at: https://www.nice.org.uk/guidance/ng96. Accessed 14 October 2018.

O'Brien, J., 1987. A guide to lifestyle planning: using the activities catalogue to integrate services and natural support systems. In: Wilcox, B., Belamy, G.T., Paul, H. (Eds.), A Comprehensive Guide to the Activities Catalogue. Brooks, Baltimore.

O'Brien, J., O'Brien, C.L., 2006. Implementing Person-Centred Planning: Voices of Experience. Inclusion Press, Toronto.

O'Hara, J., 2008. Attending to the health needs of people with intellectual disability: quality standards. Salud Pública de México 50 (2), 154–159.

Oullette-Kuntz, H., Garcin, N., Lewis, M.E.S., et al., 2005. Addressing health disparities through promoting equity for individuals with intellectual disabilities. Journal of Applied Research in Intellectual Disabilities 18 (2), 113–121.

Pridding, A., Watkins, D., Happell, B., 2007. Mental health nursing roles and functions in acute inpatient units: caring for people with intellectual disability and mental health problems—a literature review. International Journal of Psychiatric Nursing Research 12 (2), 1459–1470.

Prosser, H., Moss, S., Costello, H., et al., 1998. Reliability and validity of the Mini-PAS-ADD for assessing psychiatric disorders in adults with intellectual disability. Journal of Intellectual Disability Research 42 (4), 264–272.

Public Health England (PHE), 2016. Learning Disabilities Observatory People with learning disabilities in England 2015: Main report. Available at: https://assets.publishing.service.gov.uk/government/uploads/system/uploads/attachment_data/file/613182/PWLDIE_2015_main_report_NB090517.pdf. Accessed June 2019.

Public Heath England, 2018. All Our Health. Available at: https://www.gov.uk/government/publications/all-our-health-about-the-framework/all-our-health-about-the-framework. Accessed 14 October 2018.

Public Heath England, 2018. Learning disabilities: applying All Our Health. Available at: https://www.gov.uk/government/publications/learning-disability-applying-all-our-health/learning-disabilities-applying-all-our-health#guidance. Accessed 14 October 2018.

Regan, R., Willatt, L., 2010. Mental retardation: definition, classification and etiology. In: Knight, S.J.L. (Ed.), Genetics of Mental Retardation: An Overview Encompassing Learning Disability and Intellectual Disability. Karger, Basel.

Reiss, S., 1994. Handbook of Challenging Behavior: Mental Health Aspects of Mental Retardation. IDS, Columbia.

Reiss, S., Levitan, G.W., Szyszko, J., 1982. Emotional disturbance and mental retardation: diagnostic overshadowing. American Journal of Mental Deficiency 86 (6), 567–574.

Robertson, J., Hatton, C., Emerson, E., Baines, S., 2014. The impact of health checks for people with intellectual disabilities: an updated systematic review of evidence. Research in Developmental Disabilities 35 (10), 2450–2462.

Ross, E., Oliver, C., 2002. The relationship between levels of mood, interest and pleasure and 'challenging behaviour' in adults with severe and profound intellectual disability. Journal of Intellectual Disability Research 46 (3), 191–197.

Royal College of General Practitioners (RCGP), 2018. Health Checks for People with Learning Disabilities Toolkit. Available at: www.rcgp.org.uk/clinical-and-research/resources/toolkits/health-check-toolkit.aspx. Accessed 14 October 2018.

Royal College of Nursing (RCN), 2014. Provision of Mental Health Care for Adults Who Have a Learning Disability. Available at: https://www.rcn.org.uk/professional-development/publications/pub-004445. Accessed 14 October 2018.

Royal College of Speech and Language Therapists, 2013. Five Good Communication Standards. Available at: www.rcslt.org/news/docs/good_comm_standards.

Shalock, R.L., Borthwick-Duffy, S.A., Bradley, V.J., et al., 2010. Intellectual Disability: Definition, Classification, and Systems of Supports, eleventh ed. American Association on Intellectual and Developments Disabilities, Washington.

Shepperd, S., McClaran, J., Phillips, C.O., et al., 2010. Discharge planning from hospital to home. Cochrane Database of Systematic Reviews 1. https://doi.org/10.1002/14651858.CD000313.pub2.

Slevin, E., McConkey, R., Truesdale-Kennedy, M., Taggart, L., 2008. People with learning disabilities admitted to an assessment and treatment unit: impact on challenging behaviours and mental health problems. Journal of Psychiatric and Mental Health Nursing 15 (7), 537–546.

Sovner, R., 1996. Six models of behaviour from a psychiatric perspective. The Habilitative Mental Healthcare Newsletter 15 (3), 51–54.

Spiller, M.J., Hardy, S., 2004. Developing a guide to mental health for families and carers of people with intellectual disability. Learning Disability Practice 7 (8), 28–31.

Stirk, S., Sanderson, H., 2012. Creating Person-Centred Organisations: Strategies and Tools for Managing Change in Health, Social Care, and the Voluntary Sector. Jessica Kingsley Publishers, London.

Taylor, J.L., Hatton, C., Dixon, L., et al., 2004. Screening for psychiatric symptoms: PASS-ADD checklist norms for adults with intellectual disabilities. Journal of Intellectual Disability Research 48 (1), 37–41.

Taua, C., Farrow, T., 2009. Negotiating complexities: an ethnographic study of intellectual disability and mental health nursing in New Zealand. International Journal of Mental Health Nursing 18 (4), 274–284.

Taua, C., Hepworth, J., Neville, C., 2011. Nurses' role in caring for people with a comorbidity of mental illness and intellectual disability: a literature review. International Journal of Intellectual Disabilities 21 (2), 163–174.

Vereenooghe, L., Langdon, P.E., 2013. Psychological therapies for people with intellectual disabilities: a systematic review and meta-analysis. Research in Developmental Disabilities 34 (11), 4085–5102.

Wallace, R.A., Beange, H., 2008. On the need for a specialist service within the generic hospital setting for the adult patient with intellectual disability and physical health problems. Journal of Intellectual and Developmental Disability 33 (4), 354–361.

Werges, D., 2007. The other dual diagnosis: Intellectual disability & mental illness. NADD Bulletin 10 (5), Article 2.

Wolfensberger, W., 1972. Normalization: The Principle of Normalization in Human Services. National Institute on Mental Retardation, Toronto.

World Health Organization (WHO), 1993. International Statistical Classification of Diseases and Related Health Problems, tenth ed. WHO, Geneva.

Yildiran, H., Holt, R., 2014. Thematic analysis of the effectiveness of an inpatient mindfulness group for adults with intellectual disabilities. British Journal of Learning Disabilities 43 (1), 49–54.

Yohanna, D., 2013. Deinstitutionalization of people with mental illness: causes and consequences. Virtual Mentor 15 (10), 886–891.

Young, L., Ashman, A.F., 2004. Deinstitutionalisation in Australia part 1: historical perspective. British Journal of Developmental Disabilities 50 (98), 21–28..

USEFUL WEBSITES

American Speech-Language-Hearing Association - Augmentative and Alternative Communication (AAC), https://www.asha.org/public/speech/disorders/aac

British Institute of Learning Disabilities (BILD), www.bild.org.uk

British-Sign, www.british-sign.co.uk

Centre for Disability Research (CeDR), http://wp.lancs.ac.uk/cedr

EasyHealth (easy read formats), www.easyhealth.org.uk

Communication Matters: more than just talking, www.communicationmatters.org.uk/page/what-is-aac

Dictionary of British Sign Language, www.britishsignlanguage.com

Foundation for People with Learning Disabilities, www.mentalhealth.org.uk/learning-disabilities

Makaton Sign Language, www.makaton.org/aboutMakaton

National Association for the Persons with Developmental Disabilities and Mental Health Needs (NADD) (United States), www.thenadd.org

Mental health assessment for people with an intellectual disability (including the PAS-ADD assessment tool and associated information), www.pasadd.co.uk

Personalisation through person-centred planning, www.helensandersonassociates.co.uk/person-centred-practice/working-together-change

Personal Independence Payments, www.gov.uk/pip

Royal College of Speech and Language Therapists, https://www.rcslt.org

Sense, www.sense.org.uk

14

Forensic Mental Health Nursing

Brian McKenna, Tessa Maguire and Trish Martin

KEY POINTS

- Mental health nurses have begun to identify the knowledge, skills and attitudes required to work with forensic patients.
- There is an overrepresentation of people experiencing mental illness in criminal justice processes.
- Forensic patients are heterogeneous groups of people whose offending behaviour may or may not be related to their experiences of mental illness, or the mental illness may be a result of the offending behaviour.
- The role of forensic mental health services has progressed from mainly providing containment to providing treatment for forensic patients.
- Risk assessment, treatment and management processes continue to develop and to be used by nurses to meet the needs of patients and to ensure safety for the community.
- The role of mental health nurses in forensic and justice settings is exciting but also fraught with ethical dilemmas.
- Despite the emphasis on safety and security, the forensic mental health nurse remains focussed on recovery-oriented care (for a full discussion of recovery see Chapter 2).

KEY TERMS

custody nurse
criminalisation of the mentally ill
criminal justice system
deinstitutionalisation
diversion
fitness to plead
forensic mental health nurse
not guilty by reason of insanity
recidivism
recovery
risk assessment and management
risk factors
security
structured clinical judgement

LEARNING OUTCOMES

The material in this chapter will assist you to:

- demonstrate awareness of the needs and experiences of forensic mental health patients.
- identify specific nursing interventions for forensic mental health patients.
- describe the components of forensic mental health services.
- explain common links between mental illness and offending behaviour.
- discuss the skills, knowledge and attitudes that are central to forensic mental health nursing.
- utilise the structured clinical judgement approach to risk assessment, treatment and management.
- develop an understanding of nursing in criminal justice and forensic mental health settings.

INTRODUCTION

The context of mental healthcare is constantly changing and the proactive response of mental health nurses to such changes is reflected in the evolution of our profession. This chapter focusses on the needs and wellbeing of people experiencing acute or enduring mental illness who have been charged with a criminal offence or are suspected of committing a criminal offence (Bradley 2009). The chapter provides a description of forensic patients and overviews what is known about the relationship between mental illness and offending behaviour. For many reasons, people experiencing mental illness are overrepresented in the criminal justice system. Forensic mental health services have developed in the UK to provide containment, assessment, treatment and management of forensic mental health patients. These services have grown from the recognition that neither the criminal justice system nor the mental health system can adequately provide services for forensic mental health patients and that the two systems must work in partnership to meet the needs of patients and, at times, the need for community safety.

The criminal justice system includes the police who arrest people alleged to have committed a crime and the courts responsible for making determinations of guilt or innocence and for imposing penalties if the person is found guilty. Imprisonment and community-based sentencing options are possible penalties. When the person is thought to be experiencing mental illness, there are options for diversion from police custody, court or prison to mental health services for assessment and treatment. However, most mainstream mental health services do not have the structural security or available treatment options to contain, assess, treat and manage certain forensic mental health patients and forensic mental health services have therefore been developed.

Forensic mental health services are generally independent of the criminal justice system and are managed within the health sector. Components of forensic mental health services include services within police custody centres, prisons and courts. Secure hospitals and community services are also essential components. Forensic mental health services, which have been traditionally custodial and involved in compulsory treatment and care, are being challenged to transform to recovery-oriented services. As such, the call is to focus on the lived experience of the individual patient, with the aim that the person leads a satisfying life irrespective of the difficulties imposed by mental health needs and secure services (Simpson & Penney 2011). Balancing a person-centred approach within a custodial environment remains a problematic but essential practice priority for the contemporary forensic mental health nurse.

The term 'forensic mental health nurse' is used in this chapter to identify mental health nurses who practise in criminal justice or forensic settings, i.e. forensic secure hospitals. Similar to other health fields, there are more nurses than other specialists. Nurses working in this setting must possess the knowledge, skills and attitudes that are required to provide comprehensive care for complex forensic mental health patients. Although this chapter focusses on nursing in criminal justice and forensic mental health settings, there is no doubt that nurses in mainstream services will, at some time, work in partnership with patients to address forensic mental health needs.

Forensic mental health nurses primarily focus on forensic mental health patients—the perpetrators or alleged perpetrators of crime. This role should not be confused with the title 'forensic nurse', which is prominent in countries such as the United States. Forensic nursing practice is more (but not exclusively) focussed on the needs of victims of crime or those bringing an issue to court (including roles such as sexual assault nurse examiners) (Lawson 2008).

Nor should the role of the forensic mental health nurse be confused with that of the 'prison nurse' (sometimes referred to as a 'correctional nurse'). The forensic mental health nurse works in partnership with prisoners who have experienced serious mental illness. The prison nurse often focusses primarily on the primary physical healthcare needs of prisoners (International Association of Forensic Nurses 2015). In 2013, NHS England became responsible for commissioning all health services for people in prison in England. Guidelines have been produced to support the equivalence of physical healthcare in prisons, where patients can expect to receive the same standard of physical healthcare as people living in the community, aiming to reduce inequalities, prevent deterioration and ultimately assist in rehabilitation and reductions in reoffending (NICE 2016).

THE DEVELOPMENT OF FORENSIC MENTAL HEALTH SERVICES

Since the 1950s, mental health services have undergone major restructuring internationally in response to deinstitutionalisation. This process involved large psychiatric hospitals (or asylums) being closed down in favour of a network of mental health inpatient wards and community mental health centres to meet the needs of mental health patients.

Deinstitutionalisation is one factor that has led to the development of forensic mental health services. Prior to deinstitutionalisation, people experiencing mental illness were often admitted early in the development of their symptoms and were commonly detained for long periods of time. Being contained within the asylum may have meant that residents were protected from the consequences of many of the factors that predispose them to offend or increase their risk of offending. Such factors include lack of insight, poor understanding of early warning signs of relapse of mental illness, pro-criminal or pro-violence thinking, substance use, poor stress tolerance, lack of impulse control, poor problem solving and lack of social skills. Nurses in the asylums provided care, support and risk management that ameliorated the impact of these factors and also reduced exposure to circumstances that can lead to offending behaviour (such as poverty, social disadvantage and victimisation). Furthermore, offences might not have been reported by staff because a considerable level of disturbed and deviant behaviours were tolerated in the asylums and treated as clinical problems rather than criminal offences. When the asylums closed, increasing numbers of people experiencing mental illness who committed offences made contact with the criminal justice system. It is this social process that is referred to as 'the criminalisation of the mentally ill' (Slate et al. 2013).

The difficulty of treating forensic patients in prisons and the decreasing ability to contain them securely in mainstream services for extended periods have also contributed to the need for forensic mental health services. Forensic patients require specialised services that address both their mental health needs and offence-related behaviour (Daffern et al. 2010).

IDENTIFYING FORENSIC PATIENTS

Forensic patients have complex needs that forensic mental health nurses must thoroughly assess in order to provide holistic care in partnership with the patient and their carers. Apart from the clinical need for treatment, many patients have recovery needs related to social, cultural and adaptive malfunctioning and patterns of offending that can present as a risk to themselves or others.

The Legal Status of Forensic Patients

Prisons in England and Wales are categorised as A, B, C or D services, with category A facilities catering for prisoners who are considered to pose the highest level of risk to the public or national security. High security services are defined as being for 'people requiring treatment under conditions of high security on account of their dangerous, violent or criminal propensities' (NHS 2006), such as Ashworth, Broadmoor and Rampton. Medium security services can offer differing levels of secure care, ranging from patients on remand (awaiting their court hearing) to patients with increasing unescorted community leave as part of a predischarge programme (Joint Commissioning Panel for Mental Health [JCP-MH] 2013).

Forensic mental health services are designed to care for people with a mental disorder (including a neurodevelopmental disorder) that pose, or have posed, risks to others and where that risk is usually related to their mental disorder. People may be cared for in a secure hospital, in the community or sometimes in a mainstream prison (JCP-MH 2013). The Mental Health Act 1959 first laid out the foundations for forensic mental health services with the introduction of the 'hospital order', which allowed a mentally unwell person convicted of an offence, who would normally be imprisoned, to be admitted to hospital for treatment. In 1975, the Butler Report encouraged the development of 'regional secure units', latterly becoming known as medium security services. Since the 2000s there has been a shift away from high to medium security services; for example, in 1991 there were in excess of 1700 high security service beds and less than 600 medium security beds. However, almost 1000 high security beds have since closed and been replaced by additional medium security beds, with the independent sector providing 35% of these beds in England (JCP-MH 2013).

The following is a summary of the forensic mental health sections from the Mental Health Act (1983) that covers England and Wales.

Section 35: Remand to hospital for report on accused's mental condition

Section 36: Remand of accused person to hospital for treatment

Section 37: Powers of courts to order hospital admission or guardianship

Section 38: Interim hospital orders

Section 37/41: Restriction Order, the Secretary of State decides when a person can be given leave and when they can leave hospital

Section 47: Removal to hospital of persons serving sentences of imprisonment

Section 48: Removal to hospital of other prisoners (awaiting sentencing)

The legislation is too complex to discuss further in this section (see Chapter 4 for UK-wide mental health legislation links and further discussion around professional, legal and ethical issues).

Defendants appearing in court must be fit to plead. If mental illness prevents a person from meeting certain criteria (including having an understanding of the nature of the charge and the trial, being able to enter a plea and being able to give instructions to the legal practitioner), then that person is likely to be ordered by the court to receive treatment until they are fit to return to court. A small number of patients are never fit and other processes are put in place to ensure their treatment and supervision.

Patients are found not guilty by reason of insanity by the court when it has been proved that the person was so unwell at the time of the offence that they did not understand the nature and quality of the act (the offence) or did not know that the act was wrong. Patients who are found not guilty due to insanity are required to undertake treatment; the duration and location of the treatment will depend on the severity of the offence and the risk status of the patient.

A prisoner experiencing mental illness will require a transfer to a secure hospital for treatment if an adequate level of treatment and care cannot be provided at the prison or if the prisoner is unwilling to accept treatment. Prisoners cannot be treated involuntarily in prison, as the potential for abuse of psychiatric treatment is ever-present in prisons. Some offenders in prison who are experiencing mental illness can adhere to treatment and need an equivalent level of treatment and care that is available in the community, such as outpatient appointments with a nurse. This service may be provided by prison mental health in-reach teams. Some prisons have mental health units for the short-term assessment and treatment of prisoners. Some high-risk prisoners will be referred to either a forensic mental health hospital or a community team for assessment and treatment following release from prison.

Wherever forensic mental health nurses practise, it is their responsibility to understand the legislation that affects patients. Forensic mental health patients and their carers are sometimes confused by the legal processes and requirements. The nurse's knowledge of the law needs to be used proactively to assist forensic mental health patients and their carers to understand the function and impact of criminal justice legislation and policies and to optimise care in the context of integrating security, safety and therapeutic intent. The nurse is also required to provide information to patients and carers to ensure that they are aware of their rights.

Websites that may assist you to gain some understanding of legislation related to forensic mental health are listed at the end of the chapter.

Demographic Characteristics

Research examining forensic patients generally describes a similar population in terms of demographic characteristics: young, male, never married, low socioeconomic status, unemployed, poor educational achievement and itinerant living situations prior to conviction (Constantine et al. 2010). However, the number of imprisoned women is increasing and therefore the female forensic patient population is growing. In guidance produced for commissioners (JCP-MH 2013), it was estimated that there were around 6000 people in secure services in England; 680 in high security, 2800 in medium security and 2500 in low security establishments.

Cognitive and Social Skills

When a person's ability to think clearly and relate constructively to others is compromised by mental illness, the likelihood of antisocial behaviour including violence and offending is enhanced (Douglas et al. 2009). However, the reasons for compromised cognitive and social ability are complex and may not relate directly to mental illness. These reasons may relate to diminished learning opportunities in the context of the family, environment and culture; harsh or inconsistent parenting; delinquent peer associations; and acquired brain injury. A significant proportion of forensic mental health patients have a history of traumatic childhood experiences (Egeressy et al. 2009) and acquired brain injury (Jackson & Hardy 2011). Therefore, the development of cognitive and social skills is a recovery requirement of forensic mental health services (Chapter 24 describes social skills training in more detail). Limitations in cognitive and social skills can militate against a socially positive response to life's challenges (Chapter 25Bennett et al. 2005).

Social Disadvantage

When assessing the needs of forensic mental health patients, forensic mental health nurses must also consider the patient's sociocultural context. The influences of membership of minority disadvantaged groups and low socioeconomic status are especially important (Martin et al. 2013).

Forensic mental health patients are more at risk of victimisation compared with the general population (Wolff & Shi 2009). Victimisation includes being subjected to violence, intimidation, sexual exploitation and financial exploitation. These needs require integrated health, justice and social care agency responses in order for this population to attain acceptable levels of social functioning and quality of life (either in prison or in the community) and to avoid reoffending (Harty et al. 2009).

Violence may be the reality of high-crime neighbourhoods where people experiencing mental illness live. There is an indication that people experiencing mental illness move into, or fail to rise out of, low socioeconomic localities because of the impact of the social stigma attached to the illness (Constantine et al. 2010). The stigma, symptoms and course of the illness may prevent people from acquiring vocational qualifications and securing stable employment. Surviving on benefits can result in them living in lower socioeconomic areas, where local community norms may be more supportive of offending and there is the possibility of increased contact with others who are offenders (Slate et al. 2013).

Forensic mental health nurses need to work with those forensic mental health patients with identified sociocultural needs to help them to develop or restore protective social alliances with their family and community. Supporting social care goals and strengthening cultural identity can prevent further offending and assist with the patient's recovery.

Mental Illness and Risk to Others

The relationship between mental illness and criminal behaviour is complex and varies between individuals. Nurses need to identify the unique relationship for each person so that they can ascertain the risk and protective factors that need to be addressed in treatment and risk management strategies. Most offenders who progress from assessment to remain on the caseload of forensic mental health nurses experience serious mental illness.

A seminal 25-year study undertaken by Wallace, Mullen and Burgess (2004) found that the overall frequency of violent offences was significantly higher among people experiencing schizophrenia than among the comparison community subjects (8.2% versus 1.8%). The rate of violent offending among people experiencing schizophrenia gradually increased over the years of the study, but there was no difference in the rate of increase when compared with the comparison subjects over the same period. Most people experiencing schizophrenia are not violent and do not commit criminal offences, but rates of violence and offending are higher than for comparison community subjects.

The offences committed by patients experiencing schizophrenia reflect a range of factors that are present before, during and after periods of acute illness (Kooyman et al. 2012). These factors are presented in the section on risk assessment later in the chapter. Hodgins (2008) has attributed more serious violence to delusions leaving people fearful and frightened by those around them and with a decreased ability to control personal responses to these perceived threats. It is stated that if a person with a psychotic disorder experiences voices that command violent acts, this increases the likelihood of violence. A study by Swanson et al. (2006) found that positive symptoms of schizophrenia (such as hallucinations, delusions and disorganised thinking) increase the risk of serious violence, while negative symptoms (such as loss of energy, loss of the experience of pleasure and loss of drive) lower this risk. These international studies have found modest increases in criminal and violent behaviour with serious mental illness, but also note that there is no evidence that mental illness causes criminal behaviour; rather, several factors mediate mental illness and offending. These factors include antisocial tendencies or peers, and alcohol or drug abuse (Hodgins 2008).

Substance Use

Substance abuse is common in psychiatric populations, offender populations and the community generally (Fazel & Baillargeon 2011). (See Chapter 20 for more information about substance use and abuse and their association with coexisting mental disorders.) Forensic patients have high rates of substance abuse and these coexisting conditions have a link to offending and risk of violence (Chapter 21Hodgins 2008). Although the majority of people experiencing schizophrenia are not violent, they are four to five times more likely to be violent when substance abuse is implicated. Researchers consider that the major driver of crime and violence in people (with and without a mental illness) is substance misuse. It has been recognised that there is a high prevalence of prisoners who have a mental illness and who also abuse substances (Fazel & Baillargeon 2011).

There is substantial evidence for substance misuse being a significant risk factor for violence and aggression for patients who have a major mental disorder, particularly schizophrenia (Fazel et al. 2009). In their study examining criminal offending over a 25-year period, Wallace et al. (2004) found that people with schizophrenia and substance abuse problems contributed disproportionately to the rates of conviction. Higher rates of criminal conviction were found for mental health patients with substance abuse problems compared with those without substance abuse problems (68.1% versus 11.7%).

Substance use among forensic mental health patients has been identified as being relatively common (Miles et al. 2007; Young 2006). While the link between substance abuse and aggression/offending is widely recognised, the mechanisms are poorly understood, resulting from a complex process involving the interaction of the substances' active agents, the substance misuse, the context of the substance misuse and personal factors such as a predisposition to aggression.

FORENSIC MENTAL HEALTH SERVICES

Components of forensic mental health services include services within police custody centres, courts and prisons, as well as secure forensic mental health hospitals and community services.

Police Custody Centres

The process of entering the criminal justice system commences at the point of arrest. In a freedom of information request (2017) made to the Metropolitan Police, it was revealed that in the 12-month period prior to July 2017, 115,000 calls were made to the police regarding mental health, with a national estimate of almost £4 million being directed at mental health related incidents (College of Policing 2015). Many offences were misdemeanours and typically involved public nuisance behaviours such as urinating in a public place and survival crimes such as shoplifting or leaving a restaurant without paying (Slate et al. 2013). Management of this behaviour requires arrangements between mental health services and the police, so that forensic patients can be diverted from the criminal justice system to inpatient or community mental health services (Bradley 2009). Decisions on diversion require consideration of public safety, the safety of the offender and the seriousness of the charge and they can occur at any stage of the criminal justice process. For example, if a person experiencing a psychotic mental illness is arrested for shoplifting food in order to eat, diversion to general mental health services may be possible. However, if the charge is aggravated assault, then criminal justice processes would proceed and the person's mental health needs would be managed within the criminal justice system. In this case, the person might be remanded to prison while the court process proceeds and their mental health needs would be addressed within the prison.

In the absence of initial mental health service involvement and in cases of alleged serious offending such as violent offences, people experiencing a mental health emergency may be transported to police holding cells. The person's impaired mental health state may come to the attention of police officers, who can initiate a mental health response. Under the Mental Health Act (1983) there are police powers allowing police officers to detain a person who appears to be requiring care or control because of a mental health issue, using either a Section 135 (from inside a person's home without a warrant) or a Section 136 (in a public place) and transporting them to a place of safety for a mental health assessment. These holding powers last for 24 hours, allowing arrangements to be made for the appropriate professionals to assess the patient—often at a 136 suite at a hospital or in a police custody suite if no hospital beds are available. Across the UK, some police services employ custody nurses to work in police custody centres to assist with mental health, physical health and addiction needs (Paulin & Carswell 2010). The main mental health role of these nurses is to screen for and to identify mental illness and substance abuse as soon as possible. Following assessment, nursing interventions typically focus on managing substance intoxication, withdrawal and overdose; acute symptoms of mental illness; and self-harm and suicidal behaviour.

Custody nurses are also involved in training police on how to identify mental illness, undertake a risk assessment and relate to people experiencing mental illness. Such education can provide police with greater understanding and an increasing ability to recognise mental health problems and identify options for ensuring the safe containment of people experiencing mental illness so that they can refer them to appropriate services for assistance.

The Courts

The courts are another potential point of diversion from the criminal justice system to mental health and addiction services. In the United States and Canada, this has led to the development of 'special circumstances courts' such as mental health courts, and drug and alcohol courts. The aim of such courts is to interrupt the cycle of offending by facilitating access to treatment for those people with mental health and addiction problems (Wiener et al. 2010). Delivery of services and treatment progress are monitored through court review by the judge.

Some courts have established specialist mental health settings, others employ court liaison nurses to advise judges, lawyers and the police on issues regarding the mental health, addiction status and needs of people presenting to court (McKenna & Seaton 2007). Court liaison nurses accept referrals from the police, from lawyers who have concerns about a defendant, from judges who might stand down proceedings for referral purposes and from a variety of other sources including the probation service, mental health services, families and self-referrals. Referrals usually arise from concerns about behaviour suspected of being related to mental illness, intellectual disability, communication difficulties or alcohol and drug problems.

A police summary of facts can often be made available to the nurse before the person is interviewed and assessed. The assessment involves a mental state examination (MSE) and risk assessment. In the MSE, close attention is paid to behaviour, thoughts, feelings and ways of relating that might be indicative of the presence of mental illness. In the risk assessment, close attention is paid to the extent to which the presence of symptoms of mental illness, substance use, personality construct and the person's social circumstances might impact the level of risk that the person poses to themselves or other people. The level of risk will influence the judge's decision about where the person is to be placed and whether treatment is identified as a condition.

If the charges are minor, such as those cases involving public nuisance, the court liaison nurse may be required, at the request of the court, to facilitate the person's engagement with general or forensic mental health services, in either an inpatient or a community setting. The objective is to secure mental health service placement without the impediment of court processes and associated incarceration (McKenna & Seaton 2007). If the charges are serious, such as violent offending or sex offending, the judge may request a forensic psychiatric or psychological assessment. These reports generally provide comment on issues of fitness to plead and whether the person was mentally impaired at the time of the offence. The report may also make suggestions about treatment options for the person.

Court liaison roles have some unique challenges for nurses, including functioning within a 'ritual bound environment complicated by competing professions and protocol' (McKenna & Seaton 2007, p. 6). Mental health nurses are trained to function in mental health services where a relatively structured environment provides a frame of reference to guide their practice. In contrast, the court is not a clinical environment but is the domain of court officials, the police, defence parties, prosecution parties and probation services. Each has its own language and philosophical approach that may hamper attempts to focus on mental health. Nurses working in the courts (or any part of the criminal justice system) must recognise the potential for enculturation to criminal justice values (see the later section on multidisciplinary team involvement). Nurse's Story 14.1 by Kevin Seaton describes how court liaison nurses need to negotiate both the legal and the mental health systems and make sense of their competing demands in order to achieve the best outcomes for their patients.

NURSE'S STORY 14.1

Kevin Seaton, Court Liaison Nurse

I have been employed in the court liaison service for 14 years. Before becoming a court liaison nurse, I had never entered a court and had no dealings with the criminal justice system. On my first day on the job, I helped assess a young man who had been arrested after an unprovoked attack on his neighbours with a knife. He believed they were aliens who had implanted a computer chip in his brain. We had to transfer this man to a secure forensic mental health unit for further assessment and treatment.

I thought to myself, what have I let myself in for? I knew nothing about the court process, court protocol, how to address a judge or, more importantly, how to translate a mental state examination (MSE) into a letter to the court that the judge would understand. As a court liaison nurse I found myself caught between the police who want to convict, the defence lawyers who want the charges withdrawn and the judge who wants advice on the mental health and risk status of the defendant and guidance as to where they should be placed. I really struggled trying to make sense of the court process, the criminal legislation and trying to do the 'right' thing for the patient/defendant.

I was only 2 weeks into the role when I found myself in court supporting a mentally ill defendant. The aim, supported by the lawyers and the judge, was to seek bail to the local general mental health facility under mental health legislation. Unfortunately, there were no beds in the region. When this was explained to the judge with the suggestion of the alternative of a further remand in prison for 2 days to allow a bed to be secured, the judge's retort was vehement: 'Don't expect me to look after your mental cases in prison. You find a bed.' I was so embarrassed being spoken to like that in a full courtroom. But I also felt that I should have somehow been able to 'find the bed' this person needed, and by not doing so I had failed to provide care for this person.

These are the sorts of challenges you are presented with when working in the courts. Although initially they made me uncomfortable, the challenges quickly helped me to understand the different agendas in the court context, through which the court liaison nurse is required to stay impartial. The skill is to provide clinical information that is accurate, with a clear rationale as to why certain recommendations are made. Possible responses from the judge need to be anticipated with alternative suggestions being preplanned. Sound knowledge of legislation and criminal justice processes is imperative.

Court liaison nurses need to be competent and confident not only in their MSE abilities, but also in the recommendations that arise from these assessments. The MSE must also be accompanied by a thorough assessment of risk to self and others.

Court liaison nurses are independent autonomous practitioners, often working in relative professional isolation outside the usual comfort zone of a hospital setting. The court setting is alien territory, working alongside non–health professionals who have a unique professional language and etiquette, which the nurse has to learn to become effective. No senior medical staff are readily on hand for advice and assistance. Peer clinical supervision is imperative. We see and hear horrific details of offending, so support and guidance from colleagues who understand the role and its demands are critical for both competent clinical practice and our own wellbeing.

The work is both challenging and rewarding. Over the years I have had to hone my clinical skills to enable me to practise at a level of autonomous practice I would not have thought possible 14 years ago. I have had to learn to speak and write in a 'legalistic' language rather than just 'nurse clinical speak'. I get to wear nice professional clothes (no jeans in court!) and work and talk with professionals outside the mental health setting. Judges acknowledge me and listen to and respect my opinion. The stress is high, the hours of work long, but I would work nowhere else.

(*Source*: Adapted from McKenna, B., Seaton, K., 2007. Liaison services to the courts. In: Brookbanks, W., Simpson, A., (Eds) Psychiatry and the law. LexisNexis, Wellington.)

Prison

There are some forensic patients for whom diversion from court is untenable because of the serious nature of their offending or other risk factors or for whom sentencing to prison is required. Epidemiological studies of prison populations internationally have indicated that there is a two- to fourfold increase in the prevalence rates of those experiencing psychotic illness and major depression in prison compared with the general community (Fazel & Seewald 2012). It is suggested that the number of people in the criminal justice system affected with mental illness ranges from 39% in police custody up to 90% in prison. Additionally, there is also evidence to suggest that mental disorders such as personality disorders and psychotic disorders are more prevalent in the prison population than in the general population. Prisons often have on-site mental health facilities able to manage these patients, however, in some cases it may be appropriate for patients to be transferred to specialist mental health secure services (NICE 2017).

The reasons for the high prevalence rates of mental illness in prisons are complex and hotly debated. The overrepresentation of forensic patients may reflect that some offending is truly higher among some forensic mental health patients or that their offending is more easily detected or that they are less able to defend themselves during court proceedings. It is also the case that when some people are imprisoned, their psychological wellbeing is adversely affected by life in prison. Regardless of the reason, prisons have assumed the roles of acute mental health units and detoxification units by default. For the work of a nurse within this context, see Nurse's Story 14.2 by Nathan Bruce.

Within the prison context, there are also high rates of offenders experiencing mild to moderate mental illnesses (such as anxiety and lower grade depression), alcohol abuse, drug abuse and problem gambling. A number of prisoners will experience anxiety and depression as a result of imprisonment. These mental health needs are primarily addressed by GPs and nurses employed by the prisons, often supplemented

NURSE'S STORY 14.2

Nathan Bruce, Prison-Based Mental Health Nurse

At first glance it's extremely austere, a place where the emphasis on rules and security is literally inescapable. Seventeen secure doors, innumerable closed-circuit cameras, two metal detectors, three iris scanners, a few flights of stairs and long corridors, and the pervading unpleasant bodily odours that one comes to expect whenever hundreds of men are stacked into concrete cells occupying the footprint of a small city apartment block. This is the location where I begin work each day, walking to my shared desk space, within a maximum security men's prison.

When looking at this group of men through a forensic mental health nursing lens, with time it becomes apparent that the prison merely serves as a solid structure that concentrates and contains a microcosm of the wider community's most vulnerable and marginalised groups. Though every patient is unique, you don't have to look hard to see the links between cycles of mental illness, offending, social disadvantage, substance misuse and reoffending.

In spite of the oppressive physical surroundings, a term of imprisonment can provide an impetus for breaking cycles of offending and poorly managed mental illness. Prison mental health services play an important role in supporting positive life choices to help offenders achieve goals and reach their potential as part of the wider community. Like many community services, prison mental health teams have a tendency to evolve and operate in silos. Additionally, surging rates of incarceration have called for innovative models of care to provide efficient high-quality mental health services to prisoners.

It was within this context that I was introduced to the opportunity to establish one of the first nurse practitioner roles, working across a number of different sites within the expanding public prison system in Victoria, Australia. The nurse practitioner's advanced nursing role, encompassing both autonomous and collaborative aspects of direct clinical care, clearly stood out as a potentially valuable addition to the interdisciplinary team. During these early stages, service gaps have been evaluated and clinical scope of practice has been adapted to ensure the best use of a nurse practitioner's skills and availability, while undertaking specialist training and securing ongoing project funding.

It has been satisfying to use the skills and knowledge that I have developed over a number of years. Extensions to traditional prison-based mental health nursing practice that nurse practitioners bring can include autonomous assessment, diagnoses, treatment, prescribing and evaluation of interventions. The extensions to practice have led to greater patient access to care and a single point of clinical contact for many prisoners who may otherwise be bounced from one clinician to the next. This has led to more continuity of care as well as informed referrals to specialist services including inpatient admissions. Our patients, their carers and surrounding agencies appreciate the time and attention we are able to provide to them. The work can be hard but is always interesting, diverse and you never know what you may face from one day to the next.

Prisons are like most public health systems: resources are limited and demand is great. It has become necessary to operate under an interdisciplinary triaging system that assigns the most appropriate and effective resources to those with the greatest needs. My experience has been excellent, largely thanks to the support and backing of my colleagues and organisational support.

This example of a nurse practitioner programme has been overwhelmingly positive, and although these roles are still in their relative infancy, I look forward to seeing the numbers of nurse practitioners working in specialist areas like this increase over years to come.

by specialist alcohol and drug and gambling services (Dowell et al. 2009).

The number of offenders with mental health problems in prison is also increasing because of a corresponding increase in the overall prison population. This is an international phenomenon. The international mean imprisonment rate for 223 prison systems has been calculated at 144 per 100,000 population. (Walmsley 2015, p. 13).

In prison, offenders with mental health problems have the right to access mental health and addiction services equivalent to those accessible by the general population. The care and treatment of those experiencing serious mental illness (psychotic illness and major depression) may be delivered by external forensic mental health services or mainstream mental health services (in-reach services), forensic mental health services contracted to be on site or correctional health services (part of the prison service). Regardless of the model, multidisciplinary mental health teams provide assessment and voluntary treatment for prisoners.

Prison in-reach mental health nurses case-manage offenders, addressing therapeutic needs within an environment designed for custodial purposes. This results in unique challenges. Nurses frequently face access constraints as space and privacy are limited; officers may be too busy to escort a patient to an interview with the nurse; the prison may be in 'lock down' with no entry allowed into the prison and no movement allowed within the prison because of security threats; or perhaps the patient has been transferred to another location. Within the prison environment, there are often difficulties in meeting the expressed needs of offenders with mental health problems for meaningful daytime activities, psychological interventions, medication, education and multidisciplinary team expertise (Durcan 2008).

Prisons are designed to be places of punishment, retribution and deterrence and nurses working in prisons require a conscious commitment to maintain professional standards and ethical practice. The work of mental health nurses in prisons is generally not governed by mental health legislation. Small teams of nurses and sole practitioners can experience detachment from professional values. Prison regulations are at odds with what nurses can take for granted. For example, nurses are civilians in a prison and can make recommendations but not take decisions for prisoner management; nurses have limited access to prisoners out of hours when prisoners are generally locked in their cells; and giving something seemingly innocuous to a prisoner can be considered as a contraband infringement. Nurses can maintain their professional resilience and therapeutic optimism by engaging in a range of professional and organisational strategies including reflection, professional development and clinical supervision and by ensuring that they take opportunities to meet with mental health nursing colleagues.

Although nurses face challenges when working in prisons, they also experience many opportunities to practise in innovative, independent and expert ways. Nurses have key roles in many of the processes that are required for effective mental health service delivery in prisons, including:

- systematic mental health screening for mental illness at the time of reception
- ongoing mental health assessment and active treatment through a form of outpatient services
- administration of psychiatric medications in safe amounts
- a range of options in which treatment can take place—acute assessment or high-dependency needs units and rehabilitation units within correction centres
- referral processes that are required to facilitate access to psychiatric treatment outside of a prison when necessary
- systematic identification, treatment and supervision of prisoners with suicidal tendencies
- crisis intervention services
- assisting with the transition of, planning for and treatment of prisoners being transferred to other prisons or released. Post release community transition can include making referrals for accommodation, employment, substance use programmes and other necessary supports (Weiskopf 2005).

Nurse's Story 14.3 by Katherine Duffy demonstrates how nurses can contribute to the mental health of prisoners, despite the challenges of the location.

Forensic Mental Health Hospitals

Forensic mental health hospitals (and units) take a range of forms that are influenced by local legislation, policies and other services that are available. Some are stand-alone facilities, some are colocated with prisons and others are set within larger mental health services. These hospitals are able to provide specialist assessment and treatment in conditions of safety and security.

The patients who are generally found in the forensic setting are those who are:

- found unfit to plead
- found not guilty because of mental illness at the time of the offence
- referred from courts for assessment and treatment
- referred from prison because they need involuntary treatment under mental health legislation
- referred from general mental health services because they are too high a risk to be managed in a less secure environment

Forensic mental health hospitals are able to provide acute care, recovery-oriented services, continuing care and pre-discharge planning to enable the safe and successful return of patients to the referring agency or placement in the community. Primarily, the hospitals aim to assess and treat the forensic patient's mental illness, as well as to treat and manage, when present, substance use and personality disorder. There is also a need for risk assessment, treatment and management of factors related to offending behaviour. Work in

NURSE'S STORY 14.3

Katherine Duffy, Clinical Nurse Specialist in a Prison Mental Health Team

My role as a clinical nurse specialist was developed following recognition of the need for specialist psychological interventions for offenders with mental health problems. The remit I was given, as the first clinician to take this role, was to develop and implement group and individual interventions for patients on the case load. The team covers four separate prison sites including maximum security, remand and a women's facility, and as such the people in these environments have quite diverse issues and circumstances, making the role a challenging and complex one.

It became clear that one of the areas of greatest need was the vulnerable prisoners unit of one of the prisons. This tends to be the area where individuals with severe and chronic mental health issues are accommodated and often they are unable to attend the programmes that they need to meet the requirements of the parole board. This is a consequence of being unable to mix with mainstream prisoners due to their vulnerability. The requirements of the parole board often include education on mental health issues, education about the impact of drugs and alcohol on mental health and offending behaviour, and anger management. If prisoners are unable to attend these programmes, they are unable to achieve parole.

It also became clear that there is a group of prisoners with complex mental health needs who are often transferred between prison and forensic mental health inpatient units. While these individuals are inpatients, they are able to attend therapeutic programmes, which they often find extremely beneficial. Unfortunately, on their return to prison, they are unable to continue to work on issues that they have begun to address and the initial progress made by this hard work is lost.

It was decided that the first programme to be run would be a 'recovery' programme. This would address the issue of offenders in the special needs unit being unable to attend psychoeducation groups; it would also provide some continuity of care between the prison and the inpatient units.

Building on this concept of continuity of care between prison and hospital, a group was devised by the occupational therapist and me on the acute admissions unit. This was a cognitive behavioural therapy (CBT) based group to look at new ways of managing stress. The idea was that we would cofacilitate the programme in each environment, providing not only common understanding of concepts and language but also some continuity in terms of staff working with offenders. The group was a great success and we had unanimous positive feedback from participants, prison staff and the parole board. Not only are these groups now being run on a regular basis on the acute admissions unit and the vulnerable prisoners, unit, but they have also been adapted for use at the women's prison.

In addition to the development and implementation of group programmes, there has also been a huge number of referrals for individual CBT. The variety of different issues that people can present with was a little overwhelming initially. The patients have often had very difficult histories with multiple traumas throughout their lives; they also often have coexisting major mental illness and personality disorders. Many of the referrals have been for people experiencing posttraumatic stress disorder–related symptoms, depression, anxiety, obsessive compulsive disorder, hearing voices and self-injury behaviours.

I have been in this role for 2 years and no 2 days of that time have ever been the same. One thing that continues to surprise me is the motivation of the offenders that we work with. They attend weekly, having completed tasks that were set for them, and they actively engage in group activities. In fact, they are probably the most motivated group of service users I have ever worked with. Feedback such as 'If you don't learn this stuff then your mind is like an untrained monkey in the tree of life' and 'I have learned that my mental illness is like a motorcycle and drugs are the fuel that make it go', make the hard work of planning and facilitating these groups worth every minute!

NURSE'S STORY 14.4

Tony Berry, Inpatient Forensic Mental Health Nurse

A pool hall may seem an odd place for a forensic mental health nurse to be found during work hours, but not if you're Tony Berry and the people you are supporting are practising drug-refusal techniques.

'We go into pool halls and bars to practise drug-refusal skills in the real world, so service users experience the sensory effects of these environments. By ordering their own non-alcoholic drinks at the bar, the people we are supporting have to talk to bar staff and cope with this new experience of not drinking,' explains Tony.

'Before the community outing, we do a motivational interviewing group programme (You Call the Shots) and theory sessions that focus on goal setting, assertiveness training, drug-refusal skills and relapse prevention. These programmes focus on the skills and strengths of people, their communication with others, and what they need to do to cope with cravings and offers of alcohol and drugs in the community. It is a progressive thing. Once we know they have grasped the theory, we choose people who are ready for the community part. The people we are supporting are referred through the multidisciplinary team reviews.'

Tony runs the programme in his role as a forensic mental health nurse on a secure 20-bed mental inpatient recovery unit. The alcohol and drug programme was developed with the realisation that more than 90% of service users in the inpatient area had been heavily involved in alcohol and drugs in the weeks leading up to their index offence. It is part of the overall wellness and recovery programme at the facility.

(*Source*: Adapted from Te Pou, 2010. Fostering change: Tony Berry, forensic psychiatric nurse. Handover Winter pp. 5–6.)

the hospitals also supports the personal recovery of forensic mental health patients, ameliorates the factors that decrease patient's quality of life and facilitates successful reintegration into the community. Ultimately, forensic mental health hospitals are charged with the responsibility of ensuring public safety through the safe containment of patients but, more importantly, through returning patients to the community. This challenge is reflected in Nurse's Story 14.4 by Tony Berry.

CRITICAL THINKING CHALLENGE 14.1

1. What might be your response if you were assigned the care of someone who had killed another person and was found not guilty because of mental ill health (related to the patient's experience of mental illness)?
2. How could your response influence your care for this person?
3. What measures could you put in place to protect the therapeutic relationship if you were experiencing negative feelings towards this person?

Security

Forensic mental health hospitals are complex settings where the role of integrating therapy, recovery, safety and security is not well understood by justice agencies, mainstream mental health services or the community generally. Security refers to all the processes that ensure patients do not escape from the hospital or abscond from approved leave (Wilkie et al. 2014). The failure to maintain security may have implications for public safety should the patient abscond or be absent without approval. There are repercussions for the patient who escapes or absconds. They may lose leave privileges, be transferred to a more secure setting or experience delayed discharge or release. Integrating therapeutic goals with security requirements is a challenge and the mental health nurse needs to maximise therapeutic endeavour creatively within the constraints imposed by security requirements. This emphasis on safety and security has physical, procedural and relational dimensions (Department of Health 2010).

Physical security. Forensic mental health hospitals use a variety of technologies and structural elements to assist in the maintenance of physical security. These include:

- locked doors
- high walls and fences
- surveillance cameras
- locking systems
- alarms
- scanning devices such as metal detectors

Procedural security. Procedural security refers to the policies and procedures that outline the requirements to maintain security and safety. These include:

- counting patients to detect escape
- counting and safe storage of equipment, tools and implements
- searching facilities, patients' belongings and patients
- searching visitors and supervising their activities
- screening communication such as mail and telephone calls
- escorting patients on approved leave

Relational Security. This dimension of security arises out of the therapeutic relationship between the nurse and the forensic patient and involves the nurse assessing, understanding and treating the person and knowing the potential circumstances that increase a security risk. This requires the nurse to know the patient's history, risk potential, current mental health state, behaviour and stressors. Strategies must be implemented to manage any risk. Even though such requirements are intrusive and potentially demeaning, if they are carried out with an accompanying explanation and if the nurse engages with people in a respectful and empathetic manner, it helps to reduce the sense of disempowerment. It should also be noted that these security procedures do contribute to patients feeling safer as they are the most likely victims of other patients (Daffern et al. 2003).

For example, when searching a forensic mental health patient's bedroom, the nurse would be observing for frayed carpet, pieces of glass or other self-harm items, too many electrical items and cords—these observations are all concerned with safety. The cleanliness of the contents of the room, what clothing and personal items the patient has, what hobbies and personal interests are evident could relate to therapeutic goals and provide information about the patient's mental and social state. The presence of maps, large sums of money and personal identification could identify security concerns. Anything identified by the nurse can be used as an opportunity for discussion with the patient.

Nurses working within these facilities undertake assessment, assist with treatment and facilitate recovery. Effective treatment and recovery require that forensic mental health patients are given opportunities to practise and test their progress in real-life situations. Leave is therefore an important component of recovery, but approval of leave is dependent on factors such as legal status, risk assessment and the perceived contribution of leave to facilitate recovery goals. Leave from the hospital remains a vulnerable area for forensic mental health services, because political and media reactions to escapes or absconding are generally extreme. The impact on the nurses is great as they are often the escorts for patients, but the greatest impact is on the patient: not only is the absconding patient affected by having their level of security reviewed, but all patients can be affected when all leave stops or when stricter conditions of leave are applied to all patients. Nurses carry a great responsibility to protect forensic mental health patients from their own actions.

Security procedures can be invasive and some are exceedingly invasive. However, it is the way the procedures are carried out that can have the greatest impact on patients and on nurses' ongoing relationship with patients. Insensitivity can potentially damage the results of effective interpersonal work (Department of Health 2010).

ETHICAL DILEMMA 14.1

A patient's presentation, ability to meet recovery goals and risk assessment indicate that he is ready for escorted leave in the community. However, you are aware that his violent offence has attracted substantial interest from the media, including the publication of his photo. How could you balance the patient's rights for recovery in the community with the rights of the general public to feel safe?

CRITICAL THINKING CHALLENGE 14.2

Identify how nurses can integrate therapeutic, safety and security goals when undertaking the following procedures:

- searching a bedroom
- counting cutlery
- supervising a person
- supervising visits

The Community

The correct treatment, support and level of supervision are essential to assist forensic mental health patients to maximise their successful transition from prison or a forensic mental health hospital to the community. Crucial supports include early, meaningful engagement with mental health services and substance use agencies (McKenna et al. 2015). Justice agencies may also be involved if the patient is on bail or parole or another order requiring ongoing justice involvement. Assistance to address social care needs is crucial and includes the need for housing, food, financial assistance, employment and social supports (Freudenberg et al. 2005).

The planning to establish this support should commence a number of months before a person is released from custody. Agencies that will work with the patient after they leave custody should start building a relationship with them by visiting them while they are still in prison or hospital. Pre-release planning and relationship-building bring together a variety of possible supports in partnership with the patient. Through this process, it is more likely that all involved will clearly understand one another's roles and be able to demonstrate a clear commitment to the patient following release. In addition, this ensures time for trust to be established, which makes engagement more likely once the patient is in the community and recidivism less likely (McKenna et al. 2015).

Imprisoned offenders constitute a small proportion of the sentenced population, with the criminal justice system favouring community sentencing options (Elias 2009). Little is known about the rates of mental illness in this population, although literature indicates that approximately 30% of the probation caseload have had formal contact with mental health services (Brooker et al. 2008). Patients who offend and are placed on community-based orders are usually linked to general mental health services. Furthermore, general mental health services engage with patients with complex needs who may have a forensic history or patterns of behaviour indicative of potential criminal involvement. Specialist community forensic liaison roles involving mental health nurses and psychiatrists have been piloted to assist mainstream mental health services to manage this group of patients.

Specialist community forensic mental health teams have also been established to assist forensic patients transitioning to the community from forensic mental health hospitals and prisons. The model of care of these teams often involves intensive case management with the goal of eventual transfer to general mental health services. Forensic mental health community services provide assessment, consultation and ongoing treatment or shared care with general mental health services.

There are numerous sources of referral to community forensic mental health services, including forensic mental health hospitals, justice agencies (courts, prisons, community corrections or the parole boards) and legal aid centres. Forensic patients are not always well accepted by mainstream community mental health services and tend to be referred to community forensic mental health services if they have a past history of violence and other offending; high levels of anger, suspicion or hostility; poor response or nonadherence to treatment and service engagement; or substance misuse (Coffey 2012).

As case managers in community forensic mental health teams, nurses coordinate necessary services including health, legal, social, vocational, financial and accommodation services. They assist to manage mental illness, substance abuse, offending and other specific concerns, in order to facilitate clinical recovery and support personal recovery. The community care of forensic patients also requires working with families and carers. Collaboration is often required for joint management with other agencies to comprehensively address complex needs and avoid duplication in services (Coffey 2012).

THE KNOWLEDGE, SKILLS AND ATTITUDES REQUIRED OF THE FORENSIC MENTAL HEALTH NURSE

The term 'forensic mental health nurse' is applied to a nurse working in forensic mental health or criminal justice settings, rather than being a professionally recognised classification. Most mental health nurses, at some time, will provide care and treatment for patients with an offending history or at risk of offending. When a patient has committed an offence and is experiencing mental illness, the nurse is expected to apply the core knowledge, skills and attitudes of nursing generally, mental health nursing specifically and the additional or enhanced skills that are required to work effectively with forensic mental health patients. The following section considers some of the knowledge, skills and attitudes that are needed by mental health nurses providing care and treatment to forensic mental health patients in police custody centres, prisons, forensic mental health hospitals and the community.

Assessment and Management of Risk

In forensic mental health nursing, the nurse undertakes rigorous risk assessment processes with forensic patients to identify the factors that indicate risk to self or others and the protective factors that mitigate such risk. Forensic mental health risk assessment has developed considerably since Monahan (1983) argued that psychiatrists and psychologists appeared to be wrong at least twice as often as they were right in their unstructured clinical predictions of violence. We have since moved from a second generation of actuarial prediction, which often focussed on static risk factors such as gender and age that were not amenable to change, to a third generation of structured clinical judgement. The third generation of violence risk assessment has moved beyond the prediction of an adverse event to the identification of the risk factors that contribute to the likelihood of an adverse event, a focus on dynamic factors (such as nonadherence to medication) that are open to clinical modification to reduce such risk and an emphasis on protective factors, such as a strong support group, that if enhanced also diminish the potential for adverse events (Allnutt 2013). Prevention and management of offending, especially violence, have become the focus of contemporary risk assessment in forensic mental health.

Following assessment, the nurse implements evidence-based interventions to manage risk and assists forensic patients to self-manage their risk behaviours. This dynamic process requires ongoing risk assessment and adaptation of interventions according to the patient's changing risk status. All of these processes are therapeutic tasks that should occur within the context of the therapeutic relationship (Daffern et al. 2015). Risk assessment and management involve a structured clinical judgement based on a three-phase sequential process. This process encompasses gathering accurate information, understanding the person's pathway to violence and developing a pathway to safety (Evans et al. 2006). Chapter 23 is devoted to challenging behaviours, responses and risk assessment and it provides the nurse with additional guidance about how to assess and to respond to a range of confronting situations.

Gathering Accurate Information

The first phase of structured clinical judgement in risk assessment involves an understanding of the patient's historical involvement in risk behaviour through gathering accurate information about past incidents. For each event, a description must be gathered of what actually transpired. For example, in cases of violence the following factors could be identified:

- hazard identification (which event will occur?)
- imminence (how soon?)
- hazard accounting (how frequent? how serious?)
- scenarios of exposure (in what context?)
- risk characterisation (what conditions are present?)
- nature of violence (instrumental or reactive?)
- targets/victims
- weapon use (what type? how lethal?) (Carroll 2009)

This form of assessment enables an understanding of the event, but it is also necessary to assess comprehensively the range of factors that have been found to be correlated to the risk being assessed. A number of forensic risk assessment tools have been developed through extensive research and validation studies to assist in the process of structured clinical judgement. These tools are formally administered but can also be used as an aide mémoire to assist in covering the range of risk factors that need to be considered in gathering information and pattern recognition. They also enable clarification of those risk factors that are static (cannot be changed) and dynamic (can be changed through risk management). The four most-used forensic risk assessment tools are:

- The HCR-20 (Historical, Clinical and Risk 20; Webster et al. 1997). This 20-item risk assessment tool assists in articulating risk to others through historical involvement in violence and the presence of the mental health-related and situational risk factors.
- The START (Short-Term Assessment of Risk and Treatability; Webster et al. 2009). The START is an adaptation of the HCR-20 that considers more general risks beyond risk to others. It also assists in the identification and assessment of protective risk factors, which, if present, could prevent or reduce the likelihood of an adverse event.
- The Level of Service/Case Management Inventory (Andrews et al. 2008). This assessment tool identifies and measures the risk factors of offenders. The tool also assists in the identification of strategies for treatment planning and management of offenders in justice and forensic mental health settings to reduce recidivism.
- The DASA:IV (Ogloff & Daffern 2006). The DASA:IV is a structured clinical judgement tool for the 'dynamic appraisal of situational aggression' in an inpatient setting. It is designed as a guide for assessing the likelihood of inpatient aggression and is used on a daily basis. The tool takes approximately 5 minutes to complete and is usually completed by a patient's contact nurse. The DASA is intended not only to predict the risk of aggression but also to assist in managing the risk by prompting interventions (if indicated by the assessment) that may reduce the likelihood of the patient engaging in aggressive behaviour.

Risk factors considered in these tools include the items shown in Box 14.1.

Comprehensive information needs to be collected in a systematic manner. Some of the sources that help to contribute to the collection of comprehensive information about the patient are: interviews with the forensic patient, their family/carers and any person with relevant information to contribute to the process; a review of the clinical files and other documentation (e.g. legal reports, incident reports); and the use of relevant risk assessment tools.

Risk assessment requires input from the multidisciplinary team. Other health professionals contribute expertise in specific areas and criminal justice staff should also be consulted as they often have information about the patient that augments the assessment. Risk assessment is also undertaken in collaboration with the forensic mental health patient to facilitate their understanding.

CRITICAL THINKING CHALLENGE 14.3

Consider the risk assessment factors that are included in the commonly used forensic mental health risk assessment tools (see Box 14.1). Select a few factors and identify which mental health nursing strategies could be used to treat and/or manage these factors.

BOX 14.1 Risk Factors Considered in the Four Most-Used Forensic Risk Assessment Tools

- Adherence with mediation
- Antisocial attitudes
- Antisocial patterns of behaviour
- Barriers to release
- Case-specific factors
- Companions/peers
- Coping skills
- Criminal history
- Early maladjustment
- Education
- Emotional state
- Exposure to destabilisers
- External triggers
- Family/marital
- Impulsivity
- Insight
- Leisure/recreation
- Material resources
- Medication adherence
- Mental state
- Occupation
- Personal support
- Personality disorder
- Plans
- Previous violence
- Prior supervision failure
- Prison experience—institutional factors
- Psychopathy
- Recreation
- Relationships
- Responsiveness to treatment
- Rule adherence
- Self-care
- Social skills
- Social support
- Stress
- Substance use
- Young age at first violent incident

Understanding the Pathway to Violence

A detailed understanding of individual events, supported by a structured risk assessment and clinical judgement, enables the second phase of structured clinical judgement, which is the determination of the patient's pathway to violence. The factors that have been identified in the assessment are pulled together in a risk statement that allows for specific treatment and management strategies to be identified. For example: 'This person is at risk of (specific risk behaviours) when they are experiencing (specific internal factors) in the following circumstances (specific situational aspects that support the behaviour)' (Evans et al. 2006).

Developing a Pathway to Safety

Historical factors provide good information about a patient's offending, but the risk factors and attributes of the offender are usually dynamic in nature and can be altered through active treatment and management. Identification of these risk factors and attributes automatically highlights what can be done in order for a risk to be averted. Therefore, management of these factors constitutes the third phase of structured clinical judgement, which is developing a pathway to safety for the individual.

The offending risk assessment is a transparent and accountable process that aims to improve the consistency of decisions that inform treatment and risk management to prevent offending. The process is useful to determine the appropriate setting for the forensic mental health patient, to identify those patients requiring intensive interventions and to inform leave and discharge decisions. The risk assessment facilitates effective communication between the forensic mental health patient and other agencies involved and forms the basis for advice or reports for ongoing treatment and management.

Use of Coercion

Given the emphasis in forensic mental health nursing on risk assessment, risk management, security and safety, the ability to implement these processes with therapeutic intent suggests a challenge. The tension is amplified by the use of legal mechanisms that support all of these processes. It is preferable that mental health patients enter treatment voluntarily; however, some forensic mental health patients may not be competent or willing to enter such arrangements. Even then, human rights conventions such as the United Nations Convention on the Rights of Persons with Disabilities require that human dignity be upheld and support given to reinforce the patient's autonomous decision-making ability (McSherry 2013).

The therapeutic goal of legal sanctions to enforce treatment is that of beneficial outcomes for the person experiencing mental illness. Yet the paradox is that it may result in the recipient experiencing limited choice, limited autonomous decision making or limits to their ability to act on their own volition. This may in turn be detrimental to the therapeutic intent, create mistrust of those trying to help and lead to long-term difficulties of engagement with those services intended to assist.

Significant coercion is experienced by forensic patients admitted to forensic hospitals under mental health legislation (McKenna et al. 2003). Therefore, it is important that nurses understand how coercion is perceived by patients and implement strategies to reduce patients' perceptions of coercion, while attempting to achieve the goal of beneficial therapeutic outcomes. The best strategies are grounded in the therapeutic relationship, which is the cornerstone of mental health nursing practice. Irrespective of their placement in a forensic service, patients should be exposed to processes that are fair and free from the value biases and vested interests of decision makers (including nurses) and that include mechanisms for correcting bad decisions. Patients should be able to express their views and have these views considered seriously by clinicians. This open and honest dialogue should leave patients feeling that they have been treated with dignity, respect, politeness and concern. Forensic mental health patients also require accurate and relevant information about the procedures they are involved in (McKenna et al. 2006).

As soon as the door is locked or constraints are placed on a forensic mental health patient's freedom, a power dynamic is created between the nurse and that person. This power dynamic is further enhanced by the rules through which the cohesiveness of the ward community is maintained. It is inevitable that the nurse, as the main enforcer of these rules, is perceived to hold power over the forensic mental health patient. This is often a source of conflict, as patients often struggle with rules, authority and impulsivity related to antisocial beliefs and values. Within the custodial environment of a forensic mental health hospital there is limited flexibility. It is important that what little flexibility exists is framed to allow the optimal degree of choice and autonomy for patients.

Nurses can reduce patient frustration by providing explanations as to why certain rules apply and giving patients the opportunity to discuss their concerns about security requirements, rules and limits that have been imposed. Such empathic, open, honest discussions can help alleviate patient concerns. For example, a patient may request time alone at a time when staff numbers and other ward concerns make the supervision required difficult. Rather than flatly refusing this request, the nurse can express a spirit of compromise by creatively exploring other options, such as delaying the time alone to another time of the day when ward priorities are less pressing. Situations like this can escalate into conflict or they can be treated as therapeutic opportunities to assist patients to solve problems, delay gratification and show understanding of the needs of others.

The obligation of forensic mental health nurses is to consider the least restrictive alternatives in risk management and to reduce the use of restrictive interventions such as seclusion. Research in forensic mental health settings has demonstrated that such a systemic approach can reduce both the frequency of the use of seclusion and its duration (Maguire et al. 2012).

ETHICAL DILEMMA 14.2

1. How would you balance your desire to maximise the forensic mental health patient's autonomous decision-making ability with the expressions of other staff to use compulsory treatment?
2. How would you balance your desire to maximise the forensic mental health patent's autonomy with their request to reduce the medication dosage when the patient has a long history of violent offending in the context of acute symptoms of mental illness?

Safety

The need for safety in the forensic mental health hospital is crucial. Forensic mental health patients generally have a mental illness, a history of offending, personality attributes and ways of acting and reacting that heighten their potential for risk of harm to self and others. Nurses working in forensic mental health hospitals are likely to be caring for patients who consistently present with seriously challenging behaviours, including aggression and violence (Daffern et al. 2015). Aggression may be an inevitable outcome of providing treatment to involuntary forensic mental health patients, some of whom will have limited skills to manage anger provoked by the ongoing demands, expectations and conflict of inpatient treatment (Daffern 2007).

While mental illness may influence a patient's aggression, other behavioural and cognitive processes (such as recent history of substance abuse, entrenched negative attitudes, antisocial behaviour) play a significant role in increasing the potential for aggressive behaviour (Daffern, Howells & Ogloff 2007). The most common offence committed by forensic mental health patients is violence (Braham et al. 2008). Forensic mental health nurses are faced with managing behaviours that are not always related to a patient's mental state and the consequences available for such actions may be insignificant for patients who have been exposed to punitive conditions during incarceration and may have experienced mistreatment (Daffern et al. 2007).

Although there are barriers that work against nurses in forensic hospitals being able to manage forensic mental health patients safely, there are also opportunities, such as the benefits of longer admissions, resulting in reduced access to illicit substances and increased access to treatment (Daffern et al. 2007); a higher staff–patient ratio, providing the opportunity for nurses to work with patients to undertake assessment, treatment and other environmental interventions (Timmons 2010); and access to best-practice risk assessment and management tools. Martin and Daffern (2006), in their study of clinicians at one forensic mental health hospital, found that clinicians reported confidence in their ability to manage aggression in an environment where aggression is frequent. Certain organisational factors that are generally more developed in forensic mental health hospitals (such as training, competent colleagues, a physical environment that is designed to prevent and manage aggression, policies and procedures) can support a perception of safety, which may then contribute to confidence in effectively managing aggression.

Forensic mental health nurses are responsible for working with management, the multidisciplinary team, patients and families to create safe workplace cultures. This requires nurses to have a working knowledge of workplace health and safety legislation, risk management skills, involvement in the development of safety procedures and involvement in critical incident reviews that enable quality improvement in service delivery.

Promote Optimal Physical Health

Forensic mental health patients are at a high risk of developing metabolic syndrome and associated physical illnesses such as diabetes, cardiovascular disease and respiratory problems (Robson & Gray 2007). Although a key contributing factor is the use of antipsychotic medications (Graham et al. 2008), restrictions on activities and lifestyle choices in custodial environments contribute to physical health deficits. Forensic mental health nurses must contribute to an environment that promotes a healthy lifestyle through health education and health-enhancing activities. A comprehensive nursing health assessment must include physical health and the nurse must work with the patient, their family and the multidisciplinary team to develop, implement and evaluate treatment plans that promote and enhance optimal physical health. In the literature, there are examples of mental health nurses initiating healthy living programmes targeted to address physical healthcare concerns with forensic mental health patients (for example, see Prebble et al. 2011). There is also NICE (2016) guidance (NG57) on the physical health of people in prison that offers guidance to addressing the inequalities patient experience. See also Chapter 8.

THE ETHICAL DIMENSION IN FORENSIC MENTAL HEALTHCARE

For some nurses, the ability to provide care can potentially be compromised by the complex presentation of some forensic mental health patients. Antisocial personality attributes that are not pleasant to relate to may present as a contributing factor that clouds the forensic mental health nurse's ability to place moral judgement to one side—for example, when the nurse becomes the target of hostile, manipulative or threatening behaviour, or when the patient splits staff into those liked and those disliked and attempts to play staff off against each other. In forensic mental health settings, forensic mental health nurses may also encounter protest behaviour. Examples of protest behaviour include spreading faeces on self or property, refusal to speak or eat, successfully getting on the rooftop and refusing to come down or rampage involving property damage. In addition, hostage-taking and barricades are critical incidents that may occur in forensic settings (Ireland et al. 2014). These types of incidents are generally infrequent; however, they are significant events (Vollum et al. 2013). Forensic mental health nursing research has articulated the difficulties faced by nurses when confronting moral judgements concerning such behaviour. Poor judgements regarding this behaviour compromise the delivery of nursing care. For instance, framing a patient as primarily 'bad' can result in a total absence of planned care in the form of care plans for this patient (Mason et al. 2002).

It is essential that forensic mental health nurses recognise and manage their personal feelings and values related to the offences committed by forensic mental health patients. Nurses who focus on the offences and allow their feelings and values to dominate their clinical perspective of patients will be ineffective in providing care. Often, professional dissonance is experienced. Equally inappropriate is the belief that the offending behaviour is not a concern of the nurse. In such cases, nurses may choose to ignore offending behaviour because they find the personal and moral effects distressing. But by ignoring the offending behaviour, a significant forensic mental health patient need is not addressed. Offending and other antisocial behaviours distinguish patients within the forensic mental health setting. The professional response is to view offending behaviour as another need to be addressed during therapeutic engagement with the forensic mental health patient. Patients need to understand the factors associated with their offending behaviour in order to increase their personal choice and responsibility.

Nurses are involved in both individual and group processes aimed at addressing offending behaviour. However, the specific complexities of offenders, coupled with the very nature of the custodial environment, create a tension in the caring role (Austin et al. 2006). Failure to resolve this tension can lead to the adverse development of cultures of toughness (whereby intimidation and force are used to manage clinical settings), boundary violations (whereby professional relationships revert to personal, even intimate, relationships), counter-transference difficulties (whereby nurses allow personal issues to cloud the therapeutic relationship), cynicism regarding the value of the therapeutic relationship and avoidance in addressing the needs of forensic mental health patients .

Strategies to manage this tension include professional supervision, exposure to new ideas through staff development initiatives and the development of a culture of critique, which continuously scrutinises clinical decision making, practice and communication with forensic mental health patients. Mental health nurses can turn to professional codes of conduct and ethics to assist in solving ethical dilemmas. (See Chapters 1, 4 and 10 for more information about clinical supervision, professional relationships, counter-transference and other professional and ethical practice issues.)

MULTIDISCIPLINARY TEAM INVOLVEMENT

Multidisciplinary team input at all levels of service delivery is an accepted practice in mental healthcare. This includes patient and carer advisors. The multiple disciplinary perspectives, knowledge and skills enhance assessment and treatment of patients. The mental health nurse works as a member of a multidisciplinary team at the interface of the criminal justice and mental health systems and is likely to be working in teams that include criminal justice staff. These staff may include prison officers, community corrections officers, police officers, security staff, court staff, solicitors and lawyers. Other external agency staff may also join teams to support patients' mental health, social care and recovery needs, including alcohol and drug providers and staff from the non-governmental sector such as supportive accommodation providers and disability employment agencies.

Mental health nurses need to understand the politico-legal context (see Chapter 4) in which they are working. They also need to develop ways of working collaboratively and without compromising professional nursing standards with justice colleagues whose focus may not be primarily on healthcare. Nurses based in courts, prisons and police custody centres work in settings that are not health oriented and where the culture is custodial. Working effectively with the range of justice staff is best achieved when the interface between the disciplines is flexible and versatile and there is understanding of complementary interests and skills (Lazzaretto-Green et al. 2011). The nurse's stories of Kevin Seaton, Nathan Bruce and Katherine Duffy demonstrate that forensic mental health nurses can and do integrate nursing skills effectively within the framework of the criminal justice system. While effective communication can improve assessment and treatment, provide support and reduce risk, nurses must be aware of issues of

PATIENT STORY 14.1

Redemption Versus Stigma

In 2007, a part-time employee at a zoo was sacked when the media revealed to his employer that he was a patient at the local forensic mental health service. Six years earlier the man had tragically killed his mother when he was psychotically ill. The court found him not guilty for reasons of insanity and since then he had engaged well with services addressing mental health and offending-related needs. The employment was part of a recovery pathway towards successful integration into the community (Rudman 2007). In response to this event, a fellow patient wrote the following letter to the editor (New Zealand Herald), which exemplifies the stigma offenders with mental health problems experience.

Dear Editor,

One of my mother's catchphrases was 'make yourself useful'. I think every human needs to feel that they have something, however small, to contribute, to someone or to society. Even though we are all here [in a forensic mental health service] because we have violated human laws in some way, we feel this need too. Perhaps especially much because we have all done wrong: we need to make up for our bad deeds, to try to balance the scale somehow. In a recent newspaper article about prisons, the author stated that the main desire of the prison population is to be able to make up for the harm they have done to family and society. Apart from the odd psychopath, I guess most of us are not so evil that we can live easily with the harm we have done.

In this sense, being incarcerated without anything constructive to do is truly the worst punishment. There is no way to balance the scale, no way to contribute in the smallest way, no hope even of looking after ourselves, as everything is done for us, provided for us. All that are left are very long days of reliving again and again the past. This is justice I suppose, and when I was a 'normal' person I would not have cared for the emotional suffering of prisoners as long as they were away from 'good' people. Now, I am obsessed with the idea of redemption—I suppose it is hard to contemplate being consigned to the scrapheap for the rest of my natural life, just though this may be.

Watching Oprah today, she said what many others have expressed also, that you cannot fill your life with things, even with ambitions or achievements. The only way you can fill yourself with life is to give yourself away.

Making yourself useful, seeking redemption, giving yourself away—three ways to see the business of living. Easily done perhaps when we are well and free, and something that most people do as naturally as breathing; giving time, effort and care to family, friends, neighbours, work, and leisure interests. But when you have gone off the tracks, or have to struggle with mental illness, when you cannot work, when family and friends do not call any more, when your freedom has been taken away, how can you give? Yet that is the only thing to live for, and when you are sure you have no way left to give, then that must also be the end of living.

So how can we incorporate usefulness, giving and redemption into this environment? There are so many limitations, society needs to be kept 'safe' from us, and many of us have problems that separate us from 'normal' people. But we may still have potential to contribute, the will to work. I have met people here who are talented in art, music, writing, sport; whose talents are wasted in the aimlessness of daily life here. Although the staff do their best to facilitate outings and activities, the structure of the system and the limits of their time make this an uphill battle. I am told that this used to be a working farm, with inmates providing all the labour, producing and cooking their own food and doing all chores for themselves. This must have been so much healthier an environment, apart from saving the taxpayer a lot of money. Perhaps there is not the space for this now, but the small efforts at enterprise that are provided now are much appreciated by those that have the chance to participate—surely this approach could be expanded so that we are all gainfully occupied each day?

The other thought that occurs is that voluntary work could be encouraged. Many inmates are not considered a threat to others and do not need supervision—could they not try to redeem themselves and make use of any potential they have by giving of themselves in any of the hundreds of volunteer organisations that exist in the community? There are groups to suit any inclination: working with animals, youth, local or regional conservation, helping new migrants, teaching English, coaching sports, helping the infirm, disabled or dying, constructing housing for disadvantaged families—the list could go on forever.

I understand that we have to earn the right to be trusted again with any degree of liberty. But for those that are judged not to be a risk to society, who are trusted to go to the shops unescorted, there should be more opportunity to do something with that liberty, to contribute. I believe we all want to live again, to be useful, to give.

(*Source*: Rudman, B., 2007. Zoo's sacking of Burton less than a fair go. New Zealand Herald, 28 March.)

confidentiality related to healthcare and adhere to policies and legislation regarding verbal and written communication with justice colleagues.

CULTURE AND FAMILY

There is a strong need for cultural competency and cultural safety in forensic mental health nursing. This is a critical component of care in forensic mental health given the overrepresentation of migrant cultures in forensic mental health services. There is a strong awareness in forensic mental health services of the cultural needs of the communities served and the necessity for an appropriate response to these needs. Forensic mental health nurses must pay attention to cultural needs throughout the therapeutic process. Additional cultural expertise may be needed to assist this; for example, the inclusion of local cultural leaders in forensic mental health consultation processes, community outreach and recovery plans.

Central to any culture is the family. Family members have the potential to provide a vital link to the community for the patient and to promote the patient's wellbeing through supportive relationships. However, mental illness and the nature of the offence and its consequences may compromise this potential. For example, family members are more likely to be victims when perpetrators of serious violence have a mental illness (Canning et al. 2009). Furthermore, containment of the patient can have an impact on family function (emotional, financial and/or social). The nurse must be part of the multidisciplinary team endeavouring to assist in healing family relationships and maximising the potential of the family to be partners in addressing the needs of forensic mental health patients.

MINIMISING STIGMA AND DISCRIMINATION FOR FORENSIC PATIENTS

The possible outcome of patients' engagement with forensic mental health services is double stigma: criminality and mental illness. Community attitudes towards both are misinformed, ignorant and fearful. The media, through which the public becomes 'informed', tends to present offenders with mental health problems in a manner that potentially feeds into this stigma (McKenna et al. 2007). This stigma in turn impacts on identity, self-concept and self-esteem (Livingston et al. 2011). Understanding, support, education and advocacy are necessary to combat stigma and discrimination. It is crucial that forensic mental health nurses work in partnership with forensic mental health patients in this regard.

CONCLUSION

This chapter was written to assist students to explore the practice reality of forensic mental health nursing. The challenges of this practice reality are characterised by 'complexity'. This complexity relates to the needs of forensic mental health patients, the configuration of services to meet these needs and the law that dictates service provision. All of these present as challenges to forensic mental health nursing practice. However, satisfaction with nursing in this area is a direct corollary of this complexity. The challenges of the complexity can inspire nurses and create a passion for serving some of the most vulnerable and disadvantaged people in our society. The relationships nurses establish with forensic mental health patients are pivotal to this work, although there is recognition that forensic mental health patients often come to the relationship with a history of trauma, distrust and cynicism. Breaking through such barriers and meeting the challenge of recovery-oriented care are possible when nurses maintain therapeutic optimism and an ethical approach to care.

EXERCISES FOR CLASS ENGAGEMENT

Discuss the following questions with your group.

1. Explore your own responses to caring for forensic mental health patients whom the general public might consider to be 'bad' and 'mad'. Brainstorm what sort of challenges these patients might present for nursing care.
2. Which factors could influence the therapeutic relationship when the patient is also an offender?
3. The court liaison nurse or prison nurse needs to work closely with justice colleagues whose focus is not primarily on healthcare. Discuss some of the challenges you might encounter in working collaboratively with justice colleagues.
4. Brainstorm the different skills, knowledge and attributes you believe are required of the forensic mental health nurse when working in a prison, court or forensic mental health hospital setting.
5. Wherever forensic mental health nurses are working, it is their responsibility to understand the legislation that impacts on their practice. Locate from websites in your country the criminal justice legislation regarding 'unfit to plead' and 'not guilty by reason of mental illness' (or its equivalent). What are the implications of these laws for patients (i.e. where people are sent, for how long and how patients can have their legal status changed)?
6. The mental health nurse must always be thoughtful about engaging the service user's family, carers or significant others in their treatment. When a patient is also an offender, what do you think might be the needs and concerns of the family/carers/significant others? What can mental health nurses do in their work with them?

REFERENCES

Allnutt, S., Ogloff, J., Adams, J., O'Driscoll, C., Daffern, M., Carroll, A., Chaplow, D., 2013. Managing aggression and violence: the clinician's role in contemporary mental health care. Australian and New Zealand Journal of Psychiatry 47 (8), 728–736.

Andrews, D.A., Bonta, J.L., Wormith, J.S., 2008. Level of Service/Case Management Inventory. Multi-Health Systems, Toronto.

Austin, W., Bergum, V., Nuttgens, S., 2006. A re-visioning of boundaries in professional helping relationships: exploring other metaphors. Ethics and Behavior 16 (2), 77–94.

Bennett, S., Farrington, D.P., Huesmann, L.R., 2005. Explaining gender differences in crime and violence: the importance of social cognitive skills. Aggression and Violent Behavior 10, 263–288.

Bradley, K., 2009. The Bradley Report: Lord Bradley's Review of People with Mental Health Problems or Learning Disability in the Criminal Justice System. Department of Health, London. Available at: www.dh.gov.uk/en/Publicationsandstatistics/Publications/PublicationsPolicyAndGuidance/DH_098694.

Braham, L., Jones, D., Hollin, C.R., 2008. The Violent Offender Treatment Program (VOTP): development of a treatment program for violent patients in a high security psychiatric hospital. International Journal of Forensic Mental Health 7 (2), 157–172.

Brooker, C., Fox, C., Barrett, P., Syson-Nibbs, L., 2008. A health Needs Assessment of Offenders on Probation Caseloads in Nottinghamshire and Derbyshire. University of Lincoln, Lincoln.

Canning, A., O'Reilly, S., Wressell, L., Cannon, D., Walker, J., 2009. A survey exploring the provision of carers' support in medium and high secure services in England and Wales. The Journal of Forensic Psychiatry & Psychology 20 (6), 868–885.

Carroll, A., 2009. How to make good-enough risk decisions. Advances in Psychiatric Treatment 15, 192–198.

Coffey, M., 2012. Negotiating identify transition when leaving forensic hospitals. Health 16 (5), 489–506.

College of Policing, 2015. College of Policing analysis: Estimating demand on the police service. Available at: http://www.college.police.uk/News/College- news/Documents/Demand%20Report%2023_1_15_noBleed.pdf. Accessed: 15 October 2015.

Constantine, R., Andel, R., Petrila, J., Becker, M., Robs, J., Teague, G., Howe, A., 2010. Characteristics and experiences of adults with a serious mental illness who were involved in the criminal justice system. Psychiatric Services 61 (5), 451–457.

Daffern, M., 2007. The predictive validity and practical utility of structured schemes used to assess risk for aggression in psychiatric inpatient setting. Aggression and Violent Behaviour 12, 116–130.

Daffern, M., Howells, K., Ogloff, J.R.P., 2007. The interaction between individual characteristics and the function of aggression in forensic psychiatric inpatients. Psychiatry, Psychology and Law 14 (1), 17–25.

Daffern, M., Jones, L., Shine, J., 2010. Offence Paralleling Behaviour: A Case Formulation Approach to Offender Assessment and Intervention. Wiley & Sons, Chichester.

Daffern, M., Maguire, T., Carroll, A., McKenna, B., 2015. Workplace violence: a focus on the mental health sector. In: Day, A., Fernandez, E. (Eds.), Violence in Australia: Policy, Practice and Solutions. The Federation Press, New South Wales, pp. 104–116.

Daffern, M., Mayer, M., Martin, T., 2003. A preliminary investigation into patterns of aggression in an Australian forensic psychiatric hospital. The Journal of Forensic Psychiatry & Psychology 14 (1), 67–84.

Daffern, M., Ogloff, J., Ferguson, M., Thomson, L., Howells, K., 2007. Appropriate treatment targets or products of a demanding environment? The relationship between aggression in a forensic psychiatric hospital with aggressive behaviour preceding admission and violent recidivism. Psychology, Crime and Law 13, 431–441.

Department of Health, 2010. Your Guide to Relational Security: See, Think, Act. Department of Health, London.

Douglas, K., Guy, L., Hart, S., 2009. Psychosis as a risk factor for violence to others: a meta-analysis. Psychological Bulletin 135 (5), 679–706.

Dowell, A., Garrett, S., Collings, S., McBain, L., McKinlay, E., Stanley, J., 2009. Evaluation of Primary Health Care Initiatives: Summary Report, 2008. University of Otago and Ministry of Health, Wellington.

Durcan, G., 2008. From the Inside: Experiences of Prison Mental Health Care. Sainsbury Centre for Mental Health, London.

Egeressy, A., Butler, T., Hunter, M., 2009. 'Traumatisers of the traumatised': trauma experiences and personality characteristics of Australian prisoners. International Journal of Prisoner Health 5 (4), 212–222.

Elias, S., 2009. Blameless Babes. Annual 2009 Shirley Smith Address. Wellington Branch of the NZ Law Society, Victoria University, Wellington.

Evans, C., Humberstone, V., Manipoto, W., McKenna, B., Simpson, S., van Altvorst, S., Wack, R., 2006. Assessment and Management of Risk to Others: Guidelines and Development of a Training Toolkit. Mental Health Programmes, Auckland.

Fazel, S., Baillargeon, J., 2011. The health of prisoners. The Lancet 377 (9769), 965–966.

Fazel, S., Grann, M., Carlstron, E., Lichtenstien, P., Langstrom, N., 2009. Risk factors for violent crime in schizophrenia: a national cohort study of 1806 patients. Journal of Clinical Psychiatry 70 (3), 362–369.

Fazel, S., Seewald, K., 2012. Severe mental illness in 33,588 prisoners worldwide: systematic review and meta-regression analysis. British Journal of Psychiatry 200, 364–373.

Freudenberg, N., Daniels, J., Crum, M., Perkins, T., Richie, B., 2005. Coming home from jail: the social and health consequences of community reentry for women, male adolescents, and their families and communities. American Journal of Public Health 95, 1725–1736.

Graham, K., Cho, H., Brownley, K., Harp, J., 2008. Early treatment-related changes in diabetes and cardiovascular disease risk markers in first episode psychosis subjects. Schizophrenia Research 101, 287–294.

Harty, M., Tighe, J., Leese, M., Parrott, J., Thornicroft, G., 2009. Inverse care for mentally ill prisoners: unmet needs in forensic mental health services. Journal of Forensic Psychiatry and Psychology 14, 600–614.

Hodgins, S., 2008. Violent behavior among people with schizophrenia: a framework for investigations of causes, and effective treatment, and prevention. Philosophical Transactions of the Royal Society B 363 (12), 2205–2218.

International Association of Forensic Nurses, 2015. Correctional Nursing. Available at: www.forensicnurses.org/?page=correctionalnursing.

Ireland, C., Halpin, L., Sullivan, C., 2014. Critical incidents in a forensic psychiatric population: an exploratory study of motivational factors. The Journal of Forensic Psychiatry & Psychology 25 (6), 714–732.

Jackson, M., Hardy, G., 2011. ABI in the Victorian prison system. Department of Justice, Melbourne divide here Joint Commissioning Panel for Mental Health (JCP-MH) 2013 Guidance for commissioners of forensic mental health services. Available at: https://www.rcpsych.ac.uk/pdf/jcpmh-forensic-guide.pdf. Accessed: 15 October 2015.

Kooyman, L., Walsh, E., Stevens, H., Burns, T., Tyrer, P., Tattan, T., Dean, K., 2012. Criminal offending before and after the onset of psychosis: examination of an offender typology. Schizophrenia Research 140, 198–203.

Lawson, L., 2008. Forensic nursing: the maturing of a discipline. Journal of Forensic Nursing 4 (4), 147–149.

Lazzaretto-Green, D., Austin, W., Goble, E., Buys, L., Gorman, T., Rankel, M., 2011. Walking a fine line: forensic mental health practitioners' experience of working with correctional officers. Journal of Forensic Nursing 7, 109–119.

Livingston, J., Rossiter, K., Verdun-Jones, S., 2011. Forensic labelling: An empirical assessment of its effects on self-stigma for people with severe mental illness. Psychiatric Research 188 (1), 115–122.

Maguire, T., Young, R., Martin, T., 2012. Seclusion reduction in a forensic mental health setting. Journal of Psychiatric and Mental Health Nursing 19, 97–106.

Martin, T., Daffern, M., 2006. Clinician perceptions of personal safety and confidence to manage inpatient aggression in a forensic psychiatric setting. Journal of Psychiatric and Mental Health Nursing 13, 90–99.

Martin, T., Maguire, T., Quinn, C., Ryan, J., Bawden, L., Summers, M., 2013. Standards of practice for forensic mental health nurses: identifying contemporary practice. Journal of Forensic Nursing 9 (3), 171–178.

Mason, T., Richman, J., Mercer, D., 2002. The influence of evil on forensic nursing practice. International Journal of Mental Health Nursing 11 (2), 80–93.

McKenna, B., Seaton, K., 2007. Liaison services to the courts. In: Brookbanks, W., Simpson, A. (Eds.), Psychiatry and The Law. LexisNexis, Wellington, pp. 447–464.

McKenna, B., Simpson, A., Coverdale, J., 2003. Patients' perceptions of coercion on admission to forensic psychiatric hospital: a comparison study. International Journal of Law and Psychiatry 26 (4), 355–372.

McKenna, B., Simpson, A., Coverdale, J., 2006. Best practice management strategies for mental health nurses during the clinical application of civil commitment: an overview. Contemporary Nurse 21 (1), 62–70.

McKenna, B., Skipworth, J., Tapsell, R., Madell, D., Pillai, K., Simpson, A., Cavney, J., Rouse, P., 2015. Prison mental health in-reach: the impact of innovation on transition planning, community mental health service engagement and re-offending. Criminal Behaviour and Mental Health 25, 429–439.

McKenna, B., Thom, K., Simpson, A., 2007. Media coverage of homicide involving mentally disordered offenders: a matched comparison study. International Journal of Forensic Mental Health 6 (1), 57–63.

McSherry, B., 2013. Torture and ill-treatment in health care settings: lessons from the United Nations. Journal of Law and Medicine 20, 712–718.

Mental Health Act, 1983. (amended 2007) Available at: https://www.legislation.gov.uk/ukpga/1983/20/contents. Accessed: 15 October 2015.

Miles, H., Dutheil, L., Welsby, I., Haider, D., 2007. 'Just say no': a preliminary evaluation of a three-stage model of integrated treatment for substance use problems in conditions of medium security. The Journal of Forensic Psychiatry and Psychology 18 (2), 141–159.

Monahan, J., 1983. The prediction of violent behaviour: developments in psychology and law. In: Scheirer, C., James, C., Hammonds, B.L. (Eds.). Psychology and the Law. Master Lecture Series, vol. 2. American Psychological Association, Washington, DC, pp. 151–176.

National Health Service (NHS), 2006. National Health Service Act 2006. Available at: https://www.legislation.gov.uk/ukpga/2006/41/contents. Accessed: 15 October 2015.

National Institute of Health and Care Excellence (NICE), 2016. NG57 Physical Health of People in Prison. Available at: https://www.nice.org.uk/guidance/ng57. Accessed: 15 October 2018.

National Institute of Health and Care Excellence (NICE), 2017. Ng66 Mental Health of Adults in Contact with The Criminal Justice System. Available at: https://www.nice.org.uk/guidance/ng66. Accessed: 15 October 2018.

Ogloff, J., Daffern, M., 2006. The dynamic appraisal of situational aggression: an instrument to assess risk for imminent aggression in psychiatric inpatients. Behavioural Sciences and the Law 24, 799–813.

Paulin, J., Carswell, S., 2010. Evaluation of the Mental Health/Alcohol and Other Drug Watch-House Nurse Pilot Initiative. New Zealand Police, Wellington.

Prebble, K., Kidd, J., O'Brien, A., Carlyle, D., McKenna, B., Crowe, M., Deering, D., Gooder, C., 2011. Implementing and maintaining nurse-led healthy living programmes in forensic inpatient settings: an illustrative case study. Journal of the American Psychiatric Nurses Association 17 (2), 127–138.

Robson, D., Gray, R., 2007. Serious mental illness and physical problems: a discussion paper. International Journal of Nursing Studies 44, 457–466.

Rudman, B., 2007. Zoo's sacking of Burton less than a fair go. New Zealand Herald. 28 March.

Simpson, A., Penney, S., 2011. The recovery paradigm in forensic mental health services. Criminal Behaviour and Mental Health 21 (5), 299–306.

Slate, R., Buffington-Vollum, J., Johnson, W., 2013. Criminalization of Mental Illness: Crisis and Opportunity for the Justice System, second ed. Carolina Academic Press, North Carolina.

Swanson, J., Swartz, M., Van Dorp, R., Elbogen, E., Wagner, H., Rosenheck, T., Stroup, S., McEvoy, J., Lieberman, J., 2006. A national study of violent behavior in persons with schizophrenia. Archives of General Psychiatry 63, 490–499.

Te, Pou, 2010. Fostering change: Tony Berry, forensic psychiatric nurse. Handover Winter 5–6.

Timmons, D., 2010. Forensic psychiatric nursing: a description of the role of the psychiatric nurse in a high secure psychiatric facility in Ireland. Journal of Psychiatric and Mental Health Nursing 17, 636–646.

Vollum, B., Bickle, A., Gibbon, S., 2013. Incidents of hostage-taking in an English high-secure hospital. The Journal of Forensic Psychiatry & Psychology 24 (1), 6–30.

Wallace, C., Mullen, P., Burgess, P., 2004. Criminal offending in schizophrenia over a 25-year period marked by deinstitutionalisation and increasing prevalence of comorbid substance use disorders. American Journal of Psychiatry 161 (4), 716–727.

Walmsley, R., 2015. World Prison Population List, eleventh ed. Kings College, London.

Webster, C.D., Douglas, K.S., Eaves, D., Hart, S.D., 1997. HCR-20: Assessing Risk for Violence (Version 2). Simon Fraser University, Burnaby, BC.

Webster, C.D., Martin, M.-L., Brink, J., Nicholls, T.L., Middleton, C., 2009. Short-Term Assessment of Risk and Treatability (START). St Joseph's Healthcare, Forensic Psychiatric Services Commission. Port Coquitlam, BC.

Weiskopf, C., 2005. Nurses' experience of caring for inmate patients. Journal of Advanced Nursing 49 (4), 336–343.

Wiener, R., Winick, B., Georges, L., Castro, A., 2010. A testable theory of problem solving courts: avoiding past empirical and legal failures. Journal of Law and Psychiatry 33, 417–427.

Wilkie, T., Penney, S., Fernane, F., Simpson, A., 2014. Characteristics and motivations of absconders from forensic mental health services: a case control study. BMC Psychiatry 27. Open Access Online http://tinjurl.com/neevxo.

Wolff, N., Shi, J., 2009. Victimisation and feelings of safety among male and female inmates with behavioural health problems. Journal of Forensic Psychiatry & Psychology 20, S56–S77.

Young, A., 2006. Dual diagnosis and forensic care. Are the needs of service users being met? Journal of Psychiatric and Mental Health Nursing 13, 117–124.

USEFUL WEBSITES

British Psychological Society: Risk Assessment and Management, www1.bps.org.uk/system/files/Public%20files/DCP/cat-381.pdf

Mind: for better mental health: Police and Mental Health, www.mind.org.uk/information-support/legal-rights/police-and-mental-health/sections-135-136/#.W8SeZmhKjIU

Royal College of Psychiatrists: Standards for Forensic Mental Health Services: Low and Medium Secure Care, www.rcpsych.ac.uk/pdf/QNFMHS_Standards_2016%20(002).pdf

Government reoffending statistics 2013: www.gov.uk/government/collections/proven-reoffending-statistics

Royal College of Nursing: Nursing roles in forensic and justice services, www.rcn.org.uk/clinical-topics/criminal-justice-services/nursing-roles-in-criminal-justice-services

PART 4

Mental Disorders that People Experience

15

Schizophrenia and Psychotic Disorders

Katie Evans

KEY POINTS

- Schizophrenia and psychotic disorders can be among the most debilitating mental disorders prevalent in society.
- The aetiology of schizophrenia is poorly understood, although theories have been developed to explain its origins.
- Stress, trauma and circumstances can influence the development of schizophrenia and psychosis in people predisposed to a mental illness.
- Schizophrenia and/or psychosis are not inevitably life sentences and recovery is an achievable process.
- Early diagnosis and recognition of the prodromal phase of schizophrenia enable better clinical management and outcomes.
- Treatment regimens that include combined behavioural, cognitive and pharmacological interventions are likely to have better outcomes.
- Disease and stigma combine to contribute to schizophrenia's debilitating burden.
- Homelessness, poverty and schizophrenia are closely intertwined and prevalent in our society.
- Nurses are involved in longer term solutions for people who are diagnosed with schizophrenia, such as community care, housing and employment plans.
- Relapse prevention is an important strategy to encourage the person's continued recovery.
- Nurses can learn to communicate therapeutically with people in all stages of schizophrenia and psychotic disorders.

KEY TERMS

advance care planning
affect
agranulocytosis
akathisia
ambivalence
apathy
auditory hallucinations
autism
avolition
blunted affect
brief psychotic disorder
catatonia
delusion
delusional disorder
dystonic reaction (acute)
echolalia
echopraxia
hallucination
ideas of reference
incoherence
negative symptoms
neologism
paranoia
passivity
positive symptoms
prodrome/prodromal
psychosis
recovery
relapse prevention
schizophrenia
tardive dyskinesia
thought blocking
thought broadcasting
thought disorder

LEARNING OUTCOMES

The material in this chapter will assist you to:

- define the term schizophrenia.
- discuss biological and environmental theories on the development of schizophrenia.
- distinguish the presentations of the prodromal, acute and chronic phases of schizophrenia.
- identify the major pharmacological strategies in the treatment of schizophrenia, their target symptoms and their major adverse effects.
- identify nonpharmacological strategies in the treatment of schizophrenia.
- outline the role of the nurse in the care of people with schizophrenia and psychosis.
- identify education strategies that may be employed in psychoeducation of the individual and family.

INTRODUCTION

There are historical records of psychotic illness going back to 1400 BC, although there is no evidence that schizophrenia existed in its present form (Evans et al. 2003). Many modern medical terms originated in ancient Greek medicine and the Greek term 'schizophrenia' can be translated as a 'split mind', just as the term 'psychosis' is of Greek origin and is translated as 'illness of the mind' (Evans et al. 2003).

This chapter covers the ways in which schizophrenia and psychotic disorders are described, diagnosed and differentiated, noting all of the types on the schizophrenia spectrum and other psychotic disorders. Assessment and diagnosis are covered, the defining features (delusions, hallucinations, disorganisation of motor behaviour and thinking, and negative symptoms) are described and the diagnostic criteria of each major disorder are listed from the *Diagnostic and Statistical Manual of Mental Disorders*, 5th edition (DSM-5) (American Psychiatric Association [APA] 2013). This will enable the mental health professional to distinguish early psychosis because early assessment and diagnosis facilitate more successful treatment and recovery.

The disorders collectively described in the DSM-5 as 'schizophrenia spectrum and other psychotic disorders' (APA 2013, p. 125) are major mental illnesses that can have a considerable impact on the person, their family, their significant others and the community. Psychotic disorders share the common characteristic of severe disturbances in perception, cognition and thinking. While the term 'psychosis' is most strongly associated with schizophrenia, psychosis is also a feature of other disorders such as bipolar disorder, depression, dementia and delirium. People who do not have a mental disorder but who are subjected to trauma, severe stress, sleep deprivation and other adversities might experience brief psychotic episodes without being in any danger of being diagnosed with schizophrenia. Substances such as marijuana, lysergic acid diethylamide (LSD), methamphetamine and ecstasy might also cause temporary psychotic experiences or trigger a more enduring psychotic disorder.

Epidemiology and prevalence will clarify the dimensions of the disorders in the UK and the many theories that combine to explain the aetiology of schizophrenia and psychosis are examined. The development and course of the disorders, recovery, stigma and comorbid disorders are also examined. Both physical and psychological interventions are described, along with the most effective communication strategies that will assist the nurse to care for people with schizophrenia and psychotic disorders. People are cared for as inpatients and in the community, depending on their needs. Relapse prevention, community care, assisted housing and employment assistance form part of the strategy to encourage the person's continued recovery.

There is an emphasis on the most prevalent psychotic disorder, schizophrenia, and nurses are encouraged to understand schizophrenia both as a diagnostic concept and as a life experience of individual patients. This chapter takes a recovery-oriented approach to understanding psychosis and schizophrenia. We have assumed that the focus of psychiatric and mental health nursing is working with the problems experienced by patients whatever their psychiatric diagnosis. One reason psychotic disorders and schizophrenia present such a challenge relates to the age of onset, which occurs in the pivotal periods of adolescence and early adulthood when individuals are at that point in their lives when they are expected to begin to be at their most productive. The person's education is disrupted, they find themselves less able to socialise easily and therefore their ability to select a life partner can be impaired and isolation and lack of education may limit their work opportunities. The misconceptions, stigma and fear that a diagnosis of schizophrenia or psychosis generates often contribute to the person's problems.

Understanding schizophrenia and psychotic disorders can be a challenging and confronting experience. This chapter attempts to provide some insight into the conditions while articulating the role of the health professional in assisting people with these disorders to reach their optimal level of health. There is no reason to believe that a diagnosis of schizophrenia or psychosis means that the person or the mental health professional should be pessimistic about the prognosis or believe that psychosis is a chronic, irreversible condition.

HISTORICAL UNDERSTANDING

Psychotic disorders have been described in books, historical accounts and other literary sources for thousands of years, but it seems that schizophrenia did not exist in its present form until comparatively recently (Evans et al. 2003). There are better data in the historical literature to support the existence of isolated psychotic episodes rather than schizophrenia in the form that can be diagnosed by modern diagnostic systems and that encompasses early onset, hallucinations, delusions and often a degree of chronicity. Schizophrenia is thought to be of comparatively modern, possibly viral, origin and a formal identification and description of schizophrenia was eventually developed in the nineteenth century (Evans et al. 2003). Fuller evidence to support this argument can be found in Chapter 3.

Identifying and labelling the constellation of disorders now known collectively in the DSM-5 as 'schizophrenia spectrum and other psychotic disorders' commenced more than 150 years ago, when in 1856 the French psychiatrist Benedict Morel (1809–1873) used the term 'dementia praecox' (meaning precocious or early dementia) during the treatment of a young male experiencing the effects of mental illness. It took until much later, in the twentieth century, for a formal identification and description of schizophrenia to evolve (Bennett et al. 2007). In 1902 the German psychiatrist Emil Kraepelin (1956–1926) used the term 'dementia praecox' to differentiate schizophrenic illness from 'manic depression' (his term) on the basis of the course of illness (Bennett et al. 2007). Kraepelin identified that bipolar affective disorder was characterised by an episodic course with improvement in the period between episodes, while schizophrenia had a progressively worsening course with a degeneration of the brain (Bennett et al. 2007). This remains a source of debate, although it is more widely accepted today that it is possible for people who experience episodes of schizophrenia to recover and that the course is more varied than earlier believed (Bennett et al. 2007). Kraepelin's formulation of schizophrenic illness took hold in Europe, while Bleuler's (see later) was popular in the United States (Bennett et al. 2007). Morel and Kraepelin linked 'dementia' with psychotic features because they theorised that the illness was neurologically based, like forms of dementia, and that the clinical pathway led to deterioration and chronicity, similar to dementia (Sadock et al. 2009). This view was far from optimistic and the prognosis left minimal hope for the individual's recovery.

The Swiss psychiatrist Eugen Bleuler (1857–1939) coined the term 'schizophrenia' in 1911 as an amalgam of two Greek words: *schizo*, meaning 'split', and *phrenia*, meaning 'mind'. Bleuler intended the term to symbolise the schism between the external world of the individual and the internal conflict of the individual's mind (Bennett et al. 2012). Bleuler's emphasis was on the lost connections between thoughts and those between thought, emotion and will. However, there is a persistent societal belief that equates schizophrenia with a 'split personality', a sort of Jekyll and Hyde manifestation wherein an apparently 'normal' person can segue unpredictably into a person who is irrational and dangerous. Popular film and media characterisations of people with schizophrenia and psychotic disorders fail to depict accurately the manifestations of this illness and its painful effects and more often than not perpetuate the common myths and stereotypes that surround it.

To Bleuler the term symbolised the disintegration and disjointedness of the personality and its associated functions such as mood display, speech and thought. Bleuler was influenced strongly by the work of Sigmund Freud and consequently saw the illness as a disorder that involved both the mind and the personality; a functional disorder rather than an organic disorder related to neurological dysfunction (Sadock et al. 2009). While Bleuler's work has contributed significantly to understanding the clinical picture of schizophrenia, the very name and the Greek meanings of the two words that make up this name have in many respects muddied the layperson's understanding of the illness. Despite decades of publicity and education, the persistent common misunderstanding of schizophrenia is that the person has a split or multiple personality, a diagnosis that is better described as a dissociative disorder.

Kraepelin's notion that the illness has a biological basis continues to be researched and is most favoured as an explanation of causation, even if not entirely proven or understood. His rather pessimistic outlook on the course of the illness can remain valid for many individuals with schizophrenia despite major developments in the treatment of this illness although, as we will see, a person can still be in 'recovery' even though the disease has become chronic. Bleuler, on the other hand, simplified the identification of symptoms with his easily remembered 'four As':

- *Autism*: the individual's tendency to retreat into an inner fantasy world, resulting in socially isolating or withdrawing behaviours and loss of contact with reality.
- *Ambivalence*: the individual's tendency to hold opposing views and feelings simultaneously, such as love and hate, rendering meaningful decision making difficult.
- *Affective disturbance*: the individual's inability to express congruent emotions and affect.
- *Associative looseness*: the individual's gross disturbance in ability to think logically and rationally and to distinguish between related and unrelated thought processes (Sadock et al. 2009).

ASSESSMENT AND DIAGNOSIS

The schizophrenia spectrum and other psychotic disorders are defined by abnormalities in one or more of the following five domains: delusions, hallucinations, disorganised thinking (speech), grossly disorganised or abnormal motor behaviour (including catatonia) and negative symptoms (APA 2013, p. 87). The spectrum includes:

- schizophrenia
- delusional disorder
- brief psychotic disorder
- schizophreniform disorder
- substance-induced psychotic disorder
- psychotic disorder due to a medical condition
- catatonia
- schizotypal disorder (which is more fully described in the 'personality disorders' section of the DSM-5) (APA 2013, p. 87–89)

Defining Features of Psychotic Disorders

After Bleuler popularised the term 'schizophrenia', Kurt Schneider (1950s) continued the work of identifying and describing the symptoms of schizophrenia and other psychotic conditions by cataloguing what he termed the 'first rank' symptoms that were necessary to make a diagnosis of schizophrenia: auditory hallucinations; thought insertion or withdrawal; thought broadcasting; beliefs that the person's feelings and actions are imposed upon them; passivity phenomena; and perceptual delusions (Bennett et al. 2012). However, it is now recognised that these symptoms are common to all the psychotic disorders and are not specific to schizophrenia (Bennett et al. 2012).

The DSM-5 refines Schneider's six 'first-rank symptoms' making some of them broader and less specific and adding others. The key features that define psychotic disorders described in the DSM-5 (pp. 87–89) are: delusions, hallucinations, disorganised thinking, disorganised or abnormal motor behaviour and negative symptoms. The more frequently occurring symptoms of schizophrenia can also be divided into two groups:

- **Positive symptoms** are thought processes, emotions and behaviours that are exaggerations of, or additional to, what an individual experiences when they are well. Positive symptoms appear as part of the onset and experience of the illness, but are absent when the person is not experiencing the illness.
- **Negative symptoms** are absences or reductions of thought processes, emotions and behaviours that were present prior to the onset of the illness but have since diminished or are absent following the onset of the illness. The prefix 'a' means 'without' in Greek and negative symptoms include anhedonia, avolition, aphasia, anergia and alogia.

Each feature is defined in Table 15.1 and you can refer back to this list when the terms are used hereafter. The glossary at the end of the book is also a useful resource.

Diagnostic and Statistical Manual of Mental Disorders, 5th edition (DSM-5)

The DSM-5 (APA 2013) is a newly revised and highly detailed listing of mental disorders and their corresponding diagnostic criteria. Recent debate in mental health nursing has focussed on whether a categorical or a dimensional model provides the best understanding of disorders such as psychosis (Halter et al. 2013). The DSM-5 definition treats schizophrenia as a categorical diagnosis, which emphasises the ways in which people with schizophrenia are different from those with other diagnoses such as bipolar disorder. Within the categorical model diagnoses are thought to be mutually exclusive. The categorical model has been criticised because it does not reflect the wide variations seen in disorders such as schizophrenia. A different approach is the dimensional model, which emphasises that symptoms of schizophrenia and other psychotic disorders lie

TABLE 15.1 Commonly Experienced Symptoms of Schizophrenia and Psychotic Disorders

Symptom	Description
Many of the symptoms of psychotic disorders are positive (productive) symptoms	
Content of Thought	

Delusions can take different forms:
• persecutory
• somatic
• religious
• referential
• grandiose
• erotomanic
• nihilistic
• bizarre
	Fixed false beliefs that are inconsistent with one's social, cultural and religious beliefs and not amenable to change, despite conflicting evidence or argumentation.
	• The belief that the person is being harmed or harassed, conspired against, cheated, spied on, followed, poisoned or drugged, maliciously maligned or obstructed in the pursuit of long-term goals.
	• Preoccupation with the person's organs, health or bodily functions.
	• Belief that the person has become or is being influenced by religious figures in various ways.
	• Belief that gestures, comments and/or environmental circumstances are directed at the person.
	• Belief that the person has exceptional abilities, fame or wealth, some great (but unrecognised) talent or insight or has made some important discovery.
	• False belief that another person is in love with the person.
	• Conviction that a major catastrophe and destruction will occur.
	• Bizarre delusions include:
	  • thought withdrawal (thoughts 'removed')
	  • thought insertion (thoughts 'put into' the mind)
	  • thought control (body or actions controlled by others)

Ideas of reference	The belief that an insignificant or incidental object or event has special significance or meaning to that individual; for example, the perception that the newsreader on television is addressing the person.
Thought Disorder	
Disorganised thinking ('formal thought disorder') is evident when the person expresses themselves verbally	This symptom must be severe enough to substantially impair effective communication. This is evident if: • the person switches topics erratically ('derailment' or 'loose associations') • their responses to questions are unrelated (tangentiality) • their speech is incoherent or disorganised ('word salad')
Thought insertion/thought broadcasting	The feeling that the person's thoughts are being read; that people are taking the thoughts from the person's head; or that the person's feelings, impulses and actions are not the person's own but imposed by some external force.
Loosening of associations	Ideas that fail to follow one another with a logical flow and sequence; this results in shifting from one subject to another, resulting in loss of significant meaning.
Incoherence	Verbal rambling renders content impossible to understand; may present with: • neologisms (newly made-up words) • clang associations (words that sound like one another) • thought blocking (unable to express thoughts)
Perceptual Disturbances	
Hallucinations Auditory hallucinations are most common in schizophrenia and related disorders	• Vivid, involuntary perceptions that are experienced as 'normal' and occur without an external stimulus • Usually experienced as voices that are perceived as distinct from the person's own thoughts • Those that occur while falling asleep (hypnagogic) or waking up (hypnopompic) are within the range of normal experience
Other hallucinations are less common	Can involve any of the other senses such as 'olfactory' (smells), visual (sights) and tactile (touch)
Affect	
Emotional blunting	Being 'flat' or inappropriate; voice is a monotone and the face is immobile
Incongruent affect	A mismatch between the person's thoughts and their emotional expression in a given situation—for example, the person may say that they feel threatened or terrified, but appear amused by the situation.

TABLE 15.1 Commonly Experienced Symptoms of Schizophrenia and Psychotic Disorders—cont'd

Symptom	Description
Bizarre Behaviour	
Abnormal motor behaviour	Can range from agitation to child-like 'silliness', which leads to difficulties in performing activities of daily living.
Clothing and appearance	Reflects mental state: can be dishevelled, poorly groomed, quiet and immobile or screaming and agitated; may be inappropriately dressed for the occasion, environment and temperature.
Social or sexual behaviour	'Loss of ego boundaries' can cause confusion in relationships with others.
Catatonia	A marked decrease in reactivity to the environment. Behaviour includes: • resistance to instructions (negativism) • maintaining a rigid, inappropriate or bizarre posture • a complete lack of verbal and motor responses (mutism and stupor) • stereotyped repetitive movements • staring • grimacing • echoing of speech (echolalia) The person who is grossly involved in delusional thinking and preoccupation can find it difficult to relate to external stimuli.
Other presenting features: negative (deficit) symptoms	
Negative symptoms	• Diminished emotional expression (reduced facial expressions, eye contact, head and hand movements) • Avolition (decreased self-initiated purposeful activities such as work or social activities); this affects personal hygiene, attention to nutrition, occupation and work, physical activity • Alogia, manifested by diminished speech output • Anhedonia (decreased ability to experience pleasure from positive stimuli or a degradation in the recollection of pleasure previously experienced) • Asociality (apparent lack of interest in social interactions); may be associated with avolition or limited opportunities for social interactions • Poverty of ideas, which limits conversation and reduces topics or issues to think about or discuss • Anergia (loss of energy) • Loss of living skills

(*Source*: Adapted using American Psychiatric Association (APA) 2013. Diagnostic and Statistical Manual of Mental Disorders, 5th ed. APA, Washington, DC; and Sadock, B., Sadock, V.A., Ruiz, P., 2009. Kaplan and Sadock's Comprehensive Textbook of Psychiatry, 9th ed. Lippincott Williams & Wilkins, Baltimore.)

on a continuum, with many symptoms being shared by people with different diagnoses. Although it uses a categorical model for diagnosis of schizophrenia, in other respects the DSM-5 has moved towards a more dimensional approach (Tandon et al. 2013). The previous subtypes (or subcategories) of schizophrenia have been removed and the DSM-5 chapter on psychosis is titled 'Schizophrenia spectrum and other psychotic disorders'. In addition, the DSM-5 has introduced a range of dimensions of schizophrenia, further reducing the emphasis on categorical diagnosis (Pletnikov & Waddington 2015).

The benefit of a diagnostic system is that it allows clinicians to be consistent in their use of a term that describes a diagnosis, so that clinicians across the world can be more certain of diagnosing and treating mental disorders effectively. Because mental illnesses have few, if any, laboratory tests or other diagnostic procedures that can either confirm or refute a diagnosis, the means available to make psychiatric diagnoses are through detailed history taking and skilled observation. The data gained from these processes are then measured against the diagnostic criteria stated in the DSM-5 and other diagnostic systems such as the International Classification of Diseases (ICD).

Many people fear that experiencing a psychotic episode of any kind or duration means that they will inevitably be burdened with a lifetime diagnosis of schizophrenia, but that is far from the case. There are many fine distinctions that can enable different diagnoses to be made within the schizophrenia spectrum and different diagnoses imply different prognoses and treatments. We will look at three main types of disorder: brief psychotic disorder, delusional disorder and schizophrenia (plus its subtypes) and describe the main differences between them.

BRIEF PSYCHOTIC DISORDER

Brief psychotic disorder is distinctive in that it is strictly time-limited. To be diagnosed, it needs to last for more than 1 day but less than 1 month (see Box 15.1).

Prevalence, Course and Prognosis

The essential feature of brief psychotic disorder is a disturbance that involves the sudden onset of at least one of the following positive psychotic symptoms: delusions, hallucinations, disorganised speech (e.g. frequent derailment or incoherence) and grossly abnormal psychomotor behaviour, including catatonia (Criterion A). *Sudden onset* is defined as change from a nonpsychotic state to a clearly psychotic state within 2 weeks, usually without a prodrome or preceding/premonitory signs (APA 2013, p. 94). The person eventually returns to their usual level of functioning after the episode.

BOX 15.1 Diagnostic Criteria for Brief Psychotic Disorder

A. Characteristic Symptoms
Presence of one (or more) of the following symptoms. At least one of these must be 1, 2 or 3.
1. Delusions
2. Hallucinations
3. Disorganised speech (such as incoherence or frequent derailment)
4. Grossly disorganised or catatonic behaviour

Note: Do not include a symptom if it is a culturally sanctioned response.

B. Duration
At least 1 day but less than 1 month, with eventual full return to premorbid level of functioning

C. Excluding Other Diagnoses
Other illnesses including mental disorders such as mood disorders, schizophrenia or schizoaffective disorder need to be excluded. The possibility that the individual may be affected by drugs or other general medical conditions needs to be excluded. Specify if symptoms occur in response to stressful events, during pregnancy or within 4 weeks' postpartum.

(*Source*: Adapted from American Psychiatric Association (APA) 2013. Diagnostic and Statistical Manual of Mental Disorders, 5th ed. APA, Washington, DC, p. 94.)

Around 9% of initial cases of psychosis can be diagnosed as brief psychotic disorder, the most usual age of onset being the mid-30s, although it can occur in adolescence or early adulthood. Although the disorder might become chronic, it often lasts as briefly as a few days and there is the possibility of periods of recovery followed by relapse. In some circumstances, there may be no further episodes (APA 2013, p. 95).

DELUSIONAL DISORDER

Delusional disorder is quite limited in its appearance and effects. It is characterised by at least 1 month of delusions but no other psychotic symptoms (see Box 15.2).

Prevalence, Course and Prognosis

Delusional disorder is usually diagnosed in a person's late 20s or early 30s but it can occur in adolescence. The person with delusional disorder might discern that others view their beliefs as irrational, but they are unable to accept this themselves (i.e. there may be no true insight). Social, marital or work problems can result from the delusional beliefs and the person might act angrily and violently when they suffer from the persecutory, jealous and erotomanic types. The person also might become litigious and antagonistic and it is therefore not uncommon for legal difficulties to arise, particularly in the jealous type (most often males). The lifetime prevalence of delusional disorder has been estimated at around 0.2% and the most common type is persecutory (APA 2013, p. 92).

BOX 15.2 Diagnostic Criteria for Delusional Disorder

A. Characteristic Symptoms and Duration
The presence of one (or more) delusions with a duration of 1 month or longer.

B. Criterion A for Schizophrenia has Never Been Met (see Box 15.3)
Note: If hallucinations are present, they are not prominent and are related to the delusional theme.

C. Social/Occupational Dysfunction
Apart from the impact of the delusion(s) or its ramifications, behaviour is not obviously odd or bizarre and functioning has not been markedly impaired.

D. Duration
If manic or major depressive episodes have occurred, these have been brief relative to the duration of the delusional periods.

E. Other Illnesses Including Mental Disorders such as Body Dysmorphic Disorder or Obsessive-Compulsive Disorder
The possibility that the individual may be affected by drugs or other general medical conditions needs to be excluded. Specify type: e.g. erotomanic, grandiose, jealous, persecutory, mixed or bizarre.

(*Source*: Adapted from American Psychiatric Association (APA) 2013. Diagnostic and Statistical Manual of Mental Disorders, 5th ed. APA, Washington, DC, pp. 90–91.)

SCHIZOPHRENIA

Schizophrenia is a disorder characterised by a major disturbance in thought, perception, cognition and psychosocial functioning and is one of the most severe mental disorders. The DSM-5 describes the clinical presentation that needs to exist for a diagnosis of schizophrenia to be made. The diagnostic criteria are shown in Box 15.3.

Schizophrenia Subtypes Removed in the DSM-5

This textbook and slightly older literature note that the DSM viewed schizophrenia as a constellation of conditions whose common features and differences allowed subtypes to be recognised. These subtypes of schizophrenia were eliminated from the latest DSM 'due to their limited diagnostic stability, low reliability, and poor validity' (APA 2013, p. 810). However, because older literature or patient notes might still refer to these subtypes, you might need to know what they were. The subtypes of schizophrenia were designated as:

1. Paranoid: delusions or hallucinations without disorganisation of thought and/or behaviour; flat or inappropriate affect; anger; anxiety; aloofness; and argumentativeness.
2. Disorganised: disorganised speech and behaviour; flat or inappropriate affect; odd mannerisms; inability to manage activities of daily living; and impaired neuropsychological function.

BOX 15.3 Diagnostic Criteria for Schizophrenia

A. Characteristic Symptoms

Two (or more) of the following need to be present for a significant period of time during 1 month. At least one symptom must be 1, 2 or 3.

1. Delusions
2. Hallucinations
3. Disorganised speech (e.g. frequent derailment or incoherence)
4. Grossly disorganised or catatonic behaviour
5. Negative symptoms (i.e. diminished emotional expression or avolition)

B. Social/Occupational Dysfunction

A significant portion of the time level of functioning in one or more major areas, such as work, interpersonal relations or self-care, is markedly below the level achieved prior to the onset. In children or adolescents, there is failure to achieve expected level of interpersonal, academic or occupational functioning.

C. Duration

There needs to be evidence that the disturbance has existed for at least 6 months. Within this 6-month period the individual needs to display symptoms as listed in A.

D & E Excluding Other Diagnoses

Other illnesses including mental disorders such as mood disorders or schizoaffective disorder need to be excluded. The possibility that the individual may be affected by drugs or other general medical conditions needs to be excluded. If there is a history of autistic disorder or another pervasive developmental disorder, delusions and/or hallucinations need to be present for at least 1 month (or less if treatment has been successful).

(*Source*: Adapted from American Psychiatric Association (APA) 2013. Diagnostic and Statistical Manual of Mental Disorders, 5th ed. APA, Washington, DC, p. 99.)

3. Catatonic: at least two of five features: catalepsy or stupor; excessive motor activity that does not appear to be purposeful or related to external stimuli; extreme negativism or mutism; posturing, stereotyped movements, prominent mannerisms or grimacing; and echolalia or echopraxia.
4. Undifferentiated: features of schizophrenia but no other criteria met for the aforementioned subtypes.
5. Residual: negative symptoms: listlessness, problems with concentration and social withdrawal, some delusions, hallucinations, disorganised speech and/or behaviour (APA 2000).

Prevalence, Course and Prognosis

The DSM-5 states that there is a lifetime prevalence of schizophrenia of approximately 0.3% to 0.7%, although this figure is reported to vary in different countries, for different races and ethnicities and according to the origin of immigrants and the children of immigrants (APA 2013). These differences probably account for Simeone et al.'s (2015) understanding that there is a lack of consistency in findings on the prevalence of schizophrenia, although the authors also state that study design, geographical region, time of assessment, study setting, sample size and differing definitions of schizophrenia, psychosis and schizophrenia-spectrum disorders muddy the figures. There would be a difference in the figures, for example, if they were accessed from the Office of National Statistics or from inpatient mental health records of admissions, presenting difficulties in estimating the exact prevalence.

Schizophrenia tends to be more prevalent among the socially disadvantaged (Cantor-Graae 2007). The homeless population is one example where there are higher rates of the condition (Fazel et al. 2008). The genders seem to be affected differently, with males experiencing more negative symptoms, a longer duration of disorder and poorer outcomes, while females experience more mood symptoms. Briefer presentations are predictive for better outcomes for both genders (APA 2013). The median age of onset for schizophrenia is different for men and women, but it rarely occurs prior to adolescence. For males, onset is generally in the early to mid-20s, while for females it is usually in the late 20s (APA 2013). Onset can be rapid or slow and insidious, although a large proportion demonstrate a prodromal phase evidenced by a gradual deterioration in function and social withdrawal, before more obvious signs and symptoms appear and the illness becomes evident (APA 2013).

Course and outcome cannot be reliably predicted for every person, but a variable course with sometimes lengthy periods of remission and intermittent relapses is common, although the illness can become chronic in a proportion of people. Early onset is associated with poorer outcomes and later onset results in better outcomes; for most people, negative symptoms predominate later in the course of the illness (APA 2013). Factors associated with a better prognosis include:

- a good level of premorbid adjustment
- sudden and later onset
- good insight
- being female
- having identifiable triggers for episodes
- concurrent mood disturbance
- early intervention with antipsychotic medication
- good adherence with prescribed treatment
- short periods of acute illness
- higher levels of functioning between episodes
- fewer residual symptoms
- good neurological function
- family history of mood disorder but no family history of schizophrenia (APA 2013)

Development

Prodromal Phase

'Prodrome' is defined as an early or a premonitory sign or symptom of a disorder (APA 2013, p. 827). The initial markers of schizophrenia often develop in early adolescence. This development is poorly understood and even more difficult to identify (Chuma & Mahadun 2011). However, with hindsight, once the illness has become severe enough to be diagnosed, prodromal features become identifiable and significant as precursors. Negative symptoms are common in the prodromal phase and can be one of the first signs of schizophrenia when a person who has been socially active withdraws from their previous activities and routines (APA 2013). Berger et al. (2006) indicate the presence of low-grade (subthreshold) psychotic symptoms, poor functioning, depression and disorganisation as predictors of an overt psychotic episode. In addition, comorbid features such as substance abuse and depression should not be overlooked.

Because the onset of schizophrenia typically occurs during adolescence or in early adulthood, this constellation of negative symptoms interferes with schooling and the development of meaningful connections with others in a social setting. Negative symptoms cause conversations to be limited and responses to be short, often monosyllabic. This phase can be confused by parents as a fairly 'normal' one because parents are aware that adolescent children are known to need increased privacy and to seek separation from parental surveillance.

Limited social engagement means that the person finds it difficult to develop and to sustain stimulating and rewarding social relationships and partnerships at a time when most people are socialising, seeking life partners and training for their future careers. Instead of beginning to earn an income and seek personal independence, the person with schizophrenia might find themselves hospitalised or dependent on their parents for help with personal hygiene, nutrition and motivation to undertake physical activity.

NURSE'S STORY 15.1 Prodromal Phase of Schizophrenia

When I recall my school days, I think of a particular individual with whom I went to secondary school. At the time I would have described him as different rather than odd. He never fully engaged with others either individually or in a group and he certainly never initiated such engagement, yet when invited to participate in social activities he was quite capable of doing so. It seemed that, despite engaging with others, as soon as he got the chance to return to a state of detachment from the larger social group, he took it. Although the term 'odd' would be too strong a word, his whole demeanour, including how he held himself, how he dressed and what occupied his time, seemed very distant from the rest of us. When I recall his schoolwork ability, nothing exceptional comes to mind.

Years later, as a psychiatric nurse, I was witness to his admission to the psychiatric facility in which I worked. He had been diagnosed with schizophrenia. When I recall my school days with him, I now understand the reasons he appeared strange and different. There was a very good chance that he had experienced prodromal features of schizophrenia during those days at school.

Acute Phase

The characteristic psychotic symptoms of the acute phase of schizophrenia generally subside with treatment. Positive symptoms (hallucinations, delusions and disorders of thought) are usually the focus of clinical intervention and, to a large extent, they respond satisfactorily to antipsychotic medications. It is the negative symptoms (lack of motivation, blunted emotions, loss of drive, social withdrawal and inattention) that are major determinants of disability and, often, the chronicity of the person's disorder. The person with this disorder usually functions below a level that they might previously have achieved. Early manifestations might include poor or deteriorating school performance, poor social relations, decreased self-care and a failure to achieve expected developmental milestones. In addition to the decline in social and occupational performance common to the prodromal phase of the illness, the individual may present with all or some of the symptoms listed in Table 15.1.

Continuous Symptoms

The DSM-5 (APA 2013) no longer specifically refers to the 'chronic' phase of schizophrenia, instead specifying whether the symptoms are 'continuous' or in 'full' or 'partial' remission. Continuous symptoms 'fulfil the diagnostic symptom criteria of the disorder for the majority of the illness course' (APA 2013, p. 100). The course appears to be favourable in about 20% of people with schizophrenia and a small number of these recover completely. Of the other 80%, most will need help with daily living; many remain chronically ill with exacerbations and remissions of active symptoms; and others experience a course of progressive deterioration. Psychotic symptoms usually diminish over time, but negative symptoms and cognitive deficits, which are closely related to prognosis, tend to persist (APA 2013, p. 102)

The most commonly experienced symptoms in the continuous/chronic phase of schizophrenia are negative symptoms, but unlike positive symptoms, they respond poorly to conventional antipsychotic medications. Not only are neuroleptic medications largely ineffective against negative symptoms, but they could also make them worse, giving rise to the so-called neuroleptic-induced deficit syndrome (NIDS), which includes apathy, lack of initiative, indifference and blunted affect, and reduced insight into the disease (Ueda et al. 2016). Negative symptoms such as alogia and avolition leave the individual feeling numb and unable to respond to the demands of daily living. There is a significant loss of drive and the individual has difficulty initiating and completing activities. Both the illness and the treatment can introduce impairments such as difficulty learning new concepts and disturbances in attention, which further impact treatment and rehabilitation efforts since they undermine the acquisition of new skills.

AETIOLOGICAL THEORIES

Research has yet to determine the exact cause of schizophrenia and psychotic disorders, but many theories have been developed that seek to explain it. In the past, the pendulum has swung from developmental to psychodynamic to neurobiological explanations and back again, but the ultimate explanation is likely to encompass a mixture of aetiologies, perhaps differently proportioned in each case. In all probability, the cause of schizophrenia lies in a complex interaction between multiple combinations of genetic and environmental factors—for example, exposure to infection during gestation, birth or early childhood (Fuller Torrey & Yolken 2003; Brown 2006;

Venables et al. 2007), which may interfere with normal brain development and function. This complex interplay results in the constellation of behaviours collectively known as schizophrenia spectrum disorders.

The fact that the brains of people with schizophrenia differ from those without the illness is now largely undisputed and it is this altered brain development that seems to be inherited rather than the illness itself (van Os & Kapur 2009). How or why these aberrations in brain biochemistry and anatomy affect the functioning of the brain remains a mystery, as does the reason why these abnormalities appear to remain dormant until late adolescence in most individuals.

Nature Versus Nurture

A great deal of the debate that has always surrounded psychotic disorders and schizophrenia in particular concerns itself with causation. The question is asked whether the person was born that way and destined inevitably to develop the disorder or whether the person developed the disorder because of their environment or upbringing. This debate is often summarised as 'nature versus nurture' and it has yet to be settled definitively.

Advocates of the 'nurture' theory tend to blame the person's parents, specifically the mother, for their treatment of the child, which gave rise to the symptoms of schizophrenia or psychosis. The US psychiatrist Frieda Fromm-Reichmann first defined the so-called schizophrenogenic mother in 1948 (Johnston 2013; see also http://psychologydictionary.org/schizophrenogenic-mother). This type of mother was typically emotionally cold, rejecting and emotionally disturbed; a perfectionist, domineering and lacking in sensitivity; rigidly moral but seductive; and overprotective of the child who she kept in a dependent state so that she could control him or her. This parent would in theory so confuse the child with contradictory standards and expectations, or 'double-binds', that the child grew up bewildered by society's demands and unable to decipher reality or how to react to it.

However, psychiatrist Gordon Parker reviewed the schizophrenogenic mother research in 1982 and concluded that although such people existed, they were not responsible for the development of schizophrenia (Johnston 2013). The tide turned and the term was discarded. It is not surprising that the patient movement found this term objectionably stigmatising of mothers, who were often the main or sole carers of people with schizophrenia and who sought help for their children from mental health professionals only to be branded themselves as the 'cause' of their child's distress. Nowadays the role of parents is particularly hard to discuss, even when they have a significant impact on the mental health of their children. Parents can pass on genetic risk factors as well as creating a large proportion of the child's environmental setting; but clinicians are eager to respect parents' dignity and reluctant to interfere with how people choose to raise their children, provided that outright abuse is absent (Johnston 2013).

The term 'schizophrenogenic' is now, thankfully, outdated, but realistically there can be a familial predisposition to psychotic illnesses and similar behaviours and thought patterns can exist within a family network. Perhaps the pendulum has swung too far and clinicians want too strongly to 'stand apart from the psychiatrists of the mid-twentieth century and their mother-blaming beliefs' (Johnston 2013, p. 804). The risk is that separating the person with schizophrenia from their familial environment and neglecting to treat them and their context holistically risks locating the problems solely within the patient and implying that he or she alone needs to change.

The Diathesis-Stress Model

The basic assumption behind the diathesis-stress model is that individuals are exposed to stressful events in the course of their lives and that these events may precipitate symptoms in some people who have a predisposition to mental illness (Jones & Fernyhough 2007). Essential to this theory is the notion that some people are more vulnerable to mental illness than others. In the case of schizophrenia, this vulnerability may be related to genetics, environmental factors, aberrations in brain anatomy or biochemistry, or, more likely, a combination of all these things (van Heeringen 2000).

Weisman (2005) expanded the understanding of the role of family as part of an individual's environment and culture by examining the literature in this area. She asserted that a sufferer's family and home environment have the potential to affect the course of the illness. More specifically, sufferers from families that show high levels of expressed emotion (EE), typified by excessive criticism, hostility or emotional overinvolvement, do less well than sufferers from families with patterns of relating that are not high in EE. The model and its more contemporary redevelopment, known as the stress-vulnerability-protective factors model, suggests a range of appropriate actions, from targeting vulnerable but as yet asymptomatic individuals through to symptom reduction by medication (Kopelowicz et al. 2003) and possibly family therapy and counselling (Weisman 2005).

CRITICAL THINKING CHALLENGE 15.1

How might the diathesis-stress model explain the high rates of mental illness among our society's homeless population?

Social and Environmental Theories

Burns et al. (2014) conducted a global systematic review of 26 countries and found that there is a significant relationship between income inequality and the incidence of schizophrenia. They concluded that the chronic stress of living with poverty, poor social cohesion and income inequality increase the risk of schizophrenia.

Caution needs to be observed in interpreting these social patterns because there is a risk that cause and effect can be confused. Perhaps the experience of the illness results in a decline in the individual's social condition and economic disadvantage or perhaps the social disadvantages increase the likelihood of experiencing schizophrenia.

A person is more likely to be diagnosed with schizophrenia, for example, if they grow up in an urban environment, belong to a lower socioeconomic group or were born in winter or spring (McGrath & Welham 1999; Haukka et al. 2001;

Munk-Jorgensen & Ewald 2001; Suvisaari et al. 2002; van Os 2000). Research from the Northern Hemisphere strongly supports a hypothesis that people born in winter or spring are more likely to develop schizophrenia compared with the general population, but the data from the Southern Hemisphere have been less consistent. McGrath and Welham (1999) found that in the Southern Hemisphere these factors exist, but they are weaker, less prevalent and less regular, perhaps modified by other as yet unidentified variables.

Urbanisation presents a very clear and well-documented increased risk of developing schizophrenia. For example, China has recently undergone urbanisation at an unprecedented rate and scale, a process that was expected to increase the numbers of people with schizophrenia—and it did (Chan et al. 2015). As the cities doubled in size to house 600 million people, it was estimated that the numbers of people affected with schizophrenia rose from 3.09 million in 1990 to 7.16 million in 2010, a 132% increase, although the total population increased only 18% (Chan et al. 2015).

There is emerging evidence relating to the influence of traumatic life experiences in the development of psychotic disorders. The potential value of considering traumatic childhood experience as a cause of psychotic disorders or schizophrenia has been considered by researchers (Read et al. 2014; Cancel et al. 2015). Developments in understanding the impact of trauma on the brain have been studied by the international 'hearing voices' movement (www.intervoiceonline.org). Professor Marius Romme and those who experience hearing voices around the world view trauma as the origin of voice hearing (also known as auditory hallucinations) rather than seeing the voices as an aberrant symptom of schizophrenia (Longden 2013). This is an example of the emerging influence of a patient-led understanding of psychotic experience based on personal meaning.

Biological Theories

The three most commonly discussed biological causative factors are brain anatomy, genetics and brain biochemistry. It would be erroneous to consider these three factors mutually exclusive. Far more likely is the existence of a relationship between the three. For example, some as yet unidentified pattern of inheritance may predispose an individual to differences in anatomy or fluctuations in neurotransmitter biochemistry (Inta et al. 2011).

Neuroanatomical Abnormalities

Schizophrenia is often referred to as a neuropsychological disorder, which implies that the origins of the psychological disturbance lie in the neurological structure and function of the brain. Commonly, but not conclusively, modern imaging techniques reveal lower brain tissue volume and higher cerebrospinal fluid volumes (Salokangas et al. 2002). Precisely how or why these changes occur is unknown. It is commonly thought that either genetics or environmental factors during gestation are responsible for the brain abnormalities, with the effects remaining dormant until adolescence (van Os & Kapur 2009). Some research suggests that brain changes occur as a result of illness and may occur during or shortly after the first episode of psychosis (Lawrie et al. 2002). Clearly, a great deal more research between abnormal brain anatomy and schizophrenia is required and the cause/effect relationship remains inconclusive (Boos et al. 2011).

Fuller Torrey and Yolken (2003) have studied the parasite *Toxoplasma gondii* infection, which is an important cause of abortions and stillbirths in pregnant women. The organism is borne by cats and it can cross the placenta and infect the fetus, causing congenital symptoms of toxoplasmosis that include abnormal changes in head size (hydrocephaly or microcephaly), intracranial calcifications, deafness, seizures, cerebral palsy, damage to the retina and mental retardation. Acute infection with *T. gondii* can produce psychotic symptoms similar to those displayed by people with schizophrenia and the authors postulate a relationship with the development of schizophrenia in later life (Fuller Torrey & Yolken 2003, p. 1375).

Genetic Predisposition

As with neuroanatomical explanations, genetic explanations are far from conclusive. What seems most likely is that an individual's genetic make-up leaves them vulnerable to the development of the illness to some degree so that a person inherits a certain level of risk for developing the illness rather than inheriting the illness itself. The person who is most at risk of developing schizophrenia is the person who shares the most genes with a person with the disorder. That is, a person with a family member with schizophrenia is at higher risk of developing the illness than a member of the general population.

The prevalence of schizophrenia is commonly accepted to be as stated in the DSM-5; that is, approximately 1% (although as we have seen, it is by no means an easy figure to calculate). This means that on average an individual has a 1 in 100 chance of developing the illness, although this average figure has been shown to vary widely, depending on a range of environmental circumstances. Studies have consistently shown that an individual is far more likely to be diagnosed with schizophrenia if another family member has also been diagnosed. If an individual has a sibling diagnosed with schizophrenia, their chances are up to 10 times higher than the average or higher in the case of twins (van Os & Kapur 2009).

The genome project was expected by many researchers to provide a definitive answer to the question of a genetic cause for schizophrenia, but at best it succeeded in proving only that some people might have a genetic predisposition to schizophrenia if other conditions such as their lifestyle, health, stress levels and inherited vulnerability predisposed them to it (www.genome.gov/10001772). The search for the 'Holy Grail' of a genetic explanation for schizophrenia is seductive because the cure would be simplified should it be found to be a mere matter of clipping or replacing the gene or genes that are the cause of untold worldwide suffering.

Biochemical Differences

Chemicals known as neurotransmitters responsible for the transmission of nerve impulses across the synapse have also been thought to be responsible for the development of schizophrenia. The most discussed theory relating to brain biochemistry involvement in schizophrenia relates to an abnormal amount or action of the neurotransmitter dopamine in the brain of the person diagnosed with schizophrenia (van Os & Kapur 2009). This theory is often referred to as the dopamine hypothesis and the theory is a mixture of known facts and hypotheses. Antipsychotic medications such as quetiapine act by blocking some of the dopamine receptor sites in the brain and therefore the amount of effective dopamine is reduced (Seeman 2009). These medications also reduce symptoms such as hallucinations and paranoia. Certain other substances, amphetamines in particular, increase the dopamine action and contribute to the development of psychosis in individuals with no history of psychosis (Thirthalli & Benegal 2006). Antipsychotic medications have an effect on positive symptoms such as delusional thinking and hallucinations, so perhaps dopamine excesses may be responsible for the positive symptoms in schizophrenia and psychotic disorders. But negative symptoms are not produced by stimulants such as amphetamines, which are associated with dopamine excesses. These dopamine-blocking agents are effective in treating only some aspects of the illness. It is logical to assume therefore that the dopamine hypothesis only partially explains the symptoms commonly seen in schizophrenia.

Serotonin, another commonly found neurotransmitter, may also be significant in the development of schizophrenia (Sumiyoshi et al. 2008). A broad group of drugs collectively known as the atypical antipsychotics, including clozapine, olanzepine and respiridone, block both serotonin and dopamine receptors and have been shown to be more effective in the treatment of schizophrenia and other psychoses. Lieberman et al. (2005) found that typical antipsychotics might increase and atypical antipsychotics decrease basal ganglia volumes. This suggests that typical antipsychotics such as haloperidol might have effects on brain morphology due to their neurotoxicity and that newer atypical antipsychotics such as olanzapine are more neuroprotective.

COMORBIDITY

Rates of comorbidity with substance-related disorders are high in schizophrenia. Substance abuse is prevalent among people experiencing chronic schizophrenia, with tobacco, caffeine, cannabis and alcohol being common substances of abuse (Andrews et al. 2014). Substances, in particular stimulants, can worsen the symptoms of psychosis (Sara et al. 2014). In one study of 51 people with schizophrenia presenting in hospitals, community mental health facilities and emergency departments, 51% had concurrent substance use disorders; more than 80% of these also had cannabis disorders (Sara et al. 2014).

The assessment and management of substance abuse or misuse are part of the nurse's role because research identifies substance use in populations diagnosed with schizophrenia as being associated with more frequent hospitalisations, deterioration in self-care, disruptive behaviour, nonadherence to treatment and suicide (Andrews et al. 2014). Of those studied by Sara et al. (2014), 59% were hospitalised with mental health problems, 52% were admitted with injury of self-harm, 18% experienced periods of homelessness and those with stimulant disorders had more admissions than those with cannabis use alone. People with schizophrenia or psychotic disorders experienced stimulant disorders at rates 10 times those of the general population (Sara et al. 2014). An associated metaanalysis of the data related to stimulant disorders in people with psychosis conducted by the same authors (Sara et al. 2015) revealed that stimulant disorders are much higher in people with psychosis than they are in the general population and that this contributes significantly to the burden of psychosis.

Anxiety disorders can coexist with schizophrenia and the rates of obsessive-compulsive disorder and panic disorder are elevated in individuals with schizophrenia compared with the general population (APA 2013, p. 105). Up to 50% of people diagnosed with schizophrenia develop depression and 10% commit suicide within the 5 years immediately following their diagnosis of schizophrenia, so there is a compelling argument for multi-focussed care (Andrews et al. 2014). Depressed mood, delusions, hopelessness, poor self-esteem and a strong sense of personal loss associated with the illness are all recognised as factors in suicidal behaviour among those diagnosed with schizophrenia (Andrews et al. 2014). The implications for practice are that diagnosis is not the end of the story: there needs to be ongoing risk and illness assessment as well as continuing support for the person's development of lasting, meaningful social connections.

Anxiety can develop in people with a schizophrenic illness as a response to decreased self-esteem, loss of control over their life, the distressing symptoms of their illness and the havoc it wreaks with social relationships and their sense of connectedness with their community (Andrews et al. 2014). If steps are not taken to identify encroaching anxiety early, low-level fears and anxieties may develop into a more severe mental disorder. Effective intervention in the prevention and/or management of comorbid disorders is a key role for nurses and they will need to use psychoeducation and skills training in addition to encouraging more effective coping strategies in their patients (Andrews et al. 2014).

INTERVENTIONS/TREATMENTS

Psychopharmacological Interventions

Chapter 25 includes a comprehensive section on antipsychotic or neuroleptic drugs, which is an excellent guide for students seeking more information about this important intervention.

Students studying mental health nursing or gaining clinical experience in specialist psychiatric facilities may find it hard to comprehend what mental healthcare achieved prior to the development of antipsychotic or neuroleptic drugs. Chapter 3 describes the era prior to the availability of effective drug treatments, when people with mental illness were accommodated in large, harsh institutions offering few effective treatments beyond confinement and little hope for recovery. Yet this was the reality until the 1950s when the first antipsychotic medications were used in treatment.

In the 1950s, a French surgeon, Henri Laborit, used the antihistamine drug chlorpromazine to reduce the amount of general anaesthesia required by his patients during surgery. The calming effect of chlorpromazine was applied to psychiatric patients and chlorpromazine became the first of many 'typical antipsychotics' or 'major tranquillisers' belonging to the phenothiazine group, which includes thioridazine, trifluoperazine and fluphenazine. They revolutionised management of the disruptive positive symptoms of schizophrenia and, although their use has been associated with problematic adverse reactions, the phenothiazines offered new hope of successful illness management and even the prospect of independent living outside the hospital setting.

In 1990, the atypical antipsychotics emerged, offering less serious adverse effects and more effective treatment of psychotic illnesses in both the early and the residual stages (Muller et al. 2002). The first of these, clozapine, had been around since the 1960s but its habit of causing bone marrow suppression and resultant agranulocytosis (a blood disorder characterised by severe depletion of white blood cells, rendering the body almost defenceless against infection) ruled it out as a drug with widespread practical application. Recent technology has made monitoring and detection of blood dyscrasias more reliable so that the benefits of using this drug can outweigh the risks, provided that regular blood tests are undertaken. Other drugs commonly referred to as atypical antipsychotics include respiridone, amisulpride, quetiapine and olanzapine.

The primary goal of antipsychotic drug administration is to control the positive symptoms of schizophrenia, particularly delusional thinking, bizarre behaviour, hallucinations, agitation and feelings of paranoia. While the typical antipsychotic medications are effective at combatting these positive symptoms, they are less effective at targeting negative symptoms such as emotional blunting, avolition, loss of energy and social withdrawal. In fact, these drugs can make such features worse in some cases.

However, the atypical antipsychotics, named 'atypical' because they contrast with the more conventional drugs such as chlorpromazine and thioridazine in their action and pharmacology, are also effective against negative symptoms. The broader action of atypical antipsychotics has contributed to their use as the first choice in recovery-oriented treatment, which aims to facilitate the individual's return to life much as it was prior to the onset of the illness. This is particularly the case with clozapine (Asenjo Lobos et al. 2010).

The nurse's role is to monitor the efficacy and adverse side effects of medications, respond with any necessary interventions, ensure that medical staff are advised of the impact (or perhaps lack of it) that the medication is having on the individual and provide information to the person and their support persons about the medication.

The adverse effects of antipsychotics can include peripheral nervous system effects such as dry mouth, headache, constipation, urinary hesitancy, photophobia, decreased lacrimation (tear production) and sexual dysfunction in males and females. Central nervous system effects include sedation, parkinsonian effects, akathisia and lowered seizure threshold. Severe adverse effects include neuroleptic malignant syndrome, tardive dyskinesia, agranulocytosis and acute dystonic reaction (spasm). Other unwanted side effects include photosensitivity, retinal deterioration, weight gain and hormonal interference.

Chapter 25 incorporates a useful table of the side effects of typical antipsychotic medications, and Table 15.2 lists things that the nurse can do to help the person who is experiencing some of the more common side effects.

Medication Adherence

The second goal of psychopharmacology is to prevent the relapse of the illness and that requires strict medication adherence. The period in which maintenance doses of medication will be required varies from individual to individual. The general guidelines suggest that for an individual who has experienced a single episode of psychosis, medication may be required for 1 year at least. In situations of subsequent relapse the medication period is longer, with the optimal period of time unclear (Gaebel et al. 2010).

Pharmaceuticals used to treat schizophrenia or psychosis can cause many adverse reactions, which add another burden of disability to the individual who is already experiencing one of the most debilitating mental illnesses (van Os & Kapur 2009). Against such a backdrop, many individuals choose to be noncompliant. To continue taking medication that causes a wide range of unpleasant adverse reactions long after the symptoms of the illness have gone can take a large leap of faith. It is no surprise that many individuals cease taking their antipsychotic medication over the long term. Also, some individuals with psychotic disorders do not have the insight to see that there is a relationship between medications and wellness, but they do see the unpleasant side effects, so they cease taking their medication. Furthermore, some individuals cannot understand the reasons for taking medication or the frequency with which they need to take it. In some cases clinicians have not provided the necessary education for their patients to be well informed about their medication regimen. Some clinicians treat patients in an authoritarian and paternalistic way and never achieve a genuine cooperative therapeutic relationship.

The use of long-acting depot drugs requiring just one injection every week or every couple of weeks can assist in compliance because it removes the element of choice about whether or not to take medication. A therapeutic alliance between the individual and their health professional based on mutually agreed goals and shared choices is an even better way to ensure compliance (Gray et al. 2010). Box 15.4 outlines educational guidelines helpful in increasing patients' understanding of their medication regimen.

Non-Psychopharmacological Treatment

Psychopharmacology is usually the first-line treatment for schizophrenia and psychotic disorders because it is effective in managing the positive symptoms that are so disruptive to the person and the environment in which they live. Any interventions occurring at an acute stage should be simple, straightforward and aimed at reducing the person's anxiety and confusion. However, as soon as the person is able to concentrate without the severe distractions of delusions, hallucinations or disorganised thought processes, some psychological interventions can be initiated very effectively concurrently with medications.

Cognitive Behavioural Therapy

Cognitive behavioural interventions are ideally suited to the individual in the later stages of recovery or as maintenance

TABLE 15.2 Adverse Effects of Antipsychotic Medications and Nursing Interventions

Adverse Effect	Nursing Intervention
Weight gain, especially with clozapine, olanzapine and chlorpromazine	Stress the importance of activity and exercise and accompany the person, if possible, to overcome anergia. Assess current dietary intake and suggest modifications if required.
Parkinsonian effects: blank mask-like expression, drooling, tremor, muscle rigidity, stiffness and shuffling gait	Reassure the person that these adverse reactions subside with time. Monitor for parkinsonian effects and administer anticholinergics as prescribed and prn.
Akathisia ('restless leg syndrome') disturbs both sleep and rest with the incessant urge to move the limb and to change position	Report this to the medical practitioner who might need to review the antipsychotic if adverse reactions cannot be tolerated. Anticholinergics might ameliorate adverse reactions.
Neuroleptic malignant syndrome: serious and life threatening; usually develops quickly but could occur any time the person is taking a higher potency typical antipsychotic (e.g. haloperidol)	This is a medical emergency with a mortality rate of 20%–30%. Symptoms are hyperthermia, severe motor rigidity, disturbances in levels of consciousness, cardiovascular functioning, blood pressure, sweating, pyrexia, hypotension, tachycardia, stupor and muscular rigidity. Cease antipsychotic drug immediately and refer to a medical practitioner. Nursing care consists of vigilance for the syndrome in those who are taking high-potency drugs such as haloperidol, hydration, monitoring and reduction of body temperature.
Tardive dyskinesia (TD; 'late-occurring movement disorder'), a devastating, irreversible adverse reaction to long-term conventional antipsychotic medication (e.g. haloperidol) but less frequently atypical antipsychotics	Effects range in severity from mild to incapacitating and include: uncontrollable coarse tremor; spasm-like movements of the body, arms and legs; rolling the tongue; and smacking the lips. TD continues after cessation of antipsychotics and is often made worse by the administration of antiparkinsonian drugs such as benztropine. Refer involuntary movements to the medical practitioner to cease, lower or taper off the dose and assess.
Acute dystonic reaction (spasm) muscle spasms in body, trunk and neck (opisthotonos and torticollis); eyes can roll up uncontrollably (oculogyric crisis); life threatening when muscles of the larynx spasm and occlude the airway	This is a medical emergency demanding swift nursing intervention. Acute dystonic reactions respond swiftly to intravenous, intramuscular or oral (route depends on the level of acuity) administration of antiparkinsonian drugs such as benztropine, followed by careful observation. In the case of laryngeal spasm, the patient may require airway support and oxygen therapy until it resolves.

BOX 15.4 Education Guidelines

Patient education guidelines prior to commencement of antipsychotic medication include the following:

- Take the medication as prescribed.
- There is a likelihood that the medication will be needed for a significant length of time.
- Antipsychotic medications commonly cause adverse reactions and these can be discussed with the mental health professional.
- Some medications cause sedation and fatigue, so great care must be taken when driving or operating heavy machinery.
- Medication will need to be reviewed if the patient becomes pregnant.
- Medications interact with alcohol. Alcohol is best avoided when taking these medications.
- Do not mix illicit drugs (amphetamines, narcotics, etc.) with antipsychotics.
- If a dose is missed, wait until the next dose is due. Don't double up.
- Do not stop taking the medication as soon as you feel well. These medications are necessary to maintain good health.
- Not taking medication as prescribed creates the risk of relapse.
- Regular blood tests may be required if clozapine has been commenced.

when they are well. The underlying assumption behind cognitive behavioural therapy (CBT) is that individuals can positively influence their symptoms by changing their behaviour and thinking. Moreover, the symptoms currently experienced are the result of habits in thinking and behaviour learned in the past and have a detrimental effect in the present (Turkington et al. 2002). The approach to therapy is therefore to unlearn the destructive ways of the past and to replace them with more constructive approaches for the future.

CBT has no adverse effects, unlike antipsychotic medication, and has the potential to improve an individual's quality of life long after treatment ceases (Bechdolf et al. 2010). A person who hears frightening hallucinations while travelling on public transport may discover that listening to music through headphones and a portable device can drown out the voices and no-one can detect that they are talking to 'voices' if they speak into a mobile phone. In addition, the person can be encouraged to view the hallucinations as part of an illness that can be managed and that these voices are harmless. People experiencing delusional thinking can be encouraged to explore the content of these delusions. Delusional thinking may involve the belief that the neighbours are spying on them and the person might be encouraged to modify their thinking so that they view their neighbours' actions as being motivated by concern rather than malice. Getting to know and trust the neighbours could be a solution. It must be acknowledged that, because of the nature of delusional thinking, this approach may or may not be successful and in all likelihood success might take a significant amount of time to achieve.

Many individuals with schizophrenia labour under the stigma associated with the illness and as a result have poor self-esteem. CBT focusses on the person's strengths and abilities, which in turn improves self-esteem and goal achievement. There has long been a belief that schizophrenia and psychosis, along with other mental illnesses, may be a maladaptive and destructive response to poorly managed levels of stress (Sadock et al. 2009). This belief forms the basis of the diathesis-stress model of causation. CBT is effective in identifying stressors in an individual's life, ways of avoiding excessive stress and solutions to various unavoidable stressful situations. Chapter 24 provides more detail about individual interpersonal therapies in general, and CBT in particular.

CRITICAL THINKING CHALLENGE 15.2

Why is cognitive behavioural therapy (CBT) likely to be more successful in the later stages of recovery of schizophrenia than earlier in the treatment?

Supportive Psychotherapy

People who suffer from schizophrenia experience additional impairments apart from the illness process. These impairments relate largely to issues of everyday life, which the unaffected person seems to carry out with relative ease. Impairments arising from schizophrenia include an impaired ability to perceive one's external social environment accurately, resulting in feelings of threat or peril; diminished ability to relate to others socially and to maintain relationships; poor self-esteem; and failure to experience the range of normal emotions. The role of supportive psychotherapy in managing impairments arising from schizophrenia is considered to be just as important as treating the symptoms of the disease and is central to any treatment regimen. The treatment approach in supportive psychotherapy is based on the establishment of a therapeutic relationship that addresses individual needs. This reality-oriented approach enables the individual to explore aspects of their beliefs that are based in reality.

Nursing Interventions

Effective Communication

Nurses have the most frequent and regular contact with the person experiencing psychosis or schizophrenia, their family and other support people, so nurses are in the best position to assist them with stressors, provide education and establish a therapeutic relationship. Nurses can learn effective communication strategies that will enable them better to 'be with' the person with schizophrenia or psychotic disorders. For example, the advice offered by the Hearing Voices Network (www.hearing-voices.org) could be useful if the person is distracted by their symptoms, experiencing difficulties with attention and concentration, and/or distressed and isolated. This advice includes:

- Respect the person's privacy.
- Keep your conversations brief.
- Give one message at a time and don't offer too many choices.
- Check that the person has understood what you have said and that you have understood what they have said.
- Do not dismiss them, even if what they are saying sounds unusual or does not make sense to you.
- Recognise that what the person says seems very real to them.
- Listen respectfully to what they are saying.
- Avoid arguing or getting into a debate unless safety is an issue.

More supportive nursing interventions that could help the person with symptoms of schizophrenia or psychotic disorders are listed in Table 15.3.

TABLE 15.3 Supportive Nursing Interventions

Issue	Nursing Response
Delusional thinking	• Assess the risk the delusional thinking poses to self or others and take appropriate action to prevent such a threat, for example continuous close observation or use of prn antipsychotic medication. This action is designed to reduce the chances of the person acting on the delusional thinking. • Attempt to understand the content of the delusional thinking. Delusional thinking often provides a clue to themes occurring in the person's thinking. It also acknowledges that you believe the delusions are real to the person. This conveys a concerned understanding and assists the development of trust. • Don't reinforce delusional thinking by agreeing with the ideas presented but at the same time don't argue or attempt to prove the belief is false by using logic. Delusions are by definition not amenable to argumentation and you risk antagonising the person. • Provide a quiet and peaceful environment if delusional thinking is increasing, and reduce or eliminate environmental factors that appear to be stimulating delusional thinking such as television or radio.
Auditory hallucinations	• Assess the extent and content of auditory hallucinations. • If the hallucinations are commanding certain actions, assess the degree to which these commands compel the person to act. Assess especially the impact of such commands on personal safety. Such hallucinations may pose threats to safety and require accurate assessment and immediate nursing intervention by way of prn medication and close observation. • Reassure the person that hallucinations are a part of the illness and cannot be heard by others. • Identify with the person activities that appear to stimulate hallucinations and devise ways of coping with such situations. • Identify with the person actions that reduce the impact of hallucinations, such as listening to music through headphones. • Use prn medication strategically when hallucinations are most distressing.

TABLE 15.3 Supportive Nursing Interventions—cont'd

Issue	Nursing Response
Fear/anxiety/ paranoia	• Assess the level of fear, anxiety or paranoia experienced. • Reassure the person that the environment is safe and that no harm will come to them. • Be aware of your own behaviour and how it could be misinterpreted. Ensure that your approach is quietly confident and mindful of the person's need for generous personal space. • Don't touch the person, as this could be interpreted as threatening. • Don't whisper or laugh in the person's presence, as this may be misconstrued as ridicule. • Use prn medication strategically when fear/anxiety/paranoia is escalating and distressing.
Disordered thinking	• Assess the content and extent of disordered thinking. • Assess the degree to which thought disorder affects the person's activities of daily living. • Speak using clear, unambiguous language to facilitate clearer understanding. • Assess the effectiveness of medications in the reduction of disordered thinking. • Remember that diversional activities may need to be tailored to the individual's ability, given the difficulties experienced as a result of disordered thought. Going for a walk may be more appropriate than a game of Scrabble. • Assess the impact that the level of environmental stimuli is having on the person's ability to think clearly and modify the level of stimuli as needed.
Lack of insight	• Assess the person's level of understanding of the illness and the situation they are currently facing. • Provide information about the illness in a way that is appropriate to the person's level of wellness. • Reinforce the need to take antipsychotic medication according to medical instructions. One of the most common factors in nonadherence of medication regimens is lack of insight. This has a major impact on the person's prognosis.
Poor personal hygiene	• Assess the person's ability to assess and to cope with their hygiene needs. Their current level of personal hygiene might be useful as an indicator. • Encourage/remind the person to meet their hygiene needs to the best of their ability. Because patients have such difficulty in thinking clearly at times, personal hygiene is often neglected. A good level of personal hygiene would decrease the likelihood of the person experiencing harmful social rejection. • Offer tactful assistance to help the person to meet their hygiene needs.
Inadequate nutritional intake	• Assess hydration and nutritional status. • Assess the degree to which poor nutritional intake is related to paranoid delusional thinking. Often patients have a fear that their food is poisoned or contaminated. This can be overcome by a number of nursing actions, which may include the person assisting in the preparation of their food or using prepackaged tamperproof food.

NURSE'S STORY 15.2

Amina

I was 18 when I started mental health nursing at a clinic in Manchester in the 1970s. A friend had started her training there and she said that her job was simply to talk to people all the time; it sounded wonderful after being in an office where we weren't allowed to talk at all! The clinic was an unusually progressive place with no locked wards and nurses were expected not to spend time in the office unless they were writing reports at the end of the day, but to be relating to the patients all throughout the day. It sounded simple: we played cards, chess, basketball or tennis, walked and went to the movies with the patients. We dispensed medications, talked, listened and built relationships. I was not an extrovert but I had to overcome that and approach people who were alone or agitated or angry or burrowed under the bedclothes and sometimes bluntly rejecting.

The most confronting patients were those who were actively psychotic because they were different from anyone I had ever before encountered. Psychotic patients were also acutely attuned to feelings, so any fearfulness or avoidance on my part would be quickly detected and rejection, sometimes abuse, would ensue. Experienced nurses said that it was not the symptoms but the underlying feelings that I needed to respond to: after all, if the person thought that they were being watched, their thoughts were being interfered with by others, or the voices in their head were saying abusive things about them, they would probably feel vulnerable, fearful and defensive. Instead of reasoning or arguments, what they needed was humanity and consideration and to be helped to feel more safe and secure. We call it 'reflection' and 'empathy' nowadays, and it always worked.

In our second year, I was assigned my own group of patients in the day hospital: I learned to conduct large and small therapy groups; to play basketball with my group and dispense their medications; to do relaxation therapy and report my progress to expert supervisors to be supervised and learn supervision in my turn. In my third year, I staffed the clinic's drop-in sessions where people could walk in and talk about their problems, without the restrictions of an appointment. I also performed crisis assessment and follow-up visits to discharged patients in the community, with the domiciliary team.

Professional relationships among the staff from the psychiatrists to the students were the most democratic and mutually helpful that I have ever known and that equality was reflected in our relationships with the patients. Students were continuously and ungrudgingly mentored by registered nurses who taught us everything they knew: medications and how to check for com-

Continued

NURSE'S STORY 15.2—cont'd

pliance and side effects; how to run a group so that people felt safe and supported; how to interpret devastating personal attacks as symptoms of the patient's distress; how to encourage a person to talk or just 'be with' them silently if they didn't want to interact; how to work on different levels simultaneously and turn a card game into a comfortable, inclusive therapy session.

I believe that the most revelatory skill I learned was how to suppress the expectation that a 'conversation' should be two-way; to be receptive to confidences without being judgemental and without letting myself, my feelings, my beliefs and my needs intrude. I often reflect upon the hands-on education I received and contrast it with what we teach and students learn nowadays in universities, and some aspects of the change continue to disturb me. Nurses develop a better academic understanding but receive a narrower and shallower mental health skills base in the 'comprehensive' undergraduate education system. We delivered more holistic care and we were more competent in the past before occupational therapists, social workers and psychologists took over many of the roles once performed by mental health nurses. Yet the patient today is represented by recovery and patient empowerment movements, so they at least are often better served despite a national health service that seems to accept lowered standards of care for people in the interests of economy.

Early Detection and Prevention

There are innovative programmes that concentrate on the early detection of psychosis because research has shown that early intervention and treatment are productive of better long-term outcomes. The early intervention approach aims to shorten the course and decrease the severity of the initial psychotic episode, in order to limit damage to personal identity, social networks and role functioning (McGorry et al. 2000). The Early Intervention in Psychosis (EIP) service is a multidisciplinary mental health service that aims to provide support and treatment to people who are experiencing, or at high risk of developing, psychosis. This support usually lasts for approximately 3 years, with the defining characteristic of an EIP service being a strong ethos of hope and whole team commitment to enabling recovery. This is undertaken through the provision of individually tailored interventions based on current evidence-based practice in the field (National Institute for Health and Care Excellence [NICE] 2016). The key components of an EIP service are:

- Prompt assessment by a practitioner competent in recognising first episode psychosis
- Staff active in building trust and confidence
- Good quality information to help people understand psychosis and their treatment options
- A care coordinator skilled in working in EIP services also able to support people with their social care issues, e.g. housing, debt management, educational or employment needs
- Relapse prevention work
- Options for psychological and pharmacological interventions
- Support where required for families and carers
- Physical health checks
- Regular risk monitoring, crisis and contingency plans
- Care for any coexisting conditions, e.g. depression, anxiety, substance misuse, etc.

The core aims of the EIP services are to reduce the duration of any untreated psychosis or to prevent transition to psychosis for people with an at-risk mental state (NICE 2016).

Advance Care Planning

Acute deterioration might require that mental health services respond to crises including suicidality, severe neglect, cognitive disorganisation and risk of harm to the patient or to others. Once a mental health crisis has developed, options for negotiated care become limited, with a greater likelihood that the patient will be hospitalised and treated under mental health legislation. Advance care planning is a means of avoiding coercive interventions by recording patients' care preferences. It may take the form of an advance directive, which documents the patient's wishes in the event of a mental health emergency (Weller 2010). An advance decision, sometimes referred to as an advance decision to refuse treatment or a living will, is a decision a person can make that allows them to refuse a specific type of treatment at some time in the future. This has to be made at a time when the person has mental capacity, allowing for a person's wishes to be known if they are unable to communicate them in the future. Other forms of advance care planning are crisis plans, wellness recovery and action plans (WRAP) and advance statements. Advance care plans are negotiated with patients when their acute symptoms have reduced and they are able to communicate their care preferences.

An advance care plan might specify medication the patient does or does not wish to receive, who should be contacted for support and which strategies have been found helpful in past crises. Patients need to be supported in developing their advance care plan, usually by a friend or family member. They may also wish to involve their lawyer. The plan should be discussed with the patient's treatment team and a copy should be kept in the patient's file. Nurses can assist patients to initiate advance care plans and can advocate for advance care plans to be incorporated into the patient's treatment plan. Nurses also need to be aware of the content of patients' advance care plans and of their ethical responsibility to respect the choices recorded (Wareham et al. 2005). Clinicians are not bound by advance care plans, but every attempt should be made to provide care that is in keeping with the patient's expressed wishes.

Relapse Prevention

Schizophrenia is usually an episodic disorder, relapsing and remitting with periods of acute psychosis alternating with periods of relative stability. Up to 40% of all people suffer a relapse within a year of being hospitalised (Lamberti 2001), so it is essential to be able to detect the early signs of a potential relapse and put measures in place to prevent it if possible. Lamberti (2001) was an early pioneer in the field of relapse prevention in schizophrenia and his work is seminal. Lamberti found that the key to relapse prevention was working closely with families

BOX 15.5 Early Signs Questionnaire for Identifying Relapse in People with Schizophrenia

NAME_______________________DATE__________

Compared with last week, has there been an increase in any of the following symptoms?

	YES/NO	
1. Problems with sleep	____	____
2. Problems with appetite	____	____
3. Depression	____	____
4. Problems with concentration	____	____
5. Restlessness	____	____
6. Tension or nervousness	____	____
7. Use of alcohol	____	____
8. Use of street drugs (includes marijuana)	____	____
9. Hearing voices or seeing things that others can't hear or see	____	____
10. Less pleasure gained from things you usually enjoy	____	____
11. Feeling people were watching you, were against you, or were talking about you	____	____
12. Preference for being alone and/or been spending less time with other people.	____	____
13. Arguments with others	____	____
14. Inability to get your mind off of one or two things	____	____
15. Problems with attention to grooming and personal hygiene	____	____
Have any other symptoms appeared or increased?	____	____

If so, what were they?____

Did anything specific happen last week that upset you? ____ ____

If so, what was it?____

Have you been taking your medication as it is prescribed for you?

(*Source*: Lamberti, J.S., 2001. Seven keys to relapse prevention in schizophrenia. Journal of Psychiatric Practice July, 253–259. Early Signs Questionnaire. Copyright Dr Marvin Herz. Reproduced with permission.)

and other supports, who are often more likely than patients to detect the onset of relapse. Unfortunately, family and carers are often overlooked as allies in patient care.

Relapse prevention involves a number of steps: the establishment of a therapeutic relationship and ongoing education, identification of the early signs of relapse, monitoring for signs of relapse and intervening early when or if these signs are observed. It is important to engage the person, their family and their supports in the process and to have a positive relationship to ensure accuracy and honesty (Andrews at al. 2014). As in the case of advance care planning, if nurses are able to identify and record a person's characteristic early signs of relapse, these will be valuable for future reference both for relapse prevention and advance care planning processes because timely and appropriate interventions help reduce the number and intensity of relapses experienced.

Early Warning Signs

When open-ended questions were found to be inadequate to identify the early signs of relapse in people with schizophrenia, Lamberti (2001) administered the short questionnaire reproduced in Box 15.5.

Family and Carers

Sometimes families have suffered from the patient's behaviour when they were unwell in the past and they prefer to be marginally involved (or not involved at all) in the patient's care planning. Family members can have mixed feelings about their relative's mental disorder and, conversely, sometimes the patient has suffered abuse from a family member and would not wish that person to be involved with their treatment.

Relatives and the person with schizophrenia or a psychotic illness might all have to deal with conflicting emotions, but O'Brien and Cole (2004) found that in general relatives found exclusion to be a source of stress and they would rather be included in the person's care than not. Kennedy et al. (2009) concluded that more education should be offered to carers, relatives and guardians in the early stages of psychotic disorders because the patient might be too acutely unwell to offer meaningful feedback and psychotic disorders are stressful for both the patient and their support systems. Make an effort in every case to find out the help that relatives and carers want from the treating team, as well as the level of contribution they are prepared to commit, since their knowledge and resources are vital to care planning if their cooperation and involvement can be secured. Families and caregivers might benefit from education about coping strategies that work, problem solving, communication skills and the impact of medication (Andrews et al. 2014). Family psychoeducation programmes are both highly effective and very much underutilised (Lamberti 2001).

LIVING WITH SCHIZOPHRENIA

Schizophrenia is both enormously debilitating to the individual and costly to society. The costs of schizophrenia in Western countries have been found to be between 7% and 12% of the gross national product (GNP) and healthcare systems are underfunded and, in most cases, unable to cope with the burden (Chong et al. 2016).

Experiencing psychosis can raise profound questions about life and self. Despite the importance of existential and/or spiritual concerns to people who experience psychosis—such as the person's individual meaning of psychosis—there is an absence of these concerns being addressed in the literature (Geekie 2013). Questions such as the individual's relationship to God and whether the person's psychotic experience has been sent by God and, if so, whether it was a punishment for being a bad person, are not uncommon (Geekie 2013).

In Patient Story 15.1 Matthew talks about how he found validation for his experiences in the hearing voices movement, which is an example of the emerging influence of patient-led understandings and involvement. The Hearing Voices Network reasons that psychotic experiences need to be understood from the perspective of their personal meaning for the patient and supports theories that traumatic

PATIENT STORY 15.1

Matthew

I had used illicit drugs since my early teens, I had lived overseas and experienced homelessness, and I could see little future in my life when at the age of 21 I went with my mother to see a GP. The GP was concerned about my focus on suicide, sense of hopelessness and reported drug use, so following liaison with the mental health team, he arranged for a direct admission to a psychiatric hospital. Although I had many friends growing up, I had few functional relationships in my life at this time and my family was very concerned about my wellbeing. They had little knowledge about mental health problems at this stage.

Although I was assessed by a consultant psychiatrist and a nurse, I felt that the nurse heard me most clearly and appeared to be less concerned by my diagnosis and more concerned with who I might be and the experiences that might have contributed to my condition. I was started on antipsychotic and antidepressant medication and discharged 6 weeks later to my mother's home, with planned GP follow up.

One of the friends I made in hospital killed himself shortly after I left hospital, and not long after this I made an attempt on my own life. I told people I was hearing voices saying that I was worthless and should kill myself. I also heard the voice of a man saying that he was watching me through video cameras at all times, and I became very frightened.

Several admissions followed, during which I had stopped using illicit drugs, yet I still heard derogatory voices and felt a sense that the world and myself were being controlled by an external 'force'. I was suicidal and I tried to kill myself, following through on a plan I had made. Other frightening psychotic experiences included seeing a cat who I believed attempted to kill me, which led to my imprisoning myself for 3 days until I knew that the cat had gone. I experienced a sense of being an incompetent human being and searched for potential explanations for my experiences, exploring my sexuality and seeking religious justifications.

I was admitted to hospital five times, but I felt that the nursing and medical teams never discovered what caused my experiences of psychosis. My unusual realities were considered to be part of a biomedically informed rationale for a psychotic disorder and the possibility of my suffering from schizophrenia was not excluded. Nurses spent a lot of time with me in the unit but they were task oriented. I believe that they could have used basic mental health nursing skills, such as building a therapeutic relationship, to develop a more meaningful understanding of the events that contributed to my experiencing psychosis.

Treatment focussed on medications and electroconvulsive therapy (ECT). I was prescribed a concoction of antipsychotic, antidepressant and mood stabiliser medications. I feel now that as my primary workers, nurses could have been more assertive in identifying for me the side effects of my medication and their negative impact. A proactive approach on their part might have prevented or addressed a number of the difficulties and problems that arose. I gained 50 kg in 18 months probably due to medication, a poor diet and reduced exercise, and I became increasingly socially isolated: all of which were perceived by nursing staff as the usual negative symptoms of a psychotic illness. No-one talked about recovery and the concept of a positive personal and clinical journey was not easy to imagine.

During my fifth admission I commenced 2 years of psychotherapy because medication and hospitalisation had not led to an improvement in my symptoms. I went to live in a nurse-led housing community of eight residents with mental health problems, where the person-centred emphasis was less upon diagnosis and disease and more upon the acceptance of my own experiences and reality, and support for my journey towards my future. I made a number of friends in the mental health system and that mutual acceptance between peers proved to be a significant factor in making sense of the whole experience, and finally, in accepting myself.

Over time the voices and other psychotic phenomena impacted my life less, and I worked with a psychiatrist to reduce, then stop, all medications. I worked as a volunteer then found paid employment before moving into my own accommodation.

Since the 4-year period when I was 'treated' by the mental health system for a psychotic disorder I have spent 15 years following my life journey: being part of a beautiful family as a husband and a father to three children, and developing a successful career in business. Especially valuable in helping me to interpret the cause of the voices that I experienced has been the 'hearing voices' approach towards making sense of and understanding psychosis.

experiences are the origin of voice hearing (Longden 2013). See Useful Websites for the details of the Hearing Voices Network.

The importance to mental healthcare of recognising the patient's experience has led to service users being involved in undergraduate mental health nurse education. It is essential that academic roles are facilitated for people with a lived experience of mental health problems if the mental health system is to be peopled with nurses who understand the patient experience (Byrne et al. 2012). The best reason to involve patients in nurse education is to produce practitioners who will deliver appropriate and improved outcomes for patients and their carers and there are increasing numbers of patients making this contribution.

For example, Louise Byrne has a lived experience of significant mental health challenges and is employed at the Central Queensland University, Australia, as an academic, teaching nursing students about recovery. Students evaluated her teaching and contribution highly, believing that their attitudes and beliefs about patients had changed, their own self-awareness had been enhanced and their grasp of concepts such as the therapeutic relationship, stigma, hope and recovery had been strengthened (Byrne et al. 2012).

Debra Lampshire is employed as an academic within Auckland University, New Zealand, and she utilises her personal experience of recovery from a psychotic disorder and her involvement with mental health services, placing a strong emphasis on recovery and individualised care (Schneebeli et al. 2010). Lampshire's perspective was evaluated by students as being normalising and challenging stereotypes about mental health service users and reducing the fears students had about working with people who experience mental health problems. Lampshire writes prolifically about her experiences and the strengths-based ways in which recovery can be facilitated in people with enduring symptoms of psychosis (Randal et al. 2009). The 'recovery model' that Lampshire and her colleagues devised postulates that when people use the same unsuccessful coping methods to deal with trauma and challenges, each failure makes the person weaker and more vulnerable. Crises need to be treated as opportunities to identify triggers, develop new skills, increase strength and build resilience (Randal et al. 2009). See Chapter 24 for more information about the strengths-based model.

For many people who have experienced a harsh outcome to their battle with schizophrenia or psychotic illness, especially the homeless and the destitute, access to much-needed healthcare remains a major issue. Of those who can access mental health services, many experience difficulties arising from the often serious and debilitating adverse effects of medications required to manage their illness. Adherence with treatment is often problematic and many choose to cease taking medication, which often results in a return to severe mental illness and repeated admissions. This tragic pattern is often referred to in mental health contexts as the 'revolving-door syndrome', often with negative connotations.

Homelessness

Having a safe home that is conducive to a sense of security and wellbeing is an essential human need, yet this need is not met for a great number of individuals with schizophrenia, the most common serious mental illness among the homeless (Buhrich et al. 2003). Studies have shown that mental illness and homelessness are interrelated in a number of ways. An illness like schizophrenia exhibits positive symptoms that can result in the disruption of home life and the destruction of relationships. Positive symptoms may affect the relationship between an individual with schizophrenia who is a tenant and the owner of a property, in some cases resulting in eviction of the individual with the disorder. Negative symptoms often affect the individual's ability to form and maintain attachments with others (Corcoran et al. 2011). Coupled with negative symptoms is the inability to work, which may result in failure to meet commitments associated with tenancy and housing repayments.

However, this is not the only way in which mental illness and homelessness are related. For some, mental illness develops after the person becomes homeless and is probably associated with the immense stress associated with the conditions of homelessness: frequent assaults, rapes, robberies, malnourishment, lack of support and lack of access to health services. Clearly, suffering from schizophrenia and being homeless is destructive. According to the literature, the death rate for those who find themselves in both situations is four times that of the general population and twice that of those experiencing schizophrenia but who have a home (Folsom & Jeste 2002). The great challenge for mental health policy makers and clinicians is to provide comprehensive healthcare to the homeless mentally ill and to promote access to housing and health agencies for individuals suffering from schizophrenia.

Work

Work, education and socioeconomic status are key aspects of most people's lives and those who have experience with schizophrenia often suffer significant disruption and disadvantage. Lack of employment opportunities represents a form of social exclusion facing those experiencing the effects of schizophrenia. Unemployment rates are very high in people who experience psychoses and of those who are engaged in employment a significantly large period of time is lost to sick leave. There is a great need for research into the area of the beneficial effects of work on those who experience schizophrenia, as well as the factors that either facilitate or inhibit finding work or returning to work. Often the transition back into work is easier if voluntary work is undertaken initially. There is disability discrimination legislation that may have a bearing on the type of assistance the workplace is required to undertake. In most cases, the employer is responsible for the provision of a workplace that is both safe and free from adverse responses from the employer and other employees. This is often difficult given the societal stigma that a disorder such as schizophrenia carries.

Labelling and Stigma

The stigma associated with mental illness is profoundly debilitating to the individual with schizophrenia and people who experience it say that the effects of stigma are as bad as the effects of the illness itself. Mental illness continues to bring a sense of shame on the individual and often their family and the family is often blamed for its development. In Western society, despite major education campaigns, people still consider individuals diagnosed with schizophrenia as unpredictable and dangerous. Although violence is associated with the diagnosis and is often the reason for hospitalisation, the incidence is very small. Prison populations continue to have a disproportionate number of individuals diagnosed with serious mental illnesses such as schizophrenia (Rautanen & Lauerma 2011). Studies of international prison populations indicate that between 10% and 15% of offenders have a serious mental illness and they are up to four times as likely to be experiencing psychotic illness than a person in the general community (Fazel & Seewald 2012). There could be mitigating circumstances; for example, a shoplifter might offend because of lapses of memory and concentration, or confusion due to a psychotic episode, or comorbid drug or alcohol use. Nonetheless, the existence of an association between serious mental illness and crime contributes to the stigma experienced by the mentally ill (Volavka & Citrome 2008).

The news media have an enormous influence on the way people view mental illness, and even when no harm is intended, the words 'schizophrenic', 'crazy' or 'insane' are inappropriately used as terms of description. SANE Australia maintains the StigmaWatch website, which highlights instances of mockery or vilification such as occasions on which people who have committed violent or horrible crimes are stated by news media to have a mental illness before any diagnosis has been made (see www.sane.org/mental-health-and-illness/facts-and-guides/reducing-stigma). SANE Australia believes that these repetitive references add to the general public's confusion and lack of clarity about mental illness.

While medical and nursing organisations and governments attempt to demystify the illness, various media portrayals often use the term 'schizophrenic' to describe difficult and socially inappropriate behaviours that happen in the community. The term is used by the layperson as a way of conceptualising aberrant behaviour that they may not fully understand. This is a means of explaining behaviours that they find difficult or impossible to understand by any other means.

When an individual is experiencing psychotic behaviour (such as hallucinations and delusions) in a way that affects others in the community (intrusive or aggressive), the media tend to sensationalise such events to titillate the public. Furthermore, Nairn (2005) analysed mass media in a study and found that few ever reported the views of those with mental illness. According to Nairn, patients' views are seldom heard (see also Box 15.6). Lee (2002) notes that even if psychiatric stigmas are concealed, they remain a constant source of psychic pain to individuals diagnosed with schizophrenia. In the depths of their illness the individual rarely has the opportunity to concentrate on societal norms such as appropriate dress, social etiquette and personal hygiene because of the intensity of their symptoms. In addition, some of the medications used to treat schizophrenia have unsightly adverse effects, which serve to identify and alienate further the individual experiencing the illness.

BOX 15.6 A Thought From a Patient

I have a vision that goes like this: in this new century, mentally ill people will have the science, the organised voting strength and the means to leave our ghettos of isolation behind us. We will finally join with the mainstream community, where we'll be able to live as individuals and not as a group of people who are known and feared by the names of our illness (Steele & Berman 2001, p. 252). Steele, K., Berman, C., 2001. The Day the Voices Stopped: a Memoir of Madness and Hope. Basic Books, New York.

General Health

Chapter 8 was added to this book to highlight the importance of the physical health of mental health patients and to expand on this topic, so coverage here will be brief but nonetheless essential.

To live with the experience of schizophrenia is to experience poorer physical health and have a life expectancy that is significantly shorter than the prevailing average of the society to which the affected individual belongs. In some cases individuals with schizophrenia live up to 15 years less than peers without schizophrenia (van Os & Kapur 2009). Fontaine et al. (2001) stress that early death stems largely from suicide, while Bradshaw et al. (2005) explain loss of life as arising from poor physical health (natural causes). The DSM-5 agrees with Bradshaw and colleague's summation and lists the reasons for a reduced life expectancy in people with schizophrenia: weight gain, diabetes, metabolic syndrome and cardiovascular and pulmonary disease are more common in people with schizophrenia than in the general population (APA 2013).

A study by Morgan et al. (2014) collected data from 1642 participants with psychotic disorders to present estimates of 'treated prevalence and lifetime morbid risk of psychosis, and to describe the cognitive, physical health and substance use profiles of participants' (p. 2163). The results were alarming and the study concluded that people with psychotic illness needed a comprehensive, integrative recovery model to improve their health and quality of life. The investigators found that 60.8% of the participants had metabolic syndrome, 65.9% were smokers, 47.4% were obese, 32.4% were sedentary, 49.8% had a lifetime history of alcohol abuse and/or dependence and 50.8% had lifetime cannabis abuse/dependence (Morgan et al. 2014). 'People with psychosis continue to experience poor physical health, even though many of their risk factors are modifiable and despite public health campaigns aimed at these very risk factors (Morgan et al. 2014, p. 2171).

Very similar results were found by Mitchell et al. (2013) when they conducted a metaanalysis of publications examining medical comorbidity and cardiovascular risk factors in individuals with schizophrenia. The highest rates of metabolic syndrome were found in those prescribed olanzapine (Mitchell et al. 2013, p. 306). Obesity is known to be compounded by drugs such as clozapine, which can be responsible for significant weight gain (van Os & Kapur 2009). Laugharne et al. (2016) surveyed psychiatrists to find out what they did to discover and to treat metabolic syndrome in their patients who were prescribed antipsychotic drugs. Fewer than one-third responded: of these, 55% had no established routine to screen for metabolic syndrome and 13% said they did not know how to detect it; fewer than 50% checked patients' weight, fasting glucose or lipids; and basic monitoring equipment was absent in 50% of cases. Nonetheless, 83% of respondents admitted a medico-legal responsibility to monitor for the condition (Laugharne et al. 2016). Other related issues are considered to be the patient's responsibility, such as poor engagement in health maintenance behaviours (e.g. cancer screening and exercise), cigarette smoking and poor diet (APA 2013, p. 105).

THE RECOVERY APPROACH

Chapter 2 is devoted entirely to a very comprehensive coverage of the recovery approach in mental healthcare. This section will therefore take the form of a more personal approach to recovery, highlighting the experiences of people who have written about their recovery from schizophrenia. Stories of recovery and research studies increasingly represent psychosis as 'recovery-able' (Young et al. 2015). Long-term studies of recovery have shown that 75% of people with a diagnosis of schizophrenia will experience a recovery journey that includes living life in an independent way (Torgalsbøen & Rund 2010).

There is not a great deal of agreement among health professionals about how recovery should be measured or who makes the decision whether or not recovery has been achieved, but patients would probably say that it is not the health professional's place to decide this, but rather the patient's. The traditional medical view of recovery takes into account the disappearance of symptoms, with or without the need to adhere to a regimen of antipsychotic medication, with the individual sufficiently well to reengage with their social environment (Borg & Davidson 2008). This is a typical (but naive) description of recovery: a normally well person becomes sick, takes the medication and in a short space of time returns to the activity as if nothing has happened. In such a scenario, the concepts of cure and recovery are interchangeable. This is far too simple a story line for something as complex as schizophrenia.

The currently developing understanding considers symptom management as well as the individual's view of their current and future circumstances. Built largely on the work of William Anthony, who is considered to be a pioneer in this field, this understanding takes into account not only symptoms and their possible cessation, but also a process whereby the individual, previously incapacitated by symptoms either partially or totally, moves beyond the illness experience, reassesses their goals and aspirations, optimistically takes into account a new set of capabilities and accepts that, with or without the continuation of symptoms, they are no longer the person they once were (Anthony 1993).

Personal recovery is a journey that any person experiencing distress in psychosis should be supported to experience. The recovery movement has its origins in the civil rights and other social justice movements. The core principles of self-determination, citizenship and the importance of individuals experiencing freedom to be the person they are and live the life they choose are especially relevant to psychotic disorders and schizophrenia.

Recovery from a mental disorder does not imply that all of the symptoms of the disorder have been extinguished. Recovery from mental disorder is described as a deeply personal and unique experience that represents a journey rather than an end point and different people choose to adopt different approaches to it. Sutton (2004) describes two styles of recovery, one being 'integration', where the disorder is examined and accepted, and the other being 'sealing over', where the patient might choose not to examine the disorder and its implications because that would be too distressing.

de Jager et al. (2015) also investigated the lived experience of recovery in 'voice hearers' and their findings were similar to Sutton's, although framed in slightly different terms. The two main styles of recovery detailed in their research were:

1. Turning towards/empowerment, in which the person examined their experience of voices and developed a normalised account of voices, built voice-specific skills, integrated their voices into their daily life and developed a transformed identity; this was considered to be the 'more robust' approach.
2. Turning away/protective hibernation, which concentrated on survival and the importance of medication in recovery.

The authors explain that when a person is in a stage where their mental health is poor, they are exhausted and despairing. Some people are more inclined to 'batten down the hatches', turn away and become more reliant upon medication. However, others are more likely to recognise that the voices are integral parts of themselves and turn towards them, interacting with the voices in healthier ways and negotiating lower doses of medication (de Jager et al. 2015). It seems important that nurses understand that there is no single mode of recovery, instead getting to know the person and their own chosen style so that they can be actively engaged in the process.

Mark Vonnegut, a paediatrician in the United States and the son of the writer Kurt Vonnegut, rejects the option of turning away from or concealing the disorder, despite the stigma this could entail for him as a doctor and a public figure:

"There are many people who fully recover from major psychotic episodes and go on to live full rich lives. Most of them choose to keep quiet about it. In the middle of my illness when I was far from sure that I would survive, I made a promise to remember and tell the truth as best I could about whatever it was that was happening to me. I think it helped" (Vonnegut 2010, p. 374).

Long-term studies of recovery have shown that with recent advances as many as 75% of people diagnosed with schizophrenia will recover sufficiently to return to an acceptable level of independent living and recommencement of roles (Torgalsbøen & Rund 2010).

Traditionally, expertise and knowledge have been viewed as being held by the health professional, with the health professional guiding the somewhat passive and less knowledgeable patient. The concept of recovery requires the stance that the health professional 'cares with' rather than 'cares for' the patient. The individual telling their story becomes the expert and the health professional becomes the learner. Together, the individual's personal experience and the health professional's specialist knowledge assist in forging a path to recovery.

CONCLUSION

Schizophrenia and psychotic disorders are severe and often debilitating illnesses that affect a significant proportion of the population. These disorders often occur at the outset of the person's adult life, altering their expectations of normal productive work, study and relationships and severely altering their perceptions, behaviour, mood, thinking ability and social and occupational functioning. They deliver a major impact on national health expenditure and are among the most expensive of all illnesses facing Western economies.

Despite their prevalence and impact, schizophrenia and psychotic illnesses have yet to be fully understood. They continue to be erroneously associated with 'split personality' or 'multiple personality' and individuals with schizophrenia or psychotic disorders are often mistrusted, feared and discriminated against. Aetiology is a melange of causes including social and environmental, anatomical and biochemical: all are current foci of research and theory development. The relationship between stress and schizophrenia is a further area of theory development and stress management is often included in patient education and illness management.

Modern mental health treatments at least offer hope, whereas in the past, prior to effective drug-based therapies, there was none. Effective treatment for schizophrenia now includes a range of medications as well as a variety of nonpharmacological treatments. Modern drugs such as the typical and atypical antipsychotics enable a great number of individuals diagnosed with schizophrenia to recover from their illness. Nonpharmacological therapies such as CBT enable individuals to learn about their illness and ways of living with its effects. Both forms of therapy can minimise the symptoms of schizophrenia and prevent further relapses.

The patient with lived experiences movement has greatly influenced the ways in which the aetiology, terminology, prognosis and recovery from schizophrenia and psychotic disorders are viewed. The strong advocacy of capable patients is necessary when the stigma of violence and dangerousness is overemphasised by a great many in society, compounding the difficulties faced by individuals experiencing the clinical manifestations of these illnesses.

Nurses play an important role in assisting individuals experiencing schizophrenia to recover from the illness, maintain their health and achieve their optimal level of wellness. Nurses use the information gained from mental status assessment, including both subjective and objective data, to plan and to implement care designed to assist individuals to predict and prevent relapse and to take responsibility for their own style of recovery. The great challenge of improving the lives of those who experience these illnesses is far from over. Understanding schizophrenia and psychotic disorders, the symptoms and the ways in which the people who experience the disorders can be treated enables the nurse to assist in meeting this challenge.

EXERCISES FOR CLASS ENGAGEMENT

1. You are nursing a patient diagnosed with paranoid schizophrenia in an inpatient treatment facility. The individual expresses the belief that the water is poisoned and consequently refuses to drink.
   - Devise strategies that may assist the patient to drink the volume required to maintain physical health.
2. A patient believes that you and the other nurses involved in their care are assassins. How will you respond to this expression of belief?
   - Brainstorm this issue in small groups, then conduct it as a role play.
3. Make a list of adverse reactions to antipsychotic medications that are considered to be extrapyramidal. Share your list with the group. Then brainstorm with the group to develop as many strategies as you can that could contribute to greater levels of medication adherence in a person diagnosed with schizophrenia and treated with antipsychotic medication.
4. Nurses have an educative and supportive role in assisting people in their transition back to work.
   - How might nurses assist in this process?
   - Who would require education and support?
   - What information would be required in an education programme designed to assist the individual's return to work?
5. There appears to be a historical, ingrained societal perception that individuals with schizophrenia are violent or otherwise dangerous. In the past, attempts have been made to explain the behaviours of society's most dangerous members as having a basis in mental illness (for example, the random killings by Martin Bryant at Port Arthur, Tasmania, in 1996). While those with illnesses such as paranoid schizophrenia can be and sometimes are responsible for violence and aggression when they believe that someone is trying to harm them, the reality is that people who suffer from psychoses are at greater risk of becoming the victims of violence (Hiday et al. 2002).
   - What are some of the reasons why people with mental illness continue to be feared?
   - Reflect on your own fears that you hold/have held as you think about your exposure to mental health nursing.
   - Identify some occasions where popular film or television has perpetuated the stigma attached to sufferers of mental illness.

ACKNOWLEDGEMENT

This chapter has been adapted from the work of Murray Bardwell and Richard Taylor in previous editions of this book.

REFERENCES

American Psychiatric Association (APA), 2000. Diagnostic and Statistical Manual of Mental Disorders: DSM-IV, TR, fouth ed. APA, Washington D.C.

American Psychiatric Association (APA), 2013. Diagnostic and Statistical Manual of Mental Disorders, fifth ed. APA, Arlington, V.A.

Andrews, G., Dean, K., Genderson, M., Hunt, C., Mitchell, P., Sachdev, P., Trollor, J., 2014. Management of Mental Disorders. In: Clinical Research Unit for Anxiety and Depression, fifth ed. University of New South Wales School of Psychiatry, Darlinghurst, N.S.W.

Anthony, W., 1993. Recovery from mental illness: the guiding vision of the mental health service system in the 1990s. Psychosocial Rehabilitation Journal 16 (4), 11–23.

Asenjo Lobos, C., Komossa, K., Rummel-Kluge, C., Hunger, H., Schmid, F., Schwarz, S., Leucht, S., 2010. Clozapine versus other atypical antipsychotics for schizophrenia. Cochrane Database of Systematic Reviews 11.

Bechdolf, A., Knost, B., Nelson, B., Schneider, N., Veith, V., Yung, A.R., Pukrop, R., 2010. Randomised comparison of group cognitive behaviour therapy and group psychoeducation in acute patients with schizophrenia: effects on subjective quality of life. Australian & New Zealand Journal of Psychiatry 44 (2), 144–150.

Bennett, C., 2012. Developmental disabilities and psychiatric disorders. In: Meadows, G., Grigg, M., Farhall, J., McDermott, F., Fossey, E., Singh, B. (Eds.), Mental Health in Australia: Collaborative Community Practice, third ed. Oxford University Press, Melbourne.

Bennett, C., Fossey, E., Farhall, J., Grigg, M., 2007. Schizophrenia and related disorders. In: Meadows, G., Singh, B., Grigg, M. (Eds.), Mental Health in Australia: Collaborative Community Practice, second ed. Oxford University Press, Melbourne.

Bennett, C., Fossey, E., Farhall, J., Grigg, M., Jeffs, S., Sundram, S., 2012. Schizophrenia and related disorders. In: Meadows, G., Grigg, M., Farhall, J., McDermott, F., Fossey, E., Singh, B. (Eds.), Mental Health in Australia: Collaborative Community Practice, third ed. Oxford University Press, Melbourne.

Berger, G., Fraser, R., Carbone, S., McGorry, P., 2006. Emerging psychosis in young people. Part 1. Australian Family Physician 35 (5), 315–321.

Boos, H., Cahn, W., van Haren, N., Derks, E., Brouwer, R., Schanck, H., Hulshoff, P., Kahn, R., 2011. Focal and global brain measurements in siblings of patients with schizophrenia. Schizophrenia Bulletin 17, 1–12.

Borg, M., Davidson, L., 2008. The nature of recovery as lived in everyday experience. Journal of Mental Health 17 (2), 129–140.

Bradshaw, T., Lovell, K., Harris, N., 2005. Healthy living interventions and schizophrenia: a systematic review. Journal of Advanced Nursing 49 (6), 634–654.

Brown, A., 2006. Prenatal infection as a risk factor for schizophrenia. Schizophrenia Bulletin 32 (2), 200–202.

Buhrich, N., Hodder, T., Teesson, M., 2003. Schizophrenia among homeless people in inner Sydney: current prevalence and historical trends. Journal of Mental Health 12 (1), 51–57.

Burns, J.K., Tomita, A., Kapadia, A.S., 2014. Income inequality and schizophrenia: increased schizophrenia incidence in countries with high levels of income inequality. International Journal of Social Psychiatry 60 (2), 185–196.

Byrne, L., Happell, B., Welch, T., Moxham, L., 2012. 'Things you can't learn from books': teaching recovery from a lived experience perspective. International Journal of Mental Health Nursing 22 (3), 195–204.

Cancel, A., Comte, M., Truillet, R., Boukezzi, S., Rousseau, P.F., Zendjidjian, X.Y., Sage, T., Lazerges, P.E., Guedj, E., Khalfa, S., Azorin, J.M., Blin, O., Fakr, E., 2015. Childhood neglect predicts disorganization in schizophrenia through grey matter decrease in dorsolateral prefrontal cortex. Acta Psychiatrica Scandinavica 1–13.

Cantor-Graae, E., 2007. The contribution of social factors to the development of schizophrenia: a review of recent findings. Canadian Journal of Psychiatry 52 (5), 277–286.

Chan, K.Y., Zhao, F., Meng, S., Demaio, A.R., Reed, C., Theodoratou, E., Campbell, H., Wang, W., Rudan, I., 2015. Urbanization and the prevalence of schizophrenia in China between 1990 and 2010. World Psychiatry 14 (2), 251–252.

Chong, H.Y., Teoh, S.L., Bin-Chia Wu, D., Kotirum, S., Chiou, C.F., Chaiyakunapruk, N., 2016. Global economic burden of schizophrenia: a systematic review. Neuropsychiatric Disease & Treatment 12, 357–373.

Chuma, J., Mahadun, P., 2011. Predicting the development of schizophrenia in high-risk populations: systematic review of the predictive validity of prodromal criteria. The British Journal of Psychiatry: The Journal of Mental Science 199, 361–366.

Corcoran, C., Kimhy, D., Parrilla-Escobar, M., Cressman, V., Stanford, A., Thompson, J., David, S., Crumbley, A., Schobel, S., Moore, H., Malaspina, D., 2011. The relationship of social function to depressive and negative symptoms in individuals at clinical high risk for psychosis. Psychological Medicine 41 (2), 251–261.

de Jager, A., Rhodes, P., Beavan, V., Holmes, D., McCabe, K., Thomas, N., McCarthy-Jones, S., Lampshire, D., Hayward, M., 2015. Investigating the lived experience of recovery in people who hear voices. Qualitative Health Research 1–15.

Evans, K., McGrath, J., Milns, R., 2003. Searching for schizophrenia in ancient Greek and Roman literature: a systematic review. Acta Psychiatrica Scandinavica 107, 1–8.

Fazel, S., Khosla, V., Doll, H., Geddes, J., 2008. The prevalence of mental disorders among the homeless in western countries: systematic review and meta-regression analysis. PLoS Medicine 5 (12), 1670–1681.

Fazel, S., Seewald, K., 2012. Severe mental illness in 33,588 prisoners worldwide: systematic review and meta-regression analysis. British Journal of Psychiatry 200, 364–373.

Folsom, D., Jeste, D., 2002. Schizophrenia in homeless persons: a systematic review of the literature. Acta Psychiatrica Scandinavica 105 (6), 404–413.

Fontaine, K., Heo, M., Harrigan, E., Shear, C., Lakshminaravanan, M., Casey, D., Allison, D., 2001. Estimating the consequences of anti-psychotic induced weight gain on health and mortality rate. Psychiatry Research 10 (3), 277–288.

Fuller Torrey, E., Yolken, R.H., 2003. Toxoplasma gondii and schizophrenia. Emerging Infectious Diseases 9 (11), 1375–1380.

Gaebel, W., Riesbeck, M., Wölwer, W., Klimke, A., Eickhoff, M., von Wilmsdorff, M., et al., 2010. Relapse prevention in first-episode schizophrenia: maintenance vs intermittent drug treatment with prodrome-based early intervention. Results of a randomized controlled trial within the German Research Network on Schizophrenia. The Journal of Clinical Psychiatry 72 (2), 205–218.

Geekie, J., 2013. Clients' understandings of psychotic experiences. In: Read, J., Dillon, J. (Eds.), Models of Madness: Psychological, Social and Biological Approaches to Psychosis. Routledge, London.

Gray, R., White, J., Schulz, M., Abderhalden, C., 2010. Enhancing medication adherence in people with schizophrenia: an international programme of research. International Journal of Mental Health Nursing 19 (1), 36–44.

Halter, M.J., Rolin-Kenny, D., Dzurec, L.C., 2013. An overview of the DSM-5: changes, controversy, and implications for psychiatric nursing. Journal of Psychosocial Nursing and Mental Health Services 51 (4), 30–39.

Haukka, J., Suvisaari, J., Varilo, T., 2001. Regional variation in the incidence of schizophrenia in Finland: a study of birth cohorts born from 1950 to 1969. Psychological Medicine 31 (6), 1045–1053.

Hiday, V., Swartz, M., Swanson, J., et al., 2002. Impact of outpatient commitment on victimization of people with severe mental illness. American Journal of Psychiatry 159 (8), 1403–1411.

Inta, P., Meyer-Lindenberg, A., Gass, P., 2011. Alterations in postnatal neurogenesis and dopamine dysregulation in schizophrenia: a hypothesis. Schizophrenia Bulletin 37 (4), 674–680.

Johnston, J., 2013. The ghost of the schizophrenogenic mother. AMA Journal of Ethics 15 (9), 801–805.

Jones, S.R., Fernyhough, C., 2007. A new look at the neural diathesis–stress model of schizophrenia: the primacy of social-evaluative and uncontrollable situations. Schizophrenia Bulletin 33 (5), 1171–1177.

Kennedy, M., Dornan, J., Rutledge, E., O'Neill, H., Kennedy, H.G., 2009. Extra information about treatment is too much for the patient with psychosis. International Journal of Law and Psychiatry 32, 369–376.

Kopelowicz, A., Liberman, R., Wallace, C., 2003. Psychiatric rehabilitation for schizophrenia. International Journal of Psychology and Psychological Therapy 3 (2), 282–298.

Lamberti, J.S., 2001. Seven keys to relapse prevention in schizophrenia. Journal of Psychiatric Practice July 253–259.

Laugharne, J., Waterreus, A.J., Castle, D.J., Dragovic, M., 2016. Screening for the metabolic syndrome in Australia: a national survey of psychiatrists' attitudes and reported practice in patients prescribed antipsychotic drugs. Australasian Psychiatry 24 (1), 62–66.

Lawrie, S., Whalley, H., Abukmeil, S., et al., 2002. Temporal lobe volume changes in people at high risk of schizophrenia with psychotic symptoms. British Journal of Psychiatry 181 (2), 138–143.

Lee, S., 2002. The stigma of schizophrenia: a transcultural problem. Current Opinion in Psychiatry 15 (1), 37–41.

Lieberman, J.A., Tollefson, G.D., Charles, C., Zipursky, R., Sharma, T.N., Kahan, R.S., et al., 2005. Antipsychotic drug effects on brain morphology in first-episode psychosis. Archives of General Psychiatry 62 (4), 361–370.

Longden, E., 2013. The voices in my head. Available at: www.ted.com/talks/eleanor_longden_the_voices_in_my_head/transcript?language=en.

McGorry, P., Krstev, H., Harrigan, S., 2000. Early detection and treatment delay: implications for outcomes in early psychosis. Current Opinion in Psychiatry 13, 37–43.

McGrath, J.J., Welham, J.L., 1999. Season of birth and schizophrenia: a systematic review and meta-analysis of data from the Southern Hemisphere. Schizophrenia Research 35 (3), 237–242.

Mitchell, A.J., Vancampfort, D., Sweers, K., van Winkel, R., Yu, W., De Hert, M., 2013. Prevalence of metabolic syndrome and metabolic abnormalities in schizophrenia and related disorders—a systematic review and meta-analysis. Schizophrenia Bulletin 39 (2), 306–318.

Morgan, V.A., McGrath, J.J., Jablensky, A., Badcock, J.C., Waterreus, A., Bush, R., Carr, V., Castle, D., Cohen, M., Galletly, C., Harvey, C., Hocking, B., McGorry, P., Neil, A.L., Saw, S., Shah, S., Stain, H.J., Mackinnon, A., 2014. Psychosis prevalence and physical, metabolic and cognitive co-morbidity: data from the second Australian national survey of psychosis. Psychological Medicine 44 (10), 2163–2176.

Muller, M., Wetzel, H., Eich, F., et al., 2002. Dose-related effects of amisulpride on five dimensions of psychopathology in patients with acute exacerbation of schizophrenia. Journal of Clinical Psychopharmacology 22 (6), 554–560.

Munk-Jorgensen, P., Ewald, H., 2001. Epidemiology in neurobiological research: exemplified by the influenza–schizophrenia theory. British Journal of Psychiatry 178 (40), 30–32.

Nairn, R., 2005. People never see us living well: an appraisal of the personal stories about mental illness in a prospective print media sample. Australian and New Zealand Journal of Psychiatry 39 (4), 281–287.

National Institute for Health and Care Excellence (NICE), 2016. Implementing the Early Intervention in Psychosis Access and Waiting Time Standard: Guidance. Available at: https://www.england.nhs.uk/mentalhealth/wp-content/uploads/sites/29/2016/04/eip-guidance.pdf. Accessed: 9 October 2018.

O'Brien, L., Cole, R., 2004. Mental health nursing practice in acute psychiatric close-observation areas. International Journal of Mental Health Nursing 13, 89–99.

Pletnikov, M., Waddington, J. (Eds.), 2015. Modeling the Psychopathological Dimensions of Schizophrenia: From Molecules to Behavior. Academic Press, Cambridge, MA.

Randal, P., Malcolm, W., Stewart, M., Proverbs, D., Lampshire, D., Symese, J., Hamer, H., 2009. 'The recovery model': an integrative developmental stress–vulnerability–strengths approach to mental health. Psychosis 1–12 August.

Rautanen, M., Lauerma, H., 2011. Imprisonment and diagnostic delay among male offenders with schizophrenia. Criminal Behaviour and Mental Health 21 (4), 259–264.

Read, J., Fosse, R., Moskowitz, A., Perry, B., 2014. The traumagenic neurodevelopmental model of psychosis revisited. Neuropsychiatry 4 (1), 65–79.

Sadock, B., Sadock, V.A., Ruiz, P., 2009. Kaplan and Sadock's Comprehensive Textbook of Psychiatry, ninth ed. Lippincott Williams & Wilkins, Baltimore.

Salokangas, R., Cannon, T., Van Erp, T., et al., 2002. Structural magnetic resonance imaging in patients with first episode schizophrenia, psychotic and severe nonpsychotic depression and healthy controls: results of the Schizophrenia and Affective Psychoses (SAP) Project. British Journal of Psychiatry 181 (43), 58–65.

Sara, G.E., Burgess, P., Malhi, G., Whiteford, H., Hall, W., 2014. Stimulant and other substance use disorders in schizophrenia: prevalence, correlates and impacts in a population sample. Australian and New Zealand Journal of Psychiatry 48 (11), 1036–1047.

Sara, G.E., Large, M.M., Matheson, S.L., Burgess, P.M., Malhi, G.S., Whiteford, H.A., Hall, W.D., 2015. Stimulant use disorders in people with psychosis: a meta-analysis of rate and factors affecting variation. Australian & New Zealand Journal of Psychiatry 49 (2), 106–117.

Schneebeli, C., O'Brien, A., Lampshire, D., Hamer, H., 2010. Service user involvement in undergraduate mental health nursing in New Zealand. International Journal of Mental Health Nursing 19, 30–35.

Seeman, P., 2009. Glutamate and dopamine components in schizophrenia. Journal of Psychiatry Neuroscience 34 (2), 143–149.

Simeone, J.C., Ward, A.J., Rotella, P., Collins, J., Windisch, R., 2015. An evaluation of variation in published estimates of schizophrenia prevalence from 1990–2013: a systematic literature review. BioMedCentral Psychiatry 15, 193–207.

Steele, K., Berman, C., 2001. The Day the Voices Stopped: a Memoir of Madness and Hope. Basic Books, New York.

Sumiyoshi, T., Bubenikova-Valesova, V., Horacek, J., Bert, B., 2008. Serotonin(1A) receptors in the pathophysiology of schizophrenia: development of novel cognition-enhancing therapeutics. Advances in Therapy 25 (10), 1037–1056.

Sutton, D.L., 2004. Relapse signatures and insight: implications for CPNs. Journal of Psychiatric and Mental Health Nursing 11, 569–574.

Suvisaari, J., Haukka, J., Lonnqvist, J., 2002. Seasonal fluctuation in schizophrenia. American Journal of Psychiatry 159 (3), 500.

Tandon, R., Gaebel, W., Barch, D.M., Bustillo, J., Gur, R.E., Heckers, S., Van Os, J., 2013. Definition and description of schizophrenia in the DSM-5. Schizophrenia Research 150 (1), 3–10.

Thirthalli, J., Benegal, V., 2006. Psychosis among substance users. Current Opinion in Psychiatry 19 (3), 239–245.

Torgalsbøen, A., Rund, B., 2010. Maintenance of recovery from schizophrenia at 20-year follow-up: what happened? Psychiatry: Interpersonal and Biological Processes 73 (1), 70–83.

Turkington, D., Kingdon, D., Turner, T., 2002. Effectiveness of a brief cognitive–behavioural therapy intervention in the treatment of schizophrenia. British Journal of Psychiatry 180, 523–527.

Ueda, S., Sakayori, T., Omori, A., Fukuta, H., Kobayashi, T., Ishizaka, K., Saijo, T., Okubo, Y., 2016. Neuroleptic-induced deficit syndrome in bipolar disorder with psychosis. Neuropsychiatric Disease and Treatment 12, 265–268.

van Heeringen, K., 2000. A diathesis stress model of suicidal behavior. Crisis: Journal of Crisis Intervention and Suicide 21 (4), 192.

van Os, J., 2000. Social influences on risk for disorder and natural history. Current Opinion in Psychiatry 13 (2), 209–213.

van Os, J., Kapur, S., 2009. Schizophrenia. Lancet 374 (9690), 635–645.

Venables, P., Liu, J., Raine, A., et al., 2007. Prenatal influenza exposure and delivery complications: implications for the development of schizophrenia. Family and Community Health 30 (2), 151–159.

Volavka, J., Citrome, L., 2008. Heterogeneity of violence in schizophrenia and implications for long-term treatment. International Journal of Clinical Practice 62 (8), 1237–1245.

Vonnegut, M., 2010. Personal reflections on diagnosis. Journal of Mental Health 19 (4), 373–375.

Wareham, P., McCallin, A., Diesfeld, K., 2005. Advance directives: the New Zealand context. Nursing Ethics 12 (4), 349–359.

Weisman, A., 2005. Integrating culturally based approaches with existing interventions for Hispanic/Latino families coping with schizophrenia. Psychotherapy 42 (2), 178–197.

Weller, P., 2010. Psychiatric advance directives and human rights. Psychiatry, Psychology and Law 17 (2), 218–229.

Young, S., Snyder, M., Schactman, L., 2015. Early recovery from psychotic spectrum disorder within a therapeutic community: significance and effects. Psychosis 7 (1), 37–47.

USEFUL WEBSITES

Division of Clinical Psychology at Leicester University in the United Kingdom publishes a handy reference book, *Understanding Psychosis and Schizophrenia*, available free online, that has a collection of useful websites and is an excellent informative resource that includes help for clinicians as well as self-help resources, recovery stories and resources, patient accounts and a comprehensive reference list, https://www.bps.org.uk/what-psychology/understanding-psychosis-and-schizophrenia

Hearing Voices Network, www.hearing-voices.org

www.intervoiceonline.org.

www.hearing-voices.org

Human Genome Project (HGP) was an international research effort to sequence and map all of the genes—together known as the genome—of our species, *Homo sapiens*. Completed in April 2003, the HGP gave us the ability, for the first time, to read nature's complete genetic blueprint for building a human being; see the website for fascinating insights into our genetic inheritance, www.genome.gov/10001772

Psychology Dictionary is a comprehensive source of definitions written by psychiatrists and psychologists, a useful tool for looking up specialised terms, http://psychologydictionary.org

SANE, www.sane.org.uk

- StigmaWatch seeks out instances of stigma perpetuated in the news and print media: www.sane.org/mental-health-and-illness/facts-and-guides/reducing-stigma
- Discussion regarding schizophrenia: www.sane.org/mental-health-and-illness/facts-and-guides/schizophrenia

Second Life virtual world was utilised in a study by Australian Professor Peter Yellowlees designed as an educational tool to simulate the frightening experiences of hallucinations associated with mental illness in order to develop greater understanding among nonsufferers, www.youtube.com/watch?v=P4-PUF3ScL0

Surviving Schizophrenia is a video in which Elyn Saks, Debra Lampshire and Paris Williams, all world experts on mental health, use their personal experiences and work in their respective fields to debunk the myths and stigma surrounding schizophrenia, http://attitudelive.com/documentary/surviving-schizophrenia

Voice hearer and psychologist Eleanor Longden talks about her journey back to mental health and makes the case that it was through learning to listen to her voices that she was able to survive, www.ted.com/talks/eleanor_longden_the_voices_in_my_head

16

Mood Disorders

Peter Athanasos

KEY POINTS

- There are key nursing principles and interventions for working with people experiencing a mood disorder.
- Major depression is associated with an increased risk of attempting and committing suicide.
- As with all mental health disorders, the establishment of a therapeutic relationship is critical to treatment success.
- Mood disorders are responsive to a variety of psychological, sociocultural and biological interventions.
- Antidepressants and mood stabilisers are the major classes of medication used in the treatment of mood disorders.

KEY TERMS

affect
bipolar disorder
cyclothymia
egocentric
elation
gene–environment interaction
grief
hypomania
impulsivity
major depressive disorder
mania
medication collaboration
mood
persistent depressive disorder
perinatal depression
postpartum depression
postpartum psychosis
psychomotor retardation
psychotherapy
somatisation
therapeutic use of self

LEARNING OUTCOMES

The material in this chapter will assist you to:

- describe behaviours associated with mood disorders.
- describe cognitive (thinking) changes associated with mood disorders.
- understand communication changes associated with mood disorders.
- describe mood changes associated with major depressive disorder and bipolar disorder.
- describe changes in physical functioning associated with mood disorders.
- explain the reasons for nursing interventions and the expected patient responses.
- outline cognitive, social and biological theories that contribute to the understanding of the aetiology (origin) of mood disorders.
- explore nursing interventions for patients who want to self-harm and suicide.
- understand the basic mechanisms of antidepressants and mood stabilisers.
- examine the nature of medication collaboration.
- outline psychotherapies such as self-help interventions, cognitive behavioural therapy and group therapy.
- describe the therapeutic use of self.
- recognise some of the personal challenges arising for nurses working with people who are experiencing major depressive disorder and bipolar disorder.

INTRODUCTION

This chapter examines the nature of mood disorders. It also explores mental health assessment, interventions, knowledge and attitudes that nurses need to work effectively with people with mood disorders. A holistic view is essential because mood disorders affect all aspects of daily living.

Depression and elevated mood commonly occur in many mental disorders. This chapter considers disorders where the change in mood predominates and is disabling. When a person has a mood disorder, the changes they experience are more intense and persistent than those most people experience in their day-to-day lives and may affect functioning both at work and at home. The person experiences a range of disturbances in behaviour, cognition, communication and physical functioning.

This chapter addresses major depressive disorder (major depression), bipolar disorder (bipolar disorder 1 and 2), postpartum depression and depression associated with ageing. It also makes a distinction between major depressive disorder (major depression) and feeling sad.

The key to working effectively with someone with a mood disorder is a collaborative relationship characterised by openness and respect. This is emphasised throughout the chapter. The collaborative relationship is an essential part of counselling and pharmacotherapeutic interventions. At all times, the nurse must be a partner in the patient's recovery.

EPIDEMIOLOGY

Mood disorders are a common form of mental illness and cause much distress. The Mental Health and Wellbeing in England Adult Psychiatric Morbidity Survey (NHS Digital 2014) figures showed that 2% of the population screened positive for bipolar disorder, with no significant difference in the rates for men and women; however, it was noted that a diagnosis of bipolar was more common in younger age groups (3.4% in people aged 16–24 years and 0.4% in people aged 65–74 years). Rates of depression rose from 4.7% in 2007 to 6.6% in 2014.

A systematic review of data and statistics from European Union (EU) countries, Iceland, Norway and Switzerland found that 27% of the adult population had experienced at least one mental disorder in the previous year (WHO 2014). Every year about 1 in 15 people suffer from major depression in the European region. If anxiety and all forms of depression are included, nearly 4 out of 15 people are affected (WHO 2014). The problem is complex: 32% of people affected by a mental health disorder had one additional disorder, 18% had two and 14% had three or more (WHO 2014).

What do these statistics mean? A central question is whether the frequency of mental health disorders is rising, or whether they are better recognised or whether people are more willing to acknowledge that they have these disorders: it is difficult to tell. However, mood disorders and other mental health disorders represent an enormous burden of ill health in our society. As nurses, we have an obligation to develop our knowledge, to improve our skills and to help our patients however we can.

DEPRESSION

Depressive symptoms may range from mild and transient, such as 'feeling blue', to very severe, where there is extraordinary sadness, dejection and an inability to take pleasure in activities. It is important to recognise that, depending on life events, periods of transitory sadness and grief are part of normal human functioning and are not disease states. If the depressive symptoms are persistent and interfere in most areas of a person's life (e.g. work, school, home), then the person might be diagnosed with *major depressive disorder* (major depression) (see Box 16.1). If the patient reports milder depressive symptoms that have lasted for at least 2 years (that is, milder and lasting longer than major depression), their illness could be characterised as *persistent depressive disorder*. Persistent depressive disorder is more common than major depressive disorder. It can be considered an exaggeration of ordinary unhappiness. The patient may complain of feeling low, feeling hopeless (pessimism), fatigue, decreased concentration, decreased or increased sleep and/or decreased or increased appetite (American Psychiatric Association [APA] 2013).

Major Depressive Disorder Features

Major depressive disorder (major depression) is characterised by at least one of two features (depressed mood or loss of interest or pleasure) alongside five other symptoms, which may include fatigue or lack of energy, anhedonia, negative thinking, psychomotor agitation or retardation, disturbed sleep, feelings of worthlessness or excessive guilt, difficulty concentrating and recurring thoughts of death and suicide (APA 2013). Major depressive disorder often goes unrecognised when the patient presents with a range of physical ailments. It is one of the primary causes of self-harm and suicide and may have a profound effect not only on the patient but also on their family and friends. A number of features central to major depression differentiate it from milder forms of depression. These include alterations in appearance, behaviour, mood, affect, thinking, speech, perception and biological symptoms. These alterations are described below. Patients may exhibit some, but not necessarily all, of these symptoms.

Appearance and Behaviour

The person with major depression often has decreased interest in their grooming or cleanliness. The person may once have worn make-up or shaved every day, but now wears soiled clothes, has unwashed hair and has lost interest in their appearance. Major depression involves a lowering of interest in grooming from the base level that was characteristic of the person. The person may also appear tired and older looking (Schweitzer & Parke 2007).

Psychomotor retardation is a slowing of mental and physical activity. The person may move more slowly, think more slowly and exert more effort in performing the simplest of tasks. In contrast, some people may exhibit psychomotor agitation, which is a morbid increase in movement or action, often accompanied by a subjective feeling of restlessness. Frequently, the patient finds it hard to remain still for an extended period of time and may pace around the room (Gelder et al. 2005).

Mood and Affect

The patient is usually miserable and anguished. The low mood they experience is pervasive, unlike the feelings of sadness we all experience from time to time. The patient may describe feeling hopeless, worthless and powerless to do anything about their life.

Most patients experience some form of sleep disturbance. However, their patterns may vary. Some have difficulty getting off to sleep (initial insomnia), others wake up too soon (middle or terminal insomnia), while others may have diffuse insomnia, a form of difficulty sleeping that is not associated with any specific stage of sleep. It is the patient's experience of changes to their usual pattern that is important. Some patients experience

BOX 16.1 Major Depressive Episode

Criteria for a Major Depressive Episode

A. Five (or more) of the following symptoms have been present during the same 2-week period and represent a change from previous functioning; at least one of the symptoms is either (1) depressed mood or (2) loss of interest or pleasure.

Note: Do not include symptoms that are clearly attributable to another medical condition.

- Depressed mood most of the day, nearly every day, as indicated by either subjective report (e.g. feels sad or empty) or observation made by others (e.g. appears tearful). Note: In children and adolescents, can be irritable mood.
- Markedly diminished interest or pleasure in all, or almost all, activities most of the day, nearly every day (as indicated by either subjective account or observation).
- Significant weight loss when not dieting or weight gain (e.g. a change of more than 5% of body weight in a month), or decrease or increase in appetite nearly every day. Note: In children, consider failure to make expected weight gains.
- Insomnia or hypersomnia nearly every day.
- Psychomotor agitation or retardation nearly every day (observable by others, not merely subjective feelings of restlessness or being slowed down).
- Fatigue or loss of energy nearly every day.
- Feelings of worthlessness or excessive or inappropriate guilt (which may be delusional) nearly every day (not merely self-reproach or guilt about being sick).
- Diminished ability to think or to concentrate or indecisiveness, nearly every day (either by subjective account or as observed by others).
- Recurrent thoughts of death (not just fear of dying), recurrent suicidal ideation without a specific plan or a suicide attempt or a specific plan for committing suicide.

B. The symptoms cause clinically significant distress or impairment in social, occupational or other important areas of functioning.

C. The episode is not attributable to the physiological effects of a substance or another medical condition.

Criteria for a Major Depressive Episode with Mixed Features

A. Full criteria are met for a major depressive episode and at least three of the following manic/hypomanic symptoms are present during the majority of days of the current or most recent episode of depression:

1. Elevated, expansive mood.
2. Inflated self-esteem or grandiosity.
3. More talkative than usual or pressure to keep talking.
4. Flight of ideas or subjective experience that thoughts are racing.
5. Increase in energy or goal-directed activity (either socially, at work, at school or sexually).
6. Increased or excessive involvement in activities that have a high potential for painful consequences (e.g. engaging in unrestrained buying sprees, sexual indiscretions or foolish business investments).
7. Decreased need for sleep (feeling rested despite sleeping less than usual: to be contrasted with insomnia).

B. Mixed symptoms are observable by others and represent a change from the person's usual behaviour.

C. For individuals whose symptoms meet full episode criteria for both mania and depression simultaneously, the diagnosis should be manic episode with mixed features.

D. The mixed symptoms are not attributable to the physiological effects of a substance (e.g. a drug of abuse, a medication or other treatment).

(*Source*: Reprinted with permission from the Diagnostic and Statistical Manual of Mental Disorders, 5th ed. American Psychiatric Association.)

hypersomnia (sleeping for large amounts of the day). Early morning wakening is often indicative of a more severe form of depression, while initial insomnia is more typical of milder states (Schweitzer & Parke 2007). The mood is often worse in the morning, with pessimistic thoughts about the coming day and a focus on past perceived failures. As the day wears on, the person's mood may become lighter. They may withdraw both socially and emotionally from contact with others. A marked decrease in pleasure or interest in previously enjoyed activities is indicative of major depression (Gelder et al. 2005).

Thinking and Speech

The depressed person may become increasingly egocentric. They focus on themselves and fail to realise that others may have needs as well. A gloomy, negative outlook pervades all their thinking. The person thinks of themselves as incompetent, unlovable and a failure. They may also think of the world as incompetent and unlovable. Others will be thought of as uncaring and unhelpful. The depressed person's thinking becomes catastrophic and their emotional state is crippled with inappropriate guilt.

Poor concentration and poor memory are important characteristics of major depression. The person may have difficulty reading or focussing on a problem. They become immobilised by the cognitive difficulties involved in making a simple decision. Their outlook becomes dominated by negative self-absorption, poor energy and a lack of interest in others. They rarely initiate a conversation. When asked a question, they take a long time to answer and then give a short and perfunctory reply.

The spectrum of thinking of the depressed person also narrows. The person focusses on negative thoughts and ideas to the exclusion of all else. These thoughts and ideas become repetitive and fixed and the rumination eventually interferes with ordinary thought processes.

In thinking about the present, the person will see the unhappy side of everything that happens. They will be convinced that others think of them as a failure and if something positive happens, they will attribute it to a lucky chance that will never happen again.

In thinking about the past, the person will be consumed with inappropriate guilt, often over a small matter. They may feel that they have let someone down and contributed to their misfortune. They may not have considered these matters for many years but in the midst of their depression these thoughts will come flooding back and overwhelm them.

In thinking about the future, their outlook will be unremittingly grim. They foresee catastrophe in their work, failure in their relationships with family members and friends and an inevitable deterioration in their physical health. This preoccupation with a bleak future and a sense of doom often leads to thoughts of death and suicidal ideation and should be considered with care (Gelder et al. 2005).

Perception

Major depression may also be accompanied by delusions and hallucinations. While people with milder forms of depression may suffer from feelings of inappropriate guilt, some people with major depression will experience delusions of guilt (feeling guilty over completely imaginary matters). The same themes that present as inappropriate emotions in milder forms of depression are present in a more severe, psychotic form in major depression, for example feelings of worthlessness, failure or incompetency. When hallucinations are present, they usually manifest as negative, derisory voices echoing the nihilistic themes of 'you're a failure, you're incompetent, you're evil' and so on.

Biological Symptoms

Sleep disturbances and, in particular, problems in falling asleep and early morning waking are common features. Patients may also feel unrefreshed in the morning when they wake. Fatigue, lack of appetite, decreased sexual interest and decreased attention to hygiene are all common signs of major depression. Significant loss of weight is also a possible indicator of major depression. A proportion of the population will not describe a depressed mood. Rather, these depressed people will describe a range of pain conditions or other physical symptoms. This is called somatisation. See Table 16.1 for nursing interventions for major depression.

CRITICAL THINKING CHALLENGE 16.1

1. Why do you think people are so reluctant to admit that they are depressed and need help?
2. What would be your first reaction if you were diagnosed with depression, commenced on weekly counselling and were prescribed antidepressants?

Aetiology of Depression

Biopsychosocial Model of Causation

There is unlikely to be only one factor that is wholly responsible for depression; rather, it is a combination of interacting factors that cause the illness. This combination of factors is called the biopsychosocial model of causation.

Genetic factors and the gene–environment interaction. In the last 5 years our understanding of the gene–environment interaction has changed dramatically by means of

TABLE 16.1 Nursing Interventions for Patients With Major Depression

Intervention	Rationale
Be genuine and honest with patients. Accept them for who they are (both negative and positive aspects).	• Depressed people have chronically low self-esteem. • Genuine acceptance by others is a first step to recovery.
Treat anger and negative thinking as symptoms of the illness, not as personally targeted at the nurse.	• Depressed people are often negative and angry. • By identifying that negativity and anger are aspects of the illness, the nurse can encourage the patient to move on from these issues to express more appropriate emotions.
Never reinforce hallucinations, delusions or irrational beliefs.	• It is not appropriate to agree with the patient's perceptual abnormalities. Equally, arguing that they do not exist serves little purpose. • The nurse should state their perception of the situation. • The nurse should state that there is a discrepancy between what is perceived by the patient and what is perceived by the nurse. • The nurse should then steer the conversation to discussing real people and real events.
Spend time with withdrawn patients, even if no words are spoken.	• Withdrawn people are still very aware of where they are and who they are with. • Simply by spending time with withdrawn patients, the nurse can help the patient to emerge from their isolation by providing a nonthreatening one-on-one relationship, practising assertive interactions and providing positive regard.
Make positive decisions for patients if they are unwilling to make decisions for themselves (e.g. it is time to get out of bed).	• Depressed people can have difficulties making even the simplest of decisions. • By using problem-solving techniques (i.e. identifying options and the advantages and disadvantages of each option and exploring the consequences of taking these actions) the nurse can guide the patient to appropriate decisions.
Express hope that patients will get better. Focus on their strengths, however small these seem.	• By identifying their strengths and giving them hope and positive regard, the nurse encourages patients to regain a sense of self-worth.
Identify and involve patients in activities where they can enjoy success.	• It is important for patients to feel good about themselves. • By involving patients in activities that they can accomplish, they may begin to improve their sense of self-worth.

(*Source*: Adapted from Keltner, N., 2007, Depression. In: Keltner, N., Schweke, L., Bostrom, C., (Eds) Psychiatric Nursing. Mosby Elsevier, St Louis; Videbeck, S., 2009. Psychiatric Mental Health Nursing, 5th ed. Lippincott Williams & Wilkins, Philadelphia, PA.)

genome-wide association studies. A genome-wide association study is a large-scale examination of many common genetic variants in tens of thousands of different people to see whether any variant is associated with a trait.

This is our current understanding: five psychiatric disorders (major depression, bipolar disorder, schizophrenia, autism spectrum disorders and attention deficit disorder) share much of the same genetic pattern. This genetic pattern interacts with prenatal environmental factors (e.g. mother has an infectious disease, uses prescribed and nonprescribed drugs, has nutritional deficiencies or undergoes stress during pregnancy) and postnatal environmental factors (e.g. childhood maltreatment, poor socioeconomic status, poor living conditions, family conflict) to produce changes in the brain (brain plasticity) that lead to a general psychiatric disease vulnerability (Sullivan et al. 2012; Cross-Disorder Group of the Psychiatric Genomics Consortium 2013; Serretti & Fabbri 2013). This phenomenon is called pleiotropy and it involves one gene influencing multiple seemingly unrelated disorders. We do know that there is a common genetic pattern. What we do not know is how this common genetic pattern interacts with the prenatal and postnatal factors to produce the specific psychiatric illnesses. That is the next direction of research and, if achieved, will be the most profound advance in our understanding of psychiatry.

Neurochemical factors, hormonal systems, circadian rhythms and the immune system. The idea that depression is a result of a complex interaction among neurotransmitters and other systems in the brain originated in the 1960s. It should be emphasised that major depression is not simply a consequence of low levels of serotonin or other neurotransmitters (monoamines) in the brain. This was the 'monoamine hypothesis' and originated in 1965. By the 1980s, researchers had concluded that this approach was too simplistic (Hillhouse & Porter 2015). It is likely that monoamines modulate a range of other neurobiological systems to produce major depression. The more we learn, the more complex we realise the systems are.

Neurotransmitter systems (serotonin, noradrenaline, gabaminergic and glutamatergic) impact hormonal systems to produce major depression (Goldberg et al. 2014; Haase & Brown 2015; Horowitz & Zunszain 2015). Important among these systems are the hypothalamic–pituitary–adrenal (HPA) axis (which controls the release of cortisol and thyroid hormones) and the overall circadian rhythms (the body's 24-hour cycle of brainwave activity, hormone production and cell regeneration). The immune system by way of proinflammatory cytokines (to produce an inflammatory response) may underpin many of these mechanisms (Haase & Brown 2015; Horowitz & Zunszain 2015).

Sex differences. It has long been established that women are more than twice as likely to develop depression as men (Weissman & Klerman 1977; Nolan-Hoeksema 2002). This sex difference occurs across cultures (Weissman et al. 1996). The theories that have been proposed to explain this range from biological (hormonal and genetic) to social and psychological factors (Weissman & Klerman 1977; Nolan-Hoeksema 2002; Valentino et al. 2011; Moieni et al. 2015). Male and female differences in immune system responses to stress and in turn the initiation of depression are likely to be important (Moieni et al. 2015). Women may be more sensitive to the social environment and show greater inflammatory activity in response to stress. When this inflammatory response occurs, they feel more social disconnection and experience a depressed mood (Moieni et al. 2015).

Bipolar Disorder

Although the name *bipolar disorder* suggests two categories of symptoms—depression and mania—it does not require a depressive episode for the diagnosis to be made. There are individuals suffering from bipolar disorder who have never had a depressive episode. In general, the disorder is characterised by a cycling between depression and normal mood and mania. This may occur over periods of time from days to weeks to months.

Mania is characterised by three main features: persistently elevated mood, which may be one of elation or irritability; increased activity; and poor judgement (see Box 16.2). Mania is less common than depression. Again, it is

BOX 16.2 Manic Episode

Criteria for a Manic Episode

A. A distinct period of abnormally and persistently elevated, expansive or irritable mood and abnormally and persistently increased goal-directed activity or energy, lasting at least 1 week and present most of the day, nearly every day (or any duration if hospitalization is necessary).

B. During the period of mood disturbance and increased energy or activity, three (or more) of the following symptoms (four if the mood is only irritable) are present to a significant degree and represent a noticeable change from usual behaviour:
1. Inflated self-esteem or grandiosity.
2. Decreased need for sleep (e.g. feels rested after only 3 hours of sleep).
3. More talkative than usual or pressure to keep talking.
4. Flight of ideas or subjective experience that thoughts are racing.
5. Distractibility (i.e. attention too easily drawn to unimportant or irrelevant external stimuli), as reported or observed.
6. Increase in goal-directed activity (either socially, at work, at school or sexually) or psychomotor agitation (i.e. purposeless non–goal-directed activity).
7. Excessive involvement in activities that have a high potential for painful consequences (e.g. engaging in unrestrained buying sprees, sexual indiscretions or foolish business investments).

C. The mood disturbance is sufficiently severe to cause marked impairment in social or occupational functioning or to necessitate hospitalization to prevent harm to self or to others or there are psychotic features.

D. The episode is not attributable to the physiological effects of a substance (e.g. a drug of abuse, a medication, other treatment) or to another medical condition.

(*Source*: Reprinted with permission from the Diagnostic and Statistical Manual of Mental Disorders, 5th ed. American Psychiatric Association.)

important that the illness does not go unrecognised because as the illness progresses, the patient may become less inclined to accept treatment, and the consequences of the illness, such as increased activity and poor judgement, may lead the person to engage in potentially dangerous behaviours such as driving a car unsafely, engaging in risky sexual practices or acting violently. There is significant disruption to normal functioning with mania: the person may experience delusions and hallucinations and may need to be hospitalised. The symptoms of mania must be present for a week for a diagnosis to be made. Hypomania has similar symptoms to mania, with the following exceptions: there is no significant impairment in social or occupational function; there are no psychotic features; and there is generally no need for hospitalisation (Gelder et al. 2005). A mixed episode is where there are symptoms of both a manic and a depressed episode for at least a week.

The *Diagnostic and Statistical Manual of Mental Disorders*, 5th edition (DSM-5) (APA 2013) classifies bipolar disorder into bipolar 1 disorder and bipolar 2 disorder. *Bipolar 1 disorder* is defined by one or more manic or mixed episodes. *Bipolar 2 disorder* is characterised by hypomania and a depressive episode. A mixed episode is where features of mania and depression such as agitation, anxiety, fatigue or irritability occur simultaneously or in short succession. Examples are racing thoughts during a depressive episode or tears during a manic episode. There is ongoing debate as to whether bipolar 1 and bipolar 2 represent distinct forms of the condition or simply differences in severity (Ball et al. 2010). Broadly speaking, bipolar 1 disorder is a more serious and less common condition that bipolar 2 disorder.

Bipolar Disorder Features

There are a number of features central to bipolar disorder, including alterations in appearance, behaviour, mood, thinking and speech, perception and biological symptoms. These alterations are described below.

Appearance and Behaviour

In appearance the person with mania may wear colourful clothing and too much make-up. When their condition is more severe they may be dishevelled and malodorous. They are often distractible, which leads to them initiating and then leaving unfinished a series of activities. As they become more manic, their behaviour may become more disorganised and they have trouble completing even the simplest tasks (Gelder et al. 2005).

The behaviour of a person with mania is characterised by four main factors: increased activity, impulsivity, disinhibition and inflated ideas. The increased activity, often for long periods, leads to physical exhaustion. People with mania may spend excessively and dramatically increase their intake of drugs and alcohol. They may become sexually hyperactive and disinhibited. As a result, their behaviour is considered inappropriate by others. It is important to remember that such activities are often out of character for the person and may later cause embarrassment and problems at work, in their social circle and at home.

Mood

The person's mood is elated. They may appear as euphoric and excessively optimistic and display infectious gaiety. At other times they may be irritable and aggressive. These changes may vary throughout the day but there is not the same clear pattern of change in outlook as is associated with depression.

Thinking and Speech

The person's thoughts are unusually rapid, abundant and varied. Their speech reflects these rapid changes in thoughts and this is described as pressure of speech. As they become more activated, their speech may consist of puns, jokes, rhymes and irrelevancies. At the next level they exhibit looseness of associations between ideas and their ability to concentrate diminishes. At its most severe, acute manic speech is indistinguishable from the speech of someone with acute schizophrenia.

Most patients experiencing mania have delusions—the person thinks their ideas are novel, their opinions profound and their work of outstanding genius. Their delusions often have a religious, persecutory or paranoid flavour. They believe that they are extremely wealthy or powerful and become irritable when their thoughts are challenged.

Perception

Auditory and visual hallucinations might occur with mania. Their content is congruent with the person's fluctuations in mood. For example, the patient may hear voices that have religious or persecutory content when they are in a negative mood and that praise them excessively when their mood is positive.

Biological Symptoms

When in a manic episode, patients have little time for sleep. They may wake very early, feeling energetic, become active and disturb others. This increased activity may lead to exhaustion. In some cases, appetite increases and they may consume food quickly, with little concern for social etiquette. In other cases, the person is too distracted to take interest in eating. Libido increases and may bring with it recklessness and behaviour that is out of character (Gelder et al. 2005). See Table 16.2 for nursing interventions for patients with mania.

Aetiology of Bipolar Disorder

Biopsychosocial Model of Causation

Like depression, our basic understanding of what causes bipolar disorder has not changed for many years. Genetics combines with psychosocial factors to produce a mental illness. For more detail please see the biopsychosocial model of causation for depression, as this is the same model that explains bipolar disorder. We know genetics combines with psychosocial factors to produce a mental illness. However, we do not know how it happens or how this interaction causes a specific mental illness.

TABLE 16.2 Nursing Interventions for Patients With Mania

Intervention	Rationale
Speak in a calm, supportive tone.	• Using this tone of voice encourages the patient to respond positively, not defensively. • A clear, calm tone discourages the patient's need to engage in power struggles. The tone conveys to the patient that they are supported and that events are under control.
Give firm, simple directions and comments. Setting limits might be required.	• Patients with mania have flight of ideas and pressure of speech and are easily distracted. • The nurse needs to take control of the situation by politely but firmly interrupting excessively talkative patients. This is particularly important when the nurse is leading a group and the manic patient is disrupting others.
Do not argue or engage in debate about the rules and limits of the ward.	• Argument and debate may encourage a power struggle between the nurse and the patient. It may also provoke the patient to become defensive. • It is more appropriate simply to state the ward policy and then move on.
Never reinforce hallucinations, delusions or irrational beliefs. Reinforce reality and redirect conversation.	• The same policies apply to patients with mania as to depressed patients. • It is not appropriate to agree with the patient's perceptual abnormalities. Equally, arguing that they do not exist serves little purpose. • The nurse should state their perception of the situation. • The nurse should state that there is a discrepancy between what is perceived by the patient and what is perceived by the nurse. • The nurse should then steer the conversation to discussing real people and real events.
Always respond to legitimate complaints.	• Patients with mania may often make many frivolous complaints. • However, nurses must always respond to legitimate complaints appropriately, to defuse irritability and to develop trust.

(*Source*: Adapted from Keltner, N., 2007. Depression. In: Keltner, N., Schweke, L., Bostrom, C., (Eds) Psychiatric Nursing. Mosby Elsevier, St Louis; Videbeck, S., 2009. Psychiatric Mental Health Nursing, 5th ed. Lippincott Williams & Wilkins, Philadelphia, PA.)

Neurochemical Factors

The genetic–environmental interaction produces changes in neurochemical systems. The monoamine hypothesis for depression was originally extended to account for bipolar disorder. It was argued that, as decreases in monoamines (the neurotransmitters serotonin, noradrenaline and dopamine) caused depression, increases in these same monoamines caused mania. This was supported by evidence that drugs such as cocaine and amphetamines stimulate dopamine activity and mimic the symptoms of mania (Manji & Lenox 2000). However, as with depression, while neurotransmitter imbalances are important, the process is more complex than a simple increase or decrease in monoamines (Hillhouse & Porter 2015). There are many neurotransmitter systems involved and the origin of bipolar disorder remains in the complex interplay between genetic make-up and environmental factors.

Hormone Systems and Circadian Rhythms

There has been significant research into imbalances in the HPA axis and the pituitary gland as a central marker in bipolar disorder. Cortisol and thyroid hormone levels have been found to be elevated in patients during manic episodes and even when patients are in remission from the illness (Salvadore et al. 2010; Havermans et al. 2011; Young 2014). Other researchers have found differences in structural brain function (blood flow from one part of the brain to another) during elevated mood compared with periods of normal functioning (Gonul et al. 2009; Eker et al. 2014).

Circadian rhythms are likely to be important. One of the prominent features of the manic stage of bipolar disorder is a lack of sleep. In particular, patients with bipolar disorder are sensitive to disturbances in their 24-hour circadian cycles and this is a prominent feature of their illness, during both manic and depressive episodes (Schulz & Steimer 2009; Pinho et al. 2015).

CRITICAL THINKING CHALLENGE 16.2

Many patients describe hypomania as an intoxicating state that gives rise to ceaseless energy and great pleasure. At what stage do these patients need treatment?

OVERVIEW OF CAUSATION

One of the most important concepts to consider when reviewing the causal factors of depressive mood disorder and bipolar disorder is that of cause and effect. Are disruptions in circadian rhythms, differences in structural brain structure and function, dysregulated thyroid hormone levels and increased cortisol a reflection of the bipolar illness or are they the cause? Most evidence suggests that they are certainly a marker (i.e. they occur when the illness occurs) for the illness but further than this we are not sure.

PERSISTENT DEPRESSIVE DISORDER AND CYCLOTHYMIA

There are milder, longer lasting versions of the illnesses of major depression and bipolar disorder called *persistent depressive disorder* (known as dysthymia in the DSM-IV-TR) and *cyclothymia*. Persistent depressive disorder describes a chronic mild depression. In contrast, cyclothymia describes a chronic bipolar disorder, with milder depressive symptoms

CASE STUDY 16.1

Patient With Bipolar Disorder

Sarah's husband pleaded with her to go with him to the local community mental health centre to find out what was wrong. She was 39 years old, sporadically unemployed and had been functioning inconsistently for a number of years. During the past week Sarah had been partying all night with some new friends of hers and shopping during the day. She was an attractive woman, fast talking, cheerful and casually flirtatious. She easily became irritable when challenged.

About 5 years before, Sarah had experienced some mild depressive symptoms. She was listless, had trouble getting out of bed and experienced intermittent insomnia and loss of appetite. This lasted for 2 months and then Sarah became well again.

Two years later, Sarah's father died. She had been very close to her father and felt his death harshly. She believed that she had not been a good enough daughter. Sarah's husband saw a dramatic change in his wife after her father's death. She had 3 weeks of remarkable energy, hyperactivity and euphoria. She would stay awake cleaning the house every night. She had a strong sexual interest in her husband and was bright, self-confident company. This was then followed by 1 week where she could barely lift herself out of bed. She slept for long periods and complained of exhaustion.

When Sarah was in one of her energetic periods, she was bright, energetic and brimming with self-confidence. She had worked in a car yard for many years and had months when she was the most successful dealer among her coworkers. She would spend excessively during these energetic periods, on such things as clothes and shoes.

However, towards the end of her energetic periods she became irritable and caustic and she received complaints from her customers. Following these episodes, she would go to bed for weeks at a time to try to deal with symptoms of depression. She would not shower during these periods and would eat very little.

With the support of her husband, she agreed to seek counselling from her local community health centre. She was referred to a mental health nurse practitioner who performed a complete biopsychosocial assessment.

Sarah was very concerned about what was happening to her. She made and kept appointments to see her nurse practitioner over the next 2 weeks. During the counselling sessions, Sarah's mental health history and present mental state were explored. After much discussion, Sarah agreed to commence on a course of mood stabilising medication and a series of counselling sessions.

Sarah was able to discuss with the nurse practitioner the grief and guilt she felt following the death of her father. She was also able to discuss some of the frustrations she felt in her relationship with her husband. The medication she was taking moderated the moods she was experiencing. She missed the elation she felt when she was 'high' but did not miss her irritable moments that accompanied her highs or the lows she was subject to.

Her relationship with her husband improved. While her sales record at the dealership never quite achieved the records she once had, her success was steady.

and milder elevated symptoms. A diagnosis of major depressive disorder requires a minimum of 2 weeks of symptoms and a manic episode (the diagnostic criteria for bipolar 1 disorder) requires 1 week of symptoms. In contrast, a diagnosis of persistent depressive disorder or cyclothymia requires 2 years of symptoms (APA 2013).

CHILDBIRTH AND MOOD DISORDERS

Postpartum 'Blues'

The birth of a child is generally seen as a happy event. However, many women and some men experience bouts of irritation, anxiety and tearfulness after the birth of their child. Postpartum 'blues' are a transient disturbance in mood, characterised by lability (the tendency for mood to alter quickly), sadness, dysphoria and subjective confusion (Bailara et al. 2006). The mother may burst into tears and be puzzled by such uncharacteristic weeping. Somewhat incongruously, these feelings are often interrupted by happy feelings (Bailara et al. 2006). These symptoms may occur in as many as 50% to 70% of women and some men (as well) and usually resolve on their own (Miller et al. 2006).

A number of explanations have been proposed for postpartum 'blues': physical exhaustion, the stress of childbirth, awareness of the increased responsibility that motherhood (and fatherhood) brings and changes in women's hormone regulation and immune system function (Miller et al. 2006; Groer & Morgan 2007; O'Keane et al. 2011; Shelton et al. 2015). The maternal HPA axis undergoes changes during pregnancy. As the baby develops, there is a gradual increase in placental corticotrophin-releasing hormone (CRH). At birth there is an abrupt withdrawal of this placental CRH and the maternal HPA axis must reequilibrate abruptly in the days after delivery. This reequilibration of hormone systems may be the basis of the 'baby blues' (O'Keane et al. 2011).

The main nursing intervention is education and support for the new mother and father. If the symptoms last for more than 2 weeks, the patient needs to be assessed for postpartum depression.

Perinatal Depression

It is important always to remember that mental illness is one of the leading causes of maternal death in the UK (Jones et al. 2014). Perinatal (antenatal [before birth]) and postpartum (after the birth) depression are characterised by a depressed mood, excessive anxiety, insomnia and change in weight. If the illness is untreated, it may last from months to years. Between 10% and 15% of women will develop depression during their pregnancy and this may be life threatening to both the mother and the child (Kim et al. 2010). Counselling is the first-line treatment of depression. However, not everyone will respond to a single treatment, in which case medication may be prescribed, either by a medical officer or a nurse practitioner. Antidepressants are not generally associated with major congenital malformations but there may be some risk and this should be considered in the context of pregnancy (Kim et al. 2010). Some women may relapse with depression as a result of ceasing medication on confirmation of pregnancy and caution should be recommended. The causes of postpartum depression are similar to the causes of depression in all ages and are likely to have their origins in the antenatal period. These causes include heredity, a history of previous depression, adverse events, adverse social conditions, difficult relationships and social isolation (Patton et al. 2015).

Psychotherapeutic Interventions

Nursing interventions for postpartum depression include regular counselling and education for the mother. These can be provided as part of the regular postpartum care of mother and child or as additional visits as required. It is also important to work with the significant other in the relationship. This is often the child's father, but not necessarily so. This person may be the main support person and mood changes can occur for this person as well as for the mother, with significant impact on the family unit. Several factors may be involved: added responsibility, diminished sexual outlet and decreased attention from the mother. Regular counselling and education are good nursing interventions in this instance (Dennis 2005).

Postpartum Psychosis

Postpartum psychosis is a rare psychotic disorder in women who have recently given birth. It is a psychiatric emergency. The prevalence in the general population is 1 to 2 cases per 1000 childbirths (Bergink et al. 2015). The onset is usually rapid and occurs within 2 weeks of delivery. The early symptoms of the illness often include insomnia, mood fluctuations and obsessive concerns about the newborn. More severe symptoms follow, including delusions, hallucinations and disorganised behaviour (Bergink et al. 2015). Postpartum psychosis generally has a clinical presentation, family history and longitudinal illness course that overlaps markedly with bipolar disorder and some authors consider it a bipolar spectrum illness and not a primary psychotic disorder. Others suggest that it may not be related to bipolar disorder and that it has a distinctly different risk profile and expression (Zonana & Gorman 2005; Bergink et al. 2011; Bergink et al. 2015).

The delivery process is a stress that may cause the development of the major mood disorder. Similarly, the factors that have been proposed for the postpartum 'blues' may be the stressor for the major mood disorder—that is, physical exhaustion, the stress of childbirth, awareness of the increased responsibility that motherhood brings and changes in women's hormone and immune system function (Zonana & Gorman 2005).

GRIEF AND MOOD DISORDERS

Grief can be considered the normal psychological process that a person goes through following the death of a loved one. Bowlby (1980) describes four phases of normal response to the death of a spouse, family member or loved animal:

- *Shock and protest*: a numbing of emotions and disbelief punctuated by outbursts of intense distress, panic or anger. This may last from a few hours to a week.
- *Preoccupation*: a yearning for and searching preoccupation with the loved one. This may last for weeks or months. A variety of symptoms accompany these feelings, including insomnia and restlessness. Anger towards the loved one for leaving or unresolved issues is not uncommon. In time, this yearning diminishes and is replaced by disorganisation and despair.
- *Disorganisation*: when the patient begins to accept the loss of the loved one and begins to establish a new identity independent of the loved one, there is disorganisation of previous emotions and despair diminishes. The patient may begin to accept that they are now a widow or widower.
- *Resolution*: the patient begins to rebuild their life, there is a decrease in sadness and an enjoyment of life returns. The patient reorganises themselves.

Importantly, where is the point at which grief ceases to be grief and should be described as major depressive disorder? Patients with major depressive disorder often become fixed in the disorganisation and despair stage of the grief response and cannot move on. However, it is important to recognise that it is normal to show signs of depression following the bereavement of a spouse or close family member. When normal grief causes persistent lowering of mood and significant impairment in social functioning, it may have become a depressive illness. In the most recent version of the DSM (APA 2013), the 'bereavement exclusion', a condition that prevented a diagnosis of depression in a recently bereaved person, was removed from the diagnostic criteria for major depression. For a discussion of the issues involved, see Box 16.3.

OLD AGE AND MOOD DISORDERS

One in five older people living in the community and 40% of older people living in care homes are affected by depression (Mental Health Taskforce [MHT] 2016) Major depression is also the most prevalent psychiatric disorder among community dwelling older adults in the United States and it is a major health problem (Chou & Cheung 2013; Manetti et al. 2014). Major depression is often difficult to detect in the elderly because many of the symptoms associated with major depression are also associated with common medical illnesses or symptoms of dementia (Alexopoulos et al. 2002; Small 2009). For instance, it has been estimated that perhaps as many as 50% of patients with Alzheimer disease also suffer from depression, which increases the burden on families even further (Lyketsos & Olin 2002). There is often a poorer prognosis (diagnosis and treatment) because it is perceived that older people have less need of treatment and so are more reluctant to seek help (Manetti et al. 2014).

Symptoms associated with late-onset depression include marked sleep difficulties, hypochondriasis and agitation. While there are many adverse consequences for the patient's

BOX 16.3 Removal of the 'Bereavement Exclusion' From the Diagnostic Criteria for Major Depressive Disorder

People who have recently experienced bereavement will naturally feel a keen sense of loss and sadness and may also experience disturbed sleep, changes in appetite and other changes in their psychosocial functioning. Many of these naturally occurring responses are similar to symptoms of depression. Grief and depression share some common features. For these reasons, the previous version of the DSM (the DSM-IV-TR) (APA 2000) advised clinicians to refrain from making a diagnosis of major depressive disorder in people who had experienced a bereavement in the past 2 months. The rationale was that in a recently bereaved person, grief should not be confused with a mood disorder. However, an unintended consequence of the 'bereavement exclusion' was that people who were clinically depressed *and* who had experienced a recent bereavement were not treated for depression. The authors of the DSM-5 have argued that removal of the bereavement exclusion will make it easier for people who are clinically depressed *and* who have experienced a recent bereavement to receive treatment. However, others have argued that the bereavement exclusion should stay, as removing it will result in the medicalisation of grief (for a discussion covering both sides of this controversy, see Flaskerud 2011). To guard against the possible medicalisation of grief, the DSM-5 advises clinicians to distinguish between normal grief and changes in mood, thinking and behaviour that are more consistent with a mood disorder.

health if depression goes untreated, no matter what their age, there are particular dangers for the elderly (Chou & Cheung 2013). For example, Schulz et al. (2002) found that depression could double the risk of death in older people who had had a heart attack or stroke, as it impedes their ability to recover.

Baldwin (2000) describes a number of factors that may influence the presentation of depression in older people. These include an overlap between the symptoms of the physical disorder and the somatic (physically expressed) symptoms of depression, the tendency of older people to minimise a complaint of sadness and instead complain of a physical illness, newly presenting neurotic symptoms such as severe anxiety or obsessive compulsive symptoms (which 'mask' depression), any act of deliberate self-harm and behavioural disturbances such as alcohol abuse or shoplifting, which may all reflect underlying depression (Baldwin 2000). Older adults with depression sometimes present with cognitive deficits similar to those seen in dementia but that, unlike those of dementia, resolve when the person's mood lifts.

MEDICAL CONDITIONS AND DRUG REACTIONS

Many medical conditions or drug reactions can produce symptoms identical to those found with major depression or bipolar mood disorder. It is important for nurses to consider that while the patient presents with something resembling a mood disorder, there may be an organic cause. See Box 16.4 for a list of medical conditions that cause depression and mania and Box 16.5 for a list of drugs known to cause depression.

BOX 16.4 Medical Conditions That Cause Depression and Mania

Neurological Disorders
- Parkinson disease
- Dementia
- Multiple sclerosis
- Anaemia
- Organic brain lesions, especially frontal lobe (mania)

Endocrine Disorders
- Hypothyroidism
- Thyrotoxicosis (mania)
- Cushing syndrome (mania)

Virus Infections
- Influenza

Vitamin Deficiencies
- Vitamin B_{12}
- Folate

BOX 16.5 Drug Reactions That Cause Depression and Mania

Drugs That Can Precipitate Depression Include:
- antihypertensives, especially reserpine and methyldopa
- corticosteroids and possibly sex hormones
- levodopa
- digitalis
- certain cytotoxics
- certain antimalarials
- sulfonamides
- antipsychotics
- cholesterol-lowering drugs

Drugs That Can Instigate a Manic Episode Include:
- corticosteroids
- antidepressants
- levodopa
- lysergic acid diethylamide (LSD)
- cocaine
- amphetamines (Gill 2007)

SUICIDE

Suicide is a serious risk in many kinds of depression. People with a range of mental illnesses commit suicide; however, recurrent depression carries the highest risk for suicide (Qin 2011). Approximately one-third of all people who commit suicide experience depression (Goldney & Beautrais 2007). The suicide act occurs more frequently at the onset or, paradoxically, at the resolution of a depressive episode. Goldney and Beautrais (2007) suggest that those who have resolved their depression then have the energy to carry out the act of suicide and dread a recurrence of their misery. Their anguish at the prospect of more depression is all-consuming.

Suicide and intentional self-harm are important on two levels: they are major public health issues and are devastating on a personal level. Suicide rates in England have been steadily rising, peaking in 2014 with 4882 deaths (MHT 2016).

The Gender Paradox in Suicidal Behaviour

There are gender differences in suicidal behaviour, with men three times more likely than women to take their own lives (MHT 2016).

Why are women more likely to self-harm while men are more likely to commit suicide? This is known as the gender paradox in suicide behaviour (Canetto & Sakinofsky 1998). Is it a function of method? Women who attempt suicide tend to use less violent means such as overdosing, which can be less successful. On the other hand, men often use more violent methods such as hanging, which have a higher chance of success. It has been suggested that appearance is important. In the US, firearms may be used, men are much more likely to shoot themselves in the head and shots to the head are generally more conclusive. Do changing gender roles play a part? Do men feel impotent and decide it is better to die than live as (they see themselves) failures? It is difficult to know and more research is required (Schrijvers et al. 2012).

On an individual, family and community level the effects of suicide remain devastating.

> **CRITICAL THINKING CHALLENGE 16.3**
>
> You are taking care of a patient who has a history of self-harming. You are following the protocol recommended in the area in which you work (i.e. 15-minute observations for the patient who is at risk). The patient is showing no signs that they will self-harm, but while you are not with the patient, the patient self-harms. How responsible are you for the patient's actions?

THE ART AND SCIENCE OF MENTAL HEALTH NURSING

Mood disorders can profoundly change a person's life. Patients often need intensive support. Medication may help lift a patient out of the most severe part of their illness—this is the 'science' of mental health nursing. Yet psychotherapy, alone or in combination, should be thought of as an equally important factor—this is the 'art' of mental health nursing. Medication and psychotherapy are complementary and much less effective in isolation. Mental health nurses need both the art and the science to provide the best care that we can.

Importantly, the science (medication) and the art (psychotherapy) must be considered a collaboration between the patient and the nurse. The nurse should not be thought of as doing something 'to the patient' as much as 'with the patient'. There is limited value in any therapy if the patient is not engaged and the best engagement involves an active collaboration.

Psychotherapy

There are many psychotherapeutic approaches that nurses can use. Some involve years of specialised study and subsequent practice as a nurse counsellor. Others involve the simple act of listening to patients telling their story. Both approaches can be very effective. Some important examples of psychotherapy include patient-motivated interventions, cognitive behavioural therapy, group therapy and therapeutic use of self. (For a summary of psychotherapies, see Chapter 24.) It is very important to remember that most comparative studies of different psychotherapies have the same major finding: it is the quality of the relationship between the counsellor and the patient that is most therapeutic, not the specific psychotherapy used.

Patient-Motivated Interventions

Patient-motivated interventions recognise the importance of empowering the patient to make their own choices to improve their health and wellbeing. There are different types of patient-motivated interventions available. Commonly, they involve an interview and basic education about self-management with a nurse. From there, the patient takes this information away (e.g. books, CDs, DVDs, computer programs) and practises the self-management techniques at home. The interventions are often based on cognitive behavioural principles. The patient usually benefits if family members and significant others are included in the process. The patient may then be reviewed face to face, by telephone or even via e-mail. There should be easy access to follow up if relapse of the illness occurs (Lovell & Gellatly 2009).

Cognitive Behavioural Therapy

Cognitive behavioural therapy (CBT) is a common psychological approach to understanding and treating psychological disorders, addressing other types of abnormal behaviour and adjusting to life-changing events. It is supported by a large body of research evidence. There are a number of cognitive behavioural approaches but they share the following attributes: they involve a collaborative relationship between the patient and the therapist and they are based on the principle that psychological distress is largely because of disturbances in the cognitive (thinking) process. If a patient is able to change the way they think about themselves (self-statements), there will be a corresponding change in their behaviour. The therapies are generally time-limited and focus on specific target problems (Corey 2012).

Group Therapy

Group therapy is a form of psychotherapy where the therapist treats a small group of patients rather than a single patient. It can refer to any form of therapy delivered to a group, such as cognitive behavioural therapy, but it is usually applied where the group process is utilised as the mechanism of change. The group process involves the development, exploration and examination of interpersonal relationships in the group. Through this group process, group members develop social skills and achieve a greater level of self-awareness, which they then apply to situations outside the group (Corey 2011).

Therapeutic Use of Self

As nurses, when we counsel our patients and do it effectively, we are practising the therapeutic use of self. Patients in mental health services are often very distressed and frightened about what is happening to them. They may feel that they have no control over their moods. They are often worried about being rejected or being seen as 'crazy'. When we listen to our patients in a thoughtful, sensitive manner, with genuine interest, their worth as a human being is confirmed. A therapeutic relationship is formed between us and the patient and this helps the patient to get better. Through this process of building a therapeutic relationship we may instil 'hope' in our patients that things will get better (Geldard & Geldard 2011).

There are a number of basic counselling skills that we can use to enhance this therapeutic process. These are known as listening with interest or active listening, reflection of content and feeling, summarising and closure:

- *Listening with interest* is where we listen in such a way that the patient recognises that we are totally focussing our attention on what they are saying and understanding them. Such listening can have a very positive effect on someone who is confused and worried about what is happening to their mood and mental state, often referred to as active listening.
- *Reflection of content* or paraphrasing is where we pick out the most important details of what the patient is saying and reexpress it in our own words rather than using the patient's words. Reflection of content communicates to the patient that we understand what they are saying.
- *Reflection of feelings* is where we reflect back to the patient how they are feeling and, again, this can be a powerful tool in the right context. When used appropriately, the patient realises that we are empathising with them and have at least some idea of their emotional journey (Geldard & Geldard 2011).
- *Summarising* involves pausing in the counselling session and summarising what has been covered. In this way, the patient is better able to see a clear picture of their situation. Closure occurs when the counselling session is finished, the session is summarised a final time and the patient feels as comfortable as possible with the progress.

These basic principles of counselling are described in Nurse's Story 16.1 about a depressed young man.

PHARMACOLOGY

The main classes of medication used to treat major depression and bipolar disorder are antidepressants and mood stabilisers. When psychotic features are evident (with either major depression or bipolar disorder), an antipsychotic may be required. Selective serotonin reuptake inhibitors (SSRIs) are the more popular class of antidepressants and sodium valproate is one of the most popular mood stabilisers. For further discussion of all these classes of medication, refer to Chapter 25.

Antidepressants

The main groups of antidepressants are SSRIs (e.g. fluoxetine [Prozac]) or citalopram (Cipramil), selective noradrenaline reuptake inhibitors (e.g. reboxetine [Edronax]), dual serotonin and noradrenaline reuptake inhibitors (e.g. venlafaxine [Effexor] or tricyclic antidepressants (e.g. amitriptyline [Triptafen]) and monoamine oxidase inhibitors (MAOIs) (e.g. phenelzine [Nardil] or moclobemide [Manerix]) (see Box 16.6). These drugs have not been shown to differ substantially in their effectiveness, but they do differ in their side-effect profiles (Lehne 2013). See Chapter 25 for a discussion about the side effects of these drugs.

At present, the first-line pharmacological treatment for depression is the SSRIs. This class of drugs was first introduced in 1987 and has since become the most commonly prescribed group of antidepressants. These drugs are as effective as tricyclic antidepressants but do not cause hypotension, sedation or anticholinergic effects such as dry eyes, dry mouth, blurred vision, constipation and urinary retention. However, SSRIs do have a range of other side effects that may be very distressing, including sexual dysfunction (difficulty achieving orgasm) and akathisia (restless leg syndrome). Antidepressants generally have a long half-life (i.e. the time taken for the drug to be broken down to half). This means that in general antidepressants can be taken once a day. With SSRIs patients tend to improve within 3 to 5 weeks of treatment. If therapy is discontinued, the process should occur slowly, as sudden cessation may lead to restlessness, insomnia, anxiety and nausea (Lehne 2013).

Mood Stabilisers

The term 'mood stabiliser' describes a group of drugs, not a specific pharmacological class. These drugs help prevent the recurrence of bipolar affective disorder and can also be effective in treating the acute episodes of mania and depression that occur with the illness. The main mood stabilisers are lithium carbonate and the antiepileptic drugs, including sodium valproate, carbamazepine and lamotrigine. Interestingly, these same three drugs may be effective in four different disorders: bipolar disorder, epilepsy, chronic pain/neuralgia and migraine headaches (Lehne 2013). They have a common sodium channel-blocking effect and enhanced gamma-aminobutyric acid (GABA) function. These drugs stabilise the underlying irregular firing of neurons that contributes to each of these illnesses.

Sodium valproate and lithium have different effect profiles. Sodium valproate is one of the most popular agents for the long-term treatment of bipolar disorder. It has a greater safety margin for dosing than lithium carbonate (therapeutic index), fewer side effects and, compared with carbamazepine, interacts with fewer other medications (Lehne 2013). Lithium has been shown to be effective at treating the manic stage of bipolar disorder but less effective with the depressed stage. Large

NURSE'S STORY 16.1

A Depressed Young Man

Luke had been the main support for his family since his father died when Luke was 15 years old. He lived with his mother and two younger sisters in an inner-city suburb and worked in the warehouse of a local supermarket.

His mother had suffered from depression for as long as Luke could remember. Antidepressants and counselling from their local priest seemed to help his mother, but much of the time Luke worked, paid the bills, cooked the meals and organised his sisters for school each day. His position at the supermarket had some flexibility and he would pick his sisters up from school and then return to work in the evening when his family was settled.

The eldest daughter, aged 14 years, had called into the local health centre, concerned that her mother had become 'unwell' again. She asked whether a nurse could come to their house to see her. That's where I came in.

When I arrived at their house the next day, I was surprised to find Luke at home and still in his dressing gown. He told me that his mother had remained in bed for these last 2 weeks and was eating poorly. He was worried for her. His mother and I talked, I made an assessment and then spent the next half hour organising her admission to an acute mental healthcare ward.

While we waited for the ambulance, I sat down with Luke. He seemed very flat. There was little animation in his voice. I asked him why he wasn't at work and he replied rather vaguely that he just wasn't feeling very well. It was obvious that he didn't want to talk and so we sat for a little while in silence. The ambulance eventually came and before I left I made an appointment to catch up with him a week later.

I had known Luke superficially for a number of years in the context of providing care for his mother. I suspected that he was under strain but had hoped that he was coping. I had never seen him so flat before and sensed he was in some distress. My first priority was to visit him regularly to try to develop a therapeutic relationship. This was partly in the context of planning for his mother's discharge from hospital but also because I wanted to engage with him and develop a sense of trust between us. I hoped that he would open up and talk about how he felt. This happened very slowly. Much of the time we would sit quietly together each time I visited. At all times I tried to be as genuine and honest with him as I could. As a consequence, he gradually opened up to me.

Luke described how he had lost his appetite and felt constant fatigue. He was also irritable much of the time with the long hours at work and burdens at home. He recognised his irritability and hated himself for it. He didn't like being irritable with his family. He'd had a girlfriend for a couple of months the year before, but there was little time in his life to devote to another relationship and it soon ended. He then found himself lacking energy and more irritable than before.

As Luke talked about how he was feeling I took the major points he was making and reflected them back to him. I reflected the content of what he was saying. He seemed relieved that I understood the practical nature of his problems. At other times I briefly reflected I understood how he was feeling. Again he seemed relieved that I understood his emotional state.

At times during our interactions Luke was angry with himself. At other times he turned his anger on me. I realised he wasn't targeting me personally and that it was a symptom of his illness. He would always apologise after the anger had passed and we would be relaxed with each other again. At the end of each session I would summarise what we had talked about and conclude by making a time to see him again. This enabled him to reflect on what we had discussed and confirmed with me that I had understood his issues and understood how he felt and that we would talk again.

As always, I expressed hope to him that his spirits would lift. I tried to instil hope. I focussed on what a good, caring son and brother he was. He regularly visited his mother in hospital. I also praised him on how his sisters were turning out with his help. They were well-respected at the school and getting good marks in their studies.

My counselling seemed to help. At each stage it was a collaborative relationship. After much discussion about the positives and negatives of pharmacotherapy, Luke decided he wanted to trial some antidepressants. He commenced them, his mood lifted further and he admitted he was sleeping properly for the first time in months.

However, it was when his mother returned from hospital that Luke seemed to make big improvements. Luke had missed his mother keenly. She was brighter and able to help more around the house and with the two girls. Luke himself seemed to be coping better and was taking less time off from work. He had also mentioned during my last visit that he was thinking of getting in touch with his ex-girlfriend to see if she wanted to spend some time with him.

On my final visit a couple of weeks later, it was obvious that he was better. He'd recently gained a promotion at work and his girlfriend was coming around that night for dinner with his family. He thanked me for my efforts over the past couple of months and spoke in positive terms about his future. I was glad.

randomised studies have found that lithium treatment was more effective at preventing suicide and slightly more effective in general than sodium valproate (Kessing et al. 2011). Overall, worldwide clinical experience confirms the benefits of both of these drugs in reducing relapse rates of bipolar disorder. See Box 16.7 for common side effects of sodium valproate.

Medication Collaboration

Psychotropic medication often needs to be taken over a long period of time to reduce the symptoms of the disease and prevent relapse. Patients who regularly take their medication as instructed are often described as being compliant or adhering to the medication. Unfortunately, this implies that patients who do not take their medication are somehow failing. There may be a number of reasons why patients may not wish to take their prescribed medication. For example, the side effects may be interfering with their quality of life; the patient may have poor education as to why they should take their medication; and the medication may not be effective. Collaboration between the patient and the nurse is the most valuable approach to encourage appropriate adherence to medication. A good strategy to encourage adherence to medication is for

BOX 16.6 Antidepressant Drugs

Selective Serotonin Reuptake Inhibitors (SSRIs)
- sertraline (Lustral)
- paroxetine (Seroxat)
- fluvoxamine (Faverin)
- fluoxetine (Prozac)
- escitalopram (Cipralex)
- citalopram (Cipramil)

Selective Noradrenaline Reuptake Inhibitors
- reboxetine (Edronax)

Serotonin and Noradrenaline Reuptake Inhibitors
- venlafaxine (Effexor)

Tricyclic Antidepressants
- amitriptyline (Triptafen)
- imipramine (Tofranil)

Monoamine Oxidase Inhibitors
- phenelzine (Nardil)
- moclobemide (Manerix)

Atypical Antidepressants
- nefazodone (Serzone)
- mirtazapine (Zispin)

BOX 16.7 Side Effects of Sodium Valproate

- Stomach upset
- Hand tremors
- Increased appetite
- Weight gain
- Hair loss

both the patient and the nurse to have a solid knowledge of the medications (effects and side effects), the implications of discontinuing treatment and the potential options. A good knowledge of the pharmacology of these medications also ensures that both the patient and the nurse can properly monitor for signs that the medications are becoming toxic, becoming ineffective or are being therapeutic.

HOSPITALISATION

As with all mental illnesses, hospitalisation may be required when the illness is not responding to treatment and it is considered that more intense and more frequent clinical attention is required. Hospitalisation may also be required when the risk of harm to the patient or others is considered too high for the patient to be left in the community (e.g. injury as a result of neglect such as not eating or drinking, injury as a result of suicide or self-harm or injury as a result of assault to others or the patient). One criticism is that inpatient mental health units, with shorter and shorter average length of stays, largely perform a risk management function rather than any substantial therapeutic purpose. A response to that criticism is that people do become very unwell at times in spite of strong community involvement and need hospitalisation. As with most things, the best system uses properly resourced community services as well as inpatient services.

ELECTROCONVULSIVE THERAPY

Electroconvulsive therapy (ECT) involves the administration of an electric current to the head of an anaesthetised patient to produce seizure activity while motor effects (uncontrolled movements of the torso and limbs) are prevented with a muscle relaxant. ECT is a treatment for depression in the following circumstances:

- When an urgent response is needed—this can occur when the patient's life is threatened in a severe depressive disorder by a refusal to drink or eat or when the patient is experiencing treatment-resistant, intense suicidal ideation.
- For a resistant depressive disorder, following failure to respond to treatment with antidepressant medication. It can also be effective for treatment-resistive psychosis or for neuroleptic malignant syndrome where antipsychotics are contraindicated.

ECT works more quickly than antidepressant drugs, although the outcome after 3 months is similar (Payne & Prudic 2009). A common programme is several times a week over a 3- to 6-week period. The patient is given general anaesthesia and therefore they have no memory of the experience. Adverse effects include a brief period of headache following treatment and memory and cognitive impairment. Many patients report a persistent loss of memory regarding events that occurred during the ECT course and the weeks and months before the course (Sackheim 2014). It should be noted that cognitive impairment and memory loss also occur with depressive disorder.

In recent years, there has been renewed focus on the problems of cognitive impairment and the overall utility of ECT has been questioned (Payne & Prudic 2009). One option may be the use of 'ultrabrief ECT', which may have less of a deleterious effect on cognitive function than ECT (Loo et al. 2008; Sienaert et al. 2010). Unfortunately, it may also be less effective (Spaans et al. 2013).

At present, although its use remains controversial, ECT is widely accepted as an effective intervention in the treatment of resistant major depression and a range of other mental health conditions (Eschweiler et al. 2007). As always, and wherever possible, the decision to perform ECT should be based on consultation between the patient, the patient's significant others, nursing staff and medical staff (Leiknes et al. 2012).

CONCLUSION

Variations in mood are a natural part of life. They indicate that a person is connecting with the world around them. Extremes in mood are associated with normal reactions such as joy, ecstasy, grief, loss and despair. When these extremes in mood become debilitating and disordered, patients require our help.

Mood disorders are one of the most common groups of mental disorders in the community. This chapter has drawn on a range of mental health sources to provide a brief overview of our present understanding of mood disorders, their signs and symptoms and a variety of postulated aetiologies. Particular conditions associated with mood disorders have been considered, including the nature of childbirth, grief, old age, self-harm and suicide.

Practical nursing interventions have been described, with an emphasis on caring for the patient holistically and not as an abstract illness. Other major therapeutic interventions described include medication collaboration and psychotherapy. The biomedical approach, including pharmacology, is the 'science'. Psychotherapy, including therapeutic use of self, is the 'art'. The best approach combines both the art and the science of mental health nursing to care for people with mood disorders. It cannot be overestimated how important it is to work with the patient in a collaborative approach for best outcomes.

EXERCISES FOR CLASS ENGAGEMENT

Changes in mood are a normal and vital part of human existence. They affect all aspects of our lives. When they become disabling they become mood disorders. There are a great many questions that can be asked with regard to the nature of mood disorders. Working in groups, discuss the following questions:

1. Why do you think there has been an increase in the incidence of depression worldwide?
2. What evidence is there to support the following theories?
   - Depression is a reflection of the increased stress and pressures of modern living.
   - There is greater recognition among health professionals of the nature and frequency of mood disorders and depression.
   - Contemporary populations are weaker and less resilient in comparison with earlier generations.
3. If a person is depressed, how much responsibility should they have to take to improve their mood? How much is it beyond their control? How much should they blame it on physiological reasons? Should you ever say to a patient 'I'm sure you'll get over it' or 'You need to take some responsibility for your low mood'?
4. Some people with bipolar disorder claim that they are able to adjust their medication so that their mood is always a little elevated. What are the positive and negative aspects of this practice? If you had bipolar disorder, would you prefer to have a slightly elevated mood or a 'normal' mood? If a patient told you that was what they were doing or wanted to do, what would you say to them?
5. Suicide attempts and self-harm are acts usually committed in the context of a mood disorder. This is usually major depression or the depressive phase of a bipolar disorder illness. Could suicide ever occur without an accompanying mood disorder? That is, can suicide ever be a rational decision, in response to intolerable circumstances (e.g. existence in a concentration camp or euthanasia in the context of intolerable pain or inoperable tumour), without an accompanying mood disorder? Or would there always be an underlying depressive condition?

REFERENCES

Alexopoulos, G.S., Borson, S., Cuthbert, B.N., Devanand, D.P., Mulsant, B.H., Olin, J.T., Oslin, D.W., 2002. Assessment of late life depression. Biological Psychiatry 52 (3), 164–174.

American Psychiatric Association (APA), 2000. Diagnostic and Statistical Manual of Mental Disorders, fourth ed. APA, Washington. Text revision.

American Psychiatric Association (APA), 2013. Diagnostic and Statistical Manual of Mental Disorders, fifth edition. APA, Washington.

Bailara, K.M., Henry, C., Lestage, J., Launay, J.M., Parrot, F., Swendsen, J., Sutter, A.L., Roux, D., Dallay, D., Demotes-Mainard, J., 2006. Decreased brain tryptophan availability as a partial determinant of post-partum blues. Psychoneuroendocrinology 31 (3), 407–413.

Baldwin, R., 2000. Mood disorders in the elderly. In: Gelder, M., Lopez-Ibor, J., Andreasen, N. (Eds.), New Oxford Textbook of Psychiatry. Oxford University Press, Oxford.

Ball, J., Manicavasagar, V., Mitchell, P., O'Kearney, R., 2010. Mood disorders. In: Rieger, E. (Ed.), Abnormal Psychology: Leading Researcher Perspectives. McGraw-Hill, Sydney.

Bergink, V., Burgerhout, K.M., Koorengevel, K.M., Kamperman, A.M., Hoogendijk, W.J., Lambregtse-van den Berg, M.P., Kushner, S.A., 2015. Treatment of psychosis and mania in the postpartum period. American Journal of Psychiatry 172 (2), 115–123.

Bergink, V., Lambregtse-van den Berg, M.P., Koorengevel, K.M., Kupka, R., Kushner, S.A., 2011. First-onset psychosis occurring in the postpartum period: a prospective cohort study. Journal of Clinical Psychiatry 72 (11), 1531–1537.

Bowlby, J., 1980. Attachment and Loss, 3: Loss, Sadness and Depression. Basic Books, New York.

Canetto, S.S., Sakinofsky, I., 1998. The gender paradox in suicide. Suicide and Life-Threatening Behavior 28 (1), 1–23.

Chou, K.L., Cheung, K.C., 2013. Major depressive disorder in vulnerable groups of older adults, their course and treatment, and psychiatric comorbidity. Depression and Anxiety 30 (6), 528–537.

Corey, G., 2011. Theory and Practice of Group Counselling, eighth ed. Brooks/Cole, Belmont, CA.

Corey, G., 2012. Theory and Practice of Counselling and Psychotherapy, ninth ed. Brooks/Cole, Belmont, CA.

Cross-Disorder Group of the Psychiatric Genomics Consortium, 2013. Identification of risk loci with shared effects on five major psychiatric disorders: a genome-wide analysis. Lancet 381 (9875), 1371–1379.

Dennis, C.L., 2005. Psychosocial and psychological interventions for prevention of postnatal depression: systematic review. British Medical Journal 331 (7507), 15.

Eker, C., Simsek, F., Yilmazer, E.E., Kitis, O., Cinar, C., Eker, O.D., Coburn, K., Gonul, A.S., 2014. Brain regions associated with risk and resistance for bipolar I disorder: a voxel-based MRI study of patients with bipolar disorder and their healthy siblings. Bipolar Disorders 16 (3), 249–261.

Flaskerud, J., 2011. Grief and depression: are they different? Issues in Mental Health Nursing 32 (5), 338–340.

Eschweiler, G.W., Vonthein, R., Bode, R., Huell, M., Conca, A., Peters, O., Mende-Lechler, S., Peters, J., Klecha, D., Prapotnik, M., DiPauli, J., Wild, B., Plewnia, C., Bartels, M., Schlotter, W., 2007. Clinical efficacy and cognitive side effects of bifrontal versus right unilateral electroconvulsive therapy (ECT): a short-term randomised controlled trial in pharmaco-resistant major depression. Journal of Affective Disorders 101 (1–3), 149–157.

Geldard, D., Geldard, K., 2011. Basic Personal Counselling. A Training Manual for Counsellors, seventh ed. Pearson/Prentice Hall, Sydney.

Gelder, M., Mayou, R., Geddes, J., 2005. Mood disorders. In: Gelder, M., Mayou, R., Geddes, J. (Eds.), Psychiatry, third ed. Oxford University Press, Oxford, pp. 97–118.

Gill, D., 2007. Hughes' Outline of Modern Psychiatry, fifth ed. John Wiley & Sons, Chichester, UK.

Goldberg, J.S., Bell Jr., C.E., Pollard, D.A., 2014. Revisiting the monoamine hypothesis of depression: a new perspective. Perspectives in Medicinal Chemistry 6, 1–8.

Goldney, R., Beautrais, A., 2007. Suicide and suicidal behaviour. In: Bloch, S., Singh, B. (Eds.), Foundations of Clinical Psychiatry, third ed. Melbourne University Press, Melbourne.

Gonul, A.S., Coburn, K., Kula, M., 2009. Cerebral blood flow, metabolic, receptor, and transporter changes in bipolar disorder: the role of PET and SPECT studies. International Review of Psychiatry 21 (4), 323–335.

Groer, M.W., Morgan, K., 2007. Immune, health and endocrine characteristics of depressed postpartum mothers. Psychoneuroendocrinology 32 (2), 133–139.

Haase, J., Brown, E., 2015. Integrating the monoamine, neurotrophin and cytokine hypotheses of depression--a central role for the serotonin transporter? Pharmacology & Therapeutics 147, 1–11.

Havermans, R., Nicolson, N.A., Berkhof, J., deVries, M.W., 2011. Patterns of salivary cortisol secretion and responses to daily events in patients with remitted bipolar disorder. Psychoneuroendocrinology 36 (2), 258–265.

Hillhouse, T.M., Porter, J.H., 2015. A brief history of the development of antidepressant drugs: from monoamines to glutamate. Experimental and Clinical Psychopharmacology 23 (1), 1–21.

Horowitz, M.A., Zunszain, P.A., 2015. Neuroimmune and neuroendocrine abnormalities in depression: two sides of the same coin. Annals of the New York Academy of Sciences.

Jones, I., Chandra, P.S., Dazzan, P., Howard, L.M., 2014. Bipolar disorder, affective psychosis, and schizophrenia in pregnancy and the post-partum period. Lancet 384 (9956), 1789–1799.

Kessing, L.V., Hellmund, G., Geddes, J.R., Goodwin, G.M., Andersen, P.K., 2011. Valproate v. lithium in the treatment of bipolar disorder in clinical practice: observational nationwide register-based cohort study. British Journal of Psychiatry 199 (1), 57–63.

Kim, D.R., O'Reardon, J.P., Epperson, C.N., 2010. Guidelines for the management of depression during pregnancy. Current Psychiatry Reports 12 (4), 279–281.

Lehne, R., 2013. Pharmacology for Nursing Care, eighth ed. Saunders Elsevier, St Louis.

Leiknes, K.A., Jarosh-von Schweder, L., Hoie, B., 2012. Contemporary use and practice of electroconvulsive therapy worldwide. Brain and Behavior 2 (3), 283–344.

Loo, C.K., Sainsbury, K., Sheehan, P., Lyndon, B., 2008. A comparison of RUL ultrabrief pulse (0.3 ms) ECT and standard RUL ECT. International Journal of Neuropsychopharmacology 11 (7), 883–890.

Lovell, K., Gellatly, J., 2009. Self-help. In: Norman, I., Ryrie, I. (Eds.), The Art and Science of Mental Health Nursing. A Textbook of Principles and Practice. Open University Press/McGraw-Hill, Maidenhead, Berkshire, UK.

Lyketsos, C.G., Olin, J., 2002. Depression in Alzheimer's disease: overview and treatment. Biological Psychiatry 52 (3), 243–252.

Manetti, A., Hoertel, N., Le Strat, Y., Schuster, J.P., Lemogne, C., Limosin, F., 2014. Comorbidity of late-life depression in the United States: a population-based study. American Journal of Geriatric Psychiatry 22 (11), 1292–1306.

Manji, H.K., Lenox, R.H., 2000. The nature of bipolar disorder. Journal of Clinical Psychiatry 61 (Suppl. 13), 42–57.

Mental Health Taskforce (MHT), 2016. The Five Year Forward View for Mental Health. Available at: https://www.england.nhs.uk/wp-content/uploads/2016/02/Mental-Health-Taskforce-FYFV-final.pdf. Accessed: 17 October 2018.

Miller, R.L., Pallant, J.F., Negri, L.M., 2006. Anxiety and stress in the postpartum: is there more to postnatal distress than depression? BMC Psychiatry 6, 12.

Moieni, M., Irwin, M.R., Jevtic, I., Olmstead, R., Breen, E.C., Eisenberger, N.I., 2015. Sex differences in depressive and socioemotional responses to an inflammatory challenge: implications for sex differences in depression. Neuropsychopharmacology 40 (7), 1709–1716.

National Health Service Digital Survey – National Statistics, 2014. Mental Health and Wellbeing in England Adult Psychiatric Morbidity Survey 2014. Available at: https://assets.publishing.service.gov.uk/government/uploads/system/uploads/attachment_data/file/556596/apms-2014-full-rpt.pdf. Accessed: 17 October 2018.

Nolan-Hoeksema, S., 2002. Gender differences in depression. In: Gotlib, I., Hammen, C. (Eds.), Handbook of Depression. Guilford, New York, pp. 492–509.

O'Keane, V., Lightman, S., Patrick, K., Marsh, M., Papadopoulos, A.S., Pawlby, S., Seneviratne, G., Taylor, A., Moore, R., 2011. Changes in the maternal hypothalamic-pituitary-adrenal axis during the early puerperium may be related to the postpartum 'blues'. Journal of Neuroendocrinology 23 (11), 1149–1155.

Patton, G.C., Romaniuk, H., Spry, E., Coffey, C., Olsson, C., Doyle, L.W., Oats, J., Hearps, S., Carlin, J.B., Brown, S., 2015. Prediction of perinatal depression from adolescence and before conception (VIHCS): 20-year prospective cohort study. Lancet 386 (9996), 875–883.

Payne, N.A., Prudic, J., 2009. Electroconvulsive therapy: part I. A perspective on the evolution and current practice of ECT. Journal of Psychiatric Practice 15 (5), 346–368.

Pinho, M., Sehmbi, M., Cudney, L.E., Kauer-Sant'anna, M., Magalhaes, P.V., Reinares, M., Bonnin, C.M., Sassi, R.B., Kapczinski, F., Colom, F., Vieta, E., Frey, B.N., Rosa, A.R., 2015. The association between biological rhythms, depression, and functioning in bipolar disorder: a large multi-center study. Acta Psychiatrica Scandinavica 133 (2), 102–108.

Qin, P., 2011. The impact of psychiatric illness on suicide: differences by diagnosis of disorders and by sex and age of subjects. Journal of Psychiatric Research 45 (11), 1445–1452.

Salvadore, G., Quiroz, J.A., Machado-Vieira, R., Henter, I.D., Manji, H.K., Zarate Jr., C.A., 2010. The neurobiology of the switch process in bipolar disorder: a review. Journal of Clinical Psychiatry 71 (11), 1488–1501.

Sackheim, H.A., 2014. Autobiographical memory and electroconvulsive therapy: do not throw the baby out. Journal of ECT 30 (3), 177–186.

Schrijvers, D.L., Bollen, J., Sabbe, B.G., 2012. The gender paradox in suicidal behavior and its impact on the suicidal process. Journal of Affective Disorders 138 (1–2), 19–26.

Schulz, P., Steimer, T., 2009. Neurobiology of circadian systems. CNS Drugs 23 (Suppl. 2), 3–13.

Schulz, R., Drayer, R., Rollman, B., 2002. Depression as a risk factor for the non-suicide mortality in the elderly. Biological Psychiatry 52 (3), 205–225.

Schweitzer, I., Parke, G., 2007. Mood disorders. In: Bloch, S., Singh, B. (Eds.), Foundations of Clinical Psychiatry, third ed. Melbourne University Press, Melbourne.

Serretti, A., Fabbri, C., 2013. Shared genetics among major psychiatric disorders. Lancet 381 (9875), 1339–1341.

Shelton, M.M., Schminkey, D.L., Groer, M.W., 2015. Relationships among prenatal depression, plasma cortisol, and inflammatory cytokines. Biological Research for Nursing 17 (3), 295–302.

Sienaert, P., Vansteelandt, K., Demyttenaere, K., Peuskens, J., 2010. Randomized comparison of ultra-brief bifrontal and unilateral electroconvulsive therapy for major depression: cognitive side-effects. Journal of Affective Disorders 122 (1–2), 60–67.

Small, G.W., 2009. Differential diagnoses and assessment of depression in elderly patients. Journal of Clinical Psychiatry 70 (12), e47.

Spaans, H.P., Kho, K.H., Verwijk, E., Kok, R.M., Stek, M.L., 2013. Efficacy of ultrabrief pulse electroconvulsive therapy for depression: a systematic review. Journal of Affective Disorders 150 (3), 720–726.

Sullivan, P.F., Daly, M.J., O'Donovan, M., 2012. Genetic architectures of psychiatric disorders: the emerging picture and its implications. Nature Reviews Genetics 13 (8), 537–551.
Valentino, R.J., Reyes, B., Van Bockstaele, E., Bangasser, D., 2011. Molecular and cellular sex differences at the intersection of stress and arousal. Neuropharmacology 62 (1), 13–20.
Weissman, M.M., Bland, R.C., Canino, G.J., Faravelli, C., Greenwald, S., Hwu, H.G., Joyce, P.R., Karam, E.G., Le, C.K., Lellouch, J., Lepine, J.P., Newman, S.C., Rubio-Stipec, M., Wells, J.E., Wickramaratne, P.J., Wittchen, H., Yeh, E.K., 1996. Cross-national epidemiology of major depression and bipolar disorder. JAMA 276 (4), 293–299.
Weissman, M.M., Klerman, G.L., 1977. Sex differences and the epidemiology of depression. Archives of General Psychiatry 34 (1), 98–111.
World Health Organization (WHO), 2014. Global Health Estimates 2014 Summary Tables: Disability Adjusted Life Years 2000–2012. WHO, Geneva. Available at: www.euro.who.int/en/health-topics/noncommunicable-diseases/mental-health/data-and-statistics.
Young, A.H., 2014. The effects of HPA axis function on cognition and its implications for the pathophysiology of bipolar disorder. Harvard Review of Psychiatry 22 (6), 331–333.
Zonana, J., Gorman, J.M., 2005. The neurobiology of postpartum depression. CNS Spectrums 10 (10), 792–799, 805.

USEFUL WEBSITES

Bipolar UK, www.bipolaruk.org
Headspace, www.headspace.com
SANE, www.sane.org

17

Personality Disorders

Michelle Cleary, Toby Raeburn

KEY POINTS

- Personality disorders are common conditions, with borderline personality disorder being the most likely of these disorders that nurses will encounter in their practice.
- A wide range of terms are used to describe personality disorders. Section 2 of the *Diagnostic and Statistical Manual of Mental Disorders*, 5th edition (DSM-5) (American Psychiatric Association [APA]), groups personality disorders into three broad clusters: (A) odd or eccentric; (B) dramatic, emotional or erratic; and (C) anxious or fearful. In acknowledgement of the diagnostic complexity of personality disorders Section 3 of DSM-5 presents a refined group of seven disorders designed to guide future research and improve the acceptance of personality disorders as a homogenous group.
- Personality disorders are characterised by pervasive, maladaptive behaviours.
- Personality disorders are not caused by another psychiatric disorder but may coexist with another psychiatric disorder.
- Effective nursing care of patients with a personality disorder involves developing a therapeutic relationship and setting clear boundaries.
- There are a range of psychosocial treatments that help improve patients' quality of life.
- Staff education and clinical supervision help nurses to reflect on their practice and to gain insight and understanding into patients' behaviour.

KEY TERMS

antisocial personality disorder
avoidant personality disorder
borderline personality disorder
dependent personality disorder
dialectical behaviour therapy (DBT)
engagement
histrionic personality disorder
limit-setting
narcissistic personality disorder
obsessive-compulsive personality disorder
paranoid personality disorder
personality disorder
personality traits
schizoid personality disorder
schizotypal personality disorder
self-harm
stigmatisation

LEARNING OUTCOMES

The material in this chapter will help you to:

- discuss personality.
- identify the main characteristics of each of the three clusters of personality disorders.
- develop an understanding of responses that nurses and other healthcare professionals may experience when working with people who have a personality disorder.
- identify effective nursing approaches to work with people who have a personality disorder.

INTRODUCTION

People with a personality disorder exhibit feelings, thoughts and behaviours that interfere markedly with their ability to get close to others and to achieve success at work and socially. They are unlikely to seek treatment to change their personality, although they frequently present for help with depression, anxiety and substance abuse. Nurses caring for people with a personality disorder need appropriate education and training to be able to engage therapeutically with these patients.

This chapter describes how personality disorders are categorised and identifies the defining characteristics of each according to the *Diagnostic and Statistical Manual of Mental Disorders*, 5th edition (DSM-5) (American Psychiatric Association [APA] 2013). It also discusses some of the challenges faced in making a diagnosis of personality disorder. It focusses in particular on assessing and intervening in borderline personality disorder (BPD), a cluster B disorder, because it is the disorder nurses are most likely to encounter in practice. For people using psychiatric services, the prevalence of BPD is greater than 20% in community patient populations and around 40% for inpatient populations (National Health and Medical Research Council [NHMRC] 2012).

THE PERSONALITY-DISORDER CONTINUUM

Each of us has a personality and a common sense understanding of what that means. We may describe others as 'outgoing', 'assertive', 'withdrawn' or 'shy', for example. Sometimes the terms that we choose to describe ourselves are not the ones that would be chosen by those who know us. Some individuals have personalities that seem to draw people to them—they may be described as charismatic, outgoing, friendly, good team players, helpful or kind. Others seem to have difficulty attracting others or maintaining relationships—they appear to be unreceptive, cold, aloof, isolative, eccentric or perhaps moody, aggressive or reckless. Our personality may be thought of as the expression of our feelings, thoughts and patterns of behaviour that evolve over time. Genetics, family, life events, culture and the society we live in all contribute to shaping our personality. Personality manifests via our general disposition, behavioural patterns and approach to the world and is especially evident during interactions with others.

It is our range of enduring and recognisable personality characteristics that makes us unique and enables us to respond to the experiences that life presents us with. Features that distinguish one person's personality from another's may be apparent in one's outlook on life, the way we respond and adapt to challenges and how circumstances are interpreted (Kern etal. 2014). Different historical periods, societies and cultures support or discourage some personality types. For example, people raised in regimes such as the former East Germany, where the secret police network was widespread and intruded into families, would be more likely to be secretive, suspicious of others and unforthcoming. Similarly, cultures that are group-oriented may endorse mutual friendliness, sharing and fitting in at the expense of competitiveness and individualism.

Enduring aspects or features of our personality are referred to as *personality traits* and these traits are what differentiate us from one another. Social mores provide unwritten boundaries for what constitutes a 'normal' personality trait. For example, if a student expresses concern at having to present their work to the class because they are shy and public speaking makes them nervous, most people would understand their difficulties. With perseverance and support, most students will incrementally gain confidence and participate in tutorials regardless of some level of continuing discomfort. However, some individuals are so averse to public speaking that they will eventually avoid social situations where this might be required of them, to the extent of dropping out of an interesting course or a good job or from contact with friendship groups. Such extreme behaviour is beyond what is socially regarded as shyness. The personality trait has moved beyond normal boundaries to a point where it may be understood in terms of psychopathology. Some individuals display personality traits that seem to be beyond the scope of what is considered reasonable as observed by their behaviour and attitudes to others and this creates practical and social problems for them and others in activities of daily living.

When these personality manifestations interfere significantly with a person's life or the lives of those close to them, the person may be diagnosed with a *personality disorder*. As with personality types, traits associated with personality disorders are often apparent in childhood and persist through adolescence to adulthood. The difference is largely of degree: the characteristics associated with a personality disorder are more inflexible and are underpinned by low self-esteem. The person's responses to stressors are maladaptive and include self-centredness and lack of empathy for others. The characteristics of people with a personality disorder involve extreme and persistent problems across emotional, interpersonal, behavioural and cognitive domains, as well as difficulties with sense of self (Bateman 2012; Feigenbaum 2010).

The questions for anyone involved with a person displaying extreme, persistent behaviours that ultimately work against their own interests relate to determining which behaviours are problematic for the person and others and what can be done. The challenge for nurses, and indeed for anyone involved with such an individual, lies in determining appropriate behaviour, given that norms relating to behaviour are socially and culturally constructed. When is the expression of someone's personality to be considered disordered? Case Study 17.1 about Jodie can help us to consider these questions.

Jodie's ongoing belief in John's inevitable realisation of their future together and her inability to draw on more functional and appropriate coping skills indicate that something is seriously amiss. She may be exhibiting the features of a personality disorder. In order to determine whether this is so, a psychosocial history and assessment would have to be carried out to

CASE STUDY 17.1

Jodie

Jodie is 28 years old and has never moved out of her parental home. She is particularly attached to her mother. Jodie works as an administrative assistant for a small law firm where she is considered to be very good at her job. She has been reliable and highly productive. For a number of years Jodie has had a romantic fixation on John, the senior partner in the firm. Despite John's ongoing lack of romantic interest in her, the considerable age difference between them and the fact that they have no interests in common, Jodie believes that he does really love her. She knows she is in love with him and that they are meant to be together. She talks at length about him to her work mates. At times Jodie becomes very tearful and upset when speaking about John, and Laura, the office manager, has sent her home for a day of sick leave. Jodie cannot understand why John does not see how perfect they are for each other and she blames him for her inability to work on these occasions.

The situation reached a crisis point at the firm's Christmas party. Everyone from the office was treated to a dinner cruise with food, wine and music. Initially, Jodie appeared to be having a great time, laughing, flirting and expending a lot of energy on trying to get John to dance with her. After a while, however, Laura noticed that Jodie was missing and she found her sitting alone, crying and sobbing, 'Why won't he come to his senses? How can he do this to me?' Jodie was clutching some tablets and told Laura that she had already swallowed a handful and she refused to say what they were. The boat had to return prematurely and an ambulance was called. The guests felt uncomfortable and fell silent. Some were angry, while others were confused. In Jodie's opinion, it was John's fault that the cruise party was ruined.

enable clinicians to ascertain Jodie's behavioural patterns over time because one suicide attempt does not necessarily mean that the person has a diagnosable personality disorder.

CLASSIFICATION OF PERSONALITY DISORDERS

While each of the personality disorders described in the DSM-5 (APA 2013) has particular characteristics, they also have certain features in common. Personality disorders are recognised by enduring patterns of behaviour that are often damaging to the individual and others and are nearly always characterised by maladaptive and inflexible ways of coping with stress (such as Jodie's response to John's disinterest in her). People with a personality disorder often have an intense impact on those around them (some of Jodie's work mates may condemn her actions and others such as Laura may feel very sorry for her).

Section 2 of the DSM-5 groups personality disorders into three clusters: A, B and C. Cluster A is composed of the disorders of an odd or eccentric nature; cluster B includes dramatic, erratic and emotional disorders; and cluster C comprises the anxious and fearful group (APA, 2013). Table 17.1 summarises the disorders covered by each cluster along with the diagnostic criteria used in clinical settings. However, assessment and diagnosis of personality disorders are challenging because a person who exhibits symptoms of one type of personality disorder invariably also exhibits symptoms of other disorders. In an effort to address the difficulty of categorically defining people's problems as one personality disorder or another, the DSM-5 has introduced new information contained in Section 3 that seeks to guide research that may improve the clarity and evidence base for personality disorders. The simplified suggested classifications reduce the number of personality disorder types to seven (see Table 17.2).

TABLE 17.1 Criteria for Classification of the Personality Disorders

Cluster A (Odd or Eccentric)	Criteria
Paranoid personality disorder	The person: • has expectations of being harmed or exploited without sufficient reason • is preoccupied with unjustified doubts • is unwilling to confide in others • perceives hidden, demeaning or threatening messages in innocent remarks or comments by others • tends to bear grudges • perceives attacks upon their character or reputation that are not apparent to others • suspects their spouse or partner of infidelity
Schizoid personality disorder	The person: • neither enjoys nor desires close relationships • prefers solitary activities • has little interest in sexual activity • is indifferent to either praise or criticism • shows emotional frigidity
Schizotypal personality disorder	The person: • exhibits evidence that they are experiencing ideas of reference • expresses odd beliefs and thinking in their speech and is odd in their appearance • shows evidence of some paranoid ideation • has social anxiety • lacks a social network/friends
Cluster B (Dramatic, Erratic and Emotional)	**Criteria**
Antisocial personality disorder	The person: • is at least 18 years old • may have expressed a conduct disorder before 15 years of age • exhibits a disregard for the law • exhibits reckless, aggressive, deceitful and impulsive behaviour • does not show remorse • is unable to sustain employment/study
Borderline personality disorder	The person: • is terrified of abandonment and actively attempts to avoid it • experiences intense and unstable moods • forms intense and unstable relationships • experiences disturbances of identity • engages in impulsive self-destructive behaviours • exhibits recurrent suicidal behaviour • experiences chronic feelings of emptiness and transient paranoia

Continued

TABLE 17.1 Criteria for Classification of the Personality Disorders—cont'd	
Cluster A (Odd or Eccentric)	**Criteria**
Histrionic personality disorder	The person: • craves being the centre of attention and engages in self-dramatisation and/or uses physical appearance to attain this • displays inappropriately sexually seductive behaviour • uses speech to impress others but is lacking in depth • is prone to exaggeration and dramatic expression of emotion • tends to exaggerate the degree of intimacy that they share with others • tends to be easily led by others
Narcissistic personality disorder	The person: • brims with self-importance and grandiosity • is preoccupied with fantasies of success, power, genius and/or beauty • has a profound belief that they are special and therefore exude a sense of entitlement (i.e. are deserving of special treatment and favours) • displays arrogance • needs to be admired • lacks empathy • tends to exploit others for their own benefit
Avoidant personality disorder	The person: • fears disapproval, rejection and ridicule and so avoids occupations and social situations where this may occur • avoids intimate relationships due to the same fears • is preoccupied with the fear of shame, rejection and ridicule • is embarrassed and/or anxious in social situations • feels inferior • is very reluctant to take risks
Dependent personality disorder	The person: • is unable to make decisions or initiate projects without considerable advice, reassurance and direction • has difficulty with expressing disapproval • experiences discomfort when alone and fears isolation • lacks confidence and will go to extraordinary lengths to obtain support from others • has an urgent need to establish a new relationship for support and care when an existing relationship ends
Obsessive-compulsive personality disorder	The person: • is preoccupied with details, rules, schedules and organisation; perfectionism interferes with the completion of tasks • is overly conscientiousness, inflexible, rigid and stubborn • tends to hoard possessions and is reluctant to spend • tends to prefer to work rather than socialise
Personality Disorder not Otherwise Specified	**Criteria**
	• The person displays features of more than one disorder, without meeting the full criteria in one or more areas of functioning.

(*Source*: Adapted from American Psychiatric Association (APA) 2013. Diagnostic and Statistical Manual of Mental Disorders, 5th ed. APA, Washington DC.)

TABLE 17.2 Classification Suggestions for Future Research of Personality Disorders	
Classification	**Criteria**
Schizotypal personality disorder	People who exhibit eccentric behaviour, distort communication with others and are uncomfortable in close relationships may exhibit chronic mistrust and negative interpretations of others' action.
Antisocial personality disorder	People who disregard and persistently violate the rights of others.
Borderline personality disorder	People who struggle with emotional regulation and impulsiveness.
Narcissistic personality disorder	People who chronically overestimate their own importance and lack empathy towards others.
Avoidant personality disorder	People who struggle socially due to persistent feelings of inadequacy, hypersensitivity towards the views of others.
Obsessive-compulsive personality disorder	People preoccupied with order and control.
Personality disorder trait specified	When a personality disorder is considered present, but the criteria for a specific personality disorder are not fully met.

(*Source*: Adapted from American Psychiatric Association (APA) 2013. Diagnostic and Statistical Manual of Mental Disorders, 5th ed. APA, Washington DC.)

Some of the criteria in Tables 17.1 and 17.2 overlap and there are many patients who could be diagnosed with more than one personality disorder. In the past, the most common clinically documented personality disorder diagnosis was that of the residual category, 'Not otherwise specified', which means that the clinician cannot decide between two or more possibilities (Horn etal. 2014). This may not reflect a limitation in the clinician's diagnostic ability, but rather a realistic acknowledgement that the styles of interaction with someone with a personality disorder can change noticeably under different circumstances.

PROBLEMS OF DIAGNOSIS

While the layperson might be excused for believing that diagnoses are clear-cut, the nurse should be aware that all psychiatric diagnoses lack clarity in some situations and overlap at times and debates about whether a given person has a specified disorder are often legitimate. Psychiatry is an inexact science and the optimal approach to treatment is not always clear even when a definitive personality disorder diagnosis can be made (Tyrer etal. 2015). As in previous editions, the DSM-5 (APA 2013) issues a cautionary statement to clinicians regarding the interpretation of its diagnostic categories; indeed, they are advised that specific diagnostic criteria serve only to inform professional judgement, not to override it. This is especially the case in personality disorder, where the diagnosis is often argued heatedly.

Historically, psychiatric diagnoses have often become pejorative labels, where those bearing the descriptors have been prejudged and stereotyped, especially by health professionals (Flaskerud 2012; Tyrer etal. 2015). At different times, hysteria and BPD have been used to evaluate people negatively. As a result, people have felt that they were treated negatively because of their diagnosis (Horsfall etal. 2010). The current diagnosis of BPD is tantamount to negative labelling because it is experienced as unhelpful and stigmatising. Nursing staff often hold negative feelings and perceptions about this patient group (Westwood & Baker 2010). It is therefore important that nurses work in partnership with patients in a person-centred, recovery-oriented way to avoid actively or passively assisting the patient to internalise stigma (Horsfall etal. 2010).

The current taxonomy of personality disorders, alongside the use of checklists and abstract diagnostic criteria, is generally considered inadequate because it leads to narrow, subjective assessments that ignore life events, the person's history and their social circumstances (Kim & Tyrer 2010; Tyrer etal. 2015). A series of articles published in the *Lancet* in 2015 relates to personality disorder, including classification and assessment (see www.thelancet.com/series/personality-disorder).

PATIENT STORY 17.1

Alice

Alice had recently been reviewed by a psychiatrist who diagnosed her with borderline personality disorder and referred her to the DBT programme coordinated by Sharon, a mental health nurse at a metropolitan community mental health centre. Alice is a 27-year-old single mother who lives with her 14-month-old son Sam at a friend's place. Alice reported separating from her partner Daryl 12 months before. Following separation there had been numerous problematic conflicts that had resulted in a restraining order being taken out by Daryl against Alice, with allegations of abusive behaviour. In spite of court orders to stay away from Daryl, Alice had recently abused Daryl at his home and this event had led the court to refer Alice to a psychiatrist for diagnoses and any suggested treatment.

Developmentally, Alice described growing up with both her parents but not being close to either of them. She stated that her parents would often attend Alcoholics Anonymous and if she had to nominate a parent that she would share more personal characteristics with, then this would be her mother. She recalled being disengaged from studies and being suspended once during primary school. Her parents separated when she was 12 years old and in secondary school she frequently rebelled against her mother, truanting, experimenting with cannabis and cutting her wrists for 'fun'.

She met her ex-partner Daryl 3 years ago and during the course of the relationship idealised him as a partner and father. She had been pregnant twice, miscarrying the first pregnancy, and she recalled developing depressive symptoms after that. She reported feeling intensely connected to her baby son Sam. Alice found it hard to provide descriptions about her emotional state but stated that since her separation, she had felt intense betrayal by Daryl. She described her previous relationship with Daryl 'like two sides of a 50 pence coin, at times he was gorgeous and all I could wish for and at other times he was just plain lazy'.

She described Daryl as a gentle person who 'wouldn't harm a fly' but stated that when they argued she would often fly into rages that culminated with her either hitting him or throwing a piece of household furniture such as her mobile phone. Following her rage episodes, she often found that apart from the damage to furniture she struggled to recollect what the incident had been about and also her thoughts and emotions during the argument. She also described times when she felt detached and numb to situations around her and generally struggled to provide a cohesive, explanatory narrative about her life.

Alice stated that in recent times she had frequently felt in a state of worry, mostly about day-to-day difficulties, being unsupported and about how other people regarded her. She described frequently feeling numb, experienced low energy and motivation and had started superficially cutting her wrists and upper arms to 'feel alive again'. She stated she hoped things would soon improve as she had been taking a daily antidepressant prescribed by her psychiatrist. There were no suicidal or homicidal thoughts and although there were difficulties with falling asleep because of thinking about the stress in her life, there were no symptoms suggestive of hypomania.

EPIDEMIOLOGY

Personality disorders are considered to be reasonably common. Huang etal. (2009) investigated the prevalence of DSM-IV personality disorder clusters in 13 countries (*n*= 21,162) using the International Personality Disorder Examination. They estimated the prevalence to be 6.1% for any personality disorder and 3.6%, 1.5% and 2.7% for clusters A, B and C, respectively. They found rates of personality disorders were higher among males (cluster C), people who were separated or divorced (cluster C), the unemployed (cluster C), the young (clusters A and B) and the poorly educated (clusters A, B and C) (Huang etal. 2009).

It has been estimated that more than half of patients with a history of attempted suicide and half of all psychiatric outpatients have a personality disorder (Ansell etal. 2015; Soloff & Chiappetta 2012). Kim and Tyrer (2010) report that 40% or more of community mental health patients have a coexisting personality disorder, while in tertiary psychiatric services and prisons prevalence rates are estimated to be between 70% and 90%. Many patients who require long-term, assertive treatment have a personality disorder alongside a substance abuse, anxiety, mood or psychotic disorder (Newton-Howes etal. 2010). When patients have a psychosis and a personality disorder, the latter might not be diagnosed, which may explain some of the engagement and treatment difficulties that contribute to poor outcomes (Newton-Howes etal. 2010).

In both men and women, the prevalence of personality disorders appears to decrease with age (Cooper etal. 2014; Debast etal. 2014; Samuels etal. 2002). As currently classified, evidence shows that personality disorder affects around 6% of the world population, with no consistent variation or differences between countries (Cloninger & Svrakic 2008; Tyrer etal. 2010). Other reviews of epidemiological studies in different populations achieved consistent estimates of personality disorders: the median prevalence rate for 'any personality disorder' was 10.65% and the mean rate was 11.39%, indicating that 1 in 10 people have a diagnosable personality disorder (Lenzenweger 2008). Lamont and Brunero (2009) reviewed studies of prevalence rates of personality disorder and found they ranged from 5% to 10% (1 in 10 in the United States and 1 in 20 in the UK).

The most common and most complex personality disorder encountered in the clinical setting is BPD. The prevalence of BPD in other countries among the general population is estimated at approximately 1% to 4% and prevalence rates of BPD among people who use psychiatric services is estimated at up to 23% for outpatients and up to 43% for inpatient populations (NHMRC 2012). Among adolescents, BPD rates have been estimated at around 1% to 14% (NHMRC 2012).

AETIOLOGY

The causes of personality disorder are not known and there is a range of theories. Research consistently reveals that people who have experienced childhood physical, emotional or sexual abuse or emotional neglect, as well as those raised in families characterised by withdrawal or violence, are much more likely to display behaviours consistent with a personality disorder diagnosis than those who have not been abused or neglected (NHMRC 2012). Contemporary aetiological explanations are predicated on a combination of biological, psychological and social risk factors, including heredity, life experiences and environmental factors that determine whether or not personality traits become rigid and show potential to undermine the self. Cloninger and Svrakic (2008, p. 471) suggest that it is reasonable to assume that the 'temperament and character components of personality disorder are all moderately heritable'. There is some tentative support for a genetic basis for BPD (Leichsenring etal. 2011), as well as support for the view that it results from a combination of adverse biological and environmental events/factors (NHMRC 2012). Recent research shows that about half of the symptoms of BPD (the most frequently studied personality disorder) are long-term and characterological in nature and the other half are acute and usually respond well to treatment (Crawford etal. 2011; Zanarini 2009; Zanarini etal. 2007).

ASSESSMENT

People are rarely admitted to inpatient mental health settings simply because of their personality disorder. Rather, they are admitted because of conditions coexisting with their disorder, such as anxiety, depression or substance misuse, or for assessment due to extreme behaviours, including self-harming or those with suicidal intent. Impulsive behaviours, self-harming and abuse of drugs and alcohol tend to bring people with personality disorders into contact with healthcare services. Very often their admissions are accompanied by a sense of drama/crisis, broken relationships and the consequences of struggling to cope with the stresses of life.

Research reveals that large numbers of people in general psychiatric samples have a coexisting personality disorder (see Friborg etal. 2013; Friborg etal. 2014). Individuals with a diagnosis from cluster A, odd and eccentric personality disorders, are the least likely to seek treatment. Those with cluster C, anxious and fearful disorders, require treatment more frequently. It is those with cluster B, dramatic and emotional personality disorders, who most frequently find themselves the recipients of care by mental health clinicians. When the characteristics of people who have these disorders are reviewed, it is easy to appreciate why this may be so. Reckless behaviour, impulsivity, sexual risk taking and self-harming and self-mutilating behaviour tend to bring them into contact with legal and/or healthcare services. Other behaviours that may draw attention include shoplifting and abuse of drugs and alcohol.

Skodol etal. (2011) note that although symptoms vary in severity, people with personality disorders commonly present as being devoid of concern for others and as extremely egocentric; they will also lie to explain or to excuse their own behaviour or to gain sympathy. Given that these people characteristically have no or little insight into their problems, they have a pronounced tendency to blame others for problems of their own making, which further impairs their already strained relationships with others. Since they also tend not to learn from their mistakes in their relationships and in other aspects of life, they often repeat these errors over and over. For example, people with BPD fear being abandoned, yet they continue to behave in ways that tend to drive others away. This, coupled with the fact that their tolerance for emotional pain is low, inevitably leads many to experience low self-esteem, which they may deal with by self-medicating with alcohol or other drugs or indulging in self-harming behaviour such as cutting or they may develop eating disorders or be sexually promiscuous.

These maladaptive behaviours are all examples of ways in which these patients may deal with the feelings they experience. The areas that need to be assessed include drug and alcohol use, self-harm or mutilation, suicidal ideation and/or attempts, instances of aggression or violence, unexplained visible injuries to the body, sexual activity and family and workplace relationships. An established pattern in one or more of the high-risk behaviours, such as illicit drug abuse or violence, may indicate that the patient has come to the attention of the police. Outstanding fines or impending legal proceedings further complicate the lives of people with a personality disorder.

One of the greatest difficulties for people with a personality disorder is attachment—satisfying emotional involvement with others—to people in general and health professionals in particular (Koekkoek etal. 2010). Hence, the central challenges for clinicians are engagement and building rapport (Crawford etal. 2009), which depend on establishing a therapeutic relationship with the patient by being open minded, self-aware, patient and persevering. This means that engagement, the therapeutic relationship and assessment are ongoing. Box 17.1 provides key assessment points for a patient with a personality disorder in crisis.

Initial assessment should exclude conditions such as hyperthyroidism, Cushing syndrome, mood or anxiety disorder, posttraumatic stress disorder, substance abuse or an organic disorder that may explain some symptoms. If an organic cause is suspected, further investigations may be ordered and, in some cases, testing blood alcohol levels and a drug screen may be indicated. Indeed, substance or alcohol abuse often coexists with personality disorders and with BPD in particular (Di Pierro etal. 2014; Whitbeck etal. 2015). Taking a drug (legal or illegal, prescribed or over the counter) or withdrawing from one is likely to change the person's mental status and behaviours. Aggression, agitation or changing mood states (lability) as a result of withdrawal may be misinterpreted as signs of personality disorder; side effects of steroid abuse may manifest similarly. The single most significant criterion for differentiating between medical conditions, substance abuse and side effects of prescription medication is a comparison of the patient's presenting behaviour with their usual ongoing behaviour. Personality disorders are characterised by pervasive long-term patterns of behaviour, whereas other conditions usually involve abrupt inconsistent behavioural changes.

BOX 17.1 Crisis Assessment of a Patient With a Personality Disorder

- Determine the current level of risk/violence to self or others.
- Discuss the current treatment plan and strategies being used as part of that plan.
- Find out what strategies and supports they have used to deal with previous crises.
- Ask about drug and alcohol use.
- Help the patient to manage their anxiety and distress by focussing on the current problem.
- Encourage them to work with staff to identify short-term changes that they can make.

This risk assessment is only part of a broader assessment.

(*Source*: Adapted from National Collaborating Centre for Mental Health (NCCMH) 2009. Borderline personality disorder: treatment and management. National Clinical Practice Guideline Number 78. The British Psychological Society and The Royal College of Psychiatrists, Leicester.)

The nurse needs to be aware of all these potentialities when assessing and caring for individuals with a personality disorder. Assessment is a continuous process that often requires lengthy interviews, drawing on high-level communication and listening skills, and keen observation. It needs to be holistic, taking into account the patient's present relationships as well as childhood experiences and traumatic events. Even then, the findings may be considered provisional, at least until further corroborating material is gathered. (See Chapter 22 for further discussion of assessment.)

Furthermore, given the multicultural nature of contemporary society, it is very important for the nurse to be sensitive to cultural differences. A behaviour that seems incongruent to a nurse of Anglo-Celtic origin may in fact be the norm for the cultural background of the patient. For example, in some cultures interactions between women and men, the young and the elderly, are governed by certain conventions that serve to maintain respect and mirror the power differentials in relationships. Their behaviours, such as eye contact, physical proximity and taking turns during interactions, may be different from what you are accustomed to and your behaviours may seem odd to them.

CRITICAL THINKING CHALLENGE 17.1

Think about the community you live and work in and identify some examples of cultural diversity. Can you incorporate this knowledge usefully into your own nursing practice?

INTERVENTIONS: WORKING WITH PEOPLE WITH A PERSONALITY DISORDER

Service providers report patients with BPD to be moderately or very difficult to work with effectively (Cleary etal. 2002; Westwood & Baker 2010), but increasing evidence is emerging for the effectiveness of a range of treatment modalities that will make it easier to work with patients (NHMRC 2012; Stoffers etal. 2012). Change is likely to be slow and piecemeal and nurses need personal resilience and staying power, as well as highly developed interpersonal communication skills, to work productively with people with a personality disorder. Developing a therapeutic relationship underpins all of the treatment approaches. Trust is fundamental, conveying hope and optimism and being respectful during all interactions. To develop an optimistic and trusting relationship it is important to work with people in 'an open, engaging and non-judgmental manner, and [to] be consistent and reliable' (National Collaborating Centre for Mental Health [NCCMH] 2009, p. 99). The needs and preferences of the person should also be taken into account so that people with a personality disorder have the opportunity to make choices about their care and treatment in an informed manner (NCCMH 2009).

Research by McGrath and Dowling (2012) on psychiatric nurses' responses towards patients with a diagnosis of BPD revealed the following four themes:

- challenging and difficult
- manipulative, destructive and threatening behaviour
- preying on the vulnerable, resulting in splitting staff and other service users
- boundaries and structure

The theme of 'challenging and difficult' related to the symptoms that people with BPD display, along with the perception that they seldom take responsibility for their behaviours. Staff were often pessimistic about patients' prognosis and therefore felt helpless and hopeless. The theme of 'manipulative, destructive and threatening behaviour' referred to the perception that people with BPD often have hidden motivations and commonly use violent or self-harming behaviour to elicit responses from others, including nurses. 'Preying on the vulnerable, resulting in splitting staff and other service users' referred to patients with BPD who were perceived to have manipulated relationships between staff and/or other patients. The final theme of 'boundaries and structure' described nurses' need for strong boundaries when working with people with BPD. Overall, it was common for nurses to struggle with feelings of anger, frustration and fear while delivering care to people with BPD (McGrath & Dowling 2012).

Thus, there is a need for clearer principles to guide practice as well as further training and education (e.g. motivational techniques, trauma, supervision) to improve the skills of professionals (Fanaian etal. 2013; McGrath & Dowling 2012). To work effectively with people with a personality disorder, clinicians need to consider the following 'preventable errors', which they can potentially change in themselves:

- loss of professional objectivity and perspective, often characterised by strong emotions (positive or negative) termed countertransference (see Chapter 24)
- perpetuating the myth that a person with a personality disorder cannot recover, which is stigmatising and can create a self-fulfilling prophecy
- giving direct advice on personal and social problems, which can create dependence, noncompliance or resentment (Cloninger & Svrakic 2008, p. 477; Lawn & McMahon 2015)

Self-Harm

Self-harm is one behaviour that is especially difficult for nurses to countenance, to cope with and to work with. People with various personality disorders may exhibit these behaviours, but one of the main reasons that BPD has become a negative and stigmatising label is that self-harm is more prevalent among people with this diagnosis. Self-harming behaviours include, but are not limited to, cutting the skin of the wrist, head banging, deep scratching with or without an implement and self-burning with cigarettes. These self-harming behaviours are also a significant risk factor for suicide (Crawford etal. 2009).

Self-harming behaviours are confronting and distressing and undoubtedly contribute to negative attitudes towards patients with BPD and feed into stigmatisation (Commons Treloar 2009; Fanaian etal. 2013; Koekkoek etal. 2010; Purves & Sands 2009). Understanding the reasons for self-harm may help nurses and other mental health clinicians to face their own human reactions of disbelief, horror, fear or shock and to interact with patients in more humane, professional and therapeutic ways. In other words, increased understanding of both the patient and the self are required to work effectively with this group of patients.

Patients' reasons for self-harming include:

- regaining some self-control
- providing emotional relief
- relieving tension build-up
- alleviating feelings of emptiness
- escaping flashbacks and returning to reality
- expressing forbidden anger against self and/or others
- releasing self-hatred arising from experiencing violence
- decreasing alienation from others (Booth etal. 2014; Turner etal. 2012)

Research shows that self-harm is a strategy used by some patients to attempt to deal with overwhelming emotional distress and pain (Feigenbaum 2010; Holm etal. 2009; Holm & Severinsson 2008; Holm & Severinsson 2011). As Feigenbaum (2010, p. 115) succinctly states, from a patient's perspective self-harm is 'the solution not the problem'. Needless to say, many clinicians continue to see self-harm as the problem, not a part of the solution, and with good treatment as a temporary or interim solution. The reality is that expecting patients to give up self-harming actions can precipitate intense panic and anxiety, as they are effectively being asked to give up a tried and true way of managing rage, shame and alienation from self and others that works for them (Holm & Severinsson 2008).

Research suggests that patients with a diagnosis of BPD have higher rates of childhood sexual and physical abuse than other clinical populations (Commons Treloar 2009; Leichsenring etal. 2011). Holm and Severinsson (2008) reiterate the fact that even though rates are difficult to pin down, 40% to 80% of people with BPD have experienced repeated emotional, sexual or physical trauma and/or emotional neglect in their childhood. According to Leichsenring etal. (2011) approximately 39% of people with BPD have a comorbid diagnosis of posttraumatic stress disorder.

BOX 17.2 Principles for Working With People With a Personality Disorder

- Explore treatment options with a hopeful, optimistic recovery orientation.
- Bear in mind that many will have experienced abuse, rejection and/or stigma.
- Ensure that the patient is actively involved in solving problems and making choices.
- Involve the patient in setting limits and determining consequences.

Remember that patients often live with a high level of risk and clinicians need to avoid 'assuming' all responsibility for risk.

(*Source*: Adapted from National Collaborating Centre for Mental Health (NCCMH) 2009. Borderline personality disorder: treatment and management. National Clinical Practice Guideline Number 78. The British Psychological Society and The Royal College of Psychiatrists, Leicester.)

Experiencing childhood sexual assault and beatings, witnessing violence against their mother, suffering torture, teenage rape and relentless ridicule and living with addicted parents whose interests and focus are frequently elsewhere are all examples of a recipe for indelible trauma. These ongoing abuses can result in boundary confusion, fear, impulsivity, shame, self-hatred, powerlessness, guilt, an incoherent sense of self, emotional chaos and other out-of-control feelings (Koekkoek etal. 2010; Vermetten & Spiegel 2014). Acknowledging and empathising with the effect that trauma may have had in the lives of people with personality disorders is therefore essential. There are national practice recommendations for the provision of trauma-informed care for mental health services and these principles include: promoting safety; role-modelling interpersonal relationships that heal; understanding culture; advocating for patient control, choice and autonomy; understanding trauma and its impact; sharing power; inspiring hope and supporting recovery; integrating care; and sharing power and governance (see Bateman etal. 2013; Cleary & Hungerford 2015). Principles for treating a patient with a personality disorder are listed in Box 17.2.

Crisis Intervention

Crisis intervention and stabilisation are the first priorities in responding to acute distress in people with BPD (NHMRC 2012). Dealing with the presenting problem that has precipitated the admission or emergency home visit (if possible) is a good beginning, as this may fix something practical and/or calm the person sufficiently to be able to engage adequately with them. Nurses need to involve the person with a personality disorder in all decision making so that decisions are based on an explicit, joint understanding and the person is encouraged to consider the various treatment options and consequences of the choices they make (NCCMH 2009). Goal-setting and problem solving should start as soon as the person is calm enough to communicate and to negotiate with.

Limit-Setting

As these patients have underdeveloped self-control in a range of social, emotional and behavioural domains, clear limit-setting is also among the first priorities, as patients need to know exactly which behaviours are acceptable in the therapeutic relationship, which are not and what the consequences of rule breaking are. Limit-setting provides a degree of externally reinforced control over the behaviours patients have difficulty controlling. There must be consensus among team members as to how behaviours are to be managed. Clear and frequent communication among team members will assist in this regard. Firm, fair and consistent limit-setting enacted with a non-judgemental attitude should be continually strived for.

Limit-setting aims to offer patients a degree of control over their behaviour. Whenever limit-setting is employed, the patient should know in advance the behaviours expected, as well as the consequences for breaches. As far as is practicable, the person should be involved in setting these limits and determining the consequences. When limit-setting is carried out consistently by a team that communicates well, patient behaviours of seduction, dependency, rejection, agenda setting, collusion and staff splitting may be avoided (Fanaian etal. 2013). In a hospital setting, the use of time-out (where the patient is offered monitored time in a quiet, private, low-stimulus environment until the urge to self-harm passes) has been found to be a useful tool in practice, as it encourages the patient to attempt to deal with maladaptive behaviours in a more positive and acceptable way.

Self-Management

It is clear from this discussion that nurses and other members of the healthcare team face a range of personal, interpersonal and professional challenges that are not easy to address constructively for either themselves or patients. Some of the personal–professional tensions to be acknowledged, reflected upon and managed carefully are:

- flexibility and adaptability to individual needs as regards control and safety
- emotional connection as regards functional professional objectivity
- calmness in the face of anxiety-creating patient behaviours
- believing patients' stories versus disbelief that such things can happen
- developing trust in a situation of fear

A trusting and optimistic relationship is the cornerstone for working effectively with patients with a personality disorder. This is why education and clinical supervision are essential (Lawn & McMahon 2015; NCCMH, 2009). Interestingly, Zanarini (2009) says that any interactive treatment modality can be effective, provided it is done by a reasonable person with a thoughtful, insightful and caring approach, which means that learning a specific technique is not the key, but understanding the patient and ourselves is.

Interactive Therapies

Given that many patients with a personality disorder are prone to treatment nonadherence (for a range of reasons), the challenges for both patient and clinician are obvious. In a systematic review of 25 studies of treatment for people with a personality disorder, the noncompletion rate was 37% and a range of patient and environment factors were associated with this (McMurran etal. 2010). Thus, active engagement of patients is crucial. Crawford etal. (2009) studied engagement and retention in 10 specialist services for people with a personality disorder (1186 referrals) and found that although most patients became involved, men and younger people were less likely to complete the package of care.

NURSE'S STORY 17.1

Sharon's Story

Sharon, the mental health nurse leading the dialectical behaviour therapy (DBT) programme at the community health centre, felt an immediate empathy for Alice because she was a single mother herself. Sharon engaged Alice in regular one-to-one therapy and psychotherapy using a DBT approach and provided oversight for group sessions run by a psychologist at the centre. Sharon also monitored Alice's continuation on the antidepressant medication that had been prescribed by the referring psychiatrist.

Early in therapy Sharon encouraged Alice to make a commitment to avoid further visits to Daryl's home to facilitate her grieving and allow adaptation to her role as a single mother. Alice agreed to this commitment and immediately warmed to Sharon's empathetic approach, telling her that she was, 'The best counsellor I've ever met . . . way better than the psychiatrist who is only interested in what pills I am taking'. While Sharon appreciated Alice's enthusiasm, she was aware of the way that people with personality disorders can exhibit dependent traits and so made a mental note to reflect on and discuss Alice's case during her monthly clinical supervision session.

Despite Alice's enthusiasm and assurances, within a couple of months she began returning to Daryl's home abusing him in moments of stress. This led to further police involvement and culminated in a court order for Social Services to become involved in the custody of Alice's son. Sharon found the weeks when Alice behaved this way extremely difficult because she couldn't stop thinking about the relationship problems and custody battles she had experienced with her previous partner. Sharon often found herself drinking extra wine and struggling to sleep after workdays that involved such sessions with Alice.

Overall, therapy proved to be such slow progress that Sharon often felt as if they were taking a step back for every two steps forwards. However, after 2 years of support, Alice slowly developed more mature and adaptive emotional regulatory skills by virtue of the demands of being a single mother, a role to which she remained committed. She slowly became more aware of her tendency to idealise others and her fears of rejection. She continued to battle with urges to act impulsively when she became angry but got involved in a women's gymnasium that appeared to be providing a healthier outlet for her feelings. As she observed incremental improvements in Alice, Sharon also found reflecting on Alice's case self-enlightening as she continued to learn more about her psychotherapeutic capacity through clinical supervision.

Cognitive behavioural therapy (CBT) uses aspects of both cognitive therapy (which targets unhelpful beliefs) and behavioural therapy (which aims to change non-constructive or damaging behaviours). CBT aims to help people to develop more effective coping mechanisms by equipping them with strategies that promote realistic ways of thinking about and responding to everyday situations (Matusiewicz etal. 2010). Research generally supports the conclusion that CBT is an effective treatment modality for people with a range of personality disorders (Matusiewicz etal. 2010).

Dialectical behaviour therapy (DBT) is similar to CBT and research shows that it is useful for people with BPD (Koekkoek etal. 2010). DBT actively incorporates social skills training. The focus of this therapy is: (1) the attenuation of parasuicidal and life-threatening behaviours; (2) the attenuation of behaviours that hinder therapy; and (3) the attenuation of behaviours that frustrate the patient's ability to improve their quality of life. Essentially, this therapy, developed by Linehan (1998, 2000), conceptualises people with personality disorders as having significant problems regulating their emotions and behaving in accordance with social norms, often as a result of unsupportive, socially chaotic or traumatic life histories (Harned etal. 2012). DBT involves an intensive, highly structured approach to treatment including both individual and group sessions that focus on strengths identification and overcoming negative coping habits. Therapy teaches new skills and facilitates practice of replacement behaviours in a range of social contexts. Common components of a DBT program include:

- individual therapy focussed on strengths identification, reflecting on recent challenges and using the therapist–patient relationship as a template for practising new coping skills
- group therapy and teaching sessions focussed on four core themes of interpersonal effectiveness, distress tolerance, emotion regulation and mindfulness
- role playing: behaviour rehearsals practised in either individual or group therapy sessions
- homework, often involving practising social skills in real-life contexts
- telephone therapy: unlike many other approaches, telephone contact between therapist and patient is encouraged in between individual sessions (Booth etal. 2014; O'Connell & Dowling 2014).

DBT has a growing body of evidence, including randomised controlled trials and systematic literature reviews, that suggest it can be useful for a range of personality disorders (McMain etal. 2014; O'Connell & Dowling 2014; Pasieczny & Connor 2011).

Mentalisation is a psychodynamic approach that incorporates cognitive techniques and aims to teach patients to strengthen their capacity to recognise, understand and name emotional states in themselves in order to address their difficulties with affect, interpersonal functioning and impulse control (Bateman & Fonagy 2009). Bateman and Fonagy (2008) evaluated mentalisation-based treatment and partial hospitalisation for people with BPD in comparison with general psychiatric outpatient care 8 years after participation in a randomised controlled trial and 5 years after treatment completion. The treatment comprised individual and group psychotherapy within an integrated and structured programme specifically for people with BPD. Patients who had 18 months of mentalisation-based treatment remained better than those receiving treatment-as-usual (Bateman & Fonagy 2008).

A different psychoanalytically oriented package, day hospital therapy, has been shown to decrease hospital admissions and increase social skills and adjustment (Binks etal. 2006). Koekkoek etal. (2010) developed a pilot programme for people with BPD based on preventive admissions. By guaranteeing admission beforehand, the patients had a greater sense of safety and control and significantly decreased crisis admissions.

Another psychodynamically based outpatient programme, using schema-focussed therapy ('integrative cognitive therapy'), was set up in four community mental health centres in the Netherlands (Giesen-Bloo etal. 2006). It relied on the development of a therapeutic relationship and targetted daily life challenges and managing childhood trauma. Changes were achieved via a repertoire of cognitive, behavioural and experiential processes (Giesen-Bloo etal. 2006). Although there are too few data to be overconfident, these results indicate that the complex problems of people with BPD are amenable to more than the one-treatment modality.

Therapeutic Community

An approach sometimes used in correctional and substance rehabilitation programmes is the 'therapeutic community' approach (see also Chapter 5). Samuel etal. (2011) describe a therapeutic community as a setting where a conscious effort is made to ensure that the potential of all patients and staff is used to create a social environment that is conducive to personal development. Such an approach aims to minimise hierarchical power relationships so that there is equality between patients and staff in relation to decisions concerning treatment and the running of the community. At present, there are few facilities with the staff and the necessary commitment to the philosophy of a therapeutic community. However, the main aspects of such approaches that are beneficial for people with a personality disorder are an ethos of mutual respect, group negotiations of rules, support for all (staff and patients), open constructive communication and an inclusive atmosphere of interpersonal consistency, reliability and safety.

Team Nursing Approaches

Reflecting on the challenges of caring for a person with personality disorder McNee and colleagues (2014) recommend a team-based nursing approach. Adopting a coordinated approach to care tailored to specific individual patient needs, with clearly delineated roles for nursing staff, can enable more effective care. Tredget (2001) describes an example of this as 'triumvirate nursing'. Triumvirate nursing refers to nurses working in teams of three, each with equal responsibility for the provision of care to the patients assigned to them. Two nurses conduct sessions with the patient, while the third nurse functions as an 'outsider' and facilitates debriefing after each intense or detailed interaction. Tredget describes this role as the clinical coordinator role, as this nurse aims to analyse and to explore constructively issues that have arisen for either the nurses or the patient during the therapy sessions. This provides a professional forum for dealing with emotional concerns and support and facilitates reflective practice. The nurses' roles are interchangeable, so that no single nurse is always the clinical coordinator. For this system to work well, staff numbers and rostering are key issues. This intense approach (like the therapeutic community) aims to support nurses in their emotionally demanding work and ensure that the patient experiences a cohesive, consistent and hopeful treatment regimen.

Interventions for personality disorder and co-occurring mental illness should be integrated and wherever possible the same therapist/treatment team should provide treatment for both the personality disorder and the co-occurring mental illness (NHMRC 2012). If this is not possible, the therapist or service providing treatment for the co-occurring condition should collaborate with the clinician responsible for managing the BPD (NHMRC 2012). Team-based approaches need to be supported by high-quality training and education that supports staff development in areas such as engagement skills, communication skills and the ability to use reflection, so that all team members are able to apply a similar understanding and skill set and provide therapeutic care (Bowen & Mason 2012).

Pharmacological Interventions

Reviewers of treatments conclude that there is limited evidence to justify the use of medication for people with a personality disorder (Duggan etal. 2008; NHMRC 2012; Paris 2008). However, doctors do use some psychotropic medications to ameliorate symptoms and enable some patients to undertake the therapies described above. Particular symptoms targeted include mood dysregulation (selective serotonin reuptake inhibitors), impulsivity (mood stabilisers, anticonvulsants, carbamazepine), limited sociability (atypical neuroleptics) and cognitive distortions (atypical neuroleptics) (NHMRC 2012; Paris 2008). Chapter 25 provides more information about these medications.

EDUCATION OF HEALTH PROFESSIONALS FOR ATTITUDINAL CHANGE

Commons Treloar (2009) developed an education programme aimed to change clinicians' attitudes towards people who self-harm. This short, lecture-based programme targets health professionals who have contact with patients with BPD. Commons Treloar (2009) used case studies of three groups of clinicians to explain the theory and practice. These three groups consisted of: (1) a control group, without extra informational input; (2) a group educated about the DBT approach to treatment; and (3) a group involved in a psychoanalytic explanation of self-harm mechanisms. Both the DBT and the psychoanalytic content produced significant attitudinal improvements in participants; however, only the psychoanalytic group maintained their positive changes 6 months after the programme. Why would this be?

A cognitive behavioural approach or theoretical commonsense conceptualisation of self-harming actions 'implies a level of consciousness by patients in their use of self-harm to relieve distress and cope with an aroused affective state' (Commons Treloar 2009). In other words, clinicians benefit from an understanding of unconscious mechanisms because they explain more fully what is happening inside the patient and that their actions are not deliberately destructive but have a rhyme and reason that stands outside objective seeing-is-believing or commonsense perceptions. Such theoretical reasoning, particularly with clinical examples as with Commons Treloar's programme, is more likely to encourage clinicians' compassion, rather than frustration and patient blaming (Koekkoek etal. 2010).

CRITICAL THINKING CHALLENGE 17.2

Has reading this chapter changed your attitude towards people who self-harm? If so, how? If not, why not?

CONCLUSION

People diagnosed with personality disorder present major challenges for mental health service providers. Nurses and others need training, education and staff support to deal with the challenges posed by this patient group. Some of the new treatments emerging show evidence of efficacy and in the not-too-distant future it is reasonable to hope that personality disorder will be better defined, identified and appropriately managed without stigma (Kim & Tyrer 2010). There is also a need to develop best-practice programmes that can be integrated into clinical practice by nonspecialised health professionals (Koekkoek etal. 2010). In fact, Gunderson (2009) advocates developing centres of excellence for personality disorders to support new generations of clinicians and researchers, as has been previously developed for treating patients with other psychiatric disorders. Studies need to be developed around structured and systematic strategies to provide empirical evidence upon which to base practice.

EXERCISES FOR CLASS ENGAGEMENT

1. Reread Case Study 17.1 on Jodie and discuss the following questions with your group.
   - Which possible diagnoses would you consider for Jodie?
   - What other information would be needed to make a diagnosis?
   - Which potential problems might a patient like Jodie present for nursing staff in terms of her treatment?

2. When you arrive for your evening shift you receive a handover for a new patient. The patient is a 21-year-old female who has been admitted as an inpatient via the emergency department following an apparent suicide attempt. Her name is Kylie. Both her forearms are bandaged and you are told that Kylie has self-inflicted significant, though not life-threatening, wounds. It seems that her self-harming was a response to the break-up of her relationship with her partner. The relationship was only 6 weeks old. You talk to Kylie and find that despite your misgivings due to her self-harming, you easily establish rapport with her. You are about the same age and it turns out that she was in your younger brother's class at school. You feel buoyed by the experience, especially given the negative comments the other staff made about her at handover. When you return from your tea break, you find Kylie in tears. She says, 'Thank God you're back! You're the only one who has any time for me. That other old bag won't even let me have my things and she won't let me go to the shop! Can you make sure that you're always assigned to be my nurse?'

   As a group, discuss the following questions.
   - What should you do?
   - How should you respond to the patient? State exactly the words you would use when speaking to the patient.
   - Are the issues different for you depending on your own gender?
   - Would you approach the staff member involved?
   - How would you describe the behaviour exhibited here?
   - Which DSM-5 cluster is the patient's behaviour indicative of?
   - Suggest ways in which this patient could be effectively treated:
     - as an inpatient
     - as an outpatient

3. Your brother has been seeing a new girlfriend for several weeks. One night, over the family dinner table, he says that he is finally going to 'meet the parents'. He's not too worried; he hasn't had any problems with his friends' parents before and he's actually curious because his girlfriend has not really told him much about them other than that her mother is a nurse who works part time in a medical centre and her father works for the government.

   Two nights later you get the report. He says, 'Her oldies are weird.' He goes on to describe the following: each time after the telephone is used, the mother cleans it with antibacterial spray; there was a whiteboard on the kitchen wall that was ruled into columns detailing a variety of schedules and rosters; the father, who only came out of his home office to eat and then returned to his office, berated the mother for smearing the gravy on the side of his dinner plate; the dog wasn't allowed inside; and they all had to say grace before eating. He says he has never seen anything like it. He asks for your opinion.

   Discuss the following questions as a group.
   - What does this story tell you about the girlfriend's family?
   - What does it tell you about your brother?
   - How might you explain his response to some of the things he observed?
   - Do you agree with your brother's assessment of the family?
   - What is the difference between a personality trait or traits and a personality disorder?

REFERENCES

American Psychiatric Association (APA), 2013. Diagnostic and Statistical Manual of Mental Disorders, fifth ed. APA, Washington DC.

Ansell, E.B., Wright, A.G., Markowitz, J.C., Sanislow, C.A., Hopwood, C.J., Zanarini, M.C., Yen, S., Pinto, A., McGlashan, T.H., Grilo, C.M., 2015. Personality disorder risk factors for suicide attempts over 10 years of follow-up. Personality Disorders: Theory, Research, and Treatment 6 (2), 161.

Bateman, A., Fonagy, P., 2008. 8-year follow-up of patients treated for borderline personality disorder: mentalization-based treatment versus treatment as usual. American Journal of Psychiatry 165 (5), 631–638.

Bateman, A., Fonagy, P., 2009. Randomized controlled trial of outpatient mentalization-based treatment versus structured clinical management for borderline personality disorder. The American Journal of Psychiatry 166 (12), 1355–1364.

Bateman, A.W., 2012. Treating borderline personality disorder in clinical practice. American Journal of Psychiatry 169 (6), 560–563.

Bateman, J., Henderson, C., Kezelman, C., 2013. Trauma-Informed Care and Practice: Towards a Cultural Shift in Policy Reform Across Mental Health and Human Services in Australia. A National Strategic Direction, Position Paper and Recommendations of the National Trauma-Informed Care and Practice Advisory Working Group. Mental Health Coordinating Council, Sydney.

Binks, C., Fenton, M., McCarthy, L., Lee, T., Adams, C.E., Duggan, C., 2006. Psychological therapies for people with borderline personality disorder. Cochrane Database of Systemic Reviews 1. CD005652.

Booth, R., Keogh, K., Doyle, J., Owens, T., 2014. Living through distress: a skills training group for reducing deliberate self-harm. Behavioural and Cognitive Psychotherapy 42 (2), 156–165.

Bowen, M., Mason, T., 2012. Forensic and non-forensic psychiatric nursing skills and competencies for psychopathic and personality disordered patients. Journal of Clinical Nursing 21 (23–24), 3556–3564.

Cleary, M., Hungerford, C., 2015. Trauma-informed care and the research literature: how can mental health nurses take the lead to support women who have survived sexual assault? Issues in Mental Health Nursing 36, 370–378.

Cleary, M., Siegfried, N., Walter, G., 2002. Experience, knowledge and attitudes of mental health staff regarding clients with a borderline personality disorder. International Journal of Mental Health Nursing 11 (3), 186–191.

Cloninger, R., Svrakic, D., 2008. Personality disorders. In: Fatemi, S., Clayton, P. (Eds.), The Medical Basis of Psychiatry. Humana Press, Totowa, NJ, pp. 471–483.

Commons Treloar, A.J., 2009. Effectiveness of education programs in changing clinicians' attitudes toward treating borderline personality disorder. Psychiatric Services 60 (8), 1128–1131.

Cooper, L.D., Balsis, S., Oltmanns, T.F., 2014. Aging: empirical contribution. A longitudinal analysis of personality disorder dimensions and personality traits in a community sample of older adults: perspectives from selves and informants. Journal of Personality Disorders 28 (1), 151.

Crawford, M., Price, K., Gordon, F., Josson, M., Taylor, B., Bateman, A., Fonagy, P., Tyrer, P., Moran, P., 2009. Engagement and retention in specialist services for people with personality disorder. Acta Psychiatrica Scandinavica 119 (4), 304–311.

Crawford, M.J., Koldobsky, N., Mulder, R., Tyrer, P., 2011. Classifying personality disorder according to severity. Journal of Personality Disorders 25 (3), 321–330.

Debast, I., van Alphen, S.P., Rossi, G., Tummers, J.H., Bolwerk, N., Derksen, J.J., Rosowsky, E., 2014. Personality traits and personality disorders in late middle and old age: do they remain stable? A literature review. Clinical Gerontologist 37 (3), 253–271.

Di Pierro, R., Preti, E., Vurro, N., Madeddu, F., 2014. Dimensions of personality structure among patients with substance use disorders and co-occurring personality disorders: a comparison with psychiatric outpatients and healthy controls. Comprehensive Psychiatry 55 (6), 1398–1404.

Duggan, C., Huband, N., Smailagic, N., Ferriter, M., Adams, C., 2008. The use of pharmacological treatments for people with personality disorder: a systematic review of randomized controlled trials. Personality and Mental Health 2 (3), 119–170.

Fanaian, M., Lewis, K.L., Grenyer, B.F., 2013. Improving services for people with personality disorders: views of experienced clinicians. International Journal of Mental Health Nursing 22 (5), 465–471.

Feigenbaum, J., 2010. Self-harm—the solution not the problem: the dialectical behaviour therapy model. Psychoanalytic Psychotherapy 24 (2), 115–134.

Flaskerud, J.H., 2012. DSM-5: implications for mental health nursing education. Issues in Mental Health Nursing 33 (9), 568–576.

Friborg, O., Martinussen, M., Kaiser, S., Øvergård, K.T., Rosenvinge, J.H., 2013. Comorbidity of personality disorders in anxiety disorders: a meta-analysis of 30 years of research. Journal of Affective Disorders 145 (2), 143–155.

Friborg, O., Martinsen, E.W., Martinussen, M., Kaiser, S., Øvergård, K.T., Rosenvinge, J.H., 2014. Comorbidity of personality disorders in mood disorders: a meta-analytic review of 122 studies from 1988 to 2010. Journal of Affective Disorders 152, 1–11.

Giesen-Bloo, J., Van Dyck, R., Spinhoven, P., Van Tilburg, W., Dirksen, C., Van Asselt, T., Kremers, I., Nadort, M., Arntz, A., 2006. Outpatient psychotherapy for borderline personality disorder: randomized trial of schema-focused therapy vs transference-focused psychotherapy. Archives of General Psychiatry 63 (6), 649–658.

Gunderson, J.G., 2009. Borderline personality disorder: ontogeny of a diagnosis. American Journal of Psychiatry 166 (5), 530–539.

Harned, M.S., Korslund, K.E., Foa, E.B., Linehan, M.M., 2012. Treating PTSD in suicidal and self-injuring women with borderline personality disorder: development and preliminary evaluation of a dialectical behavior therapy prolonged exposure protocol. Behaviour Research and Therapy 50 (6), 381–386.

Holm, A.L., Berg, A., Severinsson, E., 2009. Longing for reconciliation: a challenge for women with borderline personality disorder. Issues in Mental Health Nursing 30 (9), 560–568.

Holm, A.L., Severinsson, E., 2008. The emotional pain and distress of borderline personality disorder: a review of the literature. International Journal of Mental Health Nursing 17 (1), 27–35.

Holm, A.L., Severinsson, E., 2011. Struggling to recover by changing suicidal behaviour: narratives from women with borderline personality disorder. International Journal of Mental Health Nursing 20 (3), 165–173.

Horn, E.K., Bartak, A., Meerman, A.M., Rossum, B.V., Ziegler, U.M., Thunnissen, M., Soons, M., Andrea, H., Hamers, E.F., Emmelkamp, P.M., 2014. Effectiveness of psychotherapy in personality disorders not otherwise specified: a comparison of different treatment modalities. Clinical Psychology & Psychotherapy 22, 426–442.

Horsfall, J., Cleary, M., Hunt, G.E., 2010. Stigma in mental health: clients and professionals. Issues in Mental Health Nursing 31 (7), 450–455.

Huang, Y., Kotov, R., De Girolamo, G., etal., 2009. DSM-IV personality disorders in the WHO World Mental Health Surveys. British Journal of Psychiatry 195 (1), 46–53.

Kern, M.L., Della Porta, S.S., Friedman, H.S., 2014. Lifelong pathways to longevity: personality, relationships, flourishing, and health. Journal of Personality 82 (6), 472–484.

Kim, Y.-R., Tyrer, P., 2010. Controversies surrounding classification of personality disorder. Psychiatry Investigation 7 (1), 1–8.

Koekkoek, B., Van Der Snoek, R., Oosterwijk, K., Van Meijel, B., 2010. Preventive psychiatric admission for patients with borderline personality disorder: a pilot study. Perspectives in Psychiatric Care 46 (2), 127–134.

Lamont, S., Brunero, S., 2009. Personality disorder prevalence and treatment outcomes: a literature review. Issues in Mental Health Nursing 30 (10), 631–637.

Lawn, S., McMahon, J., 2015. Experiences of care by Australians with a diagnosis of borderline personality disorder. Journal of Psychiatric and Mental Health Nursing 22 (7), 510–521.

Leichsenring, F., Leibing, E., Kruse, J., New, A.S., Leweke, F., 2011. Borderline personality disorder. The Lancet 377 (9759), 74–84.

Lenzenweger, M.F., 2008. Epidemiology of personality disorders. Psychiatric Clinics of North America 31 (3), 395–403.

Linehan, M.M., 2000. Commentary on innovations in dialectical behavior therapy. Cognitive and Behavioral Practice 7 (4), 478–481.

Linehan, M.M., 1998. An illustration of dialectical behavior therapy. Session: Psychotherapy in Practice 4 (2), 21–44.

Matusiewicz, A.K., Hopwood, C.J., Banducci, A.N., Lejuez, C., 2010. The effectiveness of cognitive behavioral therapy for personality disorders. Psychiatric Clinics of North America 33 (3), 657–685.

McGrath, B., Dowling, M., 2012. Exploring registered psychiatric nurses' responses towards service users with a diagnosis of borderline personality disorder. Nursing Research and Practice 601918. https://doi.org/10.1155/2012/601918.

McMain, S.F., Guimond, T., Streiner, D.L., Cardish, R.J., Links, P.S., 2014. Dialectical behavior therapy compared with general psychiatric management for borderline personality disorder: clinical outcomes and functioning over a 2-year follow-up. American Journal of Psychiatry 169 (6), 650–661.

McMurran, M., Huband, N., Overton, E., 2010. Non-completion of personality disorder treatments: a systematic review of correlates, consequences, and interventions. Clinical Psychology Review 30 (3), 277–287.

McNee, L., Donoghue, C., Coppola, A.-M., 2014. A team approach to borderline personality disorder: Linda McNee and colleagues describe how helping one patient to overcome difficulties led to the development of a staff training package to improve outcomes. Mental Health Practice 17 (10), 33–35.

National Collaborating Centre for Mental Health (NCCMH), 2009. Borderline Personality Disorder: Treatment and Management. National Clinical Practice Guideline Number 78. The British Psychological Society and The Royal College of Psychiatrists, Leicester.

National Health and Medical Research Council (NHMRC), 2012. Clinical Practice Guideline for the Management of Borderline Personality Disorder. National Health and Medical Research Council, Melbourne.

Newton-Howes, G., Tyrer, P., Anagnostakis, K., Cooper, S., Bowden-Jones, O., Weaver, T., 2010. The prevalence of personality disorder, its comorbidity with mental state disorders, and its clinical significance in community mental health teams. Social Psychiatry and Psychiatric Epidemiology 45 (4), 453–460.

O'Connell, B., Dowling, M., 2014. Dialectical behaviour therapy (DBT) in the treatment of borderline personality disorder. Journal of Psychiatric and Mental Health Nursing 21 (6), 518–525.

Paris, J., 2008. Clinical trials of treatment for personality disorders. Psychiatric Clinics of North America 31 (3), 517–526.

Pasieczny, N., Connor, J., 2011. The effectiveness of dialectical behaviour therapy in routine public mental health settings: an Australian controlled trial. Behaviour Research and Therapy 49 (1), 4–10.

Purves, D., Sands, N., 2009. Crisis and triage clinicians' attitudes toward working with people with personality disorder. Perspectives in Psychiatric Care 45 (3), 208–215.

Samuel, D.B., LaPaglia, D.M., Maccarelli, L.M., Moore, B.A., Ball, S.A., 2011. Personality disorders and retention in a therapeutic community for substance dependence. The American Journal on Addictions 20 (6), 555–562.

Samuels, J., Eaton, W.W., Bienvenu, O.J., Brown, C.H., Costa, P.T., Nestadt, G., 2002. Prevalence and correlates of personality disorders in a community sample. The British Journal of Psychiatry 180 (6), 536–542.

Skodol, A.E., Bender, D.S., Oldham, J.M., Clark, L.A., Morey, L.C., Verheul, R., Krueger, R.F., Siever, L.J., 2011. Proposed changes in personality and personality disorder assessment and diagnosis for DSM-5 part II: clinical application. Personality Disorders: Theory, Research, and Treatment 2 (1), 23–40.

Soloff, P.H., Chiappetta, L., 2012. Subtyping borderline personality disorder by suicidal behavior. Journal of Personality Disorders 26 (3), 468.

Stoffers, J.M., Völlm, B.A., Rücker, G., Timmer, A., Huband, N., Lieb, K., 2012. Psychological therapies for people with borderline personality disorder. Cochrane Database of Systemic Reviews 8 (2).

Tredget, J., 2001. The aetiology, presentation and treatment of personality disorders. Journal of Psychiatric and Mental Health Nursing 8 (4), 347–356.

Turner, B.J., Chapman, A.L., Layden, B.K., 2012. Intrapersonal and interpersonal functions of non-suicidal self-injury: associations with emotional and social functioning. Suicide and Life-Threatening Behavior 42 (1), 36–55.

Tyrer, P., Mulder, R., Crawford, M., etal., 2010. Personality disorder: a new global perspective. World Psychiatry 9 (1), 56–60.

Tyrer, P., Reed, G.M., Crawford, M.J., 2015. Classification, assessment, prevalence, and effect of personality disorder. The Lancet 385 (9969), 717–726.

Vermetten, E., Spiegel, D., 2014. Trauma and dissociation: implications for borderline personality disorder. Current Psychiatry Reports 16 (2), 1–10.

Westwood, L., Baker, J., 2010. Attitudes and perceptions of mental health nurses towards borderline personality disorder clients in acute mental health settings: a review of the literature. Journal of Psychiatric and Mental Health Nursing 17 (7), 657–662.

Whitbeck, L.B., Armenta, B.E., Welch-Lazoritz, M.L., 2015. Borderline personality disorder and axis I psychiatric and substance use disorders among women experiencing homelessness in three US cities. Social Psychiatry and Psychiatric Epidemiology 50 (8), 1285–1291.

Zanarini, M.C., 2009. Psychotherapy of borderline personality disorder. Acta Psychiatrica Scandinavica 120 (5), 373–377.

Zanarini, M.C., Frankenburg, F.R., Reich, D.B., Silk, K.R., Hudson, J.I., McSweeney, L.B., 2007. The subsyndromal phenomenology of borderline personality disorder: a 10-year follow-up study. American Journal of Psychiatry 164 (6), 929–935.

USEFUL WEBSITES

National Institute for Health and Care Excellence, Personality Disorders Overview, http://pathways.nice.org.uk/pathways/personality-disorders

National Institute for Health and Care Excellence, Borderline Personality Disorder: Treatment and Management, www.nice.org.uk/guidance/cg78

National Institute of Mental Health, Borderline Personality Disorder, www.nimh.nih.gov/health/publications/borderline-personality-disorder/index.shtml

National Health and Medical Research Council, Clinical Practice Guideline for the Management of Borderline Personality Disorder, www.nhmrc.gov.au/guidelines-publications/mh25

Royal College of Psychiatrists, Personality Disorders, www.rcpsych.ac.uk/healthadvice/problemsdisorders/personalitydisorder.aspx

18

Anxiety, Trauma and Stress-Related Disorders

Anna Elders

KEY POINTS

- Anxiety is a necessary emotion that functions to protect us by eliciting a number of stress responses in the face of a stressor or threat.
- Anxiety can become problematic in itself, whereby symptoms of an anxiety disorder may develop with significant impact on functioning and quality of life.
- The majority of people presenting with anxiety disorders receive treatment within primary care settings; however, anxiety disorders have a high level of comorbidity with substance use, depressive disorders and suicidality.
- Up to 75% of people experience at least one traumatic event within their lifetime. Reactions to trauma vary from short-term anxiety, insomnia and mood changes to symptoms of posttraumatic stress disorder.
- Psychological interventions such as cognitive behavioural therapy and acceptance and commitment therapy have good evidence bases for treating symptoms of anxiety, trauma and stress-related disorders. Combined psychological and pharmacological treatment may be warranted in more severe and complex presentations.
- Nurses provide assessment, psychoeducation, socioeconomic support and psychological interventions for people with anxiety, trauma and stress-related disorders.
- A strong, collaborative therapeutic working relationship is the basis of nursing care for people with anxiety, trauma and stress-related disorders.

KEY TERMS

avoidance behaviours
chronic stress
cognitions
emotional dysregulation
fear
fear responses
hyperarousal
hypervigilance
hypothalamus–pituitary–adrenal (HPA) axis
intrusive anxious thoughts
posttraumatic stress disorder
psychoeducation
psychological interventions
psychopathology
rumination
screening
stepped care
stress response
stressor
trauma-informed care

LEARNING OUTCOMES

The material in this chapter will assist you to:

- understand anxiety from evolutionary, adaptive and functional perspectives.
- consider the aetiology of stress and anxiety and their mechanisms of action.
- be aware of the demarcation between anxiety as a normal stress response and anxiety disorders.
- be aware of the diagnostic symptoms and characteristics of specific anxiety disorders.
- understand the considerations in making an assessment of a person presenting with anxiety.
- gain knowledge of available nursing interventions and wider treatments for alleviating the distress and symptoms of anxiety disorders.

INTRODUCTION

In order to clinically define and to understand what an anxiety disorder is, it is first necessary to consider anxiety as it naturally occurs within the human experience: as an evolutionary, inbuilt survival trait that allows for the identification and development of necessary responses to potentially dangerous stimuli (Malan-Muller et al. 2013). Anxiety can be defined as a future-oriented mood state associated with cognitive, physiological and behavioural reactions designed to reduce the level of perceived danger within a stimulating situation (Craske et al. 2009). Commonly known as the fight/flight/freeze response, such stress-based reactions are essential in the face of the numerous dangerous situations human beings can experience over a lifetime.

TABLE 18.1 Key Features of Specific Anxiety, Trauma- and Stress-Related Disorders

Disorder	Key Features
Panic disorder (PD)	• Recurrent unexpected panic attacks, in the absence of triggers • Persistent concern about additional panic attacks and/or maladaptive change in behaviour related to the attacks
Agoraphobia	• Marked, unreasonable fear or anxiety about a situation • Active avoidance of feared situation due to thinking that escape might be difficult or help unavailable if panic-like symptoms occur
Specific phobia	• Marked, unreasonable fear or anxiety about a specific object or situation, which is actively avoided (e.g. flying, heights, animals, receiving an injection, seeing blood)
Social anxiety disorder (SAD)	• Marked, excessive or unrealistic fear or anxiety about social situations in which there is possible exposure to scrutiny by others • Active avoidance of feared situation
Generalised anxiety disorder (GAD)	• Excessive, difficult-to-control anxiety and worry (apprehensive expectation) about multiple events or activities (e.g. school/work difficulties) • Accompanied by symptoms such as restlessness/feeling on edge or muscle tension
Obsessive–compulsive disorder (OCD)	• Obsessions: recurrent and persistent thoughts, urges or images that are experienced as intrusive and unwanted and that cause marked anxiety or distress • Compulsions: repetitive behaviours (e.g. hand washing) or mental acts (e.g. counting) that the individual feels driven to perform to reduce the anxiety generated by the obsessions
Adjustment disorder (AD)	• Development of emotional or behavioural symptoms occurring within three months of the onset of a stressor (not including normal bereavement) • Distress is noted to be out of proportion to the severity or intensity of the stressor
Posttraumatic stress disorder (PTSD) and acute stress disorder (ASD)	• Exposure to actual or threatened death, serious injury or sexual violation • Intrusion symptoms (e.g. distressing memories or dreams, flashbacks, intense distress) and avoidance of stimuli associated with the event • Negative alterations in cognitions and mood (e.g. negative beliefs and emotions, detachment) as well as marked alterations in arousal and reactivity (e.g. irritable behaviour, hypervigilance)

(*Source*: Adapted from Katzman, M.A., Bleau, P., Blier, P., Chokka, P., Kjernisted, K., Van Ameringen, M., 2014. Canadian clinical practice guidelines for the management of anxiety, posttraumatic stress and obsessive-compulsive disorders. Released under Open Access, Creative Commons Attribution License.)

Anxiety can move from a response that ensures survival and protects functioning to one that creates ongoing levels of distress and impairment within a person's life. Considering anxiety and fear responses on a continuum and within a theoretical framework assists us to normalise anxiety and work alongside patients to make better assessments as to whether an anxiety disorder may be present.

This chapter examines the complex interactions that occur during an anxiety response before considering the pathological nature of anxiety as it presents in the form of common anxiety disorders. Different anxiety, trauma and stress-related disorders are explored in terms of the reinforcing elements of each and the most common symptoms and treatments. A concise overview of symptoms is provided in Table 18.1 later in the chapter. The chapter also explores some of the internal triggers and reinforcing elements of anxiety, such as how we attend to and appraise risk within our environment. These appraisals are partly shaped by past experiences and the developed memories and cognitions associated with significant events (Craske et al. 2009), as well as our genetic and environmentally shaped temperaments.

Trauma and childhood adversity are experiences that can create lasting impacts on survivors' neurobiological development and lifelong functioning, potentially leading to significantly increased risk of physical illness, social problems and mental health conditions such as anxiety disorders (Anda et al. 2010; Faravelli et al. 2012). Being able to view anxiety through a trauma-informed lens can help us to consider the origins and function of anxiety for individuals presenting to health services. This enables us to choose treatments and interventions that may be most acceptable and efficacious for each individual.

AETIOLOGY OF STRESS, FEAR AND ANXIETY

Stress, fear and anxiety are normal internal experiences that occur in response to a stressor. A stressor can be defined as any internal or external stimulus that promotes a stress response within a person. Historically, humans have been exposed to numerous life-threatening situations on a regular basis, from tribal warfare to naturally occurring environmental hazards such as famine. When we study the role that stress, fear and anxiety play in human evolution, we begin to see a system containing inbuilt mechanisms that allow for early recognition, physiological priming and behavioural adaptation in the face of danger. For the purposes of survival, the human brain developed the capability to learn and to store information to aid timely responses in the face of threats. Human behaviour is shaped by our stress response system and it is this system that is implicated in the development of anxiety disorders and most other mental health disorders.

The physiological response to stress is a complex myriad of feedback mechanisms involving nearly every system of the body. The initial processes of a stress response are contained within the hypothalamus, which is located in the central nervous system (CNS). Incoming sensory information is sent

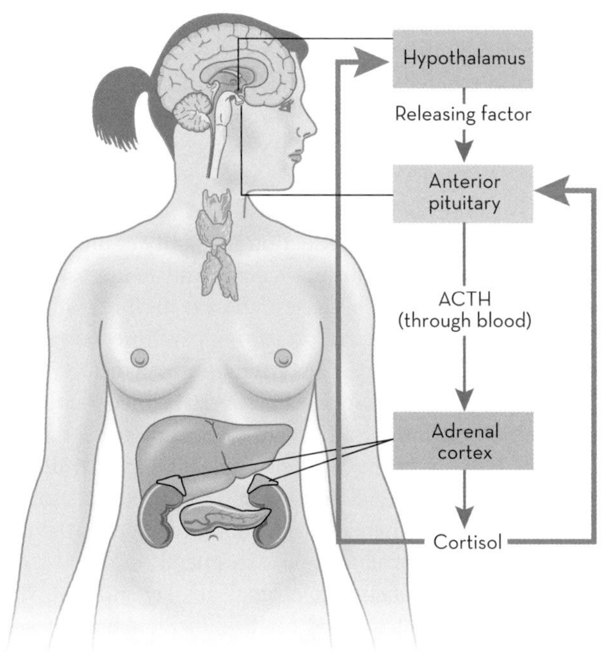

Fig. 18.1 The hypothalamic–pituitary–adrenal axis. *ACTH*, Adrenocorticotrophic hormone. (*Source*: Adapted from Simon, D.P., PhD. 2015 The science of stress and addiction: A mini-review of the research, Part 1. Available at: https://drsimonsaysscience.org/2015/03/22/the-science-of-stress-and-addiction-a-mini-review-of-the-research-part-1.)

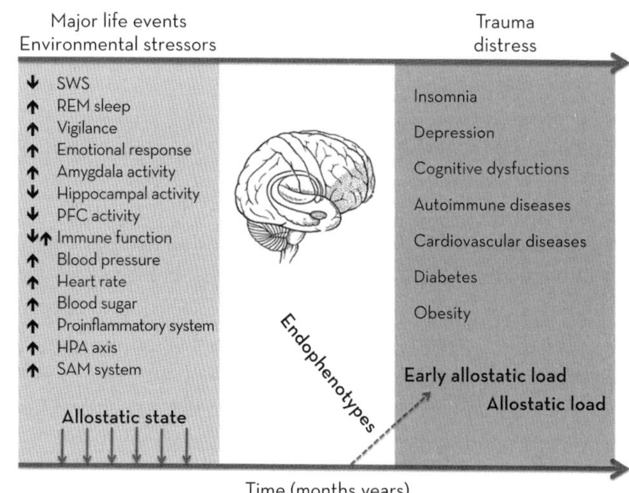

Fig. 18.2 The brain as core structure of the effect of allostatic state and allostatic load. Major life events and environmental stressors can create an allostatic state (imbalance) within pivotal centres of the brain such as the hypothalamus, the prefrontal cortex and the amygdala due to increased adaptive responses to stress (indicated in the left side grey column). If maintained over months or years, this can create an allostatic load (wear and tear), increasing susceptibility to insomnia, mental health disorders, cardiovascular disease, diabetes and so on. *HPA*, Hypothalamic–pituitary–adrenal; *PFC*, prefrontal cortex; *REM*, rapid eye movement; *SAM*, sympatho–adreno–medullary; *SWS*, slow wave sleep. (*Source*: Palagini, L., Baglioni, C., Ciapparelli, A., Gemignani, A., Riemann, D., 2013. REM sleep dysregulation in depression: state of the art. Sleep Medicine Reviews 17[5], 377–390.)

directly to the amygdala for a rapid preparatory response. At the same time, information is processed against stored memories in the hippocampus. This process allows us to ascertain the level of risk and prepare for further physiological and behavioural responses. The sympathetic nervous system (SNS) is activated, while the pituitary gland receives messages via neurotransmitters that signal the adrenal glands to release the stress hormone, cortisol. Cortisol exhibits a stimulating action on the body's systems such as the cardiovascular system, which constricts blood vessels to direct blood, glucose and energy reserves to the major muscle groups involved in the fight or flight response. Cortisol is thought to play an important role in supporting coping by reducing retrieval of emotionally arousing memories (Faravelli et al. 2012). This limits the risk of a person giving up due to feeling defeated and overwhelmed during stress. The system responsible for these responses is the hypothalamic–pituitary–adrenal axis, or HPA axis (see Fig. 18.1). The HPA axis plays other important roles such as being part of our immune response in the face of infection and assisting in the regulation of glucose levels during times of stress.

Exposure to high levels of stress, such as those experienced through childhood abuse, is associated with heightened stress responses (Leonard 2005; Faravelli et al. 2012), identifying early trauma as a significant contributor to the development of psychopathology.

Chronic stress, such as that experienced during an enduring, traumatic stressor like an abusive relationship, also leads to hypersecretion of cortisol and sustained SNS response (Leonard 2005). Sustained SNS activity and excessive systemic exposure to cortisol have been shown to result in the development of both physical illness and psychopathology because of the production of an ever-increasing and difficult-to-manage allostatic load (see Fig. 18.2) or the wear and tear on our stress systems, causing damaging effects on systems such as the CNS and cardiovascular system.

Differing responses to stressful life experiences can be understood as a combination of individual genetic (nature) and environmental (nurture) differences. Genetic vulnerability has been shown to contribute greatly to the presence of depression and anxiety symptoms in children up until the age of 7 years. However, environmental factors (positive or negative) are also known to be important predictors of the presence and stability of symptoms throughout adolescence and adulthood (Nivard et al. 2015).

Chronic stress can thereby be thought of as a direct contributor to the development of difficulty in mental health and general wellbeing. Stress is initially activated by real-life crises and adversity; however, it can continue years after the alleviation of these triggering events through the fear generalisation process. Fear generalisation is a process that supports survival through the ability to retain fear information and fear responses in the face of a similar future threat. In chronic stress, however, the limbic system becomes hypersensitive and more reactive, increasing and expanding the experience of risk and threat in a person's environment and thereby creating a generalisation of fear.

In the course of our lives, each of us develops belief systems and associated cognitive or thinking styles that help us to make sense of ourselves, others, the world and our future, helping to guide decision making and event processing. These cognitions develop as a result of both early and later life experiences gained from the environment in which we grow up, as well as our individual temperament and genetic personality characteristics. These cognitive styles play an important role in the development of reactive mood states, or affects, and are important factors in the generation of stress (Riskind et al. 2013). Hammen's (1991) stress generation effect refers to the contribution that our cognitive vulnerabilities (depressive thinking styles, hopelessness and rumination) make towards increasing the likelihood of experiencing negative events with catastrophic perceptions, thereby generating further stress and anxiety. A potentially vicious cycle then develops of anxious physiological reactions, anxious thinking, anxious feeling and anxious doing, all perpetuating each other and increasing the risk of developing pathological anxiety, emotional dysregulation and disorders such as depression. Genetic vulnerability, exposure to stressful events and patterned responses to those events explain how our usually functional and adaptive anxiety responses can become seriously debilitating when coupled with early experiences of stress and adversity and anxious temperamental traits, leading to the potential development of psychopathology.

? CRITICAL THINKING CHALLENGE 18.1

How do you currently deal with stress and anxiety? How do you feel about these particular internal experiences and how do you behave and think towards them when they come up? What things do you do that provide long-term support for yourself? Which approaches produce more obstacles or perhaps get you a bit stuck in a vicious cycle? How could you harness some of the more helpful responses you have had towards anxiety within your own practice when something happens that makes you feel anxious?

ANXIETY DISORDERS

Anxiety symptoms are commonly experienced as high levels of fear with thoughts of imminent danger and perception of risk, escape/avoidance behaviours and notable physiological arousal on presentation of an anxiety trigger. In a clinical sense, the term 'anxiety disorder' is applied following a diagnostic reasoning process in which symptoms of anxiety and related distress causing significant impairment in functioning and quality of life are recognised.

The majority of people experiencing anxiety disorders receive treatment within the primary care setting. Recognition of anxiety disorders in primary care, however, is known to be poor (Davis et al. 2008) and as such it is believed that only a small number of people receive treatment, most being offered pharmacological options (National Institute for Health and Care Excellence [NICE] 2014). Symptoms of anxiety disorders are frequently missed in people with commonly presenting major depressive symptoms, which have much higher rates of detection and gain a larger focus for treatment (NICE 2014). This presents a challenge for those living with pathological symptoms of anxiety as well as for healthcare systems because anxiety disorders are associated with high service usage as a result of the chronically disabling nature of the symptoms that can arise (Johnson & Coles 2013).

People with anxiety disorders often delay seeking treatment, a delay thought to be partly caused by avoidant behavioural coping styles. Johnson and Coles (2013) report that people with an anxiety disorder can show a significant delay in treatment seeking (9–20 years) compared with mood disorders (6–8 years) and substance use disorders (5–9 years). This delay can result in ongoing distress, impairment in functioning and considerable reduction in quality of life.

Anxiety disorders contribute significantly to the risk of self-harm and suicide, partly because of the way in which symptoms impair coping in the face of presenting psychosocial stressors (Hawton et al. 2013). Anxiety as an emotion can distort perceptions, leading to the person feeling overwhelmed, fearful and hopeless. Although there are no fail-safe treatments for anxiety disorders, there are many options available that provide hope and relief of symptoms. Screening and assessment for anxiety disorders and other mental health conditions should therefore be a necessary part of all nursing assessments.

The demarcation between 'normal' anxiety and that which may be considered 'disordered' can be difficult to make if we do not obtain all the information to make an informed assessment. Collaboration and a good therapeutic relationship and rapport are therefore imperative in assisting nurses to perform a sound assessment. The context or environment in which a patient is experiencing anxiety provides a basis on which to formulate possible precipitating and perpetuating factors, essential for consideration during assessment and treatment. Anxiety disorders can lead to misinterpretations of presenting triggers; for example, a person's catastrophic response to noticing a change in their heart rate may lead them to believe that they are going to die of a heart attack. On the other hand, symptoms of anxiety disorders can appear in response to dangerous external stimuli, such as generalised anxiety in relation to emotional or physical abuse from a violent partner.

Salkovskis (1996) provides a helpful illustration for understanding the role that perception of danger plays in the development and intensity of anxiety (see Fig. 18.3). Our interpretation of the world, others and ourselves, dictates our emotional, physiological, cognitive and behavioural responses. Many symptoms of anxiety disorders can be understood in terms of their functional significance for survival in relation to the level of threat perceived by the individual. Any potential threat is processed through an estimation of the likelihood that such an event will occur and if so, how catastrophic it would be for the person. Internal coping resources are considered alongside any external support/rescue that may be available. When

Anxiety is proportional to the perception of danger; that is

$$\frac{\text{perceived likelihood it will happen} \times \text{perceived 'awfulness' if it did}}{\text{perceived coping ability when it does} + \text{perceived rescue factors}}$$

Fig. 18.3 Anxiety and perceptions of danger. (*Source*: Salkovskis, P.M., [Ed.] 1996. Frontiers of Cognitive Therapy. Guilford Press, New York.)

the likelihood of catastrophic danger seems high without sufficient protection from self and others, we experience high levels of anxiety and fear, resulting in a cascade of survival-focussed responses until a sense of safety returns.

Salkovskis' model (1996) also provides a way of understanding our processes of threat assessment in terms of the impact of previous catastrophic experiences and developed cognitive styles. When we have lived through trauma, we use these experiences along with other life experiences to perceive and to respond to future situations. If our sense of self has been impacted so that we no longer feel capable of protecting ourselves and we do not trust others to come to our aid, we feel less in control and therefore more vulnerable. These factors are often at play in the experiences of those living with high levels of anxiety. They can wreak havoc on a person's functioning, reducing their behaviours to those that reduce the immediate risk and provide protection from perceived danger rather than those that will help them to engage in a meaningful valued life. These safety behaviours then reinforce anxiety as the person begins to act as if there is significant threat in the present and/or future, thereby continuing an internal physiological stress response and reinforcing the perceptions the person may currently be living with. It is these physiological, behavioural, emotional and cognitive experiences that form the basis for the diagnostic symptoms of anxiety and other mental health disorders (Schmidt 2012).

CRITICAL THINKING CHALLENGE 18.2

Many people experience mild symptoms of anxiety disorders throughout life because of the number of significant life stressors that come their way. What are the benefits of making a diagnosis of an anxiety disorder versus using a more normalising approach for mild presentations? When can a diagnosis be helpful and when might it not be?

EPIDEMIOLOGY OF ANXIETY DISORDERS

In a 2007 survey by the Office of National Statistics, a snapshot of anxiety disorders over a 1-week period in England showed 4.4% generalised anxiety disorder, 3.0% posttraumatic stress disorder (PTSD), 1.1% panic disorder and 1.1% obsessive compulsive disorder (NICE 2014). In 2013, it was reported that there were 8.2 million people diagnosed with anxiety in the UK (Fineberg et al. 2013). Females are almost twice as likely to be diagnosed with anxiety disorders as men, with anxiety disorders particularly common among young women aged 16 to 24 years (McManus et al. 2016). The Adult Psychiatric Morbidity Survey (2016), which reports on data gathered in 2014, suggests that 39% of adults (16–74 years) in England with conditions such as anxiety or depression were accessing mental health services, which is a 24% increase since the survey had last been conducted in 2007 (McManus et al. 2016).

COMORBIDITY

Comorbidity in anxiety disorders is so prevalent that it is often considered the rule, rather than the exception. Lifetime prevalence rates of comorbidity within anxiety disorders have been shown to be as high as 80%, with a strong correlation with depressive disorders (Katzman 2014); however, anxiety–anxiety comorbidity (presentation of more than one anxiety disorder) is very common (American Psychiatric Association [APA] 2013) and has been shown to be associated with earlier age of onset and greater chronicity of symptoms (Hofmeijer-Sevink et al. 2012).

It is important to consider the heightened anxiety seen with many mental health disorders. Given that anxiety is a common human experience, it is understandable that it is heightened in the face of any challenge to mental wellbeing, whether clinically diagnosable as an anxiety disorder or not. Studies have shown that people diagnosed with schizophrenia show clinically significant anxiety symptoms at rates between 16% and 85% (Hartley et al. 2013). Comorbid anxiety disorders have been shown to be related to positive symptoms of schizophrenia; for example, suspiciousness and paranoia appear correlated with social anxiety and panic (Hartley et al. 2013). Anxiety has also been shown to be related to an increase in the number of hospitalisations among people with schizophrenia (Cosoff & Hafner 1998). These findings support the need for therapeutic interventions for anxiety in those with a primary diagnosis of schizophrenia and other mental disorders.

Diagnoses such as social anxiety disorder, panic disorder and generalised anxiety disorder (GAD) may occur with substance abuse disorders (APA 2013), with substance use considered by some patients to be a potential way of self-medicating to manage anxiety symptoms. Anxiety disorders are also known to occur with other severe mental disorders such as bipolar disorder and have been commonly associated with personality disorders (APA 2013). Box 18.1 provides recommendations for increasing awareness of anxiety disorders.

BOX 18.1 Recommendations for Increased Awareness of Anxiety Disorders

- Become familiar with the main features of anxiety disorders, posttraumatic stress disorder and obsessive-compulsive disorder and with the main symptoms that distinguish between them.
- Develop systematic questions to ask about the nature, severity, duration, distress and associated impairment in patients with anxiety symptoms, to decide whether an anxiety disorder, posttraumatic disorder or obsessive-compulsive disorder is present.
- Become familiar with the fluctuating nature of symptoms in patients with anxiety disorders, and with the tendency for symptoms to change in nature over time.

(*Source*: Baldwin, D.S., et al. 2014. Evidence-based pharmacological treatment of anxiety disorders, post-traumatic stress disorder and obsessive-compulsive disorder: a revision of the 2005 guidelines from the British Association for Psychopharmacology. Journal of Psychopharmacology. 28,403– 439.)

ASSESSMENT AND DIAGNOSIS

The first step in undertaking any nursing assessment of the person with anxiety is to support the development of rapport and a therapeutic working relationship. (For further discussion of assessment, see Chapter 22) When people experience crises and difficulties with their mental health, engagement with services can initially heighten their anxiety because of uncertainty regarding outcomes, experience of self-stigma and feared judgement from others as well as exposure to fear-inducing stimuli through the initial assessment and treatment processes. Becoming adept with the skills of engagement and conveying a sense of unconditional positive regard supports patients to begin to have a sense of safety and trust. This in turn supports patients to begin to open up about their current and historical experiences. Gaining an understanding of these experiences helps build a picture of predisposing aspects and precipitating and perpetuating factors, as well as assisting in determining the presence of anxiety.

Trauma and childhood adversity are all too common in society today. For this reason, trauma screening should be incorporated into assessment of service users to ensure that any presenting trauma is considered and assessed regarding contribution to presenting symptoms. This is particularly pertinent for refugee communities who seek help because of the extremely high rates of trauma in these populations. Trauma screening does not assess exactly what happened to the person but gathers enough information to ascertain that trauma has occurred, which in itself can provide a context for better understanding about what people may be experiencing and why. When trauma is disclosed, assessment should focus on whether there is any present risk of harm to the person and screening should be conducted for symptoms of PTSD following on from the trauma (see later information on PTSD within this chapter).

In Nurse's Story 18.1 Karen Jones describes her use of assessment skills to develop an understanding of a patient's anxiety and to plan effective intervention.

Conducting a thorough nursing assessment includes reviewing relevant psychosocial information, enabling exploration of current fear-inducing stimuli such as financial threats, physical danger or significant losses (employment, relationships, health status, acculturative stress). This enables consideration of levels of anxiety and described cognitions and coping mechanisms from the point of view of actual threat versus perceived threat, to detect any distortions that may be present or anxiety that may be considered a normative response to abnormal stressors.

General screening questions have been recommended to ensure that health professionals provide patients with an opportunity to disclose any aspects of anxiety that are becoming problematic (see Box 18.2). Questioning relating to anxiety needs to be simple, time specific and inclusive of both an experience of heightened anxiety and a behavioural change such as avoidance.

Exploring the impact of anxiety symptoms on quality of life and functioning helps when considering whether a clinically significant level of anxiety is being experienced. Exploring triggers to anxiety (including significant historical triggers) assists in understanding precipitating factors and therefore the themes of fear that anxiety may centre on. Nurses need to be aware that a person may experience multiple triggers that may change or generalise over time, depending on the type of disorder the person is experiencing.

New migrants and refugees often experience major stress in adapting to a new country and culture and many may have suffered trauma prior to departure from their home country. Engaging with them may take longer because of language barriers and there may be misunderstandings about what services can and cannot provide if the person has little experience of the healthcare system. This is where nurses can utilise the benefits of integrated care with other social and healthcare service providers, as they uncover issues that may present obstacles to the treatment of anxiety, such as housing or physical illness.

Anxiety should be assessed in terms of experience and intensity in relation to a number of different settings and roles to explore whether a pervasive pattern exists or whether

NURSE'S STORY 18.1

Karen Jones

Karen Jones is a practice nurse working in a large general practice in a semi-rural area.

I recall working with a man in his 40s who was so anxious he wasn't sleeping or eating at all and couldn't sit still. He described walking around with earmuffs on his head to try to block noise, which he felt was worsening his anxiety. The man took 1 year off work and felt unable to drive or participate in his usual daily life, including caring for his two young children due to his hyperanxious state and lack of concentration. This took a real toll on his family, as his wife was required to take over running the household and his children did not understand what had happened but noticed their father had completely withdrawn into himself. Through thorough assessment and ongoing support from his GP, practice nurses and primary mental health services, it was established that certain changes occurring within his workplace were the cause of his anxiety. A combination of medication and cognitive behaviour therapy assisted him in identifying coping strategies, enabling him to recover and regain the ability to get back into his life. A variety of further resources were also accessed to support the patient and his family, including help from a social worker, financial support and guidance in accessing educational and self-help websites.

BOX 18.2 General Screening Questions

During the past 2 weeks how much have you been bothered by the following problems:

- Feeling nervous, anxious, frightened, worried or on edge?
- Feeling panicked or being frightened?
- Avoiding situations that make you anxious?

(*Source*: Reprinted with permission from the Diagnostic and Statistical Manual of Mental Disorders, Fifth Edition, (Copyright © 2013). American Psychiatric Association. All Rights Reserved.)

anxiety is experienced in reaction to a particular stress-inducing trigger (such as flying). Intensity of anxiety can be assessed reasonably easily via questioning and use of a rating scale, such as 'How anxious do you feel on a scale of 0 to 10, where 0 means no notable anxiety and 10 means disabling anxiety?' Questions assessing the presence of physiological arousal (e.g. tachycardia, sweating, hyperventilation) and behavioural responses (avoidance of triggers or other described behaviours to reduce anxiety and promote sense of safety) can also assist in determining whether anxiety could be considered problematic.

Assessment of other presenting issues or difficulties such as depressive mood states, alcohol and drug abuse, psychotic symptoms or mood lability helps ascertain the presence of possible comorbid disorders. Equally, anxiety should be assessed if one of these presents as the primary disorder because of the high levels of comorbidity with anxiety disorders. Assessment should include special consideration of the patient's health history, particularly conditions known to cause anxiety (e.g. Graves disease) and those that are negatively affected by anxiety (e.g. hypertension).

It is important to be aware of the different cultural presentations and beliefs about anxiety that people may present with. In some cultures, symptoms may present more somatically, such as physical symptoms experienced throughout the body (e.g. pain and other symptoms such as nightmares), or intrusive thoughts may be perceived as being caused by spiritual or supernatural experiences (Hinton 2012). It is important to gain the patient's perspective and attempt to understand the cultural context from which they come. This can assist in developing a shared understanding and approach to treatment that could incorporate interventions that support their beliefs and needs as well as those that may arise from a clinical viewpoint. Cultural advisors working within or outside clinical services can be extremely helpful in bridging the cultural–clinical gap and ensuring that care remains acceptable and culturally inclusive and safe for the patient. Finally, the prevalence of self-harm and suicidal ideation and behaviours in anxiety disorders has been previously discussed: it is imperative that nurses become comfortable asking about these issues in order to assess any risk of harm that may be present. In the following section symptoms of the different anxiety disorders are outlined. A summary of key features is provided in Table 18.1.

Assessment Tools

There are several assessment tools available for general use by nurses that can assist in screening for anxiety disorders. A few examples are given here, many of which are self-administered and available for free use and download via the internet. Most of the tools mentioned can be used within any health care setting and are sensitive for detecting mild to severe presentations, although in themselves they do not determine the diagnosis. Outcomes from such assessments need to be viewed together with historical and current information to ensure a thorough diagnostic reasoning process. Experienced nurses, particularly those in autonomous roles such as clinical nurse specialists and nurse practitioners, are able to diagnose anxiety disorders. Other nurses can provide essential support in gathering information that may help clarify any eventual diagnoses made.

GAD-7

The GAD-7 (Spitzer et al. 2006) is a seven-question self-report assessment tool designed to screen and to measure severity of any presenting symptoms of excessive worry and generalised anxiety. Scores of 5, 10 and 15 are considered cut-off points for mild, moderate and severe anxiety, respectively. Scores above 10 indicate that further assessment is required to enable exploration as to whether a diagnosis of GAD may be present.

Yale-Brown Obsessive-Compulsive Scale (Y-BOCS)

The Y-BOCS (Goodman et al. 1989) is a lengthy, comprehensive measure of the severity and type of symptoms of OCD. The assessment asks the patient to consider symptom occurrence in the week prior to assessment, providing an average occurrence and thus an indication of both symptom presence and severity. Questions also explore pertinent information such as time spent on symptoms, interference with day-to-day functioning, distress, level of control and resistance to symptoms. The Y-BOCS requires a reasonable degree of experience to administer, as it is carried out as a semi-structured interview with some clinical judgement required through questioning and observation and information collected from significant others.

Impact of event scale: revised (IES-R)

The IES-R (Weiss & Marmar 1996) is a 22-item, short self-report tool designed to measure symptoms following exposure to a trauma that may indicate the presence of PTSD. Questions aim to measure the presence of the major cluster of symptoms of PTSD: intrusive re-experiencing, hyperarousal and persistent avoidance (see information on PTSD within this chapter).

ANXIETY DISORDERS

Generalised Anxiety Disorder

GAD is a debilitating condition characterised by constant, excessive worry in which a person becomes consumed by everyday situations and issues. GAD is considered a persistent, chronic disorder accompanied by somatic complaints, restlessness, irritability, insomnia, fatigue and hyperarousal symptoms that arise because the person is in a constant state of alertness as a result of incessant worrying and anxiety (APA 2013). Those struggling with GAD have ongoing difficulties attempting to control their worrying and find that it disrupts their day-to-day functioning because of the intrusive nature of their thoughts.

In comparison with other anxiety disorders, GAD has been found to cause the most interference with life in general population studies, with almost half (48%) of responders in one study stating that it impacted considerably in at least four domains of their life (McEvoy et al. 2011). Despite this, GAD is often not well recognised in primary care because people may present with more complaints about their physical health and mood rather than anxiety symptoms, which can then be overlooked (Baldwin et al. 2014).

People with GAD may worry about numerous issues or events ranging from major issues such as their career, health and finances to minor issues such as completing housework or day-to-day life. Worry easily shifts from one concern to another. The major demarcation between experiencing normal worries of life and GAD centres on the generalised nature of the worry, disruption to functioning, the duration and the amount of distress caused and the physiological symptoms that often accompany the worry (APA 2013).

Lifetime prevalence of GAD is relatively common, with lifetime prevalence rates of 4% to 7% (Hoge et al. 2012). People who receive a diagnosis often report that they have always been a worrier and therefore part of the proposed vulnerability to GAD is having an anxious temperament (APA 2013). Interestingly, however, the mean age of onset is in later life, around 33 years of age (McEvoy et al. 2011; Wells 2006), indicating that vulnerability is long-lasting and has the potential to lead to a disorder after many years. Parental over-protection during childhood has also been identified as a risk factor and there are noted inherent genetic risks (APA 2013). These factors increase the prevalence of the comorbidity of GAD with other anxiety and depressive disorders that share similar predisposing risk factors. Major depressive disorder (MDD) commonly occurs alongside GAD (Baldwin et al. 2014), often producing a more chronic and debilitating range of symptoms. Drawing on data from a national epidemiological survey carried out in the United States, Blanco et al. (2014) explored the comorbidity of GAD with major depressive disorder and other psychiatric conditions. Comorbidity was found in 90.2% of study participants identified as having GAD, with 85.5% of these participants presenting with concurrent symptoms of MDD (Blanco et al. 2014). It is important to note that differences in expression of anxiety symptoms have been identified within certain cultures, with some people presenting with more somatic complaints while others experience more cognitive symptoms (APA 2013).

International and local guidelines for treatment of GAD indicate a stepped-care approach with education and active monitoring in the first instance; nonfacilitated self-help, guided self-help or psychoeducational group work as a second step; individual psychological intervention using cognitive behavioural therapy (CBT) or applied relaxation or pharmacological treatment such as a selective serotonin reuptake inhibitor (SSRI) as a third step; and a combination of both psychological and pharmacological intervention as a fourth step (NCCMH 2011). Patient Story 18.1 provides an account of how one patient developed strategies to help manage an anxiety disorder.

PATIENT STORY 18.1

Getting to Know my Anxiety

Anxiety is like a vicious cycle. Quite often I don't know when it is going to hit; however, I am beginning to know the warning signs: feeling more tense and on edge, getting irritable with my family, feeling something just isn't right and feeling more driven to have things 'just so'. I notice my thoughts race a lot faster and it is harder to enjoy things or be as present in the moment because I'm either thinking about something I have to do or worrying about something I've done and whether it was right or not.

My anxiety comes partly from my temperament (I've always been quite sensitive and worried as a kid), partly from my lifestyle (I don't always get a good balance between work and life) and from experiences in my childhood. I grew up with a parent who worried a lot. The older I get, the more I can see my parent's worries in the way that I see the world when anxiety descends.

The biggest aids for me in managing my anxiety better have certainly been knowledge about how it works and what goes on in my body and general ways in which to identify and look after how I am feeling. I know at these times I need what I think of as an internal hug. To acknowledge that I'm literally all worked up inside and I need to regulate myself. Quite often, stopping and paying attention to this gets me a considerably long way in feeling better. I don't try to fight it anymore. I don't even need to necessarily rationalise what is happening—I know myself well enough now to understand as soon as I notice it that there are processes at work that are almost never directly to do with the current situation I'm in. The next step for me is certainly about lifestyle changes. I protect my sleep (when I don't sleep I know I will struggle a lot more the next day), I try not to take too much on all at once and I look after my diet, trying to avoid foods that throw my energy levels all over the place. I try to acknowledge what I'm achieving and be compassionate when I'm struggling. I realise I'm always going to have to keep up this self-care and awareness. I can't change my temperament; however, I do find that as I get older and accept myself more that I'm not struggling with myself and with life's curveballs as much.

Obsessive-Compulsive Disorder

OCD involves a recurring experience of anxiety-creating intrusive cognitions (thoughts, impulses or images) that become obsessive in nature, risking dominating a person's internal world over time. Obsessive cognitions often involve themes of risk of harm to self or others, such as developing a life-threatening disease or harm coming to family members. These cognitions are experienced with significant accompanying physiological symptoms of anxiety, giving the person a real sense of danger (Wells 2006; APA 2013). In response to the obsessive cognitions and anxious bodily sensations, compulsive behaviours develop that serve the purpose of reducing the perception of harm and creating a sense of safety. Compulsive behaviours may be directly related to the obsessions, such as washing hands to prevent acquisition or transmission of disease, or totally unrelated, such as repeating phrases over and over again or tapping surfaces a particular number of times. However, the relief provided and the sense that the compulsive behaviours worked to stop the catastrophe occurring 'fuse' the compulsive behaviours to the obsessions. Thus, the more the obsessions are experienced, the more the compulsions are carried out. Unfortunately, anxiety regarding the risks posed within the obsessive content often recurs shortly afterwards as there is little resolution. Attempts to suppress the obsessions often lead to thought rebounding (recurrence of obsessional thoughts) and a cycle of further experience of obsessions and compulsions. It is the vicious nature of anxiety in OCD that often causes both an increase in symptoms and a deterioration in general day-to-day functioning, as the compulsions begin to take up larger amounts of time and the obsessive thinking is considerably disruptive to day-to-day cognitive processes.

OCD is the fourth most common mental disorder after depression, alcohol/substance misuse and social phobia, with lifetime prevalence in community surveys of 1.6%. The degree of OCD differs markedly from one person to another, with people often able to hide their OCD from family and friends. The World Health Organisation (WHO) ranks OCD as one of the most handicapping conditions by lost income and decreased quality of life (Veale & Roberts 2014). Another concerning finding is that people with OCD have higher rates of suicidal ideation, plans and suicide attempts (Wells 2006), indicating the need for timely, appropriate treatment and close monitoring for risk of harm to self.

Treatment for OCD involves a combination of medication and concurrent talking therapies because of the severity of symptoms. Exposure and response prevention, a specific type of CBT, appears to be the most successful talking therapy for OCD, with long-term improvement in symptoms reported in 75% of individuals engaging in therapy (Neziroglu & Mancusi 2014). Pharmacotherapy options include SSRIs at higher doses than prescribed for depression as a first-line treatment because of the relatively low side effects (Seibell et al. 2015).

Panic Disorder

Panic disorder (PD) is characterised by unpredictable experiences of intense, episodic surges of anxiety that occur in the form of what is described as a panic attack. During such attacks, the person experiences intense physiological anxiety symptoms such as tachycardia, sweating, shaking, dyspnoea, chest pain, dizziness, nausea, tingling and a sense of depersonalisation. Panic attacks can occur outside of PD in relation to other presentations of anxiety; however, it is the frequency of these attacks, the nonselective triggering environments in which they occur and the perpetuating, anticipatory anxiety that occurs as part of the disorder that sets apart the diagnosis of PD from other presentations that may include the experience of panic attacks.

Panic attacks reach a peak of severity within approximately 10 minutes and can last up to 45 minutes (Baldwin et al. 2014). Because of the surge of physiological symptoms, a hallmark of PD relates to the catastrophic, intrusive cognitions that arise during the event, which often include a sense of imminent death ('I'm going to have a heart attack and die') or mental health deterioration ('I'm going to lose my mind'). There may also be a fear of losing consciousness and sustaining a terrible trauma as a result ('I'll pass out and something really bad will happen to me when I'm unconscious'). As a result

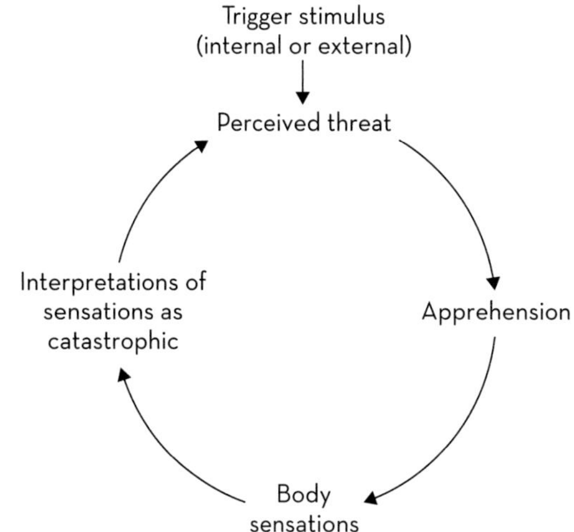

Fig. 18.4 Clark's cognitive model of panic disorder. (*Source*: Clark, D.M., 1986. A cognitive approach to panic. Behaviour Research and Therapy 24, 461–470.)

of these cognitions, during the attack people engage in rapid safety behaviours aimed primarily at seeking help, escaping the attack and avoiding anxiety symptoms in order to reduce the inherent risks they perceive. Such safety behaviours include phoning for an ambulance or presenting to medical emergency services, sitting down, body scanning for further symptoms and deterioration and taking one's pulse.

As the panic attack begins to abate (either naturally or as a response to one of the safety behaviours), the person obtains a false impression that (a) they were on the brink of a catastrophic event and (b) their safety behaviours prevented the imminent catastrophe that was occurring during the attack. This signals a major misinterpretation of anxiety symptoms, especially in those fearing death as an outcome, as anxiety is often considered secondary to the perceived problem (e.g. 'I'm going to have a panic attack and die') as opposed to the primary problem itself. As the perceived cause of the attack (heart problem, mental health illness) is sensed as imminent, there is great anticipatory anxiety regarding further panic attacks. This leads to the development of a number of preventive safety behaviours to avoid another attack or reduce any perceived risk should one occur. Such behaviours include dependency on others, body hypervigilance (body scanning for symptoms) and avoiding situations perceived as presenting a high risk of triggering an attack or that seem unsafe to be in should an attack occur.

In approximately two-thirds of PD cases, symptoms of agoraphobia develop (see later description), causing fear of public spaces and further exacerbating anxiety and avoidance behaviours (Baldwin et al. 2014). Ultimately, the more anxious and fearful a person becomes, the more vigilant they become in an attempt to prevent any future panic attacks. Unfortunately, this creates a vicious cycle of further panic attacks, anxiety and ever-increasing safety behaviours. Fig. 18.4 illustrates Clark's cognitive model of panic disorder. PD is one of the less common anxiety disorders with a prevalence rate of 1.1% in England (NICE 2014). PD has a high comorbidity rate with conditions such as depression

(Baldwin et al. 2014) and is strongly correlated with suicidal ideation, planning and completed suicide (Wells 2006). PD is linked to higher rates of help seeking (Wells 2006) because of both the accompanied fear of medical illness that can be linked to the disorder and the high rates of presentation to medical services during an attack.

Treatment for PD largely centres on the use of brief psychological interventions such as CBT. For those who struggle to access therapy, there is emerging evidence that computerised self-help can be an effective first-line alternative (Sawchuk & Veitengruber 2016). There has been conflicting evidence for use of pharmacological treatments for PD. SSRIs and benzodiazepines have shown only modest efficacy and tricyclic antidepressants, despite displaying comparable efficacy with CBT, often cause side effects that reduce adherence over longer periods of time (Royal Australian and New Zealand College of Psychiatrists [RANZCP] 2003).

Agoraphobia

Agoraphobia is characterised by generalised, consistent and significant unrealistic fear responses to exposure or anticipated exposure to public spaces such as shopping centres, crowded areas or open spaces. Common anxious cognitions associated with such exposure relate to fears that help may not be available or escape possible should the person begin to panic or experience considerable symptoms of distress. Avoidance is commonly used as a safety behaviour, thereby causing impairment in day-to-day functioning. Techniques such as distraction and dependency on others to go out are also used regularly in order to enter areas or situations that trigger anxiety.

Agoraphobia is highly comorbid with panic disorder and, up until the previous edition of the DSM, was included as a subtype of PD (PD with agoraphobia). Recent arguments have seen its separation as a distinct disorder based on findings that agoraphobia is not always preceded by panic attacks and produces significant functional limitations when experienced without symptoms of PD (Asmundson et al. 2014).

In the UK, up to 2 people in 100 have a PD, with it thought that approximately one-third will go on to develop agoraphobia. Agoraphobia is twice as common in women as in men and usually begins around 18 to 35 years (National Health Service [NHS] 2016). Despite its lower prevalence rate compared with other anxiety disorders, agoraphobia is highly correlated with suicidal ideation, plans and suicide attempts (Wells 2006), highlighting the significance of screening for suicide risk in those presenting with symptoms of agoraphobia.

Social Anxiety Disorder

Social anxiety disorder (SAD) is poorly recognised in primary medical care (Baldwin et al. 2014) and may be misconstrued as shyness and introversion (Sawchuk et al. 2015). However, SAD is linked to high levels of socially induced distress and impairment in day-to-day functioning. People with SAD often have pronounced, persistent and objectively unreasonable fears of either specific or more generalised social situations, particularly where there may be performance expectations, such as within a classroom or at a party. People with SAD often fear embarrassment, humiliation and negative judgement by others. These fears may develop as a result of past or current emotional abuse, whereby the abuse becomes internalised with a resulting development of negative, inflexible beliefs about self. In social situations, people begin to fear that others will 'discover' how useless, unworthy or ugly they believe they are, which often results in the development of safety behaviours such as social avoidance in order to reduce the risk of perceived potential judgement and rejection.

It is common for people with SAD to have considerable fear of losing control of their bowels or bladder, vomiting, blushing or shaking in social situations, all of which contribute to further anxiety about social humiliation and negative evaluations by others. Unfortunately, it is the intense focus on the self through the eyes of others and over-monitoring of the self in social experiences that appear to reinforce and perpetuate the condition. People with SAD often attempt to adapt to such cognitive intrusions by using significant avoidance strategies, such as not going to parties and avoiding social situations and social speaking. Alternatively, they may endure social or performance situations using developed safety behaviours such as conversation rehearsal, conversation redirection towards others or avoidance of interactions during attendance at such events.

By developing these safety behaviours, the person continually acts as if they are socially incompetent or at great risk of judgement and potential rejection from others. This creates further avoidance or in situ safety behaviours, bringing further focus on the self and thus anxiety that a major social faux pas is about to occur. SAD can thus have serious impacts on a person's family and romantic relationships, occupational opportunities and day-to-day functioning as it becomes both harder to make and to maintain relationships and present oneself for educational and career development opportunities.

SAD, or social phobia, affects 7% of the population and follows a chronic and debilitating course if untreated (Mayo-Wilson et al. 2014). SAD is strongly correlated with comorbid depression and drug and alcohol abuse and it is often these issues that are identified when someone presents to services for help, rather than symptoms of SAD itself (Baldwin et al. 2014). This may go some way in explaining the long delay in treatment mentioned earlier. Treatment for SAD depends on the severity of symptoms and whether comorbid conditions such as depression or another anxiety disorder are present (Sawchuk et al. 2015). A recent metaanalysis of treatment options produced a recommended optimal combination treatment, combining CBT with administration of either an SSRI or a selective noradrenaline reuptake inhibitor (SNRI) based on tolerability profiles and efficacy, with CBT showing greater enduring effect than pharmacotherapy (Canton et al. 2012). Patients with SAD without comorbidity should be offered either CBT or an SSRI/SNRI, depending on their informed preference (Sawchuk et al. 2015). Other medications such as benzodiazepines are not suggested because of the risk of developing dependence. Case Study 18.1 about Jessica describes the experience of social anxiety.

CASE STUDY 18.1

Jessica

Jessica is a 21-year-old woman with a diagnosis of dyslexia and marked anxiety in social situations. Jessica constantly fears the judgement of others and believes that when she speaks to others, they can 'hear her dyslexia' and will think she is stupid. Jessica regularly avoids social situations and, when she has to attend, has a number of safety behaviours to protect her from making a fool of herself, such as practising her replies to discussions in her head and deflecting attention by asking other people a lot of questions.

Jessica very much believes that her problem lies in her level of intellect and that her low perceived intelligence will mean that people won't want to know her when they discover this about her. Jessica is unsure how she can make any changes and is beginning to experience low moods as a result of her lack of social contact and constant anxiety.

Specific Phobia

It is common to experience transient fears of situations, animals or natural environments. However, many people develop fears that become disproportionate to the actual level of risk posed, creating the potential for the development of a specific phobia, which can have enduring impacts on functioning and quality of life. Specific phobias involve a persistent, irrational (out of proportion) intense fear reaction in the face of a specific situation, such as flying or travelling in an elevator, or in response to an object such as a particular animal or blood. The major criterion for diagnosis involves a consistently elevated anxiety response for a period of 6 months or more on presentation of the phobic stimulus, with considerable avoidance or intense fear being endured throughout exposure, causing reduction in functioning and increase in distress. Specific phobias are generally clustered into animal, situational, natural environment or blood-injection-injury subtypes. All subtypes produce similar physiological reactions; however, blood-injection-injury phobic reactions are often accompanied by a vasovagal fainting/near-fainting response as a result of a sudden increase then decrease in heart rate and blood pressure (APA 2013).

Up to 75% of people with a diagnosis of specific phobia have multiple phobias of certain objects or situations (APA 2013; Baldwin et al. 2014). In some instances, phobias can produce life-threatening dangers, such as a person with a serious medical illness refusing treatment via needles because of a blood-injury-injection phobia.

Fear of phobic objects can be experienced through direct contact, distant proximity or anticipation of contact with the stimulus and can produce a continuum of anxious responses, including panic attacks at the more severe end. The degree of anxiety experienced can be reduced/increased by the presence/absence of accompanying contextual elements of safety such as having others around or being exposed to a phobic stimulus with less perceived danger (e.g. for a person with a dog phobia, seeing a smaller dog versus seeing a bigger dog or seeing a dog on a lead across the street versus seeing a dog off the lead on the same side of the road). Longer contact with the phobic stimulus will often draw greater anxiety responses with regard to an increased perception of risk, highlighting duration of exposure as a factor in heightened anxiety.

Specific phobias typically develop between 7 and 11 years of age, although situational or natural environment subtypes have a later age of onset (APA 2013). Some phobias spontaneously remit during childhood and adolescence; however, they can persist into adulthood. It is important to assess factors around the development of phobias as phobias can occur secondary to trauma; for example, fear of the dark may develop following childhood sexual abuse that may have occurred during the night time or fear of dogs may develop after witnessing or undergoing a dog attack. Other developmental factors may include media coverage of plane crashes or storms, witnessing an incident or experiencing an intense reaction during contact with a stimulus such as having a panic attack on top of a tower.

Avoidance behaviours can have a major influence over time in terms of how people live their lives, dictating choice of home and work locations and routines. It may be a change in circumstances that leads to seeking help, such as a move that increases the person's direct contact with their phobic stimulus. Treatment of phobic disorders has been relatively under-researched in comparison with other anxiety disorders (Baldwin et al. 2014). Current treatment indications depend on the level of severity and impairment in functioning caused by the phobia. In the case of subclinical or mild symptoms, psychoeducation and monitoring are recommended to assist in normalising distress and assisting people to begin to identify their triggers for anxiety. Internationally, CBT with graded exposure to phobic stimuli is considered a first-line treatment, with use of benzodiazepines considered only in cases of acute treatment, for example if someone has a needle phobia and requires medical intervention using needles (Freidl & Zakarin 2016).

TRAUMA- AND STRESSOR-RELATED DISORDERS

The DSM-5 has seen the removal of the diagnoses of PTSD, acute stress disorder (ASD) and adjustment disorder (AD) from the anxiety disorders category and their reclassification in a new category of trauma-related disorders. (See Chapter 7 for further discussion of trauma.) This change reflects the significance of trauma as a cause of mental illness and the impact of trauma-related disorders on the lives of those affected. Another consideration in creating this new category was that for many people with trauma- and stressor-related disorders anxiety was not the most prominent feature. It is worth noting, however, that a history of trauma is common in people with a wide range of mental illnesses, not only those that are classified as trauma-related disorders.

A variety of distress responses are both common and normal following trauma, from insomnia to fear and anxiety. It is thought that approximately 25% to 30% of people who experience a traumatic event may go on to develop PTSD or develop ASD or other anxiety or affective disorders.

Posttraumatic Stress Disorder

PTSD is a disabling mental health condition that can present following direct exposure to a traumatic event or multiple traumas, either by firsthand experience or by vicarious traumatisation (witnessing a trauma, learning of a loved one's trauma or extreme/repeated exposure to details of trauma such as those gained via interviews with people who have experienced trauma such as first-responders to accidents). The types of trauma considered for the purposes of diagnosis include threatened or actual physical or sexual harm, personal violence, war, serious accidents, natural disasters and sudden, catastrophic medical events.

PTSD is characterised by symptoms located within four distinct symptom clusters (APA 2013): intrusive reexperiencing (nightmares, dissociative flashbacks, recurrent memories), hyperarousal (heightened startle response, intense physiological response to trauma recall, hypervigilance), persistent avoidance of trauma stimuli (avoiding external reminders and internal trauma-related experiences such as memories) and mood and cognitive alterations (emotional numbing, anhedonia, fear, low mood, impartial trauma memory recall, poor concentration, generalised thoughts about danger). Behavioural changes may also occur, such as sleep disturbance, increased outbursts of irritability, violence, recklessness or self-destructive behaviours. Individuals may display some symptoms with more severity, such as more severe behavioural symptoms, dysphoric mood states, dissociation or arousal (APA 2013). Symptoms typically develop within 3 months of the trauma; however, it is possible for a delayed expression of symptoms to occur months or years later (APA 2013). A diagnosis of PTSD is not made in the first month after the trauma as approximately 50% of people fully recover within 3 months, although some still experience symptoms years or even decades later (APA 2013).

Human survival partly depends on the associative learning processes that occur when we experience danger, helping us to link future fear responses and survival behaviours to encoded threat triggers. Our autobiographical memory plays an important role in processing such events, 'shelving' them in terms of time, place and other specific details to enable recall alongside other such memories for future use. In PTSD, it is hypothesised that a fault occurs during and after the trauma in terms of memory processing, resulting in the development of 'broken trauma memories' that are incomplete, inappropriately stored and containing generalised, catastrophic threat cues that later become identified with nondangerous stimuli. Trauma memories are not stored within the hippocampus alongside other autobiographical memories, so they do not produce a correct sense of placement in time when they are recalled.

The person feels that the recalled events could be happening now or may occur in the future. As a result, traumas are reexperienced rather than simply remembered. Significant avoidance strategies develop due to the emotional load and sense of danger created through reexperiencing the trauma, which often creates functional impairment in day-to-day life. The trauma is thought to create a heightened fear response within the person, triggered by the traumatic event itself and other predisposing genetic, cognitive and temperamental vulnerabilities (Zoellner et al. 2014). These and other mechanisms are thought to create the vicious cycle of PTSD, whereby the person often feels overwhelmed and struggles to function under the weight of their symptoms while expending considerable effort trying to avoid the memories that haunt them and reduce the likelihood of the trauma recurring.

In the Adult Psychiatric Morbidity Survey conducted in 2014, 3.7% of men and 5.1% of women screened positive for PTSD. Women between the ages of 16 and 24 years were most likely to screen positive (12.6%), apart from males between the ages of 55 and 64 years (McManus et al. 2016).

Rates of PTSD are shown to be much higher after exposure to specific types of interpersonal trauma; for example, in one study 50% of rape survivors were noted to have PTSD (Cooper et al. 2014). Many individuals diagnosed with PTSD report multiple trauma events alongside the identified index trauma (Kessler 2000), leading to the concept of complex PTSD, whereby individuals may experience differing symptoms secondary to experiencing different traumas. Complex PTSD symptoms relate to the impact of the enduring and/or compounding nature of multiple traumas and can cause ongoing interpersonal difficulties, emotional dysregulation, prolonged dissociative states, somatic distress/symptoms and fixed, distorted belief systems (Resick et al. 2012).

It is important to note that prevalence of PTSD has been found to be much higher for patients accessing specialist mental health services, with some studies reporting rates as high as 67.2% (Simpson et al. 2011). A large multi-site American study found that 84% of its sample of 782 reported experience of lifetime interpersonal violence, while 52% of the sample reported lifetime sexual assault. When the sexual assault was reported to occur in childhood, higher rates of further traumas into adulthood were found (Muesar et al. 2004). In addition, 34.8% of the sample met the criteria for PTSD, with high comorbidity of mood disorders and current substance abuse. Those identified with PTSD had higher rates of psychiatric readmission over the past year, poorer physical health and higher rates of hospitalisation for physical health issues in the past 6 months. These findings highlight the potentially disabling effects of PTSD on an individual's overall wellbeing.

Another consideration is the rate at which PTSD is screened for in relation to other diagnoses in clinical settings. One early study identified an alarming rate of underdiagnosis within a multi-site study containing a sample of 275 service users. Of the sample, 98% reported exposure to at least one traumatic event and 43% positively screened for PTSD. Of the 119 service users identified with PTSD, only three had the diagnosis documented in their clinical notes (Muesar et al. 1998). A later study that included 70 participants with schizophrenia (Newman et al. 2010) noted a significant effect on severity of symptoms of the disorder and increased chronicity of illness when participants had a comorbid diagnosis of PTSD. It is very concerning to note that none of the 70 participants had a diagnosis of PTSD prior to the commencement of the study (Newman et al. 2010).

PTSD has high rates of comorbidity, particularly with anxiety and affective disorders and substance abuse (APA 2013; NICE 2005). It is also important to note that any traumatic event, particularly occurring during childhood and/or of an interpersonally violent nature, increases a person's risk of suicide (APA 2013). It is therefore essential to ensure that a thorough risk assessment for self-harm is carried out. Because of the potential for ongoing trauma, assessment should also cover risk of harm from others, so that necessary protective measures can be considered.

Current international guidelines for the treatment of PTSD advise offering trauma-focussed psychological interventions such as eye movement desensitisation reprocessing (EMDR) and trauma-focussed cognitive behavioural therapy (Forbes et al. 2007; NICE 2005; Cooper et al. 2014). These specialist psychological interventions are offered by experienced health professionals (including nurses) who have undertaken training in trauma-focussed talking therapies and engage in ongoing supervision. There is little evidence to show benefit from use of pharmacological treatments, although SSRIs can be used if a patient does not wish to engage in or is not finding benefit from psychological therapies alone. SSRIS may also be used if there is a comorbid moderate-to-severe anxiety or affective disorder that would benefit from such treatment (NICE 2005).

Acute Stress Disorder

ASD is clinically very similar to PTSD, with the most notable distinguishing feature being the time required for the diagnosis to be made. ASD can be diagnosed within a month of exposure to a traumatic event, whereas PTSD is not diagnosed until after 1 month. It is important to note that people who receive a diagnosis of ASD do not necessarily go on to develop PTSD, thus one is not predictive of the other. Similarly, those who receive a diagnosis of PTSD may not have had symptoms of ASD within the first month of exposure (Australian Centre for Posttraumatic Mental Health 2013).

The evidence and guidelines for treatment of ASD are similar to those of PTSD, with trauma-focussed CBT recommended as a first-line treatment (ACPMH 2007).

Adjustment Disorder

AD is characterised by an objectively determined, significant and enduring stress response to a life stressor such as a potential or an actual serious illness or significant event. Symptoms are typically considered to involve emotional or behavioural changes such as low mood, worry, a sense of inability to cope and withdrawal from activities with accompanying impairment in social or occupational functioning (APA 2013). Life stressors that may precede the development of AD can occur once, several times or continuously and may include one or multiple stressors, such as the ending of a romantic relationship, business difficulties, socioeconomic challenges, developmental events (retirement) or ongoing illness or disability. Symptoms usually develop within 3 months of the stressor and stop within 6 months of cessation of the stressor. Diagnosis of AD following bereavement is complicated, but the diagnosis is sometimes made if grief symptoms are considered to occur at an intensity, quality and level of persistence that is considered outside the expected grief process (APA 2013).

Diagnosis of AD can be considerably challenging as it is one of the few mental health conditions that centres on causative life events that are expected to produce distress and impairment in functioning for a period of time. Differentiation between AD and a normal stress response centres on the level of severity, duration and intensity of the response in relation to the stressor (APA 2013). AD is relatively under-researched, there are few validated diagnostic tools available and it can be difficult to clearly delineate from other disorders such as MDD (Patra & Sarkar 2013), meaning there is relatively poor recognition of AD in primary care services (Casey & Doherty 2012).

AD is considered a fairly common disorder (APA 2013), although there are few epidemiological studies. Worldwide, in outpatient mental health treatment settings, the prevalence of AD is considered to be between 5% and 20% using DSM-5 criteria (APA 2013), while rates of approximately 14% have been reported in medical settings in association with physical health conditions (Kenardy 2014). One Australian study exploring postpartum mental health in men and women found that AD with features of depressive and anxiety symptoms was the most prevalent mental health condition, with 13.4% of the sample of 172 couples meeting the criteria (Wynter et al. 2013). This indicates that when AD is specifically looked for, particularly in populations considered most vulnerable (such as adults transitioning into parenthood), the disorder is both prevalent and significant in terms of possible impact on functioning for those experiencing the disorder as well as impacts on children and family members.

AD is considered a diagnosis that is found across all cultures (Patra & Sarkar 2013). Culture can play an important role in our response to life stressors and so diagnosis needs to be made carefully when the service user's culture has a different level of expectations regarding response to stressful circumstances, such as the death of a spouse or confirmation of infertility.

Treatment is predominantly targeted at supporting the individual to cope with the presenting psychological distress through cognitive behavioural therapies, mindfulness-based therapies and solution-focussed therapies (Kenardy 2014). There is no evidence to support the use of pharmacological treatments for AD. Despite this lack of evidence a significantly high level of prescriptions for antidepressants are given to patients with AD in primary care, possibly because of the misdiagnosis of symptoms as MDD (Casey & Doherty 2012).

TREATMENT AND NURSING INTERVENTIONS

Nurses have a significant role to play in supporting people experiencing high levels of anxiety or who have a history of trauma. The first and perhaps most helpful intervention we can provide is to validate the experience reported by the patient and through a thorough assessment to begin to make sense of the origins of anxiety and the purpose that it may serve in the person's life. Beginning with the assessment, nurses can provide a number of helpful interventions that can support the patient to develop a path towards peace of mind and recovery. A number of these interventions are detailed later. For an account of how a patient made use of interventions for anxiety, see Patient Story 18.2.

Psychoeducation

Psychoeducation refers to the provision of knowledge to increase a person's mental health literacy and self-awareness in order to inform future decision making. Poor mental health literacy and self-stigma have been associated with low levels of help-seeking behaviours in people struggling with their mental wellbeing (Taylor-Rodgers & Batterham 2014). Psychoeducation is a powerful therapeutic tool in the alleviation of distress caused by anxiety disorders and is considered an intervention in itself (Tursi et al. 2013). Psychoeducation can improve patient engagement, treatment outcomes and psychosocial functioning and therefore should form part of treatment during all phases of service delivery.

In the case of anxiety disorders, psychoeducation is usually provided following a thorough assessment of the person's presenting difficulties so that information can be targeted individually. Primarily, psychoeducation involves teaching people about the function and purpose of anxiety so that it can be viewed as a normal, necessary and shared human experience that does not necessarily have to be avoided or feared. Education can then be provided about heightened anxiety and specific anxiety disorders, exploring the vicious cycles that can develop in which anxiety becomes self-perpetuating. The person's own stories can be used as examples in the psychoeducation provided in order to reflect on the ways in which anxiety can become problematic, raising awareness while helping to provide a wider perspective for the person. Information about available treatments and self-directed help can assist in supporting the person to feel hopeful in seeing a way forward and can go some way in gaining informed consent for certain treatments that may be offered later.

Provision of psychoeducative materials such as self-directed learning through websites, handouts and self-help books can help people to explore information independently in a way and at a time that suits them. Nurses can prepare themselves by having a number of good-quality handouts on anxiety and different topics available within their day-to-day clinical settings to give to patients. Psychoeducation should always be provided free from unnecessary jargon and delivered along the same lines as usual clinical sessions in a well-paced, collaborative manner, allowing time for processing of information and questions.

PATIENT STORY 18.2

Learning to 'Look After' my Anxiety

I think one thing that is misunderstood about anxiety is its physical nature. It is often uncomfortable but can become quite painful at times. At my worst, my physical anxiety was at or near a panic attack level for most of the day and night for the final 2 months of my last pregnancy. My thought processes were rational, but I was unable to shut down the adrenaline and cortisol pumping through my body by trying to use calming, rational thoughts. From the moment I woke, I was acutely aware of my body and how it was feeling. It was in overdrive and hyped up to such a level of discomfort that focussing on anything else was difficult. Medication helped me sleep for 4 hours at a time, but the only time I could find peace during the day was if I was deeply engaged in an activity. Even then these moments were fleeting. My psychiatrist described me as being minute-to-minute and there were many times throughout this that I was not sure I would survive until the next minute.

Several things helped me through. I had to be busy, constantly and without question. I asked for tasks and my family kindly made jobs up if they needed to. Looking back, the tasks needed to be both physical and productive for them to distract my mind and allow some moments of peace. Puzzles were a failure as my panic easily broke through the level of distraction they provided, but actively playing with my son worked for a few minutes at a time. On one of my worst days, my psychologist told me to drive to a park on my way home and walk barefoot in the grass while focussing on nature and the feeling of the grass underneath me. I thought he was the crazy one, but I also knew I had to do it. It worked. I survived that day and all of the other days using medication, therapy, mindfulness techniques, active distraction and family support. Three years later and after eye movement desensitisation reprocessing therapy, I use only one medication instead of the six I needed at delivery, I run and I practise Pilates and try every day to look at one thing in nature very closely. I try to analyse it in detail and remind myself that the moment I am in is actually all there is.

Social Support

Social support has consistently been found to protect individuals against the potential long-term negative effects of trauma and distress by enhancing psychological protective factors, such as more positive evaluations of stressful events, using the knowledge and experience of external supports (Kazantzis et al. 2012). In contrast, lack of such support may be precipitate and perpetuate factors of distress.

Identifying the person's current level of social support can assist in interventions that may enhance required support from family, friends and the wider community. This can provide multiple benefits such as companionship, a sense of connection and increased access to resources and opportunities for engaging in activities that provide enjoyment. These aspects of life often tie in closely with our values, giving us a sense of meaning and happiness.

Unmet socioeconomic needs (housing, poverty, social isolation, etc.) can provide barriers to change and recovery, so these need to be carefully explored and considered and referrals should be made to other agencies for support where required. Integrative service approaches and concepts such as wrap-around care are designed to ensure that the individual can have their needs identified and addressed as part of a team while also allowing each service to focus on providing its own specialist interventions.

Trauma-Informed Care and Psychological Formulations

A trauma-informed approach to anxiety considers any potential trauma-based experiences that may be major predisposing factors to the current heightened state of anxiety. Taking a historical viewpoint of the person and their experiences provides further information on other possible predisposing factors, such as bullying or growing up with high levels of exposure to parental anxiety. See the assessment section of this chapter for more information on trauma screening. A trauma-informed approach seeks first to do no harm by ensuring sensitivity, choice and collaboration in all aspects of service provision. There is a strong emphasis on attempting to understand what has happened to the person as opposed to what is wrong with them.

Psychological formulations are essential in the delivery of trauma-informed care. Psychological formulations have commonly been considered a tool of psychologists, yet they are being utilised more and more by nurses. Psychological formulations provide an opportunity to understand *what* the person is experiencing through the context of *why* they may be struggling as they are. In this sense, psychological formulations are very much about meaning-making regarding difficulties with which the patient may present. The insights provided to both clinicians and the patient can assist in directing treatment that not only supports reduction in symptoms, but also provides opportunity for longer-term prevention of suffering. This effect is provided through promoting deeper changes at a core belief level that may impact perceptions and behavioural responses in the future.

Psychological formulations seek to understand the predisposing factors (what led to the development of the problem), precipitating factors (what is triggering the problem now) and perpetuating factors (what is making the problems worse). Formulations are therapeutic interventions in themselves as they clarify and communicate understanding and insight into the origins and nature of problems to both clinicians and service users. Collaborative formulations provide the potential to deepen the therapeutic relationship, align the wider clinical team and assist in empowering patients through gaining a deeper understanding of themselves. Formulations can be presented to the multidisciplinary team and family members with the consent of the patient to increase understanding and support from others. (See Chapter 22 for further discussion of formulation in the process of nursing assessment.)

Psychological Interventions

Psychological intervention is the term coined to describe the delivery of treatment designed to facilitate the modification of feelings, cognitions, attitudes and behaviours using a variety of resources such as experiments, education, psychotherapy, skills training, taught relaxation or written activities.

Internationally, psychological interventions are gaining increasing status as efficacious, evidence-based and often preferable treatment options for anxiety and trauma-related disorders and have been found to be preferred by service users as a treatment of choice (Baldwin et al. 2014; Peters 2007).

Psychological interventions can be provided as a one-off session, over a brief to long-term package of therapy (6–20+ sessions), within group treatment settings or through the use of guided self-help packages. Psychological therapy, which is the term used to refer to specific models of psychological interventions, is delivered by suitably trained health professionals, including registered nurses who adhere to evidence-based treatment protocols while engaging in specialist supervision.

Current evidence-based psychological interventions for anxiety disorders include CBT, acceptance and commitment therapy (ACT), applied relaxation and mindfulness-based stress reduction. Research generally shows that psychological therapies have more successful effects compared with waiting list controls for anxiety symptoms (Cuijpers et al. 2014).

Another important finding when considering whether to offer psychological therapy is the evidence of protection provided over a longer time period. Studies show that relapse rates are lower after an initial response to CBT with exposure than after initiation of medication (Baldwin et al. 2014). However, it is also important to consider that because of the content and focus of psychological interventions, symptoms can worsen during treatment, responses are often not immediate and difficulties can occur in ending therapy because of the significant relationship that may develop between the service user and clinician. Psychological interventions are also discussed in Chapter 24. Nurse's Story 18.2 by Kwame Okeke provides an outline of a nurse using psychological interventions in nursing practice.

Cognitive Behaviour Therapy

CBT has been shown, over a long period of time, to be an effective, evidence-based talking therapy in the treatment of a multitude of mental health conditions, particularly anxiety disorders (Schmidt 2012; Baldwin et al. 2014). Originally developed by Aaron Beck in the 1960s as a short-term treatment for depression, CBT has been modified and enhanced for a range of mental and physical health disorders, including anxiety and trauma-related disorders. Table 18.2 provides a summary of cognitive behavioural interventions, which are discussed later.

CBT is a structured psychological therapy that focusses on the collaborative establishment of a working formulation that attempts to make sense of the patient's historical experiences, developed belief systems and current-day cognitions, physiological symptoms, emotional experiences and behavioural reactions within the context of their current environment. CBT can be delivered within a brief package of care (3–6 sessions), over a longer period of time for more intensive benefits (6–20+ sessions) or pared down as part of brief, one-off psychological intervention in crisis work.

CBT generally works from a framework of proposing that our cognitions (day-to-day thoughts, core beliefs, imagery and memories) play a major role in affecting our behavioural reactions and our resulting physiological responses, as well as promoting or reinforcing our emotional states. Each of these factors has the ability to perpetuate both distress and

NURSE'S STORY 18.2

Kwame Okeke

Kwame Okeke works as a registered nurse for a community mental health team. He recently completed a postgraduate nursing paper in psychological therapies. Jerry is a pseudonym.

Jerry fills his chair, his eyes wide open, eager and willing. He has been doing this with others like me, on and off, for 10 years. I quickly notice Jerry is eager to please and open to suggestions. I must tread carefully. Jerry has anxiety. We all have anxiety; with Jerry this very natural experience has been amplified, turning life into a world of fear.

Together we talk about what isn't working in his life. His anxiety is crippling. Finding joy is close to impossible when you're trapped behind your rented curtains, frightened to come out. Joy is in a bag of chips, a bottle of fizzy.

The irrational fears are everywhere. They feel as if they are closing in. A social invitation has become a threat to Jerry: 'My friend invited me round . . . I was so angry. How dare he? He knows I can't go!' Any situation where he may come under scrutiny, Jerry fears. He fears he will come up short, like he always has, especially as a little boy trying to impress his unimpressed dad.

His thoughts are twisted: 'I can't go . . . I won't cope . . .'—from these thoughts, a cascade is launched. Anxious emotions ping through the air. His heart races, pupils dilate, muscles tense, palms sweat. These physical sensations become so severe he could fear for his heart. All of these sensations feed an old belief: 'I must stay here behind my curtain where it's safe . . . I'm not feeling good enough to leave.'

In this safe room we put words to his struggles: the thoughts, feelings and fears. Jerry's fears are spoken and heard and explored objectively. The power of the fear begins to fall away. We explore anxiety, its natural rhythm and purpose. As we explore this, he begins trusting himself to manage any negative outcome. He then exposes himself to his fears one by one. Bringing these experiences to our room to discuss, critique and learn from. Now, Jerry is able to challenge his thoughts. He uses mindfulness and relaxation to calm the physical sensations. Emotions are noticed and acknowledged.

Today, Jerry sits with a grin and an air of confidence. He was at work earlier, it wasn't easy, but it was ok. He's been visiting a friend, he'll be off soon to a family gathering and he's thinking of starting up rugby again. Today, Jerry is thoughtful about his life and the scary parts it holds, but he is not afraid.

dysfunction within the others, creating a vicious cycle that can extend to symptoms of mental health disorders. Alternatively, changes within these factors can be brought about that can support emotional regulation, physiological symptom relief, more cognitive clarity and flexibility and helpful, life-enhancing behaviours.

Cognitive approaches to difficult, distressing situations are considered dependent on early perceptions of ourselves, others, the world in general and future outcomes (our belief systems), which are shaped within our early experiences in childhood. Although CBT holds more of a present-day focus than some therapeutic approaches, careful links are established between current reactions and functioning and such early

TABLE 18.2 Components of Cognitive Behavioural Interventions

Exposure	• Encourages patients to face fears • Patients learn corrective information through experience • Extinction of fear occurs through repeated exposure • Successful coping enhances self-efficacy
Safety response inhibition	• Patients restrict their usual anxiety-reducing behaviours (e.g. escape, need for reassurance) • Decreases negative reinforcement • Coping with anxiety without using anxiety-reducing behaviour enhances self-efficacy
Cognitive strategies	• Cognitive restructuring, behavioural experiments and related strategies target patients' exaggerated perception of danger (e.g. fear of negative evaluation in social anxiety disorder) • Provides corrective information regarding the level of threat • Can also target self-efficacy beliefs
Arousal management	• Relaxation and breathing control skills can help patients control increased anxiety levels
Surrender of safety signals	• Patients relinquish safety signals (e.g. presence of a companion, knowledge of the location of the nearest toilet) • Patients learn adaptive self-efficacy beliefs

(*Source*: Katzman, M.A., Bleau, P., Blier, P., Chokka, P., Kjernisted, K., Van Ameringen, M., 2014. Canadian clinical practice guidelines for the management of anxiety, posttraumatic stress and obsessive-compulsive disorders. Released under Open Access, Creative Commons Attribution License.)

events, allowing people to gain enhanced insight and begin to make changes to their ways of thinking and living. This meaning-making is often gathered together within cognitive behavioural models or formulations, which can be specifically focussed on the type of difficulties being experienced. Sessions focus on collaborative working to continue to build on and 'test out' the developing formulation, increasing understanding of difficulties and trying out new ways of being in comparison with prior behavioural choices and cognitive frameworks. Changes to long-held belief systems and habitual ways of behaving towards distress and distressing experiences may explain the research findings on CBT's enhanced effectiveness for relapse prevention in comparison with pharmacological treatment for anxiety and depressive disorders (Baldwin et al. 2014). Patients using CBT gain the ability to identify actively and to work directly or indirectly with historical trauma and/or experiences that may drive distress and be the precipitating events that risk future health and wellbeing.

CBT has been adapted into what are considered 'third-wave' approaches, such as dialectical behavioural therapy (DBT), acceptance and commitment therapy, schema therapy and behavioural activation.

Acceptance and Commitment Therapy

Developed by Steven Hayes and colleagues in the late 1980s, acceptance and commitment therapy (ACT) takes quite a different approach to working with distress by changing the way we relate to it as opposed to challenging directly or trying to change the level of distress itself (Hayes et al. 2012). ACT predominantly works from the concept that internal experiences such as negative thoughts, distressing emotions and their accompanying physical symptoms are normal aspects of the human experience and that rather than trying to avoid or to battle to attempt to get rid of them, we can choose to accept and to work with them using mindfulness to create a more flexible, observational, present-moment focus. The approach also has a strong focus on helping people to identify with and to connect to their life values, empowering people to discover that they can make choices to live life as they wish while accepting whatever emotions, thoughts and other internal experiences show up that may have previously caused them to make choices that took them away from what they valued.

Treatment involves developing skills to improve psychological flexibility or the ability to find resiliency by developing clarity and living life steered by our values, having a flexible view of ourselves, being able to tolerate distress and difficult thoughts without being governed by them and being able to be in contact with the present moment. ACT is well evidenced now, with more than 60 randomised controlled trials providing a good empirical base in working with anxiety and other mental health conditions (Hayes et al. 2012).

CRITICAL THINKING CHALLENGE 18.3

How does anxiety operate in different mental health diagnoses such as schizophrenia, depression or eating disorders? What are the challenges that anxiety can pose to people experiencing these disorders and what might therefore be some of the shared interventions that could be helpful within these different presentations?

Transdiagnostic Treatment Approaches

Due to the increasing burden of anxiety disorders on both sufferers and healthcare systems and the need to continue improving the available interventions, a number of transdiagnostic approaches for treating anxiety disorders have emerged (Schmidt 2012). Despite the differences between the anxiety disorders, several shared vulnerabilities have been found, leading to the belief that single treatments targeting these commonalities could be efficacious and more cost-effective than targeting interventions at single disorders. Transdiagnostic treatments are considered to retain the known scientifically evidenced interventions that support their use but have been adapted to be more easily implemented across healthcare settings by different clinicians (Craske 2012).

Sensitivity to the experience of anxiety itself is one of the transdiagnostic vulnerabilities found within all anxiety disorders. Anxiety sensitivity is a fear of the arousal symptoms of anxiety and is particularly problematic in PD and PTSD. ACT is a good example of a transdiagnostic treatment that aims to reduce fear of anxiety itself through promoting acceptance of anxiety as a necessary and important human experience. In this way, if such vulnerability is noted, ACT can be utilised no matter which anxiety disorder may be diagnosed. Another good example is exposure therapy, commonly utilised as part of CBT. Exposure therapy requires the development of planned and graded experiences where the person is exposed to an identified anxiety-triggering stimulus for prolonged (40 minutes plus) and repeated periods of time in order to become desensitised to the stimulus, and in part the anxiety itself, through the process of habituation. Avoiding particular triggers is a commonly seen safety behaviour in anxiety disorders and exposure can be considered part of treatment no matter what the disorder-specific trigger may be.

Internet-Based Self-Help Treatments

The internet is being increasingly used as a resource for accessing information and self-help treatments for anxiety disorders and there are currently several very helpful websites available. Internet-based self-help is often free to access, thereby removing one barrier to seeking help. Many internet-based treatments are based on CBT and provide opportunity for self-assessment, psychoeducation, monitoring and self-directed treatment of symptoms. Some websites offer free downloads of self-help treatment manuals, while others such as SPARX (an abbreviation of Smart, Positive, Active, Realistic, X-factor thoughts; Merry et al. 2012) incorporate learning and self-help utilising CBT through an interactive gaming program targeted at supporting young people with depression.

A small number of studies have compared face-to-face psychological interventions with internet-based treatments and their effectiveness appears to be similar (Cuijpers et al. 2014) and generally better than waiting list comparisons (Baldwin et al. 2014). Despite this, it is felt there is currently insufficient evidence for the use of computerised CBT to warrant the general introduction of such an approach for anxiety disorders within countries such as the UK (Baldwin et al. 2014).

It is important to consider the notable difficulties that many people have in accessing face-to-face talking therapies in both primary and secondary care services. Internet-based treatments may be a helpful option initially for health users unable to access therapy because of costs, physical location or the availability of a therapist or for those who may not feel comfortable talking to someone directly and who may engage better with a computerised treatment. Alternatively, therapies delivered via the internet can be considered a first step for people with mild to moderate anxiety in line with stepped-care models of treatment (Earl et al. 2014).

Stepped Care

Psychological interventions are now provided in the majority of healthcare systems within a stepped-care model. The stepped-care model was originally developed by the National Institute for Clinical Excellence with the purpose of increasing access to and improving the efficiency of the delivery of psychological interventions within the UK (Earl et al. 2014). The model is beginning to be adapted within the healthcare services of other countries such as New Zealand and Australia in an attempt to ensure that evidence-based psychological interventions are available. Treatment is delivered dependent on level of symptom severity, in the least restrictive manner that is most likely to produce positive outcomes for the service user (Earl et al. 2014). Often the more severe the symptoms are, the more a combined pharmacological and psychological treatment option will be considered. However, it is still unclear whether the majority of anxiety disorders benefit from such an approach.

Cultural Support

Our culture is inherently as much a part of who we are as our mind and body. Culture can be difficult to define but it is commonly thought to comprise a set of collective values, practices, customs and traditions (Gee et al. 2014) and is not necessarily bound solely by ethnic identity. Connection to culture provides a multitude of protective factors and resilience as it gives people a sense of belonging, security and meaning, as well as helping them to find their place within their histories and in the present moment, assisting with a vision of themselves into the future.

It is essential to note that culture plays a major role in the ways in which we perceive health and wellbeing, both in ourselves and in others. Our systems typically originate from Western models of health, which naturally bring about implications and challenges for those whose own culture does not align to such models or belief systems. Healthcare systems across the UK face the challenge of attempting to provide accessible, acceptable and efficacious services to people from a variety of different cultures.

PSYCHOPHARMACOLOGY

The drivers for use of pharmacological treatments for anxiety disorders are the intensity, impact on daily functioning and duration of symptoms experienced by patients. Psychopharmacology should always be utilised through a process of obtaining informed consent once all aspects of the medication, including the side effects and adverse risks, have been discussed. Generally, medication is not a first-line approach for anxiety and trauma-related disorders given the risk of side effects and the costs involved. It has also commonly been difficult to prove the efficacy of medication in the treatment of mild anxiety disorders as assessment and monitoring of symptoms alone have often provided high placebo responses, indicating that placebo alone can play a large part in positive outcomes (Baldwin et al. 2014). Another concern is that pharmacological treatments merely target symptoms of conditions as opposed to the underlying predisposing and precipitating factors themselves, which appear to play a crucial role in the risk of relapse (Baldwin et al. 2014).

Certain psychological treatment models such as ACT challenge the attempts of medication to reduce internal experiences of anxiety. Instead ACT hypothesises that what we attempt to resist persists. ACT opts for supporting internal regulation of anxiety through acceptance and willingness to experience 'symptoms' as part of normal life. In addition, ACT supports value-based behaviours to improve quality of life. Short-term use of medication, however, can support people with more moderate to severe symptoms to engage in psychological therapies (Baldwin et al. 2014; NICE 2005) and combined use in more severe cases of GAD, for example, has been shown to be more efficacious than either treatment alone (NCCMH 2011).

It is important to note that psychotropic medications used for anxiety (apart from benzodiazepines) often do not produce an immediate response. There can be a short-term worsening of symptoms, which the patient should be prepared for in advance. Often, administration needs to continue over a long period of time to maintain initial treatment response (Baldwin et al. 2014). Choice of medication is steered by levels of evidence for efficacious use in the presenting disorders, safety in terms of side effects and any contraindications for the individual, as well as any prior positive responses with past use.

SSRIs are routinely used in the treatment of depression and affective disorders and are commonly prescribed for the treatment of anxiety and trauma-related disorders because of a comparable evidence base, broad-spectrum efficacy and high levels of tolerability in terms of side effects (Baldwin et al. 2014; NICE 2005). SNRIs have proven efficacy in anxiety disorders, particularly GAD and the acute treatment and relapse prevention phase of PD (Baldwin et al. 2014). However, SNRIs appear to be less well tolerated than SSRIs, may cause hypertension in higher doses and, if stopped abruptly, risk discontinuation syndrome, a cluster of unpleasant side effects such as dizziness, insomnia and influenza symptoms.

Benzodiazepines such as lorazepam and diazepam have some proven efficacy for short-term treatment of PD, SAD and GAD (Baldwin et al. 2014). However, because of the side effects of sedation and cognitive impairment, coupled with possible dependence in prolonged use, prescribing should be considered only for short-term crisis management unless there is significant severe impairment and distress caused by anxiety and if other treatments, including psychological therapies, have proven unhelpful (Baldwin et al. 2014).

There is a high incidence of discontinuation of medication because of concerns about dependency or tolerance to medications, but the provision of psychoeducation and information, alongside continuing monitoring of effects and risks, has been found to support adherence to prescribed pharmacological treatments (Baldwin et al. 2014). Chapter 25 contains further discussion of psychopharmacology.

CONCLUSION

Anxiety produces uncomfortable sensations such as increasing heart rate and other physical complaints. It is responsible for sending anxious intrusive thoughts into our consciousness, filled with a myriad of dangerous possibilities that can create further anxiety and fear of what might be happening now and into the future. However, anxiety is a very normal and necessary emotion and is a protective mechanism in our day-to-day lives, involving a finely tuned system that both elicits anxious responses and works to inhibit them when the danger passes.

Anxiety and trauma-related disorders can develop within a myriad of situations, being elicited following a number of predisposing and precipitating life events and factors such as temperament, early experiences and day-to-day life stressors. In themselves, anxiety and trauma-related disorders provide people with experiences that are clearly distressing and that appear to perpetuate themselves as people begin to fuse their anxious cognitions, feelings and experiences. In this way, day-to-day functioning and connectedness with values and sense of meaning in life can be jeopardised.

Treatment of anxiety and trauma-related disorders largely centres on good assessment, support and the provision of knowledge and skills that help people to begin to regulate their own emotional response systems. Psychological interventions play a large role and may be complemented with thoughtful pharmacological treatment. Nurses will be well equipped to work alongside people with anxiety disorders if they can adapt their listening, assessment and formulation skills, as well as identifying and learning psychological interventions that span different diagnoses and problems. The greatest tool we have to work with, however, is the collaborative therapeutic relationship, recognising patients' own expertise and helping them harness this expertise within their own lives.

ACKNOWLEDGEMENT

I would like to thank Dr Christina Campbell for all the help she provided in establishing the direction of this chapter.

EXERCISES FOR CLASS ENGAGEMENT

Separate the class into two groups in order to undertake a debate on the benefits of living life with a lot of anxiety versus living life with no anxiety. Allow time for each group to discuss and to devise arguments on its allocated topic and then set up a debate, either inviting an impartial group or devising one from within the class to decide which team wins the debate. Ensure that the major points of argument are written down in full view of students for discussion after the debate.

REFERENCES

American Psychiatric Association (APA), 2013. Diagnostic and Statistical Manual of Mental Disorders, fifth ed. APA, Washington, DC.

Anda, R.F., Butchart, A., Felitti, V.J., Brown, D.W., 2010. Building a framework for global surveillance of the public health implications of adverse childhood experiences. American Journal of Preventative Medicine 39 (1), 93–98.

Asmundson, G.J.G., Taylor, S., Smits, J.A.J., 2014. Panic disorder and agoraphobia: an overview and commentary on DSM-5 changes. Depression and Anxiety 31, 480–486.

Australian Centre for Posttraumatic Mental Health (ACPMH), 2007. Australian Guidelines for the Treatment of Adults with Acute Stress Disorder and Posttraumatic Stress Disorder. ACPMH, Melbourne, Victoria. Available at: www.nhmrc.gov.au/_files_nhmrc/publications/attachments/mh13.pdf. Accessed 1 July 2015.

Australian Centre for Posttraumatic Mental Health (ACPMH), 2013. Australian Guidelines for the Treatment of Acute Stress Disorder and Posttraumatic Stress Disorder. ACPMH, Melbourne. Available at: http://phoenixaustralia.org/wp-content/uploads/2015/03/Phoenix-ASD-PTSD-Guidelines.pdf. Accessed 1 July 2015.

Baldwin, D.S., Anderson, I.M., Nutt, D.J., Allgulandeer, C., Bandelow, B., den Boer, J.A., Christmas, D.M., Davies, S., Fineberg, N., Lidbetter, N., Malizia, A., McCrone, P., Nabarro, D., O'Neill, C., Scott, J., van der Wee, N., Wittchen, H., 2014. Evidence-based pharmacological treatment of anxiety disorders, post-traumatic stress disorder and obsessive-compulsive disorder: a revision of the 2005 guidelines from the British Association for Psychopharmacology. Journal of Psychopharmacology 28 (5), 403–439.

Blanco, C.S., Rudio, J.M., Wall, M., Secades-Villa, R., Reesdo-Baum, K., Wang, S., 2014. The latent structure and comorbidity patterns of generalized anxiety disorder and major depressive disorder: a national study. Depression & Anxiety 31 (3), 214–222.

Canton, J., Scott, K.M., Glue, P., 2012. Optimal treatment of social phobia: systematic review and meta-analysis (report). Neuropsychiatric Disease and Treatment 8, 203–215.

Casey, P., Doherty, A., 2012. Adjustment disorder: implications for ICD-11 and DSM-5. The British Journal of Psychiatry 201, 90–92.

Clark, D.M., 1986. A cognitive model of panic. Behaviour Research and Therapy 24, 461–470.

Cooper, J., Metcalf, O., Phelps, A., 2014. PTSD: an update for general practitioners [online]. Australian Family Physician 43 (11), 754–757.

Cosoff, S.J., Hafner, R.J., 1998. The prevalence of comorbid anxiety in schizophrenia, schizoaffective disorder and bipolar disorder. Australian & New Zealand Journal of Psychiatry 32, 67–72.

Craske, M.G., 2012. Transdiagnostic treatment for anxiety and depression. Depression and Anxiety 29, 749–753.

Craske, M.G., Rauch, S.L., Ursano, R., Prenoveau, J., Pine, D.S., Zinbarg, R.E., 2009. What is an anxiety disorder? Depression and Anxiety 26, 1066–1085.

Cuijpers, P., Sijbrandij, M., Koole, S., Huibers, M., Matthias, B., Andersson, G., 2014. Psychological treatment of generalised anxiety disorder: a meta-analysis. Clinical Psychology Review (34), 130–140.

Davis, J., Galyer, K., Halliday, T., Fitzgerald, J., Ryan, J.M., 2008. Identifying psychological distress in New Zealand primary care: the General Health Questionnaire-12 (GHQ-12) as a screening instrument. New Zealand Family Physician 35 (2), 86–90.

Earl, T., Hodgson, E., Bunting, A., Feather, J., 2014. Talking therapies in times of change. Journal of NZCCP 24, 5–24.

Faravelli, C., Lo Sauro, C., Lelli, L., Pietrini, F., Lazzeretti, L., Godini, L., Benni, L., Fioravanti, G., Talamba, G.A., Castellini, G., Ricca, V., 2012. The role of life events and HPA axis in anxiety disorders: a review. Current Pharmaceutical Design 18 (35), 5663–5674.

Fineberg, N., Haddad, P., Carpenter, L., Gannon, B., Sharpe, R., Young, A., Joyce, E., Rowe, J., Wellsted, D., Nutt, D., Sahakian, B., 2013. The size, burden and cost of disorders of the brain in the UK. Journal of Psychopharmacology 27 (9), 761–770.

Forbes, D., Creamer, M., Phelps, A., Bryant, R., McFarlane, A., Devilly, G.J., Matthews, L., Raphael, B., Doran, C., Merlin, T., Newton, S., 2007. Australian guidelines for the treatment of adults with acute stress disorder and post-traumatic stress disorder. Australian and New Zealand Journal of Psychiatry 41 (8), 637–648.

Freidl, E.K., Zakarin, E.B., 2016. Phobias. BMJ Publishing Group, London. Available at: http://bestpractice.bmj.com.

Gee, G., Dudgeon, P., Schultz, C., Hart, A., Kelly, K., 2014. Aboriginal and Torres Strait Islander social and emotional wellbeing. In: Dudgeon, P., et al. (Ed.), Working together: Aboriginal and Torres Strait Islander Mental Health and Wellbeing Principles and Practice. Commonwealth of Australia.

Goodman, W.K., Price, L.H., Rasmussen, S.A., et al., 1989. The Yale–Brown Obsessive–Compulsive Scale. I. Development, use, and reliability. Archives of General Psychiatry 46, 1006–1011.

Hammen, C., 1991. Generation of stress in the course of unipolar depression. Journal of Abnormal Psychology 100, 555–561.

Hartley, S., Barrowclough, C., Haddock, G., 2013. Anxiety and depression in psychosis: a systematic review of associations with positive psychotic symptoms. Acta Psychiatrica Scandinavica 128 (5), 327–346.

Hawton, K., Saunders, K., Topiwala, A., Haw, C., 2013. Psychiatric disorders in patients presenting to hospitals following self-harm: a systematic review. Journal of Affective Disorders 151 (3), 821–830.

Hayes, S.C., Pistorello, J., Levin, M.E., 2012. Acceptance and commitment therapy as a unified model of behaviour change. The Counseling Psychologist 40 (7), 976–1002.

Hinton, D.E., 2012. Multicultural challenges in the delivery of anxiety treatment. Depression and Anxiety 29, 1–3.

Hofmeijer-Sevink, M.K., Batelaan, N.M., van Megen, H.J.G.M., Penninx, B.W., Danielle, C.C., van den Hout, M.A., van Balkom, A.J.L.M., 2012. Clinical relevance of comorbidity in anxiety disorders: a report from the Netherlands Study of Depression and Anxiety (NESDA). Journal of Affective Disorders 137 (1–3), 106–112.

Hoge, E., Ivkovic, A., Fricchione, G., 2012. Clinical review: generalized anxiety disorder: diagnosis and treatment. The BMJ e7500.

Johnson, E.M., Coles, M.E., 2013. Failure and delay in treatment-seeking across anxiety disorders. Community Mental Health Journal 49 (6), 668–674.

Katzman, M.A., Bleau, P., Blier, P., Chokka, P., Kjernisted, K., Van Ameringen, M., 2014. Canadian clinical practice guidelines for the management of anxiety, posttraumatic stress and obsessive-compulsive disorders. BMC Psychiatry 14 (Suppl. 1), S1–S83.

Kazantzis, N., Kennedy-Moffat, J., Flett, R., Petrik, A., Long, N., Castell, B., 2012. Predictors of chronic trauma-related symptoms in a community sample of New Zealand motor vehicle accident survivors. Culture, Medicine, and Psychiatry 36 (3), 442–464.

Kenardy, J., 2014. Treatment Guidance for Common Mental Health Disorders: Adjustment Disorder. InPsych October (online). Available at: www.psychology.org.au/Content.aspx?ID=6213. Accessed 1 July 2015.

Kessler, R.C., 2000. Posttraumatic stress disorder: the burden to the individual and to society. Journal of Clinical Psychiatry 61 (Suppl. 5), 4–12.

Leonard, B.E., 2005. The HPA and immune axes in stress: the involvement of the serotonergic system. European Psychiatry 20, S302–S306.

Malan-Muller, S., Hemmings, S.M.J., Seedat, S., 2013. Big effects of small RNAs: a review of microRNAs in anxiety. Molecular Neurobiology 47, 726–739.

Mayo-Wilson, E., Dias, S., Mavranezouli, I., Kew, K., Clark, D., Ades, A., Pilling, S., 2014. Psychological and pharmacological interventions for social anxiety disorder in adults: a systematic review and network meta-analysis. The Lancet Psychiatry 1 (5), 368–376.

McEvoy, P.M., Grove, R., Slade, T., 2011. Epidemiology of anxiety disorders in the Australian general population: findings of the 2007 Australian National Survey of Mental Health and Wellbeing. Australian and New Zealand Journal of Psychiatry 45 (11), 957–967.

McManus, S., Bebbington, P., Jenkins, R., Brugha, T. (Eds.), 2016. Mental Health and Wellbeing in England: Adult Psychiatric Morbidity Survey 2014. Leeds: NHS Digital. Available at: http://content.digital.nhs.uk/catalogue/PUB21748/apms-2014-full-rpt.pdf. Accessed: 19 October 2018.

Merry, S.N., Stasiak, K., Shepherd, M., Frampton, C., Fleming, T., Lucassen, M.F.G., et al., 2012. The effectiveness of SPARX, a computerised self-help intervention for adolescents seeking help for depression: randomised controlled non-inferiority trial. British Medical Journal 344, e2598.

Mueser, K.T., Goodman, L.B., Trumbetta, S.L., Rosenberg, S.D., Osher, F.C., Vidaver, R., Auciello, P., Foy, D.W., 1998. Trauma and posttraumatic stress disorder in severe mental illness. Journal of Consulting and Clinical Psychology 66, 493–499.

Mueser, K.T., Salyers, M.P., Rosenberg, S.D., Goodman, L.A., Essock, S.M., Osher, F.C., Swartz, M.S., Butterfield, M.I., 2004. Interpersonal trauma and posttraumatic stress disorder in patients with severe mental illness: demographic, clinical, and health correlates. Schizophrenia Bulletin 30 (1), 45–57.

National Health Service (NHS), 2016. Conditions: Agoraphobia. Available at: https://www.nhs.uk/conditions/agoraphobia/. Accessed 19 November 2018.

NCCMH, 2011. Generalised Anxiety Disorder in Adults: Management in Primary, Secondary and Community Care. The British Psychological Society and the Royal College of Psychiatrists, London.

Newman, J.M., Turnbull, A., Berman, B.A., Rodrigues, S., Serper, M.R., 2010. Impact of traumatic and violent victimization experiences in individuals with schizophrenia and schizoaffective disorder. The Journal of Nervous and Mental Disease 198, 798–814.

Neziroglu, F., Mancusi, L., 2014. Treatment resistant OCD: conceptualization and treatment. Current Psychiatry Reviews 10 (4), 289–295.

National Institute for Health and Care Excellence (NICE), 2005. Post-Traumatic Stress Disorder: Management. NICE Quality Standard CG26. NICE, UK.

National Institute for Health and Care Excellence (NICE), 2014. Anxiety Disorders. NICE Quality Standard QS53. NICE, UK.

Nivard, M.G., Dolan, C.V., Kendler, K.S., Kan, K.J., Willemsen, G., van Beijsterveldt, C.E.M., Lindauer, R.J.L., van Beek, J.H.D.A., Geels, L.M., Bartels, M., Middeldrp, C.M., Boomsma, D.I., 2015. Stability in symptoms of anxiety and depression as a function of genotype and environment: a longitudinal twin study from ages 3 to 63 years. Psychological Medicine 45, 1039–1049.

Patra, B.N., Sarkar, S., 2013. Adjustment disorder: current diagnostic status. Indian Journal of Psychological Medicine 35, 4–9.

Peters, J., 2007. We Need to Talk: Talking Therapies—A Snapshot of Issues and Activities Across Mental Health and Addiction Services in New Zealand. Te Pou O Te Whakaaro Nui, New Zealand.

Riskind, J.H., Kleiman, E.M., Weingarden, H., Danvers, A.F., 2013. Cognitive vulnerability to anxiety in the stress generation process: further investigation of the interaction effect between the looming cognitive style and anxiety sensitivity. Journal of Behavior Therapy and Experimental Psychiatry (44), 381–387.

Royal Australian and New Zealand College of Psychiatrists (RANZCP), 2003. Australian and New Zealand clinical practice guidelines for the treatment of panic disorder and agoraphobia. Australian and New Zealand Journal of Psychiatry 37, 641–656.

Resick, P.A., Bovin, M.J., Calloway, A.L., Dick, A.M., King, M.W., Mitchell, K.S., Suvak, M.K., Wells, S.Y., Stirman, S.W., Wolf, E.J., 2012. A critical evaluation of the complex PTSD literature: implications for DSM-5. Journal of Traumatic Stress 25 (3), 241–251.

Salkovskis, P.M. (Ed.), 1996. Frontiers of Cognitive Therapy. Guilford Press, New York.

Schmidt, N.B., 2012. Innovations in the treatment of anxiety psychopathology. Behavioural Therapy 43, 465–467.

Sawchuk, C.N., Veitengruber, J.P., 2016. Panic Disorders. BMJ Publishing Group, London. Available at: http://bestpractice.bmj.com.

Sawchuk, C.N., Veitengruber, J.P., Olatunji, B.O., Welch, S.S., 2015. Social Anxiety Disorder. BMJ Publishing Group, London. Available at: http://bestpractice.bmj.com.

Seibell, P.J., Pallanti, S., Bernardi, S., Hughes, M.E., Hollander, E., 2015. Obsessive-Compulsive Disorder. BMJ Publishing Group, London. Available at: http://bestpractice.bmj.com.

Simpson, T.L., Comtois, K.A., Moore, S.A., Kaysen, D., 2011. Comparing the diagnosis of PTSD when assessing worst versus multiple traumatic events in a chronically mentally ill sample. Journal of Traumatic Stress 24, 361–364.

Spitzer, R.L., Kroenke, K., Williams, J.B., Löwe, B., 2006. A brief measure for assessing generalized anxiety disorder: the GAD-7. Archives of Internal Medicine 166 (10), 1092–1097.

Taylor-Rodgers, E., Batterham, P.J., 2014. Evaluation of an online psychoeducation intervention to promote mental health help seeking attitudes and intentions among young adults: randomised controlled trial. Journal of Affective Disorders Oct (168), 65–71.

Tursi, M.F., Baes, C.V., Camacho, F.R., Tofoli, S.M., Juruena, M.F., 2013. Effectiveness of psychoeducation for depression: a systematic review. The Australian and New Zealand Journal of Psychiatry 47 (11), 1019–1031.

Veale, D., Roberts, A., 2014. Clinical review: obsessive-compulsive disorder. The BMJ 348, g2183.

Weiss, D.S., Marmar, C.R., 1996. The impact of event scale: revised. In: Wilson, J., Keane, T.M. (Eds.), Assessing Psychological Trauma and PTSD. Guilford, New York, pp. 399–411.

Wells, J.E., 2006. Twelve-month prevalence. In: Oakley Browne, M.A., Wells, J.E., Scott, K.M. (Eds.), Te Rau Hinengaro: The New Zealand Mental Health Survey. Ministry of Health, Wellington.

Wynter, K., Rowe, H., Fisher, J., 2013. Common mental disorders in women and men in the first six months after the birth of their first infant: a community study in Victoria, Australia. Journal of Affective Disorders 151 (3), 980–985.

Zoellner, L.A., Pruitt, L.D., Farach, F.J., Jun, J.J., 2014. Understanding heterogeneity in PTSD: fear, dysphoria, and distress. Depression and Anxiety (31), 97–106.

USEFUL WEBSITES

Anxiety UK, www.anxietyuk.org.uk

GET Self-Help is a cognitive behaviour therapy self-help resources website that includes a free downloadable self-help CBT course, information leaflets and handouts and CBT tools for use by both clinicians and the public, www.getselfhelp.co.uk

Headspace, www.headspace.com

NICE Guideline lists of all evidence-based guidelines produced by the National Institute for Health and Care Excellence (NICE) for a range of mental health conditions, www.nice.org.uk/guidance

PTSD UK, www.ptsduk.org

SANE, http://www.sane.org.uk

19

Eating Disorders

Gail Anderson, Peta Marks

KEY POINTS

- Eating disorders are mental illnesses associated with significant morbidity and mortality.
- Anorexia nervosa has the highest mortality of any mental illness.
- Recovery is always possible and outcomes improve with early identification, intervention and appropriate treatment.
- Eating disorders can become long term. Remission and relapse of symptoms are common. Holding hope for the person is an essential part of the nurse's role.
- Psychological distress associated with the illness is high; ambivalence and resistance to treatment are part of the illness and are to be expected.
- There are many myths and stereotypes associated with eating disorders. Nurses need to be aware of their own values, attitudes and biases that may impact on their capacity to work effectively with the person.
- Disordered eating behaviours seen in anorexia nervosa and bulimia nervosa are driven by fear of weight gain.
- Disordered eating and weight-control behaviours include food restriction and avoidance, bingeing, vomiting, excessive exercise, use of appetite suppressants and diuretic and laxative abuse.
- Nurses working across all clinical settings need to be aware of who is at risk, commonly presenting circumstances and potential medical and mental health manifestations of illness and to support a person's access to treatment at the earliest possible time. Early detection and intervention improve treatment outcomes.
- Nurses working in particular clinical settings (e.g. emergency department, paediatric units, mental health and eating disorder specific services) where the illness may be more severe, more complex and/or more long term require illness-specific medical and mental health knowledge and skills to manage the biopsychosocial complexities.
- An empathic, respectful, collaborative and supportive approach by nurses and other health professionals is required.
- Nutritional rehabilitation is an essential component of recovery.
- The major therapies used to treat people with eating disorders include cognitive behavioural therapy (CBT), specialist supportive clinical management, interpersonal therapy, motivational interventions, family-based therapy and psychoeducation.
- A collaborative approach to treatment is essential and should include the person's family wherever possible and appropriate. Consistent therapeutic nursing care within a structured programme is imperative to successful inpatient treatment.

KEY TERMS

anorexia nervosa
binge eating disorder
body image disturbance
bulimia nervosa
cognitive behavioural therapy (CBT)
disordered eating
family-based therapy
weight restoration
interpersonal therapy
Maudsley family-based therapy
motivational interventions
nutritional rehabilitation
other specified feeding or eating disorder (OSFED)
psychoeducation
re-feeding syndrome
specialist supportive clinical management
therapeutic meal support
weight loss

LEARNING OUTCOMES

The material in this chapter will assist you to:

- develop an understanding of eating disorders within individual, family and social contexts.
- identify behaviours commonly associated with eating disorders.
- identify areas of health and wellbeing, including physical health, mental health, nutritional status, social and behavioural patterns, that are useful when assessing people experiencing eating disorders.

- recognise the potential medical complications associated with eating disorders.
- understand the importance of a collaborative and compassionate nursing approach to positive clinical outcome across all treatment settings.
- understand the genuine struggle with ambivalence to treatment typically experienced by a person with an eating disorder.
- describe important aspects of nursing care for hospitalised patients with anorexia nervosa.
- identify various approaches to treatment including specialist supportive clinical management, cognitive behavioural therapy, interpersonal therapy, motivational interventions, Maudsley family-based therapy, psychoeducation and pharmacotherapy.

INTRODUCTION

This chapter discusses the eating disorders as classified by the *Diagnostic and Statistical Manual of Mental Disorders*, 5th edition, (DSM-5) (American Psychiatric Association (APA) 2013) including anorexia nervosa, bulimia nervosa, binge eating disorder and other specified feeding or eating disorders (OSFED). Although the DSM-5 describes the criteria for diagnosis of specific eating disorders, symptoms are known to exist on a continuum from moderately serious, higher prevalence illnesses (e.g. bulimia nervosa and binge eating disorder) to very serious relatively low prevalence disorders (anorexia nervosa). While a person cannot be simultaneously diagnosed with anorexia nervosa, bulimia nervosa and/or OSFED, disordered eating behaviours can fluctuate between these illnesses over time.

Eating disorders are characterised by one or more seriously disturbed eating behaviours such as food restriction or recurrent episodes of uncontrolled eating and weight-control behaviours including self-induced vomiting, excessive exercising or the misuse of laxatives or diuretics. A person with anorexia nervosa or bulimia nervosa is preoccupied with their weight and their self-worth is dependent largely, or even exclusively, on their shape and weight and their ability to control them (Murphy et al. 2010).

While it is common to think of eating disorders as modern illnesses, descriptions of illnesses resembling anorexia nervosa appeared as early as the seventeenth century (Hay et al. 2014). During the late nineteenth and early twentieth centuries, people from Western societies began to focus on thinness as a representation of beauty and success. While the overall incidence of anorexia nervosa has been relatively stable over time, research shows an increase in illness in 15- to 19-year-old females (Smink et al. 2012). Bulimia nervosa and binge eating disorder were not described until the twentieth century. OSFED is a more recently defined category of eating disorder (APA 2013) and, as such, has not been well described in the research literature. However, OSFED's predecessor 'eating disorder not otherwise specified' (EDNOS), which differed from OSFED in that it included binge eating disorder, has shown that subclinical disorders can also have a significant impact on health, wellbeing, quality of life and morbidity and mortality (Arcelus et al. 2011).

Because of stigma and because eating disorders are often hidden, many people in the community who experience them do not seek treatment. As such, eating disorders are underdiagnosed, particularly in men (Strober & Johnson 2012). Nurses across all clinical settings need to develop an evidence-based understanding around the development and maintenance of illness, identifying those at risk and developing the skills required to intervene early and to work with people who have eating disorders towards their recovery. The focus is on educating the community, providing effective person-centred treatment and supporting better outcomes for individuals and their families. As with all other physical and mental health disorders, early detection and intervention improve outcomes and reduce morbidity and mortality.

Eating disorders are among the most serious and misunderstood of all mental illnesses, with myths and stereotypes significantly impacting those who experience them (Mond et al. 2006; Bannatyne & Abel 2015). Eating disorders are not lifestyle choices driven by vanity or a desire for attention. They are complex and potentially lethal illnesses that generally require long-term treatment. As well as having significant negative health effects, eating disorders are associated with significant quality of life impairment and impact on home, personal and social life (Mond et al. 2012; Mond et al. 2013) as well as having economic costs (Butterfly Foundation 2012).

CHARACTERISTICS OF EATING DISORDERS

Anorexia Nervosa

Anorexia nervosa is a complex and potentially long-term mental illness that has impairment outcomes comparable to people with schizophrenia and has the highest mortality of any mental illness (Surgenor & Maguire 2013). It is characterised by three key features: persistent restriction of energy intake; intense fear (and avoidance of) weight gain or of being 'fat'; and a disturbed perception of body weight and/or shape (DSM-5) (see Box 19.1).

Young people who develop anorexia nervosa may fail to make expected weight gains or maintain normal developmental trajectories (as opposed to losing weight). If the onset of anorexia nervosa is prepubertal, the sequence of pubertal events will be delayed or even arrested (e.g. in girls, their breasts do not develop and there is primary amenorrhoea and in boys, their genitals remain juvenile) (Royal Australian and New Zealand College of Psychiatrists (RANZCP) 2004). Patient Story 19.1 about Gabriela describes the early development of an eating disorder.

Anorexia nervosa typically begins in early to middle adolescence and starts with dieting or restricting food that is perceived to be fattening. This dietary restriction becomes more rigid and extreme as the illness progresses and is generally accompanied by worsening depressed mood, cognitive

BOX 19.1 Diagnostic Criteria for Anorexia Nervosa

A. Restriction of energy intake relative to requirements, leading to a significantly low body weight in the context of age, sex, developmental trajectory and physical health. *Significantly low weight* is defined as a weight that is less than minimally normal, or for children and adolescents, less than that minimally expected.

B. Intense fear of gaining weight or of becoming fat or persistent behaviour that interferes with weight gain, even though at a significantly low weight.

C. Disturbance in the way the person's body weight or shape is experienced, undue influence of body shape and weight on self-evaluation or persistent lack of recognition of the seriousness of the current low body weight.

Subtypes

Restricting type: During the last 3 months, the individual has not engaged in recurrent episodes of binge eating or purging behaviour (i.e. self-induced vomiting or the misuse of laxatives, diuretics or enemas). This subtype describes presentations in which weight loss is accomplished primarily through dieting, fasting and/or excessive exercise.

Binge eating/purging type: During the last 3 months, the individual has engaged in recurrent episodes of binge eating or purging behaviour (i.e. self-induced vomiting or the misuse of laxatives, diuretics or enemas).

Specify Current Severity

The minimum level of severity is based, for adults, on current body mass index (BMI) (see later) or, for children and adolescents, on BMI percentile. The ranges below are derived from the World Health Organization categories for thinness in adults; for children and adolescents, corresponding BMI percentiles should be used. The level of severity may be increased to reflect clinical symptoms, the degree of functional disability and the need for supervision.

Mild: BMI ≥ 17 kg/m^2
Moderate: BMI 16–16.99 kg/m^2
Severe: BMI 15–15.99 kg/m^2
Extreme: BMI ≤ 15 kg/m^2

(*Source:* American Psychiatric Association (APA), 2013. Diagnostic and Statistical Manual of Mental Disorders, 5th ed. APA, Washington, DC. Reprinted with permission.)

PATIENT STORY 19.1

Gabriela

Gabriela is a 16-year-old in sixth form, living with her parents and sister who is 17 and doing her A Levels. Gabriela has lost a significant amount of weight over the past few months by engaging in restrictive eating and excessive exercise behaviours. She was previously sporty, sociable and a high academic achiever, but this year she has struggled with changes to her peer group at school, as well as bullying by exclusion and having shame-inducing comments posted to her Facebook page, which has caused her to feel anxious, embarrassed, sad and very distressed at times. Her mother, a dietician, has tried to help Gabriela to stabilise her weight loss, but this has been ineffective. The GP found that Gabriela was at least 8 kg underweight and medically unstable (low body temperature, low pulse, blood pressure changes on standing and an irregular Electrocardiogram (ECG)) and referred her immediately to the local hospital emergency department for further assessment.

Triage nurse: I've got a 16-year-old anorexic in bed 5 who is medically unstable for you to see . . . You know, I really don't get people who starve themselves to be beauty queens . . .

Psychiatric liaison mental health nurse: You know, I've actually never met someone with an eating disorder who started out wanting to be a supermodel—that's pretty much a myth. Mostly, it's a way of managing a whole host of underlying psychological issues and once the starvation kicks in, the illness gains momentum and spirals out of control. Did you know anorexia nervosa has the highest mortality rate of any mental illness?

Triage nurse: Really? I don't know how anyone could not want to eat! Surely it's as simple as going home and just eating properly. They're all manipulative if you ask me.

Psychiatric liaison mental health nurse: If only it *were* that simple . . . unfortunately, once people get caught in the starvation syndrome, they find it really difficult to stop and all their behaviours are protective of the illness and make it worse. Have you ever heard about the starvation experiment?

Learning Point

Stigma and discrimination can impact a practitioner's attitude and approach, which in turn impacts a patient's help-seeking behaviour and potentially their health outcome. It is important to share your knowledge with other health practitioners in an effort to dispel some of the myths and stereotypes that surround the eating disorders.

A Note About Language

Referring to someone as 'anorexic' or 'bulimic' focusses the attention on the disorder, rather than the person, which is the antithesis of a person-centred approach. This is a *person* who happens to be *experiencing* an eating disorder. Disorder-focussed language implies that the illness is an integral part of the person, rather than an unwelcome interloper that is having a profound physical and mental health effect on the person and that can be treated. Use the person's name, describe them as a 'person with an eating disorder' and always externalise the illness.

impairment, increasing anxiety and obsessive-compulsive features. Common weight-controlling behaviours include excluding entire food groups, excessive exercise, self-induced vomiting or purging and, less commonly, the use of appetite suppressants or diuretics.

The person experiencing anorexia nervosa often feels that their identity becomes synonymous with the eating disorder and through the disorder they experience a sense of control over their environment or satisfaction at achievement of weight loss goals. This is despite the significant nutritional compromise and life-threatening medical complications (affecting most major organ systems) experienced as a result of weight loss and malnutrition and the often debilitating psychological distress that accompanies the illness (Mehler & Brown 2015).

There are real feelings of body weight and shape distortion, where the person feels globally overweight or focusses on particular body parts (particularly, buttocks, thighs or abdomen) as being 'too fat'. Because the idea of weight gain is seen as an unacceptable failure of self-control, regardless of how thin a person with anorexia nervosa may become, there remains an overwhelming fear of becoming fat, a desire to lose more weight and an increasing preoccupation with strategising for continued weight loss.

The essential criteria defined in the DSM-5 (APA 2013) for anorexia nervosa and its two subtypes are listed in Box 19.1.

Bulimia Nervosa

Bulimia nervosa is characterised by regular, overwhelming urges to over-eat (binge), followed by the use of compensatory behaviour to avoid weight gain such as self-induced vomiting, excessive exercise, food avoidance or laxative misuse. The public perception of a 'binge' as presented in magazines and in the media is inaccurate. In fact, a 'binge' is defined as eating an excessive amount of food that is definitely larger than most individuals would eat, over a similar period of time, under similar circumstances. There is always a sense of lack of control associated with binge eating (APA 2013, p. 345). Patient Story 19.2 about Chris describes a patient presenting to their GP with a request for laxatives, but where the issue is disordered eating and elimination patterns.

One of the main triggers for binge eating is hunger and a cycle is often established where food is restricted during the day and binge eating behaviour occurs in the evening (usually in secret or as inconspicuously as possible). Other triggers can be interpersonal stressors, intense emotions, boredom or negative feelings related to self-worth, body weight and shape. Binge eating continues until the person is uncomfortably or painfully full and leads to feelings of guilt, self-recrimination and self-disgust. Fear of weight gain triggers vomiting or other compensatory behaviours, further reinforcing the person's poor sense of self-worth and, because they resolve to do better with 'dieting' the next day, helps maintain the bulimic cycle.

The key feature distinguishing bulimia nervosa from anorexia nervosa (binge eating/purging type) is weight: people with bulimia nervosa are likely to have normal or near-normal body weight (Fairburn & Harrison 2003). People with bulimia nervosa are less likely to require inpatient hospitalisation; however, that does not mean that bulimia nervosa is a harmless illness. In fact, the fluid and electrolyte disturbances created by purging can create serious and potentially fatal medical problems (e.g. cardiac arrhythmias, oesophageal tears, gastric rupture).

The essential criteria for bulimia nervosa and its subtypes are defined in the DSM-5 (APA 2013) and listed in Box 19.2.

PATIENT STORY 19.2

Chris

Chris is a 25-year-old who presented to the GP for a laxative prescription, as his usual doctor was unavailable. He had been having problems with abdominal pain, said he was constipated and requested a stronger laxative. He had tried most over-the-counter laxatives but they were not effective. Chris admitted he had problems with stress, controlling his weight and managing his diet. He thought he had been suffering from food allergies. He also experienced tiredness, moodiness and erratic emotions. He was thin and pale, his weight was within the normal range and he was not clinically constipated. He had just started a new job, was not eating regularly and was skipping meals.

GP: Chris, I don't see any clinical signs of constipation when I do the examination, so let's have a think about what else might be going on. Some people who worry about constipation say they have difficulties with their eating . . . would you say that this is an issue for you?

Chris: Well yeah, I suppose you could say that. I do have some issues with food.

GP: What sort of issues in particular?

Chris: Well, mostly, I don't handle stress very well and I guess I have a pretty erratic diet.

Learning Point

Asking about disordered eating behaviours in a matter-of-fact, non-judgemental way is important for early identification and intervention. The SCOFF is a simple evidence-based screening tool that involves five simple questions:

S Do you make yourself Sick because you feel uncomfortably full?
C Do you worry you have lost Control over how much you eat?
O Have you recently lost Over 6 kg in a 3-month period?
F Do you believe yourself to be Fat when others say you are too thin?
F Would you say Food dominates your life?

An answer of 'yes' to two or more of the questions indicates the need for a more comprehensive assessment around eating and dieting practices. In addition, asking the next two questions has been shown to indicate a high sensitivity and specificity for bulimia nervosa (which is more common in older adolescents and young adults):

1. Are you satisfied with your eating patterns?
2. Do you ever eat in secret?

(*Source:* Hill, L.S., Reid, F., Morgan, J.F., Lacey, J., 2010. SCOFF, the development of an eating disorder screening questionnaire. International Journal of Eating Disorders 43(4):344–351.)

BOX 19.2 Diagnostic Criteria for Bulimia Nervosa

A. Recurrent episodes of binge eating. An episode of binge eating is characterized by both of the following:
  1. Eating, in a discrete period of time (e.g. within any 2-hour period), an amount of food that is definitely larger than most people would eat during a similar period of time and under similar circumstances.
  2. A sense of lack of control over eating during the episode (e.g. a feeling that one cannot stop eating or control what or how much one is eating).

B. Recurrent inappropriate compensatory behaviour in order to prevent weight gain, such as self-induced vomiting, misuse of laxatives, diuretics, or other medications, fasting or excessive exercise.

C. The binge eating and inappropriate compensatory behaviours occur, on average, at least once a week for 3 months.

D. Self-evaluation is unduly influenced by body shape and weight.

E. The disturbance does not occur exclusively during episodes of anorexia nervosa.

Specify Current Severity

The minimum level of severity is based on the frequency of inappropriate compensatory behaviours (see later). The level of severity may be increased to reflect other symptoms and the degree of functional disability.

Mild: An average of 1–3 episodes of inappropriate compensatory behaviours per week

Moderate: An average of 4–7 episodes of inappropriate compensatory behaviours per week

Severe: An average of 8–13 episodes of inappropriate compensatory behaviours per week.

Extreme: An average of 14 or more episodes of inappropriate compensatory behaviours per week

(*Source:* American Psychiatric Association (APA) 2013. Diagnostic and Statistical Manual of Mental Disorders, 5th ed. APA, Washington, DC. Reprinted with permission.)

Binge Eating Disorder

Binge eating disorder is characterised by recurrent episodes of binge eating without the compensatory behaviours that people who experience bulimia nervosa use to avoid weight gain. Binge eating disorder is less common but much more severe than overeating. Like bulimia nervosa, there is a lack of self-control during the binge eating and marked distress (guilt, disgust, depressed mood) after a binge (APA 2013, p. 350). Binge eating disorder can occur in people who are normal weight, overweight or obese (that does not mean that all people who are obese engage in binge eating). People who are obese and who have binge eating disorder experience greater functional impairment, poorer quality of life, greater subjective distress and psychiatric comorbidity than those who do not. Overall, binge eating disorder is associated with significant psychiatric comorbidity comparable with anorexia and bulimia nervosa.

BOX 19.3 Binge Eating Disorder: Level of Severity

Mild: 1–3 binge eating episodes per week
Moderate: 4–7 binge eating episodes per week
Severe: 8–13 binge eating episodes per week
Extreme: 14 or more binge eating episodes per week

(*Source:* Reprinted with permission from the Diagnostic and Statistical Manual of Mental Disorders, Fifth Edition, (Copyright © 2013). American Psychiatric Association. All Rights Reserved.)

Level of severity for binge eating disorder is defined in the DSM-5 (APA 2013) and listed in Box 19.3.

Other Specified Feeding or Eating Disorder

At times, people experience eating disorders that cause clinically significant distress or impairment in important areas of functioning (e.g. social, occupational) but that do not meet the full criteria for diagnosis as an eating disorder; for example, a person who meets all of the criteria for anorexia nervosa, but whose weight is within or above the normal range, or someone who meets all the criteria for bulimia nervosa or binge eating disorder except the criteria around frequency of binge eating/compensatory behaviours. OSFED also includes purging disorder where a person purges without binge eating and night eating syndrome.

The essential criteria for OSFED are defined in the DSM-5 (APA 2013, p. 354) and listed in Box 19.4.

INCIDENCE AND PREVALENCE

Eating disorders affect people across all age and cultural groups and across the socioeconomic spectrum. Incidence and prevalence rates are difficult to determine because most people who experience an eating disorder do not seek treatment and often go undiagnosed. Based on UK hospital admissions 2012 to 2013, the eating disorders charity BEAT estimated that there were over 725,000 people with an eating disorder in the UK, with approximately 90% of those people being female. However, a community-based study suggests that 25% of people with an eating disorder are male (NICE 2017). Although eating disorders can develop at any age, it is important to note that the risk is highest for young men and women between 13 and 17 years of age (National Institute for Health and Care Excellence [NICE] 2017). For disorder-specific information on incidence and prevalence, see Table 19.1.

Eating Disorders in Males

Nurses need to be very aware of overlooking illness, or risk of illness, as a result of stereotyping; for example, while 65% of people who experience eating disorders are female (and 90% of those with anorexia nervosa are female), eating disorders also occur in men, older women, people from non-Western countries and people who are obese (Hoek 2014). In fact, males are increasingly affected (Strother et al. 2012). The gender ratio changes according to age and type of eating disorder or disordered eating behaviour. For example, in prepubertal

BOX 19.4 Other Specified Feeding or Eating Disorder

This category applies to presentations in which symptoms characteristic of a feeding and eating disorder that cause clinically significant distress or impairment in social, occupational or other important areas of functioning predominate but do not meet the full criteria for any of the disorders in the feeding and eating disorders diagnostic class. The other specified feeding or eating disorder category is used in situations in which the clinician chooses to communicate the specific reason that the presentation does not meet the criteria for any specific feeding and eating disorder. This is done by recording 'other specified feeding or eating disorder' followed by the specific reason (e.g. bulimia nervosa of low frequency).

Examples of presentations that can be specified using the 'other specified' designation include the following:

A. *Atypical anorexia nervosa:* All of the criteria for anorexia nervosa are met, except that despite significant weight loss the individual's weight is within or above the normal range.
B. *Bulimia nervosa* (of low frequency and/or limited duration): All of the criteria for bulimia nervosa are met, except that the binge eating and inappropriate compensatory behaviour occurs, on average, less than once a week and/or for less than 3 months.
C. *Binge eating disorder* (of low frequency and/or limited duration): All of the criteria for binge eating disorder are met, except that the binge eating occurs, on average, less than once a week and/or for less than 3 months.
D. *Purging disorder:* Recurrent purging behaviour to influence weight or shape (e.g. self-induced vomiting, misuse of laxatives, diuretics, or other medications) in the absence of binge eating.
E. *Night eating syndrome:* Recurrent episodes of night eating, as manifested by eating after awakening from sleep or by excessive food consumption after the evening meal. There is awareness and recall of the eating. The night eating is not better explained by external influences such as changes in the individual's sleep–wake cycle or by local social norms. The night eating causes significant distress and/or impairment in functioning. The disordered pattern of eating is not better explained by binge eating disorder or another mental disorder, including substance use and is not attributable to another medical disorder or to an effect of medication.

(*Source:* American Psychiatric Association (APA), 2013. Diagnostic and Statistical Manual of Mental Disorders, 5th ed. APA, Washington, DC. Reprinted with permission.)

children, eating disorders occur almost as frequently in males as in females (Gonzales et al. 2007) and while bulimia nervosa is more common in females, recent research has found only small to moderate gender differences in frequency of eating disorder behaviours such as binge eating and the use of excessive exercise to control weight (Weltzin et al. 2012).

Concern regarding the potential increased incidence of eating disorders in men has arisen because of the increasing focus on appearance among men in Western societies. While the impact of underweight role models on the prevalence of disordered eating among men over time is yet to be studied, some early observations can be made. In contrast to the popular 'thin ideal' of female beauty, young men experience two conflicting social pressures—to 'bulk up' *and* to look slim—and males therefore generally pursue lean and muscular bodies, rather than a thinner physique (Strother et al. 2012). Behaviours such as excessive exercising, dieting, bingeing, purging and steroid use are not uncommon among young males and there is an increased prevalence of eating disorders in certain subgroups of males who are vulnerable to weight and shape concerns, such as wrestlers, homosexual men (Strother et al. 2012) and athletes (Muise et al. 2003). One study (O'Dea & Abraham 2002) investigated eating, weight, shape and exercise behaviours in young men and found that one in five men worried about their weight and shape, followed rules about eating and restricted their food intake; and while 9% reported disordered eating, none of the population studied had sought treatment. The incidence rate for anorexia nervosa in males has been reported to be below 1 per 100,000 people per year (Hoek 2006).

Muscle dysmorphia, a condition most prevalent in males, is characterised by a preoccupation with muscle size and build and the persistent belief that the person's muscles are too small. In contrast to people with anorexia nervosa who feel fat when they are in fact thin, people with muscle dysmorphia feel ashamed of looking small when they are actually well built (Grieve 2007; Pope et al. 2000).

It is believed that significant differences exist between males and females in terms of predisposing, precipitating and perpetuating factors for an eating disorder. For example, males who have an eating disorder are more likely to have been premorbidly mildly to moderately obese, whereas women tend to have a normal weight history but *feel* fat before losing weight; males with bulimia nervosa, binge eating or binge eating disorder are less likely to engage in vomiting or laxative abuse and more likely to use excessive exercise as a compensatory behaviour than women; and men report that anger can trigger a binge, whereas suppressing anger is a more likely trigger for women (Strother et al. 2012).

The clinical features of eating disorders specific to males, and associated with malnutrition, include a decrease in spontaneous early morning erections and nocturnal emissions, lower testosterone levels and higher rates of comorbid depression.

Eating Disorders in Children and Adolescents

It is important for nurses in all clinical settings to understand that children with eating disorders can get 'sicker quicker' than adults. Emaciation and medical complications can occur more rapidly because young people have lower energy stores and dehydrate more quickly (Royal College of Psychiatrists [RCP] 2012) and rapid weight loss in children is more likely to result in life-threatening complications (Madden et al. 2009).

TABLE 19.1 Incidence, Prevalence and Epidemiology of Various Eating Disorders

Dieting and Body Image Concern	Extreme Dieting/ Disordered Eating	Binge Eating Disorder	Other Specified Feeding and Eating Disorders	Bulimia Nervosa	Anorexia Nervosa
Eating habits, body composition and eating behaviours are established in childhood and adolescence, mostly continuing into adulthood. Most eating disorders start with dieting behaviours. The more extreme the dieting behaviours, the higher the likelihood of an eating disorder developing. High-frequency dieting and early onset of dieting are associated with poorer physical and mental health, more disordered eating, extreme body dissatisfaction and more frequent general health problems (Tucci et al. 2007; Kenardy et al. 2001). 68% of 15-year-old girls are on a diet (Kenardy, 2001) despite the fact that dieting contributes to weight gain over time and perpetuates unhealthy attitudes towards food, weight and shape (Patton et al. 1997; Kenardy et al. 2001). Many adolescent boys/young men are increasingly concerned with 'bulking up' and/or with dieting. Women who diet frequently are 75% more likely to experience depression than those who don't (Mond et al. 2006). Obesity has increased by 75% in children over the last three decades.	Adolescent girls who engage in *moderate dieting* practices are five times more likely to develop an eating disorder, and those who engage in *extreme dieting* are 18 times more likely to develop an eating disorder than someone who doesn't diet (National Eating Disorders Collaboration [NEDC] 2010). Extreme dietary practices include fasting, crash dieting, vomiting, using diet pills and laxative abuse. Between 1995 and 2005, prevalence of disordered eating behaviours doubled among males and females aged 15+ (NEDC, 2012). International studies have shown disordered eating in 7.1% and 13.4% of 9–14-year-old boys and girls, respectively (Treasure et al. 2010). One in five people with obesity also have disordered eating.	BED begins in late adolescence/early 20s (Kessler et al. 2013). Lifetime prevalence of BED in the general population is estimated in 2.5%–4.5% of females and 1%–3% of males (NEDC 2010). Risk factors include obesity (this is also a complication of BED), childhood overweight, strict dieting, a history of depression, anxiety and low self-esteem (CEDD 2008). Most people with BED are overweight or obese.	OSFED includes disorders that don't quite meet the diagnostic criteria for AN (all other criteria but weight in the normal range), BN or BED (all other criteria but less frequent behaviours and/or duration of illness less). OSFED also includes purging disorder and night eating syndrome. OSFED are the most common eating disorders seen in most outpatient settings, primary care settings and community health settings, both for adolescent and adult populations. Estimates up to 10% of the population. Importantly, subclinical syndromes are associated with considerable medical complications, morbidity and mortality: the severity of psychopathology and degree of secondary psychosocial impairment is comparable to AN and BN. Medical complications including osteoporosis and cardiac arrhythmias, and in some studies mortality, have been demonstrated to occur at similar levels as in AN.	Lifetime prevalence in females is 0.9%–2.1% and in males is <0.1%–1% (NEDC 2010). Partial-syndrome BN is thought to have a prevalence of about 5.4% among young females. BN usually onsets between 16 and 18 years, although more cases are being reported in the younger adolescent years. Prepubertal cases have been reported, as have first-onset cases in women in their 60s, although these are rare. Earlier onset bulimia nervosa (age 15 years or younger) has been associated with higher rates of deliberate self-harm and familial depression.	One in every hundred adolescent girls develops AN. It is highly prevalent when compared with other serious diseases in the at-risk population and is the third most common chronic disease (Lucas et al. 1991). It is the 10th leading cause of burden of disease and injury in females aged 15–24 years in Australia and has the highest mortality rate of any mental illness, with one in five deaths of those with AN a result of suicide (Arcelus et al. 2011). In 15–24-year-old females the standardised mortality rate is 12 times the annual rate from all causes (Sullivan 1995). Lifetime prevalence for females is 0.3%–1.5% (some studies say 4.3%) including partial-syndrome AN (Lewinsohn et al. 2000) and 0.1%–0.5% in males. AN can onset at any age; the ages 13–18 years are high risk for onset and two peak ages at which onset of the illness is most likely are 14 and 16 years. Rates of adolescent AN have increased over the past 50 years and age of onset has decreased (Madden et al. 2009). The ratio of females to males with AN is between 10:1 and 20:1, although in prepubertal cases it is closer to 3:1.

AN, Anorexia nervosa; *BED*, binge eating disorder; *BN*, bulimia nervosa; *OSFED*, other specified feeding and eating disorders.

(*Source:* MHFOD. Course: Eating Disorders. 2014. Produced by Cadre Pty. Ltd. and the Psychosocial Research Centre of the University of Melbourne for the Project Steering Committee, on behalf of the Mental Health Workforce Advisory Committee (MHWA). Copyright: Cadre Pty. Ltd., Sydney.)

Children under 12 years of age who present with an eating disorder may present with similar psychological symptoms as adolescents and adults. However, they are less likely to report fear of fatness or weight gain, less likely to appreciate just how severe the illness is, more likely to present with nonspecific symptoms, more likely to be boys and more likely to have lost weight rapidly (Hay et al. 2014). They are also less likely to vomit or abuse laxatives and more likely to be diagnosed with an unspecified feeding or eating disorder (Hay et al. 2014).

Early and more aggressive nutritional rehabilitation is needed for children and adolescents with eating disorders to prevent potentially irreversible complications affecting development, such as stunted growth, delayed pubertal maturation and irreversible and long-term effects on bone accretion, as well as structural and morphological changes in different organ systems and chronicity of illness (Campbell & Peebles 2014; Kohn et al. 2009). As brain development is now known to continue almost into the third decade of life, the negative impact on brain structure and functioning from childhood anorexia nervosa is of great concern (Kohn et al. 2009).

Unlike adults, children should continue to grow in height during the course of treatment. Therefore, height should be measured every 3 months. As accurate height measures are needed to determine healthy weight ranges, goal weights should also be reassessed regularly to reflect any linear growth. Early restoration of nutrition helps ensure that a child reaches their full growth potential.

Unless they are medically compromised, adults with an eating disorder who require hospitalisation are usually admitted to an adult psychiatric unit. Children and adolescents, on the other hand, usually require admission to a developmentally appropriate, specialist medical setting staffed by paediatricians, child psychiatrists and nurses who understand the different physiological and psychosocial developmental needs of children and young people.

RISK AND PROTECTIVE FACTORS

It can be hard to understand how eating disorders develop and are then maintained. The experience is different for everyone; however, there are a number of factors that increase a person's vulnerability to developing an eating disorder. Some of these are modifiable risk factors, others are not. For example, being female, 10 to 25 years old and living in an industrialised society are the top three unmodifiable risk factors; genetic predisposition, a perfectionistic temperament and a history of traumatic life experiences are also unmodifiable. Dieting, disordered eating behaviours and excessive exercise, as well as body dissatisfaction, are modifiable risk factors—variables that are potentially a focus for targeted prevention activities (Paxton 2012). In terms of risk, high-frequency (or severe) dieting is the strongest predictor for the development of an eating disorder and early onset of dieting is associated with poorer physical and mental health, more disordered eating, extreme body dissatisfaction and more frequent general health problems (Tucci et al. 2007; Stice et al. 2011).

A number of risk factors are described below. Remember, though, that most young people are exposed to many of these factors and do not develop an eating disorder; it is therefore likely that an intricate interplay exists between the risk and protective factors and that the illness develops in a unique way for each individual.

Biological and Genetic Factors

Anorexia nervosa, bulimia nervosa and binge eating disorder are all familial (Mazzeo & Bulik 2009) and there is a significant body of research emerging around anorexia nervosa, in particular, which shows inherited vulnerability is a necessary component of the disorder (Strober & Johnson 2012). First-degree relatives of people who have had anorexia nervosa are around 10 times more likely to develop the disorder than someone from the general population and significantly more likely to develop an eating disorder in general. There is also a relationship between maternal depression and later anorexia nervosa in young people (Bulik et al. 2007).

While genetic research is still in its early stages, genetic factors are thought to account for more than 50% of the risk (Bulik et al. 2007) and molecular genetic studies have begun to identify chromosomal regions and genes that may contribute to the vulnerability for developing an eating disorder (Klump et al. 2009). In particular, serotonin and dopamine pathways have been studied; serotonin is involved in weight regulation, eating behaviour, mood and the development of eating disorders and dopamine has been implicated in weight loss, amenorrhoea, hyperactivity, obsessive-compulsive behaviour, repulsion to food and distorted body image (Bulik et al. 2007). Low levels of serotonin activity have been associated with impulsivity and may predispose a person to developing bulimia nervosa, whereas high levels have been associated with rigidity and constraint and may predispose to anorexia nervosa.

Alterations of central nervous system serotonin activity may directly affect eating behaviours, as well as other psychiatric symptoms such as depression and obsessive-compulsive symptoms. In fact, there is compelling evidence emerging around shared genetic factors in the development of comorbid depressive symptomatology and eating disorder, with dysregulation of the serotonergic pathways impacting on both depressive and eating disorder symptoms (Rodgers & Paxton 2014). Leptin, leptin secretion and leptin resistance have also been studied because of the complex relationships that exist around the mechanisms responsible for the regulation of food intake and the knowledge that exists around the role of leptin in obesity. However, this is only one part of a very complex picture and the research is as yet inconclusive (Stachowicz et al. 2013).

Also likely to be important are epigenetic changes to DNA structure that are not encoded by the DNA sequence itself but that nonetheless result in enduring changes in gene expression and that are transmitted to subsequent generations (Hay et al. 2014). Biological issues, such as those occurring as a result of dietary restriction and disordered eating or of excessive exercise, as well as weight loss associated with physical illness or the presence of an illness such as diabetes mellitus that requires dietary restriction, also increase the risk of developing an eating disorder.

Individual Psychological Factors

Cognitive behavioural theories have been proposed to account for the development and maintenance of eating disorders; that is, the restriction of food and other characteristic behaviours are related to the person's need to feel in control of life. The sense of control experienced reinforces the overvaluation of restrained eating, as well as the underlying body shape and weight concerns (Lavender et al. 2013). From a *psychodynamic theory perspective*, issues of separation and autonomy, involving enmeshed relationships and difficulties with the expression of anger and psychosexual development, are described (APA 2006).

A number of common personality traits can often be found in people with anorexia nervosa including low self-esteem, perfectionism, obsessionality, alexithymia and intimacy concerns, along with a sense of not feeling in control of one's life. A range of emotion regulation difficulties are also common, including feelings of guilt, disgust and shame, avoidance and negative problem solving, engaging in external comparison and submissive behaviours, worrying and ruminating and using emotional suppression to avoid conflict (Oldershaw et al. 2015).

Personality traits more common to people with bulimia nervosa include impulsivity, mood lability and self-criticism (Merlotti et al. 2013). Bulimia nervosa and binge eating disorder have been understood as manifestations of impulsivity, difficulties with emotional regulation and the experience of dissociative states, as a self-harming behaviour or even as an addictive behaviour (Lavender et al. 2015; Gearhardt et al. 2013; Curtis & Davis 2013). Urban living has been identified as a risk factor for bulimia nervosa but not for anorexia nervosa (Van Son et al. 2006).

Childhood adversity such as neglect, physical and sexual abuse and other traumatic experiences (for example, criticism, teasing, bullying about weight and shape, loss and grief) have all been associated with the development of eating disorders (Sweetingham & Waller 2008; Caslini et al. 2016). Interventions aimed at enhancing a strong sense of self-efficacy and identity and a focus on resilience and wellness are important to help children, adolescents and adults to cope with life pressures (Wand 2015).

Sociocultural and Environmental Influences

'Culture has consistently been recognised as an essential and significant factor in the cause, course and outcome of eating disorders'. In fact, early descriptions named them 'culture-bound' syndromes, describing them as belonging to Western European, American and other 'Westernised' countries like the UK (Pike et al. 2014, p. 436). However, the broader cross-cultural literature is now documenting the increasing prevalence of eating disorders in non-Westernised countries across Asia and the Middle East regions, where increased 'industrialisation, urbanisation, and globalisation' is occurring (p. 437). Eating disorders also seem to be increasing among ethnic minority groups in already developed nations such as the UK (Pike et al. 2014).

Sociocultural influences include unrealistically thin media images, the stigmatisation of fatness and the increasing use of plastic surgery, as well as valuing thinness over other personal qualities. Low self-esteem and concerns about appearance and body image are exacerbated for many young people by social and cultural pressures to conform to a particular thin ideal of beauty. Comparing one's body with others (such as peers, family or media personalities) and appearance-related teasing are recognised as factors contributing to body dissatisfaction, dieting and symptoms of disordered eating. For middle-aged women, menopausal status and anxiety around ageing are also associated with body image dissatisfaction (Selvec & Tiggerman 2011; Menzel et al. 2010). The importance of psychological function in regard to an individual's vulnerability to these types of sociocultural and environmental influences may be significant (Rogers et al. 2010).

Currently, pressure is being continually applied to the fashion, media, marketing and advertising industries to encourage the employment of models with a greater diversity of more realistic weight and body shapes. The French government has recently joined Israel, Spain and Italy in legislating against excessively underweight models working in the fashion industry. It will be interesting to see whether this pressure has any impact on lowering future incidence and prevalence rates of eating disorders.

Engaging in sports, hobbies or careers where body weight, shape and appearance are emphasised (e.g. modelling, gymnastics, body building and ballet dancing) should be considered high-risk environments, particularly for those in the at-risk population (Treasure et al. 2010).

Interpersonal Relationships

Family Relationships

There is no research evidence that proves a causative link between family functioning and the onset of eating disorders. In fact, the proportion of people with eating disorders whose families have relationship problems is thought to be about the same as in the general population (RANZCP 2009). Families need reassurance that they did not cause the eating disorder and are not to blame. Nurses need to be aware that the support and understanding that a person's family can provide are very often vital to the recovery process.

On the other hand, negative paternal comments and dieting have been known to influence self-esteem, body image and the eating behaviours of children. Family influences such as high conflict around meal times (Bulik et al. 2007), modelling eating-disordered behaviours (e.g. dieting, compulsive exercise) and eating disorder attitudes (e.g. body dissatisfaction) can be problematic. Differential parenting styles, for example where one parent is over-involved and the other is passive (Freeman 2002), and families where there is difficulty expressing and resolving conflict or who are overly controlling are more likely in cases of anorexia nervosa.

Bulimia nervosa is more likely to develop when family systems are chaotic (Hamilton 2007), where there is family discord, lack of consistency, lack of warmth and emotional connection to the child. Families of people with bulimia nervosa have also been shown to have higher rates of substance abuse, affective disorder and certain personality traits such as perfectionism (Lilenfeld et al. 2000).

Peer and Other Important Relationships

Adolescence is a time when the relationships that develop within peer groups begin to overshadow the importance of family for many young people. Peer groups that have a high level of body-related competitiveness or where there is pressure to diet or to be thin and people of influence (such as a weight-focussed coach or personal trainer) can reinforce the overvaluation of appearance that some young people experience and to which they are vulnerable. Peer groups who diet together and compare body weight and shape are extremely influential for young people. In particular, bullying or teasing around appearance is related to shame and body dissatisfaction (Sweetingham & Waller 2008).

It is important to consider the impact of all peers, including friends and connections that young people have in their online community. The increasing use of social media by young people means they are particularly vulnerable to online disinhibition (e.g. saying and doing things in an online space that they would not do in person and may later regret), which may be benign (e.g. revealing personal things about themselves) or toxic (e.g. engaging with pornography, developing rapid, false intimacy) (Suler 2004). Access to and impact of relationships developed in the context of the 'pro Ana' (pro-Anorexia) movement are also particularly influential and potentially dangerous, where 'tips and tricks' of weight loss are shared and the 'community' support each other to maintain focus and motivation on extreme thinness (Harshbarger et al. 2008).

Prevention and Protective Factors

Given the significant life impact, illness severity and treatment complexity of eating disorders, prevention is an important public health goal (Yager & O'Dea 2008). Protective factors operate by reducing the impact of risk factors and, like other mental illnesses, eating disorder protective factors can be individual, familial and/or environmental and they can be universal or targeted. For example, individual protective factors may include good social and emotional skill development (emotional wellbeing) including assertiveness, being self-directed and having a positive coping style, i.e. developing resilience. Media literacy and the ability to process media images critically are also important. Protective family factors may include family connectedness, being part of a family where the emphasis is on recognising strengths and skills unrelated to weight and appearance (rather than being weight and physical appearance focussed) and a harmonious, consistent, parenting approach. One of the simplest and best protective behaviours for families, across eating disorders and a range of other mental health concerns, is to have shared family meals (Dunifon & Cook 2012). From an environmental and sociocultural perspective, a climate where a range of body shapes and sizes are accepted, where performance is valued over physical attractiveness and where relationships (e.g. peers, teachers, community members) are supportive and caring, rather than competitive and critical, may be protective (Watson et al. 2010; Paxton 2012).

CRITICAL THINKING CHALLENGE 19.1

1. How would you describe a 'normal' interest in body image and dieting versus an obsessive interest?
2. Is your answer different for males and females?
3. Does age affect what you consider to be 'normal'?
4. Severe dieting is the single biggest risk factor for the onset of an eating disorder. There is also a focus on preventing obesity and a high incidence of dieting behaviour in the community. How might it be possible to balance these messages of risk and prevention?
5. To what extent would your own values about weight and shape influence your approach to a person suffering with an eating disorder?

PHYSICAL HEALTH

The protein calorie malnutrition seen in anorexia nervosa affects every organ in the body and the related medical complications can be life threatening. Acute complications of anorexia nervosa include bradycardia and cardiac compromise, hypotension, hypothermia, electrolyte disturbance (generally associated with purging or dehydration), gastrointestinal motility disturbances, renal problems, infertility and perinatal complications (Miller et al. 2005; NICE 2017). Measures of weight or body mass index are not necessarily good indicators of the degree of potential medical compromise. People who lose weight rapidly can become medically compromised at higher weights than those who lose weight slowly over time.

The abnormalities seen in a person with bulimia nervosa, particularly electrolyte disturbances, are usually related to frequent vomiting or laxative and diuretic misuse. Binge eating disorder carries similar medical risks and long-term consequences to those seen in obesity, such as hypertension, high blood cholesterol, heart disease and increased risk of diabetes and stroke.

Most of the medical complications of anorexia nervosa, with the exception of osteoporosis, can be reversed with restoration of adequate nutrition and maintenance of a healthy weight range. However, the long-term effect of malnutrition on cognition and brain structure and functioning requires further research.

Cardiovascular Effects

Cardiac and cardiovascular irregularities caused by malnutrition include bradycardia, hypotension and cardiac arrhythmias. Electrocardiogram (ECG) abnormalities, including a prolonged QTc interval and nonspecific ST segment depression or T wave changes, can be associated with electrolyte

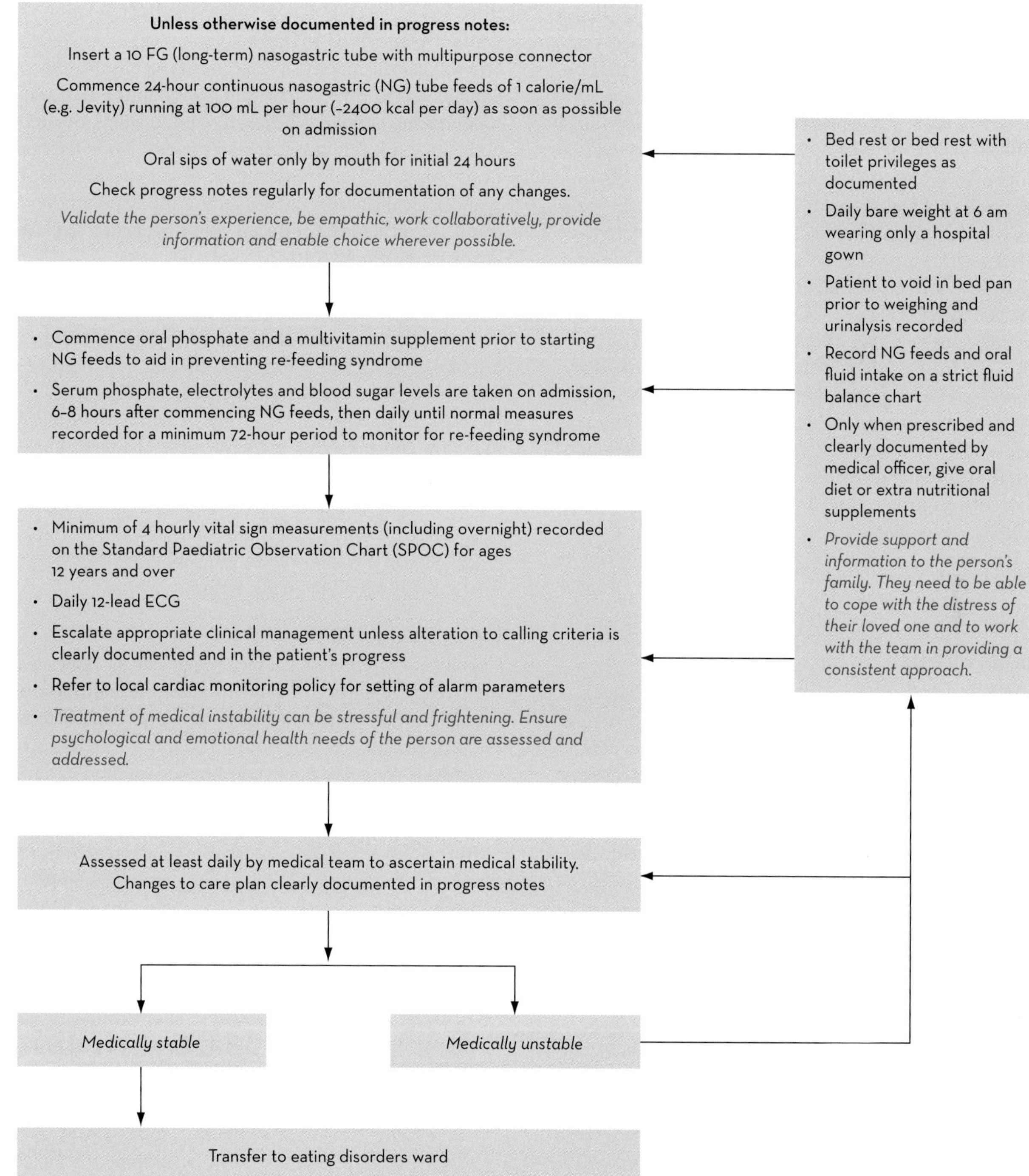

Fig. 19.1 Example of a flowchart for adolescent eating-disordered patients who are medically unstable and require cardiac monitoring (*Source:* Adapted from Anderson, G., Squire, J., Clarke, S., Kohn, M., 2015. Caring for medically unstable adolescents with anorexia nervosa requiring cardiac monitoring. Policy. Western Sydney Local Health Network, Westmead Hospital, Sydney.)

disturbances as well as malnutrition. As cardiac arrest can result from arrhythmias, hospitalisation and cardiac monitoring are recommended for patients with bradycardia or a prolonged QTc interval on ECG (see Fig. 19.1).

Electrolyte Abnormalities

Electrolyte abnormalities, including low potassium, chloride and sodium levels, are more common in the purging subtype of anorexia nervosa and in bulimia nervosa. Frequent vomiting can result in metabolic alkalosis and hypokalaemia, whereas laxative misuse can lead to metabolic acidosis, hyponatraemia and hypokalaemia.

Renal Dysfunction

Reduced glomerular filtration rate, elevated serum urea nitrogen and hypovolaemia can occur in both anorexia and bulimia nervosa. Reduced urine production can indicate severe dehydration or progressive renal insufficiency. Associated renal failure is sometimes seen in adult patients, especially in those whose illness has become chronic.

Gastrointestinal Effects

People who severely restrict their dietary intake over time describe feeling bloated or full even after eating small amounts of food, which can indicate shrinking of the stomach or delayed gastric emptying. Binge eating, on the other hand, can lead to gastric dilation and, in rare cases, stomach rupture or death (RANZCP 2004).

Diarrhoea can be a sign of laxative abuse, while constipation can result from inadequate food (and fibre) intake, dehydration or decrease in gastric motility. It should be noted that laxatives used by patients can include those found in common household food supplies, such as artificial sweeteners, chewing gum and diet drinks.

Recurrent vomiting can lead to enlarged parotid and salivary glands, oesophagitis or oesophageal or gastric tears. Abdominal pain or involuntary regurgitation of food can be associated with both the trauma and the frequency of vomiting.

Endocrine Effects

Amenorrhoea in anorexia nervosa is a result of the effects of protein–calorie malnutrition on central regulatory structures such as the pituitary gland and the hypothalamus, in combination with decreased secretion of a hormone secreted by fat cells in the body called leptin (Kohn et al. 2009). Decreased serum testosterone levels and accompanying loss of libido are commonly found in underweight males. Women with bulimia may have irregular menstrual periods.

Thyroid function (in particular, T_3 levels) may be depressed in low-weight patients with anorexia nervosa and is consistent with clinical findings such as dry skin and brittle hair, fatigue and cold intolerance.

Musculoskeletal Effects

Osteopenia, osteoporosis and associated risk of fractures are common in longstanding and severe cases of anorexia nervosa (Grinspoon et al. 2000; NICE 2017). Irreversibly decreased bone mineral density is associated with prolonged malnutrition, low oestrogen levels and amenorrhoea for longer than 6 months and decreased muscle mass. A dual-energy X-ray absorptiometry (DEXA) scan is generally ordered to assess bone mineral density when a woman with an eating disorder has experienced amenorrhoea for longer than 6 consecutive months. Linear growth retardation can occur in children when the onset of the disorder occurs before closure of the epiphyses.

Dental and Oral Effects

Dental erosion and subsequent caries can occur with recurrent self-induced vomiting. Riboflavin deficiency may cause fissures of the lips, especially in the corners of the mouth, and iron and zinc deficiencies cause glossitis and loss of taste sensation (Royal College of Psychiatrists [RCP] 2005).

Skin/Integument Effects

Protein–calorie malnutrition leads to loss of subcutaneous fat. Lanugo, a fine, downy hair that grows on the face and body, is often seen. Lanugo is believed to be an adaptation to loss of body fat and it functions to help preserve body temperature. Cool hands and feet with bluish discolouration (peripheral cyanosis), calluses on the dorsum of the dominant hand as a result of repeated self-induced vomiting, brittle nails and dry skin are commonly seen.

Neurological Effects

Structural changes in the brain including loss of brain volume, cerebral atrophy and ventricular dilation have been reported in malnourished and emaciated patients (Klump et al. 2009; Fairburn & Harrison 2003; Rome & Ammerman 2003) and there are concerns that some of these changes persist even after nutritional rehabilitation. Loss of brain white matter (composed mainly of omega-3 fatty acids) is also profound as this affects brain structure and function (Kohn et al. 2009). Severe electrolyte imbalances can lead to abnormal electrical discharges in the brain and seizures.

Cognitive Changes

Cognitive and emotional functioning deficits associated with the biological impact of protein–calorie malnutrition include impaired concentration, memory and comprehension and a pervasive preoccupation with food and weight-related issues. In children and adolescents, poor concentration can lead to difficulties keeping up with schoolwork and special consideration should be requested from education departments for important exams.

The profound effects on cognitive function and, in particular, executive functioning impair the person's ability to engage in psychological interventions. This impairment underscores the need for nutritional rehabilitation to a minimum healthy weight in order to enhance effective use of psychotherapeutic interventions and ultimate emotional and psychological recovery.

Refusing care, being ambivalent about engaging in treatment and denying the severity of illness are common, even when the person is seriously unwell. These are aspects of the eating disorders that can seriously challenge a health practitioner's skills and test their patience. It is important for nurses to understand that the person is not trying to be purposefully difficult; these behaviours are part of the disorder. In rare situations, where the illness places the person in a life-threatening position (e.g. they are extremely depressed or expressing delusional beliefs about not needing to eat) and they are unwilling or unable to agree to treatment, legal intervention should be considered, including involuntary hospitalisation under mental health legislation (see Chapter 4) or, for children and young adolescents, notification to social services whose role is to promote the safety and wellbeing of children. A person's values and sense of identity change in response to anorexia nervosa and, while they may understand or appreciate this in terms of the illness, their capacity to make an informed decision about treatment will be an important consideration for clinicians (Ayton et al. 2008).

How restrictive practices are used is of fundamental importance. While it may be necessary to mandate treatment, implicit coercion should never be used. Restrictive and coercive practices can be experienced as traumatic and reduce the person's feeling of control over their own life. They can also retraumatise a person and reduce the likelihood of them voluntarily engaging with and seeking help from health services in the future. There is a difference between a therapeutic intervention and an intervention that is implemented for safety under emergency circumstances. While many people with anorexia nervosa who are treated involuntarily and their families later agree that involuntary treatment was necessary, being treated involuntarily is not therapeutic in and of itself. However, if the intervention is to be seen as something helpful, as opposed to punitive and coercive, the focus should be on providing care and treatment in a collaborative manner with the person and their family. As always, using the least restrictive treatment context is always the goal (Hay et al. 2014).

MENTAL HEALTH

The psychological and emotional aspects of eating disorders are significant and can be devastating for the person and their family. There are four aspects of mental health that need to be considered.

First, the underlying psychological and emotional issues that may have been important in the aetiology of the illness have to be considered. These might be related to the individual risk factors outlined earlier and are the issues need to be addressed over longer-term treatment.

Second, most people with eating disorders experience comorbid mental health issues and lifetime comorbidity is high, particularly with major depressive disorder, anxiety disorder, posttraumatic stress disorder, obsessive-compulsive disorder, substance abuse/dependence and personality disorder (especially obsessive-compulsive personality disorder). Anxiety disorders frequently predate the onset of an eating disorder and anxiety may also develop or worsen as treatment progresses and weight is restored. Substance misuse is also a significant issue, occurring particularly in people who engage in binge eating and/or purging as part of their clinical picture (Glasner-Edwards et al. 2011). This includes the use of legal and illicit substances such as alcohol, tobacco, amphetamines, methamphetamines and the typical drugs used for weight loss, such as caffeine, emetics, diet pills (teas/herbs), diuretics and laxatives. Some studies support a familial relationship between substance use disorders and eating disorders and monitoring for substance misuse throughout treatment is recommended (though it is less likely in children and adolescents) (Herzog et al. 2006; Piran & Gadalla 2007). Comorbid mental health problems increase the complexity of treatment for an eating disorder. Moderate to high agitation and distress and comorbid mental illness may increase the person's risk and indicate that hospitalisation is required.

Third, the cognitive and psychological effects of starvation and the symptoms of the illnesses themselves can complicate the mental health picture. For example:

- Symptoms of depression such as low mood, irritability and social withdrawal are common in very underweight people and are the result of malnutrition. These symptoms do not necessarily warrant a separate diagnosis of major depression as they often reverse with nutritional rehabilitation.
- Obsessive-compulsive behaviours (see Chapter 19) might be observed, particularly in people with anorexia nervosa, and usually take the form of repetitive counting and ritualistic eating patterns such as chewing food a certain number of times or not allowing different foods on the plate to touch. Again, unless the condition predated the onset of the eating disorder, the obsessive-compulsive symptoms tend to resolve with nutritional rehabilitation.

Fourth, the increased anxiety and emotional distress that accompanies treatment (requiring weight gain, normalising eating and addressing underlying psychological issues) can be harrowing for the person and their family. Supportive nursing interventions including validation, empathy, externalising the illness and working collaboratively with the person and their family are therefore important (Rodgers & Paxton 2014; O'Brien & Golding 2003; Kaye et al. 2004; Hay et al. 2014).

From a mental health perspective, the high prevalence of suicidality experienced by people who have eating disorders is most worrying. In particular, anorexia nervosa is associated with high rates of suicide. Self-injurious behaviours are also common in people with eating disorders: they are more frequent in adolescents with eating disorders, those with comorbid mental health problems and those whose eating disorder includes binge and purge symptoms (Kostro et al. 2014). Asking the person about suicidal ideation and active self-harm is essential. Questions like, 'Have things been so bad with the eating that you have wanted to harm yourself in any way?' will not trigger the person towards suicidal or self-harming behaviours. More likely, the person will be relieved to know that someone understands how severe the disorder has become and how bad they are feeling. Nurses need to respond to all expressions of suicidality in this very high-risk group.

ASSESSMENT

A comprehensive multidisciplinary assessment will determine whether the criteria for diagnosis of a specific eating disorder are met and identifies symptoms and behaviours that require intervention in the individual's treatment programme. This is also the opportunity for health practitioners to establish rapport with the person and to get to know them as an individual. A collaborative approach to assessment and treatment planning is an important part of engaging the person with recovery. It is important that screening tools are not used as the sole method to determine whether a person has an eating disorder (NICE 2017). Patient Story 19.3 about Poppy talks about assessment of a young person with an eating disorder.

PATIENT STORY 19.3

Poppy

Poppy is 17 years old. Her mother is worried about her weight loss and lack of interest in food over the past few months. Poppy has always been thin, but the weight loss began when life stresses made her feel fairly sad some months before and she says she simply lost her appetite. Poppy discovered that she felt better if she didn't eat and has avoided doing so even when she does occasionally feel hungry. When she has been forced to eat, Poppy complains of feeling sick and usually vomits. There are no underlying medical problems. Poppy does well at school but finds socialising difficult and describes herself as 'a loner'. She lives with her mother, younger brother and stepfather and sees her father every second weekend as she has done since she was three. She has a close relationship with all three caregivers who are on reasonably amicable terms. Poppy says her main worry is her dad, who is still single and has recently been drinking heavily, which makes her feel sad and worried. She has been wondering if she should move in with him because she feels sorry for him and bad that he is all alone when she's not there.

Health practitioner: I'm not 100% sure what to do with someone who has an eating disorder . . . I don't tend to see them. She looked OK to me, but her mother said she's basically been eating less than 500 calories a day (2090 kilojoules) for weeks.

Eating disorder support service: What is her BMI? What were her observations?

Health practitioner: Oh, I got her weight, she's 45 kg, but I didn't get a height. She said she felt fine.

Learning Point

All practitioners will at some stage see people who have eating disorders or who are engaging in disordered eating behaviours. Many clinicians do not feel that they have enough experience or knowledge to identify when a person is experiencing an eating disorder or how to manage emerging issues with eating, so they feel uncomfortable asking questions that may identify a problem. People with eating disorders, especially people with anorexia nervosa (or emerging disorder), are at high risk in terms of their own health and safety, and the sooner the illness or the risk is identified, the better the outcome for the person.

Physical Assessment

The physical assessment, including blood chemistry, urinalysis and ECG, helps detect any significant medical complications. It is also important to exclude other causes of weight loss. A medical examination includes weight and height measures, vital signs, cardiovascular and peripheral vascular function, metabolic status, dermatological manifestations and evidence of self-harm (APA 2006).

Medical complications develop at higher weights in those who lose weight rapidly and recording the history of highest and lowest weights since the onset of the eating disorder helps assess the rapidity and course of weight loss. It is also useful to note any significant relationships between life events and weight loss as this gives insight into potential contributing factors that can be addressed in treatment. In adults, height and weight are used to calculate BMI (see Box 19.5), which helps determine the degree of starvation. Children and adolescents younger than 16 years of age are assessed on percentage of ideal body weight or gender-specific standardised growth charts. Rather than asking the child or adolescent to undress, sexual or pubertal development can be assessed by asking them to point to the diagrammatic picture most closely matching their own body development on the Tanner stages rating scales that accompany standardised child growth charts.

BOX 19.5 Calculation of Body Mass Index

To calculate body mass index (BMI), divide the person's weight (in kilograms) by their height (in metres squared). For example, a person who is 163 cm (1.63 m) tall and weighs 55 kg would have a body mass index of 20.70, which is within the normal range.

To calculate:

$$1.63 \times 1.63 = 2.656$$

$$55 \div 2.656 = \text{a BMI of } 20.70$$

An online calculator is available at: https://www.nhs.uk/live-well/healthy-weight/bmi-calculator

Mental Health Assessment

The mental health/psychiatric assessment will confirm the specific diagnosis, identify comorbid mental illness and exclude possible differential diagnoses such as major depression, which can present as loss of appetite and weight loss, without the body image disturbance and fear of weight gain seen in eating disorders. Other aspects of the person's mental health status that influence the clinical course and outcome will be assessed, including mood and anxiety, substance use, motivation to engage with treatment, personality traits and family support (Hay et al. 2014).

A mental state assessment should be conducted and cognitive changes that may have occurred due to starvation should be identified, in particular, slowed thought processes, short-term memory impairments, changes in cognitive flexibility, difficulty with attention and poor concentration (Hatch et al. 2010).

Psychosocial factors that should be reviewed in the mental health assessment include the person's family history (including eating disorders and other mental illness in family members), attachment and developmental issues, any interpersonal problems or relationship issues that particularly impact the person, as well as trauma or significant life events (Hay et al. 2014).

Denial of illness and minimisation of symptoms are common in people with anorexia nervosa and can complicate the assessment process (Couturier & Lock 2006). Parents or carers of children and adolescents are generally interviewed as part of the assessment process to help validate findings and provide a family history that is helpful in identifying risk and protective factors.

Body Image Assessment

It is common for attitudes towards one's own body to develop during childhood and early adolescence and for dissatisfaction with body image to increase during adolescence and into young adulthood. These negative perceptions can be maintained throughout adulthood.

From an assessment point of view, it is useful to understand the person's perception of their weight during childhood and to identify any significant events that might have triggered negative responses to body image, such as teasing, bullying or criticism about weight or body shape. Assessing the degree and nature of body image disturbance and fear of weight gain assists in diagnosis, in understanding the severity of the disorder and in guiding treatment. Assessment of body image has several components:

1. *Body image distortion:* a multidimensional phenomenon consisting of perceptual disturbance, cognitive-affective and behavioural components, in which people describe their body or parts of it as large or fat despite concrete evidence to the contrary (Schneider et al. 2009).
2. *Body image dissatisfaction:* a disturbance of cognition and affect that leads to a negative evaluation of physical appearance. Body image dissatisfaction may be considered 'normative' because it is highly prevalent in the general community, not just in people with eating disorders. However, this does not mean it is benign. Even in women without eating disorders, body image dissatisfaction is associated with significant quality of life impairment, particularly around mental health, psychosocial functioning and physical health (Mond et al. 2013).
3. *Body-related avoidance:* avoidance behaviours can be personal or situational. Avoiding confrontation with one's own body (e.g. by not looking in mirrors or avoiding taking baths where the body is clearly visible) is thought to be related to body image distortion (Vossbeck-Elsebusch et al. 2014). Body-related avoidance behaviour significantly contributes to body size overestimation. Situational avoidance involves avoiding environments or social situations that provoke anxiety about the body, such as going to the beach.
4. *Body checking behaviours* such as feeling bones, weighing oneself many times a day or only looking at one part of the body may also be assessed.

Simple questions that can provide insight into the person's body image include:

'When I look at you, I can see that you are very thin. How do you see yourself?'

'People often *feel* fat, even when they are not. How do you feel about your body?'

'Some people weigh themselves many times a day, do you do this?'

'When you look in the mirror, do you focus on one particular part of your body, or look at your body as a whole?'

'What weight do you think is the right weight for you? What weight would you like to be?'

CRITICAL THINKING CHALLENGE 19.2

1. Think about your personal body image, weight and shape perception. What has influenced how you feel about these aspects of yourself?
2. Do you believe that your body image has been affected more by your individual temperament or by family, cultural and social issues?
3. To what extent have images in the mass media affected your body image?
4. How might your own body image, weight and shape perceptions impact how you provide nursing care and a therapeutic relationship with a person who has an eating disorder?

Nutritional and Exercise Assessment

A dietician on the multidisciplinary team usually performs a comprehensive nutritional assessment. The dietary history is used to identify specific deficiencies and should include information about the person's nutritional (food and fluid) intake, as well as any behaviours designed to reduce or control appetite (e.g. caffeine, smoking), alcohol use, use of supplements (e.g. vitamins, herbal preparations) and frequency of self-measurement of weight (RCP 2005). Energy input and output are assessed, including the amount and types of food eaten and avoided, and the degree of any compensatory behaviours including over exercising, bingeing and purging used to control weight gain. Many people with anorexia nervosa and sometimes people with bulimia nervosa avoid whole food groups (typically meat protein, dairy products or carbohydrates). Because of the person's beliefs about uncontrollable weight gain, some foods can be considered 'fear foods'.

Excessive exercise is a significant issue in 30% to 70% of people with eating disorders, more commonly in those with anorexia than bulimia nervosa. It can be used as a compensatory behaviour to avoid weight gain or as a weight loss mechanism. Excessive exercise can be identified where a person experiences negative emotionality (e.g. intense guilt) when exercise is missed or postponed or where hard exercise is focussed primarily on influencing weight or shape (Mond & Calogero 2009) (instead of on enjoyment). Asking people what the goal of their exercise is will help determine if it is excessive and associated with the eating disorder.

Assessing Disordered Eating Behaviours and Rituals

Disordered eating behaviours commonly seen in people with anorexia nervosa are driven by fear of weight gain. In inpatient settings, nurses can assess the extent of the person's struggle with food when observing mealtime behaviours. Box 19.6 provides examples of some frequently observed eating abnormalities.

People with eating disorders sometimes utilise excessive amounts of some condiments or foods that they perceive may be of benefit in terms of weight loss. For example, a common addition to meals is chilli sauce which, in the absence

BOX 19.6 Examples of Eating-Related Abnormal Behaviours

- Refusing to eat
- Cutting out particular foods (e.g. cake, cheese, chocolate) or whole food groups (e.g. carbohydrates, fats)
- Cutting up food into tiny pieces and then eating the pieces individually, or by colour, or in groups of numbers (e.g. two peas followed by two pieces of carrot)
- Attempting to remove any oil and fats from food (e.g. pressing food into absorbent serviettes and scraping butter from sandwiches)
- Restricting food so as to eat the same thing every day
- Fear of touching food or having different food groups touch on the plate
- Eating painfully slowly and without enjoyment
- Constantly fidgeting at the table: this could be related to anxiety or to the physical hyperactivity that can be activated by starvation
- Obsessive kilojoule counting and/or measuring of all food quantities
- Leaving the table during or immediately after the meal, usually to purge or throw away food hidden during the meal
- Excessive use of diet foods or diet products
- Excessive preoccupation with the preparation and serving of food to others, but not eating it
- Avoiding eating with others in a social context

of concrete evidence, the person may believe increases their metabolic rate. Large quantities of fluid can help suppress hunger and it is not unusual for a person with an eating disorder to drink copious amounts of diet drinks, coffee or water if they perceive this as helpful in avoiding weight gain. Secretive consumption of water just prior to being weighed (water loading) often occurs in an attempt to give a false impression of weight gain.

Hunger is the strongest trigger for binge eating and people with bulimia nervosa commonly skip breakfast and lunch and then binge eat at night in response to the body's hunger signals. Bingeing can be spontaneous or planned and it can occur in a ritualistic manner; for example, the binge might occur at the same time and place every day or it might only happen on certain nights of the week when there is no-one else around or the binge might progress with foods in a particular order. It can cause great anxiety to a person if their planned binge episode is prevented or interrupted or events outside their control impact them carrying out the ritual. Some people with bulimia will, over time, choose food that is easily regurgitated or food that is economical if they cannot finance their binges (which can be very expensive). A binge episode is usually terminated in response to one or more of the following: abdominal fullness, distension and pain, running out of food or social interruptions.

Self-induced vomiting usually follows a binge episode and techniques used to induce vomiting include putting fingers or another implement such as a toothbrush down the throat or spontaneous regurgitation after eating. Signs that vomiting may be occurring in people with anorexia nervosa include weight loss or no weight gain despite apparent adherence to a prescribed nutritional programme, leaving the dining table immediately after a meal to go to the shower or toilet or the smell or presence of vomit in the toilet, sink or shower.

Diuretic and laxative abuse tends to be ineffective in achieving real weight loss. Diuretics cause fluid loss and laxatives work on the large bowel in which only approximately 12% of the nutrition from food is absorbed and therefore most nutrition is absorbed in the small bowel before the laxatives act.

It is important for nurses to approach discussing disordered eating behaviours and rituals sensitively and in a matter-of-fact and non-judgemental way. The person may be deeply embarrassed by some of their behaviours, which they may perceive as disgusting; they may also be protective of the behaviours as part of the disorder or worried that they will be forced to change what they are doing immediately, causing massive weight gain. Asking questions about disordered eating behaviours can be made less threatening by using statements that indicate that other people also experience similar issues; for example, 'Many people who experience an eating disorder do things that they feel help them to control their eating or weight, such as vomiting or using other ways of getting rid of food. Has this ever been something that you have tried?'

Family Assessment

There is no evidence that proves families cause eating disorders (Le Grange 2010). In fact, blaming family members is harmful and could impair their desire, willingness and capacity to participate actively and constructively in the process of treatment and recovery. What is helpful, though, is to assess the quality of family relationships, the level of support available within the family, the way family members communicate with each other, family attitudes towards eating and appearance and the effect the eating disorder has on family and social relationships. A family history of eating disorder, mental illness or substance use may have implications for treatment. During the assessment, be aware that many families and carers are emotionally exhausted by their own struggle to help their family member to manage the eating disorder and that feelings of guilt, failure, anger, blame and fear are common.

Family involvement has been identified in the literature as useful in reducing both medical and psychiatric morbidity, particularly for younger patients with a short duration of eating disorder (Le Grange 2010). There is some contention in the literature as to the reported efficacy of family-based treatment (see the debate generated around Strober 2014). What is not in contention is that engaging parents and families of children and adolescents during the assessment stage is essential, as their ongoing support of treatment and, for some, participation in family therapy may prove essential in optimising the outcome for the young person. Working with family members to develop their skills has been shown to increase feelings of efficacy and to reduce the impact of the eating disorder in terms of anxiety and psychological distress (Macdonald et al. 2010).

While family involvement is strongly encouraged, confidentiality issues must be taken into account for both adolescents and adults and these should be clearly discussed during the assessment period. The decision to involve families, spouses and/or partners of adult patients should be made in consultation with the patient.

The importance of the nurse's role in supporting families through the treatment process cannot be overstated and is discussed later in the chapter. At the family assessment stage, it can be useful to provide information about the eating disorder and to help family members to understand the challenges and opportunities that are associated with the disorder.

TREATMENT AND RECOVERY

Treatment for people with eating disorders, as with other mental illnesses, should be provided within a recovery framework (Hay et al. 2014). This includes taking a holistic approach:

- recognising and embracing the person's capacity to recover, including their strengths and skills
- maximising self-determination and self-management practices
- working with families
- providing evidence-informed treatment, therapy and support focussed on maximising mental health and physical health outcomes
- supporting positive risk taking wherever possible
- providing care in the least restrictive treatment context
- promoting safety

There is no doubt that eating disorders can be challenging to treat, but recovery is always possible and should be the goal. On average, the recovery process is likely to take around 5 to 7 years, with remission and relapse of symptoms often occurring during this time. The illness duration can range from less than 1 year in children and adolescents who are identified and treated early to a long-term or lifetime of illness.

Several studies have explored the treatment experience from the perspectives of both people with eating disorders (Malson et al. 2004; Zugai et al. 2013) and nursing staff (Ramjan 2004; Ryan et al. 2006; Tierney 2008). These studies highlight the complexity of treatment and some of the frustrations experienced by both patients and healthcare professionals.

Services available for treating people with eating disorders include outpatient and day patient programmes and inpatient care in both medical and psychiatric settings. Determining the most appropriate treatment service will depend on the person's age and their physical and mental health, as well as the availability of expert local healthcare providers. A multidisciplinary team approach is needed because medical and nursing care, nutritional rehabilitation, psychological therapy and, particularly in children and adolescents, family-based therapy are all integral parts of treatment.

The priorities for treating people with anorexia nervosa have been described by the RANZCP as:

- engaging with the person through the use of a non-judgemental, inclusive, empathic and nonthreatening approach
- engaging with the person's family and enlisting their support in appealing to the 'healthy' part of their loved one
- medical stabilisation and addressing medical complications
- reversing the cognitive effects of starvation
- providing structured psychological treatment, including support and psychoeducation, building the therapeutic relationship in the first instance and later when the person is sufficiently stabilised from a medical/cognitive perspective in terms of the effects of starvation, individualised therapies (Hay et al. 2014)

The Royal College of Psychiatrists (2010) MARSIPAN guidelines also identify the tasks of an inpatient team working with patients with anorexia nervosa who are very sick as being:

- safely re-feeding the person
- avoiding re-feeding syndrome and underfeeding
- managing the behavioural issues that arise during treatment
- using compulsory treatment where necessary
- managing family concerns
- working collaboratively to provide medical and mental healthcare in the most appropriate setting (e.g. medical healthcare for medical stabilisation and mental healthcare when medically stable)

People with anorexia nervosa rarely seek treatment of their own accord; when they do, fear and ambivalence about complying with treatment are always present, largely because the eating disorder gives the person a sense of identity, control and accomplishment that they do not otherwise feel. Ambivalence and resistance to treatment are not purposefully designed to aggravate healthcare professionals; they are the tricky aspects of the illness that nurses (and others) need to address by collaborating with the person.

People with bulimia nervosa who seek treatment are generally managed in primary care by a psychologist specialising in working with people with bulimia nervosa and a GP through an outpatient eating disorder clinic or a day patient programme. The aims of treatment have been described by the APA (2006) as:

- reducing and eliminating (where possible) binge eating and purging behaviours
- treating the physical complications of the illness
- supporting and enhancing the person's ability to restore healthy eating patterns and engage fully with treatment
- providing information and education about normal eating (including healthy nutrition and eating patterns)
- helping the person to assess and to address the psychological aspects of the illness (including their thoughts, feelings, attitudes, beliefs, motives, conflicts)
- treating a co-occurring mental health issue, including anxiety or mood disorder, and addressing issues such as impulse control, emotion regulation and other self-esteem and behavioural issues that contribute to the maintenance of the illness
- engaging with the person's family to enlist their support; providing family therapy/counselling where possible and appropriate
- engaging in relapse prevention

PATIENT STORY 19.4

Lizzie

Lizzie is a 24-year-old woman who has been admitted to the acute mental health unit for the third time in 18 months. She has a 10-year history of anorexia nervosa and although she has spent most of the last 10 years out of hospital and has completed her university studies, she has not been able to achieve a healthy weight since she was first diagnosed. Lizzie has been having individual psychotherapy on and off for the past 5 years and is estranged from her family. Two years ago Lizzie was sexually assaulted on the way home from the library one night. She has been extremely unwell since that time.

When Lizzie is admitted, she had lost all the weight she put on at the last hospital admission. She is very medically compromised, tearful, defeated and psychologically unwell, requiring one-to-one nursing care. She struggles desperately with the eating disorder and, by her own admission, tries to hide food, tampers with the nasogastric tube (even though she has agreed to have it inserted) and sabotages the programme that is developed for her by exercising in secret when she gets an opportunity. Lizzie says that she wants to recover, but feels like nobody can help her.

Nursing Response Option 1

The nursing staff in the handover roll their eyes when they hear that Lizzie is back. 'What a surprise . . . She's never going to get better. I don't know why we bother! I don't know why she bothers! She's such a difficult patient.'

Nursing Response Option 2

The nursing staff in the handover empathise with Lizzie's struggle. They know how difficult she is finding recovery and they are cognisant of the trauma that she has experienced and the toll the illness is taking on her physical and mental health. They understand that recovery from anorexia nervosa can be a long-term process. They are keen to know why the discharge plan didn't adequately support Lizzie to maintain her weight after discharge. They are determined to support Lizzie to pick up the pieces and they hold hope for her recovery. 'Lizzie must be feeling so defeated being back here so soon. I wonder what happened when she left here last time? She was sounding so positive and seemed determined to keep her weight up. It's going to be really important for us to be focussed on what she wants to achieve while she's here and to try to work out how to support her better when she's back in the community'.

Self-Reflection

1. If you were Lizzie, who would you prefer to work with on your admission plan, the nurses with response 1 or the nurses with response 2? Who would you be more likely to open up to, to share your feelings with?
2. How do you think Lizzie would feel returning to a unit where response 1 was the prevailing atmosphere? Response 2?
3. Reflect on your own attitudes and values around the eating disorders. How might they impact on someone you were working with?

People with binge eating disorder are generally treated on an outpatient basis. The aims of treatment include normalising eating patterns, reducing or eliminating binge episodes, stabilising weight within a healthy weight range, effectively treating any underlying psychopathology and preventing relapse.

Hospitalisation

People with an eating disorder are generally admitted to hospital when they require nursing care. They may be at imminent risk of serious medical sequelae or complications of the illness, they may be experiencing significant mental health symptoms associated with the illness or outpatient treatment may not be working (Hay et al. 2014). Patient Story 19.4 about Lizzie describes the experience of presenting to the emergency department with an eating disorder.

People with anorexia nervosa or OSFED are more likely to become medically compromised and require hospitalisation than those with bulimia nervosa. Box 19.7 lists some of the medical indications for hospitalisation. Other indications for admission include significant risk of self-harm, psychiatric symptoms or comorbidity requiring hospitalisation, and severe family dysfunction or abusive relationships.

Prior to or early in the admission, the person's healthy weight range will be calculated (see the section 'Monitoring weight gain' later in this chapter). This will establish the likely discharge weight and provides an opportunity for other goals of admission to be developed in collaboration with the person. Inpatient programmes generally consist of either a short-term admission for medical stabilisation or a longer admission for weight restoration and normalisation of eating. Restoration of weight to a minimum healthy BMI is recommended as this

BOX 19.7 Medical Indications for Hospitalisation

- Children: heart rate <50 bpm
- Adults: heart rate <40 bpm
- Children: blood pressure <80 mmHg systolic and 50 mmHg diastolic
- Adults: blood pressure <90 mmHg systolic and 60 mmHg diastolic
- Postural systolic blood pressure drop >20 mmHg
- Temperature <35.4°C
- Cardiac rhythm or conduction disturbance, e.g. prolonged QTc interval (>450 ms) on ECG
- Severe electrolyte abnormalities
- Acute dehydration
- Weight <75% of predicted ideal body weight
- Arrested growth and development in children and adolescents
- Medical complications with insulin-dependent diabetes or at-risk pregnancy
- Uncontrollable bingeing and purging
- Acute psychiatric emergency

ECG, Electrocardiogram.

facilitates the person's ability to engage cognitively in ongoing outpatient psychotherapy. A brief admission for 24 to 48 hours for medical stabilisation only is not conducive to recovery and will likely result in rapid readmission with the person in a worse physical or psychological condition (CEDD 2015).

Inpatient programmes aim to provide a structured yet nurturing environment that includes behavioural modification strategies targeted towards weight gain and challenging and addressing abnormal eating behaviours (Kohn et al. 2009). Behavioural programmes are usually based on rewarding progress such as safe eating and weight gain with increased physical activity. An activity 'level system', through which the patient progresses, usually incorporates strict bed rest while the person is physically compromised, bed rest with toilet privileges, ambulation on, then off, the ward and then increasing time out of hospital to practise normal eating behaviours in the home and community environment. When the person is medically stable, increasing levels of supervised activity/physiotherapy, including stretching and strengthening exercises, help the person to regain muscle and bone health. For children and adolescents, ongoing school education during hospitalisation is incorporated into the inpatient programme whenever possible.

It is essential for patients, families and staff to have realistic expectations and clear goals for the admission. It is important for everyone in the family to understand that the hospital process is just one part of the recovery process: no-one leaves hospital 'cured' from an eating disorder—recovery can be a long process involving ongoing weight restoration, normalisation of eating patterns and talking therapy. Ideally, when someone leaves hospital they are medically stable, on the way towards weight restoration and, as a result, have a greater cognitive capacity to engage effectively with a psychotherapeutic intervention, be that individual or family-based (or both).

Like any mental illness, recovery from an eating disorder is a challenging personal journey that takes time and courage. It requires self-knowledge, self-compassion and the support of friends, family and health professionals. Relapse of symptoms and two or more admissions to hospital are not uncommon. To avoid the person feeling defeated and like a failure or becoming helpless and institutionalised after several admissions, it is particularly important that every hospitalisation involves collaboratively developing a plan for the admission that includes clearly defined goals. Some units develop patient contracts outlining goals and expected progress/behaviour during the admission. The usual caveat is that the person will be discharged if they are not making good progress during the hospitalisation. In order that this kind of contract does not feel punitive, nurses need to work very closely with the person to help them achieve their goals. They also need to be mindful of their approach and how important this is to how a person feels about the admission and what they can achieve. Nurses need to be aware of any attitudes, beliefs or values that they hold that may impact (or impair) their clinical efficacy.

Nutritional Rehabilitation

Re-feeding or nutritional rehabilitation is indicated whenever there is evidence of protein–calorie malnutrition. The cornerstones of nutritional treatment are education, meal planning, establishing regular eating patterns and discouraging dieting (American Dietetic Association [ADA] 2006). Everyone with an eating disorder will be fearful of excessive weight gain, particularly in the early stages of eating normally and the nurse should provide reassurance that the aim is to increase weight only to a minimum healthy weight where the body can begin to function normally. The person is encouraged to eat a wide variety of foods and 'fear foods' are introduced slowly, with nursing staff providing reassurance and encouragement and validating the difficulty of recovery.

An experienced dietician works collaboratively with the person to develop a meal plan designed to achieve a prescribed weekly weight gain (RCP 2005). Someone who is suffering from binge eating disorder may benefit from a behavioural weight-management programme incorporating a low-kilojoule diet to assist with weight loss and reduction of bingeing. Meal plans will include regular meals and snacks and nutritional supplementation may be required for malnourished patients who are struggling with their intake. These are given either as a drink or via a nasogastric tube. Nasogastric tube feeding is usually considered when the person is medically compromised and cannot eat sufficient food to reverse the medical complications and achieve adequate weight gain.

To prevent the growth and developmental consequences of malnutrition, emphasis is placed on re-feeding children and adolescents to a minimum healthy weight. When initiated, it has been suggested that nasogastric feeds should initially be given continuously over a 24-hour period to avoid low blood sugar levels from the effects of delayed insulin phase and metabolic changes and that the supplemental feed should contain less than 40% carbohydrate (Kohn et al. 2011). Once the person starts eating adequate amounts of food during the day, the nasogastric feed can be given overnight and then stopped. People's reactions to nasogastric feeds are varied (Neiderman et al. 2001). Some express relief that they do not have to eat what they perceive to be enormous amounts of food required for weight gain and view positively the fact that the initial responsibility for weight gain has been taken away from them (Abraham & Llewellyn-Jones 2001). Others struggle with the invasive nature of the tube and the lack of control they feel they have over their nutritional intake. Supporting them to cope with the distressing thoughts that accompany nutritional rehabilitation is an important role for the nurse. Regardless of how they are delivered, nutritional supplements are given for the shortest possible time; ultimately, the person needs to re-learn how to eat food normally.

Nursing Care of People who are Medically Unstable

Nurses working with people who have severe and complex eating disorders and who are medically unstable require both medical and mental health knowledge and skills. Medical resuscitation and stabilisation of any medical instability always take priority if the patient has been admitted to hospital with life-threatening complications. If the patient is bradycardic on admission, continuous cardiac monitoring and daily 12-lead ECGs are recommended. Four-hourly vital sign measures including heart rate, temperature and blood pressure are recorded until normal readings are sustained for a minimum of 72 hours. Overnight vital sign measurements, taken when the body is most at rest, provide invaluable insight into the body's ability to maintain homeostasis. Nasogastric supplemental feeds administered either continuously or overnight are vital in reversing medical instability when patients are unable to consume sufficient kilojoules orally.

Examples of nursing responsibilities in this situation include:

- monitoring the patient's physical safety and containment
- documenting vital signs and acting as per local protocols when vital signs indicate medical instability
- empathising with the person and validating their experience
- initiating and encouraging the prescribed re-feeding process and documenting eating behaviours
- inserting and ensuring the patency of any nasogastric tubes and acting to prevent the patient from tampering with feeds
- monitoring for clinical signs of re-feeding syndrome (see the following section)
- talking with the person about their emotional response to admission and providing therapeutic support and psychoeducation to help contain the anxiety and distress of both the patient and their family
- administering any prescribed medication, including Sandoz phosphate, which is given as a prophylaxis to very malnourished patients to prevent re-feeding syndrome in the first week or two of commencing the re-feeding process

Every service treating people with eating disorders needs to have clear guidelines for managing medical instability. The flow chart in Fig. 19.1 provides an example of best-practice guidelines for managing an adolescent with anorexia nervosa who is medically unstable and requires cardiac monitoring (adapted from Anderson et al. 2015).

Re-Feeding Syndrome

Re-feeding syndrome is a rare but potentially fatal complication that can occur in the first 1 to 2 weeks of commencing re-feeding for people who are severely malnourished. It is important for nurses in all clinical settings to be vigilant for the signs and symptoms of re-feeding syndrome, which is a medical emergency that can be variable, unpredictable and may occur without warning (Khan et al. 2011).

Re-feeding syndrome involves disturbances in insulin and serum electrolytes, specifically changes in phosphate, potassium and magnesium, vitamin deficiencies and sodium and fluid retention. If serum phosphate levels drop significantly, especially during the first week of re-feeding, this can cause cardiac, neurological and haematological complications and sudden death (Ornstein et al. 2003; Kohn et al. 2011). Electrolyte abnormalities should be monitored daily until they have stabilised within normal ranges.

Most importantly, nurses need to be aware of who is particularly at risk and need to monitor the person's physical and mental state appropriately. People with eating disorders who are particularly at risk of re-feeding syndrome include those who have:

- severe malnutrition, particularly where it has been prolonged
- rapid weight loss greater than 1 kg per week over several weeks
- a very low BMI (less than 14, although the syndrome has been reported in outpatients with a BMI around 16)
- abnormal electrolytes prior to re-feeding
- a history of severe dietary restraint or not eating for a week or more
- vomiting, laxative misuse or bingeing
- concurrent medical conditions such as diabetes, infection or major organ failure (RCP 2005)

During the first 1 to 2 weeks of re-feeding, nurses monitor for clinical signs of re-feeding syndrome, such as confusion, delirium or other mental status changes, seizures, cardiac arrhythmias, fluid retention and oedema and ensure that prophylactic phosphate and vitamin and mineral supplements are administered. If signs of re-feeding syndrome become evident, urgent medical consultation should be sought in order to normalise electrolyte levels and prevent cardiovascular and other organ system failure and death. Prophylactic phosphate supplements, carefully prescribed rates of re-feeding and daily monitoring of electrolyte levels during the first 1 to 2 weeks of starting re-feeding minimise the risk of a patient developing re-feeding syndrome. Ideally, the patient will ultimately obtain all their vitamin and mineral requirements through food, but initially vitamin and mineral supplements are routinely prescribed.

ETHICAL DILEMMA 19.1

Asha, a 28-year-old woman with a 12-year history of anorexia nervosa, is admitted with severe medical complications as a result of malnutrition. This is Asha's fifth admission over the past 18 months, during which time she has spent only 6 months in total at home. All her admissions have targeted weight gain, normalising oral food intake and supporting individual therapy. The last two admissions were considered 'unsuccessful' by staff due to Asha's 'noncompliance' with the programme and she discharged herself from hospital at a low BMI. While she has moments of wanting to recover, weight gain distresses Asha so much and she is so entrenched in her rituals and behaviours in her home environment that she is unable to maintain any gains she has made during the admission. Her mother has given up work to look after Asha and is feeling overwhelmed and depressed about her daughter's illness. During the most recent admission, Asha seems to feel more hopeless than ever. She is refusing nasogastric tube feeds and has requested that she be allowed to go home to die.

ETHICAL DILEMMA 19.1—cont'd

Questions

1. What rights would health professionals have to enforce nasogastric feeding of Asha? Check the relevant mental health legislation.
2. Is it ethical to enforce treatment when the person clearly doesn't want to endure any more?
3. Is it fair to refuse treatment when a person's family wants to continue trying for recovery?
4. It is part of the role of the healthcare team to hold hope for recovery, when the person is unable to hold hope for themselves. How can the healthcare team ensure that they maintain positivity, that they work collaboratively to set realistic goals and that they hold hope when a person with long-term illness is struggling?

The following principles (from Goldner et al. 1997) might help guide your discussion:

- *The potential risk of the condition:* assess the degree to which failure to deliver treatment will result in premature death from the physical or psychological complications of the disorder.
- *Beneficence:* estimate the likely benefit of imposed treatment. Short-term results from re-feeding are considered beneficial and can lead to an improved quality of life. In an acute crisis the intervention of re-feeding can be life-saving.
- *Nonmaleficence:* evaluate the intent to avoid harm. Goldner et al. (1997) stress the importance of evaluating the physical risks of all interventions and the negative psychological effects of imposing treatment against the person's wishes when considering the enforcement of treatment. It is also important to ask who will carry the burden of care for the person and whether it can be rightfully expected that they will do so. This might be particularly important in situations where adults have endured numerous re-feeding episodes and the family has cared for the person only to watch them go through the agonising relapse into starvation.

Nursing considerations also include monitoring the person's weight daily for the first week and then less frequently (to identify sudden shifts in fluid balance); assessing the person's respiratory status, which is important for preventing respiratory failure; assessing the person's cardiovascular status, including circulatory volume (pulse rate, intake/output, peripheral or presacral oedema); ensuring laboratory values are monitored daily for 3 to 7 days in those who are at risk; monitoring blood glucose every 4 to 6 hours as determined by the patient's stability; being aware of any medications that can impede the repletion of electrolytes; and working with other team members to ensure that medical and dietetic considerations are also addressed. (See MARSIPAN: Management of Really Sick Patients with Anorexia Nervosa guidelines. https://www.rcpsych.ac.uk/docs/default-source/improving-care/better-mh-policy/college-reports/college-report-cr189.pdf?sfvrsn=6c2e7ada_2)

Ongoing Inpatient Nursing Care

Being in hospital can be very frightening for people with eating disorders and they are generally very anxious. Remember that they will nearly always be ambivalent about treatment (this is part of the illness) and they will be particularly worried about gaining weight, even if they accept that this is what they need to do to regain their health. Ambivalence may manifest as outright resistance to treatment and it is very important for nurses to anticipate that this will be the case, from the outset, and work with the person to help them contain the anxiety and distress they are feeling, promoting a safe and emotionally nurturing milieu and working collaboratively *with* the person, *against* the illness. Using a rigid, authoritarian or paternalistic approach is the best way to ensure that the person clings more staunchly to the illness and is often the basis for feelings of frustration that nurses can develop when working with people who have eating disorders.

Specialist supportive clinical management (McIntosh et al. 2006), group counselling and psychoeducation for patients and their families are therapies commonly used by nursing staff working in specialist eating disorders services. Ryan et al. (2006) identified three constructs of inpatient nursing care for patients with an eating disorder: (1) 'loving' or empathetic support; (2) discipline, surveillance and authoritative containment; and (3) constant and ever-present care. Ramjan (2004) studied nurses working in two medical wards and identified three major themes for specific difficulties that nurses need to overcome: (1) struggling for understanding; (2) struggling for control; and (3) struggling to develop therapeutic relationships. Similarly, Zugai et al. (2013) found that the style of interactions between nurses and patients is significant in terms of the person's experience of being in an inpatient setting and of their weight gain during hospitalisation. All three of these studies reflect the complexity of nursing care for eating-disordered inpatients and the need for constant awareness of countertransference issues (see Chapter 24)

Some keys to effective nursing care of inpatients with anorexia nervosa include:

- physical care of the person
  - identifying and acting to reverse signs and symptoms indicating medical instability
- psychological and emotional care of the person
  - understanding that disordered eating behaviours are driven by fear of weight gain and overwhelming anxiety
  - working with the person and their family to develop skills to contain their anxiety and distress
  - facilitating and encouraging motivation to change, rather than imposing or enforcing behavioural changes; getting to know the person, their plans for the future, hopes, dreams and desires will help them (and you) to see the bigger picture . . . is the eating disorder consistent with their goals for the future?
- coordination of the individualised 'programme'
  - balancing the need for the person to comply with the behavioural programme that has been established and encouraging the necessary nutritional rehabilitation, while simultaneously developing a collaborative, trusting and therapeutic relationship with the patient

- providing supportive meal supervision designed to achieve nutritional rehabilitation, normalised eating behaviours and reduction in compensatory behaviours
- consistently adhering to the plan of care and appropriate limit-setting within the context of the individual's prescribed programme
- ensuring that all limits set are not arbitrary but have a clear and transparent purpose and are discussed and agreed upon with the person at the outset

Professional aspects of working with a person who has an eating disorder include:

- maintaining clear professional boundaries, which includes not being over-involved or dismissive and under-involved
- developing and regularly reviewing an evidence-based local behavioural program for patients that is achievable for nurses within their specific work environment
- having realistic expectations regarding what can be achieved during a hospital admission given the complexity and chronicity of the illness; this includes the awareness that relapse and readmission are common and are not a sign of failure but an opportunity to review the relapse plan
- being aware of countertransference issues and receiving adequate professional supervision and support
- enjoying the challenge of caring for individuals with an eating disorder and assisting them to understand and care for themselves in more healthy ways
- maintaining positive regard for people with eating disorders in the face of their ambivalence and resistance to treatment

Therapeutic Relationships

Effective nursing management requires the development of a therapeutic relationship *with* the person and *against* the eating disorder. Without this, it is likely that the person will see the eating disorder as their ally or their only friend, and feel that their parents, friends and health practitioners are all against them. The therapeutic relationship is enhanced by validating the person's experience ('recovery is really hard'), empathetic discussion, consistent positive regard, reassurance, motivational enhancement and supporting the person to develop new insights and accept change. Nurse's Story 19.1 describes the experience of providing nursing care for adolescents with anorexia nervosa.

Positive regard for the person can be displayed by 'externalising' the eating-disordered thoughts and behaviours as separate from the person; for example, 'Is "the anorexia" making it really difficult for you to eat today?', 'I know it's hard for you to eat when "the anorexia" is telling you not to. How can I best help you to fight "those eating disorder" thoughts?' Putting this distance between the illness and the person is a very important first step towards helping the person see that the things they value (e.g. health, friendships, doing well at school, having a great career) are incompatible with the long-term maintenance of an eating disorder. It is also very useful for families to learn to identify and to externalise the person's disordered eating thoughts and behaviours as part of their illness rather than as wilful behaviour on the part of their child or family member.

NURSE'S STORY 19.1 **Working with Adolescents who Have Anorexia Nervosa**

When I first started working with adolescents who have anorexia nervosa I was scared that I would say or do the wrong thing. I didn't understand the complexity of the illness or why it was so difficult for them to eat normally and maintain a healthy weight.

Previously, I had always tried to meet my patients' needs and advocate for them, but I could see that if I supported the disordered eating behaviours, I would collude with the illness and the patients would only lose more weight. When I first tried to talk to them about the behaviours, they would lie to me or get angry and I initially found this hard to understand and quite frustrating.

Luckily, I work with a great team and was able to learn 'on the job'. My senior nursing colleagues spent a lot of time teaching me about the illness and about how the behaviours I was seeing were not directed at me personally but rather reflected the strength of the anorexic thoughts and the person's overwhelming fear of change.

I realised that I wasn't responsible for making them gain weight. Rather I tried to understand what it was like for them to experience the illness, work collaboratively with them to see the illness for what it is and help them to increase their motivation to recover. I soon found that by taking a different approach, I could encourage patients to manage their fears better and start taking responsibility for making small, but positive changes in their behaviours.

Now that I understand just how difficult it is for people who experience eating disorders to change, I am better able to support them in managing their anxiety, I am better at working collaboratively and I am able to gain the person's trust, so that they communicate honestly with me.

Along with a greater understanding of people who experience eating disorders came a sense of confidence in my role as a nurse and a feeling of satisfaction with my job, rather than frustration.

I enjoy my work with these young people now and feel that I am making a positive difference in their lives.

Unless a particular situation is life threatening, confrontation and invasion of privacy (e.g. observing a patient in the bathroom) are generally unnecessary and are destructive for both the development of therapeutic relationships and the promotion of the person's self-responsibility and motivation for change. Even if these behaviours are necessary, it is possible to address them in a collaborative (rather than demoralising) way and to provide choice wherever possible. For example, 'Lucy, I know that you find it difficult to resist the eating disorder when it demands you exercise in the shower. I'd like to help you regain control of that. Let's look at the options . . .'

Food avoidance and the use of compensatory behaviours will be reflected to a great extent in the person's pattern of weight gain (and in their blood and urine test results). Generally, if they fail to gain the expected amount of weight each week in hospital, they have either restricted their oral intake or participated in compensatory behaviours. Invading privacy or engaging in confrontation will result in an angry eating-disordered response rather than encouraging positive growth and motivation for change. The following statement is an example of a comment that would lead to an angry eating-disordered response: 'Lucy, it's pretty clear by your weight loss that you've been cheating on the programme. You're never going to get out of here if that's your approach.' Taking control of eating and ceasing compensatory behaviours are ultimately the responsibility of the patient. The goal for nurses is therefore not to enforce change but gradually to encourage the person's motivation to change by exploring and challenging their individual perspective on, and experience of, their disordered eating behaviours. For example: 'Lucy, your weight has gone down today and I'm wondering if we can talk about that? Usually, weight loss is either from not eating enough, or from exercising or vomiting. I'm wondering if you have felt so bad in the last few days, or you've been struggling with the eating disorder, that you've been doing any of those things?'

Younger children, however, may need a more directive approach than adolescents and adults, especially when they have not yet developed abstract thought processes. For example: 'Imogen, your weight has gone down and we need to address that . . . because to get better, you need to get back into a healthy weight range. I've noticed you haven't been finishing all your meals. You need to do that to get better. How can we help you to make sure that you finish all your meals?'

Normalising Eating Patterns

The first step in achieving a healthy eating pattern is to eat regularly throughout the day. The dietician will plan with the person what they need to eat at every meal and snack. The meal plan will be individualised and takes into consideration the person's tastes, their cultural background, their physical needs and their clinical picture. It will also identify portion sizes and gradually introduce foods that have been avoided. The aim is that the diet will include all the food groups and that fear foods have been habituated (CEDD 2015).

Meal times are usually very stressful for people with an eating disorder. Nurses can help by providing therapeutic meal support, having clear boundaries around expected mealtime behaviours and acting as a role model for healthy eating behaviour. Leichner and colleagues (2005) defined meal support as 'a form of emotional support provided to a person struggling with an eating disorder before, during and after meals and snacks'. The goals of meal support are to help the person to normalise their eating behaviours, begin the process of weight gain or at least ensure weight maintenance, reintroduce the concept of eating as a pleasant social experience, assist the person to address and to decrease food rituals and to increase their ability and confidence in making healthy food choices and eating a 'normal' amount (Leichner et al. 2005). When a patient engages in ritualistic behaviours (see Box 19.6), the nurse discusses these behaviours with them, validating their difficulty with eating, praising positive efforts and offering encouragement to eat normally during the next meal. Adequate after-meal support (which may include distraction, mindfulness practice, encouragement and re-engaging with the person around their values and what is important to them) and praise for effort encourages the continued development of normal eating behaviours.

People with an eating disorder are encouraged to eat breakfast, lunch, dinner and three snacks each day. Main meals are generally to be eaten within 30 minutes and snacks within 15 to 20 minutes. Nurses generally record the amount of food eaten and document the person's eating behaviours and any other pertinent observations. This information is particularly helpful for the multidisciplinary team when planning interventions for ongoing care.

Caring for patients in a specialist eating disorders unit enables the development of a supportive dining room milieu where patients can also encourage each other. Taking the person to a café for coffee and eating out in public can provide further exposure to, and experience with coping in, social eating situations. Discharge planning should also involve returning to the home environment and/or eating out with family and friends. The person needs to practise eating in their normal environment and nurses can support people to plan and prepare for these experiences.

Binge Eating and Purging Behaviours: The 3-Hour Rule

People who have eating disorders need to understand that if they under-eat or restrict their food intake, have lost an understanding of hunger and satiety or engage in non-hungry eating, then working with the team to set up a regular eating pattern and introducing the 3-hour rule will be important. The 3-hour rule simply means eating something every 3 hours and eliminating dieting (Fairburn et al. 1993). Since hunger is the primary trigger for binge eating, maintaining consistent intake is the first step in ceasing binge/purge behaviours. Establishing a pattern of eating something every 3 hours often creates anxiety and fear of rapid, uncontrolled weight gain in many patients. Nurses need to reassure the person that research and clinical experience demonstrate that this does not occur.

Monitoring Intake and Feelings

Monitoring dietary intake is important and diet plan monitoring is an important tool for the dietician and the team. Food monitoring helps identify food/eating patterns and gives the person and the team an overview of what and how much the patient is really eating. In hospital, monitoring will generally be done by the nursing staff, but the person may also do this themselves, provided the record is accurate.

Monitoring the person's thoughts and feelings in response to their dietary intake can also be a helpful tool for nurses and other health professionals to review with patients. These forms ask the person to identify their thoughts and feelings in association with their eating or restricting behaviours—exposing how the person responds to emotions like guilt, anger and sadness through their intake, and identifying how the eating disorder bullies them into behaving in a certain way.

Monitoring Weight Gain

The person's minimum healthy target weight range (a BMI of 20–25 for adults or 100% ideal body weight for children and younger adolescents) is calculated at the beginning of treatment. Ultimately, the return of ovulation and a normal menstrual cycle reflects a healthy minimum weight for young adult females. In most females of reproductive age, a normal menstrual cycle usually requires having a minimum of 20% to 22% body fat mass (as measured using a DEXA scan).

Most treatment facilities aim for an average weekly weight gain of 1 to 2 kg in inpatient settings and 0.5 kg in outpatient settings. The frequency of weighing or monitoring expected weight gain varies between treatment settings, but twice a week is sufficient to monitor and to reward progress.

In an outpatient setting any team member can undertake monitoring of weight gain, but in the hospital environment it is generally the responsibility of the nurse. Patients are usually weighed early in the morning wearing only a hospital gown and before consuming any food or drink. At times, patients who are struggling use techniques to increase their weight falsely, including drinking large amounts of water just prior to weighing and hiding weights on their person. Therefore, patients are usually asked to empty their bladder just prior to weighing and urinalysis will suggest water loading (if the specific gravity is <1.010) or purging (if a pH of 8–9 is recorded). A sudden increase in weight or an increase that is inconsistent with the observed eating behaviour will alert you that weight manipulation may be occurring and discussion should ensue about possible behaviours that may account for this. A random (unexpected/spot) weight measurement can be undertaken outside the normal weighing time if there is concern that the person is manipulating their real weight.

It is important to remember that if someone is attempting to manipulate their weight, they are doing so out of fear and distress and because they are really struggling with the ambivalence that the eating disorder generates. They will probably be feeling very anxious that their behaviours will be detected, but at the same time, will be relieved when the secret is out. Nurses need to respond in a very sensitive, respectful and empathic way when discussing these issues with the person to avoid them feeling humiliated, judged and hopeless. For example: 'I can see by this spot weigh that your weight is actually quite a lot lower than what it was yesterday. I'm guessing that you have felt really worried about weigh days because you've been struggling so much with the eating . . . is that right? Can you tell me what you've been doing to keep your weight measurements going up?'

Psychotherapeutic Techniques and Treatments

There is limited evidence about the most appropriate psychotherapeutic techniques and treatments for eating disorders; however, there is broad clinical consensus internationally. NICE (2018) guidelines state that people with an eating disorder should have a discussion with a professional about their options for psychological treatment. The following examples are options for psychological treatment of anorexia nervosa in adults: individual eating-disorder-focussed cognitive behavioural therapy (CBT-ED); Maudsley Anorexia Nervosa Treatment for Adults (MANTRA); specialist supportive clinical management (SSCM) (NICE 2017). Recent published systematic reviews of evidence-based treatments include Wade et al. (2013) regarding eating disorders, Watson and Bulik (2013) regarding anorexia nervosa, Hay et al. (2009a) regarding bulimia nervosa and Iacovino et al. (2012) regarding binge eating disorder. Examples of some of the psychotherapeutic techniques and treatments currently used in the management of people with an eating disorder are discussed later. In clinical practice, a combination of these therapies or other psychotherapies not described (such as psychodynamic psychotherapy, dialectical behaviour therapy and narrative therapy) may be used. (For a review of various models of psychotherapy, see Chapter 24.) When considering therapy for an eating disorder, the person's medical status, age, family supports and cognitive capacity, the duration of illness and the accessibility of services are all taken into account.

Specialist Supportive Clinical Management

Specialist supportive clinical management (SSCM) is a relatively recent and promising approach in the psychotherapeutic management of people with anorexia nervosa. It combines features of supportive psychotherapy and clinical management to establish a 'supportive therapeutic context'. The person is encouraged to explore issues that impact on and promote change and they are encouraged to make changes actively to core symptoms, e.g. by increasing their weight, eating less restrictively and decreasing the use of inappropriate compensatory behaviours (McIntosh et al. 2006). The process focusses on facilitating normal eating, weight restoration and psychoeducation about anorexia nervosa, alongside addressing other life issues that may be identified by the person as relevant to the eating disorder (McIntosh & Jordan 2009).

Supportive psychotherapy is a generalised therapy that has been used in the treatment of people with eating disorders. Techniques such as active listening, verbal and nonverbal attending, using open-ended questioning, encouraging reflection, providing reassurance and praise are key. Advice giving and therapist self-disclosure are also used. Bloch (2006) argues that supportive psychotherapy is a skill that should be used by every mental health professional. Specific components of supportive therapy described by Bloch include reassurance, explanation, guidance, suggestion, encouragement and permission for catharsis or sharing of pent-up feelings such as fear, grief, sorrow, concern and frustration.

Cognitive Behavioural Therapy for Eating Disorders

Cognitive behavioural therapy (CBT) is the rational disputation of a person's beliefs combined with behavioural experiments that function to help the person confirm alternative beliefs (Hay et al. 2009b) (see Chapter 24). CBT for eating disorders (CBT-ED) is structured to focus on the processes associated with maintenance of the eating disorder. It uses a variety of cognitive and behavioural interventions but uses strategic behaviour change to modify thinking, rather than the direct cognitive restructuring usual in other forms of

CBT. CBT-ED is delivered in three stages. The first stage involves engaging the person in treatment and change, jointly creating the formulation, establishing self-monitoring practices, weekly weighing, establishing regular patterns of eating and providing education to the person and significant others. Stage two is brief and incorporates a review of stage one and planning for stage three. The final stage is the main body of treatment, where the over-evaluation of shape and weight, dieting rules, interpersonal problems, perfectionism and self-esteem issues are addressed. The focus here is on eliminating dieting, problem solving and modifying thoughts that link body and weight with self-esteem, as well as relapse prevention and developing skills to manage stressors (Murphy et al. 2010; Surgenor & Thornton 2000).

There is only tentative evidence that CBT is effective for relapse reduction after weight restoration in anorexia nervosa and it is not an appropriate treatment for those with anorexia nervosa who are not weight restored (Chakraborty & Basu 2010). However, evidence for the use of CBT with people who have bulimia nervosa is strong (when used to address the cycle of dieting, binge eating and purging or other extreme weight-control behaviours) (Chakraborty & Basu 2010; Cooper 2005). CBT has also been developmentally adapted for adolescents with binge eating disorder (Fairburn et al. 1993; Schapman-Williams et al. 2006) and bulimia nervosa (Fairburn et al. 1993; Lock 2005).

MAUDSLEY ANOREXIA NERVOSA TREATMENT FOR ADULTS

The Maudsley Anorexia Nervosa Treatment for Adults (MANTRA) is an effective therapy tailored to the specific needs and characteristics of people with anorexia nervosa. Treatment targets:

- a thinking style characterised by rigidity, detail focus and fear of making mistakes,
- an inexpressive, avoidant emotional and relational style,
- positive beliefs about the utility of anorexia for the person, and
- a response of close others characterised by high expressed emotion and enabling of and accommodation to the illness.

Adults are usually offered 20 sessions with a trained practitioner, weekly for the first 10 and then 10 flexible sessions to be agreed on what works best for the patient. Sometimes people have up to 10 extra sessions, decided on a case-by-case basis and the severity of the symptoms. The goal of MANTRA is to help people to understand the causes of anorexia and focus on what is important to them personally, encouraging behaviour change on their terms. Treatment is based around a workbook that covers, for example, nutrition, symptom management and behaviour change. The focus is on empowering the person to develop a 'non-anorexic identity'. If desired, family or carers may be able to be involved in the therapy if the patient feels it will be of value to them (NICE 2017; Kings College 2018).

Interpersonal Therapy

Interpersonal therapy (IPT) for people with eating disorders is based on the premise that interpersonal difficulties result in the development of disturbances in self-esteem and mood, which then give rise to eating disorder symptoms (Rieger 2009). IPT is a structured, time-limited psychotherapy that focusses on resolving interpersonal difficulties and encouraging the development of affirming relationships, thereby providing a viable alternative to the eating disorder in attaining positive self-esteem, affect and problem-solving skills. The symptoms of the eating disorder are not themselves the focus of therapy (Surgenor & Thornton 2000, p. 108). IPT appears to have long-term efficacy for those with bulimia nervosa and people with binge eating disorder (Reas & Grilo 2014; McIntosh et al. 2005).

Motivational Interventions

Motivation has been seen as a key issue for people with eating disorders. In particular, a person's motivation to change at the outset of treatment has been thought to be helpful in predicting outcome (Clausen & Jones 2014). Motivational interventions typically target denial, ambivalence and resistance to change. They are commonly used with people who have eating disorders, either prior to them participating in other psychological interventions or as a key element of other therapies (Waller 2012). However, a recent review of motivational interventions in people with eating disorders (Knowles et al. 2013) demonstrated that motivation-enhancing interventions in eating disorders is not well supported by the current evidence base. It is therefore important for nurses to understand the person's motivation and where that person is at in terms of their motivation. Delivering interventions that are targeted towards a person in the action stage are likely to be ineffective if the person is precontemplative and denying that there is a problem. Collaboration with the person and targeting issues that the person sees as important are essential.

Psychoeducation

Psychoeducation involves providing information about the eating disorder to enable the person with an eating disorder to have a better understanding of the illness and its effects and to develop more effective coping strategies to overcome difficulties they are experiencing. Rome and Ammerman (2003) suggest that adherence with nutritional rehabilitation may be improved when the person is given an explanation of how and why their physical symptoms are manifesting. It is much easier for people with eating disorders to change the eating disorder behaviours when they understand the interplay between the behaviours and the illness and their dual role in keeping them trapped.

Some examples of psychoeducation used by nurses include discussion of:

- the short- and long-term medical and psychological effects of starvation
- the biological factors that regulate weight, which includes discussion of how dieting largely works against the body's weight regulators, causing stress to both physical and psychological functioning

- the physical side effects of vomiting and laxative and diuretic abuse
- the binge/purge cycle and how it affects self-esteem; nurses can help the person to identify and to manage cues for bingeing and purging behaviours, learn distraction or relaxation techniques to decrease the urge to vomit immediately after meals and understand the benefits of eating regularly throughout the day, thereby reducing the physical and psychological drive to binge in the evenings
- the importance of establishing a healthy pattern of exercise based on muscle strengthening and bone health rather than focussing on burning up calories/kilojoules for weight control
- the effects of stress and techniques for coping with stress and anxiety (e.g. relaxation techniques, mindfulness practice)

Psychoeducation on an individual or a group basis can also be extremely useful for engaging parents and family members in the treatment programme, increasing their understanding of the complexity of the illness, developing realistic expectations and facilitating useful strategies to better manage the person's disordered eating behaviours. The more informed families are, the less anxious or blaming they become and the more open they will be to making positive changes that can support and improve the person's health outcome.

There are a large number of web-based resources available for families, which provide parent and carer support programmes throughout the UK (see Useful Websites).

Family Therapy

There is moderate research to support family therapy as an effective treatment for younger children and adolescents who live with their families and whose have experienced anorexia nervosa for less than 3 years (Hay et al. 2014; Couturier et al. 2012). The focus of family therapy approaches varies, but the general theme is that the family are involved in treatment and support weight restoration and recovery. Models of family intervention have been developed for adults and couples, but these have not been evaluated. Family therapy is the treatment of choice for most children and adolescents with anorexia nervosa, but it is not demonstrably effective for those over 18 years of age (Hay et al. 2014).

As outlined earlier, families play an important role in the assessment and treatment of young people with eating disorders. Unless contraindicated, families are best placed to support their loved one to manage the burden of the illness. Families need to understand the illness and be involved and engaged as an important resource by the treating team. To facilitate change, families need to develop effective coping strategies for managing the behaviours that support and maintain the illness and to adopt interactional patterns that accommodate the young person's normal growth and development.

Sometimes, families can inadvertently reinforce the eating disorder (particularly as the person's distress around eating is so intense) by giving into, accommodating or colluding with, the anorexic behaviours (Treasure et al. 2003; Treasure et al. 2007). If families of children and adolescents are not engaged with and committed to the treatment programme or are unable to work together to provide clear, firm boundaries regarding food and disordered eating behaviours, relapse is more likely.

One particular model of family therapy designed for children and adolescents with anorexia nervosa is the anorexia-nervosa-focussed family therapy for children and young people (FT-AN) (NICE 2017). Another is Maudsley family-based therapy (MFBT), which has proven to be very effective for some families (Lock et al. 2006). This therapy is delivered in three phrases. The first phase involves the parents taking control of their child's eating until 90% of ideal body weight is achieved; the second phase involves the family gradually giving control over eating back to the young person while continuing to supervise them until they reach their healthy weight range; and the final phase involves supporting the young person to address any unresolved individual concerns, as well as assisting the family to return to the normal family life cycle by addressing any unresolved family or marital interactional problems (Rhodes & Wallis 2009).

Self-Help Programmes

Guided self-help is a form of treatment where the person is offered the use of an evidence-based self-help treatment manual (usually CBT based) delivered in combination with professional guidance by a therapist with skills and experience in eating disorders. People with anorexia nervosa do not benefit from this type of approach, but those with bulimia nervosa or binge eating disorder can (NICE 2017; NICE 2018). Many self-help books and internet resources are available for people with eating disorders. However, it is important to note that while unguided self-help (use of self-help without a supportive and experienced therapist) may be effective for people with binge eating disorder, it has poor outcomes in comparison with guided self-help for people with bulimia nervosa (Hay 2013).

Over recent years, therapists have also sought to capitalise on new communication technologies to enhance the reach of prevention interventions, to increase access to treatment, to extend the frequency or length of therapy and to improve the impact of existing therapeutic approaches). One systematic review of treating people with eating disorders over the internet (Aardoom et al. 2013) found that internet-based treatment was more effective for those with less comorbid psychopathology, binge eating as opposed to restrictive problems, and individuals with binge eating disorder as opposed to bulimia nervosa.

Pharmacotherapy

Pharmacotherapy is not used as a first-line treatment for people with anorexia nervosa and medication should not be offered as the sole treatment for anorexia nervosa (NICE 2017). Evidence for pharmacological treatment is weak, but low-dose antipsychotics (e.g. olanzapine) may be helpful for some people to reduce anxiety, rumination and obsessive thinking (Hay et al. 2014) and have shown promise in diminishing thought intrusions and distorted body image (Brambilla et al. 2007; Mondraty et al. 2005). Selective serotonin reuptake inhibitors (SSRIs) are not indicated in the acute or maintenance stages of anorexia nervosa for young people (Hay et al. 2014). The potential role of anxiolytics and antidepressants is best assessed after nutritional rehabilitation in low-weight patients with anorexia nervosa, as food and nutritional rehabilitation can be the best 'medicine' for improving mood.

Pharmacotherapy has been shown to be a helpful adjunctive treatment, with CBT-ED, for people with bulimia nervosa (Hay et al. 2014; Hay & Claudino 2012). Antidepressant medication, specifically fluoxetine hydrochloride, which is an SSRI, can be effective in reducing bingeing and purging (bulimia nervosa) and bingeing in those with binge eating disorder (Shapiro et al. 2007). If psychological therapy is not readily available, there is evidence to support pharmacological treatment for people with bulimia/binge eating disorder. However, the first-line treatment for both disorders is therapist-led CBT or CBT-ED (Hay et al. 2014).

OUTCOME

Mortality for people with eating disorders, particularly those with anorexia nervosa, is significantly elevated (Arcelus et al. 2011). Mortality from anorexia nervosa remains the highest for any psychiatric disorder (APA 2006; Hoek 2006) and the risk of premature death is 6 to 12 times higher in women with anorexia nervosa compared with the general population (Academy for Eating Disorders 2012). Crude mortality is generally reported to be around 10%, with suicide or medical complications, including organ failure and electrolyte imbalance leading to cardiac arrest, being the most common causes of death.

The general consensus is that only 50% of adult patients with anorexia nervosa have good outcomes (normal weight and eating, and return of reproductive functioning); 30% continue to have partial or residual features such as ongoing body image problems, low BMI and other interpersonal problems; and 20% have very poor outcomes. It is therefore very important for all health practitioners to identify those at risk of illness and those presenting with eating disorder-related complaints as soon as possible.

Recovery rates among adolescents have been reported as slightly better, with up to 70% recovering, 20% having improved outcomes and 10% to 20% developing chronic anorexia nervosa (Steinhausen 2002). It is possible that the greater focus on weight and nutritional restoration for children and adolescents influences this higher recovery rate. However, Halvorsen et al. (2004) report that 41% of adolescent patients who had sufficiently recovered so that they no longer had an eating disorder diagnosis did have an Axis I diagnosis, most commonly depression or an anxiety disorder. Psychological symptoms associated with a poorer outcome include depression, mood disorder, anxiety disorders and poor social functioning. A longer duration of illness and substance abuse are also associated with poorer outcomes (Berkman et al. 2007).

Considerable variability occurs in the course of bulimia nervosa, but approximately 30% of affected people maintain recurrent binge eating and purging behaviours at long-term follow up (Keel et al. 1999, 2003). Remission and relapse of symptoms are common. One study concluded that the probability of remission at 60 months was 74% for bulimia nervosa and 83% for people with eating disorders not otherwise specified (a term that has been removed in the DSM-5 but that principally refers to people with a diagnosis of OSFED), while the probability of relapse among those in remission was 47% for bulimia nervosa and 42% for EDNOS (Grilo et al. 2007). Depression, substance use and poor impulse control were clearly associated with poorer outcomes (Berkman et al. 2007).

THE IMPORTANCE OF A STRONG NURSING PRESENCE

Nurses in all clinical settings are ideally placed to make a significant impact on the health and mental health of the many children, young people, women and men who experience eating disorders. Nurses have the medical and mental health skills required to work holistically and collaboratively, to empathise, to validate and to support people with eating disorders through this complex and challenging life experience. Recovery is always possible, at any stage of the illness. What is required is that as nurses, we are kind and hold hope for the person when they are not able to hold hope for themselves, we understand the difficulties the person is experiencing in their struggle to recover, we support families who are frightened and bewildered and questioning themselves and we critically reflect on our own practice to ensure that we are offering high-quality evidence-informed practice that supports the person's recovery and optimises their outcome. Working with people who have eating disorders is a rewarding professional experience. These are complex illnesses that stretch our knowledge and skills and require us to reflect on the impact of our values and attitudes on our nursing practice.

The following is an extract from a letter written by a recovering young adult:

> *It's now been six years since I was first diagnosed with anorexia nervosa. I know I still have many years ahead to learn about life and to learn from my mistakes and experiences, but this recovery process has taught me so much about confronting myself, challenging myself and training my mind to think positively and it does work. Thank you for firmly confronting my disorder when I couldn't and for hanging in with me, keeping me alive and supporting me long enough for me to finally get to the point where I feel strong enough as a person to not need or want this illness any more.*
>
> Private communication with the author (GA).

CONCLUSION

This chapter has provided an introduction to the major eating disorders encountered in nursing practice and has included a focus on psychological factors, medical complications, assessment and treatment. Eating disorders are complex, multidimensional illnesses that encompass a range of psychological and physical health issues. Although there is a relatively low but increasing incidence of eating disorders, the severity of impact of these disorders in terms of quality of life, morbidity and mortality is high. Many sufferers encounter difficulties in accessing appropriate services and this difficulty, coupled with the shame, denial and ambivalence to treatment commonly associated with these disorders, can result in delayed treatment. This is of particular concern because of the known effectiveness of early treatment in preventing or reducing progression to severe and chronic illness.

What of the future? In modern Western societies there seems to be an ever-increasing concern with body image, weight, shape and appearance for both women and men. For some this leads to severe distress, disruption and diagnosis with one of a growing list of disorders including the eating disorders. A greater emphasis on primary prevention strategies, particularly targeting the self-esteem, body image and resilience of the very young, both males and females, is needed.

A multidisciplinary approach to treatment of eating disorders is crucial and nurses committed to caring for people with an eating disorder have much to contribute in both inpatient and community treatment settings. Patients are admitted to hospital when they require 24-hour nursing care. In order that optimal care is provided, it is essential that nurses understand and develop skills to manage the biopsychosocial complexity of these very challenging illnesses.

More research is needed for a better understanding of the relative importance of biological and psychosocial risk and protective factors and to continue developing more effective psychological therapies. The outcome data show that new therapeutic treatments need to be developed to enhance outcomes and decrease the high levels of associated morbidity and mortality. Furthermore, more emphasis needs to be placed on early and more aggressive nutritional rehabilitation to enable those with an eating disorder to engage cognitively in therapeutic psychological interventions. Nurses are in a key position to undertake research designed to understand eating disorders better and to promote evidence-based effective nursing strategies that will enhance care and outcomes.

EXERCISES FOR CLASS ENGAGEMENT

1. In a group, discuss the influence of the media, marketing, the advertising industry and popular role models on the development of eating disorders among young women and men.
2. Discuss the reasons why body image dissatisfaction tends to increase during adolescence.
3. Do an internet search for Ancel Keys' 1950s Starvation Study. Identify the physical, psychological, social and emotional aspects that relate to starvation, which people with eating disorders commonly experience. Some people think that eating disorders are self-inflicted and purposeful or that they are a type of personality disorder. Having reviewed this study, which aspects of it challenge these kinds of assumptions?
4. Working with the person to find their strengths is a very important part of recovery from an eating disorder. Make a table with two columns. In one column, list the self-defeating thoughts that a person with an eating disorder may experience. In the other column, suggest alternatives that are self-supporting behaviours and thoughts.
5. 'Fat talk' has been said to be a common motif of female culture, particularly with young women in developed countries. Girls and women are encouraged to aspire to the thin 'ideal' body type and often say self-disparaging things or communicate with others around this theme. Consider the following commonly heard statement: 'I feel so fat today.' This expression is made more commonly by young women than men and is repeated over and over. But, in fact, the person is actually feeling another emotion, such as worry, guilt, anger or frustration. The expression of emotion is covered up by referring instead to an outward physical presence (being fat). So 'fat talk' is actually a metaphor for a feeling. When this notion is identified as a metaphor, it is possible for it to be challenged and replaced. What are some more productive metaphors or statements that you could suggest young women could make to help them to express their emotions more accurately (Nizette et al. 2013)?
6. Some health practitioners say that people with eating disorders engage in manipulative and 'splitting' behaviour. We know that 'splitting' is actually a process whereby a team of practitioners fails to be consistent or to work collaboratively towards shared goals. We also know that words such as 'manipulative' can be very damaging and labelling. How will you protect yourself against taking up judgemental and nontherapeutic language and ideas when you are working as a clinical nurse?

REFERENCES

Aardoom, J.J., Dingemans, A.E., Spinhoven, P., Van Furth, E.F., 2013. Treating eating disorders over the internet: a systematic review and future research directions. International Journal of Eating Disorders 46 (6), 539–552.

Abraham, S., Llewellyn-Jones, D., 2001. Eating Disorders: The Facts. Oxford Medical Publications, Sydney.

Academy for Eating Disorders, 2012. Eating Disorders. Critical Points for Early Recognition and Medical Risk Management in the Care of Individuals with Eating Disorders, second ed. Available at: www.aedweb.org.

American Dietetic Association (ADA), 2006. Position of the American Dietetic Association: nutritional intervention in the treatment of anorexia nervosa, bulimia nervosa and other eating disorders. Journal of the American Dietetic Association 106 (12), 2073–2082.

American Psychiatric Association (APA), 2006. Practice Guideline for the Treatment of Patients With Eating Disorders, third ed. APA, Washington, DC.

American Psychiatric Association (APA), 2013. Diagnostic and Statistical Manual of Mental Disorders, fifth ed. APA, Washington, DC.

Anderson, G., Squire, J., Clarke, S., Kohn, M., 2015. Caring for Medically Unstable Adolescents with Anorexia Nervosa Requiring Cardiac Monitoring. Policy. Western Sydney Local Health Network, Westmead Hospital, Sydney.

Arcelus, J., Mitchell, A.J., Wales, J., Nielsen, S., 2011. Mortality rates in patients with anorexia nervosa and other eating disorders. A meta-analysis of 36 studies. Archives of General Psychiatry 68 (7), 724–731.

Ayton, A., Keen, C., Lask, B., 2008. Pros and cons of using the mental health act for severe eating disorders in adolescents. European Eating Disorders Review 17 (1), 1–81. https://doi.org/10.1002/erv.887.

Bannatyne, A.J., Abel, L.M., 2015. Can we fight stigma with science? The effect of aetiological framing on attitudes towards anorexia nervosa and the impact on volitional stigma. Australian Journal of Psychology 67, 38–46. https://doi.org/10.1111/ajpy.12062.

Berkman, N.D., Lohr, K.N., Bulik, C.M., 2007. Outcomes of eating disorders: a systematic review of the literature. International Journal of Eating Disorders 40 (4), 293–309.

Bloch, S., 2006. Supportive psychotherapy. In: Bloch, S. (Ed.), An Introduction to the Psychotherapies, fourth ed. Oxford University Press, Oxford, pp. 215–235.

Brambilla, F., Garcia, C.S., Fassino, S., et al., 2007. Olanzapine therapy effects in anorexia nervosa: psychobiological effects. International Clinical Pharmacology 22 (4), 197–204.

Bulik, C.M., Slof-Op't Landt, M.C.T., van Furth, E.F., Sullivan, P.F., 2007. The genetics of anorexia nervosa. Annual Review of Nutrition 27, 263–275.

Butterfly Foundation, 2012. Paying the Price: The Economic and Social Impact of Eating Disorders in Australia. Available at: http://thebutterflyfoundation.org.au/wp-content/uploads/2012/12/Butterfly_Report.pdf. Accessed: 30 September 2015.

Campbell, K., Peebles, R., 2014. Eating disorders in children and adolescents: state of the art review. Pediatrics 134 (3), 582–593.

Caslini, M., Bartoli, F., Crocamo, C., Dakanalis, A., Clerici, M., Carra, G., 2016. Disentangling the associations between child abuse and eating disorders: a systematic review and meta-analysis. Psychosomatic Medicine 78 (1), 79–90. https://doi.org/10.1097/PSY.0000000000000233.

Centre for Eating & Dieting Disorders (CEDD), 2008. Online Learning for Health Care Professionals. CEDD, Sydney.

Centre for Eating & Dieting Disorders (CEDD), 2015. CEDD Online Training for Health Professionals. Available at: www.cedd.org.au.

Chakraborty, K., Basu, D., 2010. Management of anorexia and bulimia nervosa: an evidence-based review. Indian Journal of Psychiatry 52 (2), 174–186. https://doi.org/10.4103/0019-5545.64596.

Clausen, L., Jones, A., 2014. A systematic review of the frequency, duration, type and effect of involuntary treatment for people with anorexia nervosa, and an analysis of patient characteristics. Journal of Eating Disorders 2, 29.

Cooper, M., 2005. Cognitive theory in anorexia nervosa and bulimia nervosa: progress, development and future directions. Clinical Psychology Review 25, 511–531.

Couturier, J., Kimber, M., Szatmari, P., 2012. Efficacy of family-based treatment for adolescents with eating disorders: a systematic review and meta-analysis. International Journal of Eating Disorders 46 (1), 3–11.

Couturier, J.L., Lock, J., 2006. Denial and minimization in adolescents with anorexia nervosa. International Journal of Eating Disorders 39 (3), 212–216.

Curtis, C., Davis, C., 2013. A qualitative study of binge eating and obesity from an addiction perspective. Eating Disorders: The Journal of Treatment and Prevention 22 (1), 19–32.

Dunifon, R., Cook, E., 2012. Parenting in Context: Do Family Meals Really Make a Difference? Cornell University Policy Analysis and Management. Available at: www.human.cornell.edu/pam/outreach/upload/Family-Mealtimes-2.pdf.

Fairburn, C., Harrison, P.J., 2003. Eating disorders. Lancet 361 (9355), 407–416.

Fairburn, C., Marcus, M.D., Wilson, G.T., 1993. Cognitive behavioural therapy for binge eating and bulimia nervosa: a comprehensive treatment manual. In: Fairburn, C.G., Wilson, G.T. (Eds.), Binge Eating: Nature, Assessment and Treatment. Guilford Press, New York, pp. 361–404.

Freeman, C., 2002. What Causes Anorexia Nervosa? Overcoming Anorexia Nervosa. University Press, New York.

Gearhardt, A., White, M.A., Masheb, R.M., Grilo, C.M., 2013. An examination of food addiction in a racially diverse sample of obese patients with binge eating disorder in primary care settings. Comprehensive Psychiatry 54 (5), 500–505.

Glasner-Edwards, E., Mooney, L.J., Marinelli-Casey, P., Ang, A., Rawson, R., et al., 2011. Bulimia nervosa among methamphetamine dependent adults: association with outcomes 3 years after treatment. Eating Disorders 19 (3), 259–269. https://doi.org/10.1080/10640266.2011.566149.

Goldner, E.M., Birmingham, C.L., Smye, V., 1997. Addressing treatment refusal in anorexia nervosa: clinical, ethical and legal considerations. In: Garner, D., Garfinkel, P. (Eds.), Handbook of Treatment for Eating Disorders, second ed. Guilford Press, New York, pp. 450–461.

Gonzales, A., Kohn, M.R., Clarke, S.D., 2007. Eating disorders in adolescents. Australian Family Physician 36 (8), 614–619.

Grieve, F.G., 2007. A conceptual model of factors contributing to the development of muscle dysmorphia. Eating Disorders 15 (1), 63–80.

Grilo, C.M., Pagano, M.E., Skodol, A.E., et al., 2007. Natural course of bulimia nervosa and of eating disorder not otherwise specified: 5-year prospective study of remissions, relapses, and the effects of personality disorder psychopathology (CME). Journal of Clinical Psychiatry 68 (5), 738–746.

Grinspoon, S., Thomas, E., Pitts, S., et al., 2000. Prevalence and predictive factors for regional osteopenia in women with anorexia nervosa. Annals of Internal Medicine 133 (10), 790–794.

Halvorsen, I., Andersen, A., Heyerdahl, S., 2004. Good outcome of adolescent onset anorexia nervosa after systematic treatment: intermediate to long-term follow up of a representative country sample. European Child and Adolescent Psychiatry 13 (5), 295–306.

Hamilton, J., 2007. Eating disorders in preadolescent children. The Nurse Practitioner 32 (3), 44–48.

Harshbarger, J.L., Ahlers-Schmidt, C.R., Mayans, L., Mayans, D., Hawkins, J.H., 2008. Pro-anorexia websites: what a clinician should know. International Journal of Eating Disorders 42 (4), 367–370.

Hatch, A., Madden, S., Kohn, M., et al., 2010. Anorexia nervosa: towards an integrative neuroscience model. European Eating Disorders Review 18, 165–179.

Hay, P., 2013. A systematic review of evidence for psychological treatments in eating disorders: 2005–2012. International Journal of Eating Disorders 46 (5), 462–469.

Hay, P., Bacaltchuk, J., Kashyap, P., 2009a. Psychological treatments for bulimia nervosa and binging (review). The Cochrane Database of Systematic Reviews 4, CD000562.

Hay, P., Chinn, D., Forbes, D., et al., 2014. Royal Australian and New Zealand College of Psychiatrists clinical practice guidelines for the treatment of eating disorders. Australian and New Zealand Journal of Psychiatry 48 (11), 977–1008. https://doi.org/10.1177/0004867414555814.

Hay, P., Darby, A., Quirk, F., 2009b. Cognitive behavioural therapy for bulimia nervosa and related bulimic eating disorders. In: Paxton, S., Hay, P. (Eds.), Interventions for Body Image and Eating Disorders. IP Communications Melbourne, pp. 23–43.

Hay, P.J., Claudino, A.M., 2012. Clinical psychopharmacology of eating disorders: a research update. International Journal of Neuro-Psychopharmacology 15, 209–222.

Herzog, D.B., Franko, D.L., Dorer, D.J., et al., 2006. Drug abuse in women with eating disorders. International Journal of Eating Disorders 39 (5), 364–368.

Hoek, H.W., 2006. Incidence, prevalence and mortality of anorexia nervosa and other eating disorders. Clinical Opinion in Psychiatry 19 (4), 389–394.

Hoek, H.W., 2014. Epidemiology of eating disorders in persons other than the high-risk group of young Western females. Current Opinion in Psychiatry 27 (6), 423–425.

Iacovino, J.M., Gredysa, D.M., Altman, M., Wilfley, D.E., 2012. Psychological treatments for binge eating disorder. Current Psychiatry Reports 14 (4), 432–446. https://doi.org/10.1007/s11920-012-0277-8.

Kaye, W.H., Bulik, C.M., Thornton, L., Barbarich, N., Masters, K., 2004. Comorbidity of anxiety disorders with anorexia and bulimia nervosa. American Journal of Psychiatry 161, 2215–2221.

Keel, P.K., Dorer, D.J., Eddy, K.T., et al., 2003. Predictors of mortality in eating disorders. Archives of General Psychiatry 60 (2), 179–183.

Keel, P.K., Mitchell, J.E., Miller, K.B., et al., 1999. Long-term outcome of bulimia nervosa. Archives of General Psychiatry 56 (1), 63–69.

Kenardy, J., Brown, W.J., Vogt, E., 2001. Dieting and health in young Australian women. European Eating Disorders Review 9 (4), 242.

Kessler, R.C., Berglund, P.A., Chiu, W.T., Deitz, A.C., Hudson, J.I., Shahly, V., Aquilar-Gaxiola, S., Aloso, J., Angermeyer, M.C., Benjet, C., Bruffaerts, R., et al., 2013. The prevalence and correlates of binge eating disorder in the World Health Organisation World Mental Health Surveys. Biological Psychiatry 73 (9), 904–914.

Khan, L.U.R., Ahmed, J., Khan, S., MacFie, J., 2011. Review article: refeeding syndrome. A literature review. Gastroenterology Research and Practice 2011, 6. https://doi.org/10.1155/2011/410971.

King's College London, 2018. Maudsley Model of Anorexia Nervosa Treatment for Adults (MANTRA) Introduction Workshop. Available at: https://www.kcl.ac.uk/ioppn/news/special-events/maudsley-model-of-anorexia-nervosa-treatment-for-adults-mantra.aspx. Accessed: 23 November 2018.

Klump, K.L., Bulik, C.M., Kaye, W.H., et al., 2009. Academy for eating disorders position paper: eating disorders are serious mental illnesses. International Journal of Eating Disorders 42 (2), 97–103.

Knowles, L., Anokhina, A., Serpell, L., 2013. Motivational interventions in eating disorders: what is the evidence? International Journal of Eating Disorders 46, 97–107.

Kohn, M., Madden, S., Clarke, S., 2011. Refeeding in anorexia nervosa: increased safety and efficiency through understanding the pathophysiology of protein calorie malnutrition. Current Opinion in Pediatrics 23, 390–394.

Kohn, M., Madden, S., Clarke, S., Anderson, G., 2009. Inpatient treatment issues for children and adolescents with anorexia nervosa. In: Paxton, S., Hay, P. (Eds.), Interventions for Body Image and Eating Disorders. IP Communications, Melbourne, pp. 119–139.

Kostro, K., Lerman, J.B., Attia, E., 2014. The current status of suicide and self-injury in eating disorders: a narrative review. Journal of Eating Disorders 2, 19.

Lavender, J.M., Wonderlich, S.A., Crosby, R.D., Engel, S.G., Mitchell, J.E., Crow, S., Peterson, C.B., Le Grange, D., 2013. A naturalistic examination of body checking and dietary restriction in women with anorexia nervosa. Behaviour Research and Therapy 51 (8), 507–511.

Lavender, J.M., Wonderlich, S.A., Engel, S.G., Gordon, K.H., Kaye, W.H., Mitchell, J.E., 2015. Dimensions of emotion dysregulation in anorexia nervosa and bulimia nervosa: a conceptual review of the empirical literature. Clinical Psychology Review 40, 111–122.

Le Grange, D., 2010. Family-based treatment for adolescents with bulimia nervosa. The Australian and New Zealand Journal of Family Therapy 31 (2), 165–175.

Leichner, L., Hall, D., Calderon, R., 2005. Meal support training for friends and families of patients with eating disorders. Eating Disorders 13 (4), 407–411.

Lewinsohn, P.M., Striegel-Moore, R.H., Seeley, J.R., 2000. Epidemiology and natural course of eating disorders in young women from adolescence to young adulthood. Journal of the American Academy of Child & Adolescent Psychiatry 39 (10), 1284–1292.

Lilenfeld, L.R., Stein, D., Bulik, C.M., et al., 2000. Personality traits among currently eating disordered, recovered and never ill first degree relatives of bulimic and control women. Psychological Medicine 30 (6), 1399–1410.

Lock, J., 2005. Adjusting cognitive behaviour therapy for adolescents with bulimia nervosa: results of case series. American Journal of Psychotherapy 59 (3), 267–281.

Lock, J., LeGrange, D., Forsberg, S., et al., 2006. Is family therapy useful for treating children with anorexia nervosa? Results of a case series. Journal of the American Academy of Child and Adolescent Psychiatry 45 (11), 1323–1328.

Lucas, A.R., Beard, C.M., O'Fallon, W.M., Kurland, L.T., 1991. 50-year trends in the incidence of anorexia nervosa in Rochester, Minn.: a population-based study. The American Journal of Psychiatry 148 (7), 917–922.

Macdonald, P., Murray, J., Goddard, E., Treasure, J., 2010. Carer's experience and perceived effects of a skills based training programme for families of people with eating disorders: a qualitative study. European Eating Disorder Review 19 (6), 475–486.

Madden, S., Morris, A., Zurynski, Y.A., et al., 2009. Burden of eating disorders in 5–13-year-old children in Australia. Medical Journal of Australia 190, 410–414.

Malson, H., Finn, D.M., Treasure, J., et al., 2004. Constructing 'the eating disordered patient': a discourse analysis of accounts of treatment experiences. Journal of Community Applied Social Psychology 14 (6), 473–489.

Mazzeo, S.E., Bulik, C.M., 2009. Environmental and genetic risk factors for eating disorders: what the clinician needs to know. Child and Adolescent Psychiatric Clinics of North America 18 (1), 67–82.

Mehler, P.S., Brown, C., 2015. Anorexia nervosa: medical complications. Journal of Eating Disorders 3, 11. https://doi.org/10.1186/s40337-015-0040-8.

Menzel, J.E., Schaefer, L.M., Burke, N.L., Mayhew, L.L., Brannick, M.T., Thompson, J.K., 2010. Appearance-related teasing, body dissatisfaction, and disordered eating: a meta-analysis. Body Image 7 (4), 261–270.

Merlotti, E., Mucci, A., Volpe, U., Montefusco, V., Moteleone, P., Bucci, P., Galderisi, S., 2013. Impulsiveness in patients with bulimia nervosa: electrophysiological evidence of reduced inhibitory control. Neuropsychobiology 68, 116–123.

McIntosh, V., Jordan, J., 2009. Specialist supportive clinical management for anorexia nervosa. In: Paxton, S., Hay, P. (Eds.), Interventions for Body Image and Eating Disorders. IP Communications, Melbourne, pp. 75–94.

McIntosh, V., Jordan, J., Carter, F., et al., 2005. Three psychotherapies for anorexia nervosa: a randomised controlled trial. American Journal of Psychiatry 162 (4), 741–747.

McIntosh, V., Jordan, J., Luty, S.E., et al., 2006. Specialist supportive clinical management for anorexia nervosa. International Journal of Eating Disorders 39 (8), 625–632.

Miller, K.K., Grinspoon, S.K., Ciampa, J., et al., 2005. Medical findings in outpatients with anorexia nervosa. Archives of Internal Medicine 165 (5), 561–566.
Mond, J.M., Calogero, R.M., 2009. Excessive exercise in eating disorder patients and in healthy women. Australian and New Zealand Journal of Psychiatry 43, 227.
Mond, J.M., Hay, P., Rodgers, B., Owen, C., 2012. Quality of life impairment in a community sample of women with eating disorders. Australian and New Zealand Journal of Psychiatry 46, 561–568.
Mond, J.M., Mitchison, D., Latner, J., Hay, P., Owen, C., Rodgers, B., 2013. Quality of life impairment associated with body dissatisfaction in a general population sample of women. BioMedCentral: Public Health 13, 920. https://doi.org/10.1186/1471-2458-13-920.
Mond, J.M., Robertson-Smith, G., Vetere, A., 2006. Stigma and eating disorders: is there evidence of negative attitudes towards anorexia nervosa among women in the community? Journal of Mental Health 5, 519–532. https://doi.org/10.1080/09638230600902559.
Mondraty, N., Birmingham, C.L., Touyz, S., et al., 2005. Randomised controlled trial of olanzapine in the treatment of cognitions in anorexia nervosa. Australasian Psychiatry 13 (1), 72–75.
Muise, A.M., Stein, D.G., Arbess, G., 2003. Eating disorders in adolescent boys: a review of the adolescent and young adult literature. Journal of Adolescent Health 33 (6), 427–435.
Murphy, R., Straebler, S., Cooper, Z., Fairburn, C.G., 2010. Cognitive behavioural therapy for eating disorders. Psychiatric Clinics of North America 33 (3), 611–627. https://doi.org/10.1016/j.psc.2010.04.004.
National Eating Disorders Collaboration (NEDC), 2010. Eating Disorders Prevention, Treatment & Management: An Evidence Review. Available at: www.nedc.com.au/nedc-publications.
National Eating Disorders Collaboration (NEDC), 2012. Eating Disorders in Australia. Available at: www.nedc.com.au/eating-disorders-in-australia.
National Institute for Health and Care Excellence (NICE), 2017. Eating Disorders: Recognition and Treatment [NG69]. Available at: https://www.nice.org.uk/guidance/ng69/chapter/Context. Accessed: 20 November 2018.
National Institute for Health and Care Excellence (NICE), 2018. Eating Disorders: Quality standard [QS175]. Available at: https://www.nice.org.uk/guidance/qs175. Accessed: 20 November 2018.
Neiderman, M., Farley, A., Richardson, J., Lask, B., 2001. Nasogastric feeding in children and adolescents with eating disorders: toward good practice. International Journal of Eating Disorders 29, 441–448.
Nizette, D., McAliste, M., Marks, P., 2013. Stories in Mental Health: Reflection Inquiry Action. Elsevier, Sydney.
O'Brien, A.J., Golding, C.G., 2003. Coercion in mental healthcare: the principle of least coercive care. Journal of Psychiatric and Mental Health Nursing 10, 167–173.
O'Dea, J.A., Abraham, S., 2002. Eating and exercise disorders in young college men. Journal of American College of Health 50 (6), 273–278.
Oldershaw, A., Lavender, T., Sallis, H., Stahl, D., Schmidt, U., 2015. Emotion generation and regulation in anorexia nervosa: a systematic review and meta-analysis of self-report data. Clinical Psychology Review 39, 83–95.
Ornstein, R., Golden, N., Jacobson, M., et al., 2003. Hypophosphatemia during nutritional rehabilitation in anorexia nervosa: implications for refeeding and monitoring. Journal of Adolescent Health 32 (1), 83–88.
Patton, G.C., Carlin, J.B., Shao, Q., Hibbert, M.E., Rosier, M., Selzer, R., Bowes, G., 1997. Adolescent dieting: healthy weight control or borderline eating disorder? Journal of Child Psychology and Psychiatry 38, 299–306.
Paxton, S., 2012. Modifiable risk factors that can be translated into prevention or resilience. In: Alexander, J., Treasure, J. (Eds.), A Collaborative Approach to Eating Disorders. Routledge, UK.
Pike, K.M., Hoek, H.W., Dunne, P.E., 2014. Cultural trends and eating disorders. Current Opinion 27, 436–442. https://doi.org/10.1097/YCO.0000000000000100.
Piran, N., Gadalla, T., 2007. Eating disorders and substance abuse in Canadian women: a national study. Addiction 102 (1), 105–113.
Pope, H., Phillips, K., Olivardia, R., 2000. The Adonis Complex. How to Identify, Treat, and Prevent Body Obsession in Men and Boys. Touchstone, Simon & Schuster, New York.
Ramjan, L.M., 2004. Nurses and the 'therapeutic relationship': caring for adolescents with anorexia nervosa. Journal of Advanced Nursing 45 (5), 495–503.
Reas, D.L., Grilo, C.M., 2014. Current and emerging drug treatments for binge eating disorder. Expert Opinion on Emerging Drugs 19 (1), 99–142. https://doi.org/10.1517/14728214.2014.879291.
Rhodes, P., Wallis, A., 2009. The Maudsley model of family therapy for anorexia nervosa. In: Paxton, S., Hay, P. (Eds.), Interventions for Body Image and Eating Disorders. IP Communications, Melbourne, pp. 58–74.
Rieger, E., 2009. Interpersonal psychotherapy for eating disorders. In: Paxton, S., Hay, P. (Eds.), Interventions for Body Image and Eating Disorders. IP Communications, Melbourne, pp. 217–233.
Rodgers, R.F., Paxton, S.J., 2014. The impact of indicated prevention and early intervention on co-morbid eating disorder and depressive symptoms: a systematic review. Journal of Eating Disorders 2, 30.
Rogers, R.F., Sales, P., Chabrol, H., 2010. Psychological functioning, media pressure and body dissatisfaction among college women. European Review of Applied Psychology 20 (2), 89–95.
Rome, E.S., Ammerman, S., 2003. Medical complications of eating disorders: an update. Journal of Adolescent Health 33 (6), 418–426.
Royal Australian and New Zealand College of Psychiatrists (RANZCP), 2004. Australian and New Zealand clinical practice guidelines for the treatment of anorexia nervosa. Australian and New Zealand Journal of Psychiatry 38 (9):659–670.
Royal Australian and New Zealand College of Psychiatrists (RANZCP), 2009. Anorexia Nervosa: Australian Treatment Guide for Consumers and Carers. Available at: www.ranzp.org.
Royal College of Psychiatrists (RCP), 2005. CR130 Guidelines for the Nutritional Management of Anorexia Nervosa. Royal College of Psychiatrists, London.
Royal College of Psychiatrists (RCP), 2012. Junior MARSIPAN: Management of Really Sick Patients under 18 with Anorexia Nervosa. Council Report CR168. Royal College of Psychiatrists, London.
Royal College of Psychiatrists (RCP), 2010. MARSIPAN: Management of Really Sick Patients with Anorexia Nervosa. Council Report CR 162. Royal College of Psychiatrists and Royal College of Physicians, London.
Ryan, V., Malson, H., Clarke, S., et al., 2006. Discursive constructions of 'eating disorders nursing': an analysis of nurses' accounts of nursing eating disorder patients. European Eating Disorders Review 14 (2), 125–135.
Schapman-Williams, A.M., Lock, J., Couturier, J., 2006. Cognitive-behavioural therapy for adolescents with binge eating syndromes: a case series. International Journal of Eating Disorders 39 (3), 252–255.
Schneider, N., Martus, P., Ehrlich, S., Pfeiffer, E., Lehmkuhl, U., Salbach-Andrae, H., 2009. The assessment of body image distortion in female adolescents with anorexia nervosa. Eating & Weight Disorders 14 (2–3), e128–e136.

Selvec, J.H., Tiggerman, M., 2011. Predictors of body dissatisfaction and disordered eating in middle-aged women. Clinical Psychology Review 31 (4), 515–524. https://doi.org/10.1016/j.cpr.2010.12.002.

Shapiro, J.R., Berkman, N.D., Brownley, K.A., et al., 2007. Bulimia nervosa treatment: a systematic review of randomised controlled trials. International Journal of Eating Disorders 40 (4), 321–336.

Smink, F.R.E., van Hoeken, D., Hoek, H.W., 2012. Epidemiology of eating disorders: incidence, prevalence and mortality rates. Current Psychiatry Reports 14, 406–414.

Stachowicz, M., Janas-Kozik, M., Olszanecka-Glinianowicz, M., Chudek, J., 2013. The role of leptin in eating disorders: current views. Psychiatria Polska 47 (5), 897–907.

Steinhausen, H.-C., 2002. The outcome of anorexia nervosa in the 20th century. American Journal of Psychiatry 159 (8), 1284–1293.

Stice, E., Marti, C.N., Durant, S., 2011. Risk factors for onset of eating disorders: evidence of multiple risk pathways from an 8-year prospective study. Behaviour Research and Therapy 49 (10), 622–627.

Strober, M., 2014. Proposition: family based treatment is overvalued. Advances in Eating Disorders, Theory, Research and Practice 2 (3), 264–299.

Strober, M., Johnson, C., 2012. The need for complex ideas in anorexia nervosa: why biology, environment, and psyche all matter, why therapists make mistakes, and why clinical benchmarks are needed for managing weight correction. International Journal of Eating Disorders 45, 155–178.

Strother, E., Lemberg, R., Stanford, S.C., Turberville, D., 2012. Eating disorders in men: underdiagnosed, undertreated and misunderstood. Eating Disorders: The Journal of Treatment and Prevention 20 (5), 346–355.

Suler, J., 2004. The online disinhibition effect. Cyberpsychology & Behaviour 7 (3), 321–326.

Sullivan, P., 1995. Mortality in anorexia nervosa. American Journal of Psychiatry 153, 1073–1074.

Surgenor, L., Thornton, C., 2000. Eating disorders and disturbed body image: a view from psychology. In: Gaskill, D., Sanders, F. (Eds.), The Encultured Body: Policy Implications for Healthy Body Image and Disordered Eating Behaviours. QUT, Kelvin Grove, Queensland, pp. 106–118.

Surgenor, L.J., Maguire, S., 2013. Assessment of anorexia nervosa: an overview of universal issues and contextual challenges. Journal of Eating Disorders 1, 29.

Sweetingham, R., Waller, G., 2008. Childhood experiences of being bullied and teased in the eating disorders. European Eating Disorders Review 15 (5), 401–407. https://doi.org/10.1002/erv.839.

Tierney, S., 2008. The individual within a condition: a qualitative study of young people's reflections on being treated for anorexia nervosa. Journal of the American Psychiatric Nurses Association 13, 368–375.

Treasure, J., Claudino, A.M., Zucker, N., 2010. Eating disorders. The Lancet 375, 583–593.

Treasure, J., Gavan, K., Todd, G., et al., 2003. Changing the environment in eating disorders: working with carers/families to improve motivation and facilitate change. European Eating Disorders Review 11 (1), 25–37.

Treasure, J., Smith, G., Crane, A., 2007. Skills-Based Learning for Caring for a Loved One With an Eating Disorder: The New Maudsley Method. Routledge, UK.

Tucci, J., Mitchell, J., Goddard, C., 2007. Modern Children in Australia. Australian Childhood Foundation, Melbourne.

Van Son, G., Van Hoeken, D., Bartelds, A., et al., 2006. Urbanisation and the incidence of eating disorders. British Journal of Psychiatry 189 (6), 562–563.

Vossbeck-Elsebusch, A.N., Waldorf, M., Legenbauer, T., Bauer, A., Cordes, M., Vocks, S., 2014. Overestimation of body size in eating disorders and its association to body-related avoidance behaviour. Eating & Weight Disorders 20 (2), 173–178. https://doi.org/10.1007/s40519-014-0144-1.

Wade, T., Byrne, S., Touyz, S., 2013. A clinician's quick guide of evidence-based approaches. Number 1: eating disorders. Clinical Psychologist 17 (1), 31–32. https://doi.org/ 10.1111.cp.12004.

Waller, G., 2012. The myths of motivation: time for a fresh look at some received wisdom in the eating disorders? International Journal of Eating Disorders 45, 1–16.

Wand, T., 2015. Recovery is about a focus on resilience and wellness, not a fixation with risk and illness. Australian and New Zealand Journal of Psychiatry 49 (12), 1083–1084.

Watson, H., Bulik, C., 2013. Update on the treatment of anorexia nervosa: review of clinical trials, practice guidelines and emerging interventions. Psychological Medicine 43 (12), 2477–2500. https://doi.org/10.1017/S0033291712002620.

Watson, H., Elphick, R., Dreher, C., Steele, A., Wilksch, S., 2010. Eating disorders prevention, treatment and management: an evidence review. National Eating Disorders Collaboration. Available at: www.nedc.com.au/files/pdfs/NEDC_Evidence%20Review_Final.pdf.

Weltzin, T.E., Conrnella-Carlson, T., Fitzpatrick, M.E., Kennington, B., Bean, P., Jeferies, C., 2012. Treatment issues and outcomes for males with eating disorders. Eating Disorders 20 (5), 444–459.

Yager, Z., O'Dea, J., 2008. Prevention programs for body image and eating disorders on University campuses: a review of large, controlled interventions. Health Promotion International 23 (2), 174–189. https://doi.org/10.1093/heapro/dan004.

Zugai, J., Stein-Parbury, J., Roche, M., 2013. Effective nursing care of adolescents with anorexia nervosa: a consumer perspective. Journal of Clinical Nursing 22, 2020–2029.

USEFUL WEBSITES

BEAT Eating Disorders, www.beateatingdisorders.org.uk/?gclid=EAIaIQobChMIopHn_ubq3gIVw-d3Ch0H-8Qb-EAAYAiAAEgI2f_D_BwE

Journal of Eating Disorders, Open Access, Peer-Reviewed Journal Publishing Leading Research in the Science and Practice of Eating Disorders, www.jeatdisord.com

MARSIPAN Guidelines: Management of Really Sick Patients with Anorexia Nervosa, https://www.rcpsych.ac.uk/docs/default-source/improving-care/better-mh-policy/college-reports/college-report-cr189.pdf?sfvrsn=6c2e7ada_2

MIND Eating Problems, https://www.mind.org.uk/information-support/types-of-mental-health-problems/eating-problems/#.W_gZg-j7TIU

National Eating Disorders Collaboration (NEDC), National Eating Disorders Collaboration (NEDC), http://nedc.com.au/

NHS Eating Disorders, https://www.nhs.uk/conditions/eating-disorders/

20

Substance Use and Comorbid Mental Health Disorders

Peter Athanasos

KEY POINTS

- Excessive alcohol consumption is the cause of a wide range of health harms including the major cause of road accidents, domestic violence, public violence, crime, liver disease and brain damage. It contributes to family breakdown and broader social dysfunction.
- Fifty-eight percent of adults in England (over 16 years) had drunk alcohol in the previous week in 2017, which was similar to 2016 but lower than 2007 (National Health Service [NHS] 2018).
- There were 5507 alcohol-specific deaths in England in 2016, which was 4% higher than 2015 and an increase of 11% on 2006 (NHS 2018).
- Alcohol is associated with liver disease, pancreatitis, some cancers, diabetes, epilepsy, motor vehicle accidents and a range of social problems such as neglect and abuse.
- There is a considerable degree of coexistence between substance use disorder (particularly alcohol) and other mental health disorders.
- Psychoactive drugs can cause harm through intoxication or addiction. They are classified as depressants, stimulants, hallucinogens or mixed effect drugs.
- Specific assessment tools and criteria are used for people who present with a substance disorder or who have a comorbid disorder.
- Interventions include harm reduction, management of the intoxicated patient, detoxification, early interventions and brief interventions.
- Accurate assessment and appropriate management of a patient with a comorbid disorder are essential.
- Treatment for comorbidity patients can include pharmacological and psychological interventions to reduce substance use.

KEY TERMS

abstinence
alcohol and other drugs use
alcohol use disorders
anxiety disorders
assessment
cannabis
coexisting disorder
comorbidity
dependence
detoxification
drug use disorders
comorbid disorder
harm reduction
harmful use
hazardous use
illicit
injecting drug use
interventions
intoxication
lactation
parenting
pharmacodynamics
pharmacokinetics
physical dependence
pregnancy
problematic substance use
psychoactive drugs
psychological dependence
psychosis
risk
substance misuse
substance-related disorders
therapeutic use
tolerance
toxicity
withdrawal

LEARNING OUTCOMES

The material in this chapter will assist you to:

- discuss the incidence and impact of substance-related disorders and comorbid disorder diagnosis in the UK.
- describe the pharmacokinetics and pharmacodynamics of psychoactive drugs.
- identify the importance of undertaking a drug and alcohol assessment for all mental health patients.
- describe a range of interventions that can be used for patients with a coexisting substance use disorder and a mental illness.
- apply your knowledge of the nursing process to the patient who is dependent on alcohol and other drugs.
- critically analyse the range of treatment services available for patients with a comorbidity diagnosis.

INTRODUCTION

Wherever nurses work they will come across people who have substance use problems. These substances are either legal or illegal, depending on local laws and customs. In the same way, wherever nurses work they will come across people with mental health problems. We may have times in our own lives when we experience mental health or substance use problems. If we understand the nature of these problems, we can offer the best care possible.

This chapter explores issues of substance use, substance-related disorders and coexisting disorders (mental health problems and substance use problems) in the UK. It highlights the costs of drug and alcohol use to the person, family and community. The pharmacology of psychoactive drugs is explored, terms are defined and the diagnostic criteria for substance disorders are presented. The skills needed to ask the right questions and to provide a comprehensive drug and alcohol assessment are detailed. Specific interventions such as early interventions, brief interventions and harm reduction are explored. The assessment and treatment of patients who are intoxicated or withdrawing from substances is described.

The final section of the chapter discusses comorbid diagnosis. The phenomenon is often referred to as 'dual diagnosis'. However, this is a misleading description as many patients present with a range of co-occurring conditions of varying pathology (Drake & Wallach 2000; Mills et al. 2008). The final section examines the significance of comorbid diagnosis, why people with a mental illness use alcohol and other drugs, treatment models and interventions. You will find additional information and specific nursing interventions for comorbid diagnosis in other relevant chapters.

EPIDEMIOLOGY

The problems of substance use disorders comorbid with mental health disorders have been gaining in prominence in drug and alcohol services, mental health services, gambling services and general health services over the last 30 years (Lai et al. 2015). There is strong evidence that substance use disorders occur more frequently among people with mental health disorders than among the general population (Regier et al. 1990; Menezes et al. 1996; Kessler 2004; Merikangas & Kalaydjian 2007; Rosenthal et al. 2012; Lai et al. 2015). This has contributed to the high burden of disease for these comorbid disorders worldwide (Lai et al. 2015).

There are causal relationships between alcohol consumption and more than 200 types of disease and injury. A significant proportion of the alcohol disease burden is due to road accidents, violence and suicides. Overall, 5.1% of the global burden of disease and injury is attributable to alcohol as measured in disability adjusted life years (World Health Organization [WHO] 2014a). There is also a proven causal relationship between harmful use of alcohol, a range of mental and behavioural disorders, other noncommunicable conditions and injuries (WHO 2014b).

Alcohol consumption causes death and disability relatively early in life. Globally, in the 20 to 39 year age group approximately 25% of the total deaths are attributable to alcohol (WHO 2014b). There are significant gender differences in the prevalence of substance use and dependence, with lifetime prevalence of exposure for all categories of substances higher for males than for females in almost all societies and cultures (Degenhardt & Hall 2012; Steingrimsson et al. 2012; Lev-Ran et al. 2013).

Globally, fewer people use illicit drugs than use alcohol (roughly one-tenth), while tobacco use is far more widespread, and so its contribution to disease burden is greater than that for alcohol or illicit drugs (Degenhardt & Hall 2012). Compared with other countries, the UK has one of the highest rates of burden of disease attributable to illicit drug dependence, along with the USA, Russia and Australia and among the highest prevalence of opioid dependence worldwide (Degenhardt et al. 2013).

Overall, alcohol use in England is declining. In 2017 58% of adults (16+ years) in England had drunk alcohol in the previous week, which was similar to 2016 but lower than 2007. In 2016/17 there were 337 thousand estimated admissions where the main reason for admission to hospital was attributable to alcohol, which is 1% lower than in 2015/16; however, 17% higher than in 2006/7. There were also 5507 alcohol-specific deaths in England in 2016, which was 4% higher than 2015 and an increase of 11% on 2006 (NHS 2018). Across the whole of the UK, the annual amount of alcohol sold per adult (16+ years) rose from 9.53 litres of pure alcohol in 1986/87, peaked at 11.73 litres in 2004/05, before dropping to 9.65 litres in 2012/13 (National Institute of Health and Care Excellence [NICE] 2015).

In 2017 to 2018 there were 268,390 adults in contact with drug and alcohol services, a 4% reduction from the previous year, with the largest proportion (53%) being people in treatment for opiates. There was an increase (18%) in people being treated for crack cocaine since the year before—which was a considerable increase on the year before that (44%). This rise in treatment numbers was seen in all age groups except those over 65 years. These latest figures suggest a 10% increase in the number of people using crack cocaine since 2011 to 2012, which is thought to be due in part to the changes in purity, affordability and patterns of distribution (Public Health England [PHE] 2018). In 2017 to 2018 there was a 16% decrease in the number of people seeking help for problems related to new psychoactive substances (NPS) or 'legal highs', which have been around since approximately 2008/2009 and are under the control of the Drugs Act 1971 or subject to the Psychoactive Substances Act 2016 (PS Act), the most well known being mephedrone. People who start treatment are more likely (25%) to be homeless, which has increased from 6% in 2013 to 2014 (Home Office 2016). Cannabis (also known as marijuana, weed, pot, dope or grass) is the most widely used illegal drug in the UK (NHS 2017).

SUBSTANCE USE AND GAMBLING

A high level of association exists between problem gambling and drug, alcohol and mental health disorders. A 2011 systematic review of international research on comorbid disorders in problem gambling found that more than one-quarter (28%) of problem gamblers had a lifetime alcohol use disorder and 17% had a lifetime illicit drug use disorder (Lorains et al. 2011). Problem gamblers with lifetime alcohol dependence reported greater lifetime gambling severity, displaying addictive behaviour across multiple domains and reported personality styles characterized by hopelessness, impaired control and resistance to externally motivated treatment approaches (Lister et al. 2015).

Pregnancy, Lactation and Parenting

There is irrefutable evidence that alcohol is a teratogen (able to disturb the growth of an embryo or fetus) and these studies have been replicated many times (Fukui & Sakata-Haga 2009). There is no safe level of alcohol use by the mother and abstinence is recommended in pregnancy (Royal College of Obstetricians and Gynaecologists 2018). However, abstinence is not always a realistic option and in such cases the pregnant woman needs to be advised to talk to her health professional to find out the safest option if she plans to continue using substances.

The consequences of alcohol intake during lactation compared with pregnancy have not been as extensively examined. A recent review of alcohol and breastfeeding found that approximately half of all women in Western countries consume alcohol while breastfeeding (Haastrup et al. 2014). The authors found that alcohol concentrations in breast milk closely resemble those in maternal blood and therefore the amount of alcohol presented to nursing infants through breast milk is approximately 5% to 6% of the weight-adjusted maternal dose. Even in a case of binge drinking, infants would not be subjected to clinically relevant amounts of alcohol. The long-term consequences for children of alcohol misusing mothers are yet unknown, but occasional drinking while breastfeeding has not been convincingly shown to adversely affect infants who are nursing. The authors recommend that lactating women should follow standard recommendations on female alcohol consumption (Haastrup et al. 2014).

Pregnant women use significantly fewer substances than other women of child-bearing age and tend to reduce use as they progress through their pregnancy (Havens et al. 2009). The most prevalent substance used by pregnant women is cigarettes (18.9%), followed by alcohol (10%) and cannabis (3.7%). Polysubstance use is reported by 6.1% of pregnant women (Havens et al. 2009). Use of alcohol and other substances can affect the development of children from conception, after birth and across the lifespan (Taplin et al. 2015). Pregnancy can be a very good time to address maternal alcohol and other drug use. It might also be a brief window where 'the multiple intersecting and complex issues that led to substance use initiation and continuation' might be addressed (Jones & Kaltenback 2013; Taplin et al. 2015). Infants and children develop within a context of complex social and environmental conditions. These conditions influence functional and behavioural capacities. This makes it difficult to clearly ascertain a drug-specific effect on developmental processes (Bandstra et al. 2010; Taplin et al. 2015).

However, parental use of alcohol and other substances can be associated with child maltreatment and is a common characteristic of families involved with the child protection system (Taplin et al. 2015). Mothers with drug and alcohol problems who are involved with the child protection system are more likely to have mental health problems, be younger, have more children, have greater economic problems, have a history of homelessness and have fewer social supports (Nair et al. 1997; Grella et al. 2006; Gilchrist & Taylor 2009; Grella et al. 2009; Grant et al. 2011; Taplin & Mattick 2013; Laslett et al. 2014; Taplin et al. 2015). They are also likely to have greater levels of life stressors, often including trauma and abusive histories of their own, which may impact on their parenting style. Parental substance misuse may be a marker for mental health problems, which have the stronger association with child maltreatment (Dawe et al. 2006).

As Taplin et al. (2015) suggest, although evidence is limited, universal screening for alcohol and other drug use in pregnancy (including tobacco) is recommended. This reduces targeted screening of groups that are marginalised, reduces stigma and reduces the under-identification of alcohol and other drug use in pregnancy.

PHARMACOLOGY OF PSYCHOACTIVE DRUGS

Pharmacological Aspects of Addiction

When people take drugs, drink alcohol, eat, gamble, exercise or have sex there is a release of the chemical dopamine along the mesolimbic dopamine pathway in the brain (note: there are many other chemicals and pathways involved, including the noradrenaline, serotonin, glutamate and glycine systems) (Koob & Volkow 2010; Moore et al. 2014; Berridge & Kringelbach 2015). The release of dopamine along this pathway makes you feel good and 'want' more. It is a central mechanism in all animals (including humans) and is essential for survival. It communicates to the animal that this activity (chasing and eating an animal, having sex) is vital for the survival of the species and should be their focus (Miller & Gold 1993; Robertson et al. 2015). However, this ancient mechanism designed for species survival was hijacked by alternative means: humans found that drinking alcohol or using drugs also released dopamine. This is the reason why alcoholics and drug addicts can get so fixated on using the drug to the exclusion of all else. They have developed a need for dopamine release through using substances. For them it feels as though their survival is dependent on the substances they take. Broadly, the release of dopamine also underpins the behavioural addictions to gambling, exercise and sex (Nutt et al. 2015).

This psychoactive effect includes changes in mood, arousal, perception, thinking and behaviour. These drugs may be produced in a laboratory (e.g. amphetamines, ecstasy) or extracted from plants (e.g. heroin, cocaine). They can be legal (e.g. alcohol) or illegal (e.g. cannabis). They can be classified in many ways but one of the most common methods is to classify them as depressants, stimulants or hallucinogens. Some drugs have multiple actions and therefore can be placed in more than one category (Teesson & Hall 2001; Ries et al. 2014). The common effect of all psychoactive drugs, at least in early stages of use, is to produce euphoria and a change in mental state. Over a period of time many people may describe little positive effect but rather a decrease in negative effect when they use (Ries et al. 2014).

Depressants

Depressants are drugs that slow the activity of the brain. When used in small doses they can produce euphoria, relaxation or drowsiness. In larger doses they can produce a loss of consciousness similar to a deep sleep, impaired coordination, depression, coma and death by respiratory depression. Depressant drugs include ethanol (alcohol), benzodiazepines (e.g. diazepam or temazepam), opioids (e.g. codeine, morphine, heroin), solvents and inhalants (Galanter et al. 2015).

Stimulants

Stimulant drugs increase activity in the nervous system and increase the body's level of arousal. Small doses increase awareness and concentration and decrease fatigue. Increasing amounts produce irritability, nervousness and insomnia. At high doses some people experience delusions and hallucinations. Toxic doses lead to convulsions and death via heart attack (myocardial infarction), stroke (cerebrovascular accident) or muscle meltdown (rhabdomyolysis). Stimulants include amphetamines (commonly known as speed), methamphetamines (commonly known as crystal meth or ice), D-amphetamine (dexamphetamine) and methylphenidate (Ritalin), as well as cocaine, nicotine, caffeine and 3,4-methylenedioxymethamphetamine (MDMA, commonly known as ecstasy) (Ries et al. 2014; Harro 2015).

Hallucinogens

Hallucinogens (also called psychedelics) share properties with depressants and stimulants. However, their specific function is to distort perception and consequently induce hallucinations (auditory, tactile and visual). In small doses, some hallucinogens reduce inhibitions and cause the user to become relaxed and feel more sociable. Hallucinogens include lysergic acid diethylamide (LSD), psilocybin (magic mushrooms) and mescaline (part of the Mexican cactus peyote). Some amphetamine derivatives such as MDMA (ecstasy) are chemically related to mescaline and have both stimulant and hallucinatory properties. These drugs may be placed in both categories for classification purposes (Galanter et al. 2015).

Cannabis

Although cannabis is commonly placed with the hallucinogenic group of drugs, it is often difficult to classify in pharmacological terms as it has a mixture of mood, cognitive, motor and perceptual effects and does not clearly belong with any one drug class (Kaufmann et al. 2010; Kleinloog et al. 2014). Cannabis taken in low doses produces a mixture of stimulatory and depressant effects; at high doses the effects are mainly depressant. The effects of cannabis include euphoria, relaxation and a feeling of well-being, as well as perceptual distortions such as altered time sense. Memory, cognition and skilled task performance are impaired, although many users may feel confident and highly creative. Other physical effects include tachycardia, vasodilation and hypotension (Kleinloog et al. 2014; Martin-Santos et al. 2012).

Cannabis stimulates the appetite and is also an anti-emetic; people who have taken cannabis often experience 'the munchies', where they feel hungry and crave certain foods. As with all psychoactive drugs, the effects vary between people depending on the amount taken, the manner of administration, the frequency of use, concurrent use with other drugs, past exposure and the environment in which the drug is used (Kleinloog et al. 2014).

Emerging Psychoactives

The class of drugs known as emerging psychoactives, NPS or 'legal highs' (see Table 20.1) is structurally similar but not identical to psychoactive drugs that are currently available but illegal, such as methamphetamines, cannabis, ecstasy and depressants (Burns et al. 2014b). These substances are constantly being developed and modified to stay ahead of legal restrictions. They are available both 'on the street' and via the internet. Internet websites such as 'The Silk Road 1.0 and 2.0' and others continue to grow as a source of mail-box-delivered psychoactives. Although the original websites have been closed down and the operators prosecuted by law enforcement authorities, other websites have quickly arisen to supply the market (Burns et al. 2014a). This conceivably means that millions of drugs that have not been invented yet are potentially illegal (Davies 2012; Burns et al. 2014b).

Determining the toxicity of this emerging class of drugs is challenging because it consists of many different types of substances that vary in their psychological and physiological effects and the drugs may be combined (Weaver et al. 2015). All alcohol and other drug use entails risk and when substances are purchased over the internet without quality control, the risk is increased (Davies 2012; Burns et al. 2014a; Weaver et al. 2015).

DIAGNOSIS FOR SUBSTANCE USE

Substance use exists on a spectrum that ranges from abstinence to occasional use to harmful use to addiction. Occasional use may not cause problems or may even be beneficial. In general, the more often the substance is used and the greater the amount used, the more severe the health consequences, psychosocial consequences and risk of dependence.

DIAGNOSTIC AND STATISTICAL MANUAL OF MENTAL DISORDERS, 5TH EDITION (DSM-5)

The *Diagnostic and Statistical Manual of Mental Disorders*, 5th edition (DSM-5) (American Psychiatric Association [APA]

TABLE 20.1 Emerging Psychoactives

Drug	Similar to	Examples	Source
Synthetic cathinones	Stimulants (e.g. amphetamines and ecstasy)	Mephedrone, methadrone, methylone, meow, M-Cat, 'drone', 'bath salts', 'plant food'	Khat plant
2C agents	Stimulants with some hallucinogenic effect (e.g. amphetamines and ecstasy)	2C1, 2CB, 2CT, NBom	Chemically derived
Piperazine derivatives	Primarily hallucinogenic with some stimulant activity (e.g. less potent lysergic acid diethylamide [LSD])	'Party pills', BZP	Chemically derived
Synthetic cannabinoids	Cannabis	K2, 'Gold', 'Spice'	Derived from cannabis plant. Specifically modified variations on the proportions of naturally occurring delta-9 tetra-hydro-cannabinol and cannabadinol
Bromo-dragon FLY	Long-acting hallucinogen of several days duration (e.g. LSD)	Bromo-dragon FLY	Derived from cannabis plant. Specifically modified variations on the proportions of naturally occurring Delta-9 tetra-hydro-cannabinol and cannabadinol
Benzofurans	Ecstasy	Benzofurans	Chemically derived

(*Source:* Musselman, M.E., Hampton, J.P. 2014. Not for human consumption: a review of emerging designer drugs. Pharmacotherapy. 34, 745–757.)

2013) is used widely for classifying mental health, drug and alcohol disorders. In contrast to the previous DSM-IV TR, the DSM-5 does not use the terms 'dependence', 'addiction' or 'substance abuse' as the authors have determined that these terms can be very confusing and judgemental. Rather, the DSM-5 describes substance use disorder (referring to drugs or alcohol) and then determines the severity of the disorder by the number of symptoms present (see Box 20.1). The DSM-5 also describes intoxication and withdrawal in relation to specific substances. Alcohol dependence is defined in ICD-10 and DSM-IV in categorical terms for diagnostic and statistical purposes as being either present or absent, but in reality dependence exists on a continuum of severity. It is clinically helpful to subdivide dependence into categories of mild (scoring 15 or less on the Severity of Alcohol Dependence Questionnaire; SADQ) which does not usually require assisted alcohol withdrawal, moderate (SADQ score of between 15 and 30) which usually requires assisted alcohol withdrawal which can typically be managed in the community and severe (SADQ score 30+) which requires assisted alcohol withdrawal typically carried out in an inpatient or residential setting (NICE 2011). See Boxes 20.2 and 20.3 for more information about how to recognise and manage intoxication and Box 20.4 for diagnostic criteria for alcohol withdrawal.

Intoxication

Problems can occur from once-off use (e.g. intoxication or bingeing), regular use (e.g. financial, relationship, memory and physical impacts) and addiction (e.g. withdrawal, craving, conflict) (Thorley 1982). Nurses need to manage intoxication correctly because it complicates assessment and patient management, even when it is not life threatening. Intoxication

BOX 20.1 DSM-5 Criteria for Substance Use Disorder

Substance use disorders span a wide variety of problems associated with substance use. There are 11 criteria:

1. Taking the substance in larger amounts or for longer than was intended
2. Wanting to cut down or stop using the substance but not managing to
3. Spending a lot of time getting, using or recovering from use of the substance
4. Cravings and urges to use the substance
5. Not managing to do what you should at work, home or school because of substance use
6. Continuing to use, even when it causes problems in relationships
7. Giving up important social, occupational or recreational activities because of substance use
8. Using substances again and again, when it is physically hazardous
9. Continuing to use, even when you know you have a physical or psychological problem that could have been caused or made worse by the substance
10. Needing more of the substance to get the effect you want (tolerance)
11. Development of withdrawal symptoms, which can be relieved by taking more of the substance.

The DSM-5 allows clinicians to specify how severe the substance use disorder is, depending on how many symptoms are identified. Two or three symptoms indicate a mild substance use disorder, four or five symptoms indicate a moderate substance use disorder and six or more symptoms indicate a severe substance use disorder

(*Source:* Reprinted with permission from the Diagnostic and Statistical Manual of Mental Disorders, Fifth Edition, (Copyright © 2013). American Psychiatric Association. All Rights Reserved.)

BOX 20.2 DSM-5 Criteria for Alcohol Intoxication

Diagnostic criteria

A. Recent ingestion of alcohol.

B. Clinically significant problematic behavioural or psychological changes (e.g. inappropriate sexual or aggressive behaviour, mood lability, impaired judgment) that developed during, or shortly after, alcohol ingestion.

C. One (or more) of the following signs or symptoms developing during, or shortly after, alcohol use:

1. Slurred speech
2. Incoordination
3. Unsteady gait
4. Nystagmus
5. Impairment in attention or memory
6. Stupor or coma

D. The signs or symptoms are not attributable to another medical condition and are not better explained by another mental disorder, including intoxication with another substance.

(*Source:* Reprinted with permission from the Diagnostic and Statistical Manual of Mental Disorders, Fifth Edition, (Copyright © 2013). American Psychiatric Association. All Rights Reserved.)

BOX 20.3 General Principles of Managing Intoxication

- Maintenance of airways and breathing is of paramount importance to the comatose patient.
- Any patient presenting as incoherent, disoriented or drowsy should be treated as per head injury until proven otherwise.
- Intoxicated patients must be kept under observation until their intoxication diminishes.
- A thorough physical and mental status examination will reveal the level of a patient's intoxication to provide baseline information.
- Patients who appear intoxicated may be suffering from other conditions, so if the intoxication does not diminish with falling serum drug levels, the patient must be assessed for other possible causes of their condition. If an apparently intoxicated person cannot walk, stand or get up from a chair they must continue to be observed.
- Intoxicated patients should be treated with respect. Speak slowly and simply, treat them in a quiet place if possible, give information clearly and protect them from accidents.
- Patients who have stabilised after being intoxicated should be further assessed for any possibility of withdrawal—early identification and intervention of withdrawal management can prevent complications that may be life threatening.
- Alcohol withdrawal can occur before a zero blood alcohol reading is noted.
- Polydrug use is common, so it is important to identify and observe for the effects of more than one drug in the intoxicated person.
- Any patient presenting with seizures should be assessed for alcohol withdrawal, benzodiazepine withdrawal or stimulant intoxication, as well as other possible causes. The seizures must be treated according to policy and the patient observed for at least 4 hours postseizure, using the Glasgow Coma Scale score (see Table 20.2 later in the chapter).

(*Source:* New South Wales Ministry of Health, 2016. Clinical guidelines for nursing and midwifery practice in NSW. Identifying and responding to drug and alcohol issues. Reproduced by permission, NSW Ministry of Health. Also see: The Royal College of Emergency Medicine: Alcohol Toolkit (https://www.rcem.ac.uk/docs/College%20Guidelines/5z24.%20Alcohol%20toolkit%20(June%202015).pdf)

BOX 20.4 DSM-5 Criteria for Alcohol Withdrawal

A. Cessation of (or reduction in) alcohol use that has been heavy and prolonged.

B. Two (or more) of the following, developing within several hours to a few days after the cessation of (or reduction in) alcohol use described in Criterion A:

1. Autonomic hyperactivity (e.g. sweating or pulse rate greater than 100 bpm)
2. Increased hand tremor
3. Insomnia
4. Nausea or vomiting
5. Transient visual, tactile or auditory hallucinations or illusions
6. Psychomotor agitation
7. Anxiety
8. Generalized tonic–clonic seizures

C. The signs or symptoms in Criterion B cause clinically significant distress or impairment in social, occupational or other important areas of functioning.

D. The signs or symptoms are not attributable to another medical condition and are not better explained by another mental disorder, including intoxication or withdrawal from another substance.

Specify if: With perceptual disturbances. This specifier applies in the rare instance when hallucinations (usually visual or tactile) occur with intact reality testing, or auditory, visual or tactile illusions occur in the absence of a delirium.

(*Source:* American Psychiatric Association (APA), 2013. Diagnostic and Statistical Manual of Mental Disorders, 5th edn (DSM-5). American Psychiatric Association, Washington. Reprinted with permission.)

can mask serious illness or injury (e.g. infections, hypoxia, head injury and cerebrovascular accidents). It can also be life threatening because it can cause altered physical functioning (e.g. depressed respiration, temperature dysregulation) and disturbed mental state (e.g. panic or paranoia), which can result in accidental injuries (New South Wales Health 2013).

Dependence

Dependence can be both physical and psychological; strictly speaking, dependence is when withdrawal symptoms occur when you stop using a substance (drugs or alcohol). Physical dependence is the physical symptomatology of withdrawal as evidenced by sweating, perspiration and raised blood pressure. If a person is using regularly and that person rapidly reduces their use or stops using the drug, they are very likely to experience what is known as physical withdrawal. They are physically dependent. Psychological dependence is the withdrawal-driven craving for the substance when the person stops using the substance.

Often, physical and psychological dependence are combined, but not always. A person might be psychologically dependent on cannabis (want to smoke it all the time) but show little physical withdrawal when they stop. A patient with chronic pain who is taking opioids might go into physical withdrawal if they stop taking the opioid medication, without psychologically craving the drug. Addiction to sex or gambling is a primarily psychological dependence and there is less physical withdrawal when ceased (Nestler 2005; Koob 2015).

Tolerance

Tolerance (the need for more and more of a substance to get the same effect) can also be physiological and psychological. Physiological tolerance results from the repeated effects on the brain from daily doses of drugs such as alcohol, methamphetamines, nicotine or opioids. Brain neural circuitry involving dopamine neurons adapts to the addition of the drug and reduces the responsiveness of the dopamine receptors (among other neural circuits). This decreased responsiveness leads to tolerance for the drug and reduces the sense of pleasure or pain relief.

Psychological tolerance is the need for more of the substance to get the same sense of euphoria. For example, someone may become psychologically tolerant to gambling and need to gamble progressively more for the same effect: a nonpharmacological, purely psychological tolerance has developed. Most often, however, physical and psychological tolerance are combined (Nestler 2005; Koob 2015).

NURSE'S STORY 20.1 Working in Alcohol and Other Drug Nursing

The ultimate challenge and 'high' of working in drug and alcohol nursing is the experience of assisting a patient and seeing them creating a happier life out of what is sometimes chaos. My part in providing the information and the skills that help that process of recovery gives me a sense of wellbeing and achievement about what I do.

I am only talking about small steps here. Every small step no matter how hesitant is a cause for celebration and joy. You cannot do the patient's work for them but you can provide assistance to them on the journey they must make. That is where skill is needed. The skill is assessing where the patient is on the motivational cycle and being able to provide assistance that helps them towards their recovery, yet recognising that everyone has different recovery goals and that each person's needs are unique. So, the passion for me is in feeling that I am doing something to help people out of this mess. Even if it is only by offering my respect, recognition, skills and time.

The downside is that you cannot do it for them, and the struggle with addiction and dependence is a hard and lonely one. At those times when people give up on their goals I remind myself that these problems were a long time developing and will be a long time in being resolved, and that a step back is just that, not the end of the game.

ASSESSMENT AND DIAGNOSIS

Alcohol and drug use is common and should be considered with every patient in all settings. Specific assessment tools and criteria are available. It is important to carefully elicit alcohol and drug use to make a diagnosis so that an appropriate management strategy can be implemented. Kelleher (2007) found that, in a European setting, one in four of those attending the emergency department had substance-related injuries or illness and one in eight was in a state of clinical intoxication. The success rate in detecting these patients was disturbingly low (25%–50%). As a result, many substance use problems are misdiagnosed or remain undetected. This can have lethal consequences (Saunders & Young 2002; Hoban 2017).

Presentation and Setting

The process of assessment is dependent on the nature of the presentation and the setting. For example, people who present to an emergency department are likely to be distressed due to recent trauma experienced by themselves or loved ones. This distress should be carefully acknowledged but it must not interfere with obtaining important information about the patient's alcohol and drug use for their immediate management (Saunders & Young 2002).

Substance Use History

A patient's substance use (prescribed and nonprescribed) must be measured to determine whether the level of use may cause harm or whether withdrawal is imminent. A recent substance use history will determine the type of substance used, the level of use, the frequency of use and whether a withdrawal state could occur, so that staff can determine the patient's requirements for analgesia and any risk of infection if the person is an injecting drug user. This information is also important to identify triggers for initiating use and to prevent relapse. A developmental and family history should be documented to identify the age at which the patient first used a substance, how this use has developed over time, when the patient thought the use became problematic, when there were periods of abstinence and when there were changes in substances used (Saunders & Young 2002).

For alcohol, there is an agreed low level of consumption (less than 20 grams per day), but alcohol interacts with many medications including some herbal preparations (Holton et al. 2017). There are too many medications with the potential to interact with alcohol to be listed here, but comprehensive and up-to-date information on alcohol and medication interactions can be found in the British National Formulary (BNF) (https://bnf.nice.org.uk/drug/alcohol.html)

Taking a Substance Use History

When working with people who misuse substances, it is important to build a therapeutic relationship and engage with the person in a supportive, empathetic and non-judgemental manner. Remember to take into account that often stigma and discrimination are associated with alcohol misuse and the person may minimise the problem when they discuss their use with you. Ensure that assessments are conducted in settings that respect the person's confidentiality, privacy and dignity (NICE 2011).

In a substance use assessment it is essential to clarify the elements listed later. Individual health services or Trusts may use standard substance use assessment forms that cover each of these elements. Drug and alcohol use assessment must be quantified and documented. Systematic assessment of all patients should include a thorough examination of:

- indicators of risk
- past medical history
- psychosocial issues
- physical signs and symptoms
- mental health status
- pathology results

No single sign, symptom or pathology test is conclusive evidence of an alcohol or drug-related issue, a holistic assessment is required.

Key Elements of Assessment

The following key elements must be clarified with each patient as part of the drug and alcohol use assessment:

- type of drug
- types of beverage the patient usually consumes
- route of administration
- frequency of use
- dose
- duration of use
- time and amount of the last dose (e.g. grams of alcohol, mL and mg of methadone, grams of cannabis, etc.)

Note: It is important to ask the person if they are using more than one drug at a time, as polydrug use can significantly increase the risk involved (Saunders & Young 2002).

It can be difficult to discuss personal issues with people you do not know. However, the following hints can help make a drug and alcohol assessment flow more smoothly:

- Ensure that the environment is as quiet and private as possible.
- If it is not possible to be completely private, speak quietly so that others do not hear the patient's personal details.
- When you are interviewing the patient, note any inconsistencies in what you are being told.
- If the patient becomes angry, leave the question and rephrase it later.
- A substance use history can also be elicited from the patient's friends or family.
- If there is a discrepancy between what the patient tells you and what significant others tell you, record this and clarify details when possible.
- How you ask the questions is important. Although many patients may drink at levels higher than those recommended, do not assume that they see this as problematic. The patient may lead a very different lifestyle to yours and may not conform to what you consider to be acceptable behaviour. It is important to remain non-threatening and non-judgemental. Remember that many of the substances used are illegal and patients may be guarded about revealing the full extent of their use until they feel that you can be trusted. Remind them that the information is required for their health purposes only and is confidential.
- Considerations about the legality or illegality of substances used must not affect the therapeutic process. Remember that substance use is a health issue, not a moral one. Although illicit drugs may be involved, it is the patient's health and not the legal aspect that nurses are concerned about.
- It is always important to check with senior nursing staff about any legal issues of confidentiality and duty of care and refer to your local and the national guidelines. Failure to abide by such procedural guidelines may place you in jeopardy (Staunton & Chiarella 2013).
- Introduce drinking and substance use as a normal everyday occurrence. For example, ask: 'What is your favourite drink?' or 'What do you like to drink?' Phrase questions in a way that assumes the patient does drink alcohol and use other drugs. By asking questions in this way, it gives patients permission to talk about their substance use. For example, ask: 'When did you last drink enough to make you merry or even drunk?' rather than 'Have you ever been drunk?' which is more likely to elicit a yes/no answer, consider using open questions.
- When asking about the number of drinks consumed or the frequency of drug use, suggest a quantity towards the extreme range of the scale. For example, 'How many drinks would you normally consume in an evening? Twenty pints?' or 'How many sleeping tablets do you take at a time? Five or six?' A person is more likely to admit to a high level if you imply that such a number is not out of the question. However, you must also be careful that you do not encourage the patient to overestimate their alcohol and drug use (Allen 2003; Saunders & Young 2002).

NURSE'S STORY 20.2 **Why I work as a drug and alcohol nurse**

A question I get asked regularly, not only in the workplace but also at dinner parties, is: 'Why do you want to work with drug addicts?' To be honest I have never really been able to come up with a clear answer but I will give it a go.

I have nursed in drug and alcohol for 15 years. I enjoy the job.

A skill learned early in my career was to engage patients honestly and openly with the expectation that this would be reciprocated. I find it a great privilege to be allowed into the complex layers of drug and alcohol dependency, allowing me the opportunity to offer solutions to health and social needs. There is great scope in working with patients holistically and not merely with their first presenting issue.

I have a very strong belief that as nurses we are not in a position to judge who is worthy of healthcare. Some of my colleagues treat drug-dependent patients with little respect and understanding. Part of my job is to challenge those beliefs, address fears, educate and assist patients in receiving nondiscriminatory healthcare.

One rare gem that comes with drug and alcohol nursing is that of working with a team of people who know how to look after each other. Having a supportive team helps to build your resilience and keep balance in your life.

BOX 20.5 Signs of Current Drug Use

- Puncture marks
- Cellulitis
- Phlebitis
- Skin abscesses
- Erosion or irritation around nostrils/septum
- Irritation around mouth or nose
- Tenderness or liver pain

(*Source:* New South Wales Ministry of Health, 2016. Clinical guidelines for nursing and midwifery practice in NSW. Identifying and responding to drug and alcohol issues. NSW Ministry of Health. Reproduced by permission, NSW Ministry of Health.)

Guidelines

The area of drug and alcohol use and abuse is a complex one because of societal, political and economic factors. Evaluating alcohol use and its impact is an imprecise science. Different countries approach it in different ways and the issue is complicated by political influences and the actions of competing pressure groups.

Guidelines from the Chief Medical Officer (Department of Health 2016) that have been formulated in conjunction with all UK Governments, is that to keep health risks from alcohol to a low level no more than 14 units should be consumed per week on a regular basis. This applies to both men and women and if a person is regularly drinking as much as 14 units per week then this should be spread evenly over 3 days or more.

Illicit drugs are more difficult to quantify than alcohol because the same drug can differ vastly from dose to dose in its purity and ingredients.

Observations

An assessment of a person's physical and mental state may reveal evidence of recent substance use, such as the smell of alcohol or signs of withdrawal. A person who has misused substances for some time might have a decline in global functioning, which might be evidenced by a decline in health status and poor hygiene. An assessment should include the following:

- General appearance—look for evidence of malnutrition, in which the person can look gaunt; and for signs of agitation, which might indicate stimulant use or withdrawal from a substance. People who regularly inject drugs will often wear long sleeves and long trousers, even in hot weather, in an attempt to cover up injection marks (see also Box 20.5).
- Signs of intoxication—such as ataxia (lack of coordination of muscle movements), confused thinking, being argumentative or the smell of alcohol on the person's breath.
- Signs of withdrawal—such as tremors and sweating, particularly of the hands and face, hallucinations.
- Stigmata—such as abscesses at injection sites, inflammation of the nasal septum from snorting cocaine, bruising and scars unrelated to surgery, which might indicate accidents while under the influence of drugs and alcohol.

TABLE 20.2 Glasgow Coma Scale

Feature	Scale (responses)	Score (notation)
Eye opening	Spontaneous	4
	To speech	3
	To pain	2
	None	1
Verbal response	Oriented	5
	Confused conversation	4
	Words (inappropriate)	3
	Sounds (incomprehensible)	2
	None	1
Best motor response	Obeys commands	6
	Localises pain	5
	Flexion—normal—abnormal	4 3
	Extension	2
	None	1
Total score 3/15–15/15		

(*Source:* Rosenfeld, J.V., 2012. Practical Management of Head and Neck Injury. Churchill Livingstone, Sydney.)

- Pulse rate, blood pressure and evidence of head injury, which may indicate recent substance use

The Glasgow Coma Scale is a neurological scale that aims to give a reliable objective way of recording the conscious state of a person for initial as well as subsequent assessment and may be required for medical and trauma patients, particularly if they are intoxicated (see Table 20.2).

CRITICAL THINKING CHALLENGE 20.1

1. When assessing a patient for possible substance abuse, which of the following would alert the nurse to alcohol intoxication?
   A. pupillary constriction
   B. unsteady gait (ataxia)
   C. slurring of words
   D. a strong smell of alcohol on the person's breath
2. Which of the following would alert the nurse to possible opiate use?
   A. tremor and sweating
   B. wearing long sleeves and trousers on a very hot day
   C. inability to concentrate
   D. reddened eyes

Tests

Mental Status Examination

A mental status examination is essential (see Chapter 22), paying particular attention to:

- clouding of consciousness
- perceptual abnormalities, especially visual, auditory and tactile (e.g. believing insects are crawling under the skin) hallucinations
- thought abnormalities, especially paranoid ideation
- suicidal ideation
- altered cognition

Laboratory Tests

Laboratory tests may provide evidence of substance misuse. Physiological markers of consumption such as mean corpuscular volume (MCV) and gamma glutamyl transferase (GGT) are most widely used to verify a diagnosis of substance use. However, other reasons for alterations in these markers should always be considered. Carbohydrate-deficient transferrin (CDT) in serum and phosphatidylethanol (Peth) in whole blood are more sensitive but less commonly used indicators of excessive alcohol use (Daetwyler et al. 2012; Helander et al. 2012).

Screening Tests

Screening tests may also be used. These instruments usually take the form of self-reported questionnaires and are used for diagnostic purposes. One of the most widely used screening instruments is the Alcohol Use Disorders Identification Test (AUDIT), which is designed to screen for a range of drinking problems, particularly harmful and hazardous use. It is especially suitable for primary healthcare settings and has reliability across cultural groups and a range of specific populations. The AUDIT is a self-report measure comprising 10 items, which are scored by totalling the items (see Box 20.6). Items 1 to 8 are scored on a scale of 0 to 4 and items 9 and 10 are scored 0, 2 or 4. A score of 8 or above has frequently been used to indicate the presence of alcohol problems (Babor et al. 2001; NICE 2011). The AUDIT is in the public domain and can be used without cost.

BOX 20.6 Alcohol Use Disorders Identification Test (AUDIT) Screening Instrument

Please circle the answer that is correct for you.

1. How often do you have a drink containing alcohol?
   Never
   Monthly or less 2–4 times a month
   2–3 times a week
   4 or more times a week
2. How many drinks containing alcohol do you have on a typical day when you are drinking?
   1 or 2
   3 or 4
   5 or 6
   7 to 9
   10 or more
3. How often do you have six or more drinks on one occasion?
   Never
   Less than monthly
   Monthly
   Weekly
   Daily or almost daily
4. How often have you found that you were not able to stop drinking once you had started?
   Never
   Less than monthly
   Monthly
   Weekly
   Daily or almost daily
5. How often during the last year have you failed to do what was normally expected of you because of drinking?
   Never
   Less than monthly
   Monthly
   Weekly
   Daily or almost daily
6. How often during the last year have you needed a first drink in the morning to get yourself going after a heavy drinking session?
   Never
   Less than monthly
   Monthly
   Weekly
   Daily or almost daily
7. How often during the last year have you had a feeling of guilt or remorse after drinking?
   Never
   Less than monthly
   Monthly
   Weekly
   Daily or almost daily
8. How often during the last year have you been unable to remember what happened the night before because you had been drinking?
   Never
   Less than monthly
   Monthly
   Weekly
   Daily or almost daily
9. Have you or someone else been injured as a result of your drinking?
   No
   Yes, but not in the last year
   Yes, during the last year
10. Has a relative or friend or a doctor or other health worker been concerned about your drinking or suggested you cut down?
    No
    Yes, but not in the last year
    Yes, during the last year

(*Source:* World Health Organization (WHO) 2001 AUDIT: the Alcohol Use Disorders Identification Test. Guidelines for use in primary healthcare, 2nd ed. Available at: http://whqlibdoc.who.int/hq/2001/who_msd_msb_01.6a.pdf.)

Other widely used screening tools are: ASSIST (Alcohol, Smoking and Substance Involvement Screening Test), a questionnaire developed by the World Health Organization (WHO) that screens for all levels of problem or risky substance use in adults (WHO 2015); the SADQ or LDQ for severity of dependence; Clinical Institute Withdrawal Assessment of Alcohol Scale, revised (CIWA-Ar) for severity of withdrawal; APQ for the nature and extent of the problems arising from alcohol misuse (NICE 2011).

CASE STUDY 20.1

Helen

Helen has been a patient of community health services for approximately 6 months receiving care for a leg ulcer, which is exacerbated by type 2 diabetes. She is 63 years old and lives by herself. Her husband died approximately 12 months ago. She has one married daughter and three grandchildren, who live overseas. On previous visits Helen was well groomed, her house was clean and she seemed pleased to see the community nurse, offering her cups of tea and cakes that she had cooked. Recently, though, Helen seemed to have lost interest in caring for herself. On the last visit she appeared unkempt; her clothes were wrinkled and had food stains on them. Her hygiene was poor and the smell of urine and body odour was quite strong. The community nurse noticed two empty bottles of sherry on the table and a half-full sherry bottle. Helen was irritable and her words were slurred. She stated that she felt lonely and bored without her daughter and husband, and that 'the sherry helps me to forget'. Helen denied any previous problems with alcohol or other substances, but she did say that sherry had helped her to cope with the death of her husband, and that the doctor had then given her some pills and gradually they had made her feel better. Helen 'thinks' that she 'mostly remembers' to take her diabetes medication, but she does not know what all the fuss is about, as there is nothing wrong with her.

CRITICAL THINKING CHALLENGE 20.2

With reference to the case study about Helen (Case Study 20.1), assume that you are working in a community mental health team and have arranged to visit Helen. The community district nurse has given you Helen's history in her referral letter.

1. How will you prioritise this situation?
2. What types of assessment will you initiate?
3. What questions might you ask?
4. Who will you discuss Helen's situation with?
5. What follow-up plan might you implement?

INTERVENTIONS

Early and Brief Interventions

Studies have shown that early and brief interventions (talking to people at an early stage in their substance use) are an effective way to prevent later possible complications (Bien et al. 1993; Vasilaki et al. 2006; Wild et al. 2007; Marsh et al. 2013; Moyer & Finney 2015). Chapter 24 describes these and other interventions in more detail. Brief interventions for substance use involve sessions of 5 to 15 minutes and often include the provision of self-help materials such as pamphlets or substance use diaries. This may extend to a brief assessment and providing advice (in a one-off session), as well as assessing the patient's readiness to change (motivational interview), harm reduction and follow up. The components of brief interventions include:

- assessment
- providing feedback to the patient on risk or impairments due to drug use
- listening to the patient's concerns; advising the patient about the consequences of continued drug use
- defining treatment goals such as reducing or ceasing drug use
- discussing and implementing strategies for treatment (e.g. identifying triggers for drug use and strategies to overcome them, and offering a follow-up session) (Marsh et al. 2013)

Brief interventions are recommended for patients experiencing relatively few problems related to their substance use and who have low levels of dependence. They are also recommended for patients with a dependence on nicotine, a low-to-moderate dependence on alcohol or a low-to-moderate dependence on cannabis. Brief interventions are not recommended for patients with severe dependence. If a brief intervention consists of only one session, it should include advice on how to reduce drug use or drinking to a safer level, provision of harm-reduction information and discussion of harm-reduction strategies (Bien et al. 1993; Vasilaki et al. 2006; Wild et al. 2007; Marsh et al. 2013; Moyer & Finney 2015). Examples of resources to support in delivering brief interventions are available at NHS Health Scotland (http://www.healthscotland.scot/publications/alcohol-brief-intervention-resources).

Motivational Interviewing

Motivational interviewing (MI) using the Transtheoretical Model of Change is an intervention developed by Prochaska, DiClemente and Miller to work with patients to assess and then enhance the motivation to change their level of substance use (Prochaska & DiClemente 1984; Miller & Heather 1986; Prochaska & Velicer 1997; Miller & Rollnick 2009; Lundahl et al. 2013). MI is one of the most widely used interventions. Nurse's Story 20.3 provides a practical example of MI in action and it is discussed further in Chapter 24.

The Transtheoretical Model of Change is described by Prochaska and DiClemente (1984) briefly as follows:

- *Precontemplation.* The patient has no intention of changing. They are in 'denial' or resistant to change. The therapist works to increase the patient's awareness of the problem while consistently remaining non-judgemental and respectful. The therapist provides information and consciousness-raising at the same time. It is vitally important that the therapist does not disengage at this stage. The therapist needs to continue to try to connect with the patient and raise awareness of the dangers of their alcohol and substance use even if the patient does not initially show interest.

- *Contemplation.* The patient is aware of their problem but remains ambivalent about change. The therapist acknowledges the patient's ambivalence while working to tip the decisional balance by weighing the pros and cons of change versus the risks and benefits of continuing substance use. Responsibility for change remains with the patient.
- *Preparation.* The patient intends to change but might be confused about the best way to do so. The therapist inspires realistic hope, offers a menu of choices to help determine the best course of action and demystifies the change process. Both work to create a plan for change.
- *Action.* Actual behaviour change commences. The patient implements a collaborative, realistic plan. Both the therapist and the patient monitor the patient's progress, highlighting and valuing even small successes, and progressively problem solving.
- *Maintenance.* Behaviour change has been achieved and the patient has developed a new lifestyle. The therapist and the patient are vigilant to avoid relapse. They have realistic hopes and avoid exaggerated expectations.

Patients may slip back to a previous stage (e.g. from preparation to precontemplation) and work their way up again. This is an expected part of the process and relapses should be anticipated. The principle is to ascertain which stage of 'readiness to change' the patient is at and then to provide information and support to move them on to the next stage. If the patient understands what is occurring, they are more likely to change.

The model is a very powerful tool. Simply by discussing the stages of change with a patient, one can raise awareness of possible harms and produce long-lasting behavioural change. The model is not restricted to substance use and can be used for any self-harming behaviour including behavioural addictions (i.e. nonpharmacological) such as gambling and sex (Prochaska & DiClemente 1984; Miller & Heather 1986; Prochaska & Velicer 1997; Miller & Rollnick 2009; Lundahl et al. 2013). MI is also described in Chapter 24.

NURSE'S STORY 20.3 Using Motivational Interviewing on Thursday Afternoon in Detox—A Conversation With Isabella

Isabella, could you please tell me how you use motivational interviewing?

When we talk about motivational interviewing, we very often fall into the trap of thinking it is very formal and done in the office and it's very much the nurse/patient sitting down and talking about things, but in actual fact it's very different to that. Take Thursday afternoon in the detox unit, for example. Thursday is very often the day that patients receive benefits and payments into their accounts and you find that suddenly patients become quite agitated and edgy and they will come up to staff and say that they have to go out and pay a water bill or a phone bill or something and that it can't possibly wait. It becomes their major focus for that day, when in actual fact we know that they are going out to use. So we really need to be on our toes about motivational interviewing.

Some of the techniques that we use might be to develop discrepancy in their thinking because they are very focussed on wanting to go, so what we might do is bring them back to their initial goals. It is very useful if you were involved in their initial assessment and know what their goals were (or have read their management plan and know their goals) and can bring them back to that and say 'One of your goals was to stay here, what if you just wait a bit longer?' We often use techniques aimed at delaying the decision, so we might try distracting them. For example, around meal times we might say, 'Why don't you go and have lunch and think about this for a while and then come back and make that decision then?' This type of conversation can happen walking down the corridor, outside or even when the patient is at the door with their bags packed. You've got to be really thinking about what you're doing.

Also, if it's a Friday and they're a bit edgy and actually do leave, it triggers everyone else in the place and they start to think about their own recovery and they may begin to think that they need to go as well. So what we try to do, what we have to do, is to put those strategies in really early about what are the potential triggers for that person and look at some of the strategies that we can use on a Thursday or Friday because they may not realise when they first come in that it is going to be an issue. But we know that similar patterns will take over, so we will be thinking about that during the whole time.

Is it a difficult technique to use?

I don't think so, but in saying that, I instinctively did it for years without actually putting a name to it. It just seemed that a lot of my interactions were around negotiation—negotiating with patients around what their goals were if they seemed to be a bit off track and going back to these original goals. It's all about negotiation. A lot of us have been doing it for years before we put a name to it. I was working with it for years and it was when I started further studying I thought 'Oh, that's what it's called.' You can put it in words then and think 'Oh, that's what we are doing,' but a lot of people out there are doing it without actually realising that they're doing it. Once you learn more about it you can add more to your skills and enhance them.

For a student nurse who might be on placement and unfamiliar with an area, is it a technique they could use?

Oh, absolutely. I think if they have just a general understanding—I'm not just talking drugs and alcohol at the moment—but a general understanding of some of the issues with addiction or abuse, or with alcohol, knowing what the national standards or national guidelines are, they can use it. If they have a patient in any setting, whether it's emergency, medical-surgical, maternity or paediatric, and they detect that person may have some sort of issue with alcohol or any other drug, just a brief intervention is the starting block for any sort of motivational interviewing.

It might be the case that they detect it and bring it to the attention of the nurse. Or in a general conversation when they are washing the patient they might just gently bring it into the conversation. Or the patient might bring it up that they drink a lot. The student can ask a few more questions and say 'Have you ever thought about cutting back or stopping, or has it ever caused you any concerns or harm?' If the patient says yes, the student can contact the nurse or they might be aware of what

NURSE'S STORY 20.3 Using Motivational Interviewing on Thursday Afternoon in Detox—A Conversation With Isabella—cont'd

services are available. It would be good if students do know what services are available and can put patients in contact with them. That's a start.

It's all about developing discrepancies and that's what you can do in a brief intervention. The patient might be precontemplative if they are sitting in hospital after an accident and they might have moved over to the contemplative mode, but to get them to move over to the action stage might be where the student nurse is the key and can play a pivotal part in bringing it to someone's attention. Generally, you find that the student nurse is the one who is spending more time with patients and getting into general conversations with them. I think that's really good.

So getting someone to think about their drinking or substance use and putting some strategies in place to help them seems to be a technique that can be used with all people, not just people who are heavy alcohol or drug users?

Absolutely. It can be used with anyone. The student just needs to know the basics. If we stick with alcohol, then that means the stages of change and some of the national guidelines put out for drinking—what is acceptable and what can be seen as hazardous drinking. So the student might think, 'This is where I can step in because this could be hazardous drinking on some level. What can I do to assist this person?' It might be as simple as handing that person a brochure. If the patient turns around and says, 'No, I don't want this,' the student might hand it to them and say here is a brochure for the future. That's it. It's that easy.

So, a person doesn't have to be at 'rock bottom' before you can use this technique?

No, that seems like a very late stage. There are just so many opportunities for students to talk to patients. When they do they should be very mindful about where the patient is at and what they could possibly do to move them on. Just one brief intervention may be enough to tip the balance and move the patient on and over into action.

That sounds really good. Is there anything else?

Yes, there is, as a matter of fact. I was teaching some students this morning about brief interventions with alcohol and they were talking about the ways that they could use it. It just came up in a general conversation in primary healthcare, which emphasises that they are really thinking about these techniques.

Cognitive Behavioural Therapy

Cognitive behavioural therapy (CBT) involves identifying self-destructive thoughts ('Everything has to be perfect', 'I always do the wrong thing') and replacing them with more realistic thoughts ('Not everything has to be perfect. Not always', 'I don't always do the wrong thing. Sometimes I do good things'). By replacing self-destructive thoughts with more realistic thoughts (cognitions), emotions and behaviour should change for the better as a result. CBT may be effective for substance use and other comorbid conditions including posttraumatic stress disorder and depression (Riper et al. 2014; McGovern et al. 2015). MI and CBT are very important counselling approaches in the drug and alcohol field. More detailed explanations of these approaches are given in Chapter 24.

RELAPSE PREVENTION

There is a distinct difference between a lapse and a relapse. A lapse is a 'slip' in which the person uses a substance again, possibly a couple of times. At this stage the person may decide to keep using or learn from their lapse and stop using. A relapse occurs when a person resumes substance use and stops making an effort not to use (Marsh et al. 2013). A lapse does not always result in a relapse, and patients can be made aware of this during relapse-prevention education.

All patients should have a plan so that if they do lapse, they have support and strategies available to avoid the more dangerous relapse. A lapse should be viewed as a learning experience for both the patient and the therapist. For example: What were the triggers that led to the lapse? How did the patient manage to contain their substance use to a lapse and not relapse into old behaviours? Within a CBT or MI framework, the therapist explores the patient's underlying thoughts and feelings that resulted in the lapse. The therapist's role is to assist the patient to work through the thoughts that contributed to the lapse and replace them with less damaging thought processes for the future (Marsh et al. 2013).

For example, if a patient lapses (e.g. starts drinking alcohol following a period of abstinence) after a stressful day at work, the therapist could explore this further and show how maladaptive thought patterns triggered the lapse. The therapist could ask the patient to explain what was happening at work to cause stress and then together they could undertake structured problem solving or explore whether the patient is perhaps catastrophising, overgeneralising or thinking negatively. The introduction of more appropriate reactions to stress should help avoid future lapses. This might include options on how to deal with a stressful situation at the time, such as removing oneself temporarily from the situation, practising relaxation techniques or following other appropriate stress-reducing interventions. These are alternatives to letting the stress build up, which can result in a relapse. The therapist should seek opportunities to teach the patient how to deal with stress and feel good, rather than allowing increased stress and feelings of failure to endanger their abstinence (Prochaska & DiClemente 1984; Miller & Heather 1986; Prochaska & Velicer 1997; Miller & Rollnick 2009; Lundahl et al. 2013; Marsh et al. 2013; Bachiller et al. 2015; Riper et al. 2014; McGovern et al. 2015).

OTHER HEALING APPROACHES

There is not one approach that works for everyone. It is always best to offer a wide spectrum of treatment approaches. Residential treatment services may be effective for some people. For others, pharmacotherapy such as acamprosate (Campral) and naltrexone decreases cravings to drink alcohol. For yet other patients, a 12-step programme can be very effective; these are peer support programmes such as Alcoholics Anonymous (AA) and Narcotics Anonymous UK (UKNA); these groups are based on an abstinence philosophy (Kelly et al. 2013; Humphreys et al. 2014).

Community drug and alcohol services provide a range of interventions including individual and group counselling, pharmacotherapies (such as methadone and buprenorphine maintenance for opiate-dependent patients), CBT and MI. All of these therapeutic interventions are described more fully in Chapter 24.

Harm Minimisation and Harm Reduction

The aims laid out in the Government's 2017 Drug Strategy (Home Office 2017) were to reduce illicit and other harmful drug use and to increase the rates recovering from their dependence. The approach is balanced over four key themes:

- Reducing Demand—preventing the onset of drug use over all age groups, placing greater emphasis on building resilience and confidence in young people.
- Restricting Supply—adapting approaches to reflect the changes in criminal activity, improving and using innovative technology.
- Building Recovery—raising ambitions for full recovery outcomes for different user groups, ensuring the right interventions are provided and employing a joined-up approach to commissioning.
- Global Action—take a leading role in driving international action, targeting new initiatives on the new psychoactive substances and sharing best practice.

A major harm-reduction strategy is opioid substitution therapy. The long-acting opioids methadone (24-hour dosing) and buprenorphine (24-, 48- or 72-hour dosing) are administered as substitution treatment for heroin or other opioid addiction and are considered 'essential medicines' for this purpose (Marsch et al. 2005; WHO 2013). As substitution opioids have the potential to be diverted and intravenously injected, deterrent strategies have been introduced. Naloxone was added to buprenorphine (Suboxone) and marketed with the information that if the combination was injected, it would produce little euphoria but it would produce withdrawal symptoms and this would deter diversion (Larance et al. 2011; Yokell et al. 2011).

Unfortunately, a recent large-scale review has found that diversion rates of Subuxone film, Suboxone tablets and methadone tablets are similar (Larance et al. 2014). The authors concluded firstly that there is a need to accept that some diversion of substitution therapy will occur that current clinical delivery methods cannot control; secondly, that similar problems affect the extramedical use of other pain and psychotropic medications; and thirdly, the problems of diversion need to be weighed against the benefits to the patients and the community of supplying opioid substitution to those in need (i.e. decreases in heroin overdose deaths, lower rates of high-risk HIV activity and decreases in the amount of heroin and other nonprescribed opioids used by patients) (Larance et al. 2014). (See also Auriacombe et al. 2004; Mattick et al. 2008; Sullivan et al. 2008; Woody et al. 2008; and Schwartz et al. 2013.)

Managing an Intoxicated Patient

Patients who are aggressive or disruptive because they are intoxicated can risk their own safety and the safety of others. Intoxicated patients can be frightened, disruptive and upset. How they are approached and treated is an important part of managing intoxication. Of course not all intoxicated patients will present as agitated, some may be excessively happy and vocal, which can present its own challenges.

When dealing with an intoxicated person always approach them in a friendly and respectful manner. Authoritarian or patronising attitudes can provoke anger and aggression. If other intoxicated people accompany the patient, ask them to wait outside, because they might exacerbate the situation and distract the patient. When talking to the patient use the patient's name and use slow, distinct speech with short simple sentences. It is very important to be genuine in your approach. Be careful not to adopt a patronising tone. Do not talk down to them. Maintain eye contact, without being intrusive. Most importantly, make other staff aware of the situation for your own safety and the safety of others. (See Chapter 23 for useful skills such as anger management and aggression management and techniques for preventing violence.)

All intoxicated patients must be kept under observation. A thorough physical and mental status examination will reveal the extent of intoxication. If the intoxication does not diminish with falling blood plasma levels, the patient must be assessed for other possible causes of their condition. If the patient is unconscious, observe for airway and breathing. Vomiting is likely to occur in grossly intoxicated people and can be fatal (Warren et al. 2012; Pelissier et al. 2014) (Box 20.3).

Substance Withdrawal and Detoxification

Most people going through withdrawal have a craving to readminister the substance to reduce the symptoms. The signs and symptoms of withdrawal vary, but most of the symptoms are the opposite of what is observed during intoxication. The dose and duration of drug use affects the withdrawal process.

Detoxification (or withdrawal) is the process by which alcohol- or drug-dependent people recover from intoxication in a supervised manner so that withdrawal symptoms are minimised. It can take place in an inpatient unit or in the person's own home. The patient might be medicated or non-medicated, depending on the severity of the withdrawal and the patient's wishes. Symptoms of withdrawal range in severity from mildly uncomfortable to life threatening; however, careful assessment and management can alleviate many of the symptoms. The onset and length of withdrawal syndrome depends on the half-life of the drug taken. Nursing management of withdrawal focusses on five main areas:

- minimising progression to severe withdrawal
- decreasing risk of injury to self/others
- eliminating risk of dehydration, electrolyte and nutritional imbalance
- reducing risk of seizures
- identifying the presence of concurrent illness that masks/mimics withdrawal (Hoban 2017)

Withdrawal from psychostimulants, opioids, cannabis and combinations of drugs (polysubstance use) in the emergency department all require a similar treatment approach. This includes supportive care, monitoring of vital signs and the management of agitation by use of benzodiazepines. Benzodiazepines are particularly useful if there is a risk of seizures. If the patient is experiencing psychosis, an antipsychotic such olanzapine may be required (Musselman & Hampton 2014; Richards & Derlet 2014).

Alcohol Withdrawal

Severe alcohol withdrawal is potentially life threatening and it is important to anticipate when it might occur. Minor (mild or moderate) withdrawal usually occurs within 24 hours after the person has had their last drink and begins to experience 'the shakes'. Often the tremor is associated with hypertension, restlessness, sweating, diarrhoea, headache, difficulty sleeping, decreased appetite and anxiety. Most patients do not experience all symptoms, and for many of those who do experience some withdrawal, symptoms usually subside after 2 or 3 days of abstinence. However, for some people the symptoms are more severe; approximately 15% of chronic alcohol users will experience seizures 2 or 3 days after their last drink (Saunders & Young 2002).

Identifying those at risk of alcohol withdrawal, and monitoring the withdrawal state using a standardised assessment tool, has contributed to a substantial reduction in the complications of alcohol withdrawal. Rating scales available include the Alcohol Withdrawal Scale (AWS), the Clinical Institute Withdrawal Assessment for Alcohol (Revised) (CIWA-Ar) scale and the Short Alcohol Withdrawal Scale (Sullivan et al. 1989). Each health service will have a standard scale to use. Caution must be exercised when using withdrawal scales as in most cases one size does not fit all and reliance on completing a form does not replace the importance of observation and critical assessment of the patient's symptoms (Bostwick & Lapid 2004).

Parenteral thiamine followed by a short course of oral thiamine is prescribed for hospitalised patients. In the UK, chlordiazepoxide hydrochloride is the most commonly used treatment for alcohol withdrawal, as benzodiazepines are the most effective and least toxic intervention in treating withdrawal. The dose is titrated depending on the severity of the withdrawal according to the symptoms, and in most cases medication will be decreased after a few days and discontinued after 1 week (Saunders & Young 2002; refer to the BNF https://bnf.nice.org.uk/).

Benzodiazepines, used widely to treat anxiety and insomnia, have the potential for addiction and abuse in people with a predisposition to alcohol and drug abuse. Some patients who use benzodiazepines as well as alcohol on a regular basis will need to be withdrawn more slowly; however, use of these drugs for short periods in a controlled setting such as an inpatient unit is safe and warranted for most patients.

Less than 5% of people with chronic alcohol use who withdraw from alcohol may experience a major withdrawal syndrome known as delirium tremens (Saunders & Young 2002; NICE 2011). This syndrome occurs 3 to 10 days after the person has had their last drink. The patient may present with agitation, disorientation, high fever, paranoia and visual hallucinations (Schuckit 2009). Nursing attention for a patient experiencing delirium tremens must be vigilant. The patient should be nursed in a separate room. Intravenous fluid replacement may be required if there is severe dehydration and excessive sweating. In addition, specific electrolyte replacement (calcium, phosphate, magnesium and potassium) may be required. It is essential to reduce any agitation and the patient must be kept calm to reduce exhaustion. Oral or intravenous diazepam may be prescribed to relieve withdrawal symptoms. Antipsychotic medication such as olanzapine may also be prescribed (Ntais et al. 2005).

There are some factors that predict the likely severity of alcohol withdrawal syndrome. One is whether the patient has a long history of regular heavy alcohol use. Another is the use of other psychoactive drugs, particularly central nervous system depressants such as benzodiazepines. Furthermore, if the person has a past history of withdrawal syndrome, particularly delirium tremens or seizures, this places them at greater risk of withdrawal and withdrawal complications (Schuckit 2009). Box 20.4 outlines the DSM-5 criteria for alcohol withdrawal.

Physical Effects of Long-Term Alcohol Use

An example of the effects of harmful use is Wernicke-Korsakoff syndrome. Chronic, excessive alcohol consumption results in thiamine deficiency, which affects the central nervous system and can lead to Wernicke-Korsakoff syndrome. Wernicke encephalopathy is the acute phase of the syndrome. It causes nystagmus (involuntary, rhythmic movement of the eyes), ataxia (staggering gait) and confusion. This is reversible with thiamine therapy. Korsakoff psychosis is the chronic phase of the syndrome, resulting in short-term memory loss and confabulation (spontaneous reporting of events that never happened). Recovery from the chronic phase is usually incomplete. Irreversible alcoholic dementia (very similar to Alzheimer disease) may also occur (Latt & Dore 2014).

Comorbid Disorders

Several terms are used to describe someone who has more than one disorder concurrently; mental health, alcohol and drug nurses use the terms 'comorbid disorders', 'comorbidity', 'coexisting disorder' and 'dual diagnosis' interchangeably (Drake & Wallach 2000; Mills et al. 2008). Patients with a mental health problem are often drawn to alcohol and drugs with serious and sometimes fatal consequences (e.g. depression and alcohol, psychosis and methamphetamines, bipolar disorder and methamphetamines). There are many theories to explain comorbid diagnosis, but most fit into one of three categories:

1. *Direct causal relationship theory:* one disorder produces the other disorder. Drug use may cause mental illness. For example, a habitual cannabis user might start to experience psychosis and the psychosis becomes the predominant problem. Alternatively, a mental illness may cause the drug use. Someone with depression may drink alcohol to treat the depression. The alcohol use then becomes the most debilitating problem.
2. *Indirect causal relationship theory:* for example, depression during childhood might lead to poor school results. This in turn might lead to a less satisfying career, frustration with one's life and subsequent drinking of alcohol to treat the depression. Depression causes the drinking but in an indirect way.
3. *Common causal factors:* for example, terrible childhood experiences or a family history of mental illness and drug abuse produce both mental health and drug and alcohol problems, but one disorder does not directly initiate the other.

Prevalence rates of comorbid diagnosis vary significantly, depending on the definitions used and the populations studied. Studies indicate that substance use disorder is the most common comorbidity for people with severe mental illness, with approximately 50% of people with severe mental illness having a comorbid diagnosis (Brunette et al. 2008).

The patient is one person, not two or more separate disorders. Mental health nurses need to know about substance use and treatment, and drug and alcohol nurses need to know about mental health issues and treatment. There continues to be a 'silo' approach to treatment (i.e. mental health clinicians dealing only with mental health problems and drug and alcohol clinicians dealing only with drug and alcohol problems), which produces poor outcomes (Baker & Vellman 2007; Allsop 2008).

CASE STUDY 20.2

Maria

Presenting: Maria is an 18-year-old woman who has been referred to your community health service. She is seeking help about her drug and alcohol disorder. She has been supported by her youth worker to make contact. She lives at a youth residential care unit 1 to 2 days per week and at acquaintances the other nights. Maria has presented several times (voluntarily and involuntarily) to hospital emergency departments following emotional crises. She has suicidal thoughts and made deliberate self-harm attempts by cutting her arms and upper legs. She has also taken overdoses of prescription medication. She has no contact with her family. Her mother is in prison. She has never met her father, who was a customer of her mother when her mother was drug dealing.

Pattern: Maria has described her current drug use as 'out of control'. She has engaged in prostitution for the last 7 months to support her substance use disorder. She has been using alcohol for 4 years (a bottle of spirits once or twice per week) and methamphetamine for 6 months. On average she uses five points (a point is 0.1 of a gram of methamphetamine) over a week. Maria smokes cannabis and uses benzodiazepines most days to feel comfortable. She also uses benzodiazepines when trying to withdraw from her other drug and alcohol use. Her 21-year-old ex-boyfriend has been supplier and co-user of those substances.

Predisposing: Maria suffered childhood sexual abuse in her early years by boyfriends of her mother and by her grandfather. She experienced early childhood neglect, was removed from her mother and placed into foster care placements. She had behavioural issues at each of the placements. Presently, when faced with conflict she has poor impulse control and often engages in deliberate self-harm or violence towards others. She describes periods of isolation from people where she withdraws to her room. She has no significant positive adult relationships in her life apart from her youth workers who change regularly due to changes in funding. Her mother is in prison for drug dealing and is being treated for a bipolar disorder.

Precipitating: Maria is socially isolated. She has no peers that she considers friends apart from her ex-boyfriend who is controlling and exploitative towards her. She is highly irritable. She did not return to school following the breakdown of her last foster placement 8 months ago and has refused trying other education options as she feels that 'she does not fit in'. In the past Maria has attended school intermittently. Though of above-average intelligence, she has difficulties with literacy and numeracy.

She misses meals regularly. She has admitted to binge eating and then vomiting her food. Subsequently, she has problems with oesophageal/acidic reflux which at times has led to bleeding. Maria describes her sleep pattern as generally poor with recurrent sleep disturbances and disruptions. She averages 3 hours of sleep per night.

Perpetuating: Maria began using alcohol and drugs from the age of 13. She has increasingly been using methamphetamine. Her work at the brothel brings up memories of her early childhood trauma and she uses more methamphetamine to cope. She had several recent overnight presentations to emergency departments around the city when intoxicated or self-harming and threatening suicide. She has refused follow-up mental health services. She has forensic matters pending relating to driving under the influence of alcohol and driving without a licence.

Protective: Maria is an intelligent, attractive young woman. She has shown interest in working in a clothes store and pursuing a career in fashion. She has some insight and is seeking support with her self-harming behaviour and drug and alcohol disorder. She is ambivalent about how services can help or what to expect.

(As told by Harald Budein, Consultant Liaison Clinician)

CRITICAL THINKING CHALLENGE 20.3

With reference to the case study about Maria (Case Study 20.2), and remembering that care should always be patient-centred and strengths-based:

1. What challenges to engagement do you expect with Maria?
2. What would your treatment plan prioritise?
3. What safety considerations should you make?
4. How would you communicate these?

Ask the patient what they want to achieve and then work from there. That will facilitate engagement with Maria. The six 'P' factors (presenting, pattern, predisposing, precipitating, perpetuating and protective) are a useful way to analyse a patient's situation. Discuss these with Maria under these headings as you help her to achieve her goals.

A good comorbidity website is the free screening tool and training programme Psycheck (Lee et al. 2007; Turning Point 2015). Suggestions:

- explain to Maria motivational interviewing and the Transtheoretical Model of Change
- ask her what stage she thinks she is at
- ask how she thinks she might progress
- explain that relapse is a stage of the process

Clinical Significance of Comorbid Diagnosis

There is evidence to suggest that patients with a comorbid diagnosis do less well than those with either a single mental health problem or a single substance use problem. They are more difficult to manage due to their complex health and social needs, have higher rates of nonadherence with treatment and are more likely to be violent and to be exposed to violence (Drake et al. 2000; Teesson & Hall 2001). Patients with a comorbid diagnosis are more likely to have a chronic disability and consequently require more service utilisation (MacDonald et al. 2004). They have less access to treatment service and a greater chance of experiencing difficulties with relationships, poor employment prospects, social isolation, poor health and chronic financial difficulties (MacDonald et al. 2004). These patients often have a number of surrounding issues that combine and add to the complexity of their treatment goals and outcome, for example children placed in care due to parental substance abuse, pending legal action, housing difficulties and psychological problems (Marsh et al. 2013; Baker & Vellman 2007; Allsop 2008).

Why do People With a Mental Illness use Nonprescribed Drugs?

Several reasons have been proposed for the increase in the numbers of people with a mental illness using nonprescribed drugs. Since deinstitutionalisation, the number of people with a mental illness living in the community has increased and this exposes them to a substance-using culture that they may not have been exposed to when separated from mainstream society and living in asylums. Furthermore, an increase in the social acceptability and prevalence of substance use might contribute to higher levels of disorders. There might also be increased awareness of and interest in comorbid diagnosis, with more clinicians actively assessing their patients (Baker & Vellman 2007; Allsop 2008).

BOX 20.7 Differentiating Between a Primary Psychotic Disorder and a Substance-Induced Disorder

- Substance-induced psychotic symptoms can result from intoxication, chronic use or withdrawal.
- Intoxication with cannabis can induce a transient, self-limiting psychotic disorder characterised by hallucinations and agitation.
- Prolonged heavy use of psychostimulants (e.g. amphetamines) can produce a psychotic picture similar to schizophrenia.
- Hallucinogen-induced psychosis is usually transient, but may persist if use is sustained.
- Heavy alcohol use has been associated with alcoholic hallucinosis and morbid jealousy.
- Psychotic symptoms can also occur during withdrawal (e.g. delirium tremens) and delirious states.
- A non–substance-induced psychotic disorder should be considered when:
  - psychosis preceded the onset of substance use
  - psychosis persists for longer than 1 month after acute withdrawal or severe intoxication
  - psychotic symptoms are not consistent with the substance used
  - there is a history of psychotic symptoms during periods of abstinence greater than 1 month
  - there is a personal or family history of a non–substance-induced psychotic disorder

(*Source:* Lubman, D., Sundram, S., 2003. Substance misuse in patients with schizophrenia: a primary care guide. Medical Journal of Australia. 178(Supp May), S71–75. Reproduced with permission.)

Tobacco smoking is an important comorbidity. Nicotine is a stimulant. Features of schizophrenia include a lack of energy and a lack of pleasure in activities normally pleasurable (anhedonia). Sedation is also one of the side effects of antipsychotic medication used to treat psychosis. Stimulants provide energy (at least in the short term) and so people with schizophrenia are particularly drawn to tobacco smoking and can quickly become addicted (Baker & Vellman 2007; Allsop 2008).

Management of Patients With a Comorbid Diagnosis

Patients with a comorbid diagnosis can be very complex and difficult to treat. The nurse needs to develop the ability to distinguish between a psychotic disorder that is part of a mental illness and one that is substance induced (see Box 20.7).

Nursing staff are not always trained and educated in both areas (drugs and alcohol, and mental health) and nurses are at risk of holding negative attitudes towards patients who use alcohol and other drugs. Comorbidly diagnosed patients often evoke powerful, difficult feelings in health professionals. Some nurses are pessimistic regarding outcomes and believe that intensive time spent with these patients will produce minimal gains (Baker & Vellman 2007; Allsop 2008). Patients may be very frustrated. There is often a lack of a clear pathway for patients attempting to access services. Changes to services occur frequently as government-funded services often reorganise every few years and non-government organisation services appear and disappear according to funding variations (Cairney et al. 2015). In addition, comorbidly diagnosed patients may feel stigmatised by mental health nurses' attitudes when these are related to an abstinence model that is in direct contrast to the harm-minimisation model supported by the drug and alcohol sector (Baker & Vellman 2007; Allsop 2008).

This group of patients offers many challenges to nursing staff, as most comorbidly diagnosed patients have a range of personal and social problems and have difficulty maintaining a concurrent level of wellness in both areas. Continued drug use (e.g. cannabis) may exacerbate positive symptoms of schizophrenia and lead to admission or readmission to hospital. The key principles of drug and alcohol history-taking and assessment have been detailed under the section on assessment earlier in this chapter. Developing a collaborative therapeutic relationship is essential and the nurse needs to adopt an empathetic and non-judgemental approach. It is important to assess patients accurately and to screen them for substance use, as many patients with schizophrenia or other mental illness will often deny or understate their substance use. Once a diagnosis has been made, appropriate management combines pharmacological treatment of the psychotic episode and psychosocial interventions to reduce substance use. Ideally, a patient's mental state should be relatively stable before attempting detoxification or modifying use, although this is not always possible. Early and brief interventions can be used in both outpatient and inpatient settings. For management principles for patients with schizophrenia and substance abuse, see Box 20.8.

As with all aspects of nursing care, safety is the main concern. If a patient has been admitted to a mental health facility in a psychotic state, it is essential that the psychosis be managed. When the patient's mental state is more settled, the nurse can engage in psychosocial interventions to assist the patient with their problematic substance use. These interventions will need to be continued once the patient has been discharged from hospital. If the patient is at risk of withdrawal from one or more substances, detoxification strategies as outlined earlier in this chapter need to be implemented immediately. The patient will need to be monitored closely and appropriate medication prescribed. When the patient is more settled, the nurse can begin to explore reasons for the patient's substance use, including the relationship of the substance to the patient's psychiatric symptoms, treatment for the patient's mental illness and feelings of social isolation related to their negative symptoms.

The patient's readiness to change and their degree of commitment to treatment of both their mental illness and their substance use need to be explored (Lubman & Sundram 2003). Remember: patients may be at different stages of readiness in their problematic drug use and their mental illness, and interventions need to reflect this. For example, a patient may be at a precontemplation stage for their substance use but at an action stage for their mental illness (Baker & Vellman 2007; Allsop 2008).

BOX 20.8 Management Principles for Patients with Schizophrenia and Substance Abuse

Assessment

- Screen patients with psychosis for substance misuse.
- Determine the severity of use and associated risk-taking behaviours (e.g. injecting practices, unsafe sex).
- Exclude organic illness or physical complications of substance misuse.
- Seek collateral history—family or close supports should be involved where possible.

Treatment

- First engage the patient using a non-judgemental attitude.
- Educate the patient.
- Give general advice about the harmful effects of substance misuse.
- Advise about safe and responsible levels of substance use.
- Make individual links between substance misuse and the patient's problems (e.g. cannabis use and worsening paranoia).
- Inform the person about safer practices (e.g. safe sexual practices).
- Treat psychotic illness and monitor the patient for side effects.
- Help the patient to establish the advantages and disadvantages of current use and motivate the patient to change.
- With medical staff, evaluate the need for concurrent substance use medications (e.g. methadone, acamprosate, nicotine replacement therapy).
- Refer the patient to appropriate community services as appropriate.
- Devise relapse-prevention strategies that address both psychosis and substance misuse.
- Identify triggers for relapse (e.g. meeting other drug users, family conflict) and explore alternative coping strategies.

(*Source:* Lubman, D., Sundram, S., 2003. Substance misuse in patients with schizophrenia: a primary care guide. Medical Journal of Australia. 178(Supp May), S71–75. Reproduced with permission.)

Adopt a concrete problem-solving approach with the patient whenever possible. For example, set tasks that are readily achievable, such as keeping a daily diary of substance use or psychotic symptoms. During the sessions, focus on specific skills to deal with high-risk situations. This might involve training to be assertive, a useful skill to learn if the patient needs to say 'no' to a dealer. Interpersonal skills training is often of great benefit.

People frequently become isolated from family and friends during the course of their drug use. In feeling socially isolated they frequently become vulnerable to relapse if they lack the skills to form new and healthier friendship groups. Consider the use of role play to assist the patient. Remember that a long-term perspective with ongoing intervention is required (Baker & Vellman 2007; Allsop 2008).

NURSE'S STORY 20.4 Best Practice Advice

I have found, from 25 years' experience working in a mental health unit, that very high numbers of people admitted to a mental health unit have a comorbid diagnosis or at least a problem with alcohol and/or drugs. My advice is to learn about substance misuse early, it will be an intrinsic part of your work and developing these skills will be invaluable in supporting your patients along their recovery journeys. You need to be able to deal with the whole person. The mental health nurse has a responsibility to find out more about substance abuse, even if initially that it is only how to recognise symptoms and how and when to refer to other services.

CONCLUSION

Alcohol and drug use are commonplace across the UK. Many people do not experience problems with their use, but some do and at harmful levels. People who have a coexisting drug or alcohol and mental health problem are at greater risk. There is evidence that these people experience more social problems and have less positive treatment outcomes.

As a nurse it is important to assess every patient for drug or alcohol use and to offer timely and effective treatment. Careful assessment is the key to offering the best management to comorbidly diagnosed patients and to identifying those patients who are at risk of harm. These patients may not have been diagnosed previously. Treatment might take the form of brief interventions that can be offered in the drug or mental health setting. Alternatively, drug and alcohol and mental health services might need to find ways of working together to offer appropriate services to these patients.

Rates of tobacco use are high among patients with a comorbid diagnosis, and interventions should be made available to assist patients in reducing or ceasing their tobacco use. Alcohol is still the most used substance and nurses need to undertake an accurate history and to follow area health service protocols to minimise the risk of withdrawal.

Despite the high prevalence of comorbid diagnosis, there is little evidence about the nature of best practice for this patient group. However, early recommendations from the research literature suggest that a programme that treats both disorders concurrently, with preference given to an integrated model of treatment, is most beneficial. Patients should be matched with treatments that work for them; there should be an emphasis on the relationship between the nurse and the patient; and services should work together to offer a holistic approach. Patients are not separate diagnoses: they are a single person.

Patients who have a mental health problem do not necessarily have a substance use problem and, conversely, patients of drug and alcohol services do not necessarily have a mental health problem. However, many patients who use treatment services do have a comorbid diagnosis. Before any intervention is offered, it is imperative that all patients undergo an adequate substance use assessment and a mental status examination.

EXERCISES FOR CLASS ENGAGEMENT

1. Discuss the following five questions with your group.
   - What would you do if you were working on a ward or in a community setting where there were negative attitudes and feelings towards patients with alcohol and drug disorders? Would you challenge your colleagues or refrain from commenting? What would you do if their attitudes impacted on patient care? When would you challenge and what could you do?
   - How would you feel if you observed another nurse drinking vodka during a lunch break when you were both working together on a ward? What would you do?
   - The senior nurse on the ward invites you out for lunch at a nearby hotel. The senior has two strong alcoholic drinks in succession and the two of you return to the ward. You are due to be assessed by your senior later that week. Do you report your senior?
   - Are you aware of your own negative attitudes and feelings that might impede your interactions and therapeutic response to a patient with a substance-related disorder? If you have such attitudes, how would you overcome them to establish a therapeutic relationship with the patient?
   - What role does the Nursing and Midwifery Council (NMC) have in responding to a complaint about a nurse using substances when on duty?
2. A 36-year-old man is admitted with the following signs and symptoms: T 38.1, P 106, R 28, BP 189/93, profuse perspiration and tremulousness. He appears highly agitated. A mental status examination reveals confusion, disorientation and visual and tactile hallucinations. His partner advises that he had been a heavy drinker, but he stopped 2 days ago. What substance-induced disorder is the patient experiencing?
   A. substance-induced psychosis
   B. alcohol withdrawal syndrome
   C. delirium tremens
   D. substance-induced anxiety disorder
3. When the nurse does an initial admission interview on a patient being admitted for detoxification, which of the following areas is it critical to assess?
   A. type(s) of drug used
   B. family history
   C. reason for admission
   D. physical history

REFERENCES

Allen, J., 2003. Assessment of alcoholic patients: advances and future challenges. Recent developments in alcoholism. In: Galanter, M., Begleiter, H. (Eds.), Lagressa D Research on Alcohol Treatment, vol. 16. Kluwer Academic, New York, pp. 13–24.

Allsop, S., 2008. Drug use and Mental Health: Effective Responses to Co-Occurring Drug and Mental Health Problems. IP Publishing, Melbourne.

American Psychiatric Association (APA), 2013. Diagnostic and Statistical Manual of Mental Disorders, fifth ed. American Psychiatric Association, Washington (DSM-5).

Auriacombe, M., Fatseas, M., Dubernet, J., Daulouede, J.P., Tignol, J., 2004. French field experience with buprenorphine. American Journal on Addictions 13 (Suppl. 1), S17–28.

Babor, T., Higgins-Biddle, J., Saunders, J., Moteiro, M., 2001. The Alcohol Disorders Identification Test. Guidelines for Use in Primary Care, second ed. World Health Organization, Geneva.

Bachiller, D., Grau-Lopez, L., Barral, C., Daigre, C., Alberich, C., Rodriguez-Cintas, L., Valero, S., Casas, M., Roncero, C., 2015. Motivational interviewing group at inpatient detoxification, its influence in maintaining abstinence and treatment retention after discharge. Adicciones 27 (2), 109–118.

Baker, A., Vellman, R., 2007. Clinical Handbook of Co-Existing Mental Health and Drug and Alcohol Problems. Routledge, Taylor & Francis, London.

Bandstra, E.S., Morrow, C.E., Mansoor, E., Accornero, V.H., 2010. Prenatal drug exposure: infant and toddler outcomes. Journal of Addictive Diseases 29 (2), 245–258.

Berridge, K.C., Kringelbach, M.L., 2015. Pleasure systems in the brain. Neuron 86 (3), 646–664.

Bien, T.H., Miller, W.R., Tonigan, J.S., 1993. Brief interventions for alcohol problems: a review. Addiction 88 (3), 315–335.

Bostwick, J., Lapid, M., 2004. False positives on the clinical institute withdrawal assessment for alcohol-revised: is this scale appropriate for use in the medically ill? Psychosomatics 45 (3), 256–261.

Brunette, M.F., Asher, D., Whitley, R., Lutz, W.J., Wieder, B.L., Jones, A.M., McHugo, G.J., 2008. Implementation of integrated dual disorders treatment: a qualitative analysis of facilitators and barriers. Psychiatric Services 59 (9), 989–995.

Burns, L., Roxburgh, A., Bruno, R., Van Buskirk, J., 2014a. Monitoring drug markets in the internet age and the evolution of drug monitoring systems in Australia. Drug Testing and Analysis 6 (7–8), 840–845.

Burns, L., Roxburgh, A., Matthews, A., Bruno, R., Lenton, S., Van Buskirk, J., 2014b. The rise of new psychoactive substance use in Australia. Drug Testing and Analysis 6 (7–8), 846–849.

Cairney, I., Galletly, C., de Crespigny, C., Liu, D., Moss, J., Procter, N., 2015. Stopping the run-around? A study of services for people with comorbid mental health and substance use disorders in northern Adelaide. Australasian Psychiatry 23 (3), 233–235.

Daetwyler, C., Schindler, B., Parran, T., 2012. The Clinical Assessment of Substance Use Disorders. MedEdPORTAL, National Institutes of Drug Abuse. Available at: www.mededportal.org/publication/9110.

Davies, B., 2012. Dangerous drugs online. Australian Prescriber 35 (1), 32–33. https://doi.org/10.18773/austprescr.12012.18009.

Dawe, S., Frye, S., Best, D., Moss, D., Atkinson, J., 2006. Drug Use in The Family: Impacts and Implications for Children. Australian National Council on Drugs, Canberra.

Degenhardt, L., Hall, W., 2012. Extent of illicit drug use and dependence, and their contribution to the global burden of disease. Lancet 379 (9810), 55–70.

Degenhardt, L., Whiteford, H.A., Ferrari, A.J., Baxter, A.J., Charlson, F.J., Hall, W.D., Freedman, G., Burstein, R., Johns, N., Engell, R.E., Flaxman, A., Murray, C.J., Vos, T., 2013. Global burden of disease attributable to illicit drug use and dependence: findings from the Global Burden of Disease Study 2010. Lancet 382 (9904), 1564–1574.

Department of Health, 2016. UK Chief Medical Officers' Low Risk Drinking Guidelines. Available at: https://assets.publishing.service.gov.uk/government/uploads/system/uploads/attachment_data/file/545937/UK_CMOs__report.pdf. Accessed: 23 November 2018.

Drake, R.E., Wallach, M.A., 2000. Dual diagnosis: 15 years of progress. Psychiatric Services 51 (9), 1126–1129.

Fukui, Y., Sakata-Haga, H., 2009. Intrauterine environment-genome interaction and children's development (1). Ethanol: a teratogen in developing brain. Journal of Toxicological Sciences 34 (Suppl. 2), SP273–S278.

Galanter, M., Kleber, H., Brady, K., 2015. The American Psychiatric Publishing Textbook of Substance Addiction, fifth ed. American Psychiatric Publishing, Washington.

Gilchrist, G., Taylor, A., 2009. Drug-using mothers: factors associated with retaining care of their children. Drug and Alcohol Review 28 (2), 175–185.

Grant, T., Huggins, J., Graham, J., Ernst, C., Whitney, N., Wilson, D., 2011. Maternal substance abuse and disrupted parenting: distinguishing mothers who keep their children from those who do not. Children and Youth Services Review 33 (11), 2176–2185.

Grella, C.E., Hser, Y.I., Huang, Y.C., 2006. Mothers in substance abuse treatment: differences in characteristics based on involvement with child welfare services. Child Abuse & Neglect 30 (1), 55–73.

Grella, C.E., Needell, B., Shi, Y., Hser, Y.I., 2009. Do drug treatment services predict reunification outcomes of mothers and their children in child welfare? Journal of Substance Abuse Treatment 36 (3), 278–293.

Haastrup, M.B., Pottegard, A., Damkier, P., 2014. Alcohol and breastfeeding. Basic & Clinical Pharmacology & Toxicology 114 (2), 168–173.

Harro, J., 2015. Neuropsychiatric adverse effects of amphetamine and methamphetamine. International Review of Neurobiology 120, 179–204.

Havens, J.R., Simmons, L.A., Shannon, L.M., Hansen, W.F., 2009. Factors associated with substance use during pregnancy: results from a national sample. Drug and Alcohol Dependence 99 (1–3), 89–95.

Helander, A., Peter, O., Zheng, Y., 2012. Monitoring of the alcohol biomarkers PEth, CDT and EtG/EtS in an outpatient treatment setting. Alcohol 47 (5), 552–557.

Hoban, C., 2017. Assessing for head injury in alcohol-intoxicated patients. Emergency Nurse 25 (5), 30–33.

Holton, A., Gallagher, P., Ryan, C., Fahey, T., Cousins, G., 2017. Consensus validation of the POSAMINO POtentially Serious Alcohol–Medication INteractions in Older adults) criteria. BMJ Open. Available at: https://bmjopen.bmj.com/content/bmjopen/7/11/e017453.full.pdf. Accessed: 23 November 2018.

Home Office, 2016. New Psychoactive Substances (Nps) Resource Pack for Informal Educators and Practitioners. Available at: https://assets.publishing.service.gov.uk/government/uploads/system/uploads/attachment_data/file/544030/6_1845_HO_NPS_Resources_Booklet_June16_v10.pdf. Accessed: 22 November 2018.

Home Office, 2017. Drug Strategy 2017. Available at: https://assets.publishing.service.gov.uk/government/uploads/system/uploads/attachment_data/file/628148/Drug_strategy_2017.PDF. Accessed: 23 November 2018.

Humphreys, K., Blodgett, J.C., Wagner, T.H., 2014. Estimating the efficacy of alcoholics anonymous without self-selection bias: an instrumental variables re-analysis of randomized clinical trials. Alcoholism Clinical and Experimental Research 38 (11), 2688–2694.

Jones, H., Kaltenback, K., 2013. Treating Women With Substance Use Disorders During Pregnancy: a Comprehensive Approach to Caring for Mother and Child. Oxford University Press, Oxford.

Kaufmann, R.M., Kraft, B., Frey, R., Winkler, D., Weiszenbichler, S., Backer, C., Kasper, S., Kress, H.G., 2010. Acute psychotropic effects of oral cannabis extract with a defined content of Delta9-tetrahydrocannabinol (THC) in healthy volunteers. Pharmacopsychiatry 43 (1), 24–32.

Kelleher, S., 2007. Health care professionals' knowledge and attitudes regarding substance use and substance users. Accident & Emergency Nursing 15 (3), 161–165.

Kelly, J.F., Stout, R.L., Slaymaker, V., 2013. Emerging adults' treatment outcomes in relation to 12-step mutual-help attendance and active involvement. Drug and Alcohol Dependence 129 (1–2), 151–157.

Kessler, R.C., 2004. The epidemiology of dual diagnosis. Biological Psychiatry 56 (10), 730–737.

Kleinloog, D., Stevens, J., Heuberger, J., Spinhoven, P., van Gerven, J., 2014. The influence of personality on the sensitivity to subjective effects of Delta9-tetrahydrocannabinol. Psychiatry Research 220 (3), 945–953.

Koob, G., 2015. Neurobiology of addiction. In: Galanter, M., Kleber, H., Brady, K. (Eds.), The American Psychiatric Publishing Textbook of Substance Abuse Treatment, fifth ed. American Psychiatric Publishing, Washington.

Koob, G., Volkow, N.D., 2010. Neurocircuitry of addiction. Neuropsychopharmacology 35 (1), 217–238.

Lai, H.M., Cleary, M., Sitharthan, T., Hunt, G.E., 2015. Prevalence of comorbid substance use, anxiety and mood disorders in epidemiological surveys, 1990–2014: a systematic review and meta-analysis. Drug and Alcohol Dependence 154, 1–13.

Larance, B., Degenhardt, L., Lintzeris, N., Bell, J., Winstock, A., Dietze, P., Mattick, R., Ali, R., Horyniak, D., 2011. Post-marketing surveillance of buprenorphine-naloxone in Australia: diversion, injection and adherence with supervised dosing. Drug and Alcohol Dependence 118 (2–3), 265–273.

Larance, B., Lintzeris, N., Ali, R., Dietze, P., Mattick, R., Jenkinson, R., White, N., Degenhardt, L., 2014. The diversion and injection of a buprenorphine-naloxone soluble film formulation. Drug and Alcohol Dependence 136, 21–27.

Laslett, A., Room, R., Dietze, P., 2014. Substance misuse, mental health problems and recurrent child maltreatment. Advances in Dual Diagnosis 7 (1), 15–23.

Latt, N., Dore, G., 2014. Thiamine in the treatment of Wernicke encephalopathy in patients with alcohol use disorders. Journal of Internal Medicine 44 (9), 911–915.

Lee, N., Jenner, L., Kay-Lambkin, F., Hall, K., Dann, F., Roeg, S., Hunt, S., Dingle, G., Baker, A., Hides, L., Ritter, A., 2007. Psycheck: Responding to Mental Health Issues within Alcohol and Drug Treatment. Australian Government Department of Health and Ageing, Canberra.

Lev-Ran, S., Le Strat, Y., Imtiaz, S., Rehm, J., Le Foll, B., 2013. Gender differences in prevalence of substance use disorders among individuals with lifetime exposure to substances: results from a large representative sample. American Journal on Addictions 22 (1), 7–13.

Lister, J., Milosevic, A., Ledgerwood, D., 2015. Personality traits of problem gamblers with and without alcohol dependence. Addictive Behaviors 47, 48–54.

Lorains, F.K., Cowlishaw, S., Thomas, S.A., 2011. Prevalence of comorbid disorders in problem and pathological gambling: systematic review and meta-analysis of population surveys. Addiction 106 (3), 490–498.

Lubman, D., Sundram, S., 2003. Substance misuse in patients with schizophrenia: a primary care guide. Medical Journal of Australia 178 (supp May):S71–75.

Lundahl, B., Moleni, T., Burke, B.L., Butters, R., Tollefson, D., Butler, C., Rollnick, S., 2013. Motivational interviewing in medical care settings: a systematic review and meta-analysis of randomized controlled trials. Patient Education and Counseling 93 (2), 157–168.

MacDonald, E., Luxmoore, M., Pica, S., 2004. Social networks of people with dual diagnosis: the quantity and quality of relationships at different stages of substance use treatment. Community Mental Health Journal 40 (5), 451–464.

Marsch, L.A., Bickel, W.K., Badger, G.J., Jacobs, E.A., 2005. Buprenorphine treatment for opioid dependence: the relative efficacy of daily, twice and thrice weekly dosing. Drug and Alcohol Dependence 77 (2), 195–204.

Marsh, A., Dale, A., O'Toole, S., 2013. Addiction Counselling. Content and Process, second ed. IP Communications, Melbourne.

Martin-Santos, R., Crippa, J.A., Batalla, A., Bhattacharyya, S., Atakan, Z., Borgwardt, S., Allen, P., Seal, M., Langohr, K., Farre, M., Zuardi, A.W., McGuire, P.K., 2012. Acute effects of a single, oral dose of d9-tetrahydrocannabinol (THC) and cannabidiol (CBD) administration in healthy volunteers. Current Pharmaceutical Design 18 (32), 4966–4979.

Mattick, R.P., Kimber, J., Breen, C., Davoli, M., 2008. Buprenorphine maintenance versus placebo or methadone maintenance for opioid dependence. Cochrane Database of Systemic Reviews (2), CD002207.

McGovern, M.P., Lambert-Harris, C., Xie, H., Meier, A., McLeman, B., Saunders, E., 2015. A randomized controlled trial of treatments for co-occurring substance use disorders and post-traumatic stress disorder. Addiction 110 (7), 1194–1204.

Menezes, P.R., Johnson, S., Thornicroft, G., Marshall, J., Prosser, D., Bebbington, P., Kuipers, E., 1996. Drug and alcohol problems among individuals with severe mental illness in south London. British Journal of Psychiatry 168 (5), 612–619.

Merikangas, K.R., Kalaydjian, A., 2007. Magnitude and impact of comorbidity of mental disorders from epidemiologic surveys. Current Opinion in Psychiatry 20 (4), 353–358.

Miller, N.S., Gold, M.S., 1993. A hypothesis for a common neurochemical basis for alcohol and drug disorders. Psychiatric Clinics of North America 16 (1), 105–117.

Miller, W., Heather, N., 1986. Treating Addictive Behaviors: Processes of Change. Plenum Press, New York.

Miller, W.R., Rollnick, S., 2009. Ten things that motivational interviewing is not. Behavioural and Cognitive Psychotherapy 37 (2), 129–140.

Mills, K., Deady, M., Proudfoot, H., Sannibale, C., Teeson, M., Mattick, R., Burns, L., 2008. Guidelines on The Management of Co-Occurring Alcohol and Other Drug and Mental Health Conditions in Alcohol and Other Drug Treatment Settings. National Drug and Alcohol Research Centre, University of New South Wales, Sydney.

Moore, T.J., Glenmullen, J., Mattison, D.R., 2014. Reports of pathological gambling, hypersexuality, and compulsive shopping associated with dopamine receptor agonist drugs. JAMA Internal Medicine 174 (12), 1930–1933.

Moyer, A., Finney, J.W., 2015. Brief interventions for alcohol misuse. Canadian Medical Association Journal 187 (7), 502–506.

Musselman, M.E., Hampton, J.P., 2014. Not for human consumption: a review of emerging designer drugs. Pharmacotherapy 34 (7), 745–757.

Nair, P., Black, M.M., Schuler, M., Keane, V., Snow, L., Rigney, B.A., Magder, L., 1997. Risk factors for disruption in primary caregiving among infants of substance abusing women. Child Abuse & Neglect 21 (11), 1039–1051.

National Health Service, 2017. Cannabis: the Facts. Available at: https://www.nhs.uk/live-well/healthy-body/cannabis-the-facts/. Accessed: 22 November 2018.

National Health Service (NHS) Digital, 2018. Statistics on Alcohol: England. Available at: https://digital.nhs.uk/data-and-information/publications/statistical/statistics-on-alcohol/2018. Accessed: 22 November 2018.

National Institute of Health and Care Excellence (NICE), 2015. Alcohol: Preventing Harmful use in the Community [QS83]. Available at: https://www.nice.org.uk/guidance/qs83. Accessed 22 November 2018.

National Institute of Health and Care Excellence, 2011. Alcohol-use disorders: Diagnosis, Assessment and Management of Harmful Drinking and Alcohol Dependence [CG115]. Available at: https://www.nice.org.uk/guidance/cg115. Accessed: 22 November 2018.

Nestler, E.J., 2005. Is there a common molecular pathway for addiction? Nature Neuroscience 8 (11), 1445–1449.

Ntais, C., Pakos, E., Kyzas, P., Ioannidis, J.P., 2005. Benzodiazepines for alcohol withdrawal. Cochrane Database of Systemic Reviews 20 (3), CD005063

Nutt, D.J., Lingford-Hughes, A., Erritzoe, D., Stokes, P.R., 2015. The dopamine theory of addiction: 40 years of highs and lows. Nature Reviews Neuroscience 16 (5), 305–312.

Pelissier, F., Lauque, D., Charpentier, S., Franchitto, N., 2014. Blood alcohol concentration in intoxicated patients seen in the emergency department: does it influence discharge decisions? Journal of Studies on Alcohol and Drugs 75 (6), 937–944.

Prochaska, J., DiClemente, C., 1984. The Transtheoretical Approach: Crossing Traditional Boundaries of Therapy. Dow/Jones Irwin, Homewood, Ill.

Prochaska, J., Velicer, W., 1997. The transtheoretical model of health behaviour change. American Journal of Health Promotion 12 (1), 38–48.

Public Health England (PHE), 2018. Adult Substance Misuse Statistics from the National Drug Treatment Monitoring System (NDTMS) 1 April 2017 to 31 March 2018. Available at: https://assets.publishing.service.gov.uk/government/uploads/system/uploads/attachment_data/file/752993/AdultSubstanceMisuseStatisticsfromNDTMS2017-18.pdf. Accessed: 22 November 2018.

Regier, D.A., Farmer, M.E., Rae, D.S., Locke, B.Z., Keith, S.J., Judd, L.L., Goodwin, F.K., 1990. Comorbidity of mental disorders with alcohol and other drug abuse. Results from the Epidemiologic Catchment Area (ECA) Study. JAMA 264 (19), 2511–2518.

Richards, J.R., Derlet, R.W., 2014. Beta-blocker and antipsychotic treatment of toxicity from so-called designer drugs. Pharmacotherapy 34 (8) e159–160.

Ries, R., Fiellin, D., Miller, S., Saitz, R., 2014. American Society of Addiction Medicine: Principles of Addiction Medicine. Wolters Kluwer, Philadelphia.

Riper, H., Andersson, G., Hunter, S.B., de Wit, J., Berking, M., Cuijpers, P., 2014. Treatment of comorbid alcohol use disorders and depression with cognitive behavioural therapy and motivational interviewing: a meta-analysis. Addiction 109 (3), 394–406.

Robertson, C.L., Ishibashi, K., Mandelkern, M.A., Brown, A.K., Ghahremani, D.G., Sabb, F., Bilder, R., Cannon, T., Borg, J., London, E.D., 2015. Striatal D1- and D2-type dopamine receptors are linked to motor response inhibition in human subjects. Journal of Neuroscience 35 (15), 5990–5997.

Rosenthal, R.N., Nunes, E.V., Le Fauve, C.E., 2012. Implications of epidemiological data for identifying persons with substance use and other mental disorders. American Journal on Addictions 21 (2), 97–103.

Royal College of Obstetricians and Gynaecologists, 2018. Alcohol and Pregnancy. Available at: https://www.rcog.org.uk/globalassets/documents/patients/patient-information-leaflets/pregnancy/pi-alcohol-and-pregnancy.pdf. Accessed: 22 November 2018.

Saunders, J., Young, R., 2002. Assessment and diagnosis. In: Hulse, G., White, J. (Eds.), Cape G Management of Alcohol and Drug Problems. Oxford University Press, Melbourne.

Schuckit, M., 2009. Alcohol use disorders. The Lancet 373, 492–501.

Schwartz, R.P., Gryczynski, J., O'Grady, K.E., Sharfstein, J.M., Warren, G., Olsen, Y., Mitchell, S.G., Jaffe, J.H., 2013. Opioid agonist treatments and heroin overdose deaths in Baltimore, Maryland, 1995–2009. American Journal of Public Health 103 (5), 917–922.

Staunton, P., Chiarella, M., 2013. Law for Nurses and Midwives, seventh ed. Elsevier, Sydney.

Steingrimsson, S., Carlsen, H.K., Sigfusson, S., Magnusson, A., 2012. The changing gender gap in substance use disorder: a total population-based study of psychiatric in-patients. Addiction 107 (11), 1957–1962.

Sullivan, J., Sykora, K., Schneiderman, J., et al., 1989. Assessment of alcohol withdrawal: the revised clinical institute withdrawal assessment for alcohol scale (CIWA-AR). British Journal of Addiction 84, 1353–1357.

Sullivan, L.E., Moore, B.A., Chawarski, M.C., Pantalon, M.V., Barry, D., O'Connor, P.G., Schottenfeld, R.S., Fiellin, D.A., 2008. Buprenorphine/naloxone treatment in primary care is associated with decreased human immunodeficiency virus risk behaviors. Journal of Substance Abuse Treatment 35 (1), 87–92.

Taplin, S., Mattick, R.P., 2013. Mothers in methadone treatment and their involvement with the child protection system: a replication and extension study. Child Abuse & Neglect 37 (8), 500–510.

Taplin, S., Richmond, G., McArthur, M., 2015. Identifying Alcohol and Other use During Pregnancy. Outcomes for Women, their Partners and their Children. Institute of Child Protection Studies, Australian Catholic University, ACT.

Teesson, M., Hall, W., 2001. Substance-related disorders. In: Meadows, G., Singh, B. (Eds.), Mental health in Australia: Collaborative Community Practice. Oxford University Press, Melbourne.

Thorley, A., 1982. The effects of alcohol. In: Plant, M. (Ed.), Drinking and Problem Drinking. Junction Books, London, pp. 23–64.

Turning Point, 2015. Psycheck Screening Tool and Training Manual. Available at: www.psycheck.org.au/index.html. Accessed: 1 June 2015.

Vasilaki, E.I., Hosier, S.G., Cox, W.M., 2006. The efficacy of motivational interviewing as a brief intervention for excessive drinking: a meta-analytic review. Alcohol 41 (3), 328–335.

Warren, O.U., Sena, V., Choo, E., Machan, J., 2012. Emergency physicians' and nurses' attitudes towards alcohol-intoxicated patients. Journal of Emergency Medicine 43 (6), 1167–1174.

Weaver, M.F., Hopper, J.A., Gunderson, E.W., 2015. Designer drugs 2015: assessment and management. Addiction Science & Clinical Practice 10, 8.

Wild, T.C., Cunningham, J.A., Roberts, A.B., 2007. Controlled study of brief personalized assessment-feedback for drinkers interested in self-help. Addiction 102 (2), 241–250.

Woody, G.E., Poole, S.A., Subramaniam, G., Dugosh, K., Bogenschutz, M., Abbott, P., Patkar, A., Publicker, M., McCain, K., Potter, J.S., Forman, R., Vetter, V., McNicholas, L., Blaine, J., Lynch, K.G., Fudala, P., 2008. Extended vs short-term buprenorphine-naloxone for treatment of opioid-addicted youth: a randomized trial. JAMA 300 (17), 2003–2011.

World Health Organization (WHO), 2013. WHO Model List of Essential Medicines. Available at: http://apps.who.int/iris/bitstream/10665/93142/1/EML_18_eng.pdf. Accessed: 22 November 2018.

World Health Organization (WHO), 2014a. Global Health Estimates 2014 Summary Tables: Disability Adjusted Life Years 2000–2012. WHO, Geneva. Available at: www.euro.who.int/en/health-topics/noncommunicable-diseases/mental-health/data-and-statistics. Accessed: 22 November 2018.

World Health Organization (WHO), 2014b. Global Status Report on Alcohol and Health. WHO, Geneva. Available at: www.who.int/mediacentre/factsheets/fs349/en. Accessed: 22 November 2018.

World Health Organization (WHO), 2015. ASSIST (Alcohol Smoking and Substance Involvement Screening Test). Available at: www.who.int/substance_abuse/activities/assist/en. Accessed: 1 June 2015.

Yokell, M.A., Zaller, N.D., Green, T.C., Rich, J.D., 2011. Buprenorphine and buprenorphine/naloxone diversion, misuse, and illicit use: an international review. Current Drug Abuse Reviews 4 (1), 28–41.

USEFUL WEBSITES

Alcohol brief intervention resources NHS Health Scotland, www.healthscotland.scot/publications/alcohol-brief-intervention-resources

Alcoholics Anonymous UK, www.alcoholics-anonymous.org.uk

British National Formulary (BNF), https://bnf.nice.org.uk/

Cochrane Library, evidence-based healthcare decision making, www.cochranelibrary.com
FRANK drug and alcohol support, www.talktofrank.com
GamCare gambling support, www.gamcare.org.uk
Glasgow Structured Approach to Assessment of the Glasgow Coma Scale, www.glasgowcomascale.org
Management of substance abuse (WHO), www.who.int/substance_abuse/activities/sbi/en/
Narcotics Anonymous UK, www.ukna.org
The Royal College of Emergency Medicine: Alcohol Toolkit, https://www.rcem.ac.uk/docs/College%20Guidelines/5z24.%20Alcohol%20toolkit%20(-June%202015).pdf
Turning Point, www.turning-point.co.uk
World Health Organization (WHO), 2001. AUDIT: The Alcohol Use Disorders Identification Test. Guidelines for use in Primary Healthcare, second ed. www.who.int/substance_abuse/publications/alcohol/en

PART 5

What Mental Health Nurses Can Do To Help

21

Mental Health Promotion, Prevention and Primary Healthcare

Tom Meehan

KEY POINTS

- The lifetime burden of disability associated with mental illness is high due to the early onset of most mental disorders.
- Mental health service provision needs to be reoriented to provide a greater focus on activities such as health promotion, illness prevention, early intervention and recovery.
- Health promotion and prevention strategies target the determinants of health, which are influenced by a complex interplay of risk factors and protective factors.
- Mental health promotion aims to increase resilience to illness by creating supportive living conditions and environments. Mental health prevention aims to reduce symptoms and mental disorders.
- Primary care services play an important role in the care of those with mental health problems, as GPs are frequently the first point of contact for people with mental illness.
- Primary healthcare in the UK is provided through an array of community-based public, private and third sector health service

KEY TERMS

early intervention
illness prevention
mental health
mental health promotion
mental illness
mental wellbeing
primary healthcare
primary mental healthcare
protective factors
recovery
risk factors

LEARNING OUTCOMES

The material in this chapter will assist you to:

- understand the relationships between promotion, prevention, early intervention and primary healthcare.
- understand the determinants of mental health and wellbeing.
- differentiate between protective factors and risk factors.
- describe the role of health promotion and illness prevention and how these activities are applied in the field of mental health.
- understand the importance of early intervention in preventing the onset of mental illness and/or reducing its impact.
- reflect on the current structure of primary mental healthcare and the different players involved.
- recognise the expanding role of nurses in the delivery of primary mental healthcare services.
- gain insights into the different services available to people with mental health problems in the primary care sector.

INTRODUCTION

In 2016, The Five Year Forward View for Mental Health for the NHS in England was created, a collaboration between the independent Mental Health Taskforce, health and care leaders, people who use the services and experts in the field. The report highlighted that mental health services have been underfunded for decades, recognising that people with mental health problems have been marginalised and stigmatised by health services, which have treated their mind and body separately. It has been acknowledged that public attitudes towards mental health are changing, with workplaces, schools and communities committed to changing the way they think about mental health (Mental Health Taskforce 2016). The report calls for there to be parity of esteem between mental and physical health for people of all ages, addressing the inequalities at local and national levels. This has brought into focus the importance of activities such as mental health promotion, illness prevention and recovery. These activities are now considered key components of a modern mental health system aimed at reducing mental illness and the burden of disease associated with it.

It is clear that many of the factors that impact on mental health and wellbeing (such as social inclusion, employment, housing and education) are outside the reach of mental health services. The need for multilevel interventions provided through a 'cross government' approach is now recognised (Mental Health Taskforce 2016).

This chapter commences with a discussion of mental illness and its impact on individuals and their communities and highlights the growing influence of the relatively new concepts of promotion, prevention, early intervention and primary care. These interrelated concepts are defined and examples provided to highlight the similarities and differences between them. The expanding role of mental health nurses in the prevention and management of mental health conditions in the primary care sector is also discussed.

MENTAL ILLNESS, MENTAL DISORDER OR MENTAL HEALTH PROBLEM?

Throughout this chapter the terms 'mental illness' and 'mental disorder' are used interchangeably. Mental illnesses and disorders are classified as clinically diagnosable conditions that have a significant impact on an individual's cognitive, emotional or social functioning. Disorders can comprise of a broad range of problems with a variety of symptoms, but are generally characterised by a combination of abnormal thoughts, emotions, behaviours and relationships with others (World Health Organization [WHO] 2018). Conditions in this category include mood disorders (such as depression and bipolar disorder), psychotic disorders (such as schizophrenia), eating disorders and personality disorders. These disorders should be differentiated from mental health problems, which can also impact on an individual's ability to function, but are unlikely to meet the criteria for mental illnesses or disorders.

MENTAL ILLNESS AND ITS IMPACT

Mental disorders impact on the lives of millions of people around the world and, if left untreated, create enormous suffering, disability and economic loss. It is thought that one in four adults will experience at least one diagnosable mental health problem in any given year, with half of all mental health problems being established by the age of 14 years. This rises to 75% by age 24 years and 1 in 10 children (5–16 years) have a diagnosable mental health problem (Mental Health Taskforce 2016).

Mental health problems are the single largest cause of disability in the UK. Approximately two million adults were in contact with specialist mental health services at some point in 2014/15, with 9 out of 10 adults being supported in primary care. For adults with more severe mental health problems, 90% were supported by community services. However, it was revealed that almost one-fifth of people who were under the Care Programme Approach had not had a formal review meeting in the previous 12 months and one-quarter of the people accessing secondary mental health services did not know who was responsible for coordinating their care (Mental Health Taskforce 2016). There is a strong association between mental illness and physical ill health. It has been estimated that the impact of physical conditions such as obesity, heart disease and diabetes can reduce life expectancy for people with psychosis by up to 15 to 20 years (Lawrence et al. 2013; Mental Health Taskforce 2016). Suicide is also a leading cause of premature death in people with mental health conditions. Despite improvements in treatment and our understanding of mental illness, suicide rates in England have been steadily rising since the 1990s after many years of decline, peaking at 4882 deaths in 2014. Suicide has become the leading cause of death in males (aged 15–49), with men three times more likely to take their own lives than women (Mental Health Taskforce 2016).

The burden associated with mental illness is high and can manifest in many different ways depending on the individual's circumstances and resilience. For example, the burden associated with mental illness may emerge from the stigma and discrimination people with mental illness frequently experience, the loneliness and low levels of life satisfaction, the impact of the illness on the person's capacity to be productive and contribute to the workplace and society and the impact on physical health (Bywood et al. 2015).

It is clear from the discussion earlier that the disability associated with mental illness is a major contributor to overall illness burden. The World Bank, in collaboration with WHO, introduced a measure of burden based on disability-adjusted life years (DALYs). The index considers ill health and years lived with a disability in addition to premature death from mental illness (WHO 2015). As such, morbidity and mortality are combined to provide a single, common metric so that one DALY is equal to one lost year of healthy life due to premature death or disability. The measure is useful in that it can be used to compare mental health mortality and morbidity across the globe.

It is predicted that by 2020 depression will be one of the largest health problems worldwide, second only to heart disease, with a major impact not only on health services but also on productivity and economic growth (WHO 2012).

The burden of mental ill health on the UK economy is high, estimated to be £105 billion a year—which equates to approximately the entire cost of the NHS (Mental Health Taskforce 2016). By the time a person deteriorates to the stage where mental health services such as acute inpatient care are required, the person is likely to have already experienced impaired functioning in many areas of their life. The illness is likely to impact on their relationships with family and friends, an inability to study or to get and keep a job, loss of income, isolation and self-neglect, in extreme cases leading to crime and homelessness.

Over recent years, public attitudes have changed, in part due to the Time to Change campaign, resulting in increased awareness and a heightened understanding of the urgent need to act on improving the experiences of people with mental ill health, both within and beyond the NHS. The Five Year Forward View for Mental Health sets out recommendations to reenergise mental health services, meeting the increasing demand and improving outcomes with a greater focus on activities such as health promotion, illness prevention, early intervention and recovery—that is, programmes that help prevent and/or intervene in the early stages of mental illness (Mental Health Taskforce 2016). The following priority actions have been identified for the NHS to achieve by 2020/21:

1. A 7-day NHS: right care, right time, right quality
2. An integrated mental and physical health approach

3. Promoting good mental health and preventing poor mental health—helping people lead better lives as equal citizens

The priority areas are underpinned by the concepts of recovery, prevention and early intervention. There is evidence to suggest that shifting resources 'upstream' to programmes focussing on early intervention and prevention will reduce the growing expenditure on 'downstream' services such as medication, acute inpatient care, rehabilitation, emergency department visits and income support (Knapp et al. 2011).

CRITICAL THINKING CHALLENGE 21.1

It is often suggested that too much money is being spent on 'treating' illness and not enough on preventing it. Why is it difficult for governments to move funding and resources from treating people with illness (i.e. hospitals) to promoting wellbeing, healthy living and illness prevention?

MENTAL HEALTH PROMOTION

Over the past 20 years, a growing body of evidence has emerged to support the use of health promotion and prevention principles in mental health practice (Beardslee et al. 2011; Jané-Llopis et al. 2005). Mental health promotion is now considered a key component of the broader concept of health aimed at assisting people to take greater control for the way they live and maintain their health (WHO 1986). Herrman (2001, p. 173) noted that the aim of health promotion is to 'keep people healthy or become even healthier'. The Mental Health Taskforce (2016) state that 'prevention matters – it's the only way that lasting change can be achieved'. It is also recognised that helping people to live fulfilled and productive lives is not the work of the NHS alone, for this to be achieved support needs to go into good parenting, education, housing and to build supportive communities that have the opportunity to forge relationships.

Risk Factors and Protective Factors

Health promotion (and illness prevention) strategies target the determinants of health, which are influenced by a complex interplay of risk factors and protective factors. *Risk factors* increase the likelihood of developing a mental health condition or increase the burden of dealing with a diagnosed condition. Risk factors include a wide range of genetic, biological, behavioural, psychological, cultural, economic and environmental factors (see Table 21.1). While a single risk factor (e.g. social isolation) may have minimal impact on an individual's ability to cope with a stressful situation, the combined effect of many risk factors such as homelessness, poverty, drug use and poor coping skills is likely to overburden the individual's coping capacity, leaving them susceptible to developing mental health problems. Exposure to risk factors over a prolonged period can have a cumulative effect and this may impact on an individual's ability to fight off a mental illness (Shaffer & Yates 2010).

Although the list of potential risk factors is extensive (see Table 21.1), the association between them and the development of mental health conditions varies. Therefore, a causal relationship should not be drawn, as some individuals may present with many risk factors yet do not go on to develop mental illness, while others may have none or few risk factors yet present with some form of mental illness.

Protective factors have the opposite effect to risk factors and enhance an individual's ability to manage stressful life events. Protective factors (such as employment, education, self-confidence, resilience and social support) act by reducing the person's exposure to risk factors and may also reduce the impact of illness when it manifests. According to Keleher and Armstrong (2006), the three most important protective factors for mental wellness are social inclusion, freedom from discrimination and violence and access to economic resources.

Resnick and colleagues (1997) found that the presence of a greater number of protective factors was instrumental in lowering the level of risk. Examples of protective factors are provided in Table 21.2. As with risk factors, a causal relationship between protective factors and better outcomes cannot be assumed. Although risk factors may be present, protective factors tend to mitigate the overall risk.

Mental health nurses frequently have to balance risk factors and protective factors. In assessing the risk of suicide in a patient with suicidal thoughts; for example, the nurse would consider risk factors such as the patient's strength of suicidal ideation, previous attempts, gender, age and access to means, and weigh these against protective factors such as the patient's social support, children in the home and religious beliefs. In health promotion initiatives, a similar process is

TABLE 21.1 Examples of Risk Factors Associated With the Development of Mental Disorders

Individual	Family	School	Life events	Community
• Poor self-esteem • Chronic illness • Poor social skills • Genetic loading for illness • Substance misuse • Insecure attachment in infancy	• Violence (in family and culture) • Marital discord in parents • Low parental involvement • Neglect and rejection • Mental disorder in parent • Harsh discipline in childhood	• Bullying • Peer rejection • Deviant peer group • School failure	• Physical/sexual abuse • Divorce in parents • Poverty in the home • Homelessness • Stress/bullying at work • Death of close family member	• Living in a disadvantaged community • Social isolation • Neighbourhood violence • Lack of health services, transport, etc. • Discrimination

(*Source:* Adapted from Commonwealth Department of Health and Aged Care, 2000. National Action Plan for Promotion, Prevention and Early Intervention for Mental Health. Mental Health and Special Programs Branch. Commonwealth Department of Health and Aged Care, Canberra, p. 16.)

TABLE 21.2 **Examples of Protective Factors Associated With the Development of Mental Disorders**

Individual	Family	School	Life events	Community
• Good attachment to family • Good problem-solving skills • Good social skills • Internal locus of control and optimism • Calm temperament	• Supportive caring parents • Stable family unit • Small family size • Strong family norms • More than 2 years between siblings	• Positive school climate • Sense of belonging • Recognition of achievement • Positive peer group involvement	• Economic security • Support at critical points in life • Good physical health • Involvement with significant other/partner	• Sense of connectedness • Attachment to community networks • Involvement in religion or other group • Strong cultural identity • Little or no community violence

(*Source*: Adapted from Commonwealth Department of Health and Aged Care, 2000. National Action Plan for Promotion, Prevention and Early Intervention for Mental Health. Mental Health and Special Programs Branch. Commonwealth Department of Health and Aged Care, Canberra, p. 15.)

conducted to assess the risk of individuals developing mental illness. For example, health promotion activities might focus on strengthening protective factors such as providing support to parents with young families or on reducing risk factors such as addressing school bullying in high-risk communities. Nurses engaged in health promotion activities must have a clear understanding of the risk factors and protective factors associated with the condition of interest.

Health promotion strategies target 'modifiable' risk and try to strengthen protective factors. While factors such as age, gender and genetics are important determinants of health, they tend to be static and cannot be modified through health promotion activities. However, factors such as lifestyle, behaviour, education, income, housing and access to health services are modifiable and are likely to be enhanced through health promotion strategies. As such, the overall goal of health promotion is to work with modifiable factors to build resilience and strengthen coping mechanisms. By way of example, the charity Mind: for better mental health (www.mind.org.uk) aims to increase awareness of mental illness and reduce the stigma associated with it. The organisation uses health promotion strategies such as education, advertising and media campaigns to promote acceptance of mental illness and encourage early access to treatment for mental health conditions. A good example of a health promotion programme in action is the £15 million campaign by Public Health England, aiming to train 1 million people in basic mental health first aid skills, a programme that aims to improve personal resilience and help people recognise and respond effectively to signs of mental illness in others (UK Government 2017). A number of providers run the courses (see Useful Websites for details).

CRITICAL THINKING CHALLENGE 21.2

1. Reflect on your own feelings about health promotion. Do you believe that mental health conditions can be prevented through health promotion initiatives?
2. Think about a patient you worked with recently: what risk factors may have contributed to their illness? What protective factors were present?

The Ottawa Charter

Many of the determinants of mental health and wellbeing (such as social inclusion, employment, housing, education) cannot be fully addressed by mental health service providers working in isolation. The need for multilevel interventions, implemented across a wide range of services and programmes, is now recognised as a means of ensuring community-wide engagement in health promotion initiatives (WHO 1986). In 1986, one of the most influential policy documents in the health promotion field, the Ottawa Charter, was developed to promote a broader focus on community engagement.

The fundamental principles outlined in the Ottawa Charter highlight the need to focus health promotion activities in five key areas: policy, supportive environments, community action, personal skills and the reorienting of health services. These are briefly described here.

- ***Building healthy public policy*** recognises that healthy public policy is broader than health and calls for investment and legislation in other sectors such as education, housing, work location and nutrition. The focus of initiatives may include human rights, reducing the impact of stigma, improving social inclusion and preventing domestic violence and crime. This principle places pressure on policy makers to consider the health of local communities and the broader population.
- ***Creating supportive environments*** advocates for the development of supportive environments such as at home, in schools and in the workplace. This is particularly important in mental health as the development of mental illness is closely related to how an individual interacts with their environment and their wider social network. Initiatives may include strengthening families, addressing bullying in schools and workplaces, and helping young people to access peer support.
- ***Strengthening community action*** focusses on encouraging communities to be actively involved in local initiatives so as to set priorities, plan interventions and implement these to achieve better mental health outcomes. Initiatives are usually implemented at the local level and examples include drought support to farmers, initiatives to prevent suicide in a local community and initiatives to increase exercise in children.
- ***Developing personal skills*** assists individuals to improve personal and social competence through better education

and information. Barry and Jenkins (2007) noted that improved personal skills such as self-awareness, self-efficacy, self-esteem and problem solving assist people to cope better with life and have more control over their life and environment. The Positive Parenting Program (Triple P) (www.triplep.net) provides a good example of a health promotion initiative designed to help families work together to create a harmonious, stable and supportive home environment. The programme works with parents to build their confidence and knowledge in caring for children and young adults. The programme has been found to be effective in addressing behavioural, emotional and developmental problems in children (Sanders 2008).

- ***Reorienting health services*** promotes the need for mental health services to move beyond a focus on acute care and treatment to a focus on promotion, prevention and early intervention. This calls for a greater emphasis on treating the person in a holistic way and not just the illness. However, the reorientation of health services requires service providers to adopt new thinking and refined skills and attitudes (Borg & Kristiansen 2004). The move towards recovery-focussed care is an example of service reorientation. The recovery journey recognises the critical role of the patient and their 'lived experience' in securing their recovery. Mental health staff are having to replace the traditional approach of 'doing to' the patient with 'doing with' the patient.

There is considerable scope for promoting mental health within mental health services. Working with communities to improve mental health literacy, reducing self-harm and promoting a recovery orientation are examples of useful initiatives. Mental health services can also play a greater role in reducing stigma and promoting a more positive attitude to mental illness. Indeed, those who work in the mental health field have an important role to play in engaging other service providers (child welfare, disability services, housing, education and law enforcement) and promoting initiatives that impact positively on mental health (Herrman 2001).

CRITICAL THINKING CHALLENGE 21.3

1. Identify one thing you could do in your service/hospital to promote better health for patients in your care.
2. What factors prevent or hinder nurses from adopting a stronger focus on health promotion?

MENTAL ILLNESS PREVENTION

While mental health promotion aims to build capacity and resilience in individuals and communities, mental illness prevention aims to decrease the extent and severity of mental illness by reducing risk factors and enhancing protective factors. It can be difficult in practice to identify whether a programme centres on promotion, prevention or early intervention, as initiatives and programmes frequently include some elements of all three. Indeed, illness prevention frequently employs health promotion activities to secure positive outcomes for individuals and communities. The WHO defines the distinction between health promotion and illness prevention as follows:

> *Mental health promotion aims to promote positive mental health by increasing psychological wellbeing, competence and resilience, and by creating supportive living conditions and environments. Mental disorder prevention has as its target the reduction of symptoms and ultimately of mental disorders. It uses mental health promotion strategies as one of the means to achieve these goals (WHO 2004, p. 7).*

Prevention in the mental health context has emerged from the successful implementation of preventive interventions in the field of infectious diseases. The principles of illness prevention have now been expanded to include noninfectious and more chronic conditions. The overall aim of prevention in the mental health context is to reduce the number of new people diagnosed with mental illness (incidence) as well as the number of people already diagnosed with mental illness (prevalence). In keeping with mental health promotion initiatives, prevention interventions are relevant to people at all levels regardless of their mental health status. Illness prevention interventions can occur at different stages in the illness process and are frequently classified on a continuum from primary (before the onset of illness), to secondary (during an episode of illness) and tertiary (following an episode of illness) (Mrazek & Haggerty 1994, p. 23) (see Table 21.3).

TABLE 21.3 Illness Prevention at the Different Stages of Illness Development

Stage	Intervention
Primary prevention	Designed to prevent the number of new cases with a mental disorder (incidence). Interventions can target the whole community (universal), at-risk groups (selected) and individuals at very high risk or already presenting with early indications of mental illness (indicated). These three categories (universal, selective and indicated) underscore the concept of 'primary prevention' as described by Caplan (1964). Working with schools to reduce bullying is an example of primary prevention.
Secondary prevention	Designed to reduce the number of existing cases (prevalence) through early intervention and effective treatment. Secondary prevention strategies can be applied throughout the lifespan from childhood to old age. Intervening early in the treatment of people diagnosed with psychosis is an example of secondary prevention.
Tertiary prevention	Tertiary prevention targets the burden of illness on an individual's life and overall functioning. The aim is to reduce the impact of mental illness through rehabilitation and relapse prevention strategies. An example is teaching life skills to people with schizophrenia to prevent homelessness.

(*Source:* Adapted from Mrazek, P., Haggerty, R., 1994. Reducing Risks for Mental Disorders: Frontiers for Preventative Intervention Research. National Academies Press, Washington, DC, p. 23.)

The underlying assumption of health prevention is early intervention in order to prevent the development of a given condition or reduce its impact. One of the difficulties with this public health approach in the mental health field is the difficulty in recognising the onset of illness. The progression of mental disorders such as schizophrenia from a state of being symptom free to being symptomatic is not always linear or obvious (Herrman 2001). As a consequence, it can be difficult to implement early intervention strategies. Nonetheless, there is now evidence to suggest that many mental, emotional and behavioural problems can be prevented before they take hold (Beardslee et al. 2011). Even when a disorder has developed, preventive strategies are likely to reduce its severity, duration and associated disability (Saxena et al. 2006).

The NHS, social care, public health and third sector organisations are increasingly seeking to take a more joined up approach to achieve the much needed improvements in mental healthcare, promotion and prevention. A statement of intent has been set out in the Prevention Concordat for Better Mental Health, which aims to support the key agencies in achieving this goal, complementing the Mental Health and Wellbeing Joint Strategic Needs Assessment (JSNA) Toolkit (Selbie 2017).

CRITICAL THINKING CHALLENGE 21.4

The 2016 Five Year Forward View on Mental Health sets out the goal to reduce suicide by 10% by 2020/21.

1. Do you think 10% is a reasonable goal?
2. In the future, more people are likely to use web-based applications to treat their stress, anxiety and depression. What are some of the advantages and disadvantages of this approach?

Early Intervention

In the mental health field, early intervention is frequently discussed alongside promotion and prevention. While the aims of promotion, prevention and early intervention are different, there are many similarities. For example, providing early treatment for a person with psychosis (early intervention) may prevent the development of a more chronic form of the disorder (prevention). Early intervention strategies are designed to reduce the duration and disability associated with a mental health condition (National Institute for Health and Care Excellence [NICE] 2016). In so doing, the aim is to reduce the duration of untreated psychosis (DUP) because the longer a person remains untreated, the greater the risk they will strain support networks and drop out of school or work (Yung 2012). There is also evidence to indicate that longer periods of untreated illness lead to poorer outcomes in terms of symptoms and later functioning (Castle 2012).

Early intervention has more of an individual rather than a community focus. The key to early intervention is intervening in supportive and sensitive ways so as to reduce the risk of negative outcomes such as helplessness, isolation and stigma (McGorry et al. 2006). However, mental health workers and indeed the broader workforce (such as police, teachers and employers) are likely to require training to identify, refer and/or treat people presenting with the early symptoms of mental illness. Early intervention in psychosis teams were introduced across the UK in 1999 by the National Service Framework, now standard care as recommended by NICE guidelines (2016). There is relatively little evidence from randomised controlled trials in the UK, which is not surprising given that early intervention is now standard care. However, there have been some UK studies conducted (Neale & Kinnair 2017), for example the Lambeth Early Onset (LEO) trial (Craig et al. 2004) and the subsequent Lambeth Early Onset Crisis Assessment Team study (LEO-CAT) (Power et al. 2007). An example of the work by the early intervention services can be seen in Box 21.1.

RECOVERY

Despite advances in treatment and the focus on early intervention over the past 20 years, the outcomes for those developing psychotic conditions remain poor (McGrath 2012). Saha et al. (2008) concluded from a systematic review of the

BOX 21.1 Overview of the Early Intervention in Psychosis (EIP) Services

EIP services provide an integrated service designed to meet the needs of young adults in the early stages of psychotic illness. There is local variation between teams regarding the age range of acceptance into EIP services. The National Institute for Health and Care Excellence (NICE) recommends that early intervention services should be open to people of all ages; however, usually services are offered to people under the age of 35 years (Rethink 2017). The services provided aid in the early identification and treatment of psychosis. This helps reduce the duration of untreated psychosis (DUP) and disruption to the functioning and ongoing development of the individual. In the absence of early treatment, the illness can intensify to a level where it interferes with the young person's ability to cope with life. The danger is that related problems such as substance abuse, unemployment and behavioural problems may develop and thus complicate treatment efforts. Aims of EIP services are to:

- explore the possible causes of psychotic symptoms and treat them
- educate the young person and their family about the illness
- reduce disruption in a young person's life caused by the illness
- support the young person and their carers through the recovery process
- restore normal developmental trajectory and psychosocial functioning
- reduce the young person's chances of having another psychotic experience

Patients receive ongoing treatment for up to 2 years by a team of qualified nurses, medical staff, clinical psychologists, occupational therapists and social workers. People experiencing a first episode psychosis should have access to an EIP service within 2 weeks of referral. A target has been set by the Five Year Forward View for Mental Health in England for 60% of people meeting this criteria to be seen by EIP within 2 weeks by 2020/21 (Mental Health Taskforce 2016).

literature that the annual recovery rate from schizophrenia was only 1.4%. This implies that for every 100 people diagnosed with schizophrenia, only one or two people per year will meet criteria for recovery (McGrath 2012). Consequently, a large majority of those with psychotic conditions such as schizophrenia will require support and treatment for protracted periods of time, possibly throughout their lives. Until interventions to successfully treat psychosis can be found, the concept of recovery will continue to offer hope and provide new meaning for those with mental illness.

'Recovery' as it applies to mental health is discussed in other sections of this book. It is revisited here to briefly highlight how the process is closely aligned to promotion, prevention and early intervention. The concept of recovery emerged more than 20 years ago in the United States (Anthony 1993) from the experience of people with mental illness who had overcome some, if not all, of their difficulties to lead rewarding and productive lives. These accounts suggest that recovery involves a process whereby the individual develops a new approach to life, 'taking responsibility for one's illness, renewing a sense of hope, being involved in meaningful activities, managing symptoms, overcoming stigma, and being supported by others' (Meehan et al. 2008, p. 178). As such, recovery suggests that while people with mental illness may continue to have struggles with their symptoms and disability, they are capable of achieving greater self-confidence and control over their lives (Meehan et al. 2008). This ability to bounce back and control important aspects of one's life are integral to mental health promotion and prevention efforts (Barry & Jenkins 2007).

Anthony (1993) was one of the founding fathers of the recovery movement in the United States. He suggests that mental health interventions across the lifespan must be guided by recovery-oriented practice. In providing health services, mental health nurses and other providers are urged to consider the uniqueness of the individual and how best to meet their needs. This requires the service provider to reach a balance between doing too little and doing too much for the patient. All service providers (mental health, housing, rehabilitation, etc.) must maintain a positive attitude towards the patient and believe that they can and will recover.

Similar strategies underpin recovery strategies in the UK where service providers are encouraged to use informed decisions and patient-centred practices.

? CRITICAL THINKING CHALLENGE 21.5

1. Reflect on your own interactions with patients: are they truly recovery oriented?
2. Do patients in your service have 'real' choices?
3. What factors operating within your service facilitate and/or hinder recovery-based practice?

PRIMARY MENTAL HEALTHCARE

As previously discussed within this book, relatively recent years have seen a reduction in hospital-based services, and resources have been redirected at community-based alternative options for people with mental illness. The focus has shifted more towards treating and supporting people in their communities rather than in hospitals, with 9 out of 10 adults with a mental health problem being supported in primary care (Mental Health Taskforce 2016). Around one in three GP appointments involves a mental health component and people with physical long-term conditions are two to three times more likely to experience mental health problems than the general population (Farmer 2017; Mental Health Taskforce 2016). It has been recognised for some time that there are strong links between long-term conditions and mental health, with it shown that innovative forms of liaison psychiatry have demonstrated that providing better support for comorbid mental health needs can reduce physical healthcare costs (Naylor et al. 2012).

Primary mental healthcare refers to mental health services and support networks that are embedded into primary care services, such as GP practices, community pharmacists, health visitors, occupational therapy, counselling services and the Improving Access to Psychological Therapy (IAPT) services (Funk & Ivbijaro 2008). The role of the primary healthcare sector across the UK has acquired a new importance as a key provider of physical and mental healthcare for people with mental illness. The GP remains the first point of contact for many of those with mental health problems and The Five Year Forward View for Mental Health sets out the NHS-funded plans to recruit up to 4500 new mental health therapists, 3000 of which are to be integrated into primary care settings. These therapists will deliver evidence-based treatment to support people with mental health problems, including those with long-term physical health conditions (Mental Health Taskforce 2016).

It should be noted that while many more people are receiving treatment through the primary care sector, those requiring specialist care for more severe problems continue to access secondary and tertiary services. Secondary services include those provided through acute inpatient units and hospitals, while tertiary services include community and residential rehabilitation programmes.

Integrating Mental Health Services Into the Primary Healthcare Sector

Mental and physical health problems are interwoven, with evidence showing that there are multidirectional links between mental and physical health and illness. Thoughts, feelings and health behaviour have a significant impact on physical health, with physical health conversely influencing mental health and wellbeing (Funk & Ivbijaro 2008). People with mental illness frequently present with comorbid physical health problems in addition to a range of social and functional difficulties. There are significant benefits from integrating mental health services into the broader primary care sector. GPs are in an ideal position to recognise not only physical health problems but also mental health problems (Andrews 2006). Services provided by the primary care sector tend to be accessible and more acceptable as they are less stigmatising and provide a 'one-stop shop' for those with complex health problems

TABLE 21.4 Advantages of Providing Mental Health Services Through Primary Healthcare	
Reduced stigma	Primary health providers are not associated with any particular condition, unlike community mental health centres. As a result, people with mental illness feel less stigmatised when they seek treatment from a primary health provider such as a GP.
Improved access to treatment	People with mental illness are likely to present with a range of physical health problems. GPs are well placed to treat physical health conditions and refer patients to specialised mental health providers for mental health problems.
Improved prevention	Providing GPs (and other primary health workers, such as school nurses) with mental health skills enables them to detect and intervene early to prevent or reduce the impact of mental illness.
Treatment is more acceptable and more accessible	Many people with mental health problems find it difficult to access treatment. Providing treatment through GPs and Urgent Care Centres enables accessibility to treatment 24 hours a day, 7 days a week, with GPs increasingly expanding their opening hours and offering more walk-in services.
Reduced burden placed on patients	There is considerable disruption to life, employment, education and family when patients have to travel long distances to access treatment. Providing mental health treatment through primary care reduces this burden.
Better outcomes	There is some evidence to suggest that the outcomes for those with common mental disorders are better when these conditions are treated in primary rather than secondary care (i.e. hospital).
Reduced burden placed on mental health services	Community mental health services in most countries are under-resourced. Having GPs and other primary care providers treat a large proportion of people with common disorders reduces the burden placed on mental health services.

(*Source:* World Health Organization and World Organization of Family Doctors (Wonca), 2008. Integrating Mental Health Into Primary Care: a Global Perspective. WHO, Geneva.)

(see Table 21.4). Meehan and Robertson (2013) found that mental health patients felt more satisfied and more willing to receive care for mental health problems from a GP clinic than a community mental health centre. Attention to physical health problems is important given that people with mental illness are likely to die 15 to 20 years younger from physical health complications induced through poor lifestyle and prolonged use of psychiatric medications (Lawrence et al. 2013; Mental Health Taskforce 2016).

Primary healthcare across the UK is increasingly being provided through a range of agencies including the NHS, private and some third sector organisations. In addition, the British Medical Association (BMA 2018) reports that NHS spending on non-NHS and independent sector provision (ISP) is growing each year, with the Department of Health budget spent on ISPs also increasing, calling for increasing transparency in the level of private provision of NHS services.

NHS England has committed to the recommendations in the Five Year Forward View for Mental Health, to transform mental health services through increasing people's access to psychological therapies for common mental health issues such as depression and anxiety. In 2015–16, 1.4 million referrals were made to IAPT services. The goal is to increase the number of people accessing IAPT services each year until 2020/21 until the programme reaches an additional 600,000 people per year thereafter. The vision is to give to mental health equal importance to physical health, to achieve the ambition of parity of esteem between mental and physical health (Mental Health Taskforce 2016) is also reinforced in the General Practice Forward View (NHS England 2016). The IAPT programme began in 2008, transforming the treatment of adult anxiety and depression in England. The programme has had high levels of success in supporting people to move forward with their lives, including returning to work and meaningful occupation of their time. Psychological therapy has been shown to improve outcomes for people experiencing a range of long-term conditions, including chronic obstructive pulmonary disorder (COPD) and diabetes (NHS England 2018). There is also strong evidence to support the use of therapies in addressing medically unexplained symptoms (MUS), which account for up to a fifth of GP consultations (Royal College of General Practitioners & Royal College of Psychiatrists 2011). See Box 21.2 for an example of what characterises an IAPT service.

People with mental illness, especially those with severe mental illness, are likely to require support services in addition to mental health services. Support services frequently include assistance with everyday living, securing a home, finding a job and managing personal care. Stable employment and housing are both factors that contribute to a person's ability to maintain good mental health and are important factors in their recovery when they have experienced mental ill health. Between 60% and 70% of people who experience common mental health problems are in employment; however, not many employees have access to specialist occupational health services. People with mental health problems are overrepresented in high turnover, low paid and often temporary or part-time work and the employment rate is unacceptably low—43% of all people with mental health problems are in employment. The Five Year Forward View for Mental Health states that employment is vital to health and calls for that to change, aiming for 29,000 more people each year to be supported to find or stay in work by 2020/21, with this increase supported by the improvement in access to IAPT services and doubling of access to Individual Placement and Support (IPS) programmes. The Work and Health Programme should prioritise investment in health-led interventions that are proven to work for people with mental health problems, creating healthy communities. Housing has also been identified as critical in the recovery and prevention of mental ill health (Mental Health Taskforce 2016).

BOX 21.2 What Characterises an Improving Access to Psychological Therapies (IAPT) Service

IAPT services are characterised by three things:

1. Evidence-based psychological therapies: delivered by fully trained, accredited practitioners. The intensity and duration of therapy is matched to the mental health problem and designed to optimise outcomes. Commissioning groups have been required to offer IAPT services that are integrated with physical care pathways since April 2018. Guidance is provided for the IAPT Pathway for People with Long-term Physical Health Conditions and Medically Unexplained Symptoms (NHS England and NHS Improvement 2018).
2. Routine outcome monitoring: ensuring that the person receiving the therapy and the clinician are both up to date with the progress the individual is making, supporting the development of a positive and shared approach to the goals of the sessions. Anonymised data is published to promote transparency in service performance and encourage service improvement.
3. Regular and outcomes-focussed supervision: ensuring that practitioners are continuously supported by to improve their practice and deliver the highest quality patient care.

(Adapted from: National Health Service England (NHS) England 2018 Adult Improving Access to Psychological Therapies programme Available at: https://www.england.nhs.uk/mental-health/adults/iapt).

Integrating Mental Health Into Primary Healthcare: What is Required?

Bywood et al. (2015) have revisited the 10 principles produced by WHO and Wonca (2008) that describe the factors that should be considered when integrating mental health and primary healthcare (see Box 21.3). These principles highlight the complexities of integrating mental health into the broader primary care sector. They promote the need for clear policy directions, training for staff, the development of positive attitudes towards people with mental illness, the need for collaboration across a number of agencies and the ability of providers to respond to people with complex mental health, social and physical health needs.

GPs treat people with a broad range of mental health problems. These tend to vary in terms of severity and level of disability. Nonetheless, Bower and Gilbody (2005) have categorised the mental health conditions commonly seen by GPs into four levels, ranging from severe mental disorders such as psychotic disorders (level 1) through to less severe disorders that tend to resolve spontaneously with support (level 4); see Table 21.5. However, GPs can treat only a proportion of the morbidity associated with mental illness given the time and resources available to them (Balestrieri 2013). Therefore, many people who consult a GP with a mental health problem are likely to be referred to psychologists and psychiatrists for specialist psychological treatment and support.

Children and young people are also a priority group for mental health promotion and prevention initiatives. One of the priority actions laid out in the Five Year Forward View for Mental Health is 'Prevention at key moments in life' and calls for the recommendations from the Future in Mind (Mental Health Taskforce 2016) to be fully implemented, creating a whole system approach that builds capacity and capability across the systems. A goal has been set for at least 70,000 more children and young people to have access to high-quality mental healthcare when they need it by 2020/21. This includes the complete roll out of Children and Young People's Improving Access to Psychological Therapies (CYP IAPT) programme across England. In order to achieve this change in the way fundamental health services are

BOX 21.3 Principles for Integrating Mental Health Into Primary Care

1. Policy and plans need to include primary care for mental health issues.
2. Advocacy is required to shift attitudes and behaviour so that both mental health and primary health sectors can work successfully together.
3. Adequate training of primary care workers is required to recognise and treat mental health conditions.
4. Primary care tasks must be limited and feasible to provide in the primary setting.
5. Health professionals and facilities must be available to support primary care.
6. Patients must have access to essential psychotropic medications in primary care.
7. Integration is a process, not an event—it takes time to secure true integration.
8. A mental health service coordinator is crucial to act as a 'bridge' between primary and mental health services.
9. Collaboration with other government non-health sectors, non-governmental organisations, community health workers and volunteers is required to ensure a holistic approach to service provision.
10. Financial and human resources are needed to support the establishment of new service models. In general, new funding is required to establish new services.

(*Source:* World Health Organization and World Organization of Family Doctors (Wonca), 2008. Integrating Mental Health Into Primary Care: a Global Perspective. WHO, Geneva, p. 34.)

TABLE 21.5 Classification of Mental Health Conditions Treated by GPs

Level	Description
1	Severe mental disorders, such as schizophrenia, bipolar and organic disorders that are associated with severe disability. These will involve input from both primary and secondary care.
2	Disorders such as anxious depression, pure depression, generalised anxiety, panic disorder and obsessive-compulsive disorder for which there are effective treatments. These can usually be managed in primary care.
3	Disorders (phobias, somatic distress, chronic fatigue) in which psychiatric medications have a more limited impact, but for which psychological therapies are available.
4	Disorders such as bereavement and adjustment disorder that tend to resolve spontaneously with support.

(*Source:* Adapted from Bower, P., Gilbody, S., 2005. Managing common mental disorders in primary care: conceptual models and evidence base. British Medical Journal. 330, 839–842.)

commissioned is required, placing greater emphasis on prevention and early identification (Mental Health Taskforce 2016).

The growing demand for mental health services is likely to create more opportunities and a greater role for mental health nurses in the delivery of care in the primary setting. Mental health nurses working alongside GPs in primary care have already demonstrated their ability to bring about significant improvements for people with severe mental illness (Meehan & Robertson 2015). Hardy and Kingsnorth (2015) demonstrated how mental health nurses were able to increase capability and capacity in primary care by educating practice nurses about mental health issues. Another example demonstrates how a mental health nurse was able to successfully coordinate, as a clinical lead, a range of clinical, housing and support providers. The aim of the project was to offer an integrated approach to reducing homelessness among people with mental illness (Prout 2015). Finally, in the United States, Trehearne et al. (2014) showed that a nurse-led collaborative care programme could be applied within primary settings for patients with complex healthcare needs and multiple comorbidities. The authors concluded:

> *Healthcare systems should consider a greater role for nurses within a collaborative care model to achieve improved clinical outcomes and more appropriate use of health services for patients with multi-morbidities*
> ***(Trehearne et al. 2014, p. 178).***

CRITICAL THINKING CHALLENGE 21.6

What actions can governments take now to ensure that people in need of mental health services will have access to services in 15 years' time?

CONCLUSION

The primary focus of mental health funding across the UK has traditionally been the treatment of mental health conditions rather than the promotion of wellness and the prevention of mental illness. However, over the past 20 years there has been a greater emphasis on early intervention and prevention of mental illness. This shift in focus has been driven largely by the introduction of financial incentives to prevent illness rather than treat it. Moreover, relocating resources to 'upstream' health promotion and prevention programmes is likely to reduce the growing expenditure on 'downstream' services such as expensive inpatient care.

The shift to community care for people with mental illness has brought into focus the importance of using primary healthcare models to provide services to people with mental illness. A primary healthcare approach acknowledges that the absence of mental illness does not mean the presence of mental health and wellbeing. It is now clear that the prevention and treatment of mental illness are well beyond the reach of mental health professionals and a host of other service providers such as housing, employment and education are frequently required. Primary healthcare principles applied to nursing practice facilitate a holistic patient-focussed approach in that social, political and environmental issues are taken into account and placed in the ambit of the nurse's awareness.

The successful integration of mental health with primary care will require the development of strategic partnerships across a wide range of organisations and sectors. The ongoing expansion of promotion, prevention and primary mental healthcare is likely to create new and exciting opportunities for mental health nurses.

EXERCISES FOR CLASS ENGAGEMENT

1. A study on bullying in schools by Cross et al. (2009, p. xxi) found that:

   Being bullied every few weeks or more often (considered to be frequent) overtly and/or covertly during the last term at school is a fairly common experience, affecting approximately one in four students (27%). Frequent school bullying was highest among Year 5 (32%) and Year 8 (29%) students. Hurtful teasing was the most prevalent of all bullying behaviours experienced by students, followed by having hurtful lies told about them.

   In small groups, use the internet to gain a better understanding of bullying in schools and the risk factors and protective factors associated with bullying in school-aged children. Then develop a health promotion plan to deal with bullying at a school of your choice. The plan should identify:
   - the target group for intervention (teachers, students, parents, etc.)
   - examples of health promotion interventions that may be useful
   - the type and content of potential interventions; has the increase of social media use changed these?
   - examples of anti-bullying programmes currently used across the UK (from an internet search)
   - how well your planned interventions match what is currently in place.
2. Internationally there have been significant reforms of mental health services over the past 20 years. Most traditional psychiatric hospitals have closed and people with severe mental illness are now supported to live in the community. David, a 58-year-old with schizophrenia, is one of the many people who moved to the community some years ago. He is currently living in a bedsit on a disability payments. Over the past month he has become increasingly suspicious of his neighbours. He has just been to see his GP and told her that he believes his neighbours are spying on him with special cameras. In small groups address the following issues:
   - Discuss the challenges facing someone like David living with severe mental illness in the community.
   - In addition to mental health services, what other services might David require?
   - What options are available to David's GP within primary healthcare to manage David's exacerbation of his schizophrenia?
   - You are one of the nurses working with David's local community mental health team. The GP has referred David to you for review and advice regarding his treatment. What would you suggest for David at this stage?
   - Once David's illness has settled, what actions would you take to help him to prevent future episodes of his illness?

REFERENCES

Andrews, G., 2006. Tolkien II: a Needs-Based, Costed, Stepped Care Model for Mental Health Services: Recommendations, Executive Summaries, Clinical Pathways, Treatment Flowcharts, Costing Structures. World Health Organization, Sydney.

Anthony, W., 1993. Recovery from mental illness: the guiding vision of the mental health service system in the 1990s. Psychosocial Rehabilitation Journal 16, 11–23.

Balestrieri, M., 2013. The management of mental disorders in the primary care setting. In: Thornicroft, G., Ruggeri, M., Goldberg, D. (Eds.), Improving Mental Health Care: the Global Challenge. Wiley-Blackwell, Chichester.

Barry, M., Jenkins, R., 2007. Implementing Health Promotion. Elsevier, Philadelphia.

Beardslee, W., Chien, P., Bell, C., 2011. Prevention of mental disorders, substance abuse and problem behaviours: a developmental perspective. Psychiatric Services 62, 247–254.

Borg, M., Kristiansen, K., 2004. Recovery orientated professionals: helping relationships in mental health services. Journal of Mental Health 13, 493–505.

Bower, P., Gilbody, 2005. Managing common mental disorders in primary care: conceptual models and evidence base. British Medical Journal 330, 839–842.

British Medical Association (BMA), 2018. Hidden figures: private care in the English NHS. Available at: https://www.bma.org.uk/collective-voice/influence/key-negotiations/nhs-funding/privatisation-report. Accessed: 23 November 2018.

Bywood, P., Brown, L., Raven, M., 2015. Improving the Integration of Mental Health Services in Primary Health Care at the Macro Level. PHCRIS Policy Issue Review. Primary Health Care Research and Information Service, Adelaide.

Castle, D., 2012. The truth, and nothing but the truth, about early intervention in psychosis. Australian and New Zealand Journal of Psychiatry 46, 10–13.

Caplan, G., 1964. Principles of Preventive Psychiatry. Basic Books, New York.

Craig, T., Garety, P., Power, P., Rahaman, N., Colbert, S., Fornells-Ambrojo, M., Dunn, G., 2004. The Lambeth Early Onset (LEO) Team: randomised controlled trial of the effectiveness of specialised care for early psychosis. BMJ 329 (7474), 1067–1070.

Cross, D., Shaw, T., Hearn, L., Epstein, M., Monks, H., Lester, L., Thomas, L., 2009. Australian Covert Bullying Prevalence Study (ACBPS). Child Health Promotion Research Centre. Edith Cowan University, Perth.

Farmer, P., 2017. Mind: Working with Primary Care to Deliver the Five Year Forward View for Mental Health. Available at: https://www.kingsfund.org.uk/sites/default/files/media/Paul_Farmer.pdf. Accessed: 23 November 2018.

Funk, M., Ivbijaro, G., 2008. Integrating Mental Health into Primary Care: A Global Perspective. World Health Organization/WONCA (World Organization of Family Doctors), Geneva.

Hardy, S., Kingsnorth, R., 2015. Mental health nurses can increase capability and capacity in primary care by educating practice nurses: an evaluation of an education programme in England. Journal of Psychiatric and Mental Health Nursing 22, 270–277.

Herrman, H., 2001. The need for mental health promotion. Australian and New Zealand Journal of Psychiatry 35, 709–715.

Jané-Llopis, E., Barry, M., Horsman, C., et al., 2005. Mental health promotion works: a review. Promotion and Education Supplement 2, 9–25.

Keleher, H., Armstrong, R., 2006. Evidence-Based Mental Health Promotion Resource. Department of Human Services, Melbourne.

Knapp, M., McDaid, D., Parsonage, T., 2011. Mental Health Promotion and Mental Illness Prevention: the Economic Case. Department of Health, London.

Lawrence, D., Hancock, K., Kisley, S., 2013. The gap in life expectancy from preventable physical illness in psychiatric patients in Western Australia: retrospective analysis of population-based registers. British Medical Journal 346, 2539.

McGorry, P., Hickie, I., Yung, A., et al., 2006. Clinical staging of psychiatric disorders: a heuristic framework for choosing earlier, safer and more effective interventions. Australian and New Zealand Journal of Psychiatry 40, 616–622.

McGrath, J., 2012. The early intervention debate. Australian and New Zealand Journal of Psychiatry 46, 681–682.

Meehan, T., King, R., Robinson, J., et al., 2008. Recovery-based practice: do we know what we mean or mean what we know? Australian and New Zealand Journal of Psychiatry 42, 177–182.

Meehan, T., Robertson, S., 2013. The Mental Health Nurse Incentive Program: perceptions of GPs and their patients. Australian Health Review 37 (3), 337–340.

Meehan, T., Robertson, S., 2015. Impact of the Mental Health Nurse Incentive Program on patient functioning. International Journal of Mental Health Nursing 24, 75–78.

Mental Health Taskforce, 2016. The Five Year Forward View for Mental Health. Available at: https://www.england.nhs.uk/wp-content/uploads/2016/02/Mental-Health-Taskforce-FYFV-final.pdf. Accessed: 21 November 2018.

Mrazek, P., Haggerty, R., 1994. Reducing risks for mental disorders: frontiers for preventative intervention research. National Academies Press, Washington, DC.

National Health Service (NHS) England, 2016. General Practice Forward View. Available at: https://www.england.nhs.uk/wp-content/uploads/2016/04/gpfv.pdf. Accessed: 25 November 2018.

National Health Service England (NHS) England, 2018. Integrating Mental Health Therapy into Primary Care. Available at: https://www.england.nhs.uk/mental-health/adults/iapt/integrating-mental-health-therapy-into-primary-care/. Accessed: 25 November 2018.

National Health Service (NHS) England and NHS Improvement, 2018. The IAPT Pathway for People with Long-term Physical Health Conditions and Medically Unexplained Symptoms Guidance is Intended to Help with Implementation and sets out the Ideal Pathway for IAPT Services. Available at: https://www.england.nhs.uk/wp-content/uploads/2018/03/improving-access-to-psychological-therapies-long-term-conditions-pathway.pdf. Accessed: 25 November 2018.

National Institute for Health and Care Excellence, 2016. Implementing the Early Intervention in Psychosis Access and Waiting Time Standard: Guidance. Available at: https://www.england.nhs.uk/mentalhealth/wp-content/uploads/sites/29/2016/04/eip-guidance.pdf. Accessed: 23 November 2018.

Naylor, C., Parsonage, M., McDaid, D., Knapp, M., Fossey, M., Galea, A., 2012. Long-Term Conditions and Mental Health: The Cost of Co-Morbidities. Available at: https://www.kingsfund.org.uk/sites/default/files/field/field_publication_file/long-term-conditions-mental-health-cost-comorbidities-naylor-feb12.pdf. Accessed: 23 November 2018.

Neale, A., Kinnair, D., 2017. Early intervention in psychosis services. British Journal of General Practice 67 (661), 370–371.

Power, P., Iacoponi, E., Reynolds, N., Fisher, H., 2007. The Lambeth Early Onset Crisis Assessment Team Study: general practitioner education and access to an early detection team in first-episode psychosis. British Journal of Psychiatry 191 (51), 133–139.

Prout, D., 2015. Mental Health Nurses Can Play a Key Role as a Clinical Lead in Partnership Projects. Australian College of Mental Health Nurses Inc., Canberra.

Resnick, M.D., Bearman, P., Blum, R.W., et al., 1997. Protecting adolescents from harm: findings from the National Longitudinal Study of Adolescent Health. Journal of the American Medical Association 278, 823–832.

Rethink Mental Illness, 2017. Early intervention. Available at: https://www.rethink.org/diagnosis-treatment/treatment-and-support/early-intervention-teams. Accessed: 23 November 2018.

Royal College of General Practitioners and Royal College of Psychiatrists, 2011. Forum for Mental Health in Primary Care: Guidance for Health Professionals on Medically Unexplained Symptoms (MUS). Available at: www.rcgp.org.uk. Accessed: 25 November 2018.

Saha, S., Barendregt, J., Vos, T., et al., 2008. Modelling disease frequency measures in schizophrenia epidemiology. Schizophrenia Research 104, 246–254.

Sanders, M., 2008. Triple P: positive parenting program as a public health approach to strengthen parenting. Journal of Family Psychology 22, 516–517.

Saxena, S., Jané-Llopis, Horsman, C., 2006. Prevention of mental health and behavioural disorders: implications for policy and practice. World Psychiatry 5 (1), 5–14.

Selbie, D., 2017. Public Health Matters: Moving Forward with The Prevention of Mental Health Problems. Available at: https://publichealthmatters.blog.gov.uk/2017/08/30/moving-forward-with-the-prevention-of-mental-health-problems/. Accessed: 21 November 2018.

Shaffer, A., Yates, T., 2010. Identifying and understanding risk factors and protective factors in clinical practice. In: Compton (Ed.), Clinical Manual of Prevention in Mental Health. American Psychiatric Publishing, Washington, pp. 29–48.

Trehearne, B., Fishman, P., Lin, E., 2014. Role of the nurse in chronic illness management: making the medical home more effective. Nursing Economics 32 (4), 178–184.

UK Government, 2017. NEWS STORY: New £15 Million Programme to Help Train One Million in Mental Health First Aid. Available at: https://www.gov.uk/government/news/new-15-million-programme-to-help-train-mental-health-first-aiders. Accessed: 21 November 2018.

World Health Organization (WHO), 1986. Ottawa Charter for Health Promotion. WHO, Geneva.

World Health Organization (WHO), 2004. Prevention of Mental Disorders. WHO, Geneva.

World Health Organization (WHO), 2012. Depression: a Global Crisis. WHO, Geneva. Available at: www.who.int/mental_health/management/depression/wfmh_paper_depression_wmhd_2012.pdf. Accessed: 10 August 2015.

World Health Organization (WHO), 2015. Metrics: Disability-Adjusted Life Year (DALY). Available at: www.who.int/healthinfo/global_burden_disease/metrics_daly/en.

World Health Organization and World Organization of Family Doctors (Wonca), 2008. Integrating Mental Health into Primary Care: a Global Perspective. WHO, Geneva.

World Health Organisation (WHO), 2018. Mental Health: Mental Disorders. Available at: http://www.who.int/mental_health/management/en/. Accessed: 21 November 2018.

Yung, A., 2012. Early intervention in psychosis: evidence, evidence gaps, criticism, and confusion. Australian and New Zealand Journal of Psychiatry 46, 7–9.

USEFUL WEBSITES

Headspace, www.headspace.com

Mental Health First, Aid England, www.mhfaengland.org

Royal College of Psychiatrists, 2018. Standards for Early Intervention in Psychosis Services, first ed, www.rcpsych.ac.uk/docs/default-source/improving-care/ccqi/quality-networks/early-intervention-in-psychosis-teams-(eipn)/epin-standards-first-edition.pdf?sfvrsn=fd9b4a0f_2

SANE, www.sane.org.uk

St John Ambulance, www.sja.org.uk (Mental Health First Aid courses)

22

Assessment in Mental Health Nursing

Anthony O'Brien, Mandy Allman

KEY POINTS

- Assessment is the first step of the nursing process and is ongoing throughout each episode of care.
- The purpose of mental health nursing assessment is to understand the mental health problems the person is experiencing and what nurses can do to help.
- Comprehensive assessment involves gathering information about multiple domains of the person's life.
- Mental health nursing assessment can involve both conversational and structured interviews, in addition to nursing observation and information from third parties.
- Standardised assessment instruments can assist in the process of assessment and in evaluating changes in patients' clinical presentation.
- Risk assessment involves weighing up static and dynamic risk factors within the context of the person's current presentation and clinical history.
- Clinical formulation is the process of developing, with the patient, a summary of the various influences on the patient's current problems, and how the patient and clinician can work towards resolving those problems.
- Physical health assessment is an integral component of assessment in mental health nursing.
- Psychiatric diagnoses are assigned using either the DSM-5 or the ICD-10 diagnostic systems. A version of the ICD-11 was released in June 2018, to allow Member States to prepare for implementation, with a view to reporting using ICD-11 from 1st January 2022.

KEY TERMS

assessment
clinical formulation
cultural assessment
diagnosis
differential diagnosis
documentation
DSM-5
ICD-10 and the planned version ICD-11 MMS
interviewing
mental health outcome measures
mental state assessment
narrative
physical assessment
risk assessment
screening
spiritual assessment
standardised assessment
strengths assessment
triage

LEARNING OUTCOMES

The material in this chapter will assist you to:

- understand the purpose and process of mental health nursing assessment.
- outline narrative and descriptive approaches to mental health nursing assessment.
- explain the contribution and limitations of standardised assessment instruments in the assessment process.
- discuss the place of physical health assessment within comprehensive mental health nursing assessment.
- conduct and document a mental state assessment.
- utilise a model of comprehensive mental health nursing assessment in clinical practice.
- discuss the place of risk assessment in clinical practice.
- identify the two major systems of classification of mental disorders.
- discuss the relationship between assessment and clinical decision making.
- describe the use of outcome measures in mental healthcare.

INTRODUCTION

Assessment is one of the most important and fundamental skills of the mental health nurse. Through assessment, we develop an understanding of patients, formulate a plan of care and contribute to the decision making of multidisciplinary teams. Assessment also tells us about the effectiveness and acceptability of mental health nursing care. A comprehensive assessment encompasses multiple aspects of patients' lives, including current and past mental health problems, family and social history, use of alcohol and other drugs, physical health and cultural and spiritual influences on mental health. Assessment focusses on problems in the patient's life, as well as the strengths and capabilities available to the patient to respond to those problems. As the patient's recovery progresses, assessment will reflect the developing understanding between the nurse and the patient, new issues in response to treatment and the patient's development of new coping skills and strategies.

Assessment is the first step of the nursing process (DeWit & O'Neill 2014) and is ongoing over the time a patient is engaged with mental healthcare. Initial assessment occurs when the patient first accesses a mental health service and has the aim of developing a shared understanding of what problems the person seeks help with, their strengths and resources, and what the mental health service can do to assist with those problems. As the nurse and the patient develop their relationship, and as initial problems are resolved, the shared understanding of the goals of care will change. Ongoing assessment helps review goals, redefine problems and strengths and develop new strategies to assist in the patient's recovery.

This chapter outlines the process of mental health nursing assessment. Assessment is explained as both a structured process in which the nurse seeks to apply professional frameworks of understanding and as an exploratory process in which the nurse and the patient review their understandings of the nature of the patient's problems and the care and treatment the patient is receiving. The aim is always one of clarifying the shared understanding that provides the basis of nursing care.

The chapter also introduces current models of assessment and the various skills of mental health nursing assessment such as taking a history, assessing mental state, using standardised assessment instruments, clinical formulation and diagnosis. As much as possible the chapter is organised to follow the standard process of psychiatric assessment, from recording the presenting problem through to formulation of a plan of care.

ASSESSMENT

Assessment is fundamental to mental health nursing and provides the platform on which nursing care is delivered (Coombs et al. 2011; National Institute of Health and Care Excellence [NICE] 2011). Nurses are the single largest group of professionals in mental healthcare and are well positioned throughout the continuum of care to make significant contributions to care delivery. Nursing assessment is carried out in a variety of settings, throughout each episode of care and at key transition points, such as discharge and admission. Assessment makes a significant contribution to diagnosis and treatment planning. Mental health nursing assessment adds to the decisions regarding care delivery carried out by nurses and other members of the multidisciplinary team. As such, nursing assessment is both an independent activity and interdependent with the treating team.

Despite the potential strengths of mental health nursing assessment there is a lack of clarity over what this actually entails in practice (Coombs et al. 2013a). Barker (2004) said that 'it is difficult to say anything concrete about psychiatric nursing assessment except to say that it is in its infancy and is often gravely misunderstood'. The published research literature does little to help here. There is evidence that nurses often gather assessment information in the course of other 'simple social activities' such as making a cup of tea (Coombs et al. 2013b). However, nurses also have difficulty in articulating a model of mental health nursing assessment. Nurses rely on the eclectic nature of nursing, their own intuition and a 'tacit, experiential model of assessment' (MacNeela et al. 2010, p. 1298) when assessing patients. This chapter provides a clear way through this maze and offers both a framework for mental health nursing assessment and a description of some of the key tasks of assessment.

To do a comprehensive assessment well, it is important that a recognised nursing assessment framework is used to identify presenting problems, strengths, health history and risks and to formulate goals for care. The completion of a robust comprehensive assessment requires the interplay of complex skills and ultimately leads to a sound diagnosis and care planning. Box 22.1 outlines the threads of mental health nursing assessment, threads that must be woven together by each clinical practitioner (see also Fig. 22.1).

CRITICAL THINKING CHALLENGE 22.1

Why is assessment considered fundamental to nursing practice? Why is it important to develop skills in assessment as a basis for any form of nursing intervention?

BOX 22.1 The Threads of Mental Health Nursing Assessment

Assessment comprises several main threads woven together:

- Process: the *way* information is gathered, including the therapeutic relationship, observation, rating instruments and informal/formal methods.
- Content: *what* information is gathered, such as definition of the presenting problem, mental health history, mental state, physical health review and substance use.
- Interpretation: the *meaning* ascribed to the above content that is jointly understood by the patient, the nurse and the treating team and informs treatment planning. Nursing and other theories help the nurse in the process of interpretation.
- Communication: this includes *articulation*—formulation, sharing of assessment information, presentation of assessment at handover, multidisciplinary team meetings and clinical review—and documentation, the *written record* of assessment findings.

The Scope of Comprehensive Mental Health Nursing Assessment

Comprehensive mental health nursing assessment involves establishing a therapeutic relationship and using that relationship to collect a range of information about the person in order to formulate a collaborative plan of care. Assessment is not limited to aspects of psychological or social functioning, or to psychiatric symptoms, but includes a wide range of information, such as developmental history, general health history, history of involvement with police (forensic history), cultural identity and spiritual beliefs. Because of the range of information included in a comprehensive mental health nursing assessment, such assessments are sometimes referred to as holistic or biopsychosocial assessments. Whether, in practice, assessments really live up to the ideals of being holistic or biopsychosocial depends in part on the nurse's theoretical and philosophical perspectives, and how these influence the interpretation of the information available.

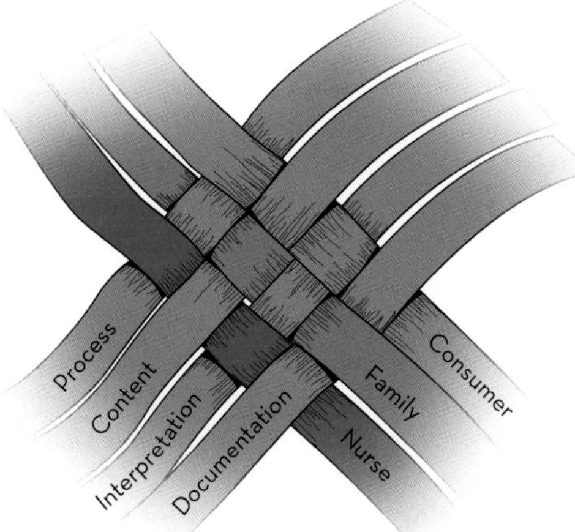

Fig. 22.1 The threads of mental health nursing assessment. (*Source:* Adapted from the Ministry of Education New Zealand, CC BY 3.0 NZ.)

While mental health nursing assessment can seem daunting, nurses can become adept over time and with experience and good professional support (see Nurse's Story 22.1). A suggestion for new graduates is to focus on developing competency in each thread of assessment. While the threads are interdependent, each also has its own skills. Focussing on individual threads will provide a transparent pathway for skill acquisition.

Professional Standards and Mental Health Nursing Assessment

In addition to being a set of clinical skills, assessment is also an obligation of mental health nurses. All mental health nurses are expected to be able to conduct a comprehensive assessment and this core skill is reflected in the Nursing and Midwifery Council (NMC 2014) standards for competence for registered nurses (of interest, new standards are due to be implemented

NURSE'S STORY 22.1 Assessment and Diagnosis From a Newly Qualified Nurse's Perspective

As a newly qualified nurse, assessment and diagnosis are utilised daily within my role as a Community Mental Health Nurse and Case Manager. This is an autonomous role where I am required to be proactive within a variety of settings, from an multidisciplinary team (MDT) meeting to liaising with third sector organisations to seek guidance and support in regards to my assigned caseload.

First and foremost, both professional and therapeutic relationships need to be established, to ensure that my assessment and nursing diagnosis is at a consistent level of professionalism to be an advocate and support person for service users on my assigned caseload.

I need to ensure that I obtain an all-encompassing view of not only the service user's mental and physical health, but also a comprehensive history and understanding of their situation. I utilise this information to assist the person on their journey to wellness, along with being able to monitor their individual progress.

On completion of my 'supernumerary' 6-week period with my preceptor I was effectively 'let loose'. Not surprisingly, around this time the enormity of 'I was now it!' struck, and I found myself doubting my ability to work within the community on my own. After in-depth discussions with my colleagues and other newly qualified graduates, I found I was not alone in feeling this way and this was considered a normal reaction. Personal acknowledgement and processing of the huge leap across a seemingly endless chasm from a final-year nursing student to registered nurse, responsible for my own caseload, was a lot to decipher.

There are a number of factors that need to be taken into account when working within the community environment, and developing the skill to identify the nuances of when patients are experiencing increased problems. I incorporate a mental state assessment within my notes, which assists in identifying specific issues in service users' presentation. No-one expects me to be an expert as a newly qualified practitioner, but I am expected to build on my core assessment skills and, as time goes on, my individual practice and professional development reflect my learning and growth.

Initially, the hardest questions I found to ask were along the lines of: 'Have you cut yourself since I saw you last?', 'Do you want to harm others?', 'Are you having thoughts of suicide?' When the answer is yes to any or all of the above, then your questioning for your assessment teases out the risk component.

As my own practice continually develops, it is apparent that a core understanding of not only the nursing process, but also a holistic health model assists to form a 'whole picture' of the person and their needs, along with input from identified key support people and agencies.

Working within a supportive environment is invaluable and this has assisted my learning and growth immensely. This is reflected in my personal growth and confidence as a Community Mental Health Nurse and Case Manager.

from 28 January 2019). In the NMC standards it is stipulated that all nurses must 'carry out comprehensive, systematic nursing assessments that take account of relevant physical, social, cultural, psychological, spiritual, genetic and environmental factors, in partnership with service users and others through interaction, observation and measurement'. The standards are applied in conjunction with The Code: Professional standards of practice and behaviour for nurses, midwives and nursing associates (NMC 2018) which has been updated in October 2018 to reflect the new responsibilities for the regulation of nursing associates.

Narrative and Descriptive Approaches to Mental Health Nursing Assessment

Mental health nursing assessment involves the use of formal and semiformal tools, as well as a range of interpersonal processes in which the nurse uses skills in therapeutic relationships to establish trust, maintain dialogue, communicate empathy and explore patients' perceptions of their problems and what will assist their recovery. It can sometimes seem that the tools of nursing assessment, such as the assessment templates provided by clinical services, dominate the assessment process due to their requirement to collect a large amount of detailed information. In addition, services usually require clinicians, often nurses, to complete risk assessment forms in which assessment information is used to establish levels of risk. Standardised assessment tools such as mood rating scales, risk scales, symptom scales and measures of cognitive functioning may appear to reduce assessment to eliciting answers to questions rather than exploring with patients the meaning of their experiences.

Mental health nursing assessment can be thought of as comprising two key tasks: collecting and interpreting assessment information (which can be assessed using standard tools and templates); and developing an understanding of each patient and their perspectives of their current situation. The *tasks* of assessment should not determine the *process* of assessment, which can include a variety of methods from conversational interviewing with its focus on the individual narrative (Brown 1995) to completion of patient—or clinician-rated assessment instruments (Barker 2004). The skilled mental health nurse combines the tasks in any assessment and is able to move between the more *descriptive* approach of seeking specific information and the *exploratory* approach of narrative enquiry. Both approaches have an important place in comprehensive assessment, and together they will yield a full understanding of each patient and contribute to the development of a therapeutic relationship.

METHODS OF MENTAL HEALTH NURSING ASSESSMENT

Mental health nursing assessment uses a range of methods including structured and conversational interviews, standardised assessment instruments, diaries, direct observation and information from third parties including friends and family and clinical records. All of these methods have a common purpose: to enhance our understanding of the person seeking mental healthcare and to help with the problems that led them to seek mental healthcare. In this section we describe the assessment methods of interviews, mnemonics, standardised assessment tools, diaries, direct observation and information from third parties.

 **CRITICAL THINKING CHALLENGE 22.2**

What methods of nursing assessment are you familiar with? How can they be used in a mental health clinical setting?

Interviews

An assessment interview can be thought of as a more or less structured conversation that has a specific goal: to elicit information about the patient and to help the nurse understand the patient's problems and develop a plan of care. While it is possible to describe a structured assessment interview as a logical series of topics—such as the presenting problem, history of mental health problems, social history and so forth—in practice assessment interviews rarely follow a prescribed course. Interviewing is a core skill of mental health nursing and requires a range of nursing skills. Interviews may be brief or lengthy, depending on the demands of the situation and on the needs of the patient. Interviews may also be formal or informal, and in practice a combination of formal and informal approaches may be necessary. Nurses need to be flexible in their approach to interviews and be ready to change their planned approach as the interview progresses. In particular, at times it may be necessary to stop an interview, for example if it proves too distressing for the patient, or if the patient is not able to concentrate on the interview process. In developing their interview skills, nurses should take opportunities to work with different colleagues from the multidisciplinary team and to observe how colleagues conduct interviews, manage the complex issues that arise and engage with patients around difficult and sensitive issues such as experiences of trauma, thoughts of self-harm and risk to self and others.

Interviews and Therapeutic Communication

Interviews should be seen as a form of nursing intervention, thus requiring all the interpersonal skills of attending, empathy, listening, reflection, paraphrasing and responding that are inherent in mental health nursing practice. In an interview the nurse is inviting the patient to share sensitive and personal information, so it is essential that the nurse approaches the interview with an attitude of respect and with a genuine interest in what the patient has to say. The nurse needs to be *available* to the patient, which means not being distracted by other commitments or obligations, and be responsive to the concerns expressed by the patient. As in any therapeutic relationship, *rapport* is essential to conducting an interview. The nurse needs to spend the initial part of the interview developing rapport and then maintain rapport as the interview progresses. Any issues of cultural or language differences need to be acknowledged as they would in any therapeutic interaction. In considering the development of interview skills, it

TABLE 22.1 Questions and Responses for Assessment Interviews

Patient Statement	Nurse's Response	Comment
I don't know where to start.	Perhaps if we begin by talking about what brought you into the (clinic/hospital/service) today?	At the commencement of the interview the patient may feel overwhelmed by the issues they are facing. A concrete question or statement can help in initiating dialogue.
I've been seeing my GP for depression, but it's not getting better.	Can you tell me more about the depression? How bad has it been?	By using the term 'depression' the nurse communicates that they are listening and are aware of the significance of the problem.
The voices are there all the time. They never leave me alone.	That sounds very difficult for you. Tell me more about the voices. What sorts of things do they say?	The nurse's responses are designed to validate the patient's experience and to encourage dialogue about the voices.
I feel so hopeless; I can't seem to do anything right.	It can feel really bad when nothing is going right for you.	This response focusses on the patient's emotional state and need to have their distress recognised.
I sometimes wish it was all over.	Are you saying that you don't want to be alive any longer?	Patients may talk indirectly about suicidal thoughts. A direct question can assist the patient to acknowledge suicidal thoughts and can be followed up with further exploration of these thoughts, including intent, available means, etc.

is helpful to review the principles of therapeutic communication outlined in Chapter 1. Some questions and responses that can be used in interviews are listed in Table 22.1.

Interview Settings

Interviews take place in a range of locations and nurses need to be able to adapt their interview skills to the setting. These settings include primary care offices, community clinics, patients' homes, emergency departments, inpatient wards, general hospital wards, courts, prisons and police stations. In planning an interview, the nurse needs to consider the safety of the patient and themselves (see later), privacy, adequate seating (especially if multiple family members are to be involved) and the availability of the interview room. Some settings, such as general hospital wards or patients' homes, may present difficulties in ensuring privacy and whenever possible an area separate from the patient's bed space should be sought. The ideal setting is a separate room that is close to other work areas and that provides adequate space and privacy.

Safety in Conducting Interviews

In arranging an interview, the nurse needs to be mindful of the patient's safety and their own. An interview can be a challenging experience for a patient, who may feel vulnerable in the presence of health professionals. Gender, ethnicity and age differences may also contribute to a patient's feeling of vulnerability. It may be advisable to invite a family member or friend to be present at the interview, although the support provided needs to be balanced against the potentially inhibiting effect on the interview process. The patient also needs to consent to the family member or friend being present, and should be asked about this in privacy so that they are able to express their preference free of any sense of obligation or coercion.

Another safety consideration is the mental state of the patient. Prior to the interview commencing the nurse will have some indication of the patient's level of distress, ability to tolerate the nurse's questions and willingness to participate in the interview. It is often advisable for a second clinician to be present, both as a means of supporting the first clinician and to respond to any difficulties that may arise. In conducting the interview, the nurse needs to continuously assess the patient's mental state and take steps if the patient becomes too distressed, including abandoning the interview. If the nurse feels threatened by the patient's attitude or behaviour (for example, the emergence of paranoid ideas or anger directed at the nurse) consideration should be given to disengaging from the interview. The nurse should always advise other team members where they will be conducting an interview and how long they expect to take. This allows colleagues to be aware of the patient and nurse's whereabouts and to be available if additional support is needed.

Managing the Interview Process

Interviews are more easily manageable if the nurse and the patient have a clear idea of the purpose and goals of the interview, the time available and the possible outcomes of the interview. Because the outcomes of an interview depend on the problems identified, their severity and the support available, outcomes should initially be stated in general terms, such as clarifying current problems and planning future care rather than, for example, deciding whether hospital admission is necessary.

Although the nurse should always have a plan for an interview, and should be clear about its purpose, the interview should begin informally. The nurse should briefly explain the purpose of the interview and provide an opportunity for the patient to make an opening statement about their current concerns. This may include discussion of any concerns the patient has about the interview, such as privacy, confidentiality, what will happen to the information collected and possible outcomes of the interview. From there, the interview can either focus on the concerns expressed by the patient or begin with background discussion that will provide a wider context for understanding the presenting issues. It is not possible to prescribe the exact order of an interview: that will very much depend on the needs of the patient at the time. The interview should begin with more general questions first and proceed to more specific questions as rapport develops and the patient's concerns become clearer. In this way the more sensitive areas of assessment can be included naturally in the interview and will seem less intrusive.

Some patients will freely discuss their concerns and may need to be provided with structure to manage issues one at a time. Others may be withdrawn or less forthcoming and may need more prompting with specific questions. The flow of the interview can be determined by the patient's responses, although the nurse does need to be aware of the need to achieve the aims of the interview. An unstructured interview that simply follows its own course, unguided by a sense of purpose, is of little use to the patient. It will not help to clarify problems or to decide an appropriate plan of care. As the interview progresses the nurse should be attentive to the verbal and nonverbal responses of the patient, and any changes in those responses as the areas of discussion change. A patient who begins with good eye contact and an open body posture may become closed, with reduced eye contact, when discussing distressing events, giving valuable clues to the intensity of the feelings involved. The nurse carries responsibility for keeping the interview 'on track' and avoiding digressions that do not help in the process of assessment. It may be necessary at some points to comment when an interview is losing focus and gently redirect the focus to the main issues.

If friends or family members are present the nurse will need to manage their participation, sometimes by encouraging comment and at other times asking that comments are limited until a more appropriate point in the interview. Interviews are designed to elicit sensitive issues from patients and it is critical that these issues are acknowledged and the patient's experience validated by the nurse. A skilled interviewer will provide opportunity to discuss important issues but will also move the interview on at some points, in order that all important aspects can be covered.

Problems in the Interview Process

With the best possible plan, and the best attempt to develop rapport, it is still possible that an interview may become 'bogged down' with limited dialogue, there may be interpersonal tension between the nurse and the patient, or the patient may have difficulty answering questions or be reluctant to discuss certain topics. There can be many reasons for problems in the interview process, and the nurse should not assume that the source of the problems is the patient. Problems may arise from cultural, age or ethnicity differences, issues of transference or countertransference (see Chapter 24), the nurse's attitude or nonverbal behaviours, as well as factors to do with the interview setting such as noise, limited time and an uncongenial environment. As in any therapeutic interaction, difficulties in the interview process should be acknowledged and discussed as part of the process. Methods to help an interview to progress include deferring topics until later, asking questions in different ways, exploring reasons for a patient's discomfort with specific topics and acknowledging that some issues are hard to discuss. It may be necessary to defer some areas of assessment to a later time. Sensitive areas such as sexuality may be difficult for both the nurse and the patient and may need to be deferred until a stronger relationship has developed. This can be acknowledged at the time of the interview so that the patient is not left feeling that these issues cannot be addressed. Finally, if the patient becomes too distressed to continue with the interview, this can be acknowledged and the interview terminated with a plan for further assessment later.

Summarising and Concluding

As the interview draws to a conclusion the nurse should begin to move the discussion towards a shared understanding of what has been achieved, clarification of presenting problems and discussion of possible interventions and further care. This can involve the nurse offering a summary or asking the patient to provide a summary. This phase of the interview is an opportunity to engage the patient in a plan of care that recognises unresolved problems and draws on the patient's strengths and supports. The nurse should indicate when the allotted time for the interview is almost up, so that the patient is able to introduce any issues not previously discussed. Friends or family members can also be invited to ask final questions at this stage. It can be helpful for the nurse to ask if there are any questions the patient wishes to raise about the assessment information, further care and so forth. Summarising can provide an opportunity to further validate the patient's concerns. It is not unusual for patients to feel that they are 'going mad' or may be about to be admitted to hospital, even if those issues have been canvassed earlier in the interview.

If the nurse feels unsure about the best course of action following an interview, they should openly discuss this with a co-interviewer and include the patient in that discussion. Acknowledging uncertainty does not need to undermine confidence in the nurse, or the clinical service, but can be an opportunity for the nurse to share different perspectives on the assessment and future plan. It is important at the end of an interview to establish what has been agreed, as well as where there may be differences between the nurse and the patient. The interview should terminate with discussion of the next step in terms of further care and confirmation of contact details.

While an assessment interview is designed to establish a broad understanding of a patient and the problems they seek help with, it is not the only assessment tool available to nurses. Even the best interviews provide only a limited range of information, and the interview needs to be supplemented with other sources of information.

Mnemonics

Mnemonics (or acronyms) are aids to memory that prompt the nurse to ask specific questions or consider specific areas of assessment. Mnemonics are nonstandardised structured assessment tools that provide a convenient reminder when undertaking an assessment. For example:

- OLDCART can be used for assessment of pain, where the letters stand for Onset, Location, Duration, Characteristics, Aggravating factors, Radiation and Timing (Chase 2015).
- The HEADSS assessment is used in youth services, where the letters stand for Home, Education, Activities, Drug and alcohol use, Sexuality and Suicide (Eade & Henning 2013). There are many variations of the HEADSS assessment format, and HEADSS can be adapted for application in your own practice.
- The SAD PERSONS mnemonic (Sex, Age, Depression, Prior suicidality, Ethanol [alcohol] abuse, Rational thinking, Support systems, Organised support system, No significant other, Sickness) can be used in assessment of suicidality (Patterson et al. 1983). This mnemonic should be used only as a prompt to memory, not as a rating instrument, as the scoring system of SAD PERSONS has no validity in predicting future self-harm (Warden et al. 2014).
- Mnemonics remind clinicians of important areas of enquiry, but do not result in a numerical score. Because they are not standardised, mnemonics may be used differently by different clinicians. You can create your own mnemonics for assessment by making a list of areas of assessment you have found to be useful, assigning a name to each area and arranging the names so that the first letters form an easily remembered term. Important assessment findings resulting from use of mnemonics identify areas for further assessment.

Standardised Assessment Tools

In some areas of mental health nursing assessment, standardised instruments are used to gain a quantified measure of some aspect of psychological or social functioning, for example mood, cognitive functioning, risk or alcohol problems. A comprehensive overview of assessment instruments is provided by Baer and Blais (2010). Of the many instruments available, nurses will use only a small number, but it is helpful to be aware of the range of instruments available and their application to clinical practice. A list of commonly used standardised assessments that nurses can incorporate into their practice is shown in Table 22.2. All the instruments listed in the table can be used by nurses in their clinical practice, although in each case training is required to ensure reliable administration of the instrument. Training can occur in formal staff development sessions or as part of supervised clinical practice. Some instruments are subject to licensing, so before using any instrument check whether your service holds the necessary licence. It is common for different NHS Trusts or private providers of mental health care to adopt specific tools for use within the services, nurses should familiarise themselves with these. An example of a comprehensive person-centred approach to psychiatric nursing assessment is the multimodal biopsychopharmacosocial (BPPS) approach. The BPPS approach structures and guides person-centred nursing assessment, formulation and care planning (Clark & Clarke 2014).

Standardisation refers to the statistical evaluation of instruments aimed at ensuring their reliability and validity. Standardised instruments can be regarded as *screening tools* that alert clinicians to a problematic area of mental health and signal the need for further assessment. An important consideration in using standardised instruments is that they should not be regarded as complete assessments: they do not replace comprehensive assessment. Instead, they augment clinical assessment by providing a uniform means of measuring one aspect of functioning. Most instruments have cut-off scores; that is, scores that indicate levels of severity, need for treatment or need for further assessment.

Standardised instruments contribute to assessment in several ways. They provide a benchmark—for example, of mood or cognitive functioning—and a basis for comparing the same area of functioning at some future time. Comparison of scores over time allows the clinician to determine any improvement or deterioration in the area measured. This can be very helpful in assessing response to medication or other interventions, or to determine whether the patient's problems are escalating, indicating a need for review of the treatment plan. Standardised measures also allow clinicians to communicate about the extent of a problem, knowing that each is using the same criteria to estimate the level of severity. Another advantage is that they remind clinicians of questions they should ask in assessment. For example, the Alcohol Use Disorder Inventory Test (AUDIT), developed by the WHO, asks 10 specific questions about alcohol use; without this tool, clinicians may not remember all 10 questions in the course of an interview.

Instruments can be either clinician rated or patient rated. Self-rated instruments enable patients to report various experiences to the nurse that they might find hard to express in words. For example, someone who is very depressed might find it difficult to verbalise their low mood, but might be able to indicate low mood on a rating form that requires only a tick. If you are using a standardised instrument, take the opportunity to discuss the instrument with the patient and use the findings to develop collaborative means of addressing significant problems. As clinical problems improve, the changes measured on a standardised instrument can provide the patient with reassurance of their improvement.

On a cautionary note, it is important to consider the conditions under which a standardised instrument is used. We all feel anxious if we feel we are being assessed, and patients may feel that the findings of an instrument will be used to show

TABLE 22.2 Standardised Assessment Instruments

Test	Purpose of Test	Description
Cognitive Functioning		
MMSE (Mini-Mental State Examination) (Folstein et al. 1975)	Measure cognitive impairment related to dementia	An 11-item test that provides a cut-off score indicating significant cognitive impairment
ACE-R (Addenbrooke's Cognitive Examination—Revised) (Larner 2013)	Measure cognitive impairment	A 26-item test that provides cut-off scores for severity of cognitive impairment; ACE-R incorporates the 11 items of the MMSE
CAM (Confusion Assessment Method) (Inouye et al. 1990)	Screen for delirium	An 11-item instrument to detect delirium; CAM measures four different areas of cognitive functioning
Substance Use		
AUDIT (Alcohol Use Disorder Inventory Test) (Babor et al. 2001)	Detect the presence of alcohol problems	A 10-item test available in clinician- or patient-rated formats; AUDIT provides cut-off scores for four levels of clinical intervention
Mood		
BDI (Beck Depression Inventory) (McPherson & Martin 2010)	Screen for clinically significant depression	A 21-item self-report of experiences of low mood, with cut-off scores for levels of depression severity; subscales can be used to assess suicidality
GDS (Geriatric Depression Scale short form) (Burke et al. 1991)	Screen for clinically significant depression in older adults	A 15-item clinician administered instrument with three cut-off scores representing different levels of depression severity
Medication Side Effects		
LUNSERS (Liverpool University Neuroleptic Side–Effect Rating Scale) (Day et al. 1995)	Identify the presence of side effects of antipsychotic medication	A 51-item clinician- or patient-administered instrument that rates areas of medication side effects on a five-point Likert scale; provides scores for seven different areas of medication side effects
Risk of Violence		
HCR-20 (Historical Clinical Risk Management Scale) (Jaber & Mahmoud 2015)	Assess risk of violence	A 20-item clinician-rated instrument that combines historical, current clinical and future risk factors
Nonspecific Mental Health Problems		
Biopsychopharmacosocial Approach (BPPS)	The BPPS approach structures and guides person-centred nursing assessment, formulation and care planning	A multimodal, multiperspective approach to the assessment of the person as a whole—addressing predisposing, precipitating and perpetuating factors
GHQ 12 (General Health Questionnaire) (Hankins 2008)	Detect risk of developing mental illness in primary care populations	A 12-item clinician-rated instrument that provides a single cut-off score indicating possible mental illness

there is something wrong with them. Anxiety about completing a rating instrument will adversely affect the results, so it is important that the nurse creates optimal conditions for using the instrument and takes account of factors such as age, literacy level, sensory deficits, pain and discomfort and the explanation provided for the use of the test.

CRITICAL THINKING CHALLENGE 22.3

Read the list of standardised assessment instruments included in Table 22.2 and consider the areas of psychological and social functioning they address. How could one of these instruments help you in performing a comprehensive nursing assessment?

Diaries

Diaries are records of important experiences that are kept by patients in between contact with clinicians. A diary might record feelings, thoughts, activity level, interpersonal interactions, food intake or other self-observations. If you are going to use a diary as part of an assessment you need to explain the purpose to the patient, clarify what is to be recorded and discuss how the diary will contribute to care. Diaries can be helpful in developing your understanding of patients as they contain information that might not be accurately remembered. They also help by actively engaging the person in their care. In addition to contributing to assessment, diaries are a therapeutic intervention as they help increase the patient's self-awareness of important areas of functioning. Mood diaries have been developed as applications for smartphones

(Foreman et al. 2011) with the additional advantage that information can be shared with a therapist or clinician.

Direct Observation

Of all the professionals involved in mental healthcare, nurses have the most direct contact with patients. In inpatient settings this can include contact in the context of activities of daily living, such as care of the bed area, meals and social activities. Other forms of contact are providing medication, involvement in therapeutic activities such as groups or teaching sessions, and discussing issues such as leave requests. In community settings nurses may have contact with patients in their homes, in community clinics or at patients' places of work. Any contact with a patient is an opportunity to make direct observations of mental state, physical health, interaction and socialisation patterns, side effects of medication and other areas. Direct observations can be 'triangulated' with the patient's self-reports, observations of other nurses or clinicians and observations of third parties such as friends or family members. Nurses can gain a great deal of information from other clinicians and from clinical notes, but there is no substitute for actually seeing, talking to and interacting with the patient. They may seem very different to the picture suggested from other sources, or from your past understanding.

Information From Third Parties

In addition to information obtained directly from the patient, nurses make use of additional information from friends and family members, other clinical services and clinical records. In obtaining information from family members you need to be mindful of confidentiality and potential conflicts between family members. Some patients welcome the involvement of their family; others prefer not to have family involved (Tambuyzer & Van Audenhove 2013). Using a collaborative approach nurses can explore the potential contribution of family members to care, and the important role played by families in supporting their loved one. Families have a unique perspective on the care of their loved one and often remind mental health clinicians that it is they who know the patient best.

From the earlier description of the methods of mental health nursing assessment it can be seen that information contributing to an understanding of the patient as a person comes from a variety of sources. These include patients, nurses' subjective and objective observations, interviews, information from rating scales and information from a range of other individuals and clinical records. No one source of information is enough on its own, and some of the information from various sources may appear to conflict. The skill of mental health nursing assessment is to use the range of information available to build a picture of the patient as a person, to develop a shared understanding of what problems the patient is seeking help with and a plan of how the nurse and other members of the multidisciplinary team can help with the identified problems.

Nurse's Story 22.2 by Antony Abbey illustrates how the scope and purpose of nursing assessment can be expanded.

NURSE'S STORY 22.2 Antony Abbey RN

Reflecting on my early exposure to assessment as a student mental health nurse in 1981, I observed it initially as a linear and two-dimensional procedure. It appeared at the time to sit definitively within the context of gathering information. Patients were on the receiving end of this activity. They (or others who knew of them) would provide information in accordance with a set of questions and observations. Nursing care, although linked to the assessment, was a discrete and subsequent step within an overall process.

I discovered along the way that assessment becomes buoyant and three-dimensional when it allows the patient to explore the less familiar and sometimes unknown corridors of their psyche. When this occurs there is an opportunity for discovery, catharsis and positive change. In this sense, assessment becomes a therapy in its own right. Good questions are enabling, as are the variety of standardised assessment tools that are available. It is also useful to approach the assessment with a comprehensive framework in mind. But we should not be restricted and contained by these tools. We should stop, open up and listen to the patient's story, picking up on cues and gently guiding, much like the style that is eloquently described by Brown (1995) in her conversational approach to the assessment interview.

Take the example of Mr C, a man in his 40s who was admitted to the general hospital with severe headache, left-sided weakness and paraesthesia. After medical causes were ruled out I was asked, within the context of my psychiatric liaison nurse role, if I could help to unravel the mystery of this presentation. Mr C's personal story was one of hard work, stoicism and battling along in the face of any adversity. Emotional expression was not a language that he knew. His narrative was also one of significant recent stressors. It was a story of loss, redundancy and housing and financial struggles. Within the safety of a confidential and nonjudgemental setting, and enabled by a conversational approach, Mr C discovered a dialectic side to his story. He discovered that he had been caged in by his emotional illiteracy and 'stiff upper lip' rule. He realised that it didn't have to be that way. Supported with a further three or four sessions, with a focus on learning the language of emotion, Mr C was freed from his rule. He was supported also with developing new tools to help him accept and deal with emotional distress so that he could perhaps be liberated from his somatic manifestation.

Mr C is now free of his neurological symptoms and is working successfully through many of the stressors that he struggled with. So for this clinician, assessment and intervention work together in partnership, but also have interchangeable properties. Assessment as a therapy is one of the most satisfying interventions that a psychiatric nurse can deliver.

(*Source:* Brown, S.J., 1995. An interviewing style for nursing assessment. Journal of Advanced Nursing 21:340–343.)

COMPREHENSIVE ASSESSMENT PROCESS

In the following section the steps of the standard process of the comprehensive assessment process are explained. Most services will have a template for initial assessment, and may have an additional template for risk assessment. The content of these templates will vary between services, so you will need to be familiar with the models used in your own service, as well as with more general assessment issues. An example of a standard template is included in Table 22.3. A comprehensive mental health assessment involves collecting a wide range of information from the patient and from other sources. The following outline incorporates examples of dialogue between the nurse and the patient, and examples of documentation. Note that the examples are provided to illustrate aspects of the assessment process and documentation, but are not a complete record of an assessment.

Identifying Information

This is the first part of the comprehensive assessment and includes key demographic information about the patient,

TABLE 22.3 Comprehensive Mental Health Assessment

Date/time/venue | **Interviewers/others present**
Referrer | **GP**
Legal status

Area of Enquiry	Question(s) to be Addressed	Rationale
Reason for referral/presentation	What does the referral letter say?	You need to know what another health professional thinks the problem is. In some cases, there may not be a referral letter.
Patient's response to referral	Does the patient agree that they need help?	You need to know the patient's perspective, especially whether they agree there is a problem. You need to know something of the relationship between the patient and the referrer. For example, does the patient think the referrer understands them?
Presenting problem	What is happening? What can we do to help? Why now?	These questions help clarify the presenting problem as the patient sees it. They also help clarify the patient's expectations of mental healthcare.
History of presenting problem	How long has this been happening? Is the problem getting worse? Or better? Have you found any way of dealing with the problem?	This helps establish the duration of the problem, any fluctuation in severity and any strategies that might be helpful. (Note: this section does not include the mental health history: see next section.)
Mental health history	Have you had problems like this before? Have you ever had problems such as very low mood, very high mood, severe anxiety, sleep disturbance, unusually (for you) severe difficulty coping with life problems? Have you ever sought professional help or counselling for mental health–related problems? Have you ever heard voices when there was no-one there? Have you had any unusual thoughts or perceptions (give examples, such as thoughts of being controlled, receiving messages from the television etc.)? Have you ever had thoughts that you would like to be dead? Or of ending your life? Have you had any hospital admissions for mental health problems? What treatment have you had, and did it help? How long did you maintain treatment for? Ask for names of medications, doses taken, benefits and side effects experienced and reasons for discontinuation. Where possible, confirm prescription patterns by consulting clinical notes or pharmacy records.	The person may have had previous mental health problems that influence their response to the current problem. The presenting problem may be part of a pattern, or it may be a break from the patient's previous coping pattern. The presenting problem may represent a worsening of a long-term problem. Exploring previous help-seeking will help you to understand the patient's attitudes to health professionals, degree of trust and strategies that have been useful in the past. Areas of enquiry involving direct questions such as thoughts of self-harm should be raised naturally in an interview or interaction if possible. If there is no opportunity to do this, you need to give a brief explanation of why you are asking (e.g. 'Some people who feel depressed have thoughts about ending their life'). Understanding the patient's experience of medication is important in considering the role of medication for the current problem.
Family history	Has anyone in your family experienced similar problems? Has anyone in your family been diagnosed with a mental illness or substance use disorder? Has anyone in your family been admitted to a mental health unit? Has anyone in your family died by suicide?	A family history of mental illness is known to be a predisposing factor. The patient's experience of a family member's mental illness will influence their expectations of help for themselves. Suicide of a family member is a risk factor for other family members.

TABLE 22.3 **Comprehensive Mental Health Assessment—cont'd**

Area of Enquiry	Question(s) to be Addressed	Rationale
Substance use history	Do you drink alcohol? What is your drinking pattern? Has your drinking increased recently? Do you use any other substances, such as marijuana, methamphetamine, cocaine, ecstasy? (Ask about recreational substances known to be prevalent in your community.) Do you smoke? How many per day? Have you tried quitting?	For a comprehensive assessment you need to know the patient's long-term and short-term drinking patterns. Consider using the AUDIT or similar alcohol or substance use screening tool. Brief screening has been shown to increase the possibility of help-seeking and behaviour change.
Medical history	Use a question and answer format to ask about illnesses, hospitalisations, injuries (especially head injuries), past and current treatment. Include childhood illnesses. Include a brief systems review (see Table 22.1). Ask whether the patient has a GP and when was the last visit. Include questions about family medical history, such as whether first-degree relatives have had illnesses such as cardiovascular disease, diabetes, hypertension or respiratory disease.	Physical health is frequently overlooked in mental healthcare. People with mental illness have high rates of physical comorbidity. Physical health problems may contribute to mental health presentations; for example, hyperthyroidism may cause anxiety; hypothyroidism may cause low mood and loss of energy. Family history is strongly linked to likelihood of illness.
Social and developmental history	Tell me about your childhood. How was your life as you were growing up? Explore areas such as number and order of siblings, past and current relationships with siblings, peer group relationships, friendships and intimate relationships. For students, enquire about study programme, achievement, stress associated with study and future plans. What is your area of employment? How long have you been in your current job? Do you enjoy your work? What are your future employment plans? Explore patterns of sexual relationships, including gender identification and gender preference. Information on marital status may already be known, but explore the quality of relationships and whether there have been recent changes or stressors.	Developmental influences are critically important in shaping personality and individual adaptive style. Understanding family and personal relationships can help in identifying sources of stress as well as support systems. Study and employment can be both a source of stress and a protective factor in helping to build a sense of the future. Areas such as sexuality are quite sensitive so any discussion needs to take into account the degree of rapport established and whether the assessment situation is an appropriate one in which to explore these issues. By attending carefully to the process and content of communication, you will develop a sense of when is an appropriate time to explore sensitive areas.
Trauma	Have you ever experienced any form of interpersonal violence or sexual assault? Have you ever been bullied at school/at work/at university? Have you ever been bullied on social media? If there is current violence, consider the vulnerability of children. For older adults, consider their vulnerability from caregivers or family members.	Trauma is known to contribute to mental illness and to limit patients' willingness to engage with professionals. Experiences of trauma may be discussed without the need for specific questioning. Most people expect to be asked about trauma, even if they find it difficult to talk about it. Making an enquiry about trauma is an opportunity to validate the patient's experience and to offer intervention. Some services have mandatory screening policies for interpersonal violence. These should be followed and incorporated into the comprehensive assessment.
Cultural/spiritual needs	What culture/s do you identify with? Do you have any specific cultural needs or preferences? Are you a spiritual person? How would you describe your spiritual beliefs? Are you religious? How would you describe your religious beliefs and practices?	Cultural and spiritual beliefs can impact on the expression of mental distress and illness. Cultural and spiritual beliefs can also offer an opportunity for the nurse and patient to engage in dialogue about what interventions are helpful and appropriate. Some services have staff specifically employed for their cultural and spiritual skills.

Continued

TABLE 22.3 Comprehensive Mental Health Assessment—cont'd

Area of Enquiry	Question(s) to be Addressed	Rationale
Forensic history	Have you ever been involved with the police? Do you have any current charges?	It is not uncommon for people with mental illness to have had contact with the police, either in response to a mental health emergency or as arrest on criminal charges. For some patients, contact with the police is a pathway into mental healthcare as an initial arrest may be diverted to mental health services.
Mental state assessment	See Pages 446-48	Mental state assessment provides a snapshot of the person's emotional and cognitive functioning at the time of the assessment. It provides an important baseline for assessing the response to intervention.
Clinical formulation/summary	See Pages 448-49	This is a summary of the significant information from the assessment, presented in narrative form. More than a list, it is an attempt to show the relationship between various past and current factors, and how they influence the likely course of the person's mental health treatment.
Risk assessment	Risk assessment draws on the information discussed earlier, but might include a risk formulation, a narrative statement of the risks identified and the factors thought to contain risk or that might exacerbate risk. See page 449 for a discussion of risk assessment.	Risk is just one area of assessment and should not be the only factor considered in developing an understanding of the patient and a plan of care. Services may have specific risk assessment and documentation protocols.
Diagnosis/problem list	A list of the major problems the patient is facing, in prioritised order. These can include psychiatric diagnoses as well as nursing diagnoses. Problems can include symptoms of mental illness, safety, accommodation issues, physical health problems, relationship problems and social problems such as employment and finances.	The problem list is an attempt to focus on a manageable number of specific issues. It does not include every problem the patient has—only those that can benefit the most from mental healthcare or from referral to another agency.
Plan	A statement of the intended actions to be taken by the clinical team and the patient. The plan should be negotiated with the patient. Actions should be stated in priority order. The plan should end with the next review date or the date of referral to another agency.	Both the nurse and the patient need to have a considered strategy for actions to be taken to address identified problems.

including name, age, gender, employment, ethnicity, main support persons, living situation and address and contact details. Although some of these details will previously have been recorded the nurse needs to ensure that they are accurate.

Example

Mr Pavlovich is a 56-year-old unemployed single European male who lives alone in his rented central city apartment. He was referred today by his GP.

Presenting Problem

The presenting problem is the issue that causes the person to present for mental healthcare. The presenting problem should always be expressed from the patient's perspective, not from the perspective of the health professional. For example, a patient may seem to be very depressed when first seen, but their reason for presenting might be expressed as 'I'm desperate. I can't go on.' In the case of a patient who does not agree that they need mental healthcare, their presenting problem might be 'They forced me to come here. I don't need to see anyone.'

Dialogue

Nurse: Mr Pavlovich, your GP has referred you for help with feelings of depression. Can you tell me how you have been feeling recently?

Mr Pavlovich: I don't know. I've been pretty down. The doctor said I should come here. He didn't know what to do with me.

Nurse: That sounds difficult for you. Have there been any other changes recently?

Mr Pavlovich: Well, I've lost weight, and I can't seem to sleep like I used to. I've been thinking, you know, it's not worth going on.
Nurse: So, quite a few things happening for you. I'd like to hear more about those problems. Have you felt that you would rather not be alive?
Mr Pavlovich: Yeah, sometimes.

Documentation
Mr Pavlovich presents today with problems of persistent low mood. His sleep has been disturbed and he has lost weight over the past 3 weeks. He has recently begun to have suicidal thoughts.

History of Presenting Problem

The history of the presenting problem is concerned with the events leading up to the assessment: the onset, duration, course and severity. Once again, it is important to try to get an understanding of the history as the patient has experienced it and not as the health professional sees it. Factors that have led to the presentation will be varied and may be positive (such as winning the lottery) or negative (for example, losing a job), as both positive and negative events can trigger mental health presentations. It is also important to focus on recent precipitants as triggers; for example, the context of a presenting problem may be long-standing marital discord but the cause for presentation may be that the spouse has left recently. In documenting the history of the presenting problem, pay attention to the chronological order of events. Patients may relate events in order of their significance, rather than in chronological order, and while the meaning and significance of events are very important, the order of events is also important in understanding how the presenting problem has developed.

Exploring the history of the presenting problem should include a review of symptoms of the most common mental illnesses such as mood disorder, anxiety, psychosis or disorders of cognition. Some symptoms will be obvious, but others might need to be elicited by asking probing questions. As much as possible these questions should be incorporated into an interview; however, you might also need to make a direct enquiry about some symptoms such as unusual perceptions. Factors of significance will not be limited to clinical factors (mood, thoughts, perceptions etc.) but will also include personal factors such as changes in relationships, interests and activities.

The nurse should consider the patient's self-help and support strategies, and how effective these have been. Patients may have used previously learned methods of stress management and distress tolerance, and may have sought support from friends and family members. Other responses can include increased use of prescribed medication, use of non-prescribed medication and use of alcohol or other drugs.

Dialogue
Nurse: Mr Pavlovich, can you tell me how long these problems have been going on?
Mr Pavlovich: Well, I've been depressed before, but I've always managed to, I don't know, pick myself up.
Nurse: So you've been able to do things to help yourself in the past but this time it's different?
Mr Pavlovich: Yeah, much worse.
Nurse: And when did you first begin to feel worse?
Mr Pavlovich: I think it started when I lost my job.
Nurse: I see, and can you remember when that was? How many weeks ago did you lose your job?
Mr Pavlovich: About 6 weeks I think, yeah about 6 weeks.

Documentation
Feelings of low mood began 6 weeks ago and are related to loss of employment. Reports previous feelings of depression but this episode is qualitatively different and described as 'much worse'. Previous coping strategies have not been successful.

Because Mr Pavlovich has disclosed thoughts suggestive of suicidality these would be specifically followed up.

Dialogue
Nurse: You mentioned that you have had thoughts about not carrying on with life.
Mr Pavlovich: Yeah, sometimes.
Nurse: That must be very difficult for you. Have you had thoughts of ending your life?
Mr Pavlovich: Yeah, I've thought of that.
Nurse: Okay, and have you got to the point where you thought you might do something to end your life?
Mr Pavlovich: I've thought about taking pills, sleeping pills or something.
Nurse: And have you acted on these thoughts? Do you have any sleeping tablets available?
Mr Pavlovich: No, but the doctor would probably give me some.
Nurse: And do you still have these thoughts of ending your life?
Mr Pavlovich: Well, if I don't get better.

Documentation
Has had thoughts of suicide and has considered means, but has not acted on these thoughts. No current plan but thoughts of self-harm still present.

Mental Health History

Information gathered for the mental health history is concerned with the patient's history of mental health concerns. It is important to ask about past attempts the patient has made to receive help for their mental health. This information should be documented chronologically. Most people will have sought help from various sources at some point in their life and it is important to be aware of this as it helps to better comprehend the nature, longevity and understanding that the person has given their concerns. Many people will ask a chemist or health-food shop for assistance with symptoms relating to mental health. Some may have been to a naturopath, chiropractor or massage therapist, others to their GP, church minister or school or university counsellor. For some people the main source of help will be family, extended family or their own cultural advisors. All of this information is valid and adds to our understanding.

It is important to ask what treatment the patient has tried and what the results were. If the patient has been prescribed medication such as antidepressants, this should be recorded along with the dose and response. Other treatments such as electroconvulsive therapy, group therapy and psychological therapy should also be included, along with the patient's response. A helpful way to explore medication is to enquire whether the patient found it helpful, how long they took the medication for and (if relevant) their reasons for discontinuing medication.

Hospital admissions and contacts with community mental health services should also be documented in this part of the assessment. If the patient has had previous admissions or periods of community care, their legal status should be recorded. Areas of risk should be explored, including past history of self-harm or suicidality, history of violence towards others and any history of victimisation, such as exposure to domestic violence or assault from others.

Dialogue

Nurse: You mentioned you have had problems with depression in the past. Can you tell me more about that?
Mr Pavlovich: Like I said, I've been down a few times but I've always been able to get myself out of it.
Nurse: So until now you've never been to a doctor for help with depression?
Mr Pavlovich: There was one time, but the doctor thought it was stress.
Nurse: So you didn't have treatment at that time?
Mr Pavlovich: No, there was no treatment.
Nurse: How long ago was that?
Mr Pavlovich: Maybe 10 years.
Nurse: So, quite a while ago. And at that time did you feel the same way you are feeling now?
Mr Pavlovich: Yeah, much the same. Not quite as bad. I couldn't go to work. But I got over it.
Nurse: At that time did you have any thoughts that you didn't want to be alive?
Mr Pavlovich: No, it wasn't that bad.

Documentation

No previous treatment for depression despite occasional periods of depression in his adult life. Recalls one episode, 10 years ago, when symptoms were comparable to current presentation. Was unable to work, but no thoughts of suicide. Saw GP but was not treated. Episode eventually resolved.

Note that this is not a complete assessment of Mr Pavlovich's suicidality, which would require further exploration, for example of protective factors and sense of hope for the future.

Substance Use History

Taking a good substance use record is essential as all substances have an effect on mental health. Some issues of substance use may have been discussed in relation to past mental health history and these areas should be explored in more detail. Rates of coexisting mental illness and substance use are very high (Gilbert et al. 2014) and substance use will complicate recovery from a mental illness. In some cases, substance use may have precipitated mental illness, or may be a factor in perpetuating mental illness. In taking a substance use history you will need to name the specific substances the patient has used. Patients may be concerned that information about use of illegal substances will be passed onto the police, so the assessment should include reassurance that the information is sought for the purposes of healthcare and will remain confidential.

In exploring substance use, patients should be asked for specific information about the level of use; for example, the statement, 'I don't drink much' could have different meanings for different people. Ask clarifying questions to establish the level and pattern of alcohol or other drug consumption. There are many useful screening tools for assisting with this assessment. Patients can be asked to complete a brief questionnaire such as the AUDIT (Babor et al. 2001). Assessment of substance use is an opportunity to explore readiness to change using a model such as motivational interviewing (Stewart 2012) and to discuss whether referral to a substance use agency might be helpful.

Dialogue

Nurse: Mr Pavlovich, I'd like to ask you some questions about drinking. This is a usual part of assessment. Are you okay with that?
Mr Pavlovich: Yeah, that's okay.
Nurse: Thanks. Can I start by asking do you drink alcohol?
Mr Pavlovich: Yes, a bit.
Nurse: Okay, how much is 'a bit'? Do you drink every day, every week?
Mr Pavlovich: Every week but every other day, not every day.
Nurse: Okay, and when you do drink, how much would you drink?
Mr Pavlovich: It's different on different days. Mostly two or three drinks, but I get a bit carried away sometimes.
Nurse: When was the last time you got carried away?
Mr Pavlovich: Last week. I can't remember much about it.
(This part of the interview would continue to explore the pattern of drinking and its consequences, in particular whether drinking had increased recently in response to low mood.)

Documentation

Describes himself as a regular drinker of moderate amounts, with occasional binges. Normally drinks 3–4 days a week. Last week had a 'big night' followed by blackout for the evening. Increasing frequency of drinking recently in an attempt to help with sleep (not usually successful). No history of withdrawal symptoms.

This section of the assessment would proceed to explore other areas such as use of recreational substances, prescribed drugs and tobacco.

CRITICAL THINKING CHALLENGE 22.4

Mental health assessment involves asking patients about areas of their lives usually considered private and personal, such as questions about sexuality, use of drugs and experiences of trauma. How comfortable do you feel about exploring these areas with patients? Why is it important that nurses are able to overcome discomfort about asking very personal questions? What are some of the risks of asking very personal questions and how can those risks be managed?

Family History

It is important to ask about the mental health history of the family, particularly close relatives such as parents, grandparents, siblings, aunts, uncles and cousins. We are interested in knowing this for two reasons. First, some of the major mental health conditions are known to have familial patterns (i.e. schizophrenia, bipolar disorder and depression). These conditions are more common in people with close relatives with the disorder (Rasic et al. 2013). Second, we know that the environment that a person grows up and lives in has impacts on their health generally and on their mental health specifically. As we grow up we all role-model our ways of living, behaving and coping on significant others around us. For example, a child raised in a family with a depressed parent who took to their bed for prolonged periods may replicate this behaviour as their way of coping with the world and this may lead to a mental health presentation.

Enquiry about family history can begin with a question such as 'Has anyone else in your family had problems like these?' The patient's answers can be explored to gain more detailed information and to gain an understanding of the patient's past and current relationships with family members.

Dialogue

Nurse: Can I ask you a few questions about your family? Has anyone in your immediate family had similar problems to yours?
Mr Pavlovich: My father used to get depressed.
Nurse: Was his experience similar to yours, do you think?
Mr Pavlovich: Yeah. There was one time when he had to stop work for a while.
Nurse: Did he need to see a doctor?
Mr Pavlovich: He saw the GP. I think he took some medication but I don't know what it was.
Nurse: Is your father still alive?
Mr Pavlovich: He died a few years ago. Doctor said it was a heart attack.
Nurse: So you've had experience of depression in your family. Have any other relatives had mental illness?
Mr Pavlovich: Not that I know of, I don't think so.

Documentation

Father sought GP treatment for episodes of depression. At one point, depression prevented work. No other family history identified.

Developmental and Social History

This area of assessment considers the stages of the patient's life and their possible influence on personality, coping style and the current problem. Understanding experiences at various life stages is an important component of comprehensive assessment. The developmental history can take a chronological approach, although some social stressors may relate to early life experiences and so may have been discussed at other stages of the comprehensive assessment process. Areas of assessment include infancy and early childhood, early family experiences, past relationships with siblings, developmental milestones, peer relationships and friendships, experiences of schooling, academic achievements and relationships with parents and caregivers. Following the life course will lead to discussion of employment, university or other study, intimate relationships and sexuality. Adult relationships are important, especially any pattern of difficulty in maintaining long-term relationships, and relationships with children. For older adults the nurse should discuss later life milestones such as retirement, socialisation patterns, relationships and illnesses, especially those that limit mobility or social functioning or that cause sensory deficits.

Dialogue

Nurse: Mr Pavlovich, how was life for you growing up? Can you tell me a little about your family?
Mr Pavlovich: I grew up in the city. There was me and my brother and sister. I was the oldest.
Nurse: And do you remember growing up as a happy time?
Mr Pavlovich: Mostly. We used to go for picnics and to visit relatives.
Nurse: Your parents got on well?
Mr Pavlovich: Yeah, they had their moments, you know, but they got on well.
Nurse: And how was school for you?
Mr Pavlovich: I did well at school. Teachers liked me because I guess I was a good kid. I liked school.
Nurse: And did you have friends at school?
Mr Pavlovich: Yeah, always had friends. Too many friends sometimes [laughs].
Nurse: Too many friends?
Mr Pavlovich: You know, I liked the social side of it.
Nurse: I see. You liked spending time with friends, but you still did well academically?
Mr Pavlovich: Yeah, it was a good time.
From here the interview would proceed to explore other areas of Mr Pavlovich's development, such as employment, intimate relationships and adult relationships.

Documentation

Oldest of three children. Grew up in the city and describes a happy childhood of social outings and contact with wider family. Parents were together and got on well. Enjoyed school and was successful academically. Describes good peer group relationships.

Trauma

Trauma is now recognised as a major contributor to the development of mental illness and as a common experience among people with mental illness (Lommen & Restifo 2009). Experiences of trauma may emerge in any clinical interaction. In many cases you will not need to make a specific enquiry about trauma, but you do need to be prepared to respond empathically to disclosures about trauma and to offer any further intervention or referral if necessary. Patients commonly feel that their experience of trauma is discounted in healthcare services, so any disclosure should be validated, together with the opportunity for further exploration. Trauma can take many forms, including bullying, physical violence, sexual assault, intimate partner violence, neglect, exposure to traumatic events such as war or military conflict, torture or refugee experiences. Trauma should be approached with tact and sensitivity. Clinicians need to be alert for indications that the patient does not currently feel safe to discuss experiences of trauma, and in such cases should leave exploration of trauma until a more appropriate time. This decision needs to be communicated to the patient, together with an explanation of how the patient can seek further help.

Dialogue

Nurse: The next area I'd like to explore is trauma, which is about whether you have had any experience of violence, abuse or exploitation. Can I begin by asking if you have ever experienced any especially troublesome incidents or events in your life?
Mr Pavlovich: Not really. Not that I can think of.
Nurse: So you've never had any experience, for example of being assaulted or bullied, that sort of thing?
Mr Pavlovich: No worse than anyone else.
Nurse: Do you mean there have been some incidents but you don't think they were significant?
Mr Pavlovich: No, I mean I've never had any experience that was that bad.
Nurse: Have you ever been involved in a serious accident?
Mr Pavlovich: No, nothing like that.

Documentation

No personal experience of trauma identified.

Note that the preceding section describes a brief, informal screen for experiences of trauma. In this case the result is negative; however, people presenting to mental health services report a high rate of traumatic experiences. Despite trauma being quite prevalent in this population, clinicians frequently do not ask screening questions, so there is no opportunity to understand the relationship between past trauma and current mental health problems.

Cultural Issues

Cultural issues can have a major impact on the expression of mental distress and illness, and on patients' engagement with mental healthcare (O'Brien et al. 2016). The populations across the UK have become increasingly culturally diverse. Assessment should identify cultural issues experienced by patients and seek to understand how these issues might impact on the expression of distress and on care and treatment. Cultural differences between clinicians and patients can be a barrier to assessment, and clinicians should consider whether the presence of a translator or cultural support person will help facilitate assessment. Clinicians should be cautious in identifying patients' cultural needs, and should check these with each patient and seek advice if unsure.

Dialogue

Nurse: Mr Pavlovich, you're a European?
Mr Pavlovich: Yes, family came here after the war.
Nurse: So that was in the 1950s?
Mr Pavlovich: Yes, they were from Croatia.
Nurse: Do you have contact with the Croatian community?
Mr Pavlovich: Yes, I grew up with it. I even tried to learn that language but it's hard when you don't get to use it. But I go to the social club sometimes.

Documentation

European male who identifies with his Croatian ancestry. Maintains contact with Croatian community.

CRITICAL THINKING CHALLENGE 22.5

Consider your own cultural beliefs and practices. How comfortable would you feel discussing these beliefs with a mental health professional? How can you help patients to feel comfortable discussing these areas as part of their mental healthcare?

Spirituality

As with culture, spirituality is increasingly recognised as an important aspect of mental health and should be considered in every comprehensive assessment (Elliott 2011). Spirituality can include membership or identification with organised religions or faith communities, or nonreligious spiritual beliefs. Spiritual beliefs are important in helping patients give meaning to their experiences of mental distress and illness. Faith communities are also significant sources of informal support. Consideration of spirituality in assessment can include the patient's developmental experience of religion, current engagement with religion and religious practices and personal belief systems. Some patients may indicate that they do not have spiritual beliefs and this expression should be respected and recorded.

Dialogue

Nurse: Mr Pavlovich, would you describe yourself as a spiritual person?
Mr Pavlovich: Well, I was brought up Catholic, but I don't go to Mass regularly.
Nurse: Some people don't attend church but still have beliefs that are important to them.
Mr Pavlovich: I still have some of the beliefs. I just don't have much to do with it.
Nurse: Would you say those beliefs are an important part of you?
Mr Pavlovich: Yes, yes I would. They are still important.

Documentation
Raised with Catholic beliefs but is not a regular church attender. Maintains spiritual beliefs that are important to him.

Forensic History

It is not unusual for people with mental illness to have had contact with the police or the legal system, and possibly contact with forensic mental health services. These aspects of the personal history may emerge spontaneously or may need to be the subject of specific assessment questions. In the context of an assessment interview, it may become clear from responses to more general questions that the patient has no history of police involvement, in which case no specific enquiry is needed. In addition to noting specific events, such as any arrests, convictions and sentencing, it is important to know the patient's current perceptions of events involving legal issues and whether there are any outstanding charges. Forensic history can help in documenting any events involving interpersonal violence and form part of risk assessment. See Chapter 14 for further discussion of forensic mental health issues.

General Health History

It is important to gather the patient's medical history to check for health problems and medical comorbidities that might be impacting on their mental health. This is a good chance to ask about medication use that might have been missed earlier in the assessment. The health history should include childhood illnesses, any current or chronic illnesses, history of head injury or loss of consciousness and known allergies. Having a systematic approach to the medical history will help avoid missing important findings. Thorough questioning may uncover health problems that you might not have considered; for example, pain is an often-overlooked problem that unless specifically asked about can go undetected and may impact greatly on a person's wellbeing. Taking a health history is also an opportunity for discussion about physical issues that might not directly impact on the person's mental health but may require attention. It is particularly important to ask about head injuries and any loss of consciousness, including general anaesthetics. Uncovering this information will add to your clinical picture and help the team to decide if seeking historical medical information is pertinent to treatment planning. It may also indicate the need for particular diagnostic tests such as computed tomography (CT) imaging of the head or psychometric assessments. People with serious mental illness have high rates of physical disorders (Welsh & McEnany 2015), so this part of the comprehensive assessment is an opportunity to reinforce important health messages such as undertaking regular exercise, smoking cessation, cardiovascular screening and sexual health screening. Discussion of physical health issues can also help in checking whether the patient is enrolled in a primary care practice and is receiving regular primary healthcare. Chapter 8 provides an extensive discussion of physical health issues experienced by people with mental illness.

Dialogue
Nurse: Mr Pavlovich, I'd like to ask you a few questions about your general health.
Mr Pavlovich: I generally keep pretty well.
Nurse: That's good to hear. Do you have any illnesses, like diabetes, heart disease, high blood pressure?
Mr Pavlovich: My blood pressure's high sometimes.
Nurse: Are you on any treatment for that?
Mr Pavlovich: No, the doctor just said I need to get a bit more exercise and cut down on salt.
Nurse: Have you ever been in hospital with an accident or illness?
Mr Pavlovich: I had a hernia operation a few years ago but that's all.
Nurse: You said your father died of a heart attack. Has anyone else in your family had heart problems?
Mr Pavlovich: I had an uncle. My father's brother. He died of a heart attack. And my grandfather was only 60 when he died. They said it was a heart attack.

Documentation
History of high blood pressure (controlled with diet and exercise). Strong family history of heart disease.

Physical Health Assessment

Like other areas of assessment described in this chapter, physical health assessment is a core skill of mental health nurses. In some research studies mental health nurses have reported that they do not feel well prepared or confident to assess physical health (Howard & Gamble 2011). However, mental health patients experience high rates of physical disorders (De Hert et al. 2011) and reduced life expectancy (Cunningham et al. 2014). In addition, mental health patients are frequently prescribed second-generation antipsychotic agents that are associated with higher risk of metabolic syndrome (Brunero & Lamont 2009). Other medications such as clozapine, lithium and sodium valproate require skills of physical health assessment to ensure safe monitoring (see Chapter 8). Sound physical health assessment skills also provide the basis for health promotion interventions in areas such as smoking cessation, exercise regimens, weight management and diet.

Physical health assessment should include a health history (see earlier), both of the patient's health and that of their immediate family, with special attention to factors that might place the patient at risk of health problems common in mental health patients, such as cardiovascular disease and metabolic syndrome. Physical health assessment should include a systems review to ensure that no areas of health problems are missed. You can use the top-to-toe assessment that you have been introduced to for physical health screening to frame your thinking and questions (see Box 22.2).

Laboratory Investigations

Laboratory investigations are part of any comprehensive assessment and have several purposes, including to understand the role of physical illness in the current presentation; to establish adherence to prescribed medication; to assess organ functioning and how it might be impacted by prescribed medication (for example, the effect of liver functioning on the half-life of benzodiazepines); to identify potentially toxic blood levels of prescribed medication (for example, lithium carbonate); and to identify any use of nonprescribed drugs. Laboratory tests are used in initial assessment and to monitor the impact of prescribed medication (for example, the development of markers of metabolic syndrome).

BOX 22.2 Review of Systems Checklist

General
- Have you noticed any changes in weight (loss or gain)?
- Have you been tired recently?
- Have you had any fever or chills?
- Have you noticed any weakness in your arms or legs, or generally?
- Have you had trouble sleeping?

Skin
- Have you noticed any rashes, lumps, itching or dryness of your skin?
- Have you noticed any changes in skin colour?
- Have you noticed any changes in your hair or nails?

Head
- Have you had headaches recently?
- Have you ever had a head injury or been knocked unconscious?
- Do you have any neck pain?

Ears
- Do you have any problems with hearing?
- Do you have ringing in your ears?
- Do you have earache?
- Have you noticed any discharge from your ears?

Eyes
- Have you noticed any changes in your eyesight?
- Do you wear glasses or contacts?
- Have you had any pain or redness in your eyes?
- Have you experienced blurred vision or double vision?
- Have you noticed any flashing lights?
- Have you noticed any specks in your vision?
- Do you have glaucoma or cataracts?
- When was your last eye exam?

Nose
- Have you noticed any stuffiness, discharge or itching?
- Do you suffer from hay fever, nosebleeds or sinus pain?

Mouth and throat
- Have you noticed any bleeding?
- Do you wear dentures?
- Have you noticed any sore tongue, dry mouth, sore throat or hoarseness?
- Have you recently had any mouth infections or sores?

Neck
- Have you noticed any lumps, swollen glands, pain or stiffness?

Breasts
- Have you noticed any lumps, pain or discharge?
- Do you regularly examine your breasts?
- When was your last breast screen?
- Are you currently breastfeeding?

Respiratory
- Have you had any cough, sputum or coughing up blood?
- Have you noticed any shortness of breath, wheezing or painful breathing?

Cardiovascular
- Have you had any chest pain or discomfort?
- Have you noticed any tightness in your chest or palpitations?
- Have you noticed any shortness of breath with activity, or difficulty breathing when lying down?
- Have you noticed any swelling of your ankles or limbs?
- Have you experienced sudden wakening from sleep with shortness of breath?

Gastrointestinal
- Have you had any difficulties with swallowing?
- Have you noticed any heartburn, changes in appetite or nausea?
- Have you noticed any change in your bowel habits?
- Have you noticed any rectal bleeding, constipation, diarrhoea, yellow eyes or skin?

Urinary
- Have you noticed any changes in urinary frequency?
- Have you noticed any urgency, burning or pain when passing urine?
- Have you noticed any blood in your urine?
- Have you experienced any incontinence or change in urinary flow?

Vascular
- Have you noticed any calf pain when walking?
- Have you noticed any leg cramps?

Musculoskeletal
- Have you noticed any muscle or joint pain, stiffness or back pain?
- Have you noticed any redness or swelling of your joints?
- Have you had any recent injuries?

Neurological
- Have you noticed any dizziness, fainting, weakness, numbness, tingling or tremor?
- Have you had any seizures?

Haematological
- Do you bruise or bleed easily?

Endocrine
- Have you noticed any difficulty with heat or cold?
- Have you noticed any sweating?
- Have you noticed that you need to drink more or less than you usually do?

Nurses should be familiar with the most commonly used laboratory tests and be able to interpret the results of tests using knowledge of the patient's general health status and the accepted range of values for the particular test. Most results are reported along with the normal range. A list of commonly used laboratory tests is included in Table 22.4; not all tests are used in every assessment, but the list here includes those most likely to be included. For a full description of laboratory tests in health assessment, see Kellerman (2011).

TABLE 22.4 Laboratory Tests for Mental Health Assessment

Test	Normal Range	Clinical Implications of Abnormal Findings
Full Blood Count		
White blood cells (WBC)	4.0–11.0 10^9/L	Infection
Red blood cells (erythrocytes)	4.3–6.0 10^9/L (M) 3.6–5.6 10^9/L (F)	Anaemia, loss of energy, low mood
Haemocrit (packed cell volume, [PCV])	0.40–0.52 (M) 0.35–0.46 (F)	Anaemia, loss of energy, low mood
Haemoglobin (Hb)	130–175 g/L (M) 115–155 g/L (F)	Anaemia, loss of energy, low mood
Platelets	150–400 10^9/L	Blood clotting disorders Haemorrhagic (low platelets) Trauma or anaemia (high platelets)
Nutritional Status		
Vitamin B_{12}	170–600 pmol/L (normal) 110–170 pmol/L (borderline)	Anaemia, loss of energy, low mood, peripheral nervous system damage
Folate	>7.0 nmol/L (normal)	Loss of energy, low mood
Electrolytes		
Sodium	135–145 mmol/L	Fluid retention (low sodium) Dehydration may indicate diabetes (high sodium) Lithium toxicity
Potassium	3.5–5.2 mmol/L	Cardiac arrhythmias, muscle cramps
Chloride	95–100 mmol/L	Dehydration
Serum creatinine	60–105 umol/L (M) 45–90 umol/L (F)	Elevated creatinine indicates renal impairment or dehydration
Bicarbonate	23–29 mmol/L (adult)	Diabetic ketoacidosis, metabolic acidosis (low bicarbonate) Vomiting, metabolic alkalosis (high bicarbonate)
Organ Functioning		
Serum triiodothyronine (T_3)	3.0–6.5 pmol/L	Low T_3 may indicate hypothyroidism and may be associated with loss of energy, low mood Elevated T_3 may indicate hyperthyroidism and may be associated with unexplained increase in energy, elevated mood, mania
Serum thyroxine (T_4)	10–20 pmol/L	Elevated T_4 may indicate hyperthyroidism and may be associated with unexplained increase in energy, anxiety, elevated mood, mania Low T_4 may indicate hypothyroidism and may be associated with loss of energy, low mood
Thyroid-stimulating hormone (TSH)	0.30–4.0 mL/L	Elevated thyroxine may indicate hyperthyroidism and may be associated with unexplained increase in energy, anxiety, elevated mood, mania Low thyroxine may indicate hypothyroidism and may be associated with loss of energy, low mood
Urea	3.2–7.7 mmol/L	Elevated levels indicate renal or liver impairment
Gamma-glutamyl transferase (GGT)	<60 (M) U/L <50 (F) U/L	Elevated GGT may indicate liver impairment or heavy alcohol intake
Alanine aminotransferase (AST)	<45 U/L	Elevated AST may indicate liver impairment or heavy alcohol intake
Metabolic Functioning and Cardiovascular Risk		
HbA1c	>41 mmol/mol	Elevated HbA1c is diagnostic for type 2 diabetes
Serum glucose[a]	3.5–5.4 mmol/L	Elevated serum glucose may indicate insulin resistance or type 2 diabetes

Continued

TABLE 22.4 Laboratory Tests for Mental Health Assessment—cont'd

Test	Normal Range	Clinical Implications of Abnormal Findings
Glucose tolerance	3.5–5.4 mmol/L	Impaired glucose tolerance may indicate type 2 diabetes
Total cholesterol	<5.0 mmol/L	High total cholesterol due to high LDL is a risk factor for vascular disease; high total cholesterol due to high HDL is a risk factor for vascular disease
HDL cholesterol	>1.00 mmol/L	High HDL is protective against atherosclerosis; low levels are a risk factor for cardiovascular disease
Triglycerides	<2.0 mmol/L	High triglycerides is a risk factor for heart disease
LDL cholesterol	<3.4 mmol/L	High LDL is a risk factor for vascular disease
Cholesterol ratio	<4.5	High cholesterol ratio is a risk factor for heart disease
Serum Levels of Psychotropic Medication		
Clozapine	1050–1800 nmol/L	Level needs to be monitored during titration and regularly once treatment is stabilised
Lithium	0.5–1.0 mmol/L	<0.5 is subtherapeutic; >1.0 is potentially toxic
Carbemazepine	17–40 μmol/L	<17 is subtherapeutic; >40 is potentially toxic
Valproic acid	350–700 μmol/L	<350 is subtherapeutic; >700 is potentially toxic
Phenytoin	40–80 μmol/L	<40 is subtherapeutic; >80 is potentially toxic

[a]Nonpregnant, fasting

F, Female; *HDL*, high-density lipoprotein; *LDL*, low-density lipoprotein; *M*, male; *HbA1c*, haemoglobin A1c.

Other Investigations

In addition to laboratory tests there are a range of other investigations that may be considered as part of a comprehensive assessment. For example, every patient should have an electrocardiogram (ECG), both to assess their baseline cardiac functioning and to identify any vulnerability to the effects of prescribed medication. Other tests that might be considered are a CT scan to exclude space occupying lesions or other pathology, magnet resonance imaging (MRI) for more detailed imaging of organs, and an electroencephalogram (EEG) to assess possible abnormalities of brain function. A range of other tests may be considered on the basis of the patient's presenting symptoms.

Mental State Assessment[a]

Mental state assessment is part of every comprehensive assessment and provides a statement of the patient's emotional and cognitive functioning at a single point in time (Huline-Dickens 2013). The importance of focussing the mental state assessment on a single point in time is that it can provide a point of comparison for future assessments. Other elements of the patient's presentation are excluded from the mental state assessment, such as social functioning, history and risk. Many elements of a mental state assessment can be integrated into routine nursing interactions such as the initial assessment interview, reviewing a plan of care or discussing recovery goals. During these interactions the nurse will be able to observe the patient's behaviour, appearance and mood and will gain a good understanding of thought content. However, some elements of mental state assessment require specific enquiry on the part of the nurse. For example, the nurse may need to ask direct questions to test their impression that a patient is disoriented or has problems with memory. Mental state assessment requires both objective observation and empathic communication. Appearance and behaviour can be objectively observed, while to assess the patient's mood the nurse will need to establish rapport and enter into the patient's emotional world. Many situational variables impact on mental state, such as an unfamiliar environment, anxiety or pain, and these can be taken into account when the findings of the mental state assessment are interpreted.

The structured format used for recording a mental state assessment does not mean that the mental state assessment requires a question-and-answer interview. In fact, the opposite is true: a supportive therapeutic conversation will probably provide most of the information required for a mental state assessment. Additional information can be elicited, if necessary, by direct questions, but these should flow naturally from the interaction with the patient. A standardised measure of cognitive functioning can be used to augment a mental state assessment. (See Table 22.1 for standardised assessments of cognitive functioning.)

There is no set format for recording a mental state assessment, but we suggest the BATOMI mnemonic as a useful means of organising the findings (Behaviour and appearance; Affect and mood; Thought and speech; Orientation, cognition and sensorium; Memory; Insight and judgement). An example of a documented mental state assessment using this mnemonic is provided in Box 22.3. The following sections outline the types of observations that can contribute to a mental state assessment.

Behaviour and Appearance

Behaviour and appearance refer to the patient's general appearance and activity. Begin with the most obvious aspects

[a]In this chapter the term 'mental state assessment' is used in preference to 'mental state examination', as the latter implies an objectified evaluation of the patient's mental state, whereas we wish to promote an understanding based on an engaged relationship.

BOX 22.3 Documentation of Mental State Assessment

The following assessment records the mental state of a woman assessed following an overdose of prescribed medication and medical treatment in the emergency department.

Behaviour and Appearance
54-year-old European woman who is attentive to interview, although a little sleepy from lingering effects of overdose. Looks older than her chronological age. Dressed in jeans and T-shirt. Is well groomed and appears well cared for. No unusual movements or mannerisms. Maintains good eye contact. Tearful at times.

Affect and Mood
Affect sad. Intermittently brighter in response to interview. Mood is objectively depressed. She describes her mood as low, rates it at 4 on a 1–10 scale where 1 is the lowest it has been. Not irritable.

Thought and Speech
Thoughts focus on recent events, and her perception that she is not well supported by family members. Returns to the theme of past long-term relationship that ended 12 months ago. Ruminates about abandonment. Limited ability to focus on problem solving in relation to current stressors. Depressive themes: loneliness, undeserving of help, lack of confidence in future. Slow rate of thought and talk. No delusional ideas expressed. No unusual perceptions. Has occasional thoughts of suicide but stresses she would not act on these. Has no specific plan. Gives involvement with grandchildren as a protective factor.

Orientation, Cognition and Sensorium
Alert and oriented to time, place and person. Is aware of the name of the hospital and her current location and the date and time of day. Accurately identifies staff by role or name. Able to perform serial sevens.

Memory
Both short- and long-term memory are intact. She remembers events of the past few days, and more distant. Able to recall 3 objects after 5 minutes.

Insight and Judgement
Identifies that her mood is currently low and has been low for several weeks. Is aware that alcohol has a disinhibiting role when her mood is low, and increases suicidal thoughts. Accepts referral to mental health service and need to review current antidepressant medication. Judgement is unimpaired when not intoxicated.

of behaviour, such as clothing, grooming and hygiene, evidence of self-care or neglect and distinguishing marks such as tattoos, piercings and notable physical features such as scars. This section also includes observations of motor activity and behaviour, such as posture, eye contact, restlessness, tearfulness, nervous mannerisms such as tremors and shaking and behaviour indicating level of interest in the interaction. Attitude towards the assessment process can be seen in appearance, responses, body language and facial expressions. Consider not only what you are observing, but how appropriate it is, taking into account the setting of the assessment. For example, in an assessment in an emergency department you might expect someone to look dishevelled and perhaps sleepy (at least initially). Anxiety about the assessment process will also influence behaviour.

Affect and Mood

Affect and mood have various definitions that sometimes conflict. Both refer to emotional state, with *mood* referring to sustained emotional state (especially as it is experienced by the individual) and *affect* referring to expressed emotion, something that can be observed by the clinician. A skilled clinician can often gauge a patient's mood, especially if a good rapport has been developed and the patient feels safe to communicate their emotional state. However, it is important that patients are given the opportunity to describe their mood. Because this may be difficult for people who are depressed, patients can be asked to rate their mood on a scale of 1 to 10, where 1 is the lowest it has ever been and 10 is the highest. Emotional state can be appropriate or inappropriate to the assessment context—for example, a patient who is elated and buoyant despite an objectively formal context such as a clinical review. Terms sometimes used to describe affect and mood are dysphoric, flat, elevated, depressed, anxious, labile (fluctuating without obvious reason) and restricted. The term 'euthymic' is often used if the patient's mood is neither happy nor sad. In assessing mood, you are using your own emotional state as a means of understanding the emotional state of the patient. Nurses who have established an empathic understanding of a patient will be best able to assess that patient's emotional state.

Thought and Speech

Thought and speech are usually described together (sometimes called thought and talk) and focus on the rate, form and content of thought, and the nature of the patient's verbal communications. It is not possible to assess thoughts directly, so thought is assessed through the indirect medium of speech. Speech is more easily observed as it is the major medium of communication. Aspects of speech are rate (speed of speech), volume, amount of speech, tone and content. Speech that is rapid or slowed, very quiet or loud, hesitant or limited may be significant in the assessment of mental state and should be recorded. For example, rapid or pressured speech might indicate mania or anxiety; quiet or hesitant speech might indicate low mood or anxiety; and loud speech might indicate anger or suspicion. It is important to note whether speech is goal directed, or circumstantial and tangential. This part of the mental state assessment (sometimes called perception) also records any delusional ideas, such as ideas of being influenced by others, paranoid ideas, thoughts that radio or television news is referring to the individual and other forms of disordered thinking. Auditory or other hallucinations are noted in this section of the assessment. It is helpful to describe the nature of voices, whether the patient feels threatened by them or whether they perform an important function for the patient, such as providing company.

Orientation, Cognition and Sensorium

Orientation is easily assessed and may not need direct questioning. Orientation refers to understanding of time, place and person and can be assessed by asking questions about whereabouts, time of day and place. Because these might seem odd questions to some patients it is important to explain that these are part of routine assessment. Cognition refers to the ability to recognise and manipulate information and to perform tasks of reasoning. General interview questions will give some evidence of cognitive functioning. Cognition can also be tested by asking the patient to perform individual tasks from standardised assessments, such as 'serial sevens' (subtracting in sevens starting from 100) or naming different common objects (e.g. pen, book, watch). Disturbances in sensorium are likely to be evident in many interactions, especially in structured interviews. Sensorium can be assessed by observing the patient's attentiveness and ability to keep focussed on tasks. Patients with an altered level of consciousness may show limited ability to attend and fluctuation in attention and awareness.

Memory

Memory involves the capacity to recall information and extends from initial registration of information to recall of information that is years old. Registration can be assessed by asking the patient to repeat back to the nurse the names of three unrelated common objects (e.g. pen, clock, tree). Short-term memory can by assessed by asking for recall of the same three objects after 5 minutes, during which time other discussion takes place. Finally, long-term (or remote) memory involves recall of years-old information such as events from childhood or adolescence.

Insight and Judgement

Insight can be a controversial area of assessment because it is sometimes interpreted as a test of whether the patient agrees with the clinician's opinion about what is happening, in particular whether or not the patient is mentally ill (Baier 2010; Diesfeld & McKenna 2007). Insight is best understood as a patient's perception of their current situation. It is not always helpful to simply record 'lacks insight', as this does not tell us what the patient believes about their problems. Judgement refers to the person's ability to act safely and with understanding of the possible consequences of their actions. A confused person may have markedly impaired judgement and hence be unsafe unless in a situation where they can be observed.

CLINICAL FORMULATION

Once all assessment information has been gathered you will have both a subjective impression of the patient as a person and a set of objective data about the patient. You will also have an understanding of the patient's perceptions of their current problems and how those problems relate to the patient's life history. Clinical formulation is the process of bringing this information together to develop an individualised explanatory account of the patient. Different models of psychological therapy often have their own model of formulation; for example, the cognitive formulation used in cognitive therapy (Persons 2012). In this section we discuss a more general model of formulation, but one that can incorporate psychological understandings of the person.

Clinical formulation is a potentially complex process, but fortunately there are several models available to assist nurses in writing clinical formulations and developing skills in this aspect of assessment. Biological, psychological and social theories help explain the relationships between the various aspects of the patient's history and presentation. Clinical formulation is not undertaken by the clinician alone, although in some literature (e.g. Selzer and Ellen 2014) this is how formulation is described. However, as Crowe et al. (2008) explain, clinical formulation is an opportunity for the nurse and the patient to discuss their different perspectives and negotiate both common understandings and differences in understandings. If the assessment has been a collaborative process throughout, there will be a strong enough relationship between the nurse and the patient to allow this negotiation to occur.

A useful model for developing clinical formulation is the 4 Ps model described by Selzer and Ellen (2010, 2014) and shown in Table 22.5. In this model the 4 Ps (predisposing, precipitating, perpetuating and protective) are used to describe factors that contributed to the development of the current problems, factors that contribute to the persistence of the problem and those that protect the person from the effects of the problem. In addition to the 4 Ps, this model allows for consideration of biological, psychological and social factors. Theoretical and philosophical understandings, such as learning theory, adaptation theory and recovery philosophy, can be used to interpret the contribution of the various factors. Using this model the clinician can focus on factors in any cell of the matrix, depending on what the significant factors are for the individual patient. With some patients there will be a greater emphasis on social factors, while with others psychological or biological factors will be more important.

Clinical formulation is written in narrative form. The clinician and the patient work together to reach agreement regarding how different aspects of the patient's history affect the current presentation. It may not always be possible to reach agreement. In such cases, the formulation is written to reflect the different perspectives of the clinician and the patient (Crowe et al. 2008). The written formulation concludes with a statement about the possible future for the patient and focusses on how strengths and protective factors can be enhanced by support from clinical services. Writing clear, clinical formulations takes practice. A typical difficulty encountered by clinicians is attempting to include too much information. Remember, the clinical history contains all the relevant information about the patient. The formulation is

TABLE 22.5 **Clinical Formulation**

FORMULATION MATRIX			
	Biological	**Psychological**	**Social**
Predisposing	Genetic Birth trauma Brain injury Illness—psychiatric, physical Medication Drugs/alcohol Pain	Personality Modelling Defences (unconscious) Coping strategies Self-esteem Body image Cognition Trauma	Socioeconomic status Culture/spirituality
Precipitating	Medication Drugs/alcohol Trauma Acute illness Pain	Stage of life Grief Loss Treatment Stressors	Work Finances Connections Relationships
Perpetuating	Any of the above factors that are continuing	Any of the above factors that are continuing	Any of the above factors that are continuing
Protective	Physical health	Engagement Insight Adherence Coping strategies Intelligence	Group belonging and affiliations Family and social relationships

(*Source:* Adapted from Selzer, R., Ellen, S., 2010. Psych-Lite: Psychiatry That's Easy to Read. McGraw-Hill, Sydney.)

a selective summary: only the most pertinent information should be included and the emphasis is on how the various factors interact.

DIAGNOSIS

A diagnosis is a definition of a problem, once all available information has been considered.

From a medical perspective, diagnosis is the process of grouping clusters of signs and symptoms into individual illness categories. A definition of diagnosis is:

1. the identification of diseases by the examination of symptoms and signs and by other investigations
2. an opinion or conclusion so reached (Collins Online Dictionary: collinsdictionary.com)

Psychiatrists in the UK tend to use the World Health Organization's International Classification of Diseases (ICD) system to diagnose mental health conditions, rather than the *Diagnostic and Statistical Manual of Mental Disorders* (DSM) (American Psychiatric Association [APA] 2013), which is more commonly used in the United States. Nurses need to be familiar with the diagnostic criteria of the more common mental illnesses and of the diagnostic reasoning process applied to making these diagnoses. An example of the DSM model of diagnosis is provided in Box 22.4, which outlines the diagnostic criteria for major depressive disorder. A full list of all diagnostic criteria is provided in the ICD-10 (WHO 1989) and the DSM-5 (APA 2013). However, a version of the ICD-11 was released in June 2018, to allow Member States to prepare for implementation, with a view to reporting using ICD-11 from 1st January 2022.

TRIAGE

Triage refers to the assessment that takes place when a patient first makes contact with a health service. A patient may present with self-harm, hearing voices, self-neglect or suicidal thoughts. Presentations may involve use of alcohol or other substances. Triage assessments may occur in the emergency department, at community mental health clinics, at ambulance call outs, in primary care settings or in patients' homes. Triage may also be conducted by telephone. The aims of triage are to establish how urgent the problem is, any immediate safety issues and the immediate priorities for health service response. One example of this is the UK Mental Health Triage Scale (Sands et al. 2016).

Questions to be addressed in mental health triage are outlined in Box 22.5. Triage is usually followed by comprehensive assessment, once immediate issues of safety have been addressed.

RISK ASSESSMENT

Risk assessment is a requirement of most mental health service providers and it is therefore important that nurses have an understanding of the language and limitations of risk assessment. However, there is controversy about the value of risk assessment (Ryan et al. 2010; Szmukler 2012; Wand 2012) and about the ability of clinicians to accurately identify patients at high risk and to predict the likelihood of adverse events occurring. The most commonly identified areas of risk are risk to self through self-harm or neglect, risk of violence to others and risk of victimisation. In inpatient settings nurses also need to assess risk of absconding.

BOX 22.4 Diagnostic Criteria for Major Depressive Disorder

A. Five (or more) of the following symptoms have been present during the same 2-week period and represent a change from previous functioning; at least one of the symptoms is either (1) depressed mood or (2) loss of interest or pleasure. (Note: do not include symptoms that are clearly due to a general medical condition.)
  A) Depressed mood most of the day, nearly every day, as indicated by either subjective report (e.g. feels sad or empty) or observation made by others (e.g. appears tearful). Note: in children and adolescents, can be irritable mood.
  B) Markedly diminished interest or pleasure in all, or almost all, activities most of the day, nearly every day (as indicated by either subjective account or observation).
  C) Significant weight loss when not dieting or weight gain (e.g. a change of more than 5% of bodyweight in a month), or decrease or increase in appetite nearly every day. Note: in children, consider failure to make expected weight gains.
  D) Insomnia or hypersomnia nearly every day.
  E) Psychomotor agitation or retardation nearly every day (observable by others, not merely subjective feelings of restlessness or being slowed down).
  F) Fatigue or loss of energy nearly every day.
  G) Feelings of worthlessness or excessive or inappropriate guilt (which may be delusional) nearly every day (not merely self-reproach or guilt about being sick).
  H) Diminished ability to think or concentrate, or indecisiveness, nearly every day (either by subjective account or as observed by others).
  I) Recurrent thoughts of death (not just fear of dying), recurrent suicidal ideation without a specific plan, or a suicide attempt or a specific plan for committing suicide.

B. The symptoms cause clinically significant distress or impairment in social, occupational or other important areas of functioning.

C. The episode is not attributable to the physiological effects of a substance or another medical condition.

(*Source*: Reprinted with permission from the Diagnostic and Statistical Manual of Mental Disorders, 5th edn. American Psychiatric Association.)
NICE Guidelines (2018) Depression in adults: recognition and management [CG90] adopted the DSM-IV diagnostic criteria; however, previous guidelines used the ICD-10.

BOX 22.5 Important Questions for Mental Health Triage

- Does the patient feel safe in their current situation?
- Is the patient at imminent risk of self-harm?
- Is the patient at risk of harming others?
- If there are risks of harm to self or others, does the patient have the means in their possession to carry out that harm?
- Is the patient likely to stay where they are or are they likely to leave?
- How soon does the patient need to be seen?
- Are there physical health problems that may be contributing to the presentation?

Risk assessment is not a separate form of assessment: it is a process that selectively draws on information obtained in the comprehensive assessment to identify the existence of risk, the level of risk and a plan to manage risk. Such an understanding will assist nurses to meet employers' expectations to assess and document risk. A very good summary of risk assessment and management, including the limitations of risk assessment, is provided by Flewett (2010). Flewett makes the important point that risk assessment and management are not about eliminating risk or about predicting the occurrence of adverse events. Rather, they are about understanding the factors that contribute to risk and working with patients to manage that risk. Nurses also need to balance awareness of risk with the positive value of risk in the lives of patients and of the value of learning from the consequences of decisions (Robertson & Collinson 2011) (positive risk taking is discussed in Chapter 23).

Risk assessment tools can assist in the assessment and documentation of risk. Commonly used instruments include the Historical-Clinical-Risk Management-20 (HCR-20) (Douglas & Reeves 2010) for assessing risk of violence and the Beck Scale for Suicide Risk (Beck & Steer 1991) for assessing suicide risk. Some services require clinicians to use a specific instrument. There does not currently appear to be a validated instrument for assessing risk of victimisation, perhaps because the risks are different for different groups—such as those at risk of intimate partner violence, youth at risk of exploitation and people with severe mental illness at risk of violent victimisation. A summary of risk factors for people with severe mental illness at risk of violent victimisation is provided by Chapple et al. (2004). In considering the use of these and other risk assessment instruments it is important to remember that standardised instruments do not replace clinical judgement in assessment (see page 433 for a discussion of the limitations of assessment instruments). Standardised instruments should not be the sole basis of clinical decision making as they are not sufficiently sensitive to identify patients at high risk or to exclude those at low risk. However, standardised instruments have the benefits that they remind clinicians of important areas of assessment, and they help ensure consistent practice across health disciplines, clinical settings and different time points.

In addition to information obtained using standardised instruments, assessment and documentation of risk should take into account the clinician's impression of risk and the collaborative formulation of risk developed with each patient. In reviewing risk instruments for adult psychiatry, Kumar and Simpson (2005) concluded that there were benefits to both actuarial methods (use of checklists and rating scales) and clinical assessment methods (understanding of the individual patient together with consideration of the known risk factors). Assessment of risk always involves static and dynamic risk factors. Static factors are those that are not subject to change, such as gender, history of risk behaviours and age of onset of mental health problems. Dynamic factors are those that are subject to change, such as age, use of substances and available supports. The most common areas of risk assessment are briefly discussed here.

Risk of Violence

Assessing risk of violence involves considering the presence of factors known to contribute to violence together with the nurse's understanding of the patient's current mental state and protective factors. An instrument such as the HCR-20 can help as a prompt, and in some cases might be the service's preferred means of risk assessment (Tully 2017). A history of previous harm to others is strongly associated with future risk, although no individual factor will provide an accurate indicator of current risk. Factors that the nurse can assess for are the patient's engagement with care, available support systems, adherence with prescribed medication, use of alcohol or recreational substances, current level of emotional arousal and ability to use strategies to self-manage anger. Engaging with the patient in relation to risk behaviours can help manage the possibility of future incidents of violence.

Risk of Self-Harm

Self-harm is a common behaviour in people with mental illness, especially those who are acutely distressed. For some patients, self-harm is a means of regulating emotional distress. Risk of self-harm can be a long-term aspect of the lives of some individuals and may fluctuate in response to situational stressors. Factors contributing to risk of self-harm are different for each individual but some common factors include low mood, a sense of abandonment and a history of self-harm. Patients with psychosis may hear voices suggesting or compelling them to harm themselves. Use of alcohol is significantly associated with self-harm, while availability of support networks is a moderating factor.

Risk of Suicide

People with mental illness have a significantly increased risk of suicide compared with the general population (Randall et al. 2014). The risk is markedly increased during transitions in care such as inpatient admission and discharge from hospital (Large et al. 2011). Comorbid substance use is another clinical factor contributing to suicide risk (Bohnert et al. 2010). Other factors associated with suicide risk are recent loss, lack of social support, sense of helplessness, a family history of suicide, a previous suicide attempt and access to means. Suicide risk is higher in men than in women, in younger and older people, and in socially disadvantaged groups. Assessment of suicide risk involves knowledge of risk factors as well assessment of the patient's presenting problem and mental state. Patients should be asked about suicidal thoughts, previous attempts, their intent to act and access to means. It is also important to assess protective factors such as support networks, engagement with treatment, personal belief systems and commitment to future plans. Suicide risk should be documented in the clinical assessment and regularly reviewed.

Risk of Neglect

Self-neglect can be a significant risk for individuals who are depressed, have paranoid ideas about others or have poor support networks. These factors may occur together. They are commonly found in older people (Day et al. 2015) but younger people are also at risk of neglect. Assessment of risk of neglect includes consideration of the patient's mood and energy level, their engagement with others and the availability of supports. Previous incidents of self-neglect indicate a higher level of risk but also provide clues as to what support or intervention might reduce risk.

Risk of Victimisation

People with mental illness are more likely to be victims of crime than others in the community. They are also more likely to have contact with the police, and while police contact may result in diversion to mental health services, it can be an aversive experience. Factors associated with risk of victimisation are female gender, homelessness, substance use, arrest in the past 12 months and poorer social functioning (Chapple et al. 2004). Assessment should include the availability of supports, use of substances and security of accommodation, each of which may be amenable to intervention.

Risk of Absconding

Absconding from inpatient mental health services can be a risk in itself if the patient needs the containment of inpatient care to maintain their safety (Muir-Cochrane et al. 2011). Absconding can also be an indicator of risk, as individuals sometimes leave inpatient services under the influence of a drive to self-harm or to harm others. Factors associated with absconding may be related to the quality of the inpatient environment or to the individual's mental state. Both sets of factors may contribute, and both are modifiable through nursing intervention. From a patient's perspective, absconding might represent an attempt to maintain their personal sense of safety. Exploring patients' reasons for absconding will help to address risk factors.

In Patient Story 22.1 Gareth Edwards provides a patient assessment of the assessment process.

CRITICAL THINKING CHALLENGE 22.6

The chapter lists many different areas of risk for you to consider. Think about one area of risk and why this might be a concern for people with mental illness. How can you help reduce this area of risk in your clinical practice?

ASSESSMENT OF STRENGTHS

Assessment of strengths considers the personal resources patients are able to access to manage their mental health concerns. Many patients have had years of experience of adversity and self-management and have developed individual and interpersonal strategies for preventing and responding to their issues. Patients who are newly presenting to mental health services will also have developed life skills that will be valuable to them in coping with their mental health challenges. As in all areas of mental health nursing assessment, developing a therapeutic relationship is essential for understanding the strengths a patient may have. At times of crisis, patients

PATIENT STORY 22.1 Assessing Assessment

I'd never been in a police cell before. Without a comparison, or a *Lonely Planet Guide to Incarceration*, I assume it was your bog standard police cell. Concrete block walls painted institutional grey with hint of drab, a formidable steel door and a thin bench and/or bed next to a half-wall discreetly housing a metal toilet. So at least I was en suite.

It was very much like a room at an airport hotel, though with possibly a little more charm.

Not exactly what most people would think of as an ideal environment for a 'health assessment'. But then assessment is different in mental health than physical health.

There's no blood tests, MRI scans or even an old man in a leather-elbowed jacket tapping your knee with a fairy hammer. Sometimes you might get a questionnaire, like those Facebook games that tell you if you are 'an extrovert who likes to stay home' or 'an introvert who likes to go out'. But mostly my assessment involved a psychiatrist looking at the way I talked and behaved and deciding if I was fit for society.

In the cell it took less than a minute. Though all it actually did was buy the system some time by sectioning me for 28 days for further assessment. Assessment then became a 24/7 activity. It's hard enough being paranoid without knowing that your every moment is under close scrutiny by people who are writing secret notes about you. Then every week there was 'the day' when you were formally assessed. My most vivid memory was sitting in the ward lounge with over a dozen strangers with clipboards and being asked 'how are you today?'.

'Er ... intimidated and overwhelmed' would have been an accurate answer.

However, assessment in mental health once you are sectioned is less about 'how are you?' and more about 'will this end up in the headlines if you are discharged?' So when asked 'how are you?' the right answer is 'not a threat to myself or others'. Once you have found a way to say and demonstrate that, you are rewarded with your freedom. And then you can really start answering the question 'how am I?'

'Health assessment' in mental health is mostly 'risk assessment'. The small 'health' portion is more like those shape-matching toys toddlers have. If it looks enough like depression, you go through the antidepressants-shaped hole. If it looks enough like mania or psychosis, you go through the antipsychotics-shaped hole. And if you don't fit the holes neatly, you are called 'complex' and pushed through anyway, like a frustrated child pushing a star-shaped block through a square-shaped hole.

And if all this sounds pretty bleak, it is. But the worst part is no-one ever does a 'final assessment' to say you are no longer ill. Like a puppy bought at Christmas time, assessment is for life.

Gareth Edwards

may feel that they have no available strategies, so it is important initially to respond to the patient's current concerns and distress before exploring strengths. Assessment of strengths involves inviting the patient to identify their individual strategies and how they have responded to life challenges in the past. Rather than being the expert, the nurse needs to ask what they can learn from the patient. Examples of individual strengths that patients may identify include pleasurable activities that provide distraction and reduce stress, the availability of family members and friends, spiritual beliefs and skills learnt in stress management and problem solving.

CLASSIFICATION IN PSYCHIATRY

There have been many attempts at developing systems of psychiatric classification. One notable early example is that of psychiatrist Emil Kraepelin in the late nineteenth century. Kraepelin's system, which included just 13 diagnoses, assumed that each mental illness is distinct rather than comprising clusters of symptoms with a significant degree of overlap.

There are two manuals of diagnoses commonly used in psychiatry: the *International Classification of Diseases and Health Related Problems* (ICD) (World Health Organization [WHO] 1989) and the DSM. Since their initial establishment, both manuals have undergone numerous revisions. The most current versions are the ICD-10 (a version of the ICD-11 was released in June 2018, to allow Member States to prepare for implementation, with a view to reporting using ICD-11 from 1st January 2022) and the DSM-5. The ICD-10 is a comprehensive manual of all known diseases, with its fifth chapter being devoted to mental and behavioural disorders, while the DSM-5 exclusively catalogues mental illnesses. The two systems are broadly similar and have become more so in their most recent editions. Both manuals are based on the assumption of distinct illnesses, although there is debate about whether such categorical systems are an accurate reflection of the human experience of distress and illness (Goldberg 2010). For a full analysis of these issues, see Zachar et al. (2014).

Apart from changes in the classification of individual disorders and categories of disorders, another major change with the introduction of the DSM-5 is the withdrawal of the multiaxial diagnostic classification system. This system required clinicians to record the presence of problems in five separate domains: mental illness, personality, physical illness, psychosocial stressors and general adaptive functioning. Although the DSM-5 still requires clinicians to record factors contributing to mental illness, the removal of the requirement to formally record such a wide range of issues is a significant loss in the current system (Kress et al. 2014).

Psychiatric diagnosis is not formally part of the practice of most mental health nurses, but it is important for nurses to have an understanding of the diagnostic process and the criteria for the most commonly used diagnostic categories. Patients may have questions about their diagnoses and nurses need to be able to respond knowledgeably to these questions. In addition, at times nurses may question the diagnosis assigned to a patient in their care and it is important that such questioning is well informed. Understanding diagnoses does not mean that nurses are practising within a biomedical model. Diagnostic models are only one of many frameworks for practice, but they are important because they form part of the common language of mental healthcare. Ethical issues associated with diagnosis are discussed in Chapter 4.

The purpose of diagnosis is to accurately group together people whose clinical symptoms are sufficiently similar, with the aim of optimising treatment and clinical outcomes for each group. Accurate diagnosis is essential to identifying optimal treatment. To assist clinicians in making diagnoses the DSM-5 provides lists of criteria and decision rules about applying those criteria in individual cases. As an example, the DSM-5 diagnostic criteria for major depressive disorder are shown in Box 22.4. This example shows that not everyone who is given a diagnosis of major depressive disorder will have the same symptoms, as only five of the nine criteria need apply. Development of the diagnostic criteria for major depressive disorder was controversial because the new criteria removed the 'bereavement exclusion', a diagnostic rule that prevented clinicians making a diagnosis if the person had experienced a bereavement in the past 2 months. Removal of the bereavement exclusion means that recent bereavement does not prevent a diagnosis of major depressive episode (Flaskerud 2011). A full list of DSM-5 diagnoses and criteria is available on the APA website (www.psychiatry.org).

Despite the statement of explicit criteria and rules in the DSM-5, diagnosis may not be clear, especially for patients new to a mental health service or with complex histories. For those reasons clinicians may defer diagnosis, assign a provisional diagnosis or make a list of differential diagnoses. A differential diagnosis is a list of possible diagnoses, any of which may eventually prove to be the final diagnosis (Baid 2006). Diagnosis should always be regarded as open to revision as clinicians' understanding of the patient develops. Clinicians should also discuss diagnosis with patients and should be prepared to share their uncertainty about diagnosis and the role of diagnosis in clinical care.

CRITICAL THINKING CHALLENGE 22.7

Psychiatric diagnosis is a process of assigning a category to a patient's unique subjective experiences and problems in living. How can you work with patients to help them understand the process of diagnosis and to consider whether their diagnosis accurately reflects their experiences?

MEASURING MENTAL HEALTH OUTCOMES

Mental health outcomes allow clinicians, managers and service funders to determine whether a service has resulted in improvement in patients' clinical and social functioning. Clinical services collect data on outcome measures using standardised instruments administered at regular points in the care pathway. The Health of the Nation Outcome Scales (HoNOS) are the outcome measures most used in services (Wing et al. 1998). Several different forms of the HoNOS are available: the scales measure outcomes in adult mental health services (HoNOS), child and adolescent services (HoNOSCA: Health of the Nation Outcome Scales for Children and Adolescents), services for older adults (HoNOS 65+), forensic mental health services (HoNOS-secure) and services for people with learning disabilities (HoNOS-LD). The HoNOS consists of 12 scales each of which measures a different aspect of mental health or social functioning. Each scale is rated from zero to four in increasing level of severity of problems. The full list of scales and scoring system is outlined in Box 22.6. For services that use HoNOS, guidelines usually require ratings to be completed on service entry, on exit and at defined points for extended periods of service provision. The ratings are completed by clinicians who have undertaken training (to ensure reliability) and who are familiar with each patient's current presentation and problems. Critics have questioned whether measuring standardised outcomes assists in mental health recovery (Lakeman 2004), a view supported by the observation that relatively few patients are aware that clinicians keep records of HoNOS ratings (Guthrie et al. 2008).

BOX 22.6 Health of the Nation Outcome Scales (HoNOS)

Scale 0–4 **Rate 9 if not known**

1. Overactive, aggressive, disruptive or agitated behaviour ☐
2. Nonaccidental self-injury ☐
3. Problem-drinking or drug taking ☐
4. Cognitive problems ☐
5. Physical illness or disability problems ☐
6. Physical with hallucinations & delusions ☐
7. Problems with depressed mood ☐
8. Other mental & behavioural problems ☐
9. Problems with relationships ☐
10. Problems with activities of daily living ☐
11. Problems with living conditions ☐
12. Problems with occupation and activities ☐

Total Score (0–48) ☐☐ ☐

1) Rate each scale in order from 1–12
2) Do not include information rated in an earlier item except for item 10 which is an overall rating
3) Rate the MOST SEVERE problem that occurred during the period rated
4) All scales follow the format:
   - 0 = no problem
   - 1 = minor problem requiring no action
   - 2 = mild problem but definitely present
   - 3 = moderately severe problem
   - 4 = severe to very severe problem

(*Source:* Health of the Nation Outcome Scales (HoNOS). Royal College of Psychiatrists, 1996.)

CONCLUSION

Assessment is one of the foundational skills of mental health nursing. Assessment begins with the person's first contact with mental health services and continues throughout the episode of care. The aim of assessment is to develop an understanding of the person and the problems that have led them to seek mental healthcare. Assessment is based on the development of a therapeutic relationship. It is both a structured process in which the nurse seeks information about many aspects of the life of the patient and a process of exploration in which patients are encouraged and supported to share their experiences with the nurse. Assessment methods include structured and conversational interviews, standardised assessment instruments and diaries recording aspects of functioning such as thoughts, feelings, activities and social interactions. A range of tools are available to assist in the process, including standard assessment templates and standardised assessment instruments. In conducting assessments nurses need to use the standard tools available as well as engage in dialogue in which patients feel safe to share significant aspects of their lives. The tools of mental health nursing assessment provide the structure for the assessment to occur, while the process of assessment allows the nurse to integrate philosophical and theoretical frameworks into the assessment.

EXERCISES FOR CLASS ENGAGEMENT

You are a newly registered nurse working in a community mental health service. One of your roles in the service is to take phone calls from health professionals and members of the public who are considering whether someone they know has a mental illness and would benefit from assessment and treatment. You receive a call from Svetlana, who describes her 19-year-old son (Ivan) as moody and irritable for the past 6 months after losing his job as a shop assistant. Soon after the loss of his job Ivan ended a 12-month relationship with his girlfriend. During the past 6 months he has been drinking excessively but will not discuss his problems with anyone in the family.

1. In mental health telephone triage, it is quite common to have limited information, and rapport with the caller may be tenuous. Refer to the section on page 449 where mental health triage is discussed. Discuss the triage nurse's phone call with Svetlana with members of your class and make a list of six questions you would want to ask at some point during the telephone interview. List the questions in order of priority. What interview skills would you use to ensure that you have the opportunity to ask these questions?
2. Svetlana tells you that Ivan does not know that she is calling as he is currently out of the house. During the telephone interview, how would you work with Svetlana to help her in discussing her concerns with Ivan and supporting him to accept a face-to-face assessment?
3. Two days later Ivan presents at the mental health clinic for a face-to-face assessment. Reflecting on the narrative and descriptive approaches to mental health assessment, how could you use each approach in your assessment of Ivan?
4. In groups of six, consider the standardised assessment instruments listed in Table 22.2. Each group should identify one instrument that could be helpful in gaining a better understanding of what is happening with Ivan and report back to the class on their chosen instrument. In their report, each group should also consider the disadvantages of using a standardised instrument.
5. The face-to-face assessment involves Ivan, his mother and several members of the multidisciplinary team. The assessment interview takes an hour and the team work with Ivan to develop a collaborative understanding of what is happening for him and what the service can do to help. A plan is agreed that you will visit Ivan at home in a week's time. After Ivan has left, the team discuss psychiatric diagnosis. Most agree that Ivan is experiencing an adjustment disorder with depressed mood. In small groups, discuss the place of diagnosis in Ivan's care. The groups should consider:
   a. Whether diagnosis is necessary in order for Ivan to receive appropriate care.
   b. What problems the diagnosis of adjustment disorder with depressed mood might cause for Ivan.
   c. On your visit next week, how you will discuss Ivan's diagnosis with him, what key questions you expect he will have and how you will respond to those questions?

REFERENCES

American Psychiatric Association (APA), 2013. Diagnostic and Statistical Manual of Mental Disorders, fifth ed. APA, Washington.

Babor, T.F., Higgins-Biddle, J.C., Saunders, J.B., Monteiro, M.G., 2001. AUDIT: The Alcohol Use Disorders Identification Test Guidelines for use in primary care. World Health Organization, Geneva.

Baer, L., Blais, M.A., 2010. Handbook of Clinical Rating Scales and Assessment in Psychiatry and Mental Health. Humana Press, New York.

Baid, H., 2006. Differential diagnosis in advanced nursing practice. British Journal of Nursing 15 (18), 1007–1011.

Baier, M., 2010. Insight in schizophrenia: a review. Current Psychiatry Reports 12 (4), 356–361.

Barker, P.J., 2004. Assessment in Psychiatric and Mental Health Nursing: in Search of the Whole Person. Nelson Thornes, Cheltenham, UK.

Beck, A.T., Steer, R.A., 1991. Manual for the Beck Scale for Suicide Ideation. Psychological Corporation, San Antonio, TX.

Bohnert, A.S., Roeder, K., Ilgen, M.A., 2010. Unintentional overdose and suicide among substance users: a review of overlap and risk factors. Drug and Alcohol Dependence 110 (3), 183–192.

Brown, S.J., 1995. An interviewing style for nursing assessment. Journal of Advanced Nursing 21 (2), 340–343.

Brunero, S., Lamont, S., 2009. Systematic screening for metabolic syndrome in consumers with severe mental illness. International Journal of Mental Health Nursing 18 (2), 144–150.

Burke, W.J., Roccaforte, W.H., Wengel, S.P., 1991. The short form of the Geriatric Depression Scale: a comparison with the 30-item form. Journal of Geriatric Psychiatry and Neurology 4 (3), 173–178.

Chapple, B., Chant, D., Nolan, P., Cardy, S., Whiteford, H., McGrath, J., 2004. Correlates of victimisation amongst people with psychosis. Social Psychiatry and Psychiatric Epidemiology 39 (10), 836–840.

Chase, S.K., 2015. The art of diagnosis and treatment. In: Dunphy, L.M., Winland-Brown, J., Porter, B., Thomas, D. (Eds.), Primary Care: The Art and Science of Advanced Practice, fourth ed. FA Davis, Philadelphia.

Clark, L.L., Clarke, T., 2014. Realizing nursing: a multimodal biopsychopharmacosocial approach to psychiatric nursing. Journal of Psychiatric and Mental Health Nursing 21, 564–571.

Coombs, T., Curtis, J., Crookes, P., 2011. What is a comprehensive mental health nursing assessment? A review of the literature. International Journal of Mental Health Nursing 20 (5), 364–370.

Coombs, T., Crookes, P., Curtis, J., 2013a. A comprehensive mental health nursing assessment: variability of content in practice. Journal of Psychiatric and Mental Health Nursing 20 (2), 150–155.

Coombs, T., Curtis, J., Crookes, P., 2013b. What is the process of a comprehensive mental health nursing assessment? Results from a qualitative study. International Nursing Review 60 (1), 96–102.

Crowe, M., Carlyle, D., Farmar, R., 2008. Clinical formulation for mental health nursing practice. Journal of Psychiatric & Mental Health Nursing 15 (10), 800–807.

Cunningham, R., Sarfati, D., Peterson, D., Stanley, J., Collings, S., 2014. Premature mortality in adults using New Zealand psychiatric services. New Zealand Medical Journal 127 (1394), 31–41.

Day, M.R., Mulcahy, H., Leahy-Warren, P., Downey, J., 2015. Self-neglect: a case study and implications for clinical practice. British Journal of Community Nursing 20 (3), 110, 112–115

Day, J.C., Wood, G., Dewey, M., Bentall, R.P., 1995. A self-rating scale for measuring neuroleptic side-effects. Validation in a group of schizophrenic patients. The British Journal of Psychiatry 166 (5), 650–653.

De Hert, M., Correll, C.U., Bobes, J., Cetkovich-Bakmas, M., Cohen, Dan, Asai, I., et al., 2011. Physical illness in patients with severe mental disorders. I. Prevalence, impact of medications and disparities in health care. World Psychiatry 10 (1), 52–77.

DeWit, S.C., O'Neill, P.A., 2014. Fundamental concepts and skills for nursing, fourth ed. Elsevier, St Louis.

Diesfeld, K., McKenna, B., 2007. The unintended impact of the therapeutic intentions of the New Zealand mental health review tribunal. Therapeutic jurisprudence perspectives. Journal of Law and Medicine 14 (4), 552–566.

Douglas, K.S., Reeves, K., 2010. Historical-Clinical-Risk Management-20 (HCR-20) violence risk assessment scheme. In: Otto, R.K., Douglas, K.S. (Eds.), Handbook of violence risk assessment. Routledge, Oxford, pp. 147–186.

Eade, D.M., Henning, D., 2013. Chlamydia screening in young people as an outcome of a HEADSS; Home, Education, Activities, Drug and alcohol use, Sexuality and Suicide youth psychosocial assessment tool. Journal of Clinical Nursing 22 (23–24), 3280–3288.

Elliott, R., 2011. Spirituality, mental health nursing & assessment. Journal of Community Nursing 25 (3), 4–10.

Flaskerud, J., 2011. Grief and depression: are they different? Issues in Mental Health Nursing 32 (5), 338–340.

Flewett, T., 2010. Clinical risk management. An introductory text for mental health clinicians. Elsevier, Sydney.

Folstein, M.F., Folstein, S.E., McHugh, P.R., 1975. 'Mini-mental state': a practical method for grading the cognitive state of patients for the clinician. Journal of Psychiatric Research 12 (3), 189–198.

Foreman, A.C., Hall, C., Bone, K., Cheng, J., Kaplin, A., 2011. Just text me: using SMS technology for collaborative patient mood charting. Journal of Participatory Medicine 3, e45.

Gilbert, C.V., Adamson, S.J., Deering, D.D., 2014. Coexisting addiction and mental health practices of a national addiction workforce. Mental Health and Substance Use 7 (2), 144–156.

Goldberg, D., 2010. Should our major classifications of mental disorders be revised? The British Journal of Psychiatry 196 (4), 255–256.

Guthrie, D., McIntosh, M., Callaly, T., Trauer, T., Coombs, T., 2008. Consumer attitudes towards the use of routine outcome measures in a public mental health service: a consumer-driven study. International Journal of Mental Health Nursing 17 (2), 92–97.

Hankins, M., 2008. The reliability of the twelve-item general health questionnaire (GHQ-12) under realistic assumptions. BMC Public Health 8 (1), 355.

Howard, L., Gamble, C., 2011. Supporting mental health nurses to address the physical health needs of people with serious mental illness in acute inpatient care settings. Journal of Psychiatric and Mental Health Nursing 18 (2), 105–112.

Huline-Dickens, S., 2013. The mental state examination. Advances in Psychiatric Treatment 19 (2), 97–98.

Inouye, S.K., van Dyck, C.H., Alessi, C.A., Balkin, S., Siegal, A.P., Horwitz, R.I., 1990. Clarifying confusion: the confusion assessment method. A new method for detection of delirium. Annals of Internal Medicine 113, 941–948.

Jaber, F.S., Mahmoud, K.F., 2015. Risk tools for the prediction of violence: 'VRAG, HCR-20, PCL-R'. Journal of Psychiatric and Mental Health Nursing 22 (2), 133–141.

Kellerman, G.M., 2011. Abnormal Laboratory Results, third ed. McGraw-Hill, Sydney.

Kress, V.E., Barrio Minton, C.A., Adamson, N.A., Paylo, M.J., Pope, V., 2014. The removal of the multiaxial system in the DSM-5: implications and practice suggestions for counselors. The Professional Counselor 4 (3), 191–201.

Kumar, S., Simpson, A.I., 2005. Application of risk assessment for violence methods to general adult psychiatry: a selective literature review. Australian and New Zealand Journal of Psychiatry 39 (5), 328–335.

Lakeman, R., 2004. Standardized routine outcome measurement: pot holes in the road to recovery. International Journal of Mental Health Nursing 13 (4), 210–215.

Large, M., Sharma, S., Cannon, E., Ryan, C., Nielssen, O., 2011. Risk factors for suicide within a year of discharge from psychiatric hospital: a systematic meta-analysis. Australian and New Zealand Journal of Psychiatry 45 (8), 619–628.

Larner, A., 2013. Addenbrooke's Cognitive Examination–Revised (ACE–R): pragmatic study of cross–sectional use for assessment of cognitive complaints of unknown etiology. International Journal of Geriatric Psychiatry 28 (5), 547–548.

Lommen, M.J., Restifo, K., 2009. Trauma and posttraumatic stress disorder (PTSD) in patients with schizophrenia or schizoaffective disorder. Community Mental Health Journal 45 (6), 485–496.

MacNeela, P., Scott, A., Treacy, P., Hyde, A., 2010. The know: cognitive and social factors in mental health nursing assessment. Journal of Clinical Nursing 19 (9–10), 1298–1306.

McPherson, A., Martin, C.R., 2010. A narrative review of the Beck Depression Inventory (BDI) and implications for its use in an alcohol–dependent population. Journal of Psychiatric and Mental Health Nursing 17 (1), 19–30.

Muir-Cochrane, E., Mosel, K., Gerace, A., Esterman, A., Bowers, L., 2011. The profile of absconding psychiatric inpatients in Australia. Journal of Clinical Nursing 20 (5–6), 706–713.

National Institute of Health and Care Excellence (NICE), 2011. Service user experience in adult mental health: improving the experience of care for people using adult NHS mental health services [CG136]. Available at: https://www.nice.org.uk/guidance/cg136/ifp/chapter/what-should-happen-during-an-assessment-at-mental-health-services. Accessed: 22 November 2018.

National Institute of Health and Care Excellence (NICE), 2018. Depression in adults: recognition and management [CG90]. Available at: https://www.nice.org.uk/guidance/cg90. Accessed: 22 November 2018.

Nursing and Midwifery Council (NMC), 2014. Standards for competence for registered nurses. Available at: https://www.nmc.org.uk/globalassets/sitedocuments/standards/nmc-standards-for-competence-for-registered-nurses.pdf. Accessed: 22 November 2018.

Nursing and Midwifery Council (NMC), 2018. The Code: Professional Standards of Practice and Behaviour for Nurses, Midwives and Nursing Associates. Available at: https://www.nmc.org.uk/globalassets/sitedocuments/nmc-publications/nmc-code.pdf. Accessed: 22 November 2018.

O'Brien, A.J., De Souza, R., Baker, M., 2016. Cultural safety. In: Barker, P. (Ed.), Psychiatric and Mental Health Nursing: the Craft of Caring, third ed. Hodder Arnold, London.

Patterson, W.M., Dohn, H.H., Bird, J., Patterson, G.A., 1983. Evaluation of suicidal patients: the SAD PERSONS scale. Psychosomatics 24 (4), 343–349.

Persons, J.B., 2012. The Case Formulation Approach to Cognitive Behavior Therapy. Guilford Press, New York.

Randall, J.R., Walld, R., Finlayson, G., Sareen, J., Martens, P.J., Bolton, J.M., 2014. Acute risk of suicide and suicide attempts associated with recent diagnosis of mental disorders: a population-based, propensity score–matched analysis. Canadian Journal of Psychiatry 59 (10), 531–538.

Rasic, D., Hajek, T., Alda, M., Uher, R., 2013. Risk of mental illness in offspring of parents with schizophrenia, bipolar disorder, and major depressive disorder: a meta-analysis of family high-risk studies. Schizophrenia Bulletin 40 (1), 28–38.

Robertson, J.P., Collinson, C., 2011. Positive risk taking: whose risk is it? An exploration in community outreach teams in adult mental health and learning disability services. Health, Risk & Society 13 (2), 147–164.

Ryan, C., Nielssen, O., Paton, M., Large, M., 2010. Clinical decisions in psychiatry should not be based on risk assessment. Australasian Psychiatry 18 (5), 398–403

Sands, N., Elsom, E., Colgate, R., Haylor, H., 2016. Development and inter-rater reliability of the UK Mental Health Triage Scale. International Journal of Mental Health Nursing 25 (4), 330–336.

Selzer, R., Ellen, S., 2010. Psych-lite: Psychiatry That's Easy to Read. McGraw-Hill, Sydney.

Selzer, R., Ellen, S., 2014. Formulation for beginners. Australasian Psychiatry 22 (4), 397–401.

Stewart, J.S., 2012. A critical appraisal of motivational interviewing within the field of alcohol misuse. Journal of Psychiatric and Mental Health Nursing 19 (10), 933–938.

Szmukler, G., 2012. Risk assessment for suicide and violence is of extremely limited value in general psychiatric practice. Australian and New Zealand Journal of Psychiatry 46 (2), 173–174.

Tambuyzer, E., Van Audenhove, C., 2013. Service user and family carer involvement in mental health care: divergent views. Community Mental Health Journal 49 (6), 675–685.

Tully, J., 2017. HCR-20 shows poor field validity in clinical forensic psychiatry settings. Evidence-Based Mental Health 20, 95–96.

Wand, T., 2012. Investigating the evidence for the effectiveness of risk assessment in mental health care. Issues in Mental Health Nursing 33, 2–7.

Warden, S., Spiwak, R., Sareen, J., Bolton, J.M., 2014. The SAD PERSONS scale for suicide risk assessment: a systematic review. Archives of Suicide Research 18 (4), 313–326.

Welsh, E.R., McEnany, G.P., 2015. Approaches to reduce physical comorbidity in individuals diagnosed with mental illness. Journal of Psychosocial Nursing & Mental Health Services 53 (2), 32.

Wing, J.K., Beevor, A.S., Curtis, R.H., Park, S.B., Hadden, S., Burns, A., 1998. Health of the Nation Outcome Scales (HoNOS). Research and development. The British Journal of Psychiatry 172 (1), 11–18.

World Health Organization (WHO), 1989. ICD-10: International Statistical Classification of Diseases and Related Health Problems, 10th revision. WHO, Geneva.

Zachar, P., Stoyanov, D.S., Aragona, M., Jablensky, A. (Eds.), 2014. Alternative Perspectives on Psychiatric Validation: DSM, ICD, RDoC, and beyond. Oxford University Press, Oxford.

FURTHER READING

Sands, N., Elsom, S., Berk, M., Hosking, J., Prematunga, R., Gerdtz, M., 2014. Investigating the predictive validity of an emergency department mental health triage tool. Nursing & Health Sciences 16 (1), 11–18.

World Health Organization (WHO), 2018. ICD-11 for Mortality and Morbidity Statistics (ICD-11 MMS) 2018 version. Available at: https://icd.who.int/browse11/l-m/en. Accessed: 22 October 2018.

USEFUL WEBSITES

Diagnostic and Statistical Manual of Mental Disorders, fifth ed. (DSM-5), www.dsm5.org

Health of the Nation Outcome Scales, www.rcpsych.ac.uk/clinicalservicestandards/honos.aspx

International Statistical Classification of Diseases and Related Health Problems 10th Revision, http://apps.who.int/classifications/icd10/browse/2016/en

Mental health assessment, www.nhs.uk (enter 'mental health assessment')

Psychiatric rating scales, www.cnsforum.com/educationalresources/ratingscales/psychiatry

Risk assessment (information about the HCR-20 instrument), http://hcr-20.com

Strengths-based assessment, www.iriss.org.uk/resources/strengths-based-approaches-working-individuals

23

Challenging Behaviour, Risk and Responses

Scott Brunero, Scott Lamont

KEY POINTS

- Challenging behaviours are common in the context of mental healthcare.
- Challenging behaviour does not mean a challenging patient.
- Challenging behaviour occurs in the context of patient distress, anxiety and past experiences of mental healthcare.
- A behaviour that is challenging to one nurse may not to be challenging to another.
- Nurses should maintain a focus on the patient as a whole person, not only the behaviour in a moment in time.
- How a nurse behaves influences how a patient will respond.
- Nurses need to practise reflectively and be mindful of their own behaviour.
- Professional supervision and ongoing professional development will assist nurses in maintaining skills to manage challenging behaviour.

KEY TERMS

aggression
agitation
challenging behaviour
difficult behaviour
empathy
legal issues
limit setting
manipulation
person centred
reflection
risk analysis
self-harm
trauma

LEARNING OUTCOMES

The material in this chapter will assist you to:

- identify and describe different types of challenging behaviour.
- develop and maintain therapeutic relationships with patients who present with challenging behaviour.
- understand nursing staff, patient and environmental factors associated with challenging behaviour.
- understand risk in the context of challenging behaviour.
- understand general principles of responding to challenging behaviour.
- identify specific approaches to managing challenging behaviour.
- become familiar with self-care concepts when responding to challenging behaviour.

INTRODUCTION

It has been argued that the nurse–patient relationship is central to nursing care. Nurses in general are in continuous and direct contact with patients and, as such, spend extended periods of time with them. Continuous contact places nurses in a unique position to develop therapeutic relationships with patients through processes of collaboration, inclusiveness, mutuality and respect. However, there may be times when the relationship nurses have with patients is tested, placing nurses in a difficult position and facing challenging behaviour (Stein-Parbury 2014).

'Challenging behaviour' is a term used by nurses to describe behaviour that disrupts relationships with others and complicates healthcare delivery—for example, aggression, manipulation, self-harm, suicide and psychosis-related behaviour. The terms 'difficult behaviour', 'problem behaviour', 'difficult patient' and 'behaviours of concern' have all been used to describe challenging behaviour (Farrell et al. 2010). Challenging behaviour occurs in inpatient units, community settings, emergency departments, general hospitals and primary care settings.

The causes of challenging behaviour are numerous and do not rest solely with the patient (Koekkoek et al. 2011a). Challenging behaviour is best seen theoretically as 'socially constructed', which means the behaviour arises because of multiple realities or reasons. How nurses interact with patients, and how nurses interpret their own thoughts, language and behaviour and understand what this means for patients sets out how we understand challenging behaviour. The approach taken in this chapter is from a social constructionist theory called 'symbolic interactionism' (Blumer 1969). Symbolic interactionism is concerned with how people create subjective 'meanings' towards objects, events and behaviours in others. It argues that people behave and interact with others based on what they believe, not just what is objectively true. People interpret one another's behaviour and through these interpretations create social relationships. This approach can help us to understand our role in interpreting what patients 'mean' when they engage in challenging behaviour and can guide us to how we should behave.

The material in this chapter will assist you to engage in healthy relationships with patients, understand the most common types of challenging behaviour encountered by nurses, be aware of antecedents to challenging behaviour, recognise when challenging behaviour is present, develop responses and strategies for managing challenging behaviour, understand what people mean when they engage in challenging behaviour and become self-aware regarding your own emotions and care needs when responding effectively to challenging behaviour.

CHALLENGING BEHAVIOUR

Types of Challenging Behaviour Within Mental Healthcare

Many challenging behaviours occur within mental health settings. A key skill of mental health nurses is to interpret and understand patients with high levels of distress, to assist them in their navigation of healthcare systems, to monitor and manage their own distress and to manage conflict in interpersonal relationships (Stein-Parbury 2014). Knowing whether a behaviour is challenging or not can be very subjective and individual; it may depend on the skill of the nurse or the social setting the nurse is in. Commonly encountered challenging behaviours that are reported in the literature include:

- aggression (verbal and physical threats, shouting, conflict, nonadherence, absconding)
- manipulation (splitting, demanding attention or that special conditions are met)
- self-harm and suicidal behaviour (cutting, ingesting poisons, overdose)

These behaviours are not mutually exclusive: they may occur in combination, or all at once, frequently or infrequently, and can be seen across the diagnostic groups in mental health settings. Nurses working within the mental health setting will experience some or a range of these challenging behaviours in the course of their clinical practice. Responding to challenging behaviour requires a wide range of nursing skills. It is therefore essential to understand the social context and circumstances in which challenging behaviour occurs (Farrell & Salmon 2010; Farrell et al. 2010).

Understanding the Context in Which Challenging Behaviour Occurs

Challenging behaviour usually occurs in the context of a multitude of factors. An understanding of the social context within which challenging behaviour occurs is essential in identifying the numerous factors that precede and influence the course of the behaviour. For example, staff and patients often have different perceptions of why challenging behaviours are present; while staff may cite patient factors, patients may site staff factors (Sambrano & Cox 2013). The reality is that a range of socially determined factors including staff, patient, environmental, cross-cultural and social factors act as precipitants of challenging behaviours (Farrell & Salmon 2010).

Staff Factors

Challenging behaviours often occur as a result of what we as nurses do or, in some circumstances, don't do. We may not always be conscious of how we are perceived by patients, or how our behaviour influences the behaviour of patients. Our knowledge, skills and attitudes and subsequent behaviours become an important aspect of preventing, mitigating and managing challenging behaviours.

Developing therapeutic relationships with patients is essential in the context of challenging behaviour. This requires commitment from you as a nurse to engage purposefully with patients in a person-centred manner: developing intimate knowledge of the patient as a person; showing respect and being courteous; actively listening to concerns, fears and frustrations; responding in an empathic manner; looking for meaning behind the behaviour (for example, frustration at being detained under the mental health act directed at members of staff; and communicating a genuine desire to help (see Chapter 1 on the effective nurse). Nurses who are unable or unwilling to facilitate effective therapeutic relationships are likely to encounter more challenging behaviours as a consequence (Stein-Parbury 2014).

Developing therapeutic relationships can be easier said than done and may be compromised by a range of personal factors. For example, nurses may have personal issues that compromise their ability to engage therapeutically. This includes the nurse's own mental health and personality style, current stressors in the nurse's life, previous experience (or inexperience) with challenging behaviour, tiredness and illness (Koekkoek et al. 2011a, 2011b). Any of these factors can contribute to an interaction style that leads to a perception that nurses are not interested or are simply ignoring the needs of patients. Furthermore, nurses who are impatient, controlling, authoritarian or coercive in their interactions with patients are less likely to build positive relationships and to achieve desirable outcomes in managing challenging behaviour (Björkdahl et al. 2010).

Patient Factors

Patients may experience challenging behaviour in the context of psychotic disorders; adjustment disorders; mood, anxiety and personality disorders; organic disorders; drug and alcohol intoxication or withdrawal; intellectual disability; brain injury; being stigmatised or marginalised; or experiences of previous trauma, or trauma-related mental healthcare. All of these can limit a patient's ability to engage purposefully in the healthcare that nurses provide.

A range of symptoms associated with psychotic disorders may increase the likelihood of challenging behaviour. Symptoms can include thought disorder, hallucinations and delusions—in particular, where patients may be paranoid, suspicious, fearful or frightened. Patients who are cognitively compromised may present challenging behaviour as a result of anxiety, confusion and disorientation. Challenging behaviour is also associated with the increased energy, disinhibition and irritability associated with mood disorders (mania), making care delivery challenging. This may lead to frustration, helplessness or catastrophic thinking and to difficulties engaging with patients. Patients with a low mood typically seen in depressive disorder may be difficult to engage in their own self-care and other daily activities, which may require constant prompting from the nurse. Patients at risk of self-harm behaviours may need close monitoring and observations of behaviour, with constant efforts to engage in dialogue. Patients with personality vulnerabilities may have a heightened perception of rejection or humiliation, particularly when healthcare concerns or requests are ignored or dismissed. Some patients may have poor impulse control as a feature of their personality, while patients with narcissistic personality styles may present with excessive demands or entitlement of nursing staff time. Factors such as fatigue, pain and physical comorbidities influence patients' quality of life and subsequently their psychological and emotional wellbeing.

If patients are not involved in discussions and planning in relation to their care, they will be unaware of what is expected of them. Mental health problems often adversely influence a person's control over aspects of their life; therefore, processes of partnership, inclusion and engagement can help mitigate some of the patient factors mentioned in this section.

Environmental Factors

Health staff in general are often unaware of the effect of the environment on the wellbeing of patients. Environmental factors become part of our contextual understanding of challenging behaviour. However, the physical environment should not be viewed in isolation from system or operational aspects such as the infrastructure, policies and procedures that govern its operation. Coercive or restrictive processes that limit inclusion and choice for patients, suboptimal communication with unclear care plans, and staff caught in a reactive bind because of busy workloads and competing systemic demands are likely to experience increased frustration and consequently the presence of challenging behaviour (Shefer et al. 2014).

Many aspects of the environments in which nurses work are beyond our control: we may practise in ageing facilities that are no longer commensurate with modern care, and capital works funding may be scarce in relation to maintenance, improvement and renovation. However, being mindful of environmental aspects is essential to understanding challenging behaviour and empathising with patients, which provides the best chance of mitigating or even preventing challenging behaviour. Frustration, high expressed emotion and anger are more likely to be present in poorly structured environments that are aesthetically unappealing, noisy and crowded, too hot/too cold, devoid of natural light and lacking in private space (dormitories versus single rooms) (Shefer et al. 2014). There is a need to balance the design of inpatient wards so as not to overstimulate aroused or agitated patients while not understimulating withdrawn or depressed patients. Person-centred design using the aforementioned attributes can lead to better cognitive, motivational and emotive processes in both patients and staff. Sensory modulation or the use of specific equipment and modification of the physical and social environment have been shown to assist patients in reducing their high expressed emotions that may lead to challenging behaviour (Sutton & Nicholson 2011).

Cross-Cultural Factors

Diverse cultures have behavioural and communication nuances that may be interpreted variously by nurses from different cultural backgrounds. Behaviours that appear challenging within one culture may be acceptable within another. Therefore, the need to be culturally aware has significant implications for nurses in the context of challenging behaviours (McCann et al. 2014). In some Asian societies it is not culturally appropriate to show overt emotional reactions in public, and in some Middle Eastern cultures women may not be allowed in the same room as a man unless accompanied by a relative. Both of these situations, if poorly managed by nurses, may be precursors to challenging behaviour (Russell et al. 2014).

Nurses need to be aware of their own cultural biases and potential misconceptions and tendency to subscribe to myths about particular cultural groups. Providing culturally congruent care in the context of challenging behaviour may give the nurse an opportunity to understand why someone is behaving the way they are, to prevent the behaviour escalating, and the knowledge to approach the behaviour with confidence (Perry et al. 2015a).

Social Factors

Mental illness in our society has been impacted by the media and public perceptions, and this has resulted in the labelling of patients with mental illness as at risk, dangerous, difficult, absconders and/or frequent flyers (Livingston & Boyd 2010). The power of these negative labels can influence how we as professionals engage with people. According to symbolic interactionist theory (Blumer 1969), when these labels are attributed to people they can consequently be adopted by them, and individuals may therefore engage in behaviour that perpetuate these labels. As nurses we must be mindful of the language we use when relating to patients and how we engage them, by not proliferating negative labels that exist more broadly in society about mental illness.

Models of Care That Can Reduce or Mitigate Challenging Behaviour

Care cultures that are risk-focussed, coercive or restrictive in nature are likely to lead to negative interpersonal relationships and dynamics, and subsequent increased prevalence of challenging behaviours. Being aware of your own identity and practice within such cultures is essential to achieving optimum care outcomes. As such, healthcare planning and models of care become prominent in mitigating challenging behaviours. Patient-focussed frameworks adopt strengths-based approaches to care. Models underpinned by such a framework seek to actively involve patients as partners in all aspects of care provision and not as passive recipients of care. Thus, shared decision making and patient-led decision making enhance goal planning, care options and subsequent outcomes. Known variously as 'person centred' or 'patient centred', such models are proposed as being 'underpinned by values of respect for persons, individual right to self-determination, mutual respect and understanding' (McCormack et al. 2013).

These models operate on the premise that only patients can understand the real experience and journey of being a patient, therefore they are the key stakeholders in planning and discussions about care and so need to be active, valued and empowered throughout. Studies exploring strengths-based approaches have identified improvements in quality-of-life indicators, confidence, self-esteem, self-advocacy and self-care (Sclafani & Piren 2010). Strengths-based approaches focus unsurprisingly on strengths, abilities and empowerment—a shift from traditional problem-based care approaches, which largely ignore strengths and positive abilities that help fulfil wellbeing. Strengths-based approaches effect more purposeful engagement with patients, help maintain a sense of control over their decision making and lead to more positive experiences of care. They may also go some way to mitigating challenging behaviour.

There are various specific patient-focussed models.

- The recovery model (or recovery approach) adopts an approach whereby the patient's potential for recovery is paramount and supported by a network of personal and professional relationships. Recovery has less of an emphasis on outcomes and instead focusses on the patient's personal journey, instilling and maintaining hope, a positive sense of self and meaning, a secure base and social inclusion within a paradigm of empowerment and flourishing (Slade et al. 2014).
- The tidal model focusses on the ebb and flow of personal human experience and aims to empower patients in their own recovery with an emphasis on the power of their own self and wisdom, as opposed to health professionals directing this (Barker & Buchanan-Barker 2010).
- Solution-focussed (brief) therapy is a goal-directed psychotherapeutic partnership that focusses on what patients want to achieve in the here and now and in the future. While the relevance of past experience is not ignored, it is not an emphasis or focal point of care (Franklin et al. 2012).
- Trauma-informed care adopts the principle that only a patient who has experienced trauma can truly understand the journey of healing. The unique skills, attributes and resilience that have enabled trauma survivors to survive are emphasised within a strengths-based framework and supported by health professionals (Hopper et al. 2010).

These patient-focussed frameworks can be adopted as collaborative models of care or as individual philosophical frameworks for interpersonal relationships with patients. In doing so, purposeful therapeutic relationships can be enhanced and salient aspects of challenging behaviour mitigated. Nurses must be mindful that in order to engage purposefully with patients, they must engage in activities that promote self-care in themselves, in order to achieve desired outcomes.

Case Study 23.1 by Irene Gallagher reflects the importance of looking beyond the external manifestation of challenging behaviour. Note the interactions between the people in Irene's story, how the nurse moved beyond the initial 'labels' given to the patient and how the nurse was able to use objects in the environment to develop a social bond or therapeutic rapport. Adaptive and flexible frameworks of care will enhance relationships with individual patients.

PREPAREDNESS FOR ENGAGING CHALLENGING BEHAVIOUR

Professional Boundaries and Challenging Behaviour

There are several principles that nurses can follow to ensure they have a solid foundation when providing care to someone with challenging behaviour: these principles start with how the nurse behaves. Nurses are bound by professional practice guidelines through their nurse registration bodies. Professional boundaries can be thought of as the space between the professional's power and the patient's vulnerability. This space needs to be observed and maintained to ensure a beneficial outcome for the patient (Stein-Parbury 2014). Table 23.1 outlines some of the differences between social and professional relationships.

So what occurs within professional relationships that makes a safe and effective practitioner? An expectation of the nurse is that they have a professional body of knowledge, skills and attitudes that can be used to improve the patient's health status. The following elements could describe a poor professional relationship: cynicism, judgemental attitudes, sexual intimacy, rudeness, being patronising, developing dependency, showing favouritism, playing one person off against another, showing minimal care, neglect or punitiveness (Stein-Parbury 2014).

Nurses' Self-Care and Challenging Behaviour

The many rewards that mental health nursing brings can be compromised by environments or relationships that have high prevalence of challenging behaviours. It may come as no surprise that for nurses to engage therapeutically in relationships with patients, they must be aware of and take care of their own emotional and psychological wellbeing. The stressful nature of nursing in general is well recognised (Fiabane et al. 2013; Perry et al. 2015b) and may be more prevalent when presented with challenging patient behaviours (Bowers 2014).

CASE STUDY 23.1 Irene Gallagher: the importance of therapeutic engagement

As a peer worker, I place great value on supporting a person with lived experience of mental distress with their own personal recovery journey, which may include fostering hope, self-determination, choice and intrinsically supporting them to connect with others in developing trusting relationships. Some may proclaim this to be the essence of the peer-to-peer relationship as mutuality and reciprocity. Having said this, I don't see that fostering relationships which support an individual's personal recovery journey belongs solely to peer workers; in fact, I have both personal experience as well as having been witness to seeing the wonderful connections that begin and unravel in the therapeutic relationship.

One such therapeutic engagement which comes to mind is a patient who had been labelled by the system as being challenging and hard to engage with; lost in their own world of what the medical profession would label as 'delusional'. This individual was in fact difficult to engage with, loud and verbally abusive to everyone around them. No-one wanted to engage with this person, staff or patients, for fear of verbal backlash or perhaps a fear of not knowing what approach to use with someone in this situation.

However, one nurse chose to find a way of working with and connecting with this person, on some different level. Curiously, I asked the nurse how she had established these connections, how was it that she was able to communicate and work with this person. Interestingly, the nurse responded by noting that she had worked out that the patient liked to have their hair brushed, and when the nurse brushed the patient's hair the patient would come into 'our' reality. From here, the two were able to communicate in a way that they were previously unable to. Similarly, the nurse discovered that a gentle touch on the patient's forearm had a similar effect and they were able to have meaningful discussions such as talking about the patient's hope and dreams for their future, what treatments worked and did not work for them during their hospitalisation.

Those around perhaps put this positive relationship down to luck; however, the reality was that this nurse had taken the time to connect with the patient, to spend quality time getting to know the individual, using the therapeutic relationship to actively engage and involve the patient in their own care. Time was taken to listen intently, to explore the patient's values and what made meaning for them, while supporting the individual to participate in their recovery journey.

Engaging in reflective practice with the nurse supported how much the nurse had gained from working in this way and prioritising the development of the therapeutic relationship for all it holds: working from an empathic approach, developing rapport and trust, and approaching the collaborative work ahead as a team with mutual understanding and respect. Everyone has that connection waiting to be found—and in this scenario, one nurse found it.

TABLE 23.1 Difference Between Social and Professional Relationships

Social Relationships	Professional
Open-ended time period	Restricted to period of care
Personal choice	Restricted choice
Both parties' needs considered	Patient's needs predominant
Multipurpose	Primary purpose is care
Sympathy	Empathy
Confiding	Confidential
Tolerant to personal limit	Professional tolerance
Inconsistent	Consistent
Judgemental	Non-judgemental
Unstructured	Structured
Personal responsibility	Professional responsibility
Personal boundaries	Professional boundaries

Recent evidence within acute settings has highlighted that nursing in general can have psychological and emotional consequences for nurses. For example, a study of 382 nurses by Perry et al. (2015b) highlighted that 14% (n = 53) reported having a history of common mental disorders (stress, anxiety, depression). In the same study, there was high prevalence of symptoms potentially indicative of mental health–related issues, with 248 (65.1%) reporting they had experienced symptoms such as headaches, severe tiredness, anxiety, sleep problems and depression sometimes or often in the previous 12 months. Maintaining your own health therefore becomes a priority in delivering optimal therapeutic care, particularly where challenging behaviours exist.

Being self-aware and able to evaluate your own actions and behaviours will help you to engage therapeutically with patients. This may be easier said than done, however, as we are often unaware of the emotional labour and stress that the competing demands involved in contemporary mental healthcare place upon us. Some individuals naturally engage in reflective thinking to enhance self-awareness, while others require some formal structure to engage in this practice. It may be that as mental health nursing is your chosen specialty, you have a natural tendency for critical thinking, challenge and reflection.

The following workload practices can help in maintaining psychological and emotional wellbeing: working collaboratively where the workload is shared and delegated appropriately; being honest and transparent about your limitations (we all have bad days) but also maintaining professional conduct; and engaging in more formal, structured processes of reflective practice and clinical supervision. Clinical supervision within mental health is a practice endorsed across all professional groups, particularly nursing. The process has a focus on personal and professional development in the context of safe and effective patient care

(Brunero & Lamont 2012). Although there is a dearth of research within this area, attention to its effects and benefits is growing and is proposed as a key feature in reducing the emotional labour associated with nursing practice. Central to clinical supervision is the opportunity for protected 'time out' from clinical activity, spent with an experienced nurse who supports and guides processes of reflection and structured discussion. Reflection involves processes of enlightenment as to what nurses do and how we behave. During these processes the nurse may reflect on what they did, why they did it and implications for patients, colleagues and wider professional and ethical practice (Brunero & Lamont 2012).

There is a role for nurses to engage each other about the emotions evoked in them: the more transparent we are about these emotions, the more adaptive and self-aware we become in engaging challenging behaviour successfully (Bailey & Clarke 2013). Reflective questioning can help you to gain some control over your response to challenging behaviour, allowing you to maintain a calm and professional manner with patients.

CRITICAL THINKING CHALLENGE 23.1

Think about a situation that you were involved in or observed that was managed well or you believe could have been managed differently. Write down some notes to the following questions:

1. What were the context and/or the key issues preceding the situation?
2. What happened? Who was involved and what was each person's role? What was the outcome?
3. Could the situation have been managed differently? If so, how?
4. What are the implications for the patient or other patients?
5. What have you learned from this situation? Have you identified any learning needs?
6. How can you incorporate your learning into future practice?

How Nurses Behave

As nurses, we need to be aware of our own expectations of a patient's behaviour. Having high levels of expectation that a patient will change their behaviour completely and quickly and/or express gratitude for your help may be unhelpful to you. How you respond to challenging behaviour can have a significant impact on the outcome of the strategies employed to reduce these behaviours. Unhelpful nursing responses include avoiding the patient and minimising the issue. Such responses may be seen with patients who are demanding of care, constantly approaching the nurse's office space or persistently phoning a nurse in a community setting. Taking the avoidance approach often leads the patient to escalate their behaviour as they feel that their needs are not being met. While nurses may not want to encourage negative behaviour, there is still a need to engage the patient in this instance.

It is important to recognise the emotions evoked in you (Dahl et al. 2012), sometimes known as 'countertransference' (for further discussion of transference and countertransference, see Chapter 24). If you respond to anger from a patient by being angry yourself or respond to manipulative behaviour by being punitive in return, these responses are unhelpful and may effect an increase in the challenging behaviour. Therefore, being aware of your own emotional responses to challenging behaviour becomes an integral part of managing these behaviours.

How to Manage Your Own Emotions

When someone is displaying challenging behaviours in any relationship you will need to be able to make sense of and manage your own emotions and behaviour (Dahl et al. 2012). The natural response we have, known as the 'fight or flight response', is often evoked when people are threatening, angry and/or manipulative, resulting in an immediate natural response to defend yourself (Roberts & Grubb 2014). Nurses should be aware that the fight or flight response is normal and you should expect it to occur. Some of the physical signs that you may experience include:

- increased pulse rate and blood pressure
- shallow, rapid respirations
- muscular tension
- dry mouth
- excessive perspiration

There are also a range of psychological symptoms that you may experience following a fight or flight response, such as:

- irritability and impatience
- frequent ruminating, worry and anxiety
- moodiness
- feeling sad or upset
- poor concentration, memory lapses
- ambivalence and feeling overwhelmed, or inability to face even minor problems

To assist you in managing your response to challenging behaviours, a self-control plan can be helpful. For example, concentrating on your breathing or counting to five before you engage someone may help you to respond in a calm and measured way. Inner dialogues are also posited as a strategy for successfully approaching challenging situations. For example, if you approach a situation with a negative attitude that things are not going to go well, this will probably influence your behaviour and resulting outcome. Be aware of what you are telling yourself or thinking to yourself. Thinking the worst, or catastrophic thinking, can lead you to behave in a negative way (e.g. 'This patient will never change' or 'I can't nurse this patient any more').

Conversely, having an inner dialogue that you can negotiate a successful resolution to a challenging situation will likely help you to utilise skills and resources in doing so. You can also take time out for a few minutes to reflect on your own behaviour: 'Am I being too angry here?' or 'Do I need to calm myself down before interacting with this patient again?' In addition, conveying how you feel and reflecting on your behaviour with a colleague can be helpful. Some specific principles and techniques for responding to challenging behaviour are presented in the following sections.

CRITICAL THINKING CHALLENGE 23.2

What might be your emotional response when someone is aggressively shouting, intimidating and demanding your attention? Can you describe in words how you would feel? What physical reaction would you have? What thoughts would go through your mind?

PRINCIPLES FOR ENGAGING A PERSON WITH CHALLENGING BEHAVIOUR

It is important to understand some general principles in interacting with someone who is displaying challenging behaviour.

Verbal Interactions

How we say things can often be more important than what we say. Using an appropriate tone of voice, the rate at which you talk and the volume and pressure in your speech can influence how you engage patients. You need to make adjustments to the 'how' of speaking. Ask yourself 'Am I speaking loud enough?', 'Am I too loud, and am I sounding threatening?' You will need to fine-tune your tone of voice as the interaction with the patient occurs, testing and retesting your approach. Linking your words with actions can give the patient a sense that you are interested in the engagement and can help maintain therapeutic rapport. Alternatively, if you show incongruence between your words and actions, the patient and others may interpret this as you being untrustworthy and lacking authenticity.

Nonverbal Interactions

Your nonverbal communication, how you hold yourself or behave, is an important aspect of engaging patients with challenging behaviours. Through body language we constantly (and sometimes unconsciously) send and receive nonverbal signals. Awareness of the nonverbal signals you are sending may be particularly useful in the management of patients with challenging behaviours. Your words might convey one message but the movements and gestures you make might convey another, potentially creating confusion, misunderstanding and an array of negative feelings. The following are some ways of nonverbally responding:

- While you are talking, try to be aware of how you are sitting or standing, the expression on your face and what your hands and legs are doing.
- Allow the patient to determine the distance between yourself and them. This may help the patient to feel some sense of control. Personal space or distance can vary according to cultural and/or personal nuances.
- Keeping a relaxed open posture with your hands visible at either waist height or below can make you appear less threatening.
- The way you make eye contact can help. It is helpful to make intermittent eye contact and to avoid prolonged staring.
- The use of appropriate facial expressions for the situation can be important: seek a balance between smiling and looking concerned. Expressions of warmth and acceptance can help.

Be mindful that your position, movements and gestures may need to vary depending on the clinical situation.

Being Flexible

Nursing people with challenging behaviours requires the ability to be flexible and engage in different approaches. Nurses are often tempted to take control, when a more helpful approach is to consider how you can help the patient to maintain or regain internal self-control—care versus control is a good mantra to be mindful of. You may be required to restructure requests and allow time for information to be processed. The goal is to engage patients with challenging behaviour with a view to managing it, without it escalating. This requires qualities such as being patient and empathic, as well as skills in redirecting and negotiating.

Active Listening

Mental health nurses use active listening skills in most of their daily work with patients. Active listening shows that we are attending to someone's needs. While you may be unsure how to respond to someone with challenging behaviours, the act of active listening starts a process of being empathic and may give you more time to formulate your response. Reflecting what the patient is saying, while taking a position of not offering advice but expressing acceptance without agreeing, may offer the patient a more comfortable position to reflect on their behaviour. Active listening demonstrates the presence of empathy and helps patients to acknowledge their emotions while enabling patients to talk about them as opposed to negatively acting on them (Stein-Parbury 2014). See Chapter 1 for a discussion of communication skills.

Demonstrating Empathy

Demonstrating a sense of openness can be achieved by disclosing our concerns and issues with the patient openly and honestly. Being empathic or entering into the feelings of the patient and trying to appreciate their point of view gives the patient a sense that you are acknowledging their concerns and trying to connect with them (Brunero et al. 2010). Respecting different points of view does not mean you agree with them; for example, 'I understand that you would like to visit your family tonight, and I can see that you are angry about not being able to do that.' This position demonstrates that you can accept someone's experience, without the need to agree with it.

Being Assertive

Being assertive is a skill that requires careful consideration so as not to appear punitive or indeed aggressive. Being assertive may involve reflecting your own experience of a person's challenging behaviour and simultaneously setting expectations about the challenging behaviour. This approach involves displaying high levels of empathy while setting clear limits or boundaries on the challenging behaviour. The following are examples of assertiveness statements that demonstrate showing empathy and setting limits in a way that is non-judgemental and therefore humanistic:

- 'You are speaking very loudly and I am finding it hard to understand how I can help you.'
- 'You seem distressed and angry . . . can we talk more when you are ready?'

Combining these assertiveness statements with statements such as 'I realise you don't want to do this' and 'I appreciate you are trying' can also be helpful. It is important to avoid argument, conflicting advice and long-winded explanations. Some situations may also require a firm and concise request about what needs to happen; for example:

- 'I appreciate you want your visitors to stay after hours but unfortunately it is hospital policy that they leave by 7.30.'
- 'I need you to spend some time in this area as your behaviour is upsetting some people.'

Initially, a patient may continue with the challenging behaviour but as you repeat your expectations your message is reinforced. Provided that your demeanour is not aggressive and your response is consistent, this offers the best opportunity to manage the challenging behaviour in a nonthreatening manner. Be mindful to acknowledge any satisfactory outcome: saying 'thank you' and showing some humility are extremely powerful tools in any nurse–patient relationship.

NURSING THE FRUSTRATED OR AGITATED PATIENT

Nurses often use the word 'agitated' to describe some of the challenging behaviours they see. Agitation can be seen as a signal that something is wrong. It can be a patient's reaction to an extremely abnormal situation. Aggression or aggressive behaviour is frequently perceived to be hostile, injurious or destructive and is often caused by frustration (Cutcliffe & Riahi 2013a). Sometimes, despite our best attempts at being empathic and actively listening, patients become frustrated and agitated. While the challenging behaviour may be directed at you as the nurse, it is not directed at you as a person. Although this difference appears subtle, the implications can be significant. By not personalising the behaviour, but rather seeing it through the eyes of your professional role, this will help you to remain objective. When someone is angry they are often unaware of their own emotional state.

An integral part of mental health nursing is the observation of patients' demeanour and interactions with others. Some physiological observations that may require early intervention include:

- flushed or red face
- gritted teeth, tense facial features
- increased muscle tone such as clenched fists
- increased motor activity such as pacing or shuffling
- prolonged eye contact or staring

Patients who are frustrated or agitated may refuse to communicate or even withdraw from you. It is on these occasions that you may be required to intervene to prevent these physiological observations from escalating into challenging behaviours (Cutcliffe & Riahi 2013b).

De-Escalation Techniques

The term 'de-escalation' is used extensively in the management of aggression. De-escalation aims to bring about resolution through effective communication techniques (not force) and its success is underpinned by an empathic, respectful and collaborative approach by the nurse. This approach involves understanding common signs of escalating behaviours and an ability to use communication skills to purposefully engage anxious, emotionally aroused or agitated individuals. Despite a lack of empirical study in this area, de-escalation training may help nurses to be better prepared and more self-aware when dealing with patients displaying challenging behaviours. Several elements of de-escalation have been identified from the literature that may be helpful in preparing you to de-escalate challenging behaviour (Price & Baker 2012; Richmond et al. 2012). These primary elements of de-escalation are outlined in Table 23.2.

Restraint and Seclusion

There may be occasions when your attempts to de-escalate are unsuccessful and consequently a decision is made to physically intervene to prevent the risks associated with challenging behaviour. It should be emphasised that physical restraint of patients is an intervention of last resort and should be carried out only by health professionals trained in safely facilitating this (Lamont et al. 2012). You should always consider whether any alternative strategies are available, implementing the least restrictive practice possible, and if so, have these been exhausted? Also, what would happen if you did nothing? These questions may be asked in the context of alleged assault when considering whether reasonable force was applied, either in a patient's best interests or as a basis for self-defence. Restraint carries with it significant risks of injury to patients and staff, and in some cases even death (Boumans et al. 2014). Seclusion also carries with it significant trauma and distress for patients and staff alike. Some guiding principles for use of safe restraint and seclusion are summarised in Box 23.1 (Clinical Excellence Commission 2015).

Nurse's Story 23.1 by Natalie Cutler illustrates the complexities, and emotional and psychological issues associated with using patient restraint and seclusion. Narrated by an experienced mental health nurse who reflected upon her early beginnings in mental health nursing, the story depicts a powerful representation of trauma associated with human interaction within the mental health specialty.

TABLE 23.2 Primary Elements of De-Escalation

Element	Skills
Characteristics of effective de-escalators	Being open, honest, supportive, self-aware, coherent, non-judgemental, empathic and confident
Ensure safe conditions for de-escalation	Knowing the level of staff support necessary while being mindful that excessive show of force can escalate Assessing environment, i.e. exits and objects that can impede or be used in a dangerous manner Encouraging movement to a quiet part of the ward
Respect personal space	Avoiding being too close as this may appear threatening; maintaining a distance that protects from a potential kick but not too distant as to appear disinterested Appearing calm when anxious, which enables better decisions; being fearful may make the person feel unsafe
Don't provoke	Having a relaxed nonthreatening posture with arms visible (not folded or behind back) Having a calm demeanour and engaging assertively, not aggressively Holding intermittent eye contact and avoiding staring
When to intervene	Early intervention is essential but unnecessary interventions are not helpful Is behaviour dangerous or impacting on others?
Establish verbal contact	Using a calm, gentle soft tone, tactful language and sensitive use of humour Being aware of body language (posture, movement, touch, facial expressions, eye contact, proximity) Active listening One person only should communicate; several people attempting to de-escalate can make things worse
Be concise	Speaking clearly and slowly as the person may be unable to comprehend information when aroused or agitated; information may have to be repeated several times.
Engage with the patient	Emphasising supporting autonomy and minimising restriction, which helps create a sense of equality Remaining connected to the person via rapport—so the person is made to feel valued and respected Avoiding punitive approaches
Identify wants and feelings	Aggression is a primitive form of communicating that a need is not being met; looking beyond the external manifestation of this and asking how you can be of help
Listen closely	Conveying through body language and verbal acknowledgement that you are interested and repeating back that you understand
Agree or accept	Validating concerns where relevant and accepting that concerns are distressing for the person (even if you may not agree with them)
Set clear limits	Being clear about what you would like to happen and that you want to help Acknowledging if you are feeling uncomfortable: humility is a very powerful tool!
Offer choices and optimism	Empowering the person can enable a sense of control over their own destiny and may give the person an acceptable 'out' from challenging behaviour Offering things perceived as acts of kindness, where relevant, such as food/drink, access to phone etc.
Debrief all involved	Helps maintain therapeutic relationship Important that the person does not feel isolated following resolution, irrespective of how this is achieved Also allows learning from situations

(*Source*: Adapted from Price, O., Baker, J., 2012. Key components of de–escalation techniques: a thematic synthesis. International Journal of Mental Health Nursing. 21, 310–319; Richmond, J.S., et al. 2012. Verbal de-escalation of the agitated patient: consensus statement of the American Association for Emergency Psychiatry Project BETA. De-escalation Workgroup. Western Journal of Emergency Medicine. 13, 17–25.)

BOX 23.1 Guiding Principles for Safe Restraint

1. Restraint is the option of last resort to manage challenging behaviour; it is to be used when other less coercive interventions are unsuccessful or inappropriate.
2. Any restriction to a patient's liberty and interference with their rights, dignity and self-respect should be kept to a minimum and should cease as soon as the patient has regained self-control.
3. Restraint and seclusion should never be used as a method of punishment. All actions undertaken by staff must be justifiable and proportional to the patient's behaviour, with the least amount of force necessary.
4. Staff must exercise reasonable care and skill to ensure the safety, comfort and humane treatment of patients in restraint or seclusion.
5. Communication and engagement should be maintained with the patient at all times, with all opportunities taken to de-escalate the situation.
6. Pain compliance should never be used when restraining someone and any direct pressure on the neck, abdomen, thorax, back or joints is to be avoided.
7. The patient's physical condition should be continuously monitored, with any deterioration, in particular to the airway, noted and managed promptly.
8. All restraints should have an appointed leader throughout the restraint to maintain safety.
9. Face-up restraint (supine) should be used where it is safe to do so. Face-down restraint (prone) should be used only if it is the safest way to protect the patient and staff. Prone restraint should be used for only the minimum amount of time necessary to administer medication and/or move the person to a safer environment.
10. Postrestraint/seclusion debrief for the patient, staff and any relevant others should be undertaken in all situations.

(*Source:* Adapted from Clinical Excellence Commission, 2015. Principles for Safe Management of Disturbed and/or Aggressive Behaviour and the Use of Restraint. Ministry of Health, Sydney)

NURSE'S STORY 23.1 Natalie Cutler, Mental Health Nursing Practice Coordinator

I've been a nurse for more than 20 years, 2 things drew me to mental health: firstly, that it was a 'frontier' with little research happening and lots waiting to be discovered. Secondly, and most importantly, I could see 'mental health' everywhere. From my previous experience as a dental nurse, I was familiar with the fear and anxiety people experienced. I became aware of how powerful human interactions could be in making people feel safe. I'd say that was my beginning as a mental health nurse, well before I'd completed any training.

Something that resonated powerfully with me when I was undertaking nurse training was the concept of the nurse as advocate. The more I learned about this, the more determined I became to actively advocate for people with mental health problems wherever I could. As a clinician, and later as an educator and manager, this has been my most valued role.

To be an effective advocate, it is important to understand one's own motivations and be vigilant to the fine balance between seeking to build another's strength versus disempowering them by seeking to 'rescue'. Continuous reflection on whose needs are being met is the key. Advocacy requires being a resource for the other person to help them achieve their goals. If assertive advocacy is required, this should ideally be activated on the request or with the consent of another person. In addition to considering the needs of people with lived experience of mental illness, mental health nursing also encompasses an awareness of one's own needs. Self-advocacy and peer advocacy thus provide the foundation for safe and sustainable practice.

Being an advocate is not always easy. This is reflected in a scenario from my early career. As a new graduate nurse, my very first placement was in an acute mental health inpatient unit. Returning from a meeting on my second day, I walked into the lounge area in time to see a large male being held on the ground by several of my colleagues. Other patients in the area looked frightened. I did not have time to process what was happening before I was commanded to 'hold his foot'. For the next 25 minutes, I was part of a team involved in restraining, medicating and ultimately secluding this man. I had no idea what had happened, why we were doing this or what I was expected to do. None of my university training had prepared me for this. I was shocked and inwardly distressed.

Shortly after, my colleagues resumed their usual activities and not much was said about the incident. What appeared routine to my colleagues left me completely bewildered. Nothing in my private life or training had prepared me to be involved in holding another person on the ground against their will. I found it hard to reconcile this 'security' function with my beginning identity as a nurse, and an advocate. This confusion has stayed with me to this day. However, it also started a career-long reflection on questions such as 'What is a nurse?' and 'Who am I as a nurse?' It also made me determined never to see restraint and seclusion as 'normal' parts of being a nurse. Consequently, I have moved towards roles that allow me to engage with patients as equals. Wherever possible I try to challenge 'the way we do things round here'. For me, being a nurse means being brave and self-aware, and providing a platform for others to have a voice.

ETHICAL DILEMMA 23.1

There is often discord between staff on how best to manage challenging behaviour. You hear shouting in the patient day area of your unit and the nurse in charge asks you to draw up some intramuscular injection sedation for a patient who is shouting. Your colleagues start to form a team to approach the patient in order to restrain him, take him to seclusion and administer the medication. You feel that the patient is just frustrated and could be de-escalated. What should you do next?

Deliberate Self-Harm and Suicide

Deliberate self-harm can be an extremely confronting challenging behaviour. Patients who harm themselves often do so in the context of a situational crisis or in relation to their lived experience of trauma, and patients often describe how deliberate self-harm is a means of managing distressing emotions. Self-harming behaviour can include injury that is either external or internal. External behaviours such as cutting, scratching, burning, picking and head banging are more common. However, internal behaviours such as swallowing objects and substances may also be seen in clinical practice. Trying to understand someone's motivations, emotional state and/or triggers for self-harming behaviour is essential. Assessment of impulsiveness, the wish to control oneself or the effort to stop oneself is also important (Lees et al. 2014).

Traumatic Experiences

Physical and sexual trauma histories strongly predict and underpin self-injury. Dissociative states or feelings of detachment from physical and emotional experience are commonly described by patients who self-harm. There may be several mediating factors in patients who self-harm, including the type of trauma, affective dysregulation, dissociation, poor modulation of aggression and/or poor impulse control. Confusion may arise when differentiating between deliberate self-harm and suicidal behaviour. Deliberate self-harm is not necessarily suicidal behaviour as there is rarely an intention to die. The behaviour may be intended as a relief from anxiety or tension or as an escape from distressing emotions rather than an attempt at suicide. The complexity is that people with self-harming behaviour may also be suicidal. Assessing suicidality in a patient who also self-harms is difficult as people often feel dysphoric with depressed mood. An issue of concern when managing deliberate self-harm is not being complacent about it; for example, this behaviour carries extensive risks, even when there is no intention to die or when a patient may have been engaging in this type of behaviour for many years (Lees et al. 2014).

Interventions

As with most of the focus in this chapter, having empathy in exploring meanings of behaviour for the patient is the best place to start. Understanding the pain during the act of self-harm and what this means to the person may help engage them in a therapeutic relationship with you. Going beyond what is in front of you (i.e. the wound or cut on the arm) and exploring the meaning and significance of the act will help you to engage the patient therapeutically. Obtaining details of incidents, thoughts, feelings, precipitating events and other ideas that occur during the self-harming behaviour demonstrates a willingness to work collaboratively with the patient. Intolerant or dismissive approaches by nursing staff often cause an increase in self-harming behaviours as the emotional distress that underpins them is not being engaged or validated (Muskett 2014).

General strategies include the patient learning anxiety management techniques, including relaxation and other distraction strategies such as pinging rubber bans on the wrist when distressed, ice blocks, throwing or hitting soft objects and/or exercising when thoughts of self-harm occur. Patients may learn about their early warning signs and make plans in advance for potentially stressful and/or difficult situations they may encounter. Encouraging patients to articulate into words, drawings or stories about these experiences may help them to understand how they are relating to the world around them (Lamont et al. 2009a, 2009b). An ongoing emphasis should be placed on developing alternatives to self-harm. Deliberate self-harm is a complex issue and treatment processes can be prolonged and unpredictable. Generally, psychotherapy is the most common treatment, with dialectical behaviour therapy having dominance in this area more recently (Eren et al. 2014).

Manipulation

Manipulation generally refers to behaviours that someone exhibits to get their needs met. This may include the following types of behaviours and actions: attempting to maintain control and power over others; playing one staff member off against another (sometimes called 'splitting'); evoking guilt and shame in others; attempting to get others to take responsibility for one's actions; and attempting to gain an advantage in interactions. Manipulation can be used by both nurses and patients. Nurses may label challenging behaviour as 'manipulative' as a way of 'understanding' the behaviour. The meaning behind the word 'manipulative' can be seen as negative, suggesting that the whole patient is bad or difficult rather than just the individual behaviour. As nurses we need to be careful how we label behaviour and the meanings that arise out of those labels (McGrath & Dowling 2012).

Influence Versus Manipulation

Generally speaking, as a nurse, you hold the power in the therapeutic relationship. As such, you need to be aware of how you exercise that responsibility. Patient–nurse collaboration and positive outcomes are more likely to be achieved by using influence rather than manipulation. The goal is encouragement and negotiation rather than coercion or manipulation, and patient involvement in decision making will provide the best opportunity for managing challenging behaviour. Always try to provide balanced, not biased, information and consider the needs and concerns of the patient, not just your own needs and concerns. Identify the manipulative behaviour and communicate this with your colleagues. It is important to maintain communication and consistency. Comprehensive documentation is important and minimising the number of staff involved with the patient may help. Be clear and direct. When setting limits on behaviour, enforce the limits but also reward and praise positive behaviour. Collaborative care plans should communicate clearly what you expect from the patient and what the patient can expect from you. A written plan may contain a set of simple statements of what you will do and what the patient will do. It may even be signed by both parties to demonstrate an agreement but it should not be considered as a contract. It is simply a negotiated agreement with another person (McCloughen et al. 2011).

> **CRITICAL THINKING CHALLENGE 23.3**
>
> A patient is displaying splitting behaviour, describing one staff member as their favourite while others are the worst they have met.
>
> 1. What would you say to the patient?
> 2. What would you say to the team?
> 3. How would you behave with the patient and the clinical team?

CLINICAL PRESENTATIONS AND CHALLENGING BEHAVIOUR

Psychosis

Some of the most complex challenging behaviours can be seen in the context of psychosis. Psychotic symptoms are seen in numerous mental health presentations. Psychosis is an impaired reality testing whereby the patient has difficulty distinguishing between what is real and what is not real. This can include perceptual disturbance (usually auditory and sometimes tactile, visual, olfactory or gustatory hallucinations), and thought disorder and delusions, where fixed beliefs are held regardless of refuting information. A severe depressive illness may include delusions that tend to match the mood state; that is, having committed a terrible sin, being worthless or a burden on family. Patients experiencing mania may have hallucinations and delusions that tend to be grandiose or religious in nature (e.g. being famous or rich or having special powers). Substance-induced psychosis, which occurs from stimulants such as cocaine and amphetamines, is often associated with paranoid delusions and may include auditory and tactile hallucinations. Alcohol withdrawal states often include visual hallucinations.

In most of these presentations, the challenging behaviour is probably related to these symptoms. For example, someone who is paranoid may fear for their wellbeing and misinterpret the actions of others, causing them to be defensive, protective and aggressive, in the interests of self preservation. This section is based on research with experienced mental health nurses working in acute mental health wards (Bowers et al. 2010) (see Chapter 15 for more on the psychotic disorders). When patients are having a psychotic experience, our response needs to provide a sense of emotional and physical safety as a basis for helping them. For some patients the experience may be frightening but for others it may be less so; we need to gauge and interpret the patient's emotional and physical response and adapt ourselves and the environment to their individual experience.

Specific Communication Techniques

The first step in engaging someone who is experiencing psychosis is to ask specific questions to elicit the content and context of what is being experienced. Once the content and context are known, you can formulate how best to respond. The following is a list of probing questions to ask patients that may elicit these aspects:

- *Hallucinations:* Are the voices inside or outside your head? Have you seen or heard anything that other people cannot sense? Have you experienced any strange tastes or smells recently? Have you had any feelings that you or things around you are not real?
- *Ideas of reference:* Have you thought that people are talking about you or laughing at you? Have you seen or heard things in magazines or on TV that refer to you or have special meaning to you? Have you received special messages in other ways?
- *Formal thought disorder (echo, insertion, withdrawal and broadcasting):* Have you heard your thoughts out loud as if they were outside your head? Have thoughts been put inside your head by someone or something else? Have you felt that your thoughts were being taken away by some outside source? Have you felt that people could read your thoughts?
- *Delusions of persecution:* Do you have trouble getting along with people? Have you felt that people are against you? Is anyone trying to harm you or plot against you?
- *Delusions of sin or guilt:* Have you felt that you have done something terrible? Is anything bothering your conscience?
- *Delusion of grandiosity:* Do you have any special powers, abilities or talents?
- *Somatic delusions:* Is anything wrong with the way your body is working?

How the Nurse Behaves

Symbolic interactionist theory (outlined earlier) should be used to guide your interactions with a patient who is experiencing a psychotic episode. Being mindful of the language and behaviour you use may help you to interpret what the experience of a psychosis means to the patient. You also need to remember that the patient is trying to interpret how you behave, in the context of their delusional beliefs and hallucinations. When a patient is suffering with hallucinations, you will need to tolerate and make allowances for their behaviour that is associated with symptoms. If the behaviour is not confronting and interfering with others, it can be tolerated, often until pharmacological treatments take their effect. If the patient is distracted by hallucinations, ensure that you do not provide too much information too fast: keep messages simple and reiterate them. You may also need to use the patient's name more often than usual, to help distract them from the hallucinations and reorientate them to you and your requests. The patient's hallucinations may include ideas about the staff and the environment and this may affect their behaviour. It is helpful to be creative and willing to try different approaches (Bowers et al. 2010).

When a patient is acutely psychotic you may need to consider who engages with them: choosing the right nurse is important. Depending on the content of the patient's delusion, it may be necessary to consider the age, gender and/or cultural background of the nurse caring for the patient as these may evoke certain responses from the patient because of their delusional thinking. For example, a patient may have a particular paranoid delusion about 'young people', so using a nurse who looks older to engage them may be a better option. The nurse needs to remember that psychotic behaviour is not a personal attack on the nurse; rather, distorted thinking has permeated through to a change in behaviour that does not allow the patient to behave appropriately.

Talking to someone who is delusional can present a range of challenges. Patients with delusional ideas are often scared and defensive and addressing the emotions surrounding the delusions can be the key to engaging them. When people are delusional we mostly do not challenge the content of their delusions: this means neither denying nor dismissing the delusional beliefs and not colluding with them. If the patient's safety or yours is compromised, however, it may be necessary to accept the content of the delusion until this emergency period is over.

Connecting with the emotional sequelae of the delusional content is the most appropriate approach. When patients experience paranoid delusions they are often frightened, even terrified for their life. A statement such as 'You look scared: what can I do to help?' may be both validating of the patient's distress and comforting because it communicates an offer of help. Engage them in a conversation that is not to do with the delusion but the emotions they are experiencing, for example 'fear'. Constant reassurance about their safety, acceptance and listening (e.g. 'It must be difficult for you to feel that way') will help you build a rapport with the patient. Be flexible in your approach and be prepared to reword how you express yourself until you arrive at the best way to gain the patient's trust.

When someone is thought disordered they are often unable to express their thoughts coherently, yet they may struggle to understand why you cannot understand them. One method of engaging patients with thought disorder is known as 'acceptance and listening'. People who are thought disordered are often trying to express something: see whether you are able to identify themes in what the person is saying; ask them to write down or draw what their needs are. You can also ask them to think about it and come back to you when they feel ready. The general ideas of reminding, prompting, keeping it simple and clarifying with the patient will help with the engagement of a patient with thought disorder.

The time of day may make a difference: that is, people may respond better to your requests at different times of the day. Looking for these windows of opportunity to engage someone is worthwhile. A patient's interpretation of the time of day may be influenced by their psychotic symptoms. The psychotic symptoms may vary throughout the day in intensity, amount and duration. The person may have hallucinations all day, or the hallucinations may be less troublesome in the late morning than in the evening. There are no uniform rules. Rather, you need to understand the patient's individual patterns of these experiences. Find a window of opportunity by observing what times of day appear the best to try to interact with the patient, when they are less distracted. Keeping observations and records of what time the person is interacting may help.

Gain an understanding of the environment. Patients may interpret the objects in their environment according to the content of their delusions and the meanings they make out of these objects may determine how they behave. Mental health nurses need to try to anticipate the meanings people may make out of objects typically found in the ward environment. Ideally, when someone is distracted by hallucinations or delusions, having an environment that is nonstimulating may help reduce distractions for them. While mental health units are purposefully designed to be low stimulus, the noise and traffic within a unit needs to be managed: asking people to keep music to acceptable levels and managing how people interact with others is part of the nursing role. Unfortunately, environments like the emergency department and to some extent community settings may be high stimulus and there is little we can do to change those locations. Try to find quieter areas in the emergency department, close the curtains or use visitor rooms to see people: this is where some creative thinking is needed to make the environment suit as best you can (Sutton & Nicholson 2011).

Giving structure to the day for a patient who is struggling to organise their thought processes may help them to feel some sense of control over their surroundings. Negotiate with the patient to set appointment times, giving them plenty of warning; for example, 'After lunch I will come and talk to you about . . .' You may need to repeat this several times when engaging them: ask them to sit down or find a place they find relaxing and always give positive feedback (e.g. 'Thank you for working with me on this').

Being with the patient can convey a sense of belonging, warmth and genuineness that can help build a positive therapeutic relationship. Simply sitting with the person, being available, introducing yourself and explaining your role and others' roles may help the patient to make sense of themselves in what can be a very confusing situation. Keep the conversation light and casual, creating a sense of normality in your talk. A focus on the person rather than the disorder is helpful. What do they like? Can you help them to achieve what they like? Concentrate on the here and now and on small issues rather than overloading them with large problems when they are acutely psychotic. An approach to engaging someone who is acutely psychotic is through joint activity, often by starting an activity yourself then inviting them to join you. They may see that what you are engaged in is safe; this role modelling helps them formulate what they are about to experience as being nonthreatening. Whenever you are trying to engage the patient, keep it at a slow pace: slow speech, short sentences and a lot of repetition may be required. When you are engaging someone with psychotic symptoms, engage with their emotions, speak clearly and avoid jargon and colloquial terms that may have various meanings to different people. Appear approachable and interested and reduce barriers by having a relaxed body language (Bowers et al. 2010).

Negative Symptoms

Patients with psychotic disorders may also suffer with negative symptoms. These can include blunting of affect, poor social drive, poverty of speech and thought, apathy, anhedonia and lack of motivation. These symptoms can be challenging for the nurse and impair the patient's ability to engage in care. The nurse needs to set realistic goals and expectations with the patient when considering these symptoms. Given the impact of these symptoms on social skills, social skills training can be used to help the patient to improve how they perceive and respond to social situations. Social skills training addresses topics such as living skills, communication and vocational skills. What we can do for negative symptoms is education, behavioural training and help with the social consequences like employment, housing and family relations. Creating a written programme for the day encouraging the patient to use this as a guide can help improve their social skills and put structure in their life. Cognitive therapy can be used to help the patient connect between what they are thinking and their negative symptoms. Socratic questioning and reasoning exercises can also help challenge and reframe negative thoughts.

Mood Disorders

Mood disorders such as depression and manic episodes can be a challenge for the nurse. Patients with a depressive illness may present as withdrawn and uncommunicative, have no interest in activities, be irritable, refuse to eat and be a challenge to motivate. Offering structure and constant reassurance is the general approach. The patient may need support and assistance with taking care of their everyday needs such as personal hygiene. Patients presenting in a manic phase of a bipolar disorder may present an absconding risk and may be boisterous and disinhibited. During this phase the patient is at risk of harm from others and the nurse needs to create a safe environment and closely monitor the patient's behaviour. The intrusive behaviour seen in manic episodes can be responded to by calmly reminding the patient about their behaviour and letting them know that other people may find their behaviour intrusive and confronting. Such reminders need to be provided while reassuring the patient that they are unwell and in a manic phase of their illness.

Cognitive Disorders

Patients with cognitive disorders often present with confusion, disorientation and wandering behaviours. These behaviours are seen in patients with traumatic brain injury, dementia and delirium and can pose a challenge to nursing care. Behavioural symptoms may include physical aggression, screaming, restlessness, agitation, wandering, sexual disinhibition and hoarding. Some of these behaviours such as physical aggression may be highly challenging, while others such as wandering behaviour may not be so challenging. The general principles of challenging behaviour discussed earlier apply here. You also need to remember that for patients with disorders such as dementia the behaviour will be long lasting. Creating an environment that the patient can accept and tolerating the challenging behaviour may be necessary. The following points can be used to help when nursing patients in this group:

- Create consistent environments.
- Try to meet patients' needs and wants.
- Reorientate patients.
- Accept that patients with cognitive impairment may feel less distressed when not directly challenged about their thinking patterns.
- Tolerate don't confront.
- Create a setting that allows for the behaviour; ensure the behaviour occurs safely.

Learning Disabilities

Patients with developmental disabilities may display self-injurious behaviour (hitting, biting) and verbal and nonverbal aggressive behaviours. Causes for these behaviours may include seeking a need for social interaction; to give a sense of control; poor perception on the part of services for their needs and wants; environmental factors such as excessive noise; poor access to items they normally enjoy; or feelings of loneliness and disempowerment. Challenging behaviour in this context may be further complicated by comorbid mental health issues. The principles outlined in the first part of this chapter apply. Keeping a structured routine, writing a daily schedule of events and trying not to change it too often are important. Often, close family and friends will know how to interact with the person best, so it is essential to engage them in any management and care planning to identify normal routine, triggers, activities of enjoyment etc. Patients with developmental disabilities often behave in very predictable ways and management of challenging behaviour can be reflected in this. Try to find out how to approach the patient and what kinds of interaction the patient likes. Take an interest in their activities and use this to try to create a dialogue. You are trying to enter the patient's world and understand their likes and dislikes. You will need to be patient, as managing challenging behaviours in this context can be more time consuming than in others.

Personality Disorders

We all have a unique personality that develops over our life time: our personality is vital and determines how we interact with the people around us. Some patients you care for may have been diagnosed with a personality disorder. Personality disorders are patterns of behaviour, mood and social interaction that the patient and others find distressing. For more details on personality disorders, see Chapter 17. Table 23.3 provides tips on how to interact with people experiencing various personality disorders.

RISK IN MENTAL HEALTH SETTINGS

This section explores risk assessment and management processes, and the controversy and debate surrounding these processes, and will provide you with practical application tips for considering risk within your practice.

There is increasing pressure on nurses and other professionals to assess, predict and manage the risk of adverse events involving mental health patients. It is unfortunate that high-profile, yet rare, events involving patients with mental health issues and subsequent media interest lead to heightened community concern around the safety of patients and others, often laying the blame on inadequate or inefficient mental healthcare. This has led to the expectation that nurses become proficient in assessing and managing risk, and in justifying their actions in terms of their risk implications. Risk therefore pervades the research literature, health service policy and practice, media and public debate, and even healthcare legislation (Allnutt et al. 2010; Fazel et al. 2012).

As a nurse, you will be expected to provide assessment in relation to some specific forms of patient-related risk. Typically, this may involve but is not limited to:

- aggression and violence
- suicide and self-harm (risk of further attempts and death)
- severe self-neglect (risk of poor physical health, infectious disease)
- sexual safety (risk of sexually transmitted infection, assault and trauma)
- exploitation/reputation (risk of harm to reputation, financial loss)
- fire safety (risk to personal safety and belongings)
- absconding (risk of further harm, prolonging hospital admission)
- noncompliance with medications (risk of relapse)

Risk has thus become an integral component of mental healthcare; however, there remains much controversy and debate around minimum expectations in practice, how best to facilitate risk assessment and management processes, and even whether the outcomes of processes are commensurate with our time and efforts.

Risk Assessment Processes

The search for reliable methods of risk assessment has led to a plethora of risk tools, instruments and algorithms that attempt to measure or predict risk behaviours. It is estimated that more than 150 structured tools exist for assessing the risk of violence alone, yet these instruments have a reported low accuracy in determining a patient's risk level (Fazel et al. 2012). Other instruments focus on suicide and self-harm. Research suggests that more than 60% of general psychiatric patients are assessed routinely for violence risk, which reflects the scale of risk assessment practice (Fazel et al. 2012; Hurducas et al. 2014). Notwithstanding, three methods of risk assessment have been prominent throughout and are commonly referred to as unstructured clinical judgement, actuarial risk assessment and structured professional judgement (Allnutt et al. 2010).

TABLE 23.3 **Personality Styles, Challenges and Engagement**

Personality Style	Challenges	Tips for Positive Therapeutic Engagement
Schizotypal	Suspicion/paranoia Interpersonal discomfort Bizarre thinking	Possible motivation for human connection
Schizoid	Social detachment Emotional aloofness	Underlying neediness and sensitivity
Paranoid	Expectations of harm/exploitation Hypersensitivity to perceived criticism Inclination to withdraw or attack	Underlying need for affirmation
Borderline	Unstable emotional and cognitive states Extremely demanding Proneness to acting out Idealisation versus denigration	Relationship seeking Responds to warmth and support
Narcissistic	Need for constant positive regard Contempt for others Grandiose sense of entitlement	Responds over time to empathy and affirmation
Histrionic	Attempts to charm and entertain Emotionally labile	Relationship seeking Responds to warmth and support
Antisocial	Controlling Tendency to lie and manipulate No empathy or regard for others Use of pseudoalliance to gain advantage	May engage in treatment if in self-interest or symptoms cause sufficient distress
Avoidant	Expectation of rejection and criticism Proneness to shame and humiliation Reluctance to disclose information	Responds to warmth/empathy Desire for relationships despite vulnerabilities
Dependent	No value placed on independence/taking initiative Submission leading to pseudoalliance	Friendly and compliant Likely to stay in treatment
Obsessive–compulsive	Need for control Perfectionist towards self and others Fear of criticism from therapist Restricted affect Stubbornness	Conscientious Will try to be a good patient

(*Source*: Bender, D.S., 2005. The therapeutic alliance in the treatment of personality disorders. Journal of Psychiatric Practice. 11, 73–87.)

- *Unstructured clinical judgement* involves a subjective clinician assessment on what factors the individual assessor believes are relevant or important in relation to a risk. Critics of this unstructured approach relate the lack of consistency and interrater reliability of such assessments, as individual assessors have different levels of experience, exposure to risk, values and interpersonal skills. These factors may influence the overestimation or underestimation of risk, which is obviously suboptimal to care provision.
- *Actuarial risk assessment* methods are known variously as mathematical, mechanical or statistical prediction, where individual factors that have been statistically associated with specific risks are measured. Therefore, individual clinical judgement is replaced by a score based on a formulaic equation, but this ignores the psychosocial dynamic factors that are associated with risks eventuating. Another limitation is that actuarial methods stop at prediction and ultimately fail to inform prevention and management. It must be noted also that any statistical significance attached to actuarial methods may be associated with specific validation samples and identified risks. For example, the majority of these methods were validated in North American prison samples and relate primarily to risk of violence.
- *Structured professional judgement* essentially integrates clinical and actuarial methods in an attempt to minimise the limitations of both methods. This approach combines empirically validated risk factors, professional experience/judgement and contemporary knowledge of a particular patient. As this approach incorporates idiosyncratic and dynamic risk factors, it is argued to have transferability across different populations and also offers provisions within the framework for prevention and management.

The Risk Debate

There has been and continues to be much debate in practice and the research literature regarding risk in mental health, with somewhat polarised views emerging. Many authors have argued the benefits of risk assessment tools in clinical practice, but there is increasing research that highlights their limitations. There is little doubt that there exist false negative predictions and unacceptably high false positive predictions which attract care provision that may not be required. It is further argued that there is greater accuracy in predicting low-risk individuals and only low-to-moderate positive predictive values for high risk of violence (Allnutt et al. 2010).

Despite research showing some association between severe mental illness and violence (between 10% and 15%), a recent metaanalysis has argued that 35,000 patients with schizophrenia identified as at high risk of violence would require incarceration in order to prevent one stranger murder, such is the low base rate (Large et al. 2011). Likewise, the same authors highlighted that despite apparent strong associations between high-risk categorisation and subsequent suicide in patients with mental health issues, the low base rate of inpatient suicide shows a predictive value of high-risk categorisation at less than 2%. Certainly efforts to develop, find or support any instrument or tool that offers 100% predictive accuracy or validity is futile and misguided, given the complex dynamic factors that influence challenging behaviours and risk. Due to the complexity involved, one must accept that there are limitations to what can be predicted and perhaps there has to be greater acceptance and realistic expectations within healthcare regarding this (Lamont & Brunero 2009).

Risk assessment, while often mandated by health services, is not a standalone practice and should be part of a dynamic and collaborative approach to assessing needs in patients, within a framework of partnership and shared responsibility. There appears to be a widespread expectation within mental health services that risk assessments are completed, yet little direction about what happens thereafter. Any structured assessment can be used to engage patients and enable greater understanding of their experiences, which is integral to therapeutic relationships. Therefore, continuous and collaborative review is recommended and relevant plans should evolve accordingly. It is when these processes are static and noncollaborative that nurses are perhaps unfairly left vulnerable and open to criticism should risks eventuate. Viewing these processes and practising within a dynamic risk continuum offers an opportunity for purposeful engagement and greater opportunity for mitigating criticism of your practice.

Risk Analysis

Risk analysis is a concept more widely used in other industries to describe a continuous and dynamic process of risk assessment, formulation, management and review. Risk assessment seeks to gather information that may influence the potential of adverse events happening, linking and contextualising past information with current circumstances (Lamont & Brunero 2009). Collaborative and corroborative information gathering inclusive of the patient and relevant others is important. Risk formulation requires that 'risk factors are identified, with collaborative predictions or judgments made, which explore the likelihood of the risk occurring, when it may be likely to occur, factors likely to increase the risk, the potential outcome of such an occurrence and appropriate interventions' (Lamont & Brunero 2009). Risk formulation moves beyond merely recording information to making professional interpretations of it. Risk management unsurprisingly involves translating the assessment and formulation into a series of clinical and psychosocial interventions that seek to mitigate or prevent the risk from eventuating. Again, these interventions should sit within a framework of collaboration involving the patient, relevant health professionals and others identified such as family and friends provided consent is present to do so. Risk review should also be a collaborative and continuous process of partnership and engagement between relevant parties, again fostering mutuality and trust.

Positive Risk-Taking

The term 'positive risk-taking' is used in this context to represent professional readiness to respect and respond to service users' own recovery goals or preferences for care. Such opportunities are perceived to be under-realised in practice, exacerbating existing power differentials between service users and professionals and sanctioning professionals to have the 'final say'.

Recovery-oriented practices adopt a position whereby patients take ownership of their own personal journey and with it ownership of associated risks. It has been identified that top-down risk-averse cultures challenge the integrity of patient engagement, involvement and empowerment (Bee et al. 2015). It is argued that such practices are currently under-realised within mental health practice, in turn maintaining power differentials and coercive practices (Bee et al. 2015). As such, cultures that do not embrace patient ownership and empowerment via philosophical frameworks and practices such as positive risk-taking will probably experience a high prevalence of challenging behaviours as a result of patient disempowerment and a lack of hope.

Consequently, the concept of positive risk-taking has been catapulted to the forefront of our decision making. Positive risk-taking involves a process of reasoning within a framework of weighing up potential benefits and harms of one choice over another. It is argued that positive risk-taking is not a negligent practice where risks are ignored or minimised; rather, situations and their potential consequences are logically and carefully considered in the context of any course of action.

A pervasive negative focus on risk can lead to defensive practices that in turn lead to often costly unnecessary interventions and care, for fear of legal recourse. By contrast, positive risk-taking involves accepting risk as part of everyday life and healthcare. Examples of positive risk-taking include discharging patients from supervised inpatient care to community follow up; unescorted leave from inpatient stays previously perceived to be too risky; pharmacology-free trials as a result of severe side effects; and nonadmission following presentation in crisis to the emergency department or crisis team visit at home. Research has demonstrated that the greatest reduction in suicide rates was found following implementation of 24-hour crisis teams (While et al. 2012) rather than from services designed to provide increased supervision in hospital environments. These are all examples of everyday positive risk-taking where, as nurses, we accept that risks are omnipresent.

Ultimately, we take risks and utilise the knowledge gained following successes or mistakes for growth and empowerment. As discussed within many chapters of this text, patient engagement, partnership and coplanning of care will enable better, safer outcomes when positively taking risks. The ability to flourish is a fundamental human right and should be supported and advocated for by nurses, as opposed to legislation, policy and practice where fear of failure and adverse events pervades.

ETHICAL DILEMMA 23.2

At the multidisciplinary team meeting, a decision is made to give a patient some unescorted time out from the unit. The patient was admitted 4 weeks ago following episodes of deliberate self-harm. The patient describes continuing suicidal ideation but with no intent or plans to act. Members of the patient's family contact you and say they are unhappy at the decision for time out, stating that it is not safe and asking for it to be withdrawn. What should you do next?

Summary of Risk in Mental Health Settings

The assessment and management of risk are inextricably linked to mental healthcare provision. While exact predictions are not possible, this area of practice is not one in which nurses should become complacent. There is no doubt that a sense of perspective and realistic expectation is required among legislators, administrators, health professionals and the wider community. However, despite ongoing debate, there remains a community, professional and moral expectation that we engage with patients around identified needs and potential risks and attempt to mitigate against these (Manuel & Crowe 2014). A collaborative, dynamic and continuous process of engagement and planning can support nurses when adverse events happen, thus removing the perceived or actual burden of individual scrutiny. Box 23.2 summarises principles for working with risk (Morgan 2004, p. 18).

THE LEGAL CONTEXT RELATING TO CHALLENGING BEHAVIOUR

When experiencing challenging behaviour, nurses need to be aware of the ethical and legal contexts in which subsequent actions and interventions are considered. Some fundamental human rights underpin our ethical conduct, common law and relevant statutes within this context.

Human Rights

Several United Nations treaties have shaped domestic and international law in relation to healthcare rights. The Universal Declaration of Human Rights (United Nations 1948) is an international document that states basic rights and fundamental freedoms to which all human beings are entitled. It consists of 30 Articles, some of which have direct relevance to healthcare provision in the context of engaging challenging behaviours:

- Article 3: Everyone has the right to life, liberty and security of person.
- Article 9: No-one shall be subjected to arbitrary arrest, detention or exile.
- Article 13: Everyone has the right to freedom of movement and residence within the borders of each state.

BOX 23.2 Principles for Working With Risk

- Risk is an everyday experience.
- Risk is dynamic and constantly changing in response to varying circumstances.
- Assessment of risk is enhanced by accessing multiple sources of information.
- Sources of information may be incomplete.
- Some sources of information may be inaccurate.
- Identification of risk carries a responsibility to do something about it—that is, risk management.
- An integral component of good risk management is risk taking.
- Decision making can be enhanced through positive collaboration.
- Risk can be minimised, but not eliminated.
- Organisations carry a responsibility to meet reasonable expectations for encouraging a no-blame culture, while not condoning poor practice.

(*Source:* Adapted from Morgan, S. 2004. Positive risk-taking: an idea whose time has come. Health Care Risk Report, 10, 18–19.)

The UK is a signatory to the Principles for the Protection of Persons with Mental Illness and for the Improvement of Mental Health Care (United Nations General Assembly 1991), which were adopted by the United Nations General Assembly in 1991. With the underpinning aim to provide a framework for improving mental healthcare globally, UN91 (as it became known) sets out basic rights-based standards for the provision of care for people with mental illness. Since its inception, UN91 principles have received criticism for not influencing the suboptimal standards of mental healthcare provision enough, with some principles offering more protection than others. Consequently, UN91 should now be read and understood in the context of the United Nations Convention on the Rights of Persons with Disabilities (known as CRPD) (United Nations 2006).

These frameworks set in place obligations on member states within common and legislative law for the protection of others and act as a reflective guide for actions. When engaging patients in any course of action that may impinge on these rights, nurses must be aware of where the law positions itself in relation to any subsequent interventions.

Common Law Issues

Duty of care and negligence are common law torts (civil wrongs) that nurses need to familiarise themselves with in the context of challenging behaviour. All health professionals must be aware that they owe a duty of care to patients and that this involves acting in a manner which accords with competent professional practice. Negligence arises when health professionals are deemed negligent in fulfilling their duty and where such a breach directly causes damage to a patient. This duty pervades throughout all care provision and is not something that is invoked by specific patient behaviours. Duty of care within this context involves maintaining safety for all and, in doing so, being aware that other torts are not being committed.

The common law tort of trespass comprises three potential trespasses to the person: assault (an intentional act by someone that creates fear of an imminent harm in another); battery (a harmful or offensive touching of another—thus a distinction is created whereby assault is associated with no contact whereas battery requires contact); and false imprisonment (the illegal confinement of an individual against their will that impinges the individual's right to freedom of movement) (Staunton & Chiarella 2013). Nurses may be open to scrutiny and sometimes litigation in the course of managing challenging behaviours, particularly when engaging in restrictive or coercive care that is unsolicited or not consented to by the patient and when the patient has a voluntary status. Involuntary status under the relevant mental health statute or substitute consent under the guardianship statute in general offers protection to nurses when managing challenging behaviours. However, this protection is not absolute and these torts may still apply if the nurse's actions are outside the relevant legal framework.

The common law doctrine of necessity sometimes referred to as 'emergency powers' allows nurses to act and administer care/treatment in any situation where a patient lacks capacity and the provision of treatment is immediately necessary to prevent serious injury or even death. Again, such practice is potentially challengeable and should be used in emergencies only, not in a consistent or planned manner. When it is anticipated that challenging behaviours may require a consistent framework for management, legislative requirements become prominent.

Legislative Frameworks

Mental health legislative frameworks, irrespective of geographical location, will generally be underpinned by similar philosophies and principles. (See Chapter 4 for further discussion of mental health legislation.) These may include least restrictive care or minimising any restrictions on civil liberty, rights, dignity and self-respect; and right to appeal (Lamont et al. 2016). Thus nurses are required to be accountable for any actions that are coercive or restrictive in the context of challenging behaviours. If engaging in nonconsensual restrictive or coercive management of patients, mental health legislation may have to be applied to do so lawfully. This not only offers protection for care and treatment that patients may not agree with but, more importantly, also affords patients with a right to appeal via independent arbitration (e.g. mental health review tribunals). Relevant guardianship legislation can also be used in this manner when protecting the health rights of patients with disabilities. Again, similar procedural requirements and criteria must be met within the various geographical jurisdictions. These procedures are essential if engaging in processes that effectively impinge on a patient's freedom of movement. Without wishing to single out any particular intervention, one such intervention that becomes prominent and requires attention within a legal context is patient restraint.

Reasonable Force

Nurses often ask what constitutes the legal definition of reasonable force in situations of patient contact and challenging behaviours. The fact is there is no simple explanation for this. Reasonable force is essentially context specific and is the amount of force deemed necessary at the time in relation to the risk presented. A unique set of conditions exists in each situation and essentially requires a professional judgement to be made. This judgement is quite rightly open to challenge and scrutiny by patients, and therefore any actions pursued by you as a nurse must be commensurate with the perceived risk. Potential alternative courses of action may be put forward when considering whether any force was reasonable and justified, in keeping with least restrictive principles of human rights and mental health legislation.

Notwithstanding the aforementioned, there will be occasions when as a nurse you feel there is no other option but to engage in physical contact and potential restraint of a patient (person to person, mechanical or chemical), either because the perceived risk is too great for verbal engagement or when this is unsuccessful. However, you must be aware of the principles outlined earlier when using restraint, as this practice should always be considered a last resort because of the danger to both the patient and staff.

CONCLUSION

Patients who engage in challenging behaviour may be struggling to gauge a sense of who they are and how they are seen in the social world of mental health services and wider society. Blumer's (1969) symbolic interactionist theory argues that humans (in our case nurses and patients) act towards things (environment, other people) on the basis of the meaning they make of those things, rather than what may be objectively true or seen at the time. These meanings are derived from social interactions that we have with others and our wider society, for example with other patients, staff and visitors in an inpatient setting. Patients and staff have a need to understand or have a greater sense of themselves in challenging situations. Our role as mental health nurses is to help patients to interpret their social world.

Nursing responses to challenging behaviours come down to your interpretation of how difficult and challenging they are. This chapter has taken you through some general principles that apply across most of the challenging behaviours that you may see in your practice. As your skills develop you will go beyond seeing these behaviours as challenging, instead seeing them as your core work as a mental health nurse. What differentiates mental health nursing from other areas of nursing is caring for patients who at times in their lives are unable to see the need for care. The skills you develop will take you beyond seeing these challenging behaviours as difficult or deliberate. Being aware of your own emotional responses to some of these behaviours will allow you to depersonalise the effects that challenging behaviours can have on you. Being able to stand back and see the wider picture of the social context that someone is in, and seeing past the behaviours you are confronted with will enable you to see the person within and the meaning behind their behaviours. Achieving this level of engagement with someone indicates that you are heading towards mastery of the skills mentioned in this chapter.

EXERCISES FOR CLASS ENGAGEMENT

1. The following link has four case scenarios that you may face in your clinical practice, which you can work through to further develop your skills (Lamont & Brunero 2013, 2014): www.inkysmudge.com.au/eSimulation/mhl.html.
2. In your class group, recall a situation where a risk was identified with a patient. Complete the risk analysis plan below from a group discussion (Morgan 1998, 2004).

Risk Analysis Plan

Categories of risk identified (single or multiple—tick relevant boxes):

☐ Aggression and violence
☐ Severe self-neglect
☐ Exploitation/reputation
☐ Absconding
☐ Suicide and self-harm
☐ Sexual safety
☐ Fire
☐ Other (specify)

Detail any historical information that may indicate the potential for risk (for example, previous history of risk behaviours/threats/ideation).

....

....

Detail any health-related factors that may contribute to the potential for risk (for example, mental health symptoms, personality factors, physical disabilities, substance abuse).

....

....

What environmental factors may contribute to risk (for example, arousal in official professional settings, access to drugs/alcohol, rejection by others, access to weapons)?

....

....

Is there any current evidence to suggest 'planned intent' to engage in risk-related behaviour?

....

....

Are there any risk factors that indicate preferred staff allocation (for example, danger to women, intimidated by men, need for two workers)?

....

....

What strengths and opportunities can you identify, from the patient and/or services, as resources to support this plan?

....

....

What barriers may hinder the implementation of this plan?

....

....

State specifically the identified risk.

....

....

Presents a risk of:

....

....

Through (behaviours/cognitions/affect):

....

....

In the context of (situations):

....

....

Early intervention signs are:

....

....

Interventions for the above circumstances:

....

....

....

....

continued

EXERCISES FOR CLASS ENGAGEMENT—cont'd

Has this plan been discussed with the patient?

....

....

Has this plan been discussed with the multidisciplinary team?

....

....

Frequency of review:

....

Additional comments (if discontinuing, specify reasons):

....

....

....

REFERENCES

Allnutt, S., O'Driscoll, C., Ogloff, J.R.P., Daffern, M., Adams, J., 2010. Clinical risk assessment & management: a practical manual for mental health clinicians. www.justicehealth.nsw.gov.au/publications/handbook-february-2011.pdf.

Bailey, R.D., Clarke, M., 2013. Stress and Coping in Nursing. Springer, New York.

Barker, P., Buchanan-Barker, P., 2010. The tidal model of mental health recovery and reclamation: application in acute care settings. Issues in Mental Health Nursing 31 (3), 171–180.

Bee, P., Brooks, H., Fraser, C., Lovell, K., 2015. Professional perspectives on service user and carer involvement in mental health care planning: a qualitative study. International Journal of Nursing Studies 52 (12), 1834–1845.

Bender, D.S., 2005. The therapeutic alliance in the treatment of personality disorders. Journal of Psychiatric Practice 11 (2), 73–87.

Björkdahl, A., Palmstierna, T., Hansebo, G., 2010. The bulldozer and the ballet dancer: aspects of nurses' caring approaches in acute psychiatric intensive care. Journal of Psychiatric and Mental Health Nursing 17 (6), 510–518. https://doi.org/10.1111/j.1365-2850.2010.01548.x.

Blumer, H., 1969. Symbolic Interactionism: Perspective and Method. Prentice Hall, Englewood Cliffs, NJ.

Boumans, C.E., Egger, J.I., Souren, P.M., Hutschemaekers, G.J., 2014. Reduction in the use of seclusion by the methodical work approach. International Journal of Mental Health Nursing 23 (2), 161–170.

Bowers, L., 2014. Safewards: a new model of conflict and containment on psychiatric wards. Journal of Psychiatric and Mental Health Nursing 21 (6), 499–508.

Bowers, L., Brennan, G., Winship, G., Theodoridou, C., 2010. How expert nurses communicate with acutely psychotic patients. Mental Health Practice 13 (7), 24–26.

Brunero, S., Lamont, S., 2012. The process, logistics and challenges of implementing clinical supervision in a generalist tertiary referral hospital. Scandinavian Journal of Caring Sciences 26 (1), 186–193.

Brunero, S., Lamont, S., Coates, M., 2010. A review of empathy education in nursing. Nursing Inquiry 17 (1), 65–74.

Clinical Excellence Commission, 2015. Principles for Safe Management of Disturbed and/or Aggressive Behaviour and the Use of Restraint. Ministry of Health, Sydney.

Cutcliffe, J.R., Riahi, S., 2013a. Systemic perspective of violence and aggression in mental health care: towards a more comprehensive understanding and conceptualization. Part 2. International Journal of Mental Health Nursing 22 (6), 568–578.

Cutcliffe, J.R., Riahi, S., 2013b. Systemic perspective of violence and aggression in mental health care: towards a more comprehensive understanding and conceptualization. Part 1. International Journal of Mental Health Nursing 22 (6), 558–567.

Dahl, H.-S.J., Røssberg, J.I., Bøgwald, K.P., Gabbard, G.O., Høglend, P.A., 2012. Countertransference feelings in one year of individual therapy: an evaluation of the factor structure in the Feeling Word Checklist-58. Psychotherapy Research 22 (1), 12–25.

Eren, N., Öğünç, N.E., Keser, V., Bıkmaz, S., Sahin, D., Saydam, B., 2014. Psychosocial, symptomatic and diagnostic changes with long-term psychodynamic art psychotherapy for personality disorders. The Arts in Psychotherapy 41 (4) 375–385.

Farrell, G.A., Salmon, P., 2010. Challenging behaviour: an action plan for education and training. Contemporary Nurse 34 (1), 110–118.

Farrell, G.A., Shafici, T., Salmon, P., 2010. Facing up to 'challenging behaviour': a model for training in staff–client interaction. Journal of Advanced Nursing 66 (7), 1644–1655.

Fazel, S., Singh, J.P., Doll, H., Grann, M., 2012. Use of risk assessment instruments to predict violence and antisocial behaviour in 73 samples involving 24,827 people: systematic review and meta-analysis. BMJ 345, e4692.

Fiabane, E., Giorgi, I., Sguazzin, C., Argentero, P., 2013. Work engagement and occupational stress in nurses and other healthcare workers: the role of organisational and personal factors. Journal of Clinical Nursing 22 (17–18), 2614–2624.

Franklin, C., Gingerich, W.J., McCollum, E.E., 2012. Solution-Focused Brief Therapy. Oxford University Press, Oxford.

Hopper, E.K., Bassuk, E.L., Olivet, J., 2010. Shelter from the storm: trauma-informed care in homelessness services settings. The Open Health Services and Policy Journal 3 (2), 80–100.

Hurducas, C.C., Singh, J.P., de Ruiter, C., Petrila, J., 2014. Violence risk assessment tools: a systematic review of surveys. International Journal of Forensic Mental Health 13 (3), 181–192. https://doi.org/10.1080/14999013.2014.942923.

Koekkoek, B., van Meijel, B., Tiemens, B., Schene, A., Hutschemaekers, G., 2011a. What makes community psychiatric nurses label non-psychotic chronic patients as 'difficult'? Patient, professional, treatment and social variables. Social Psychiatry & Psychiatric Epidemiology 46 (10), 1045–1053.

Koekkoek, B., Hutschemaekers, G., van Meijel, B., Schene, A., 2011b. How do patients come to be seen as 'difficult'? A mixed-methods study in community mental health care. Social Science & Medicine 72 (4), 504–512.

Lamont, S., Brunero, S., 2009. Risk analysis: an integrated approach to the assessment and management of aggression/violence in mental health. Journal of Psychiatric Intensive Care 5 (1), 25–32.

Lamont, S., Brunero, S., 2013. 'eSimulation' part 1: development of an interactive multimedia mental health education program for generalist nurses. Collegian 20 (4), 239–247.

Lamont, S., Brunero, S., 2014. 'eSimulation' part 2: evaluation of an interactive multimedia mental health education program for generalist nurses. Collegian 21 (1), 3–9.

Lamont, S., Brunero, S., Bailey, A., Woods, K., 2012. Breakaway technique training as a means of increasing confidence in managing aggression in neuroscience nursing. Australian Health Review 36 (3), 313–319.

Lamont, S., Brunero, S., Sharma, S., 2016. Application and implications of Mental Health Act 2007 (NSW) certificate use in acute generalist settings. Australian Health Review 40 (2), 219–224.

Lamont, S., Brunero, S., Sutton, D., 2009a. Art psychotherapy in a consumer diagnosed with borderline personality disorder: a case study. International Journal of Mental Health Nursing 18 (3), 164–172.

Lamont, S., Sutton, D., Brunero, S., 2009b. A brief report of art therapy in an inpatient mental health unit: consumer feedback and experience. Australia and New Zealand Journal of Art Therapy 4 (1), 68–74.

Large, M.M., Ryan, C.J., Singh, S.P., Paton, M.B., Nielssen, O.B., 2011. The predictive value of risk categorization in schizophrenia. Harvard Review of Psychiatry 19 (1), 25–33.

Lees, D., Procter, N., Fassett, D., 2014. Therapeutic engagement between consumers in suicidal crisis and mental health nurses. International Journal of Mental Health Nursing 23 (4), 306–315.

Livingston, J.D., Boyd, J.E., 2010. Correlates and consequences of internalized stigma for people living with mental illness: a systematic review and meta-analysis. Social Science & Medicine 71 (12), 2150–2161.

Manuel, J., Crowe, M., 2014. Clinical responsibility, accountability, and risk aversion in mental health nursing: a descriptive, qualitative study. International Journal of Mental Health Nursing 23 (4), 336–343.

McCann, T.V., Baird, J., Muir-Cochrane, E., 2014. Attitudes of clinical staff toward the causes and management of aggression in acute old age psychiatry inpatient units. BMC Psychiatry 14, 80.

McCloughen, A., Gillies, D., O'Brien, L., 2011. Collaboration between mental health consumers and nurses: shared understandings, dissimilar experiences. International Journal of Mental Health Nursing 20 (1), 47–55.

McCormack, B., Manley, K., Titchen, A., 2013. Practice Development in Nursing and Healthcare. John Wiley & Sons, Hoboken, NJ.

McGrath, B., Dowling, M., 2012. Exploring registered psychiatric nurses' responses towards service users with a diagnosis of borderline personality disorder. Nursing Research and Practice, article ID 601918. https://doi.org/10.1155/2012/601918.

Morgan, S., 1998. Assessing and Managing Risk; Practitioner's Handbook. In: The Sainsbury Centre for Mental Health. Pavilion Publishing, Brighton.

Morgan, S., 2004. Positive risk-taking: an idea whose time has come. Health Care Risk Report 10, 18–19.

Muskett, C., 2014. Trauma-informed care in inpatient mental health settings: a review of the literature. International Journal of Mental Health Nursing 23 (1), 51–59.

Perry, A., Woodland, L., Brunero, S., 2015a. eSimulation: a novel approach to enhancing cultural competence within a health care organisation. Nurse Education in Practice 15 (3), 218–224.

Perry, L., Lamont, S., Brunero, S., Gallagher, R., Duffield, C., 2015b. The mental health of nurses in acute teaching hospital settings: a cross-sectional survey. BMC Nursing 14 (1), 15.

Price, O., Baker, J., 2012. Key components of de-escalation techniques: a thematic synthesis. International Journal of Mental Health Nursing 21 (4), 310–319.

Richmond, J.S., Berlin, J.S., Fishkind, A.B., Holloman, G.H., Zeller, S.L., Wilson, M.P., Rifai, M.A., Ng, A.T., 2012. Verbal de-escalation of the agitated patient: consensus statement of the American Association for Emergency Psychiatry Project BETA De-escalation Workgroup. Western Journal of Emergency Medicine 13 (1), 17–25.

Roberts, R.K., Grubb, P.L., 2014. The consequences of nursing stress and need for integrated solutions. Rehabilitation Nursing 39 (2), 62–69.

Russell, R., Brunero, S., Lamont, S., 2014. Reflecting on transcultural care; culture care theory and mental health nursing. Austin Journal of Nursing & Health Care 1 (2), 4.

Sambrano, R., Cox, L., 2013. 'I sang Amazing Grace for about 3 hours that day': understanding Indigenous Australians' experience of seclusion. International Journal of Mental Health Nursing 22 (6), 522–531.

Sclafani, M., Piren, K., 2010. Psychiatric nursing practice and the recovery model of care. Journal of Psychosocial Nursing & Mental Health Services 48 (7), 42.

Shefer, G., Henderson, C., Howard, L.M., Murray, J., Thornicroft, G., 2014. Diagnostic overshadowing and other challenges involved in the diagnostic process of patients with mental illness who present in emergency departments with physical symptoms: a qualitative study. PLoS ONE 9 (11), e111682.

Slade, M., Amering, M., Farkas, M., Hamilton, B., O'Hagan, M., Panther, G., Perkins, R., Shepherd, G., Tse, S., Whitley, R., 2014. Uses and abuses of recovery: implementing recovery-oriented practices in mental health systems. World Psychiatry 13 (1), 12–20.

Staunton, P., Chiarella, M., 2013. Law for Nurses and Midwives. Elsevier, Sydney.

Stein-Parbury, J., 2014. Patient and Person: Interpersonal Skills in Nursing, fifth ed. Elsevier, Sydney.

Sutton, D., Nicholson, E., 2011. Sensory Modulation in Acute Mental Health Wards: A Qualitative Study of Staff and Service User Perspectives. Te Pou o Te Whakaaro Nui, Auckland.

United Nations, 1948. The Universal Declaration of Human Rights. Available at: https://www.un.org/en/universal-declaration-human-rights/. Accessed: 1 September 2015.

United Nations, 2006. Convention on the Rights of Persons with Disabilities. Available at: https://www.un.org/development/desa/disabilities/convention-on-the-rights-of-persons-with-disabilities.html. Accessed: 1 September 2015.

United Nations General Assembly, 1991. Principles for the Protection of Persons with Mental Illness and for the Improvement of Mental Health Care. Available at: www.un.org/documents/ga/res/46/a46r119.htm. Accessed: 1 September 2015.

While, D., Bickley, H., Roscoe, A., Windfuhr, K., Rahman, S., Shaw, J., Kapur, N., 2012. Implementation of mental health service recommendations in England and Wales and suicide rates, 1997–2006: a cross-sectional and before-and-after observational study. The Lancet 379 (9820), 1005–1012.

24

Therapeutic Interventions

Christine J. Palmer

KEY POINTS

- Mental health nurses use a range of therapeutic interventions when they work with people who have mental health problems and/or serious mental illnesses.
- Crisis intervention strategies are used in a range of environments and settings.
- You will be more therapeutic in a mental health context if you understand yourself.
- Being able to identify the stressors in your life will enable you to help others with their stress.
- Relaxation skills and assertiveness skills can be learned and are useful for all nurses.
- Psychotherapies include individual psychotherapy, planned short-term psychotherapy, motivational interviewing, cognitive behavioural therapy, dialectical behaviour therapy and solution-focussed brief therapy.
- Behaviour is learned, and so it can be unlearned through behaviour therapy.
- Group therapy is a cost-effective and therapeutic way to treat larger numbers of people at the same time.
- Family therapy is an intervention that works to effect change in the family system.
- Psychoeducation is a family-oriented intervention designed to empower and engage families in caring for their loved one with a mental illness.
- Person-centred ideas of recovery indicate that people will not engage with rehabilitation programmes unless they have hope for a better life.
- Social skills training helps people to learn or relearn social skills.
- Case management is a person-centred approach to working with people in the community in which the key worker assists the person to live in the community as independently as possible.
- Electroconvulsive therapy is an intervention with nursing responsibilities.

KEY TERMS

acceptance and commitment therapy (ACT)
activity groups
assertiveness skills
behaviour therapy
case management
cognitive behavioural therapy (CBT)
counselling skills
crisis intervention
dialectical behaviour therapy (DBT)
electroconvulsive therapy (ECT)
family therapy
group therapy
individual psychotherapy
instilling of hope
interviewing
motivational interviewing (MI)
planned short-term psychotherapy
psychoeducation
psychosocial rehabilitation
psychotherapy
relaxation skills
social skills training
solution-focussed brief therapy (SFBT)
stress management
telephone counselling

LEARNING OUTCOMES

The material in this chapter will assist you to:

- understand the importance of listening (as a communication skill) and its significance to therapeutic interventions.
- understand the short-term nature of crisis intervention.
- identify stressors and learn strategies for managing stress.
- differentiate between aggressive, passive and assertive response styles.
- recognise fundamental concepts related to a range of psychotherapeutic intervention strategies such as individual psychotherapy, planned short-term psychotherapy, motivational interviewing, cognitive behavioural therapy, acceptance and commitment therapy, dialectical behaviour therapy and solution-focussed brief therapy.
- describe how behaviour is learned, maintained and extinguished.
- recognise the therapeutic factors as they occur within therapy and activity groups.
- understand family-centred approaches to treatment.
- realise how psychosocial rehabilitation contributes to recovery from mental illness.

- consider how nurses can influence the recovery of people with enduring mental health problems.
- understand how working alongside or with the patient contributes to better outcomes for the individual.
- consider the ethical issues related to electroconvulsive therapy.

INTRODUCTION

This chapter provides an overview of counselling skills and a range of therapeutic interventions used by mental health nurses working with people with mental health concerns and/or serious mental illnesses. Some of the content here will require you to review material in other chapters to help your understanding. Working through this chapter will not give you the skills to be expert in any of these techniques, but it will enable you to understand some fundamental concepts. You may even begin to understand yourself better. When you are working with people with mental health concerns, having a deeper understanding of yourself will help you to be more therapeutic. One aspect of self-understanding and the understanding of others involves culture. Throughout this chapter it is important to consider the specific cultural perspective and needs of the person you are working with.

Feeling overwhelmed and unable to cope is typical of crisis (see Chapter 7). Crisis intervention requires specific skills that aim to resolve current distress and to ensure risk minimisation. Crisis intervention can occur in a range of environments or settings, and telephone counselling is just one of them.

We all experience stress and the outcomes of living stressful lives. Being able to identify the stressors in your life will enable you to better manage your own stress before you can begin to help others with their stress. There are many stress-management strategies from which to choose. This chapter considers relaxation skills and assertiveness skills. Relaxation is a simple physical skill that can be learned with practice, and assertiveness skills are particularly useful for nurses in any area of clinical specialty.

Many therapies and therapeutic endeavours have been developed to help people with their psychological problems. Among those discussed briefly here are the psychotherapies, such as individual psychotherapy, motivational interviewing (MI), cognitive behavioural therapy (CBT), acceptance and commitment therapy (ACT), dialectical behaviour therapy (DBT) and solution-focussed therapy. In addition, behaviour therapy, group therapy (including activity groups) and family therapy (including psychoeducation) are briefly reviewed.

Psychosocial rehabilitation is the term used to describe the kind of rehabilitation that is provided particularly for those with enduring mental health concerns. According to person-centred ideas of recovery from mental illness, people will not engage with rehabilitation programmes unless they have hope for a better life. While people can arrive at a sense of hope without the input of nurses, we are able to contribute to a person's sense of hope so that a more desired life can be achieved. Social skills training is also an aspect of psychosocial rehabilitation that will help people to relearn the skills they need in order to engage more actively in the communities in which they live.

Finally, this chapter considers the roles of interviewing, case management and electroconvulsive therapy (ECT) in contemporary mental health nursing. Taking a more collaborative approach to interviewing supports the orientation towards person-centred care. Case management is also a person-centred approach to working with people in the community. Case management approaches of the past focussed on management of the patient's needs, but today the emphasis is on the key worker supporting the person to develop the skills to live well in the community as independently as possible. Although ECT remains a contentious intervention, it is a valid treatment strategy with involving nursing responsibilities. While providing information on all these topics, this chapter also asks you to reflect on who you are, what you believe and what is important to you (your values).

BASIC COUNSELLING SKILLS

Many nursing students express concern about knowing what to say when confronted with another person's emotional distress. Certainly, it is possible to say the 'wrong thing' at a time when the person is feeling distressed. Usually, people don't need to hear advice about what they need to do in order to work through their distress. Most often, people in distress need to know that they are being heard and that their concerns are valid. Sometimes it will be difficult for you to be able to do this because it seems to be the natural way of nurses to want to problem solve and help people to feel better immediately. However, listening patiently is the skill that will be most helpful to you and to the people you help and this is a skill that you can perfect. When you are in doubt about how to respond, listen, listen and listen some more. Problem solving with the individual will follow.

Before you can begin to be therapeutic in your interactions with another you need to develop a relationship with that person. This is developed both verbally and nonverbally. As mentioned earlier, the ability to listen is a great starting point, as listening communicates your interest and sincerity and lets the other person know that you care. Basic listening leads on to the more advanced skill of empathy, or active listening. Empathy is your ability to reflect your understanding of the other person's experiences, behaviours and feelings from that person's point of view (Egan 1985). Egan (1985) offers a two-part formula for practising empathic responses that, initially, will sound somewhat 'clunky'. However, further practice will prove valuable in making your empathic responses both effective and natural sounding. The formula for basic empathy is:

> *'You feel . . .' (followed by the right category of emotion and the right intensity of emotion) 'because . . .' (followed by the experiences and/or behaviours that give rise to the feelings).*

For example, 'You're feeling hurt because your family hasn't come to visit you.'

Naturally, it is important to get the category and intensity of emotion right in order to be effective. However, even if you are a little wide of the person's experience, it will give them an opportunity to clarify their feelings. For example, you might say 'I can see you're feeling a bit upset with your son for treating you disrespectfully', to which the person might respond by saying 'A bit upset? I'm furious with him!' This will probably lead into further discussion about the person's feelings, helping them to make sense of what is happening for them.

Empathy needs to be focussed on what is happening in the here and now. Even if a person is talking to you about a traumatic childhood experience, it is important to empathise with their emotional response in the present. For example: 'I can see that talking about these events in your childhood leaves you feeling powerless and distressed.' This will communicate to the person that you understand what is happening for them here and now and this is likely to help them to explore this further. The skill of communicating understanding is critical in helping people to move forwards (Egan 1985).

Egan (2001) offers a three-stage model for helping that outlines specific communication skills that will support the patient's movement towards achieving desired outcomes:

- The first stage involves getting the person's story and exploring their existing situation.
- The second stage involves helping the person to identify goals and aims for the future.
- The third stage involves helping the person to develop the strategies and an action plan for goal achievement.

Ultimately, this is a problem-solving method. The difference from usual problem solving is that, during counselling processes, the solving of problems occurs over multiple sessions and through a range of techniques designed to maintain focus.

The main functions of counselling are to help the patient to enter into a relationship where they feel accepted and understood. This will help them to feel prepared to talk openly about their problems and to achieve a better understanding of their situation. Once the difficulty is clear, alternative courses of action can be discussed before making a decision about what to do. Specific action plans can then be developed and followed through with support (Burnard 2005; Dickson et al. 1989). There are also times when a situation is unlikely to change, so the person will need to accommodate and adjust to life being that way. While this is a common approach in counselling, you will also find this problem-oriented view challenged by others, such as in solution-focussed brief therapy (SFBT) outlined later in this chapter.

Counselling is delivered in a range of settings, including the acute inpatient setting, a range of community settings, in the person's home and via the telephone. Originally designed for crisis intervention services, telephone counselling is now integrated into several therapeutic approaches and is used routinely by community mental health nurses.

CRISIS INTERVENTION

What represents a crisis for one person might not have the same impact on another person, but no-one is immune to crisis (see Chapter 7). Situational life crises such as unwanted pregnancy, death of a loved one, serious physical illness and assault are frequently the cause of emotional disequilibrium or imbalance requiring crisis intervention. Being able to intervene effectively during a crisis is a critical clinical skill required by the mental health nurse.

Crisis intervention has developed as a specialty area in mental health nursing that largely involves responding to people in the community who are overwhelmed by problems or difficulties with life. Often people are referred by a primary healthcare provider (such as a GP or nurse practitioner) or by a family member. Some individuals will make direct contact, often because they have no-one else to turn to for help. However, crisis work is not limited to the community setting. Nurses might be required to work with someone in crisis in any number of settings, including a range of mental health and physical healthcare settings as well as the local community or even at the person's home.

We invariably respond to crisis with our usual ways of coping. However, because of the magnitude of the problem or a distorted perception of the problem, our usual coping behaviours might fail to resolve it. As a result, we may try other means of coping (such as alcohol or other drug abuse, eating excessively or not eating at all) and these are usually even less effective. Crisis intervention involves interrupting a maladaptive or ineffective pattern of responding and supporting the person to return to the precrisis level of functioning (Greenstone & Leviton 2002). Therefore, the focus is on current difficulties and the timeframe is brief.

Crisis intervention is quick, short term and based in the here and now (see Case Study 24.1 about Emma). 'Management of the crisis, not resolution, is the goal of crisis intervention' (Greenstone & Leviton 2002). Crisis intervention helps the person in crisis to locate or develop the resources from within or externally in order to return to the precrisis level of functioning (Myer 2001). At times, following resolution of a crisis, an individual may actually develop new coping skills that will help them to deal more effectively with future crises. Conversely, lack of resolution of a crisis may result in more disabling psychological problems and subsequent crises will not be well managed.

CASE STUDY 24.1

Emma

Emma is a 29-year-old woman who is distressed about her relationship breakdown. She had been married for 2 years before her husband began seeing another woman. He informed her 2 days ago that he is leaving her for the other woman. While talking with you about her feelings of betrayal and helplessness, she mentions that her father sexually abused her as a child. She realises that the same feelings have been generated through this experience. One of the aims of crisis intervention in Emma's case would be to stay focussed on the current issue that has precipitated the crisis, in this case the relationship breakdown. The sexual abuse issue can be dealt with at a later time and potentially over a longer timeframe.

In order to work effectively in crisis intervention, it is important to have a model to direct your actions. The model will ensure that no relevant information is missed, so the best possible outcome is achieved for the patient. There are many available models—for example, see the work of Slaikeu (1990) and the model offered by Greenstone and Leviton (2002)—but they all reflect the need to act quickly and to base interventions on an accurate assessment of the situation and of risk. Aguilera (1994) offers a simple model for assessing and managing crises. She asserts that there are three factors that, when present, defend against the development of crisis. These are the presence of social support, intrinsic coping skills (such as the ability to solve problems) and a realistic perception of the event, resulting in the belief that you can manage. Consequently, if your assessment reveals a lack in any of these areas, you would direct your interventions to meet that area of need.

Well-practised communication skills, particularly listening and helping the person to tell their story, are fundamental to crisis intervention. Without being clear about what the problem is, it is unlikely that you will be able to intervene effectively in a crisis. Crisis intervention is one time when you, as the helper, take some control and provide direction because the person in crisis is usually unable to do so for themselves. Myer (2001) suggests that we take control and determine the direction of the therapy without causing dependence. 'The more severe the reaction to the crisis situation, the more active the crisis worker must be' (Myer 2001, p. 6). The focus is on ensuring both physical and psychological safety.

Telephone Counselling

Counselling by telephone was originally designed to support people in crisis, and in those situations it usually involves a single session. It often occurs after-hours and at no cost to the recipient. In addition, telephone counselling affords anonymity to the caller at a time when the person is experiencing vulnerability. As with any counselling session, the telephone counsellor helps the person to cope with the crisis by working through feelings and by problem solving. Outcomes include resolution of the problem, referral for further treatment or, if the counselling is unsuccessful, lack of engagement. Interestingly, it has been found that most calls to crisis centre call lines are from people seeking social support rather than crisis intervention (Watson et al. 2006), which may require an adjustment to the way that telephone services are offered. Telephone counselling might also be set up for the convenience of the patient—for example, for people with physical disabilities who might otherwise have difficulty accessing an office, or as a cost-effective means to treat large numbers of people (Graham et al. 2013). In addition, some counsellors might augment face-to-face counselling sessions with telephone sessions (Rosenfield 2013; Sanders 1996).

Nurses working within community crisis teams are frequently required to counsel people by telephone. Their goal is to make an accurate assessment and to ensure safety for the caller and others. Others at risk might include a spouse or children in cases where the caller is expressing anger against them. Nurses working in psychiatric inpatient units and hospital emergency departments also perform telephone counselling, often by accident rather than design. Often people in crisis will contact these services for help when they are at a loss to know what else to do. Nevertheless, whenever you are called upon to counsel someone by telephone, you will require a recipe or process to help you work through the situation.

There are many models for crisis intervention by telephone (Egan 2001; Lester 2002; Slaikeu 1990) but they all follow a similar problem-solving plan. There needs to be initial engagement or the development of rapport through a caring, honest and open approach before the problem can be explored and analysed. The same counselling skills used for face-to-face counselling are required, but with greater emphasis on listening. Following engagement, it is important to determine the person's safety before moving on to explore their needs. Once the person's needs have been thoroughly explored, a plan of action would be developed that includes a follow-up appointment.

When working on the telephone, more frequent verbal responses are necessary. It is important to let the person know that they are being heard and that you are there, listening to the story. Typical verbal encouragers include 'uh-huh', 'yes', 'sure', 'go on', 'mmmm', 'right', 'okay', 'I see', 'do you want to say more about that?' and 'please tell me more about that'. These verbal encouragers let the person know that they are being listened to, and this enables further elaboration of the story about the current crisis.

Listening carefully is also very important. When telephone counselling, there are no visual cues to attend to so you must focus your listening skills more acutely. This enables a more accurate assessment of what the person is thinking and feeling, which enables you to reflect that understanding to the person in a truly empathic way. The telephone counsellor needs to listen for voice tone, pitch and volume and breathing noises that might indicate anxiety, grief or anger. It is important to listen for crying and other noises like snorting, groaning, grunting, sighing, laughter, sarcasm and silences (Sanders 1996). These need to be interpreted in the context of what is being said.

CRITICAL THINKING CHALLENGE 24.1

How do you make psychological contact when you don't have eye contact? Role-play a counselling session by telephone. In pairs, sit back to back or side by side and begin to work through a mock crisis situation. Begin by introducing yourself. Continue for 5–10 minutes.

Report back to the larger group:

1. What specifically helped with engagement?
2. How did you overcome the barrier of no eye contact?
3. How did you know how comfortable the patient felt?
4. How did the patient know that the counsellor was interested?

STRESS MANAGEMENT

Before considering how to manage stress, it is important to understand how stress manifests and affects the body. Among the effects of stress are increased blood flow to skeletal muscles, decreased blood flow to other organs, increased heart rate, raised blood pressure, rapid breathing and increased arousal so that vision and hearing are more acute. This is the body's way of preparing for fight or flight (Selye 1976). That is, the body prepares to fight and defend against, or flee, the stress-causing situation. For example, imagine you are walking back to your car after finishing work late at night and you hear footsteps behind you. In order to prepare you for fight or flight, all of the responses described occur. They are all essential and automatic physical responses designed to keep you alive. You will decide, based on your appraisal of the threat, whether you will flee or stay and fight.

These responses occur because adrenaline is released into the bloodstream. Stress is a normal part of life today but if we have too much stress, or if it is prolonged or too intense, we experience a range of unpleasant symptoms. These include a dry mouth, tremors, palpitations, sleep disturbance, shoulder and neck pain, irritability, indigestion, uncertainty and confusion. Having high levels of adrenaline and other hormones circulating through the body much of the time is bound to affect our functioning, as we should be in a state of hypervigilance or hyperalertness for only a brief period of time.

It is also important to consider what causes stress. It is not usually a particular event or situation that causes stress, but your perception of and reaction to the event. For example, two people coming across a dog in the street might experience the situation quite differently. One person might view the dog as 'man's best friend' and experience pleasure in seeing the animal. The other might view the dog as a potential threat, perhaps because of a dog attack during childhood, and subsequently experience fear and anxiety, resulting in stress. Also, although we all experience stress, not all stressful situations have a detrimental effect on us. This is because of a range of internal and external factors that help mediate the impact of stress. Internal factors might include effective coping skills and a relaxed personal style. External factors might include strong social support and a comfortable living environment. Nevertheless, the inability to manage stress ultimately leads to difficulties in living and, for some, mental health concerns.

Stress is ubiquitous in nursing work and seems unrelated to the area of specialisation or the country in which the nurse works (Abdollahi et al. 2014; Thian et al. 2015). Escot et al. (2001, p. 273) examined the stress levels of nursing staff working in an oncology setting and found that 'stress is primarily related to inadequate training, lack of time to deal with the psychological component of caregiving, especially terminal care, and relationships with other medical staff'. Mental health nursing can be very stressful and recent research has found that it can lead to posttraumatic stress disorder (PTSD) (Lee et al. 2015). Edwards et al. (2002, p. 213) found that 'mental health workers are likely to experience stress as a result of working closely with patients over an extended period of time'. Other workplace difficulties causing stress that these authors identified include increased workloads, increased administration, lack of resources and problems with management. McTiernan and McDonald (2015) also found that organisational stressors such as lack of resources, workload and organisational structures were more stressful than patient issues for mental health nurses working in both hospital and community mental health settings.

It is important to remember that the stresses we experience in one part of our lives, such as at work, will overlap into other parts of our lives, such as relationships. There are many opportunities for us to experience stress at work. Simply working a variety of shifts during the week can be stressful. The responsibilities that nurses are expected to take on, often without the necessary experience, also contribute to stress. Personal relationships provide their own challenges and we all experience these at some time. Before you can focus on managing stress, you need to identify what causes stress for you (see the first exercise at the end of this chapter).

Once you are aware of the major stressors in your life, you can begin to think about how to manage them or, more correctly, manage the effects of the stress you are experiencing. Remember, it is not the stress itself that is the problem; it is how you react to the stress that is crucial. According to Battison (1997, p. 24) there are four main techniques people use to manage stress. You can:

- change the situation
- increase your ability to deal with the situation
- change your perception of the situation
- change your behaviour

Notice that there is a definite call for change in your life. However, many of us find change stressful. If you have a perception or belief that change will be difficult, you are much more likely to find it stressful. If you believe that change presents opportunity, you are less likely to find it stressful. Nevertheless, if we do not change the behaviour that results in stress, stress will remain a part of our lives and we will ultimately suffer ill health—mental, physical or both.

Skills such as time management, being assertive, relaxation, yoga, visualisation, managing change, meditation and correct breathing can all be learned relatively easily, and some of these skills are addressed in this chapter. Changes to your lifestyle such as healthy eating, exercising and reducing alcohol, drug and tobacco consumption require considerable commitment. There is now significant support for the benefits of exercise for a range of mental health concerns (Beebe et al. 2005; Donaghy 2007; Fogarty & Happell 2005; Kerling et al. 2015; Rosenbaum et al. 2015; Soundy et al. 2015; Wand & Murray 2008). It is important to find out what works well for you in addition to lifestyle changes so that you can use these strategies whenever you feel the effects of stress. Bear in mind that a strategy or technique that works well for you might not be as beneficial for the next person. Try not to impose your favourite stress-reduction strategies onto others. At the end of this chapter you will find reference to websites that provide a range of exercises and materials to help you and the people you work with to manage stress and improve your lives.

BOX 24.1 Belly Breathing

- We generally take breathing for granted and are unaware of our breath. When we are stressed or feeling distressed we usually hold our breath much more than we are aware. This contributes to bodily tension. Anxiety results in rapid, shallow breathing and this also contributes to increased tension and further anxiety (see Chapter 18). Becoming aware of our breathing is an important first step in managing anxiety and distress.
- Belly breathing is a simple technique that can be readily practised wherever you are. It is a technique that teaches you to slow your breathing from the diaphragm.
- Belly breathing can be easily practised in a seated position or when lying down but when you are learning to belly breathe, practise it from the lying down position. Once you have mastered belly breathing, you will be able do it sitting down or standing up and no-one will notice. This is important for people who experience anxiety in public places.
- Make yourself comfortable using pillows. Place one hand on your belly. Inhale slowly while you count to four and expand your belly as much as you can. You should be able to feel your belly expand. Then exhale slowly to the count of four and notice the tension leaving your body. Practise for 5–10 minutes, 2–3 times each day.

We are all responsible for building on our current strengths so that we might better manage the stress that will inevitably enter our lives.

Relaxation Training

Relaxing is an excellent way to manage your body's responses to stress. It works because you cannot be both tense and relaxed at the same time. When you experience tension, relaxation is a certain way to alleviate it. It is also important to use relaxation to prevent the adverse effects of stress, not just to manage these symptoms. Relaxation can involve simply setting aside some time to sit back and listen to soothing music, read a good book or take a stroll around the park (Battison 1997). Listening to music and reading might also be done from the comfort of a hot bath and combined with aromatherapy. Learning to breathe more effectively will also lead to relaxation (see Box 24.1).

Progressive muscle relaxation (PMR, also known as deep muscle relaxation) can be carried out reasonably quickly and with great effect. It can be done independently or by following the instructions on your smart phone, tablet, computer, CD or DVD. Because PMR is a skill, it will take practice. You won't develop the skill overnight. PMR involves the progressive relaxation of the major muscles of the body while making a conscious effort to distinguish muscle tension from muscle relaxation. It has been found that PMR also relaxes the mind and internal organs (Romas & Sharma 1995). Ultimately, you will be able to relax groups of muscles at will, which can be done anywhere. PMR has been shown to be effective in treating a range of physical and psychological conditions such as headaches, depression and anxiety disorders and in preventing the effects of stress (Ayers et al. 2007; Rausch et al. 2006; Zhou et al. 2015) and even for the management of nicotine withdrawal (Limsanon & Kalayasiri 2015).

To learn how to use PMR, you need to set aside some time every day to practise. You can do this sitting in a comfortable chair, or preferably lying down. Find a quiet place where you won't be interrupted. Avoid PMR immediately after food as relaxation of the stomach may occur, resulting in delayed digestion (Patel 1991). If lying flat on the floor or bed, be sure that you let your feet flop loosely and, if in a chair, let your arms hang loosely. Above all, be sure that you are comfortable or you will find it difficult to relax. You can either follow written instructions until you have memorised them, or listen to an audio recording of the instructions—play it through each day. This way you can devote your attention to relaxation.

Before beginning muscle relaxation, it is important to take a few slow, deep breaths to prepare yourself. PMR involves working the major muscle groups, starting with the lower limbs and working through to the head (although some authors don't follow this directional flow). Begin by flexing the feet, holding the flexion for a few seconds, then releasing the tension. Focus on the difference between the tension resulting from flexion and the relaxation resulting from releasing the muscles. Repeat this action for each muscle group and take a short break between each action. Alternately tense and relax the calves, thighs, buttocks, back, chest, shoulders, hands, arms, neck, jaw, eyes (face) and forehead (Battison 1997). Finishing the session should involve acknowledging freedom from tension, resting quietly for a few minutes and counting backwards from 10. Then take a deep breath and get up quietly. To effectively help others to develop relaxation skills you need to be able to do this well for yourself. This will also lead to a belief in the benefits of relaxation.

Assertiveness Training

Assertion is about being able to communicate clearly to others and avoiding misunderstandings that might contribute to stress. Assertiveness, therefore, is a communication skill that will enhance your interpersonal effectiveness and make social situations more comfortable (Gambril 1995). As our personalities develop, we tend to learn a pattern of responding that is either passive, assertive or aggressive (see Table 24.1). At one end of the continuum, the passive person's rights are often violated by others. Being taken advantage of inevitably leads to frustration, anxiety and unhappiness. At the other end of the continuum, the aggressive person violates the rights of others and takes advantage of them. The aggressive person is generally defensive and humiliating, perhaps resulting in social isolation. The assertive person, however, protects the rights of each party and achieves goals without hurting others. This results in self-confidence and the ability to express oneself appropriately in emotional and social situations.

Central to these ways of responding is the consideration of basic human rights. We all have the basic right to be treated with respect, for example, and the right to say no without feeling guilty. Making your situation understood by others in a nonaggressive way enables you to feel comfortable without violating the rights of the other person. It is important that

TABLE 24.1 Comparing Passive, Assertive and Aggressive Styles

Passive	Assertive	Aggressive
Communicates indirectly; can have human rights violated	Communicates directly and clearly; protects own rights and the rights of others	Communicates critically and explosively; violates the rights of others
Does not achieve goals	Achieves goals without hurting others	Achieves goals at the expense of others
Allows others to make choices or decisions	Chooses for self	Intrudes on others' choices
Does not manage problems	Addresses problems and negotiates	Unwilling to listen to others and acts on problems too quickly

(*Source:* Adapted from Davis, C.M., 1989. Patient–Practitioner Interaction. Slack, Thorofare, NJ.)

your verbal and nonverbal behaviours match. Appropriate nonverbal behaviour to support your verbal message includes good eye contact, a firm voice (don't apologise or shout) and open body posture to show sincerity (Patel 1991). So, what is your communication style? Complete Critical Thinking Challenge 24.2 to develop some insight into your communication style.

? CRITICAL THINKING CHALLENGE 24.2

You've had a number of stressful situations within your family recently and so you have been unable to complete your essay on time. You approach your lecturer to ask for an extension on your essay return date. Decide which of the following responses would best describe your pattern of responding.

You would say:

- If it's okay with you . . . If it's not too much trouble . . . um, would it be okay . . . this essay that's due . . . I'm sorry . . .
- I've had a number of stressful situations lately and I'm going to need an extension on the essay. Would it be all right if I have another week to return it to you?
- Look, I can't get that essay done on time. You haven't given us enough time. You should schedule these things better.

The first response in Critical Thinking Challenge 24.2 is nonassertive or passive and the last response is aggressive. As you can see from the assertive (middle) response, the message is honest, direct and clear. The problem is clearly addressed and the desired outcome openly negotiated.

Being assertive is a skill that anyone can develop with practice. Indeed, Lee et al. (2013) taught assertion skills to people with schizophrenia who subsequently experienced significantly decreased social anxiety and greater satisfaction with interpersonal communication. Learning to be assertive means that you will have a choice about how you respond to others. It is important to be aware that you are under no obligation to be assertive all the time. When you have assertion skills, you have the choice to be assertive or to say nothing at all. Many of us have never learned to be assertive and may find it difficult to change patterns of responding that are passive or aggressive. For example, women in some cultural and religious groups learn to defer their thoughts and feelings to those of others, particularly men. These early and strong patterns of responding might be difficult to alter in the short term. However, it is important to determine what your pattern of responding is so that you can acknowledge it and work on changing specific aspects of your behaviour.

There are many types of assertion skills that can help you to handle situations you will encounter either personally or professionally. Some difficult situations can include making or refusing requests (saying 'no'), accepting and giving compliments, expressing opinions, giving negative feedback or being confrontational, initiating conversations, sharing intimate feelings and experiences with others, and expressing affection. Examples include conveying a nursing assessment to other members of the multidisciplinary team and refusing a request to care for a patient with complex needs when you are a novice nurse. Indeed, nurses' concerns about advocating on behalf of patients have been found to be a factor that supports the use of assertiveness skills in the workplace (Timmins & McCabe 2005). Many of us find it hard to refuse unwanted requests and this can make life difficult. Just as often, a person might be unable to accept a compliment without minimising it. For example, when someone says, 'You look nice today', it is important to say 'Thank you'. It is quite a different response to say, 'Thanks, but this old dress/suit belongs in a clothing bin'.

Teaching assertiveness skills to others is usually done in groups involving people who need to develop assertion skills. There are a number of workbooks available that can be used to work through and learn how to develop assertiveness skills. A simple and easy text by Davis et al. (2000) can help you to assess your interpersonal style and your difficulties before guiding you through some strategies for changing your behaviour if you see the need to do so. Once you learn some of these skills, you will be able to support others to recognise their nonassertiveness or aggressiveness and help them to learn new ways of behaving.

PSYCHOTHERAPY

Once extremely popular, psychotherapy now has to compete in a world where the biomedical approach to diagnosis and treatment prevails. The biomedical model focusses on chemical treatment and limits the consideration of a person's historical trauma. Psychotherapy, on the other hand, is concerned with 'the complex messy nature of the human experience. This includes the problematic domains of the aesthetic, the ethical, and the spiritual' (Petchkovsky et al. 2002, p. 330). The term 'psychotherapy' is used to describe a number of interpersonal models, each with its own individual philosophy and set of techniques. Examples of psychotherapeutic models include individual psychotherapy, planned short-term psychotherapy, MI, CBT, ACT, DBT and SFBT. To be able to practise any of these psychotherapies expertly, you would need to undertake a specialised programme of study that might include supervised practice, but nurses can and do regularly conduct psychotherapy.

Individual Psychotherapy

The early work of Sigmund Freud (1938/1965) revealed that much of what motivates us and influences our behaviour occurs at an unconscious level. Despite some of Freud's work being challenged over the years, this tenet still holds true and it is this understanding that underpins psychotherapy. Although psychotherapy can occur in groups, it most commonly occurs individually. The goal of psychotherapy is to effect change in the person's character, as difficulties of living are viewed as linked to childhood development of the psyche. 'Psychodynamic theory is rooted in the belief that we develop a sense of self during childhood' (Gallop & O'Brien 2003, p. 216).

Psychotherapy occurs between the patient and the therapist, usually over a lengthy period of time (time-unlimited). It provides the patient with opportunities to examine the historical experiences that have shaped who they are and influenced their life decisions. This happens when the person brings those past experiences into the present relationship with the therapist and reenacts them (transference). Transference is an unconscious process—that is, the person is unaware that they are doing it. According to Evans (2007, p. 191), 'transference is about one's fundamental ways of relating to those one loves, fundamental ways that repeat throughout one's life, although new experiences do provide the possibility for change in this pattern'. The person may begin to relate to you as the nurse in one of these patterned ways—for example, as someone who can be trusted, loved and respected. From this place, the patient may be able to talk more deeply about the things that concern them (see Case Study 24.2 about Sinead). Alternatively, the patient may respond to you as someone who is unlikeable and untrustworthy, reflecting their earlier experiences. This negative transference is quite common and needs to be immediately recognised as such, rather than taken personally.

The therapist is also responsible for recognising what they bring to the therapeutic relationship and the counter-transferences that support the patient's reenactment of earlier relationships. For example, it is important to recognise that reciprocal love or dislike for the patient is counter-transference and that expressing this would be counter-therapeutic and potentially destructive. Counter-transference can be viewed as a natural and expected response in some instances (e.g. responding as the caring and nurturing mother), but it is important to recognise this response as counter-transference, as it has the potential to be damaging to the patient. For example, an adult who struggled as a child to get confirmation of love from a parent might reenact that struggle in the patient–therapist relationship (transference). The therapist who doesn't recognise the transference and allows the patient to continue to seek affirmation (without challenging it) is demonstrating counter-transference. So, the therapist is responding to a situation that is rooted in the patient's past and causing the situation to be repeated in the present. The appropriate response on the part of the therapist would be to explore the patient's need for love and to help the patient gain insight into how this is related to experiences from an earlier time in their life.

Gallop and O'Brien (2003) argue that nurses need to deepen their understanding of psychodynamic theory, not just at the cognitive level, but also at the affective level—the level of emotions. We need to be aware that our own developmental experiences determine who we are and that we reenact our personal histories in everyday relationships, professional or personal. Much of this occurs unconsciously and puts us at risk of behaving inappropriately. 'Our history that creates the self is replayed in every interaction and decision throughout our lives. So that when we respond to our patients and they respond to us, we in the present bring with us our past' (Gallop & O'Brien 2003, p. 219). This is particularly important to acknowledge when we are working with people who are already distressed by mental health concerns and are vulnerable.

CASE STUDY 24.2

Sinéad

Sinead was a 21-year-old woman admitted to hospital due to self-harming behaviour. She had repeatedly cut her arms and body with razor blades. She said she did this because it helped with her emotional pain. It eventually transpired that when Sinead was a young girl, she had been sexually abused by a neighbour. She was deeply ashamed and embarrassed about what had happened to her and was also worried how her parents would react once they knew. Sinead's experience was validated by her parents and friends, and by the nurses working with her. Rather than staff feeling anger towards her continued self-harming, it was important for Sinead to be acknowledged as a young person struggling to manage her emotional responses to past traumatic experiences. She needed time and patience before she could begin to learn new ways of responding. Several years on, Sinead is a different person, undertaking postgraduate studies, working and having a life worth living.

Planned Short-Term Psychotherapy

Initially known as brief psychotherapy, this group of psychotherapies is now more commonly referred to as planned short-term psychotherapy. This title differentiates it from short-term therapies that are not planned. The brief therapies began in the 1960s when efforts were made to make the psychotherapeutic model of counselling available to greater numbers of people. Access to psychotherapy was limited due to the time-unlimited nature of early psychodynamic psychotherapy. However, the brief therapies expanded as it became clear that they could be very effective (Bloom 1997). Brief psychotherapies include interpersonal psychotherapy, CBT and MI. Effectiveness, efficiency and economy have therefore led to an explosion in planned short-term psychotherapies.

The goal of planned short-term psychotherapy is to manage problems in the here and now (the present). The duration of the short-term therapies ranges from a single session through to around 20 interviews, as compared with individual psychotherapy, which occurs regularly over at least a 2-year period. Short-term therapists believe that the person's presenting complaint is symptomatic of deeper psychopathology, so that ultimately, in managing current difficulties, significant psychological change also occurs (Bloom 1997). This, of course, matches the goal of the original, time-unlimited psychotherapy. Given today's fiscal environment in healthcare services improved access to less-expensive forms of treatment is welcomed. Furthermore, 'planned short-term psychotherapies are, in general, as effective and long lasting as time-unlimited psychotherapy' (Bloom 1997, p. 7).

Motivational Interviewing

MI is a relatively modern psychotherapeutic model, having been conceptualised in 1982 by Bill Miller and Steve Rollnick. It is an intervention that was initially developed for work with people with substance abuse and dependence problems (for more information on substance-related disorders, see Chapter 20). Indeed, Miller (1998) defines addiction as fundamentally a problem of motivation. You may be aware that many people with these problems tend to use the defence mechanism of denial—that is, they initially refuse to acknowledge that a problem exists. Once the person begins to acknowledge that there may be a problem, they may still be reluctant to engage in treatment. This indecision is known as ambivalence and MI essentially aims to change the substance-use problem by helping people to explore and resolve this ambivalence (Rollnick & Miller 1995).

MI is described as a directive form of counselling. It is not directive in terms of the therapist telling the patient what to do and how to behave because it is also defined as a patient-centred counselling strategy. It is directive in that it is goal directed and the therapist provides guidance in an attempt to resolve ambivalence. When the patient begins to see that there is a problem with substance use, resistance is expressed or experienced. This is normal and expected, and is accepted as part of the MI approach. The therapeutic relationship is more like a partnership where two people work together, rather than a professional relationship where the therapist is acknowledged as the expert. It is thought that the nature of this type of relationship is also empowering. This gives the patient a sense of self-control and personal power, which contributes to the recovery process (see Patient Story 24.1 by Kelly).

Rollnick and Miller (1995) differentiate what they call 'the spirit of MI' from the techniques they recommend to support it. Central to MI is the need for the therapist to resist persuading the patient to make changes in behaviour. Motivation to change is believed to come from the patient. Readiness to change, however, is a result of interpersonal interaction rather than being a personality attribute of the patient (trait). Any attempts to persuade or coerce the patient will only lead to increased resistance. The MI counselling style is described as quiet and involves guiding the patient towards considering the options and their consequences. It is not confrontational. The therapist would never tell the patient what they should be doing. According to Rollnick & Miller (1995, p. 326): 'It is inappropriate to think of motivational interviewing as a technique or set of techniques that are . . . "used on" people . . . rather it is an interpersonal style. It is a subtle balance of directive and patient-centred components, shaped by a guiding philosophy and understanding of what triggers change. If it becomes a trick or a manipulative technique, its essence has been lost.'

PATIENT STORY 24.1

Kelly

I had a difficult childhood and found myself on the streets at the age of 13 doing what I had to do to survive. I married young to a violent man and had four children. I didn't start using drugs until I was in my mid-40s when I was told that speed (methamphetamine) wasn't addictive! Before too long I was injecting it and had a £300-a-day habit. I even injected it into my neck when I couldn't find a vein in my arm. I was always chasing the dragon (trying to get that incredible elation experienced at the first taste). I was a junkie and nothing mattered more than getting my next hit. Not even my kids. Eventually I realised I had a problem so I walked down to my local GP and asked for some help. I was told they didn't work with people like me. I was stunned but I walked back further along the street to another GP and was standing at the reception desk asking if someone would see me when one of the doctors, who just happened to be standing near the desk, invited me into his office right there and then. He referred me to the mental health nurse working at that practice and I saw both of them for the next several years. She (the mental health nurse) would see me at home, even when I didn't want to see her! There were times when I wouldn't see her because I'd started using again and I was too ashamed to look her in the eye. But she kept coming back. After 10 years of addiction I've now been clean for more than 2 years. I now have a 'normal' life. I work two jobs, but more importantly, I have a pretty good relationship with my kids and a fantastic relationship with my three gorgeous grandkids. And now I've been cigarette free for almost 11 months!

The wheel of change or the Transtheoretical Model of Change, developed by Prochaska and DiClemente (1983), is used to support the philosophy of MI. The model outlines five stages related to the readiness to change behaviour—in this case, abstaining from addictive substances like alcohol:

- *Precontemplation.* The individual does not intend to change. The person is often not aware that there is a problem, and is not actively looking for an alternative life.
- *Contemplation.* There is acknowledgement that a problem exists, and so the person begins to think about change. There is a developing awareness of the advantages of change, but the disadvantages are also recognised (Prochaska 2001).
- *Preparation.* The person begins to learn new skills and gather information as the readiness to change develops. At this stage the plans are for change to take place within the next month (Finnell 2003).

- *Action.* Significant behaviour change occurs as the person begins to engage in new behaviours.
- *Maintenance.* Permanent changes in behaviour are now sought. The person works towards establishing the change, by adjusting their lifestyle and actively avoiding returning to old patterns of behaviour.

According to the philosophy of MI, the therapist guides the patient through these stages at a pace determined by the patient. Changing destructive patterns of substance abuse and dependence does not happen all at once. Motivated by relevant and meaningful goals, the change occurs progressively (Finnell 2003). As relapse is viewed as part of the process of change, a return to earlier stages in the process is considered normal.

In addition to the spirit of MI, five principles underpin the model, as outlined by Miller et al. (1992).

- *Avoid argumentation.* There should not be any confrontation or arguing with the patient. This will only result in the patient returning with argumentation and withdrawing from the therapy. If the patient were to deny having a problem with alcohol, despite the overwhelming evidence, the therapist would not argue about the evidence with the patient.
- *Express empathy.* This is considered critical to the approach. Expression of empathy gives patients the message that they are heard and understood. This is important because it is unlikely to have occurred within the family or the community. This leads to patients being more open to therapy and to sharing their stories. Patients are also more likely to be open to the gentle challenges from the therapist about their beliefs about substance use. Change occurs because patients are more comfortable in working with their ambivalence.
- *Support self-efficacy.* Supporting a person's sense of self-efficacy contributes to the patient's belief that change is possible. Self-efficacy is supported through acknowledging the person's past ability to change and by supporting the person to choose their own plan for change. Observing others who have made changes in their lives is also a powerful motivator for change.
- *Roll with resistance.* Resistance from the patient is considered normal and not to be contested. The therapist rolls with the resistance by encouraging the patient to find their own solutions to problems. Because there is no differentiation between the therapist and the patient, there is nothing for the patient to fight against. The therapist might offer new perspectives, but these are not imposed on the patient.
- *Develop discrepancy.* This involves helping patients to see the discrepancies between what they hope to achieve (their goals) and how they are currently behaving. Recognising that their actions are leading them away from, rather than towards, the achievement of their important goals provides the motivation for change.

MI has been found to be very effective, particularly where a person's suffering from the effects of the addiction has increased, as it does over time. People have changed their patterns of substance dependence after as little as 1 to 2 hours of MI; and a single session of MI prior to embarking on a rehabilitation programme has been found to double the chances of a person's abstinence continuing 3 months later (Miller 1998). This is possible because someone has actively listened to the person's problems, helped the person to acknowledge and resolve ambivalence and supported them in achieving their goal of a changed life. But problems with motivation and behaviour change are not limited to the addictions field and to mental health concerns alone. MI has been found to be effective in working with people with eating disorders (Arkowitz et al. 2015: Carels et al. 2007; Treasure et al. 2007) and sexual health concerns (Byrne et al. 2006; Weir et al. 2009), with criminal offenders (Clark et al. 2006; Arkowitz et al. 2015), in improving medication adherence (Spoelstra et al. 2015) and in improving general health (Butterworth et al. 2006; Knight et al. 2006).

Cognitive Behavioural Therapy

CBT grew out of behavioural therapy but is considered a planned short-term psychotherapeutic technique. Originally designed as a treatment approach for people with depression, CBT is now used for a range of disorders and has been found to be a cost-effective approach (Brettschneider et al. 2015; Myhr & Payne 2006; Vos et al. 2005). It is usually conducted over 16 to 20 sessions. Its premise is that there is an interrelationship between thoughts, feelings, behaviour, biology and the environment. That is, each factor influences the others. This has been understood for centuries. Blackburn and Davidson interpret here the words of the Roman emperor Marcus Aurelius who said:

> *If some external object distresses you, it is not the object itself but your judgement of it which causes pain. It is up to you to change your judgement. If it is your behaviour which troubles you, who stops you from changing it? (Blackburn & Davidson 1990, p. 16)*

In the cognitive model, our thoughts are classified into three layers: the outer layer holds our automatic thoughts; the middle layer contains our intermediate beliefs or underlying assumptions; and the inner layer stores our core beliefs. The core beliefs develop during childhood as a result of experience and the influence of significant others. CBT aims to cause change at each of these levels. The goal of treatment is to bring into conscious awareness the person's negative automatic thoughts, which are specific to certain situations, and the person's underlying assumptions, and to challenge them.

We all have negative automatic thoughts that are present when we are awake. They are responsible for many of our behaviours. An example of a negative automatic thought is: 'I can't cope.' This leads to the person behaving in a helpless way. The underlying assumption might be: 'If I can't work this out, then I'm no good.' The core belief for this person might be: 'I'm a failure.' Negative automatic thoughts are the most superficial and are more likely to be acknowledged. Once challenged, the patient learns to develop new or revised beliefs. These are considered during therapy and practised in vivo (in real life).

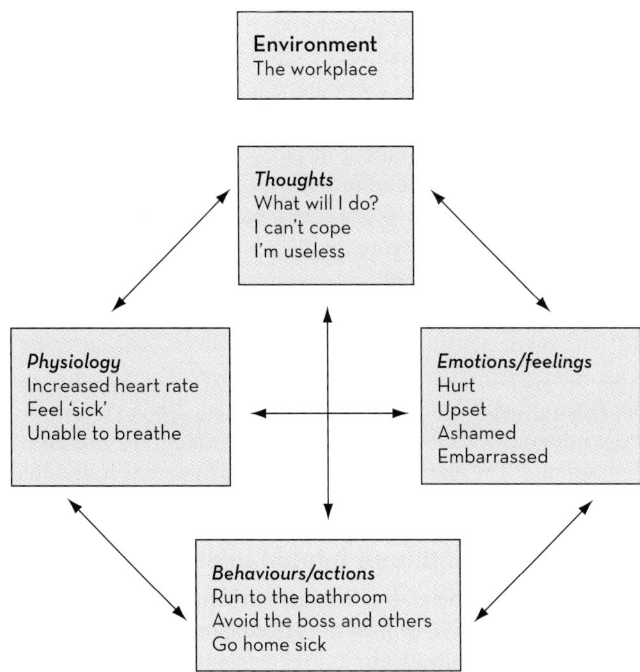

Fig. 24.1 The five-part model for problem identification using cognitive behavioural therapy (*Source*: Adapted from Padesky, C.A., Mooney, K.A., 1990. Presenting the cognitive model to patients. International Cognitive Therapy Newsletter, 6, 6–7.)

Assessment for suitability to engage with the CBT model is carried out initially. This assessment will determine whether the person might have the necessary motivation to change and the ability to engage and to problem solve. The model is prescriptive—that is, there is a distinct process for engaging in therapy using CBT. Regardless of the person's difficulties, the same specific techniques and strategies central to the model are used. These include Socratic questioning (Calvert & Palmer 2003) and homework, such as charting behaviours and mood using a visual analogue scale and keeping automatic thought records. Keeping an automatic thought record alerts the person to the negative automatic thoughts that continue to affect their feelings and behaviour, ultimately maintaining mental health problems. Homework is set after each session to ensure that the patient remains motivated and learns the skills to take over their own therapy.

Initially, patients are given an overview of CBT and shown how the five-part model (illustrated in Fig. 24.1) will be used to identify the more serious problems. Patients are asked to identify a situation that caused a strong negative emotional response in them. Then they identify their specific emotional responses to that situation as well as their cognitions, physical responses and behaviours. The fifth aspect of the model, the environment, provides the context within which these responses occurred, including culture and personal history. Organising the person's experiences into the categories of thoughts, feelings, behaviour and physical responses is fundamental to CBT (Dattilio & Padesky 1990). An example of this might be if an employee, 'Jane', received negative feedback about her work performance from her employer and had a strong emotional response. Figure 24.1 shows a description of the emotions, thoughts, actions and physical responses that occurred within the work environment for Jane during this scenario. You can see from this scenario how thoughts and feelings are inextricably linked and how they lead to behaviours that are unhelpful in living a full and satisfying life.

The therapeutic relationship in CBT is collaborative. The patient is an active participant in the process and is responsible for learning new ways of responding. There is also an emphasis on empiricism, which is the gathering of data to provide evidence to challenge current beliefs. Patients are taught to identify their dysfunctional thoughts and the therapist then tests the validity of those beliefs. For example, in the situation described earlier and in Figure 24.1, Jane believes that everyone thinks she is stupid. The therapist would ask Jane for evidence of this. It is most unlikely that Jane would have any evidence. Ultimately, patients learn to evaluate their own thoughts and manage their own responses (Dattilio & Padesky 1990).

Over many years, CBT has been found to be very effective in the treatment of depression and is now used for a range of health conditions. Its efficacy has been strongly reported for the anxiety disorders (e.g. Barlow et al. 2005; Handley et al. 2015; Rosser et al. 2004), even when delivered online with children (Rooksby et al. 2015), and for the management of medication nonadherence (Rodrigues 2007). CBT has also been found to be useful in working with people with learning disabilities (Brown & Marshall 2006) and for people requiring cancer care and palliative care (Mannix et al. 2006; Semple et al. 2006).

Acceptance and Commitment Therapy

ACT is spoken as the word 'act' rather than spelled out like DBT and CBT. ACT takes on its true meaning in this therapeutic approach because it has a philosophy about taking action to make change so that one lives a meaningful life according to one's values. Developed in 1986 by Steven Hayes, a psychologist, and emanating from behavioural therapy, ACT combines mindfulness skills with behavioural activities linked to personal values. ACT is a brief therapeutic approach that acknowledges the normal functions of the human brain that are designed to ensure our survival but that, in the modern world, undermine our coping. According to Harris (2007), we become caught in 'vicious cycles' of attempting to manage uncomfortable thoughts and feelings with strategies that ultimately become the problem.

Life is challenging and sometimes very difficult and this often causes us to have unpleasant thoughts and feelings. The human response is usually to attempt to eliminate or control those experiences, or to use 'emotional control strategies' that might cause long-term harm, such as drinking excessive amounts of alcohol. According to Harris, there are two major goals of ACT:

- Developing acceptance of unwanted private experiences which are out of personal control, and
- Commitment and action towards living a valued life (Harris 2006, p. 5).

Rather than trying to teach people how to change or get rid of unwanted thoughts and feelings, ACT aims for acceptance and accommodation of those troublesome thoughts and feelings (Kohlenberg et al. 1993).

There are six core processes in ACT. These are:

1. *Contact with the present moment:* Instead of focussing on the past or the future, this involves being fully engaged with what is happening in the here and now. Mindfulness allows us to engage fully in what we are doing 'in the moment'.
2. *Acceptance:* When we have unpleasant thoughts and feelings we automatically try to push them away or avoid them. This aspect of ACT asks you to be fully open to your experiences and this ultimately makes those experiences less uncomfortable.
3. *Defusion:* Unpleasant thoughts can become overpowering to the extent that they take on an almost tangible life of their own. Defusion involves developing strategies to recognise thoughts as simply 'mind chatter'. Relating to your thoughts in a different way will enable you to see thoughts for what they are . . . just thoughts.
4. *The observing self:* Also referred to as 'self-as-context', this is a concept that can be quite difficult to engage. Once you are able to experience yourself as more than your thoughts, feelings, memories, images or physical body, you will be better able to distance yourself from them and better able to connect with the here and now.
5. *Values:* Understanding what is important to you allows you to live a life that is meaningful to you. ACT engages you in the process of clarifying your values so that you can begin to live a life that is more committed to those values.
6. *Committed action:* Taking action is often the most difficult part for many of us but it is not possible to live a meaningful life unless you take action that is guided by your values. *Committed* action involves continuing to take action regardless of how many times you fail.

Historically, ACT has been shown to be effective across a range of conditions including depression and anxiety (Kohlenberg et al. 1993; Swain et al. 2013). More recent studies have proved ACT to be efficacious in stress management (Daltry 2015), in reducing posttraumatic stress disorder (PTSD) symptoms in adolescents (Woidneck et al. 2014), in working with people with persistent symptoms of psychosis (Bacon et al. 2014) and in improving the lives of people with cancer (Feros et al. 2013; Hulbert-Williams et al. 2015). ACT has been shown to be useful across a range of mental illnesses and in transdiagnostic or heterogeneous groups; that is, where group participants suffer from any type of illness (Pinto et al. 2015). This is because the intervention increases our capacity to respond in more flexible ways to the things that distress us and so the symptoms of psychological distress are reduced.

Dialectical Behaviour Therapy

DBT was developed by Marsha Linehan and first published in 1993. It is a therapeutic technique designed specifically to help to manage self-harming or self-injurious behaviours in people, frequently women, who meet the criteria for a diagnosis of borderline personality disorder. DBT is highly structured, goal-oriented and time-limited, and is based on a cognitive-behavioural approach paired with Eastern mindfulness practices.

The patient's involvement in DBT is voluntary. Inevitably, the person will be committed to working towards the behaviour change that is necessary to alter their difficulties, leading to a more satisfying life. This is known as the pretreatment phase of DBT. Without commitment from the patient, DBT cannot proceed. In particular, 'the patient must agree to work on decreasing parasuicidal behaviours [self-harming] and interpersonal styles that interfere with therapy and on increasing behavioural skills' (Swales et al. 2000, p. 10). The core intervention strategies involved are validation and problem solving. The main work is carried out in weekly individual therapy sessions that focus on targeted behaviours. The therapist accepts the patient as a valid human being while at the same time expecting change (dialectics). The most important behaviour to be addressed is the self-harming behaviour. Once the person learns how to better manage this behaviour, other issues are addressed.

The group therapy aspect of DBT occurs concurrently with individual therapy and involves skills training. The person with borderline personality disorder has not developed effective coping skills, and so learning how to solve problems effectively is very important. There are four groups of skills, or modules (Linehan 1993):

- core mindfulness skills (derived from Buddhist meditation)
- interpersonal effectiveness skills
- emotion modulation skills
- distress tolerance skills

As skills are learned in the group sessions they are applied in the real world and also addressed in individual counselling sessions. The therapist acts as coach to support the use of these new skills, both within sessions and over the telephone as problems arise (Wolpow 2000). It is the combination of acceptance or validation and active change or problem solving that brings about the alteration in personality style that enables people to lead more fulfilling lives.

Before considering DBT, it is important to consider what borderline personality disorder means (see also Chapter 17), especially in the context of DBT. People with borderline personality disorder can be very challenging to work with because of their personality style, which often develops as the result of a very difficult childhood. According to Linehan (1993), the experiences and responses of the child who develops borderline personality disorder were 'invalidated' or disqualified by the significant others around the child. This means that the child's experiences were not acknowledged or accepted as real. Sexual abuse is considered the ultimate form of invalidation and is frequently an aspect of the history of people with borderline personality disorder. At the same time, Linehan argues that, for these people, there exists a biological predisposition within the autonomic nervous system to react poorly to stress. Indeed, research into the neurobiological impacts of all forms of abuse confirms increased adrenocorticotropic hormone concentrations in abused women (MacMillan & Munn 2001). It is important to note that the majority of people who are given the diagnosis of borderline personality disorder are women.

The person with borderline personality disorder classically feels deeply emotionally unfulfilled, resulting in chaos and the use of maladaptive coping strategies such as substance abuse and self-harming. Linehan (1993) points out that these patients are unable to regulate their emotions (they have extreme emotional reactions to situations), have chaotic interpersonal relationships, have a disturbed sense of self and are unable to regulate their thoughts and behaviours. They lack problem-solving skills and so respond to life haphazardly. They frequently engage in self-damaging behaviours such as substance abuse, promiscuity and overeating, but the most common behaviour leading to a need for mental healthcare is self-mutilation. According to the DBT approach, the diagnosis relates to a certain pattern of behaviours and so, once these self-damaging behaviours cease, the diagnosis also no longer exists (Swales et al. 2000).

DBT was originally designed as an individual therapy approach combined with group skills training, telephone contact between sessions and a strong emphasis on therapists also receiving DBT from each other. Therapist consultation is fundamental due to the risk of therapist burnout when working so intensively with patients with such challenging patterns of behaviour. Aspects of DBT can now be applied in a range of settings using the principles of treatment rather than these specific modes (Wolpow 2000) and for a range of conditions (Linehan et al. 1999). However, success is determined by the quality of the patient–therapist relationship. In particular, the patient learns that their own needs and the therapist's needs are both important.

Solution-Focussed Brief Therapy

SFBT uses the therapeutic relationship to support the person to identify their strengths and abilities, and McAllister (2003) argues that this is an approach that is more closely aligned to the philosophy of nursing. Working in a solution-focussed way requires a shift in the way we work with people that is more closely aligned with the recovery philosophy (Chopra et al. 2009). A collaborative approach enables us to see the patient as having a view about where they see themselves now and into the future. Collaboration involves working alongside and with the person rather than assuming superior knowledge and expertise. A solution orientation assumes that the person has goals and aspirations and is capable of working towards their achievement with our support. The initial identification of clear and achievable goals is essential and these provide the ongoing focus for therapy.

Developed by De Shazer and colleagues in the United States (De Shazer 1985), the solution-focussed approach to therapy helps people to find solutions to their problems rather than dwelling on the problems. Based in the strengths approach to working therapeutically, the solution-focussed approach turns away from a problem orientation in favour of acknowledging the person's strengths and capacities. The traditional approach to people with mental health problems is to identify their problems and attempt to solve or ameliorate those problems. Inherently paternalistic, the problem-based approach positions the care provider as expert and fails to consider the person in distress as the expert in their own experience. Fundamental to the solution-focussed approach is the view that the person is capable of knowing what is best for them (Ferraz & Wellman 2008) and that the person is able to move towards the achievement of self-defined goals.

Ferraz and Wellman (2008, p. 39) provide a brief overview of the techniques involved and point out that 'the therapeutic process is structured around using questions to identify patient strengths, resources and their vision of a future when their problems are solved or at least not present'. The starting point is to find out what the person hopes to achieve and to consider what the person has already done or is doing to achieve those goals. Three specific techniques used in SFBT are outlined here.

1. The Miracle Question is a well-known technique that has developed out of SFBT (Weatherall & Gibson 2015). It is a question specifically designed to help the person to begin to see what life might be like if their goals were to be achieved. This inspires hope and optimism for the future (Ruddick 2008). According to De Shazer (1988), the Miracle Question is posed like this: 'Imagine that you go home to bed tonight and go to sleep. While you are asleep a miracle happens and that miracle is that your current problems are resolved. But, because you were sleeping when the miracle happened, you're not even aware that the miracle has happened. So, when you wake in the morning, what are the things that you will notice that will make you realise that this miracle has happened?' Talking about miracles might not suit everyone, so you might modify this slightly to talk about a 'shift in the universe' or about a magical spell if that better suits your conversational style.
2. To enable a focus on the person's strengths, one of the central tasks of SFBT is to 'Search for Exceptions'. As the nurse you would ask the person to talk about times when their problem or issue might have occurred but it didn't cause the same degree of distress that they are experiencing at the moment. Here the person is 'encouraged to describe what was different when the problem did not occur, or what they did differently' (Ferraz & Wellman 2008, p. 39). This helps the person to see that they have applied certain skills in the past that helped them and that doing this again might help them to achieve their goals.
3. Another technique specific to SFBT is 'Scaling'. A scale rated from 0 to 10 is used to help the person to visualise how they are moving towards the achievement of their goals or desired future. Zero on the scale means they are as far away as possible from achieving their goals and 10 means they have reached their goals and are living the life they had hoped for. A score better than zero suggests that the person is doing something well to move them forwards and this is worth pointing out. For example, if the person places themselves at a 4 on the scale, rather than focussing on how much more needs to be done, you would ask them

to talk about what they are doing now that helps them along (Ferraz & Wellman 2008). Identifying and reinforcing even small movements towards the achievement of goals is fundamental to the solution-focussed approach.

In their work to introduce SFBT to mental health nurses working in acute psychiatric admission units, Hosany et al. (2007, p. 689) saw this as an opportunity for nurses to engage more collaboratively with people in their care in this setting and point out that this approach 'aims to discover "what works" in a given situation, simply and practically. The focus of discussion is on solutions (not problems), the future (not the past) and on what's going well (rather than what's gone wrong).' The results of their pilot study showed that staff significantly reduced their focus on problems and used each of the three solution-focussed techniques described earlier significantly more often.

Haley (2000) provides an engaging account of how she used solution-focussed counselling with a survivor of sexual abuse. She outlines the counselling sessions and specific strategies used to help the patient achieve her goals, ultimately demonstrating that resolution of problems is possible. Atkinson and Amesu (2007) provide an interesting account of how solution-focussed approaches can be used alongside MI in helping young people to address substance use and other concerns. They outline some excellent questions to help guide the therapeutic process and to work towards change. Examples include:

- What has worked for you in the past?
- Who has helped you?
- If change is going to happen soon, what needs to happen so that change can take place, and who needs to help?
- How will you know that things are changing?
- Who would notice that things are changing and what might they say? (Atkinson & Amesu 2007, p. 34)

SFBT provides some focussed strategies that even the novice nurse can use to help a patient to move forwards. Keeping in mind the philosophical emphasis on the person's strengths and abilities will ensure that you are effective.

BEHAVIOUR THERAPY

The behavioural model developed from the early work of Pavlov at the turn of the nineteenth century and Skinner during the early twentieth century. Pavlov's early experiments involving dogs showed that involuntary behaviours can be conditioned to occur (classical conditioning) and that, ultimately, this learned response can be unlearned (extinguished). It is normal for salivation to occur in response to the presentation of food, but it is not normal for salivation to occur at the sound of a tuning fork. Pavlov paired the presentation of food with the sound of a tuning fork until eventually salivation occurred at the sound of the tuning fork without the presence of food. The dogs had been conditioned to salivate at the sound of the tuning fork. Persistent sounding of the tuning fork without the presentation of food eventually led to extinction of this learned response—that is, the dogs no longer salivated at the sound of the tuning fork.

CRITICAL THINKING CHALLENGE 24.3

What are some of your conditioned responses? For example, consider how the sound of the school bell at the end of the day results in a lightening of mood for both students and teachers! What happens when you smell toast cooking in the kitchen?

Skinner later developed the early work of Thorndike (1911, cited in Barker & Fraser 1985). He called this operant conditioning and showed that behaviours can be learned and unlearned through processes of positive and negative reinforcement. That is, behaviours can be strengthened through positive reinforcement or the presentation of rewards, and weakened through negative reinforcement involving the removal of rewards. Removing a reinforcer to a behaviour, such as walking away from a child having a temper tantrum, results in extinction of the temper tantrum behaviour. Be aware, though, that initially ignoring a behaviour will result in an increase in that behaviour before it begins to subside.

Negative reinforcement can also be used to change behaviour. When defined in behavioural terms, negative reinforcement refers to procedures designed to suppress behaviours, not the infliction of a punishment, psychological pain or harm. Negative reinforcement decreases the strength of certain behaviours rather than eliminating them (Sundel & Sundel 1993). Negative reinforcement can involve applying a negative stimulus immediately after the unwanted behaviour is performed. An example of this is when the teacher humiliates a student verbally for arriving late at class. Alternatively, negative reinforcement might involve the removal of a positive reinforcer. Examples of this include a child being placed in time-out following a temper tantrum, or a person with anorexia who loses weight, or doesn't gain weight according to a prescribed schedule, losing the privilege of calling their friends for 48 hours. To be effective, the negative reinforcement needs to be applied consistently; that is, each time the behaviour presents, the negative reinforcement is applied. Negative reinforcement is most effective when applied immediately after the undesirable behaviour. It is also important to specify alternative behaviours that are more appropriate (Sundel & Sundel 1993).

Behaviour therapy has been found to be particularly useful in explaining the development of anxieties and fears and the ways in which these are generalised to a range of stimuli. For example, a person who has a fear of spiders may well find that the fear generalises to a range of crawling insects as well as to toys and pictures of spiders. The events that occur prior to or after behaviours determine whether those behaviours will be learned, maintained or changed. For example, the presence of a spider will result in heightened anxiety. Moving away from the spider causes the anxiety to subside. Therefore, the person learns that spiders are to be feared and to avoid spiders. Unfortunately, this will result in avoidance of environments that have the potential to contain spiders, causing constriction of the person's social world.

CASE STUDY 24.3

George

George suffers from schizophrenia but is more disadvantaged by his social and panic anxiety (see Chapter 18). Using Truax's (2002) model for behavioural case conceptualisation, the reinforcers and punishments that cause his anxieties to occur and persist, resulting in increasing social isolation, are:

- *Positive reinforcement*—an increase in a consequence leads to an increased probability that panic attacks will happen in the future. For example, George's family members carry out his weekly grocery shopping and manage his finances and bill paying for him. This reinforcement increases the likelihood of George not engaging in these behaviours and increases the probability of panic attacks occurring should he engage in these behaviours.
- *Negative reinforcement*—a decrease in an uncomfortable or aversive consequence or outcome leads to increased avoidance of anxiety-provoking situations in the future. When George stays at home rather than engaging in social situations or using public transport, it reduces his anxiety, thereby increasing his avoidance of these anxiety-provoking situations.
- *Positive punishment*—an increase in a negative consequence leads to decreased engagement in anxiety-provoking situations in the future. For example, when George goes for long walks far from his home but within his street, his anxiety increases because he fears 'freaking out'. He has now limited his walks to a small radius from his home, and so his social world is shrinking even further.
- *Negative punishment*—a decrease in a consequence leads to a decreased probability that he will stay in anxiety-provoking situations in the future. For example, George is unable to use positive self-talk to manage his anxiety and is therefore unable to stay in anxiety-provoking situations. He is so certain that he will 'freak out' that he no longer puts himself at risk.

It is important to point out that in Case Study 24.3, George is not aware that his avoidance of anxiety-provoking situations actually increases his anxiety. He will not accept the idea that staying within an anxiety-provoking situation will be helpful in managing his anxiety and in preventing future panic attacks. George believes that he would 'freak out' and that this would be the most awful outcome for him. He would feel vulnerable and he might never get back home. Combined with education, staying with George and verbally supporting him to stay within the anxiety-provoking situation will show him that his most feared outcome will not be realised. Once he recognises that avoidance only worsens the situation, that he can cope with his anxiety and that terrible things won't happen to him, he can begin to change his behaviour.

In George's case, the target behaviour, the behaviour we wish to change, is the social isolation that George suffers as a result of his avoidance of anxiety-provoking situations. It is important to point out that 'the target behaviour is the behaviour to be observed and measured; it is the focus of modification' (Sundel & Sundel 1993, p. 4). The target behaviour can be the behaviour we want to increase (e.g. acceptable or appropriate social behaviour), or the behaviour we want to minimise (e.g. lying on the bed all day). George has hopes and goals that include working and living in a small beachside community. In order to achieve these goals, George needs to be able to cope with driving a vehicle or using public transport, meeting new people and widening his social world without fear of losing control.

Prior to working with George and his problems, the nurse would need to carry out a behavioural assessment. This requires George to record the triggers, both internal and external, to his anxiety, and to identify his physical, cognitive, emotional and behavioural responses. The frequency and duration of anxiety responses would also need to be recorded. This helps to identify specific cues to certain behaviours and also to determine improvement or deterioration. Treatment should address both his behavioural responses (e.g. social avoidance) and his cognitive responses (e.g. believing that he will lose control and perhaps his life). This is because his beliefs continue to limit his ability to act.

After determining what causes and maintains certain behaviours, it is possible to develop a treatment plan together that specifies goals, what will need to be done to achieve those goals, how goal achievement will be measured and a timeline for goal achievement. For example, George may set as his goal: being able to travel into the city in a car. A plan involving systematically working from sitting in a stationary car to driving short distances in the car, to travelling into the city, will need to be laid out. The plan will also need to indicate how many weeks or months this process will take.

GROUP THERAPY

Group therapy involves the engagement of two or more people in therapy at the same time. This mode of therapy is more cost effective than individual therapies because more people can be treated at once. Group counselling is also more efficient if the group is composed of people with similar problems (the homogeneous group)—for example, a psychoeducational group for families of people with schizophrenia. However, efficiency and cost effectiveness are not the most important reasons for engaging people in group therapy. There are immense benefits for people joining together with others who are experiencing the same or similar difficulties (Gerhart et al. 2015). Often benefits are derived from interactions with others in the group rather than through the therapeutic efforts of the counsellor (Byrne & Byrne 1996).

There are as many approaches that can be taken in group therapy as there are for individual therapy. Group therapy provides an opportunity for people to explore their thoughts, feelings and behaviours and the impact they have on others. This is achieved through facilitation by the therapist/nurse therapist and through feedback from other group members. Ultimately, learning occurs about relating to others. One thing that is certain is that almost everyone benefits from healthy interpersonal relationships. We are all social beings and we thrive on relating to others. An important outcome of any type of group is the relationships developed with others and the opportunity to learn better or more effective ways of relating (see Nurse's Story 24.1).

NURSE'S STORY 24.1

Facilitating a Group

I used to facilitate a discharge planning group in an acute inpatient setting. This was an open group due to the nature of the rapid turnover of patients in this setting. While I might plan for a reasonably structured group with specific goals, the members inevitably determined the direction of the group. I always began with introductions and gave each person an opportunity to identify short- and long-term goals. I also attempted to discuss any concerns about medications, accommodation, family relationships, employment and money management. However, the acuity of the mental health problems of the group members dictated the issues addressed. For example, a group member with a bipolar mood disorder and somewhat elevated in mood will inevitably find it difficult to stay 'on track'. As the group facilitator, it's important to allow everyone to participate in the group. It may be necessary to gently point out the domination by a group member or to encourage others to have some say. Despite this challenge to the group process, it enables several of the curative factors to operate. These include and are probably not limited to: universality, instillation of hope, altruism, interpersonal learning and the development of socialising techniques. So, despite the concerns of nurses that group therapy might not be effective or appropriate in an acute inpatient setting, coupled with the challenges that these groups will pose, group therapy is valuable at a range of levels, not least of which is patients having the opportunity to relate more effectively with others.

Therapeutic groups can be divided into two main categories: general-purpose groups and problem-focussed groups (Earley 2000). Addressing specific issues such as grief, sexual abuse or alcohol abuse is the goal of problem-focussed groups. They aim to impart information and provide support to people in crisis and consequently are time limited. General-purpose groups attempt to facilitate deeper character change by addressing problems that arise from the interpersonal processes that occur in groups (Earley 2000). This involves the expression of transference and counter-transference as early relationships and customary interpersonal difficulties are reenacted in the group with other group members. These processes occur unconsciously, and interactions within the group provide opportunities for other group members or the therapist to gently make the person aware of what has been happening.

Yalom (1995) determined that there are 11 curative or therapeutic factors that occur in psychotherapy groups. When a psychotherapeutic group is working effectively, these curative factors are operating and group members are benefiting from them. The factors work interdependently—that is, they do not occur or function separately but interrelate with each other. The same factors operate in every type of group but their interplay and importance can vary widely from group to group. In addition, people from within the same group can benefit from differing clusters of therapeutic factors. These factors are:

- *Instilling of hope*—people are inspired by the improvements that others have made, and the group provides opportunity for the therapist to point out the improvements people have made.
- *Universality*—entering a group enables people to see that they are not alone in their struggles. Hearing that others have the same difficulties is reassuring because people realise that their problems are not beyond solving.
- *Imparting information*—this might include learning about their illness or how to cope. Education might be an explicit or implicit part of the group.
- *Altruism*—in giving to and supporting others, group members also receive. Finding that they are valuable to others boosts self-esteem.
- *Corrective recapitulation of the family group*—the therapy group represents the family in many ways. This provides the opportunity to act out old family relationships and to recognise how earlier relationships continue to be acted out in current relationships.
- *Development of socialising techniques*—learning social skills might be an explicit part of the group or it may be more indirect, as people observe the socially acceptable behaviour of others.
- *Imitative behaviour*—group therapists influence the communication patterns in members by modelling certain behaviours such as self-disclosure or support.
- *Interpersonal learning*—the group becomes a social microcosm so that members are able to reenact interpersonal behaviours typical of their lives outside the group. Feedback from others enables them to see that their behaviours are responsible for their interpersonal difficulties.
- *Group cohesiveness*—cohesiveness is essential for the other curative factors to operate. It involves members feeling warmth and comfort in the group and feeling that they belong and are accepted and supported by others.
- *Catharsis*—this is the expression and mutual working through of strong emotions that have not been expressed previously. The group provides a safe environment for this to happen. Therefore, catharsis will occur only once group cohesiveness develops.
- *Existential factors*—these are the elements in the group process that help members to develop an understanding of their individual existences. This is more likely to occur in groups where there is a focus on thinking, talking and feeling.

Some of these factors are self-evident, while others are more subtle and take an understanding of psychotherapy to enable their facilitation and expression. Nevertheless, when setting up a group therapy programme, it is important to plan it well (Sharry 2001) and to consider the expectations or goals you have for the group. If you are the therapist you will need to decide whether it will be a closed group—that is, one that has a set number of members for a set period of time—or an open group. An open group allows different membership each time the group meets and the group membership at each session will determine to some extent the direction the group takes. Whichever type of group you facilitate, there will be a specific process of coming together or initial engagement, reaction and resistance to working, developing trust, working through issues, and termination or closure (Fehr 1999). In an open group, trust may take longer to develop as membership fluctuates.

Activity Groups

Activity groups grew out of the perceived need to occupy people during the long hospital stays of the past. Ultimately, activity groups became a part of psychosocial rehabilitation programmes and are also often part of an organised therapy programme in psychiatric inpatient units today. While the task of organising an activity programme has been taken on largely by occupational therapists, this role was historically a nursing responsibility. Given the amount of time that nurses spend with patients, nurses need to once again embrace this responsibility. Activity groups involve gathering together a group of people interested in a particular activity or those who need to develop skills in a particular area.

Examples of activity groups include those based on cooking skills, gardening, art, walking, newspaper discussion, reminiscence, and games and sporting groups. Many inpatient psychiatric units hold daily 'community meetings' designed to engage people in daily planning and organisation. Originally developed to help construct a therapeutic milieu—that is, a physical and emotional ward environment that is therapeutic and empowering for patients—these community groups might also be viewed as activity groups in some respects. Despite the perception that activity groups are not particularly challenging and that they only serve the purpose of keeping people occupied, many of Yalom's curative factors outlined earlier can operate. Not least of these are the development of socialising techniques and imitative behaviour.

FAMILY THERAPY

Family therapy developed in the 1950s from the belief that the family was responsible for causing schizophrenia. In particular, it was believed that certain communication styles within families were responsible for causing the illness (the skewed and schismatic families). A further belief centred on the communication style of the mother, the so-called schizophrenogenic mother. Although these ideas have long since been rejected, a group of interventions known as family therapy had been born (Goldenberg & Goldenberg 2000). Family therapy shifted the focus on therapy directed at unconscious material (psychotherapy) 'to a focus on the interpersonal process—that is, how family members interact with each other' (Kadis & McClendon 1998, p. 6).

Family therapy is an approach to treatment that is based on the fundamental premise that when a person has a problem, it usually involves the whole family (Eisler et al. 2007; Mellor et al. 2000). Family interactions might be causing the problem or prolonging the problem for the identified patient, or the problem or behaviours of the patient might be affecting other members of the family. Family therapists aim to effect change in the entire family system. Family therapy usually involves multiple family members, not necessarily the same family members each time, or therapy might involve a single family member (Meech & Wood 2000).

Even when therapy involves a single individual, its impact will be experienced by the wider family. This might be demonstrated through an improvement in family functioning and/or through the alleviation of symptoms (Mellor et al. 2000). Unlike individual therapists who believe that problems reside within the person, family therapists believe that 'the dominant forces within our lives are located externally, within the family' (Nichols & Schwartz 2001, p. 6). Therapy concentrates on the family and the way it is organised. Ultimately, this affects the lives of each family member in some way. That is, the whole system is affected (see Case Study 24.4 about Kurran and Devika).

Nichols and Schwartz (2001) maintain that family therapy is particularly useful in working with children who are having problems. This is because they are strongly influenced by the family and must remain within its influence. Marital problems, family feuds and difficulties that develop in people when there has been a major family transition are also particularly amenable to family therapy. Family therapy has been found to be very useful in the treatment of gambling disorders (Mladenovic et al. 2015) and eating disorders (Gelin et al. 2015), and in changing the behaviours of young people who break the law (Dakof et al. 2015). The role of the family therapist is to understand the dynamics that occur within families and to help the family members to reconsider the ways in which they interact with each other. The family therapist then motivates the family members to change.

When working with families, the problem is viewed as dysfunction in the relationship between family members. The relationship therefore becomes the focus of attention. Sometimes the person identified as 'the problem' behaves in that way in order to hold the family together. For example, consider the child who misbehaves when her parents begin fighting. The misbehaviour distracts the parents from their conflict and so further fighting is averted. The parents then work together to manage the child's problem behaviour. Ultimately, the problem is not with the child but with the marital relationship.

CASE STUDY 24.4

Kurran and Devika

Kurran and Devika have been married for 30 years. Devika has a bipolar affective disorder and had been moderately depressed for around 2 years. At around the time that Devika became well, Kurran was made redundant from his job after a very lengthy period of employment with the company. Kurran had always been the breadwinner and the caregiver in the family. Now his wife was supporting him emotionally and was independent of him. This role transition resulted in a great deal of conflict in the family. Kurran had difficulty adjusting to his new role and in accepting that his wife no longer relied on him. Their teenage daughter blamed her mother for causing the conflict. Although Devika was being held responsible for the problems, no doubt due to her history of mental health problems, essentially the expected roles of family members had been reversed and there was now confusion about how to function. The therapy concentrated on the patterns of communication within the family and on accepting that Devika was now well and functioning in different and unexpected ways.

The two-way mirror is a useful tool in family therapy. While there is a therapist in the room with the family, behind the mirror sit a number of other members of the team observing the therapy in progress. This allows immediate feedback, as the observers call in to the therapy room by telephone to give feedback or direction to the therapist and/or family. Observers may see things (communication styles, body language) that the therapist does not, so these can be communicated during the session rather than following it.

Another tool used in family therapy is the genogram, which is a graphic representation of the family and its patterns across generations. The genogram is drawn up with the involvement of the family, helping to engage all family members, as the mapping process seeks input from everyone. Enduring and broken relationships, illegitimate and legitimate children, blended and nuclear family relationships are all depicted on the same page, revealing the emotional processes of the family to both the therapist and the family members (McGoldrick et al. 1999).

Psychoeducation

Initially designed to help families develop skills to understand and cope with a family member with schizophrenia, psychoeducation is now used with families with any type of difficulty, including families with relationship problems (Goldenberg & Goldenberg 2000). In the mental health field, psychoeducation refers to the provision of information about a person's mental illness to that person and/or their family. Psychoeducation grew out of the belief that people with mental illness, particularly those with schizophrenia, are vulnerable to stress and that excessive stress in the person's life is likely to exacerbate the illness—that is, too much stress will cause the person to become unwell or to relapse. Therefore, psychoeducation is considered an intervention designed to reduce the impact of the illness on the patient. For example, it has been found to be effective in reducing the number and duration of relapses for patients with bipolar affective disorders (Colom et al. 2003).

The early work of Brown (1958, cited in Bland 1986) claimed that some families contribute to stress through the ways they communicate and behave. These families were deemed to have high levels of expressed emotion (EE) and high EE was considered detrimental to the wellbeing of the person with schizophrenia. EE was originally defined as consisting of five constructs: critical comments, hostility, emotional over-involvement, warmth and positive remarks (Jenkins & Karno 1992). Today, however, EE in families tends to be assessed only in terms of the first three, negative, constructs. The level of EE in families is determined through a face-to-face interview with family members, known as the Camberwell Family Interview. Once a family is deemed to indicate high EE, psychoeducation is considered the appropriate intervention.

Psychoeducation programmes are usually run in multi-family groups over several weeks but may also be organised around the needs of individual families. The benefit of several families coming together in a group is the sharing of information, the support they provide each other and the experience of universality—that is, the recognition that they are not alone in having these problems. Supportive family education programmes need to attempt to reinforce strengths and promote resilience. Psychoeducation will also enable families in particular to understand the medical jargon we use and to appreciate the experience from the perspective of others, including the patient. A comprehensive psychoeducation programme will provide information not only about the specific mental illness but also about the available resources in the community, as well as information on and practice in applying problem-solving skills (Palmer 1996).

Families and patients need to be provided with information about mental illness, just as they would if the diagnosis was a physical health problem. Indeed, Mullen et al. (2002) argue that family interventions need to be considered 'core business' for mental health services. When there is an emphasis on providing information to support patients and their families, they are more likely to benefit from the intervention. A collaborative approach that recognises the experiences of families and patients and their unique knowledge of the disorder will convey to them that they are not to blame and that they have something to contribute to the overall care plan. Family problems need to be viewed as normal responses to very difficult situations that tax the family's usual coping resources (Kavanagh 1992).

Providing psychoeducation to families is designed to alert them to the need to reduce stress at home and to change the ways in which they relate to the person with mental illness. This is thought to reduce relapse rates, which is argued to be a cost-effective way of managing mental illness. Ultimately, though, the psychoeducation approach designed to reduce EE in families maintains a philosophy that families are responsible for the illness, or at least are responsible for contributing to hospitalisation and subsequent healthcare costs. While historically families were blamed for directly causing mental illness, the shift to assessing EE and providing psychoeducation can be seen as a more subtle form of blaming families. Families experience considerable burden in taking care of family members with mental illness in the community. This perception of responsibility for the patient's illness has the potential to add to that burden.

PSYCHOSOCIAL REHABILITATION

Psychosocial rehabilitation is a treatment approach developed by professionals and designed for people severely disabled by long-term mental illness. Most people with enduring mental health concerns have a diagnosis of schizophrenia. However, many people with bipolar affective disorder and depression also have long-term needs (Ekdawi & Conning 1994). The cognitive and emotional problems experienced by people with enduring mental health concerns can result in social disability, which in turn results in their needing help and support to negotiate the social world (Perkins & Repper 1996). In line with the shift from inpatient to community mental healthcare, most psychosocial rehabilitation is now carried out in the community (see also Chapter 2 for issues related to patients, recovery and rehabilitation).

Psychosocial rehabilitation is the process of assisting people to tap into and learn the internal and external skills, supports and resources necessary to be successful (Vandevooren et al. 2007). Success is measured by the individual's satisfaction in living, learning and working in the environment(s) of their choice. At its most basic level, psychosocial rehabilitation seeks to help people to determine and prioritise their goals, identify the pathways for achieving those goals and develop the necessary skills and supports to achieve them (Anthony et al. 1991; Legere 2007). Rehabilitation programmes once had a 'one size fits all' approach to recovery, with mental health professionals determining what they thought people needed to do in order to return to community living. Psychosocial rehabilitation programmes today are much more person-centred, with collaboration and choice designed to help people to achieve their individual goals.

The concept of recovery from physical illness and disability does not mean that the suffering has disappeared, all the symptoms have been removed and/or functioning has been completely restored. For example, as Deegan (1988) points out, a person with paraplegia can recover even though the spinal cord cannot. Similarly, a person with mental illness can recover even though the illness is not cured. Recovery is what people with disabilities do. Treatment, case management and rehabilitation are what helpers do to facilitate recovery (Anthony 1993). It is argued that before a person actively engages the rehabilitation services offered, they need to have embarked on their personal journey of recovery (Anthony 1993). Psychosocial rehabilitation efforts designed to have a positive impact on severe mental illness can do more than leave the person less impaired, less dysfunctional, less disabled and less disadvantaged. These interventions can result in the person gaining more meaning, purpose, success and satisfaction with their life. Recovery outcomes include more subjective outcomes such as self-esteem, empowerment and self-determination. For example, art appreciation (Ketch et al. 2015) and art therapy (De Vecchi et al. 2015) have been shown to have positive impacts on mood, self-esteem, relationships and community participation.

Curtis (1997, p 16) has identified a number of recovery principles that, she argues, need to be reflected in the rehabilitation programmes we offer:

- Recovery is an active, ongoing and individual process.
- Recovery is not linear; it entails growth, plateaus, setbacks, side tracks and fast tracks.
- Recovery relates not only to the experience of symptoms, but also to the secondary assaults of stigma, discrimination and abuse.
- Hope is the most fundamental factor in recovery.
- Recovery requires the presence of people who believe in and stand by the person.
- Recovery can occur without professional intervention.
- The establishment of a sense of control or free will is critical to recovery.
- 'Remembering your track record', or learning from observing your own mental and emotional behaviour, is critical to coping.
- Self-directed coping strategies are effective and can be learned.
- Maintaining or developing connections to valued activities and people is critical to the recovery process.
- Connecting with other people on a human level is important.
- Recovery is a process of 'finding meaning in your experience'.

There are a number of possible stimulants to recovery. These may include other patients who are in recovery or recovering effectively. Books, films and therapy groups may lead to unexpected insights into possible life options. Visiting new places and talking to various people are other ways in which the recovery process might be triggered. Critical to recovery is regaining the belief that there are options from which to choose, a belief perhaps even more important to recovery than the particular option one initially chooses (Curtis 1997). Therefore, we need to structure our settings so that recovery 'triggers' are present. Boring day treatment programmes and inactive inpatient programmes are characterised by a dearth of recovery stimulants (Anthony 1993). We need more creative programming. The strongest recovery-oriented programmes identified to date are those that arise from and are operated by skilled patient providers (Curtis 1997). Chapter 2 is devoted to recovery as the context of mental health nursing practice.

The Clubhouse model offers a recovery-oriented model for psychosocial rehabilitation that emphasises partnership between members and staff (Raeburn et al. 2014) that has been shown to align well with the principles of self-determination theory (Raeburn et al. 2015). Clubhouse International declares its intention to give people with mental illness hope and the opportunity to reach their full potential. There are currently more than 300 Clubhouses operating in 33 countries around the world. Central to the daily activities within Clubhouses is the 'work-ordered day': a strategy designed to emulate real-world expectations in relation to work and structure that also offers choice and opportunities for the development of a range of social and occupational skills. Tanaka and Davidson (2015, p. 269) investigated the nature and meaning of the work-ordered day to Clubhouse members and found that it helps people to 'reconstruct a life, develop their occupational self and skill sets, and experientially learn and live what parallels a good life in the general community'. Ensuring that psychosocial rehabilitation programmes are underpinned by a recovery philosophy will enable people to develop their personal skills and healthy relationships, develop independence, engage in supported education and employment, and enhance community inclusion (Rosen & O'Halloran 2014; Drake et al. 2015).

We cannot presume to know what a person hopes to achieve in life. We are all individuals who have different desires and needs (see Nurse's Story 24.2 on goals). As nurses, we may think we know what is best for a person, but this is at best naive and at worst paternalistic. Before engaging someone in rehabilitation services, it is important to find out what they hope to achieve. A rehabilitation programme designed to be completed by everyone is unlikely to suit the needs of all people seeking to recover from mental illness.

NURSE'S STORY 24.2

Goals

Goals are integral to living. Without goals we merely react to what happens in our lives. I used to routinely invite into the classroom two people with bipolar affective disorder who lived independently in the community. They talked about their experiences with mental health services to groups of post-graduate nursing students. While one of these people valued himself according to his ability to remain employed, the other accepted that work was too stressful for him. He gained his sense of self-worth from his ability to be a good husband and a good father to his two young daughters. Although the two held different goals, their goals allowed each of them to survive and thrive in the community.

To help identify people's goals I routinely started my inpatient predischarge group therapy sessions with introductions and a request for people to identify their short-term and 5-year goals. The goals were almost always quite different from each other. For some, at this stage of their illness, a 5-year projection into the future was impossible. However, everyone has a dream and this should be tapped into, as dreams provide the impetus for goals. Furthermore, it is not our place to decide whether the goals are realistic or not. If a goal seems unachievable, it might be wise to break it down into smaller and more achievable sub-goals. I would usually say, 'That sounds like a great goal. What do you think you'll need to do to achieve that?' From there, people are able to contemplate a way forward with something to live for and work towards.

Instilling Hope

There has been a great deal of research into what helps people with long-term mental illness to recover in such a way that they can live relatively normal and productive lives despite the reemergence of symptoms of illness from time to time. It has been found that hope is considered fundamental before a person can embark on recovery. Curtis (1997) identified a number of factors considered critical to recovery reported by patients. The factor that was ranked as the most important was having 'just one person who believed in me'. This is one of the ingredients thought to be important in promoting a sense of hope. Morse and Penrod (1999) offer a process model for the development of hope following a critical life experience, such as being told that you have breast cancer or that you have a mental illness. This model was developed out of qualitative enquiry exploring emotional responses to the experience of illness.

The Morse and Penrod (1999) model has a number of overlapping phases that begin with a critical life event. People inevitably experience uncertainty, suffering, hope and the challenge of despair and, ultimately, the achievement of a 'reformulated self'. At each of these phases, a different level of knowing or perceiving is experienced:

- *Enduring*—after a critical life experience we initially focus on cultivating our powers of endurance, which involves suspending or suppressing emotions and remaining in control. We do this because we worry that we will 'lose it' or disintegrate. The level of knowing here is awareness.
- *Uncertainty*—this is evident when we recognise what has happened and know what our goals are for the future, but we are unable to choose a course of action from a range of options. This state of uncertainty paralyses hope. At this time, we simply exist in an emotional state and suffer as a result of not being able to act. When we are in a state of uncertainty, we have no other choice but to tolerate the present.
- *Suffering*—the level of knowing here is acknowledgement. We begin to grasp the situation and consequently suffer emotionally. Morse and Penrod (1999, p. 148) comment that 'the depth of the state of suffering is despair, utter hopelessness'. Out of this overwhelming emotional experience, we begin to piece together reality and develop a perception of the future. 'This process of piecing together a new future begins in small incremental pieces, eventually building to . . . acceptance of the event and identification of both a goal and the means to attain it, which eventually leads to hope' (Morse & Penrod 1999, p. 148). So suffering is viewed as integral to moving on and ultimately to repair.
- *Hope*—the level of knowing is now acceptance and we become future oriented. We are able to develop an action plan designed to achieve desired goals. When we have hope, we understand the reality of the event while also understanding the real possibility of negative outcomes. Indeed, 'bracing for negative outcomes is a powerful motivating force for developing hope' (Morse & Penrod 1999, p. 148). Supportive relationships are now sought and hope is bolstered.
- *Reformulated self*—there is now a sense of becoming a 'better person' for having suffered. This state has been labelled the 'reformulated self', where the past is accepted and we also accept that the future has been irrevocably changed and a choice is made to 'make the most of life'.

Understanding the process involved in developing a sense of hope for one's future is fundamental to helping nurses know how to respond to people during the phases of enduring, uncertainty and suffering. If these phases are acknowledged as normal or expected, we will not make the mistake of attempting to force people to have hope when they are not ready to accept it. The trauma involved in dealing with a critical life experience, such as the diagnosis of a mental illness, results in a range of responses. These responses are part of a process that is not linear—people move back and forth between these phases. Understanding this may also explain the delays for some in developing hope. These are normal responses and so should not be assessed as being part of an illness.

Deegan (1996, 1997) was diagnosed with schizophrenia at 17 years of age and is very clear about the need for health professionals to treat people with mental illness as human beings. Although this may seem like a simple thing to do, the medically dominant model of disease reinforces the notion of the person as illness. Deegan (1993, p. 9) says: 'it is as if the whole world has put on a pair of warped glasses that blind them to the person you are and leaves them seeing you as an illness'. Stocks (1995, cited in Hayne & Yonge 1997, p. 319) agrees, saying, 'once our personal identities are transformed into a psychiatric label, we are objects that are never allowed to be people again'.

It is clearly important to see the person as separate from the illness. However, there are many ways in which we maintain the view of the person as an illness. These include a tendency to focus predominantly on problems, interpreting all behaviour as part of the illness; overemphasising assessment, diagnosis and prognosis; and neglecting to engage with the person (Palmer 1999). These are all things that are likely to stifle hope. If nurses cannot accept people with mental illness as human and social beings, who else in society will? After all, we are all human beings with unique abilities, shortcomings and, often, disabilities. We are all a psychological 'work in progress' and having a mental illness does not make one 'weak' or imperfect.

Social Skills Training

The development of social skills occurs through opportunities to learn, relearn and practise them in true-to-life situations. While the word 'training' suggests a paternalistic or controlling approach, the term is used here because it remains the accepted language. There are many types of skills-training activities designed to improve problem solving and coping generally. Similarly, social skills can be learned. We are not born with them. How do you know how to greet someone in a culturally appropriate way? How do you know how to behave when you walk into a university classroom? These are behaviours that we take for granted and therefore tend not to think about before doing them. They are also examples of social skills that we have learned as we were socialised into our culture. Much of this learning took place during childhood and adolescence, and so by adulthood we pretty much have these skills well developed.

However, if you develop a mental illness during childhood or adolescence, it is unlikely that you will develop sound social skills. Mental illness can distort communication with family members and peers, and the separations that ensue if a child or an adolescent is hospitalised can disrupt family life, social life and schooling, where we learn many early social skills. If you develop a long-term mental disorder later in life, it is likely that you will have fewer opportunities to practise learned social skills, and if you do not use them, you will lose them. Social isolation often occurs for people with serious mental illness because of the stigma and discrimination that result and because it is harder to communicate with others when you have distorted thinking and sensory experiences (e.g. hallucinations). These interfere with the ability to sustain relationships and develop new ones. Social skills deficits have also been shown to be related to poor vocational (work) outcomes for people with severe mental illness (Cheung et al. 2006).

Social skills training programmes have been found to have enormous benefits in improving the lives of people with severe mental illness (Lyman et al. 2014). Much of the social skills training in mental health services focusses on working with people with schizophrenia (Bellack 2004). People with social phobia and depression also often need to learn or relearn social skills (O'Donohue & Krasner 1995). Essentially, though, most people with mental health problems will have social and interpersonal problems as part of their overall picture. A lack of attention to social skills development may have a negative impact on social functioning (Saravanamuttu & Pyke 2003).

Social skills training is centred on teaching people the skills necessary to communicate effectively with others. There are some general approaches to teaching people social skills. As with most skills training packages, social skills training is usually carried out in groups. However, there are opportunities at almost every encounter to teach skills and to reinforce those skills already taught and being practised. When we role model appropriate social skills we provide opportunities for learning. However, O'Donohue and Krasner (1995) recommend using a role model similar in presentation to the group members so that the behaviour has more relevance to them. That is, the role model for a group of adolescents learning how to present for a job interview should be an adolescent who has suffered similar life problems.

Most social skills training groups combine instruction, modelling, rehearsal and role-playing as well as coaching, feedback and reinforcement. Rehearsal and role-playing involve practising the skill once instruction has been provided. Coaching involves having an instructor or teacher help the group members to practise the skill accurately by giving feedback on performance and praise (positive reinforcement) when the skill is performed well. Homework is an essential component of training packages because without practice in the real world, the goal of improved social skills will never be achieved. That is, social skills are not simply taught, they are developed through practice and the more opportunities for practice, the more socially able the person will be.

INTERVIEWING

While the skill of interviewing might not strictly be considered an intervention, the nurse's interviewing style may have considerable impact on therapeutic outcomes. When you meet with a patient to carry out a clinical interview, you need to engage or connect with that person in the same way that you might when being therapeutic. That is, it is important to develop rapport by being open, thoughtful, caring and honest, both verbally and nonverbally. Interviewing a person to attempt to find out what is happening is likely to be viewed as threatening if the approach taken is to fire off a list of questions that seek to arrive at a medical diagnosis. As part of the process of empowering people with mental illness, the assessment process (usually undertaken via clinical interview) needs to be collaborative and shared (see Chapter 22).

It is the patient who has the knowledge or information required for them to move towards identifying problems and planning care. As nurses, we currently ask questions from a power base rather than a discovery base. However, the person is the expert in their experience of mental illness, so we can share in the discovery of an understanding of the person's experience through the way in which we ask questions. At the outset, set the scene by letting the person know that your goal is to work together with them to arrive at some conclusion regarding what is going on at the moment. You might say something like, 'Let's talk about what is happening for you. You'd probably like to get a clearer idea of what is going on and I need to hear your story so that we can better know what to do next.' Ask questions that help people to understand themselves and, through this, also arrive at some understanding of what is happening. Asking questions that recognise the expertise of the person and summarising that information represents a collaborative approach to guided discovery (Palmer 1999).

CASE MANAGEMENT

The term 'case management' carries with it certain messages. It implies that people are cases that require managing. These words are loaded towards paternalism at a time when we are encouraged to view people/patients/service users as active participants in their own care and in their recovery from mental illness. The term 'case management' is used here because it is a term used universally, but the term 'key worker' better describes the role of the case manager and is less paternalistic.

Case management describes a pattern of service delivery for people with mental illness living in the community that arose as a result of deinstitutionalisation (the term used to describe the return of people to live in the community rather than in psychiatric institutions). The key worker is often a nurse but can also be a social worker, an occupational therapist, a psychologist or a psychiatrist—that is, anyone from the multidisciplinary team. Key workers are considered to have generic skills or a core group of skills that allow them to provide a particular service to people with enduring mental health problems who are living in the community (see Nurse's Story 24.3). People with a long-term mental health problem, or whose mental illness causes them to require frequent admission to hospital, are usually assigned a key worker, sometimes without their consent. If a person does not accept the need for this type of supervision in the community, it may need to be enforced under a Mental Health Act order for community treatment. Most people, however, agree to and welcome additional support in the community.

Staff who act as key workers deliver a range of services including counselling, assistance with social and financial needs and supervision of medication (Johnston et al. 1998). In addition, key workers are responsible for ongoing mental state assessment as well as risk assessment to ensure the person's safety and the safety of the community. Because case management is often carried out in the person's own home, there is often greater contact with family members and, therefore, greater opportunity to work with families.

Early models of case management had the patient working through the key worker to access other services in the community. Although this seemed reasonable, it made the patient dependent on the key worker. Today, the patient is considered central and the key worker is just one form of community support. The patient is encouraged and supported to access other community services independently. If, for example, the patient seeks support in accessing social services, the key worker would certainly be supportive. However, unless this help was requested, the key worker would expect the patient to negotiate the community without support. The responsibility of the key worker might be to teach the negotiation and social skills necessary to do this independently. This model of case management supports patient empowerment through partnership (Howgego et al. 2003).

NURSE'S STORY 24.3

The Therapeutic Encounter

As a key worker in the community, most of my time with people was spent talking through any current concerns, from weight gain to marital difficulties. These are the personal issues that contribute to difficulties in living and they are the mental health issues that we all experience and need an active listener for. However, most of us don't have the additional burden of a serious mental illness. The therapeutic encounter is designed to provide support and to enable people to solve their problems through exploring their difficulties in greater depth. When a person has a recurrence of symptoms, we attempt to manage them (the symptoms) together in the community with more frequent visits and telephone contact. Whenever someone required hospitalisation, I would liaise with staff working in the ward and visit the person there throughout the hospitalisation. I was also involved in discharge planning and family meetings. This clearly communicated to people that I was there with them throughout the ordeals that they experienced. This is particularly important if you, as the nurse, were responsible for their admission in the first place.

Routine case management usually involves a ratio of around 20 to 30 patients per case manager (King 2009). For people who are more seriously affected by their mental health concerns, there are now teams that provide intensive case management. This involves low patient numbers with ratios of around 8 to 10 people per key worker. A cost-effectiveness analysis carried out (Johnston et al. 1998) comparing the cost of routine case management with intensive case management revealed that there were greater improvements in functioning and higher rates of engagement in treatment in the intensive case management group. However, it costs considerably more for this type of support and, for this study, there was no reduction in hospital use after 12 months of intensive support. Importantly, though, the routine case management group required four times as many visits from the community crisis team. This means that patients who have limited key worker support inevitably require more support from the community crisis team. Therefore, this study suggests that people with enduring mental illness require more intensive support than we realise, so cost savings are not realised.

ELECTROCONVULSIVE THERAPY

Invented in 1938 in Italy by two eminent psychiatrists (Ugo Cerletti and Lucio Bini), ECT was investigated at a time when a number of physical treatments were developed, including insulin coma therapy, metrazole convulsive therapy and psychosurgery. ECT is the only one of these treatments used routinely today. Much of the controversy surrounding ECT grew out of its initial indiscriminate use and abuse. At first ECT was used without anaesthetic or muscle relaxation, with many adverse effects such as fractures, pain and cardiovascular problems.

Today, however, once a person is considered a candidate for ECT—that is, the person has an illness that may respond well to ECT—a full psychological and physical assessment is carried out. Wherever possible, consent for treatment is sought from the person. If this is not possible, application of the Mental Health Act may be necessary to allow for treatment to proceed, but only pending the second opinion of another psychiatrist and only for one course of treatment (usually 12 treatments), when informed consent should be sought to continue.

ECT involves the application of two electrodes to the head, through which an electric current is delivered. The electrodes can be applied bilaterally (BL, one on each side of the head, usually in the frontotemporal region), unilaterally (UL, both on the same side of the head, usually the right) or bifrontally (BF, both on the frontal lobe). Regardless of the location of the electrodes, the treatment is almost equally effective. However, different adverse effects can be experienced and due to the more severe memory impairments experienced with bilateral placement, this positioning is now used much less frequently. According to Endler and Persad (1988, p. 26), 'unilateral ECT to the nondominant hemisphere is less stressful for the patient than bilateral; it minimises confusion and memory loss; and it is almost as efficacious as bilateral in terms of alleviating the symptoms of depression'.

Indeed, more recent studies have found that there was no difference in treatment outcomes between the three electrode placement options (Dunne & McLoughlin 2012; Kellner et al. 2010). Sienaert et al. (2009) also found no difference in efficacy between BF placement and UL placement. In response to concerns about the effects of ECT on cerebral function, a study by Ende et al. (2000, p. 941) found that ECT does not cause tissue damage and that 'there is no hippocampal atrophy, neuronal damage, or cell death induced by ECT'. Nevertheless, some research has revealed that ECT causes memory impairment that cannot be attributed to the original illness state (MacQueen et al. 2007; Watkinson 2007), while others argue that amnesia is largely temporary and confined to the period immediately following ECT (Meeter et al. 2011).

ECT is widely accepted as an effective intervention in the treatment of severe depression, although it remains controversial (Persad 2001). There is contention not only among the public regarding ECT (Teh et al. 2007), but also within the mental health professions, as many professionals question its efficacy (Barker 2003; Challiner & Griffiths 2000). However, recent publications support earlier conclusions that antidepressants and ECT are effective and safe treatments for depressed elderly patients (Salzman et al. 2002) and for people who are suicidal (Persad 2001).

In the past, ECT has been used to treat a wide range of mental disorders, including schizophrenia. An examination of both older and more recent research has revealed that ECT is as effective as antipsychotic medications in the treatment of schizophrenia, particularly with people experiencing an acute episode. When used in combination with antipsychotic medications, it has been found to be more effective than ECT or medication used alone (Keuneman et al. 2002).

Whether conducted in a general theatre or a specialised ECT suite attached to the inpatient psychiatric unit, ECT remains a physically intrusive treatment that requires specialised nursing skills. Generally, though, the role of the nurse in working with a person preparing for ECT is to support the person and to prepare them for the procedure, both physically and psychologically, just as you would for any procedure requiring a general anaesthetic. Other responsibilities for the nurse are also the same as for any operative procedure conducted under general anaesthesia. For example, you may be required to provide close observation to ensure that the person does not eat or drink prior to the procedure. You would also need to make certain that make-up and jewellery have been removed. These are basic safety measures to prevent complications and to ensure an accurate assessment of skin colour during the anaesthetic.

ECT remains a controversial intervention in psychiatry today. Much of this controversy stems from the historical use of ECT and from its representation in films such as *One Flew Over the Cuckoo's Nest* (Vermeulen 1999), as well as its depiction in the general media (Euba & Crugel 2009; Payne & Prudic 2009). This is despite substantial research and descriptive evidence testifying to its effectiveness. Those who have not observed ECT and who base their understandings on historical and media representations of it are likely to be surprised at how innocuous it is. A positive attitude to ECT has been found to be directly related to greater exposure to and knowledge about ECT (Endler & Persad 1988; Gass 1998; Grover et al. 2011). Nevertheless, concern persists because we are not entirely certain how ECT works (Burgese & Bassitt 2015) and because of the cognitive side effects experienced (Meeter et al. 2011). Ultimately, patients and families still express fears about the long-term effects of ECT on brain function, although one study found that relatives' knowledge and attitudes were positively impacted when they shared the experience of ECT with their family member (Grover et al. 2011). See Nurse's Story 24.4 for a nurse's experience regarding ECT.

REPETITIVE TRANSCRANIAL MAGNETIC STIMULATION

A less-invasive treatment known as repetitive transcranial magnetic stimulation (rTMS) was established about 15 years ago as an alternative to ECT. It has been found to be particularly effective for people with treatment-resistant depression (Paus & Barrett 2004; Holtzheimer et al. 2010; Rosenberg et al. 2010). rTMS is a procedure that uses magnetic fields to stimulate nerve cells in the brain. The magnetic field is

NURSE'S STORY 24.4

Electroconvulsive Therapy

A woman in her mid-30s with whom I had worked many years ago left a lasting impression on me regarding the efficacy of electroconvulsive therapy (ECT). She was a very attractive woman with a supportive husband and two young children. However, she suffered from major depression. When depressed she experienced feelings of hopelessness and delusions of worthlessness. She believed that she was so worthless that her family would be better off without her and that we really shouldn't bother helping her. As with any delusion, her thoughts could not be countered.

She began treatment with ECT at the usually prescribed rate of three times each week. She had a very quick recovery and I recall her saying to us not long before she was discharged home, 'Thank you for keeping me alive until I got well'. She was also overheard recommending ECT to other depressed patients in the hospital.

This was a very important lesson for me as a mental health nurse. I was able to see someone move from a very distressed and debilitated state. She had been profoundly suicidal, but came to find pleasure in her life again following ECT. While ECT has the usual risks associated with a general anaesthetic, the risk of suicide from major depression seemed to be far greater for this woman. Every person needs individual assessment when making clinical decisions about treatment and certainly current ECT research has been more explicit in relation to its adverse effects, but this experience and many others testify to its continued utility.

produced via a plastic-enclosed coil of wire that is held next to the skull. The electric current is generated across the skull and scalp without direct physical contact with the person (Cacioppo et al. 2007) and, because it is noninvasive, it does not require an anaesthetic or sedation. The magnetic pulses are similar to those experienced during magnetic resonance imaging (MRI) of the brain. rTMS is normally delivered as an outpatient intervention and is usually applied for about 40 minutes at a time, daily (Monday to Friday), for a period of around 4 to 6 weeks (Holtzheimer et al. 2010). However, Chung et al. (2015) have tested and propose a new form of TMS treatment for depression known as theta-burst stimulation (TBS), which requires only 1 to 3 minutes of stimulation and which has been found to have similar or better efficacy compared with rTMS.

There is a low rate of adverse events in rTMS, and it has been found to be safe in pregnancy (Burton et al. 2014; Sayar et al. 2014). The most common adverse effects are headache (Slotema et al. 2010) or localised skin irritation (Chung et al. 2015). While the risk for side effects is significantly better for rTMS, ECT is significantly more effective (Rasmussen 2008); however, further research is needed. Like ECT, the mechanisms of action for rTMS are unknown. (For further reading and to view an image of the figure-of-eight coil used in rTMS, go to http://en.wikipedia.org/wiki/Transcranial_magnetic_stimulation#cite_note-34).

CONCLUSION

This chapter has given some fundamental information about a number of therapeutic intervention strategies that will assist you in being with and working with people with mental illness. Some of these intervention strategies apply to specific situations or difficulties but there is always a way of working effectively with people experiencing challenging mental health concerns. Some are more technical than others and require further education and practice to master. But many of the skills outlined here can be learned and applied to the interactions you will experience now as a novice nurse and later as your experience develops.

Novice nurses frequently express their concern that they might 'say the wrong thing' and make the situation more challenging for the person in their care. If you take a caring and thoughtful approach that avoids the generous delivery of advice, it is unlikely that you will cause harm. However, if you take with you some specific skills and models for your practice, you are likely to feel more confident and to understand the goals of your interaction. It is also hoped that, through reading this chapter, you have developed a sense of the importance of responding to people with mental health concerns as valid human beings who require your support and help through a particularly troubling time.

EXERCISES FOR CLASS ENGAGEMENT

A number of exercises are presented here to help you to engage with and consolidate what you have learned from this chapter. You should discuss the issues raised with your group or class members. Some of these activities also ask you to reflect on your personal values, beliefs and actions; this greater insight into yourself will help you to be more effective in your interactions with others.

1. What are the main stressors in your life? Consider relationship problems, difficulties with children, problems with parents, financial worries, physical conditions, environmental factors, study pressures, work factors, nutrition and exercise in addition to chemical factors such as nicotine, alcohol, caffeine and other substances. Identify those that you can learn to manage and list the stressors in terms of their importance or greatest impact.
2. Using the written text from a book or an app/CD/DVD, follow the instructions for carrying out PMR, measuring your respiratory rate and heart rate before and after the exercise. Were you able to relax? What effect did the exercise have on your respiratory rate and heart rate?
3. Which of the assertion skills (making requests, refusing requests, accepting and giving compliments, expressing opinions, giving negative feedback or being confrontational, initiating conversations, sharing intimate feelings and experiences with others and expressing affection) do you find difficult to manage? Why do you think this is? Of the situations that you find difficult to manage, which one in particular presents the greatest challenge to you? How do you feel whenever you fail to manage these situations assertively?

EXERCISES FOR CLASS ENGAGEMENT—cont'd

4. Consider the kinds of life events that might cause an individual to experience crisis, such as rape, loss of a job, unplanned pregnancy or death of a loved one. How would you respond to being admitted to hospital for colorectal surgery? How would you respond to being admitted involuntarily to an acute psychiatric unit?
5. Mark is a 25-year-old single male. He has just been diagnosed with genital herpes and is extremely distressed. Although he is intelligent, has coped well with previous life crises and has good relationships with family and friends, he feels so ashamed that he cannot discuss this with anyone he knows well. He believes that life is no longer worth living as he thinks he will never have a normal sex life or a meaningful relationship again. What do you make of Mark's perception of his problem? Which interventions do you think are necessary according to Aguilera's model for crisis intervention?
6. What are your short-term goals (i.e. what do you hope to achieve over the next few weeks or months)? What is your main 5-year goal? What will you need to do over the next 5 years to achieve that goal? What is likely to interfere with your achievement of that goal? What is likely to support your achievement of that goal?
7. On a scale of 1 to 10, how near are you to achieving your goals? What are the things/choices/decisions that are helping you to achieve your goals?
8. As a group, watch the film *One Flew Over the Cuckoo's Nest*. What stereotypes are portrayed in this movie? Which of these persist today? How does the portrayal of ECT in this movie make you feel about ECT? In addition, what are your thoughts about the nurse–patient and doctor–patient relationships as portrayed for that era? How do you think a movie made today would portray these things?
9. Consider your values concerning health and wellness as well as self-determination. What issues might arise for you if you were responsible for preparing a patient for ECT against that person's wishes? How would you deal with this situation?

REFERENCES

Abdollahi, A., Talib, M.A., Yaacob, S.S., Ismail, Z., 2014. Hardiness as a mediator between perceived stress and happiness in nurses. Journal of Psychiatric and Mental Health Nursing 21 (9), 789–796.

Aguilera, D., 1994. Crisis Intervention: Theory and Methodology, seventh ed. Mosby, St Louis.

Anthony, W.A., 1993. Recovery from mental illness: the guiding vision of the mental health service system in the 1990s. Psychosocial Rehabilitation Journal 16 (4), 11–23.

Anthony, W.A., Cohen, M., Farkas, M., 1991. Psychiatric Rehabilitation. Centre for Psychiatric Rehabilitation, Boston.

Arkowitz, H., Westra, H.A., Miller, W.R., Rollnick, S., 2015. Motivational Interviewing in the Treatment of Psychological Problems, second ed. Guilford Press, New York.

Atkinson, C., Amesu, M., 2007. Using solution-focused approaches in motivational interviewing with young people. Pastoral Care in Education 25 (2), 31–37.

Ayers, C.R., Sorrell, J.T., Thorp, S.R., et al., 2007. Evidence-based psychological treatments for late-life anxiety. Psychology and Aging 22 (1), 8–17.

Bacon, T., Farhall, J., Fossey, E., 2014. The active therapeutic processes of acceptance and commitment therapy for persistent symptoms of psychosis: clients' perspectives. Behavioural and Cognitive Psychotherapy 42 (4), 402–420.

Barker, P., 2003. Barker's beat. Mental Health Practice 6 (10), 38–39.

Barker, P.J., Fraser, D. (Eds.), 1985. The Nurse as Therapist: A Behavioural Model. Croom Helm, London.

Barlow, J.H., Ellard, D.R., Hainsworth, J.M., et al., 2005. A review of self-management interventions for panic disorders, phobias and obsessive-compulsive disorders. Acta Psychiatrica Scandinavica 111 (4), 272–285.

Battison, T., 1997. Beating Stress. Allen & Unwin, London.

Beebe, L.H., Tian, L., Morris, N., Goodwin, A., Allen, S.S., Kuldau, J., 2005. Effects of exercise on mental and physical health parameters of persons with schizophrenia. Issues in Mental Health Nursing 26 (6), 661–676.

Bellack, A.S., 2004. Skills training for people with severe mental illness. Psychiatric Rehabilitation Journal 27 (4), 375–391

Blackburn, I., Davidson, K., 1990. Cognitive Therapy for Depression and Anxiety. Blackwell Scientific, New York.

Bland, R., 1986. Family Support Program. Occasional Paper 86(1). University of Queensland, Brisbane.

Bloom, B.L., 1997. Planned Short-Term Psychotherapy: A Clinical Handbook, second ed. Allyn & Bacon, Boston.

Brettschneider, C., Djadran, H., Harter, M., Lowe, B., Riedel-Heller, S., Konig, H.-H., 2015. Cost-utility analyses of cognitive-behavioural therapy of depression: a systematic review. Psychotherapy and Psychosomatics 84 (1), 6–21.

Brown, M., Marshall, K., 2006. Cognitive behavioural therapy and people with learning disabilities: implications for developing nursing practice. Journal of Psychiatric and Mental Health Nursing 13 (2), 234–241.

Burgese, D.F., Bassitt, D.P., 2015. Variation of plasma cortisol levels in patients with depression after treatment with bilateral electroconvulsive therapy. Trends in Psychiatry and Psychotherapy 37 (1), 27–36.

Burnard, P., 2005. Counselling Skills for Health Professionals. Nelson Thornes, Cheltenham, UK.

Burton, C., Gill, S., Clarke, P., Galletly, C., 2014. Maintaining remission of depression with repetitive transcranial magnetic stimulation during pregnancy: a case report. Archives of Women's Mental Health 17 (3), 247–250.

Butterworth, S., Linden, A., McClay, W., et al., 2006. Effect of motivational interviewing-based health coaching on employees' physical and mental health status. Journal of Occupational Health Psychology 11 (4), 358–365.

Byrne, A., Watson, R., Butler, C., et al., 2006. Increasing the confidence of nursing staff to address the sexual health needs of people living with HIV: the use of motivational interviewing. AIDS Care 18 (5), 501–504.

Byrne, J., Byrne, D.G., 1996. Counselling Skills for Health Professionals. Macmillan Education, Melbourne.

Cacioppo, J.T., Tassinary, L.G., Berntson, G.G., 2007. Handbook of Psychophysiology, third ed. Cambridge University Press, New York.

Calvert, P., Palmer, C., 2003. Application of the cognitive therapy model to initial crisis assessment. International Journal of Mental Health Nursing 12 (1), 30–38.

Carels, R.A., Darby, L., Cacciapaglia, H.M., et al., 2007. Using motivational interviewing as a supplement to obesity treatment. Health Psychology 26 (3), 369–374.

Challiner, V., Griffiths, L., 2000. Electroconvulsive therapy: a review of the literature. Journal of Psychiatric and Mental Health Nursing 7 (3), 191–198.

Cheung, L.C.C., Tsang, H.W.H., Tsui, C.U., 2006. A job-specific social skills training program for people with severe mental illness: a case study for those who plan to be a security guard. Journal of Rehabilitation 72 (4), 14–23.

Chopra, P., Hamilton, B., Castle, D., Smith, J., Mileshkin, C., et al., 2009. Implementation of the strengths model at an area mental health service. Australasian Psychiatry 17 (3), 202–206.

Chung, S.W., Hoy, K.E., Fitzgerald, P.B., 2015. Theta-burst stimulation: a new form of TMS treatment for depression? Depression & Anxiety 32 (3), 182–192.

Clark, M.D., Walters, S., Gingerich, R., et al., 2006. Motivational interviewing for probation officers: tipping the balance toward change. Federal Probation 70 (1), 38–44.

Colom, F., Vieta, E., Martinez-Aran, A., et al., 2003. A randomised trial on the efficacy of group psychoeducation in the prophylaxis of recurrences in bipolar patients whose disease is in remission. Archives of General Psychiatry 60 (4), 402–407.

Curtis, L., 1997. New Directions: International Overview of Best Practices in Recovery and Rehabilitation Services for People with Serious Mental Illness. New Zealand Mental Health Commission, Wellington.

Dakof, G.A., Henderson, C.E., Rowe, C.L., Boustani, M., Greenbaum, P., Wang, W., Hawes, S., Linares, C., Liddle HA., 2015. A randomized clinical trial of family therapy in juvenile drug court. Journal of Family Psychology 29 (2), 232–241.

Daltry, R.M., 2015. A case study: an ACT stress management group in a university counseling center. Journal of College Student Psychotherapy 29 (1), 36–43.

Dattilio, F.M., Padesky, C.A., 1990. Cognitive Therapy With Couples. Professional Resource Exchange, Sarasota, FL.

Davis, M., Robbins Eshelman, E., McKay, M., 2000. The Relaxation and Stress Reduction Workbook, fifth ed. New Harbinger, Oakland, CA.

Deegan, P., 1988. Recovery: the lived experience of rehabilitation. Psychosocial Rehabilitation Journal 11 (4), 11–19.

Deegan, P., 1993. Recovering our sense of value after being labelled mentally ill. Journal of Psychosocial Nursing 31 (4), 7–11.

Deegan, P., 1996. Recovery as a journey of the heart. Psychiatric Rehabilitation Journal 19 (3), 91–97.

Deegan, P., 1997. Recovery and empowerment for people with psychiatric disabilities. Social Work in Health Care 25 (3), 11–24.

De Shazer, S., 1985. Keys to Solution in Brief Therapy. WW Norton, New York.

De Shazer, S., 1988. Clues: Investigating Solutions in Brief Therapy. WW Norton, New York.

De Vecchi, N., Kenny, A., Kidd, S., 2015. Stakeholder views on a recovery-oriented psychiatric rehabilitation art therapy program in a rural Australian mental health service: a qualitative description. International Journal of Mental Health Systems 9, 11 eCollection.

Dickson, D.A., Hargie, O., Morrow, N.C., 1989. Communication Skills Training for Health Professionals: An Instructor's Handbook. Routledge, Chapman & Hall, Andover.

Donaghy, M.E., 2007. Exercise can seriously improve your mental health: fact or fiction? Advances in Physiotherapy 9 (2), 76–88.

Drake, R.E., Strickler, D.C., Bond, G.R., 2015. Psychiatric rehabilitation in residential treatment settings. Psychiatric Annals 45 (3), 114–119.

Dunne, R.A., McLoughlin, D.M., 2012. Systematic review and meta-analysis of bifrontal electroconvulsive therapy versus bilateral and unilateral electroconvulsive therapy in depression. The World Journal of Biological Psychiatry 13 (4), 248–258.

Earley, J., 2000. Interactive Group Therapy: Integrating Interpersonal, Action-Oriented, and Psychodynamic Approaches. Brunner/Mazel, Philadelphia.

Edwards, D., Hannigan, B., Fothergill, A., et al., 2002. Stress management for mental health professionals: a review of effective techniques. Stress and Health 18 (5), 203–215.

Egan, G., 1985. Exercises in Helping Skills: A Training Manual to Accompany the Skilled Helper, third ed. Brooks/Cole, Monterey, CA.

Egan, G., 2001. The Skilled Helper—A Problem-Management and Opportunity-Development Approach to Helping, seventh ed. Brooks/Cole, Pacific Grove, CA.

Eisler, I., Simic, M., Russell, G.F.M., et al., 2007. A randomised controlled treatment trial of two forms of family therapy in adolescent anorexia nervosa: a five-year follow-up. Journal of Child Psychology and Psychiatry 48 (6), 552–560.

Ekdawi, M.Y., Conning, A.M., 1994. Psychiatric rehabilitation: A practical guide. Chapman & Hall, London.

Ende, G., Braus, D.F., Walter, S., et al., 2000. The hippocampus in patients treated with electroconvulsive therapy: a proton magnetic resonance spectroscopic imaging study. Archives of General Psychiatry 57 (10), 937–943.

Endler, N.S., Persad, E., 1988. Electroconvulsive Therapy: The Myths and the Realities. Hans Huber, Toronto.

Escot, C., Artero, S., Gandubert, C., et al., 2001. Stress levels in nursing staff working in oncology. Stress and Health 17 (5), 273–279.

Euba, R., Crugel, M., 2009. The depiction of electroconvulsive therapy in the British press. The Journal of ECT 25 (4), 265–269.

Evans, A.M., 2007. Transference in the nurse–patient relationship. Journal of Psychiatric and Mental Health Nursing 14 (2), 189–195.

Fehr, S.S., 1999. Introduction to Group Therapy: A Practical Guide. Haworth Press, New York.

Feros, D.L., Lane, L., Ciarrochi, J., Blackledge, J.T., 2013. Acceptance and Commitment Therapy (ACT) for improving the lives of cancer patients: a preliminary study. Psycho-Oncology 22 (2), 459–464.

Ferraz, H., Wellman, N., 2008. The integration of solution-focused brief therapy principles in nursing: a literature review. Journal of Psychiatric and Mental Health Nursing 15 (1), 37–44.

Finnell, D.S., 2003. Use of the transtheoretical model for individuals with co-occurring disorders. Community Mental Health Journal 39 (1), 3–15.

Fogarty, M., Happell, B., 2005. Exploring the benefits of an exercise program for people with schizophrenia: a qualitative study. Issues in Mental Health Nursing 26 (3), 341–351.

Freud, S., 1938/1965. The Basic Writing of Sigmund Freud. Modern Library, New York.

Gallop, R., O'Brien, L., 2003. Re-establishing psychodynamic theory as foundational knowledge for psychiatric/mental health nursing. Issues in Mental Health Nursing 24 (2), 213–227.

Gambril, E., 1995. Assertion skills training. In: O'Donohue, W., Krasner, L. (Eds.), Handbook of Psychological Skills Training: Clinical Techniques and Applications. Allyn & Bacon, Boston.

Gass, J.P., 1998. The knowledge and attitudes of mental health nurses to electroconvulsive therapy. Journal of Advanced Nursing 27 (1), 83–90.

Gelin, Z., Fuso, S., Hendrick, S., Cook-Darzens, S., Simon, Y., 2015. The effects of a multiple family therapy on adolescents with eating disorders: an outcome study. Family Process 54 (1), 160–172.

Gerhart, J., Holman, K., Seymour, B., Dinges, B., Ronan, G.F., 2015. Group process as a mechanism of change in the group treatment of anger and aggression. International Journal of Group Psychotherapy 65 (2), 181–208.

Goldenberg, I., Goldenberg, H., 2000. Family Therapy: An Overview, fifth ed. Brooks/Cole, Belmont, CA.

Graham, A.L., Chang, Y., Fang, Y., Cobb, N.K., Tinkelman, D.S., Niaura, R.S., Abrams, D.B., Mandelblatt, J.S., 2013. Cost-effectiveness of internet and telephone treatment for smoking cessation: an economic evaluation of the iQuit study. Tobacco Control: An International Journal 22 (6), 1–7.

Greenstone, J.L., Leviton, S.C., 2002. Elements of Crisis Intervention: Crises and How to Respond to Them, second ed. Brooks/Cole, Pacific Grove, CA.

Grover, S.K., Chakrabarti, S., Khehra, N., Rajagopal, R., 2011. Does the experience of electroconvulsive therapy improve awareness and perceptions of treatment among relatives of patients? The Journal of ECT 27 (1), 67–72.

Haley, T., 2000. Solution-focused counselling with a sexual abuse survivor. Guidance and Counselling 15 (4), 18–22.

Handley, A.K., Egan, S.J., Kane, R.T., Rees, C.S., 2015. A randomised controlled trial of cognitive behavioural therapy for perfectionism. Behaviour Research and Therapy 68, 37–47.

Harris, R., 2006. Embracing your demons: an overview of acceptance and commitment therapy. Psychotherapy in Australia 12 (4), 2–8.

Harris, R., 2007. The Happiness Trap: Stop Struggling, Start Living. Exisle Publishing, Wollombi, NSW.

Hayne, Y., Yonge, O., 1997. The lifeworld analysis of the chronically mentally ill: an analysis of 40 written personal accounts. Archives of Psychiatric Nursing 11 (6), 314–324.

Holtzheimer, P.E., McDonald, W.M., Mufti, M., Kelley, M.E., Quinn, S., Corso, G., Epstein, C.M., 2010. Accelerated repetitive transcranial magnetic stimulation for treatment-resistant depression. Depression & Anxiety 27 (10), 960–963.

Hosany, Z., Wellman, N., Lowe, T., 2007. Fostering a culture of engagement: a pilot study of the outcomes of training mental health nurses working in two UK acute admission units in brief solution-focused therapy techniques. Journal of Psychiatric and Mental Health Nursing 14 (7), 688–695.

Howgego, I.M., Yellowlees, P., Owen, C., et al., 2003. The therapeutic alliance: the key to effective patient outcome? A descriptive review of the evidence in community mental health case management. Australian and New Zealand Journal of Psychiatry 37 (2), 169–183.

Hulbert-Williams, N.J., Storey, L., Wilson, K.G., 2015. Psychological interventions for patients with cancer: psychological flexibility and the potential utility of acceptance and commitment therapy. European Journal of Cancer Care 24 (1), 15–27.

Jenkins, J.H., Karno, M., 1992. The meaning of expressed emotion: theoretical issues raised by cross-cultural research. American Journal of Psychiatry 149 (1), 9–21.

Johnston, S., Salkeld, G., Sanderson, K., et al., 1998. Intensive case management: a cost-effectiveness analysis. Australian and New Zealand Journal of Psychiatry 32, 551–559.

Kadis, L.B., McClendon, R., 1998. Concise Guide to Marital and Family Therapy. American Psychiatric Press, Washington, DC.

Kavanagh, D.J., 1992. Recent developments in expressed emotion and schizophrenia. British Journal of Psychiatry 160, 601–620.

Kellner, C.H., Knapp, R., Husain, M.M., Rasnussen, K., Sampson, S., Cullum, M., McClintock, S.M., Tobias, K.G., Martino, C., Mueller, M., Bailine, S.H., Fink, M., Petrides, G., 2010. Bifrontal, bitemporal and right unilateral electrode placement in ECT: randomised trial. British Journal of Psychiatry 196 (3), 226–234.

Kerling, A., Tegtbur, U., Gutzlaff, E., Kuck, M., Borchert, L., Ates, Z., von Bohlen, A., Frieling, H., Huper, K., Hartung, D., Schweiger, U., Kahl, K.G., 2015. Effects of adjunctive exercise on physiological and psychological parameters in depression: a randomised pilot trial. Journal of Affective Disorders 177, 1–6.

Ketch, R.A., Rubin, R.T., Baker, M.R., Sones, A.C., Ames, D., 2015. Art appreciation for veterans with severe mental illness in a VA psychosocial rehabilitation and recovery center. Arts & Health: An International Journal of Research, Policy and Practice 7 (2), 172–181.

Keuneman, R., Weerasundera, R., Castle, D., 2002. The role of ECT in schizophrenia. Australasian Psychiatry 10 (4), 385–388.

King, R., 2009. Case load management, work-related stress and case manager self-efficacy among Victorian mental health case managers. Australian and New Zealand Journal of Psychiatry 43 (5), 453–459.

Knight, K.M., McGowan, L., Dickens, C., et al., 2006. A systematic review of motivational interviewing in physical health care settings. British Journal of Health Care Psychology 11 (2), 319–332.

Kohlenberg, R.J., Hayes, S.C., Tsai, M., 1993. Radical behavioural psychotherapy: two contemporary examples. Clinical Psychology Review 13 (6), 579–592.

Lee, T.-Y., Chang, S.-C., Chu, H., Yang, C.-Y., Ou, K.-L., Chung, M.-H., Chou, K.-R., 2013. The effects of assertiveness training in patients with schizophrenia: a randomized, single-blind, controlled study. Journal of Advanced Nursing 69 (11), 2549–2559.

Lee, J., Deffern, M., Ogloff, J.R.P., Martin, T., 2015. Towards a model for understanding the development of post-traumatic stress disorder and general distress in mental health nurses. International Journal of Mental Health Nursing 24 (1), 49–58.

Legere, L., 2007. The importance of rehabilitation. Psychiatric Rehabilitation Journal 30 (3), 227–229.

Lester, D., 2002. Crisis Intervention and Counselling by Telephone, second ed. Charles C Thomas, Springfield, IL.

Limsanon, T., Kalayasiri, R., 2015. Preliminary effects of progressive muscle relaxation on cigarette craving and withdrawal symptoms in experienced smokers in acute cigarette abstinence: a randomised controlled trial. Behavior Therapy 46 (2), 166–176.

Linehan, M.M., 1993. Cognitive Behavior Therapy of Borderline Personality Disorder. Guilford Press, New York.

Linehan, M.M., Schmidt, H., Dimeff, L.A., et al., 1999. Dialectical behavior therapy for patients with borderline personality disorder and drug-dependence. American Journal on Addictions 8, 279–292.

Lyman, D.R., Kurtz, M.M., Farkas, M., George, P., Dougherty, R.H., Daniels, A.S., Ghose, S.S., Delphin-Rittmon, M.E., 2014. Skill building: assessing the evidence. Psychiatric Services 65 (6), 727–738.

MacMillan, H.L., Munn, C., 2001. The sequelae of child maltreatment. Current Opinion in Psychiatry 14 (4), 325–331.

MacQueen, G., Parkin, C., Marriott, M., et al., 2007. The long-term impact of treatment with electroconvulsive therapy on discrete memory systems in patients with bipolar disorder. Journal of Psychiatry and Neuroscience 32 (4), 241–249.

Mannix, K., Blackburn, I.M., Garland, A., et al., 2006. Effectiveness of brief training in cognitive behaviour therapy techniques for palliative care practitioners. Palliative Medicine 20 (6), 579–584.

McAllister, M., 2003. Doing practice differently: solution-focused nursing. Journal of Advanced Nursing 4 (6), 528–535.

McGoldrick, M., Gerson, R., Shellenberger, S., 1999. Genograms: Assessment and Intervention, second ed. WW Norton, New York.

McTiernan, K., McDonald, N., 2015. Occupational stressors, burnout and coping strategies between hospital and community psychiatric nurses in a Dublin region. Journal of Psychiatric and Mental Health Nursing 22 (3), 208–218.

Meech, C., Wood, A., 2000. Reconnecting past, present and future lives: therapy with a young person who experienced severe childhood privation. Australian and New Zealand Journal of Family Therapy 21 (2), 102–107.

Meeter, M., Murre, J.M.J., Janssen, S.M.J., Birkenhager, T., van den Broek, W.W., 2011. Retrograde amnesia after electroconvulsive therapy: a temporary effect? Journal of Affective Disorders 132 (1–2), 216–222.

Mellor, D., Storer, S., Firth, L., 2000. Family therapy into the 21st century: can we work our way out of the epistemological maze? Australian and New Zealand Journal of Family Therapy 21 (3), 151–154.

Miller, W., 1998. Toward a motivational definition and understanding of addiction. Motivational Interviewing Newsletter 5 (3), 2–6.

Miller, W.R., Zweben, A., DiClemente, C.C., et al., 1992. Motivational Enhancement Therapy Manual: A Clinical Research Guide for Therapists Treating Individuals With Alcohol Abuse and Dependence. National Institute on Alcohol Abuse and Alcoholism, Rockville, MD.

Mladenovic, I., Lazetic, G., Lecic-Tosevski, D., Dimitrijevic, I., 2015. Treatment of pathological gambling: integrative systemic model. Psychiatria Danubina 27 (1), 107–111.

Morse, J., Penrod, J., 1999. Linking concepts of enduring, uncertainty, suffering, and hope. Image: Journal of Nursing Scholarship 31 (1), 145–150.

Mullen, A., Murray, L., Happell, B., 2002. Multiple family group interventions in first episode psychosis: enhancing knowledge and understanding. International Journal of Mental Health Nursing 11, 225–232.

Myer, R.A., 2001. Assessment for Crisis Intervention: A Triage Assessment Model. Wadsworth, Toronto.

Myhr, G., Payne, K., 2006. Cost-effectiveness of cognitive-behaviour therapy for mental disorders: implications for public health care funding policy in Canada. Canadian Journal of Psychiatry 51 (10), 662–670.

Nichols, M.P., Schwartz, R.C., 2001. Family Therapy: Concepts and Methods, fifth ed. Allyn & Bacon, Boston.

O'Donohue, W., Krasner, L., 1995. Handbook of Psychological Skills Training: Clinical Techniques and Applications. Allyn & Bacon, Boston.

Palmer, C.J., 1996. Education and Support for Families and Friends of People with Schizophrenia. Masters dissertation. Queensland University of Technology, Brisbane.

Palmer, C.J., 1999. Recovery-Focused Mental Health Nursing: a Model for the Future? Paper Presented at the Scientific Meeting of the Australian and New Zealand College of Mental Health Nurses (ANZCMHN), Tasmania, 9–12 September.

Patel, C., 1991. The Complete Guide to Stress Management. Plenum Press, New York.

Paus, T., Barrett, J., 2004. Transcranial magnetic stimulation (TMS) of the human frontal cortex: implications for repetitive TMS treatment of depression. Journal of Psychiatry & Neuroscience 29 (4), 268–279.

Payne, N.A., Prudic, J., 2009. Electroconvulsive therapy. Part II: a biopsychosocial perspective. Journal of Psychiatric Practice 15 (5), 369–390.

Perkins, R.E., Repper, J.M., 1996. Working Alongside People With Long-Term Mental Health Problems. Chapman & Hall, London.

Persad, E., 2001. Electroconvulsive therapy: the controversy and the evidence. Canadian Journal of Psychiatry 46 (8), 702–703.

Petchkovsky, L., Morris, P., Rushton, P., 2002. Choosing a psychodynamic psychotherapy model for an Australian public sector mental health service. Australasian Psychiatry 10 (4), 330–334.

Pinto, R.A., Kienhuis, M., Slevison, M., Chester, A., Sloss, A., Yap, K., 2015. The effectiveness of an outpatient acceptance and commitment therapy group programme for a transdiagnostic population. Clinical Psychologist Online 1-11.

Prochaska, J.O., 2001. Treating entire populations for behaviour risks for cancer. Cancer Journal 7 (5), 360–368.

Prochaska, J.O., DiClemente, C.C., 1983. Stages and processes of self-change of smoking: toward an integrative model of change. Journal of Consulting and Clinical Psychology 51 (3), 390–395.

Raeburn, T., Schmied, V., Hungerford, C., Cleary, M., 2014. Clubhouse model of psychiatric rehabilitation: how is recovery reflected in documentation? International Journal of Mental Health Nursing 23 (5), 389–397.

Raeburn, T., Schmied, V., Hungerford, C., Cleary, M., 2015. Self-determination theory: a framework for Clubhouse psychosocial rehabilitation research. Issues in Mental Health Nursing 36 (2), 145–151.

Rasmussen, K.G., 2008. Electroconvulsive therapy versus transcranial magnetic stimulation for major depression: a review with recommendations for future research. Acta Neuropsychiatrica 20 (6), 291–294.

Rausch, S.M., Gramling, S.E., Auerbach, S.M., 2006. Effects of a single session of large-group meditation and progressive muscle relaxation training on stress reduction, reactivity, and recovery. International Journal of Stress Management 13 (3), 273–290.

Rodrigues, L.J., 2007. A closer look: the benefits and effectiveness of CBT on a female-specific unit for treatment of bipolar disorder. Issues in Mental Health Nursing 28 (5), 533–542.

Rollnick, S., Miller, W.R., 1995. What is motivational interviewing? Behavioural and Cognitive Psychotherapy 23, 325–334.

Romas, J.A., Sharma, M., 1995. Practical Stress Management. Allyn & Bacon, Boston.

Rooksby, M., Elouafkaoui, P., Humphris, G., Clarkson, J., Freeman, R., 2015. Internet-assisted delivery of cognitive behavioural therapy (CBT) for childhood anxiety: systematic review and meta-analysis. Journal of Anxiety Disorders 29, 83–92.

Rosen, A., O'Halloran, P., 2014. Recovery entails bridging the multiple realms of best practice: towards a more integrated approach to evidence-based clinical treatment and psychosocial disability support for mental health recovery. East Asian Archives of Psychiatry 24 (3), 104–109.

Rosenberg, O., Shoenfeld, N., Zangen, A., Kotler, M., Dannon, P.N., 2010. Deep TMS in a resistant major depressive disorder: a brief report. Depression & Anxiety 27 (5), 465–469.

Rosenbaum, S., Sherrington, C., Tiedemann, A., 2015. Exercise augmentation compared with usual care for post-traumatic stress disorder: a randomised controlled trial. Acta Psychiatrica Scandinavica 131 (5), 350–359.

Rosenfield, M., 2013. Telephone Counselling: A Handbook for Practitioners. Palgrave Macmillan, London.

Rosser, S., Erskine, A., Crino, R., 2004. Pre-existing antidepressants and the outcome of group cognitive behaviour therapy for social phobia. Australian and New Zealand Journal of Psychiatry 38 (4), 233–239.

Ruddick, F., 2008. Hope, optimism and expectation. Mental Health Practice 12 (1), 33–35.

Salzman, C., Wong, E., Wright, B.C., 2002. Drug and ECT treatment of depression in the elderly, 1996–2001: a literature review. Biological Psychiatry 52 (3), 265–284.

Sanders, P., 1996. An Incomplete Guide to Using Counselling Skills on the Telephone, second ed. PCCS Books, Manchester.

Saravanamuttu, R., Pyke, J., 2003. Interaction: case managers and social skills teaching. Psychiatric Rehabilitation Journal 27 (1), 79–82.

Sayar, G.H., Ozten, E., Tufan, E., Cerit, C., Kagan, G., Dilbaz, N., Tarhan, N., 2014. Transcranial magnetic stimulation during pregnancy. Archives of Women's Mental Health 17 (4), 311–315.

Selye, H., 1976. The Stress of Life. McGraw-Hill, New York.

Semple, C.J., Dunwoody, L., Sullivan, K., et al., 2006. Patients with head and neck cancer prefer individualised cognitive behaviour therapy. European Journal of Cancer Care 15 (3), 220–227.

Sharry, J., 2001. Solution-Focused Groupwork. Sage, London.

Sienaert, P., Vansteelandt, K., Demyttenaere, K., Peuskens, J., 2009. Randomized comparison of ultra-brief bifrontal and unilateral electroconvulsive therapy for major depression: clinical efficacy. Journal of Affective Disorders 116 (1–2), 106–112.

Slaikeu, K.A., 1990. Crisis Intervention: A Handbook for Practice and Research, second ed. Allyn & Bacon, Boston.

Slotema, C.W., Blom, J.D., Hoek, H.W., Sommer, E.C., 2010. Should we expand the toolbox of psychiatric treatment methods to include repetitive transcranial magnetic stimulation? A meta-analysis of the efficacy of rTMS in psychiatric disorders. Journal of Clinical Psychiatry 71 (7), 873–884.

Soundy, A., Roskell, C., Stubbs, B., Probst, M., Vancampfort, D., 2015. Investigating the benefits of sport participation for individuals with schizophrenia: a systematic review. Psychiatria Danubina 27 (1), 2–13.
Spoelstra, S.L., Schueller, M., Hilton, M., Ridenour, K., 2015. Interventions combining motivational interviewing and cognitive behaviour to promote medication compliance: a literature review. Journal of Clinical Nursing 24 (9–10), 1163–1173.
Sundel, S.S., Sundel, M., 1993. Behavior Modification in the Human Services: a Systematic Introduction to Concepts and Applications, third ed. Sage, Newbury Park, CA.
Swain, J., Hancock, K., Hainsworth, C., Bowman, J., 2013. Acceptance and commitment therapy in the treatment of anxiety: a systematic review. Clinical Psychology Review 33 (8), 965–978.
Swales, M., Heard, H.L., Williams, J.M.G., 2000. Linehan's dialectical behaviour therapy (DBT) for borderline personality disorder: overview and adaptation. Journal of Mental Health 9 (1), 7–23.
Tanaka, K., Davidson, L., 2015. Meanings associated with the core component of Clubhouse life: the work-ordered day. Psychiatric Quarterly 86 (2), 269–283.
Teh, S.P.C., Helmes, E., Drake, D.G., 2007. A Western Australian survey on public attitudes toward and knowledge of electroconvulsive therapy. International Journal of Social Psychiatry 53 (3), 247–273.
Thian, J.H.M., Kannusamy, P., He, H.-G., Klainin-Yobas, P., 2015. Relationships among stress, positive affectivity, and work engagement among registered nurses. Psychology 6 (2), 159–167.
Timmins, F., McCabe, C., 2005. Nurses' and midwives' assertive behaviour in the workplace. Journal of Advanced Nursing 51 (1), 38–45.
Treasure, J., Sepulveda, A.R., Whitaker, W., et al., 2007. Collaborative care between professionals and non-professionals in the management of eating disorders: a description of workshops focused on interpersonal maintaining factors. European Eating Disorders Review 15 (1), 24–34.
Truax, P., 2002. Behavioral case conceptualisation for adults. In: Hersen, M. (Ed.), Clinical Behavioral Therapy: Adults and Children. John Wiley & Sons, New York.
Vandevooren, J., Miller, L., O'Reilly, R., 2007. Outcomes in community-based residential treatment and rehabilitation for individuals with psychiatric disabilities: a retrospective study. Psychiatric Rehabilitation Journal 30 (3), 215–217.
Vermeulen, J., 1999. A Personal Reflection by a Psychiatric Nurse. Electroconvulsive Therapy: History, Perception, Knowledge and Attitudes. Paper Presented at the Scientific Meeting of the Australian and New Zealand College of Mental Health Nurses (ANZCMHN), Launceston, Tasmania, 9–12 September.
Vos, T., Gorry, J., Haby, M.M., et al., 2005. Cost-effectiveness of cognitive behavioural therapy and drug interventions for major depression. Australian and New Zealand Journal of Psychiatry 39 (8), 683–692.
Wand, T., Murray, L., 2008. Let's get physical. International Journal of Mental Health Nursing 17 (5), 363–369.
Watkinson, A., 2007. ECT: a personal experience. Mental Health Practice 10 (7), 32–35.
Watson, R.J., McDonald, J., Pearce, D.C., 2006. An exploration of national calls to Lifeline Australia: social support or urgent suicide intervention? British Journal of Guidance and Counselling 34 (4), 471–482.
Weatherall, A., Gibson, M., 2015. 'I'm going to ask you a very strange question': a conversation analytic case study of the miracle technique in solution-based therapy. Qualitative Research in Psychology 12 (2), 162–181.
Weir, B.W., O'Brien, K., Bard, R.S., Casciato, C.J., Maher, J.E., Dent, C.W., Dougherty, J.A., Stark, M.J., 2009. Reducing HIV and partner violence risk among women with criminal justice system involvement: a randomised controlled trial of two motivational interviewing-based interventions. AIDS and Behaviour 13 (3), 509–522.
Woidneck, M.R., Morrison, K.L., Twohig, M.P., 2014. Acceptance and commitment therapy for the treatment of posttraumatic stress among adolescents. Behavior Modification 38 (4), 451–476.
Wolpow, S., 2000. Adapting a dialectical behaviour therapy (DBT) group for use in a residential program. Psychiatric Rehabilitation Journal 24 (2), 135–141.
Yalom, I.D., 1995. The Theory and Practice of Group Psychotherapy, fourth ed. Basic Books, New York.
Zhou, K., Li, X., Li, J., Liu, M., Dang, S., Wang, D., Xin, X., 2015. A clinical randomised controlled trial of music therapy and progressive muscle relaxation training in female breast cancer patients after radical mastectomy: results on depression, anxiety and length of hospital stay. European Journal of Oncology Nursing 19 (1), 54–59.

USEFUL WEBSITES

DBT Self Help, written by people who have been through DBT; personal stories provide powerful accounts of recovery as well as showing that distress and difficulties will continue long after effective therapy, www.dbtselfhelp.com

Electroconvulsive Therapy, https://www.mind.org.uk/information-support/drugs-and-treatments/electroconvulsive-therapy-ect/#.W_V_Mej7TIU

Headspace, provides information for young people, their families and support people, as well as evidence, information and resources for professionals working with young people, www.headspace.com

Inner Health Studio, Candi Raudebaugh is a mental health occupational therapist from Canada; she offers an array of free materials with a focus on stress and anxiety management, particularly relaxation skills, www.innerhealthstudio.com

Stephen Rollnick, offers free materials about motivational interviewing by one of the original authors of motivational interviewing, www.stephenrollnick.com

25

Psychopharmacology

Kim Usher

KEY POINTS

- Psychotropic medications play an important role in the treatment of mental illness. The nurse plays a pivotal role in medication administration, promoting adherence and educating patients about medications. It is thus important for nurses to be aware of the uses, potential side effects and interactions of these medications.
- Many psychotropic medications are linked to physical health issues such as metabolic syndrome. It is important for nurses to be aware of these problems and to assess patients prior to and during use of the medications.
- Nurses must be aware of the issues surrounding the administration of these medications to vulnerable groups such as children, pregnant women and the elderly.
- Polypharmacy is to be avoided where possible, especially the tendency to use medications from different classes at the same time. Polypharmacy with older people is not advised.
- Issues related to as-needed (prn) medication administration are of contemporary relevance.
- Nursing assessment and interventions related to psychopharmacological side effects are important knowledge for the mental health nurse.

KEY TERMS

akathisia
antianxiety medications
anticholinergic
antidepressant medications
antiparkinsonian medication
antipsychotic medication
atypical antipsychotic medication
cognitive enhancers
discontinuation syndrome
extrapyramidal side effects
medication adherence
metabolic syndrome
mood-stabilising medication
neuroleptic malignant syndrome
neuroleptic medication
Parkinson's syndrome
polypharmacy
***pro re nata* (prn) medications**
psychopharmacology
psychotropic medication
tardive syndromes
tardive dyskinesia
typical antipsychotic medication
withdrawal syndrome

LEARNING OUTCOMES

The material in this chapter will assist you to:

- describe the role of the nurse in the administration of psychotropic medications and related interventions, including medication indications, interactions, side effects and precautions.
- identify the important classes of psychotropic medication and the disorders for which they are used.
- understand the issues for patients requiring psychotropic medications.
- understand the actions, use and side effects related to antianxiety/sedative hypnotic, antidepressant, mood-stabilising and antipsychotic medications.
- understand the issues related to as-needed (prn) psychotropic medications and related interventions.
- outline the relevant legal and ethical issues related to the administration of psychotropic medications.
- understand the importance of monitoring physical health prior to and during treatment with psychotropic medications.

INTRODUCTION

This chapter provides an overview of the principles of psychopharmacology, which is the study of medications used to treat psychiatric disorders. Important information is discussed related to medication indications, interactions, side effects and precautions, patient experience and education, and the issues of adherence and as-needed or *pro re nata* (prn) medication administration.

The use of medications that have a demonstrated ability to relieve the symptoms of psychiatric disorders has become widespread since the mid-1950s. The pharmacological agents used in current psychiatric practice are the antianxiety sedatives, antidepressants, mood stabilising medications, antipsychotic medications and cognitive enhancers. Collectively, these medications are referred to as psychotropic medications and are the focus of discussion in this chapter.

Psychotropic medications can be administered using a variety of methods such as oral, intramuscular and intravenous routes. It is important to remember that psychotropic medications are just one part of the patient's treatment and on their own should not be considered a 'quick fix' or cure-all. In fact, psychotropic medications are not helpful to all people who experience the symptoms of mental illness and also have many untoward effects that can cause discomfort and distress. However, a qualitative study by Piat and Sabetti (2009) found that patients rated medication highly in regard to recovery. The patients interviewed in this study identified that recovery for them meant finding a medication that works, taking the medication while also participating in other treatment and service options, adhering to the medication regimen, being involved in choices about their medication and living without medication. It is important to remember that psychotropic medications have the potential to improve quality of life for many people. However, it is also important to be aware that these medications have the potential to cause a number of serious side effects. Mental health nurses need to be aware of these effects and develop the appropriate skills to assess and monitor for them, including physical health and related issues (see Chapter 8), and educate patients and family/carers about potential issues related to psychotropic medication.

Skilful mental health nursing encompasses an understanding of the particular pharmacological actions of the psychotropic agents as well as an empathic understanding of the potential issues for the person taking these medications (see Nurse's Story 25.1). Regardless of the treatment setting, which can range from inpatient to community, mental health nurses play a pivotal role in working with patients and their families as they grapple with the issues surrounding these medications. It is important that the nurse develops a comprehensive understanding of both the medications and their impact on an individual, as well as an understanding of the supportive and therapeutic nursing interventions that support medication adherence. For a list of commonly used terms related to psychopharmacology, see Table 25.1.

NURSE'S STORY 25.1

The Importance of Working With the Person

One day a patient thanked me for looking after him and helping him to understand more about his medications and how they worked. This came as a surprise to me as I had never been thanked in this way before and thought it was my role to help patients to better understand treatment options. While the older traditional antipsychotics were linked to many major side effects, the newer second generation are better tolerated by patients and have many less reported side effects. However, it is easy to assume that because of this, people no longer need to be informed and involved in their treatment decisions. It is important to recognise that the new antipsychotics do not provide a global effect for negative symptoms and in fact still have a number of unwanted side effects such as weight gain and metabolic disturbance. These side effects can be very distressing to the patient and some have told me they think they are even worse off than before the treatment, even though it may have helped with their psychotic symptoms.

Reflecting on the incident described above I thought about how as nurses we often act in certain ways because of our own understanding or beliefs about an illness and its origins. For example, many nurses unwittingly propagate a pessimistic attitude to patients with schizophrenia because of their belief that the disorder is caused by genetic factors. In such cases nurses may engage with patients minimally and seek instead to do activities such as medication rounds. For me, it is important to try to work with patients in ways that are free of assumptions and to focus on the needs of the patients at all times.

IMPORTANT PHARMACOLOGICAL PRINCIPLES

Supportive and therapeutic nursing interventions enable the patient to develop and maintain medication adherence and foster the patient's understanding of their medications. As the mental health nurse plays an important role in the administration of psychotropic medications, especially within psychiatric inpatient units, it is essential to have a sound working knowledge of psychotropic medications, including their pharmacology and relevant neurochemistry. This knowledge is important for the nurse when offering medication education to the patient and their family.

All medications are prescribed for particular effects or target symptoms that the prescriber hopes to change. Therefore, it is important for the nurse to be aware of the symptoms that particular medications target as well as the symptoms experienced by individual patients. The correct identification of symptoms is a key component of a thorough nursing assessment. Side effects, on the other hand, are the expression of effects for which the medication was not intended. Not all side effects are harmful, but some can be, so the nurse needs a sound working knowledge of this area of practice.

Nurses also need to be aware of polypharmacy. Polypharmacy implies the concurrent use of multiple psychotropic medications at the same time (Usher et al. 2009b). Although polypharmacy might be useful at some stage for the management of people with serious psychiatric disorders, it has negative connotations and is generally not advisable as it can increase the chance of adverse medication side effects and interactions. It can also be extremely problematic with certain groups of vulnerable people, including older people who are commonly prescribed a number of different medications concurrently (Hubbard et al. 2015).

An understanding of how psychotropic medications work is important for mental health nurses so that they can better understand the issues surrounding the prescription and administration of these medications. The neuron is the basic functional unit of the brain and the central nervous system (CNS) and all communication in the brain involves neurons

TABLE 25.1 **Commonly Used Terms**

Term	Definition
akathisia	restlessness where the person cannot stay still
anosognosia	lack of insight
antipsychotic medication	medication prescribed to reduce psychotic symptoms
ataxia	lack of voluntary coordination of muscle movement
atypical antipsychotic medication	the newer, second generation of antipsychotic medication
cogwheeling rigidity	type of rigidity seen in parkinsonism whereby the muscles respond with cogwheel-like jerks to the application of constant force in attempting to bend the limb
dystonia	state of abnormal muscle tone
extrapyramidal side effects	drug-induced movement disorders
half-life	the time until the serum level of a drug is reduced by half
iatrogenic	an effect caused by a medication or by health personnel
Parkinson syndrome	imbalance between dopamine and acetylcholine, resulting in involuntary movements, reduced movements, rigidity and abnormal walking and posture
polypharmacy	use of multiple medications simultaneously
pro re nata (prn)	as needed
serotonin syndrome	a potentially life-threatening syndrome caused by excessive brain cell activity as a result of high levels of serotonin
tardive dyskinesia	involuntary movements of the tongue, lips, face, trunk and extremities related to taking anti-psychotic medications
tardive syndrome	delayed-onset abnormal involuntary movement disorders caused by a dopamine-receptor blocking agent
typical antipsychotic medication	traditional type of antipsychotic medication

communicating across synapses at receptors. Receptors are the targets for the neurotransmitters or chemical messengers necessary for communication between neurons. The neurotransmitters acetylcholine, noradrenaline (norepinephrine), dopamine, serotonin (5HT) and gamma-aminobutyric acid (GABA) are implicated in the development of mental illness.

Psychotropic medications produce their therapeutic action by altering communication among the neurons in the CNS. In particular, they alter the way neurotransmitters work at the synapse by modifying the reuptake of neurotransmitters into the presynaptic neuron, activating or inhibiting postsynaptic receptors, or inhibiting enzyme activity (Usher et al. 2009b). Generally, the major psychotropic medications are believed to act by altering the activities of the receptors, enzymes, ion channels and chemical transporter systems involved in these processes (for further information, see Chapter 2 of Usher et al. 2009b).

IMPORTANT PSYCHOTROPIC MEDICATIONS

This section explores the most important groups of psychotropic medications in current use: the anxiolytics (antianxiety), antidepressants, mood stabilisers and antipsychotics (neuroleptics). These groups of medications are listed in Table 25.2 with common examples from a local perspective.

Antianxiety or Anxiolytic Medications

Anxiety is a common human experience that is a normal reaction to a threat of some kind. It leads to a fight-or-flight response in the individual. Anxiety is also the feature of many mental health problems. When anxiety becomes disabling, antianxiety medications may be useful (Shupikai Rinomhota & Marshall 2000). Antianxiety medications can be divided into benzodiazepines and nonbenzodiazepines. The benzodiazepines are probably the most commonly prescribed medications in the world today and are the medication of choice for the short-term treatment of anxiety states.

Benzodiazepines

Indications for use. The benzodiazepines are thought to reduce anxiety because of their potentiation of the inhibitory neurotransmitter GABA, which results in a clinical decrease in the individual's anxiety by an inhibition of neurotransmission (Usher et al. 2009b). Clinically, they are used to treat anxiety, insomnia, alcohol withdrawal, skeletal muscle rigidity, seizure disorders, anxiety associated with medical disease and psychotic agitation. Therefore, although the discussion here is primarily related to the use of these medications as antianxiety agents, they also have a sedative effect and are often used for that purpose.

Side effects. Side effects from the benzodiazepines (see Table 25.3) are common, dose related, usually short term and almost always harmless. They include drowsiness, reduced mental acuity and impaired motor performance. However, other effects such as headache, dizziness, feelings of detachment, nausea, hypotension and restlessness may also be experienced. Therefore, the patient should be warned of the risk of accidents and cautioned about driving a car or operating dangerous machinery. These medications generally do not live up to their reputation of being strongly addictive, especially if they have been used for appropriate purposes, if their use has not been complicated by other factors such as the addition of other medications and if their withdrawal is planned and gradual. However, a withdrawal syndrome can result (see Box 25.1) if ceased abruptly.

TABLE 25.2 Classification of Psychotropic Medications

Type	Medication Group	Example
Antianxiety	Benzodiazepines	• Chlordiazepoxide • Diazepam • Clonazepam • Alprazolam • Lorazepam
	• Azapirones • Beta-adrenergic blockers	• Buspirone • Propranolol
Antidepressant	Tricyclic and related medications	• Amitriptyline • Lofepramine • Trazadone
	Selective serotonin reuptake inhibitors (SSRIs) and related medications	• Fluoxetine • Paroxetine
	Noradrenaline serotonin reuptake inhibitors (NSRIs)	• Venlafaxine • Mirtazapine
	Monoamine oxidase inhibitors (MAOIs)	• Isocarboxazid • Phenelzine • Tranylcypromine
Mood stabilising	Lithium	• Lithium carbonate
	Anticonvulsants	• Carbamazepine • Valproate • Topiramate • Lamotrigine
Antipsychotic Typical (traditional)	• Phenothiazines • Thioxanthines • Butyrophenones • Diphenylbutylpiperidines	• Thioridazine • Flupenthixol • Haloperidol • Pimozide
Atypical (second generation)		• Clozapine • Risperidone • Olanzapine • Quetiapine • Ziprasidone
Sedative-hypnotic	Benzodiazepines	• Flurazepam • Temazepam
	• Cyclopyrrolones • Imidazopyrimidines	• Zopiclone • Zolpidem

TABLE 25.3 Managing Benzodiazepine Side Effects

Side Effect	Intervention
Drowsiness	Encourage appropriate activity but warn against engaging in activities such as driving or operating machinery
Dizziness	Observe and take steps to prevent falls
Feelings of detachment	Encourage socialisation
Dependency, rebound insomnia/anxiety	Encourage short-term use; educate to avoid other medications such as alcohol; plan for withdrawal

It is also important to remember that older patients are more vulnerable to side effects because the ageing brain is more sensitive to the action of sedatives (Usher et al. 2009b).

BOX 25.1 Benzodiazepine Withdrawal Syndrome

- Agitation
- Anorexia
- Anxiety
- Autonomic arousal
- Dizziness
- Hallucinations
- Insomnia
- Irritability
- Nausea and vomiting
- Seizures
- Sensitivity to light and sounds
- Tinnitus
- Tremulousness

Contraindications/precautions. Benzodiazepines should not be taken in conjunction with any other CNS depressants including alcohol. Their safety in pregnancy is not established.

Interactions. Interactions may occur with alcohol, monoamine oxidase inhibitors (MAOIs), phenytoin, antacids and agents with anticholinergic activity.

Patient education. The patient should be educated about the following:

- Driving or operating machinery should be avoided until the patient knows how they react to the medication.
- Alcohol and other CNS depressants potentiate the effects of benzodiazepines and therefore should be avoided.
- Benzodiazepine use should not be stopped suddenly.
- The use of benzodiazepines during pregnancy is not recommended.

NONBENZODIAZEPINE ANTIANXIETY MEDICATIONS

Buspirone is a potent nonbenzodiazepine anxiolytic medication with no addictive or sedative properties. It is effective in the treatment of anxiety and has no muscle relaxant or anticonvulsant properties. It is of no use in the management of alcohol or other medication abuse or of panic disorder. Generally, it takes about 3 to 6 weeks before maximum anxiolytic effects are achieved.

Propranolol is a beta-blocker that is useful in the treatment of anxiety. It blocks beta-noradrenergic receptors centrally and in the peripheral cardiac and pulmonary systems. Beta-blockers reduce certain physiological symptoms of anxiety, especially tachycardia, rather than working directly on the anxiety.

Antidepressant Medications

Depression is a disorder characterised by symptoms such as depressed mood, lack of pleasure or interest, appetite disturbance, sleep disturbance and fatigue. Depression is associated with dysregulation of neurochemicals, particularly serotonin and noradrenaline. The physiological understanding of antidepressant medication action supports this theory. Antidepressant medications enhance the transmission of these neurochemicals in a number of ways: they block the reuptake of the neurotransmitters at the synapse, inhibit their metabolism and destruction and/or enhance the activity of the receptors. The action of these medications at the synapse is immediate but it takes several weeks for antidepressants to have an effect on mood.

Indications for Use

Antidepressant medications are indicated in the treatment of persistent depressive disorders, major depression, maintenance treatment of depression and prevention of relapse, and anxiety disorders such as panic disorder and obsessive-compulsive disorder. The medications elevate mood and alleviate the other symptoms experienced as part of depression. Choice of a particular antidepressant medication will depend on its symptom profile, side effects, comorbid medical conditions, concurrent medications and risk of medication interactions, and the individual's medication history. If the patient responds to the course of treatment with a particular medication, they should continue taking the medication at the same dosage for up to 9 months. If they remain symptom free during this time, the medication will be gradually withdrawn. Patients whose depressive symptoms return after withdrawal of medication may need long-term maintenance (Usher et al. 2009b).

Side Effects

Tricyclic antidepressants. The tricyclic medications, available on the market for many years now, are clinically similar, so their effects and side effects tend to vary little between individual medications. They work primarily by serotonin and noradrenaline reuptake inhibition. The blockade of reuptake leads to extra transmitters being available for receptor binding. Side effects include sedation, dry mouth, constipation, blurred vision, seizures and urinary retention. They may also cause postural hypotension and serious cardiac problems such as heart block and arrhythmias. Because of their serious side effects these medications can lead to life-threatening consequences if taken in large quantities, such as in suicide attempts, and if this is suspected, immediate action to support life must be instigated. (Box 25.2 lists signs of overdose.) In the case of severely depressed patients where a potential for suicide is predicted, close supervision is required and when the person is not an inpatient, the dispensing of small, sublethal quantities is recommended.

Monoamine oxidase inhibitors. MAOIs were the first group of antidepressant medications discovered. They remain very effective antidepressants; however, due to their potentially serious side effects the newer antidepressant medications have mostly replaced their use. The MAOIs work by inhibiting both types of the enzyme (MAO A and B) that metabolise serotonin and noradrenaline. Patients taking these medications must avoid noradrenaline agonists, which include its dietary precursor, tyramine. Adverse effects include drowsiness or insomnia, agitation, fatigue, gastrointestinal disturbances, weight gain, hypotension and dizziness, dry mouth and skin, sexual dysfunction, constipation and blurred vision. The major concern with the use of these medications is their potential to interact with specific foods that contain tyramine and other amine medications such as those found in any cough preparation (see Box 25.3). Such an interaction can result in excessive and dangerous elevation in blood pressure, known as a hypertensive crisis.

Selective serotonin reuptake inhibitors. The selective serotonin reuptake inhibitor (SSRI) group of antidepressant

BOX 25.2 Signs of Tricyclic Overdose

- Agitation
- Confusion, drowsiness, delirium
- Convulsion
- Bowel and bladder paralysis
- Disturbances with the regulation of blood pressure and temperature
- Dilated pupils

(*Source:* Treatment Protocol Project, 2004. Management of Mental Disorders, 4th edn. World Health Organization Collaborating Centre for Mental Health and Substance Abuse, Sydney.)

BOX 25.3 Food and Medications to be Avoided by Patients Taking MAOIs

Avoid

- cheeses, especially matured cheeses
- pickled herrings, cured meats and beef extracts such as marmite
- liver and chicken livers
- whole broad beans, avocados (especially if overripe), soybean paste
- figs, especially if overripe
- large numbers of bananas
- alcoholic drinks, especially chianti and red wine
- other antidepressant medications, nasal and sinus decongestants, narcotics, adrenaline (epinephrine)
- stimulants, hay-fever and asthma medications

medications inhibits the reuptake of serotonin at the presynaptic membrane. This leads to an increased availability of serotonin in the synapse and therefore at the receptors, thereby promoting serotonin transmission. These medications are as effective as the tricyclic antidepressants but safer, as they cause less serious side effects and have decreased risk of death by overdose. While the actions and effectiveness of these medications are similar, they are all structurally different from each other, resulting in differences in their side effects. Side effects are similar to those of the tricyclic group except that they do not have the cardiovascular, sedative and anticholinergic side effects. Nausea, diarrhoea, anxiety and restlessness, insomnia, sexual dysfunction, loss of appetite, weight loss and headache are the most common side effects. They should not be stopped abruptly; the withdrawal syndrome includes symptoms such as dizziness, paraesthesia, anxiety, sleep disturbance, agitation and tremor. They should not be combined with MAOIs.

Noradrenalin serotonin reuptake inhibitors. Noradrenaline serotonin reuptake inhibitors (NSRIs) are a new class of antidepressant medications. They are considered to be more effective than SSRIs in some people. NSRIs block the reuptake of serotonin and noradrenaline, thus increasing the amount of these neurotransmitters available at the synapse. Common side effects associated with NSRIs include nausea, dry mouth, dizziness, excessive sweating, agitation and constipation.

Contraindications/precautions

Caution is warranted in the use of all antidepressant medications. Once the medications start to take effect and the patient's mood lifts, the patient may become a risk for suicide. SSRIs should not be combined with MAOI therapy. MAOIs should not be started within 1 week of tricyclic therapy and, conversely, tricyclic medications should not be commenced within 2 weeks of stopping an MAOI. The tricyclics are a special risk with depressed people because of their severe cardiac toxicity if taken in large doses. Caution is warranted in patients with cardiac disease and with older patients. Tricyclics may also impair reaction times, especially at the beginning of treatment. Alcohol may increase the sedative effects of tricyclics.

Interactions

Tricyclics. Hyperpyretic crisis, seizures or serious cardiac events may occur if administered in conjunction with MAOIs. They may prevent the therapeutic effect of some antihypertensives.

MAOIs. Hypertensive crisis may occur if administered with many other medications including adrenaline, noradrenaline, reserpine, narcotic analgesics and vasoconstrictors. Patients may also experience hypertensive crisis if tyramine-rich foods are ingested (see Box 25.3).

SSRIs. Alcohol may potentiate the effect of SSRIs. Use with cimetidine may result in increased concentrations of SSRIs in the bloodstream. Hypertensive crisis may occur if taken within 14 days of MAOIs.

Patient Education

Inform the patient of the time it will take for a marked effect to be experienced from the medication and that it is important for them to keep taking the medication even though they have not noticed an initial improvement in their condition.

Other information:

- Warn the patient of problems when driving or operating machinery if sedation is experienced.
- Tell the patient to discuss with their doctor if they become pregnant or intend to breastfeed.
- Warn the patient about the effect that alcohol may have if combined with antidepressant medication.
- Inform the patient about possible interactions with foods and other medications if taking MAOIs.

Mood-Stabilising Medications

Lithium, a naturally occurring salt, is the medication of choice for the treatment of acute mania and for the ongoing maintenance of patients with a history of mania. John Cade discovered its effectiveness as a treatment for mania in 1949. Just how lithium works is not clear, but it is known to mimic the effects of sodium, thereby compromising the ability of neurons to release, activate or respond to neurotransmitters. It does appear to reduce the sodium content of the brain, and increase central serotonin synthesis and noradrenaline reuptake (Usher et al. 2009b). A number of other medications have also been used successfully, either alone or in combination with lithium, to control the symptoms of mania. The antidepressants and a number of anticonvulsant medications have also been used very successfully to reduce mania.

Indications for Use

Lithium. Lithium is the medication of choice for the treatment of acute mania and the ongoing maintenance of people with bipolar disorder (Usher et al. 2009b). It is also useful in the treatment of unipolar depression, aggressive behaviour, conduct disorder and schizoaffective disorder.

Anticonvulsants. A number of anticonvulsant medications have been used to treat mania, especially when lithium is ineffective. These medications are now rapidly becoming the medication of choice for many patients. Carbamazepine, valproate and topiramate are examples of commonly used anticonvulsants. These medications have been found to have acute antimanic and mood-stabilising effects. Carbamazepine, valproate, topiramate (Nassir Ghaemi et al. 2001) and lamotrigine (Hurley 2002) are recommended treatments for mixed or bipolar states, secondary mania, rapid cyclers and lithium refractoriness

Side Effects

Lithium. Side effects are drowsiness, metallic taste in the mouth, difficulty concentrating, increased thirst, dizziness, headache, dry mouth, gastrointestinal upset, nausea/vomiting, fine hand tremor, hypotension, arrhythmias, polyuria, dehydration, weight gain.

Anticonvulsants.

- *Carbamazepine*—blood dyscrasias, drowsiness, nausea, vomiting, constipation or diarrhoea, hives or skin rashes, hepatitis
- *Valproate*—prolonged bleeding time, gastrointestinal upset, tremor, ataxia, weight gain, somnolence, dizziness, hepatic failure, polycystic ovary syndrome (PCOS) in women
- *Topiramate*—cognitive impairment, sedation, nausea, weight loss, dizziness, vomiting, rash, agitation, paraesthesia
- *Lamotrigine*—blurred vision, rash, nausea, ataxia, drowsiness

Contraindications/Precautions

Lithium. Lithium is contraindicated with cardiac or renal disease, dehydration, sodium depletion, brain damage, pregnancy and lactation. Care should be taken with thyroid disorders, diabetes, urinary retention and history of seizures. The therapeutic range for lithium is 0.6 to 1.2 mmol/L for acute mania and 0.6 to 0.8 mmol/L for maintenance, but more conservative levels are increasingly being used. Symptoms of lithium toxicity rarely appear at levels below 1.2 mmol/L but are common above 2.0 mmol/L (Usher et al. 2009b). Therefore, as the therapeutic and toxic levels are so close, extreme care must be taken in monitoring the patient's blood level regularly, especially during early phases of the treatment. If the level exceeds 1.5 mmol/L, the next dose should be withheld and the doctor notified. Levels are usually monitored weekly until stable and then monthly. The blood samples for testing should be taken 12 hours after the last dose when lithium has been taken for at least 5 to 7 days (Psychotropic Expert Group 2013; Usher et al. 2009b).

Anticonvulsants. Anticonvulsants are contraindicated with MAOIs and during lactation. Caution is required in older patients, people with cardiac/renal disease and during pregnancy. Before commencing carbamazepine, a range of tests should be performed, including blood film examination, electrolytes, liver and kidney function and an electrocardiogram (ECG). Carbamazepine may also interfere with the metabolism and blood concentrations of other medications, so care is needed with oral contraceptives and other medications. There is a risk of fetal malformation, so it should not be taken during pregnancy.

Valproate should not be taken with aspirin and some antipsychotics. It may enhance the effects of alcohol and other CNS depressants. Polycystic ovary syndrome is more common among women treated with valproate; symptoms tend to emerge early, often within the first few months of treatment. Women should be informed of this risk before commencing treatment.

Interactions

Lithium. Diuretics, ACE (angiotensin-converting enzyme) inhibitors, neuroleptics, nonsteroidal antiinflammatory medications, alcohol and caffeine may interfere with lithium absorption.

Anticonvulsants.

- *Carbamazepine*—erythromycin, isoniazid, oral contraceptives, theophylline, fluoxetine
- *Valproate*—may potentiate alcohol, carbamazepine, barbiturates; should not be taken with aspirin or antipsychotics
- *Topiramate*—concomitant use with lithium and valproate can cause cognitive impairment

Patient Education

Lithium.

- Educate the patient about the side effects and signs of toxicity (see Box 25.4 and Nurse's Story 25.2), and the need for regular blood level checks.
- Encourage the patient to include a regular intake of approximately 10 glasses of water every day.
- Remind the patient to take medication regularly, even when feeling well.
- Advise the patient not to operate machinery until initial drowsiness subsides.
- Discuss the risks of taking lithium during pregnancy or when considering pregnancy.

Anticonvulsants.

- Inform the patient about avoiding sudden cessation of the tablets.
- Encourage the patient to report unusual symptoms, such as spontaneous bruising, unusual bleeding, sore throat, fever, malaise, yellow skin or eyes, to the doctor.
- Remind the patient to take medications with meals if gastrointestinal upset occurs.
- Advise the patient to avoid taking alcohol or nonprescription medications without consulting the doctor.
- Explain that pregnancy must be avoided while taking the medication. Alternative methods of contraception may be required if taking valproate, as oral contraception may not be effective.

BOX 25.4 Signs of Lithium Toxicity

- *Early stages*—anorexia, nausea, vomiting, diarrhoea, coarse hand tremor, twitching, lethargy, dysarthria, hyperactive deep tendon reflexes, ataxia, tinnitus, vertigo, weakness, drowsiness
- *Later stages*—fever, decreased urinary output, decreased blood pressure, irregular pulse, electrocardiogram (ECG) changes, impaired consciousness, seizures, coma, death

Note: Lithium toxicity is a medical emergency.

NURSE'S STORY 25.2

Lithium Intoxication

An older patient was admitted to an inpatient unit for an episode of manic behaviour. She had experienced mania before and was on continuous treatment with lithium. The lithium dose was increased during the admission. The nurse returned to the ward after 2 days' leave and noticed that the patient appeared unwell, had a coarse tremor, was confused, ataxic and had myoclonic jerks. She called the doctor on call, expressed her concern and told him she would withhold the evening dose of lithium. She asked him to see the patient as soon as possible and to organise to have blood taken for a lithium level. The doctor refused to come to the ward and disagreed with the nurse's concern about the patient. He insisted she give the evening dose of the medication and said he would see the patient the next morning. The nurse refused to accept his decision and called her immediate supervisor and explained her concern for the patient's wellbeing. The medication was withheld, and an urgent blood request determined that the patient's lithium level was 2.2 mmol/L. The nurse had correctly diagnosed lithium toxicity and taken the correct action to advocate best care for the patient.

Antipsychotic or Neuroleptic Medications

The traditional neuroleptic or antipsychotic medications (also known as the typical antipsychotics) have been an important treatment for psychotic disorders since their discovery in the 1950s. These medications revolutionised the treatment of mental illness and soon became the mainstay of treatment for most psychotic disorders (Usher et al. 2009a). Each group of the typical antipsychotics appears to be equally effective for the reduction or elimination of positive symptoms of psychosis (e.g. delusions, hallucinations, motor disturbances). However, the side-effect profiles of the typical antipsychotics became cause for concern because of their effect on quality of life and their link with nonadherence.

The newer second-generation antipsychotics, commonly referred to as the atypical or novel antipsychotics, were introduced in the 1990s and have quickly become the medication of choice for psychotic symptoms (Healy 2008). These medications are better tolerated and less likely to lead to problems with medication adherence (Usher et al. 2009a). Apart from clozapine, which has superior efficacy to the typical antipsychotics, their efficacy appears to be equal to that of the typical antipsychotics (Psychotropic Expert Group 2013) but they are more effective in reducing the negative symptoms of psychosis. Clozapine, risperidone, olanzapine and quetiapine remain the most widely used examples of the second-generation antipsychotics.

The typical antipsychotics are dopamine antagonists. They primarily block the postsynaptic D_2 receptors but also exert other synaptic effects. They reduce the positive symptoms of schizophrenia. Atypicals, on the other hand, have dopamine receptor subtype 2 (D_2) and serotonin receptor subtype 2 ($5HT_2$) blocking action. They not only reduce the positive symptoms of schizophrenia, but also have an effect on the negative symptoms (such as blunting of affect, avolition and anhedonia) without the serious extrapyramidal side effects (Usher et al. 2009a, 2009b). Risperidone has the same receptor profile as clozapine but without the need for blood testing. It has low incidence of extrapyramidal symptoms (EPS).

Indications for Use

Antipsychotics are indicated for the treatment of acute and chronic psychoses, delusional disorder and severe depression where psychotic symptoms are present. Schizophrenia and schizoaffective disorders are the most common indications for antipsychotic medications. Some of the phenothiazine group has other uses, such as antiemetic in the case of prochlorperazine and the treatment of intractable hiccups in the case of chlorpromazine. Many of the antipsychotic medications, especially the lower potency ones such as chlorpromazine and haloperidol, have a prominent sedative effect. This effect is particularly conspicuous early in treatment, although tolerance usually develops quickly.

Side Effects

Typical antipsychotics. The side effects of the typical antipsychotics are varied. They can affect every system of the body and range from effects on the CNS—including movement disorders, sedation and seizures—through to potentially life-threatening side effects such as neuroleptic malignant syndrome (NMS) (see Table 25.4 for an overview of the side effects of the typical antipsychotics). The most troubling of the side effects are the extrapyramidal reactions. These result from the effects of the antipsychotic medications on the extrapyramidal motor system. This is the same system responsible for the movement disorders of Parkinson disease. Acute dystonia, parkinsonism and akathisia occur early and can be managed by a variety of medications including antiparkinsonian and benzodiazepine medications. Tardive dyskinesia generally occurs later and has no effective treatment. The Abnormal Involuntary Movements Scale (AIMS) (see Box 25.5) is a useful tool for nurses to detect movement disorders in patients. NMS, an idiosyncratic hypersensitivity to antipsychotic medications, is a rare but serious reaction that is potentially life threatening (see Box 25.6). More information on traditional antipsychotic side effects can be found in the following articles: McCann and Clark (2004), Usher et al. (2013) and Morrison et al. (2014). (See also Nurse's Story 25.3.)

Atypical antipsychotics. Atypical antipsychotics are not all pharmacologically alike so they tend to have a diverse side-effect profile (Howland 2007). They do, however, have some similar side effects such as weight gain, constipation and dizziness, and are also linked to the development of diabetes and metabolic syndrome (McDaid & Smyth 2015). Some may cause extrapyramidal side effects at higher doses, but they are not uniformly associated with parkinsonian symptoms, akathisia, dystonia or dyskinesia (Howland 2007). Seizures may also occur with too rapid a titration associated with increase in dosage. In addition, cardiac

TABLE 25.4 Side Effects of the Typical Antipsychotics

Side Effects	Key Features	Time of Maximal Risk	Interventions
CNS Extrapyramidal Side Effects			
Acute dystonic reaction	Painful muscle spasms in head, back and torso; can last minutes to hours, occur suddenly; cause fear	1–5 days	Administer antiparkinsonian medication quickly; respiratory support if needed; reassure and remain with the patient
Akathisia	Restlessness, leg aches, person cannot stay still	5–60 days	Administer antiparkinsonian medication; change medication
Neuroleptic malignant syndrome	Potentially fatal with hyperthermia, severe extrapyramidal side effects, sweating, muscle rigidity, clouding of consciousness, elevated creatine phosphokinase	Weeks, usually	Supportive therapy; cease all medications; treat with bromocriptine or dantrolene
Parkinsonism	Rigid, mask-like facial expression; shuffling gait; drooling	5–30 days; can recur even after a single dose	Administer dopamine agonist; support the patient
Seizures	Typical antipsychotics reduce seizure threshold, risk about 1% but greater with rapid titration or history of seizures	Early in treatment	May need to stop the medication, observe the patient or manipulate the medication dose
Tardive dyskinesia	Usually results from prolonged use of typical antipsychotics; stereotyped involuntary movements (tongue, lips, feet)	After months or years of treatment (worse on withdrawal)	Assess the patient often; change to atypical medications; no other treatment available
Other			
Anticholinergic	Dry mouth, blurred vision, orthostatic hypotension, tachycardia, urinary retention, nasal congestion		Observe, educate the patient; provide support where needed; may need to change medication
Endocrine	Weight gain, diminished libido, impotence, amenorrhoea, galactorrhoea		Educate the patient; reduce kilojoule intake; may need to change medication
Photosensitivity	Skin hyperpigmentation		Educate the patient to avoid sun and wear protective clothing, sunscreen and sunglasses
Sedation	May be beneficial in agitated patients; can be mistaken for cognitive slowing		Educate the patient to avoid driving or operating machinery; rest periods; adjust dose

BOX 25.5 Useful Tools for Assessing Medication Side Effects

LUNSERS

The LUNSERS (Liverpool University Neuroleptic Side Effect Rating Scale) is a useful tool for assessing side effects. It is designed for self-administration but can also be a useful tool for nurses to help detect patient reactions to changes in treatment (Morrison et al. 2000). It can be accessed in the following journal article: Day, J.C., Wood, G., Dewey, M., et al., 1995. A self-rating scale for measuring neuroleptic side effects: validation in a group of schizophrenic patients. British Journal of Psychiatry 166(5), 650–653.

AIMS

The AIMS (Abnormal Involuntary Movements Scale) is a widely used tool for use with people on long-term antipsychotic medications. It is designed to assess for signs of tardive dyskinesia. It can be accessed in the following journal article: Munetz, M.R., Benjamin, S., 1988. How to examine patients using the Abnormal Involuntary Movements Scale. Hospital and Community Psychiatry. 39(11), 1172–1177.

BOX 25.6 Neuroleptic Malignant Syndrome

NMS is a rare disorder that resembles a severe form of parkinsonism with coarse tremor and catatonia, fluctuating in intensity, accompanied by signs of autonomic instability (labile pulse and blood pressure, hyperthermia), stupor, elevation of creatinine kinase in serum, and sometimes myoglobinaemia. In severe forms it may persist for more than a week after ceasing the medication. The risk of death from this syndrome is high (more than 10%); therefore, immediate medical intervention is required if suspected.

(*Source:* Usher, K., Foster, K., Bullock, S., 2009b. Psychopharmacology for Health Professionals. Elsevier, Sydney.)

problems such as atrial fibrillation, atrial flutter or myocarditis early in treatment, although uncommon, may occur. Some of the side effects of individual medications include:

- *Clozapine*—more safety concerns than any other antipsychotic medication (Remington et al. 2013). A

NURSE'S STORY 25.3

Antipsychotic Medication Side Effects

I remember talking to a young man about the side effects he was experiencing as a result of taking a number of the traditional antipsychotics to treat schizophrenia. The experiences he described made me aware of the serious impact these medications can have on a person's life. For example, he described how the akathisia he experienced was so extreme that he felt it was no longer worth living. The choice between taking the medication, which he experienced extreme pressure to do, and experiencing the side effects (especially akathisia, which was not resolved by any other treatment), or not taking the medications and living with the symptoms of the illness, caused him a great deal of confusion and distress. He said there were many times when he considered suicide the only option, as he could see no way out of the predicament. He believed that living with the side effects caused such a poor quality of life that it was possibly not worth being alive. Similarly, he also experienced suicidal thoughts when the symptoms of the illness were at its worst. He told me how he believed the medication side effects made him recognisable by others as mentally ill. This also caused him a great deal of personal distress as he remembered times when he felt conspicuous due to the visible medication side effects. He recalled a time when he visited his sister's house, where he believed his medication side effects caused the whole family embarrassment, as the side effects drew people's attention to him and to his behaviour. This man's experience of the side effects of psychotropic medications made me realise the importance of listening to the patient's side of the treatment story and helped me to become more cognisant of the issues surrounding medication adherence.

serious adverse effect is the potential for agranulocytosis, which occurs in approximately 1% to 2% of patients. Precautions must be taken to ensure swift detection of this side effect should it occur, patient will attend a clozapine monitoring clinic at least monthly and blood tests are carried out prior to further medication being commenced.

- *Risperidone*—insomnia, agitation, anxiety, headache, postural hypotension particularly at the commencement of treatment, drowsiness, weight gain, gastrointestinal upset, sexual dysfunction and EPS.
- *Olanzapine*—drowsiness, weight gain, postural hypotension, peripheral oedema, EPS and anticholinergic side effects (dry mouth, hypotension, tachycardia).
- *Quetiapine*—mild somnolence, mild asthenia, dry mouth, limited weight gain, postural hypotension, tachycardia and occasional syncope.

Weight gain and the development of metabolic syndrome associated with the atypical antipsychotics is a serious issue (McDaid & Smyth 2015). Weight gain has been previously reported as predictable: a metaanalysis of weight change by Allison et al. (1999) found weight gain over 10 weeks of treatment with a standard medication dose, as follows: clozapine, 4.45 kg; olanzapine, 4.15 kg; risperidone, 2.10 kg; and ziprasidone, 0.04 kg—with insufficient data available to evaluate quetiapine. The weight gain usually occurs during the first 4 to 12 weeks of treatment. After the initial period the weight gain continues at a lower level over a prolonged period of time (Tschoner et al. 2007). Weight gain linked to atypical antipsychotics is typically associated with abdominal obesity and enhanced adiposity, which is linked with increased morbidity and mortality, as well as reduced quality of life (Tschoner et al. 2007). Together these changes make up what is referred to as metabolic syndrome, a cluster of metabolic abnormalities including hypertension, hyperlipidaemia, hyperglycaemia and abdominal obesity, which, when experienced together, lead to an increased risk of diabetes and cardiovascular disease. Thus weight gain and metabolic disturbance linked to the atypical antipsychotics have become a major concern for clinicians and patients (McDaid & Smyth 2015; Usher et al. 2013).

Previous studies have found the prevalence rates of metabolic syndrome in people with schizophrenia to range between 51% and 68% (John et al. 2009; Tirupati & Chua 2007). A cohort study of people prescribed clozapine (Hyde et al. 2015) found higher prevalence rates for cardiovascular and metabolic events than previous studies. The most common cardiovascular condition revealed was ECG-defined abnormalities (60%), while low high-density lipoprotein (HDL) cholesterol levels (69%) and high triglyceride levels (77%) were the most common metabolic abnormalities.

The weight gain and high rate of metabolic disturbance with the atypical antipsychotics is linked to a number of factors including impairment of the glucose metabolism system, which regulates appetite and weight management. Impairment of this system appears to be linked to the development of type 2 diabetes and dyslipidaemia (Murashita et al. 2007; Usher et al. 2006).

Metabolic syndrome is diagnosed when a person has a girth measurement higher than recommended and any two of the following: raised triglycerides, reduced HDL cholesterol, raised blood pressure and raised fasting plasma glucose. Management of the syndrome includes lifestyle changes (improving nutrition and increasing exercise), ongoing monitoring and medication for dyslipidaemia, hypertension and glucose intolerance if required. Guidelines for the assessment of metabolic syndrome include baseline screening that includes girth measurement, weight, height, body mass index (BMI), blood chemistries and family and personal history, followed by regular monitoring. Thus attention to the physical health of patients is an important nursing role. This issue is covered in more detail in Chapter 8.

Early intervention for weight gain with the atypical antipsychotics should occur when the person begins taking the medication or when medication changes are made and should target reduced kilojoule intake and increased exercise, as these have been shown to have a positive ameliorating effect on weight gain. A number of interventions have been introduced in an attempt to manage the weight gain linked to these medications. For example, lifestyle interventions, education, weight loss medications and exercise have all been implemented and evaluated. However, research to date indicates significantly greater weight reduction in lifestyle intervention groups than in pharmacological intervention groups or standard care groups (Park et al. 2011).

Nurses should ensure that patients are screened for weight gain, diet and exercise on a regular basis. Indeed, nurses are well placed to educate patients about making healthy choices in an attempt to prevent weight gain and the development of metabolic symptoms such as diabetes and cardiovascular conditions (Edwards et al. 2010). It is important for nurses to be aware of the potential for weight gain with the atypical antipsychotics and to work with patients when the medication is first introduced, rather than waiting until the weight gain becomes problematic (Park et al. 2011), as the weight gain associated with these medications is known to cause significant distress to patients (Usher et al. 2013). However, while mental health nurses recognise working with patients to manage weight gain and other medication side effects is an important nursing responsibility, they report lack of education (Brown et al. 2007) and confidence (McDaid & Smyth 2015) to do so.

Antiparkinsonian medications used to treat tardive symptoms. Antiparkinsonian medications, also referred to as anticholinergics, are used to reduce the extrapyramidal side effects or tardive side effects of antipsychotic medications. Antiparkinsonian medications with a central anticholinergic action act to reduce the symptoms associated with parkinsonism, acute dystonia and akathisia (which together make up the tardive symptoms experienced by some who take antipsychotic medications). They inhibit the action of acetylcholine and are presumed to decrease cholinergic influence in the basal ganglia and thereby help balance the effects of antipsychotic medication reduction of dopaminergic influence (Psychotropic Expert Group 2013). See Table 25.5 for examples of antiparkinsonian medications, action and side effects.

However, antiparkinsonians are not routinely administered, as many patients taking antipsychotic medication do not experience extrapyramidal effects. The antiparkinsonian medications also have their own set of unwanted effects and there is considerable intentional misuse of these medications for euphoric and sometimes hallucinogenic effects.

Contraindications/Precautions

Typical antipsychotics. Caution should be taken in administering these medications to older people and to those who are medically ill or diagnosed with diabetes. Safety in pregnancy and lactation is not clear. They are contraindicated in people with a known sensitivity to one of the phenothiazines as a cross-sensitivity is possible. People taking typical antipsychotics should avoid extremes of temperature.

Atypical antipsychotics: clozapine. People taking clozapine must be made aware of the potential risk of agranulocytosis and be monitored regularly. Because of the medication's link to agranulocytosis it is restricted to those who have not responded to at least two other antipsychotics. Clozapine can be prescribed through the Clozaril Patient Monitoring System programme only. The patient's blood should be monitored weekly for 18 weeks and monthly thereafter. An immediate differential blood count must be ordered if the patient reports flu-like symptoms. If during treatment an infection occurs and/or the white blood cell (WBC) count drops below 3500/mm^3, or drops by a substantial amount from baseline, a repeat WBC and differential count should be completed. If the results confirm a WBC count below 3500/mm^3 and/or reveal an absolute neutrophil count (ANC) of between 2000 and 1500/mm^3, the WBC and ANC must be checked at least twice weekly. If the WBC count falls below 3000/mm^3 and/or the ANC count drops below 1500/mm^3, clozapine must be withdrawn at once and the patient closely monitored. Care should be taken when using these medications with older people.

Interactions

Typical antipsychotics. Concurrent use with antidepressants, antihistamines and antiparkinsonian agents may result in additional anticholinergic effects. Antacids and antidiarrhoeals may disrupt absorption of the antipsychotic. Alcohol may cause additional CNS depression.

Atypical antipsychotics. Medications known to have substantial potential to depress bone marrow function should be avoided concurrently with clozapine. Atypical antipsychotics may enhance the effect of alcohol and other CNS depressants.

Patient Education

Typical antipsychotics. The patient needs education about the medication side effects and help with maintaining adherence. People taking typical antipsychotics should be careful in the sun and in extremes of temperature.

Atypical antipsychotics. Advice about having regular blood tests when taking clozapine should be provided. Patients should also be told the importance of seeing a doctor

TABLE 25.5 Antiparkinsonians: Action and Side Effects

Name	Action	General side effects (dose related)
Procyclidine hydrochloride	Procyclidine exerts its antiparkinsonian action by reducing the effects of the relative central cholinergic excess that occurs as a result of dopamine deficiency.	Common or very common: Constipation; dry mouth; urinary retention; vision blurred Uncommon: Anxiety; cognitive impairment; confusion; dizziness; gingivitis; hallucination; memory loss; nausea; rash; vomiting Rare or very rare: Psychotic disorder
Orphenadrine	Anticholinergic action	Delirium in older people

immediately for any flu-like symptoms while taking clozapine. Information on possible side effects and medication interactions related to atypical antipsychotic medications should be provided.

While constipation is often considered as a minor medication side effect, it is a potentially serious side effect of clozapine. In fact, there have been a number of deaths associated with constipation resulting from clozapine. Other serious outcomes include paralytic ileus, bowel obstruction and toxic megacolon (Medsafe 2007). It is essential for patients to be warned of the potential for constipation, be educated about the need to monitor bowel habits and use interventions to manage constipation (for example, drinking 6–8 glasses of water per day). (See Box 25.7 for more interventions.)

Serotonin Syndrome

Serotonin is a chemical involved in communication between nerve cells in the brain. Too little serotonin is believed to be involved in the development of depression, while too much can cause excess cell activity leading to a potentially deadly expression of symptoms known as serotonin syndrome. Serotonin syndrome may occur within hours of taking a new medication. Medications that affect any step in the serotonin metabolism or regulation pathways can provoke the syndrome. Antidepressants, especially SSRIs, are the most commonly implicated. Symptoms of serotonin syndrome include confusion, agitation, dilated pupils, headache, nausea and/or vomiting, rapid heart rate, tremor, shivering, loss of muscle coordination and heavy sweating. Prompt treatment and discontinuation of the offending medications is vital. Most situations are self-limiting if the medication is ceased quickly; however, supportive care is required until the crisis is over.

Cognitive Enhancers

Cognitive enhancers improve memory, boost energy and alertness levels and increase concentration. These medications have been studied extensively since 2010 in an attempt to improve cognitive function across a number of clinical conditions. Developmental conditions such as attention deficit hyperactivity disorder (ADHD) are treated with methylphenidate and atomoxetine (Hussain & Mehta 2011). Side effects include high body temperature; increased activity; dry mouth; euphoria; decreased fatigue, drowsiness and appetite; nausea and headaches; and increased blood pressure and respirations. Neurodegenerative disorders such as Alzheimer disease and Parkinson disease are commonly treated with acetylcholinesterase inhibitors (AChEIs) and memantine as standard practice. However, it is hard to determine whether these actually improve memory or alertness (Hussain & Mehta 2011). Side effects include nausea and other gastrointestinal upsets, and impairment of verbal and visual memory (Hussain & Mehta 2011).

BOX 25.7 Managing Constipation Side Effects Caused by Psychotropic Medications

Assess for:
- regular bowel movements
- current diet, exercise
- other medications

Advise to:
- drink at least 6–8 glasses of water per day
- increase fibre in diet
- increase exercise
- use available pharmacological products as needed

PRO RE NATA (PRN OR AS-NEEDED) ANTIPSYCHOTIC MEDICATION ADMINISTRATION

The need to rapidly reduce agitation, distress or aggression often results in the prescription and administration of a prn (or as-needed) antipsychotic medication in inpatient mental health facilities. Antipsychotics and benzodiazepines are the main classes of medications used in this way. Approximately three-quarters of inpatients receive prn medication during the course of their admission and at least half of these receive at least one dose. These medications are prescribed orally or by intramuscular injection by a doctor, but are usually administered on the initiative of the nurse (Usher et al. 2009b). Once a prn regimen is instigated, it is usually administered about 10 times per person. Generally, most prn medications are given in the first few days after admission and are most frequently administered during the evening shift, from 6 pm onwards, and at weekends (Usher et al. 2009a). It appears that peaks in prn administration coincide with regular medication and meal times.

Reasons given for administering prn medications include agitation, threatening behaviour, irritability, abusiveness, insomnia, disruptiveness, assault and request by the patient. Environmental influences have also been suggested. The study by Usher et al. (2007) proposed that the physical and psychological environment in which patients were cared for had an effect on the individual's sense of security and adversely affected their mental health, causing anxiety, agitation and frustration and ultimately aggression, which in turn affected the need to resort to prn medications.

When nurses give prn medications they are often required to decide what to give from a range of medications, as well as the amount to give and when to administer (Usher et al. 2009b; Usher et al. 2010). This allows nurses to administer psychotropic medications rapidly in acute situations or at the request of the patient. Unfortunately, while this is an area of relative autonomy for nurses, it is also an area of practice that has been criticised, with concerns raised about over-reliance on psychotropic medications, particularly prn medications. Mullen and Drinkwater (2011) claim that mental health facilities should offer a range of therapeutic options and ensure that prn medications are used sparingly and their use is monitored regularly.

The medications most often prescribed for prn administration are the typical antipsychotics, particularly medications like haloperidol. There is evidence to suggest that the benzodiazepines are just as effective as the typical antipsychotics in managing acute agitation and disturbed behaviour and should therefore be the medication of choice. However, examination of current practice indicates that this is not happening and that the typical antipsychotics are being used predominantly for prn management of psychotic disturbance (Geffen et al. 2002; Usher 2001). One study found that higher levels of prn psychotropic medications are associated with unstable staffing profiles, particularly the use of less-experienced staff, high staff turnover, the deployment of nonregular staff to the ward and staff unfamiliar with the ward. There was also evidence that cultural background influenced the administration of prescribed prn medications (Usher et al. 2009a; Usher et al. 2010).

BOX 25.8 Interventions to Help With Adherence to Medication

- Get to know the patient well.
- Help the patient to develop an understanding of why the medications have been prescribed.
- Spend time talking about medications and the decisions related to adherence.
- Ask about the side effects being experienced and offer strategies to manage side effects where possible.
- Help the patient to discuss issues related to their medications with their doctor or nurse.
- Offer dispensers to assist with organising medications.
- Provide education sessions for family or significant others.

ADHERENCE TO MEDICATIONS

Effective treatment for people with schizophrenia requires a commitment to taking medications on a regular basis. Adherence to a prescribed antipsychotic medication regimen is often an ongoing problem for patients with schizophrenia. In the past, this issue has been referred to in the literature as noncompliance. However, the term 'compliance' implies a power differential between the patient and the healthcare provider, as well as passive rather than active participation by the patient in the management of their mental health, so the accepted term is now 'adherence'.

Nonadherence, when the patient does not take their medications as prescribed, is often the cause of relapse and readmission to hospital. The issue of medication adherence is complex and multifaceted and rarely includes the voice of the patient (Happell et al. 2004). When a patient does not take their medication as prescribed, their symptoms may not improve at the rate expected. This can lead to assumptions by health professionals that the medication is not effective. In the long run, this can cause unnecessary treatment changes. However, taking these medications as prescribed can facilitate functional recovery and help prevent illness-related complications.

Causes of nonadherence are related to issues such as: medication side effects (the different side effects of the typical and atypical antipsychotic medications impact adherence differently), whereby the antipsychotic medication may have an adverse impact on the person's quality of life and may even cause more distress than the symptoms of the illness (Usher et al. 2013); anosognosia, or lack of insight into the illness and the relationship between the illness and the need to take medications; and personal preference. Against advice, people sometimes stop taking their medications and, because they do not relapse immediately, fail to see the connection between the medications and their health.

To help overcome lack of adherence with antipsychotic medications, a number of strategies have been explored (see Box 25.8). Evidence suggests that an active relationship between the nurse and the patient is essential for improving adherence (Brown & Gray 2015). Other helpful strategies to aid adherence include education about the medications and their side effects, providing medication dispensers (Clyne et al. 2011), frequent follow up and support (Brown & Gray 2015), and motivational interviewing (Kemp et al. 1996). It appears that no strategy is sufficient on its own, and a mixed approach to adherence may in fact be best. A recent study sought to explore the views of mental health staff in regard to adherence. The authors report a lack of clarity about who is responsible for adherence and a focus on personal belief rather than evidence when considering adherence strategies (Brown & Gray 2015).

Discontinuation Syndrome

Discontinuation syndrome can result from switching between or rapid withdrawal of one of the antidepressant or antipsychotic medications. Common symptoms of withdrawal include: dizziness, paraesthesia, numbness, electric-shock-like sensations, lethargy, headache, tremor, sweating, anorexia, insomnia, nightmares, nausea, vomiting, diarrhoea, rhinorrhoea, irritability, anxiety, restlessness, agitation and low mood (Read 2009), as well as hyperthermia related to clozapine withdrawal (Cerovecki et al. 2013). Rapid-onset psychosis (also called hypersensitivity psychosis) occurs in some cases of discontinuation. As well as relapse of illness, sudden withdrawal of antipsychotic medications has been linked to rare but potentially life-threatening events including NMS (Kurien et al. 2013) and withdrawal catatonia (Thanasan 2010; Wadekar & Syed 2010). Box 25.9 overviews a case of discontinuation leading to NMS and demonstrates the importance for mental health nurses to be educated and aware of the physical conditions that can occur as a result of withdrawal of psychotropic medications.

Exactly why discontinuation syndrome occurs is unclear (Salomon & Hamilton 2014), but it is thought to be linked to cholinergic and/or dopaminergic blockade and subsequent rebound (Cerovecki et al. 2013). In order to avoid discontinuation syndrome, mental health nurses have an important role to play in educating and monitoring patients (Salomon & Hamilton 2014). The important principle of education is gradual withdrawal or switching of medications. See Box 25.10 for further ways to minimise the occurrence of discontinuation syndrome.

BOX 25.9 Discontinuation Leading to NMS

A man in his 40s diagnosed with paranoid schizophrenia attended the emergency department. He reported recently discontinuing antipsychotic and antidepressant medication he had been taking for 8 years (clozapine 225 mg daily and venlafaxine XL 225 mg daily). On presentation he was perplexed, sweaty and shaking, and told the nurse he was hearing 'voices'. Assessment revealed WBC count 20,600/mL (20,600 mm^3) and CPK 17,361U, temperature 37.7°C, pulse 80–122 beats per minute and respirations 18–40 breaths per minute. He was diagnosed with NMS as a result of cholinergic rebound from clozapine and venlafaxine. He was transferred to the mental health unit and treatment included regular oral diazepam 20 mg and lorazepam 4 mg daily as needed. His mental and physical state improved gradually over the following 2 weeks. He was then recommenced gradually on clozapine and venlafaxine and his mental state improved.

CPK, creatine phosphokinase; *NMS*, neuroleptic malignant syndrome; *WBC*, white blood cell.

(*Source:* Adapted from Kurien, R., Vattakatuchery, J.J., 2013. Psychotropic discontinuation leading to an NMS-like condition. Progress in Neurology and Psychiatry. 17(5), 11–12.)

BOX 25.10 How to Avoid and Manage Discontinuation Syndrome

- Switch between or withdraw from medications slowly—taper doses.
- Plan withdrawal and monitor closely.
- Prescribe hypnotics for insomnia.
- Prescribe antianxiety agents for other symptoms.

(*Source*: Cerovecki, A., Musil, R., Klimke, A., et al., 2013. Withdrawal symptoms and rebound syndromes associated with switching and discontinuing atypical antipsychotics: theoretical background and practical recommendations. CNS Drugs, 27, 545–72.)

Patient Education

While antipsychotic medications may be associated with favourable clinical outcomes for people experiencing a mental illness, patients do not always take medications as directed. Medication adherence is associated with lower use of acute care services and greater engagement with community services (Ascher-Svanum et al. 2009). However, medication adherence has been identified as a major issue for patients. A qualitative study undertaken by Happell et al. (2004) found that patients reported a general lack of understanding about the reasons for the prescription of antipsychotic medications and their side effects. Education about the need to take medications as prescribed has been identified as a key role for nurses. However, nurses report feeling inadequately prepared to educate others about psychotropic medications and many express concern about their own knowledge deficit in regard to these medications (Brown et al. 2007). While education about medication has been proposed as an important strategy for improving adherence, education alone is not always effective. Education programmes designed for improving adherence with psychotropic medications are more effective when combined with behavioural aspects of taking medication or motivational approaches, family therapy, psychological therapy or counselling.

See Case Studies 25.1 and 25.2 for an example of nonadherence and nursing responses.

CASE STUDY 25.1

Nonadherence to Psychotropic Medications (Part A)

Tony was first diagnosed with paranoid schizophrenia 5 years ago. His symptoms were exacerbated by poor adherence to prescribed medications and 'self-medication' with cannabis. Despite it being objectively clear that cannabis use made him more paranoid, Tony felt that it helped him relax and was dismissive of education about harm minimisation or abstaining.

The main hurdle to adherence with prescribed medication for Tony was denial. Tony did not accept his diagnosis; consequently, he did not accept his treatment. If we accept that a diagnosis of schizophrenia would provoke a sense of loss (e.g. normalcy, altered levels of independence, reevaluated life goals, decreased acceptance), we may be able to understand the denial as a component of grief. Tony certainly displayed other classic stages of grief, most notably anger (at his treating psychiatrist) and bargaining (with his community case manager re postponing or cancelling administration of depot medications).

Other contributing factors to Tony's nonadherence were the illness itself—paranoia is a barrier to building trust and rapport with clinicians; lack of education/understanding about the illness and its treatment; and the side effects of the prescribed medications.

CASE STUDY 25.2

Nonadherence To Psychotropic Medications (Part B)

A management plan was developed to address the factors contributing to Tony's nonadherence. Tony's outpatient care was assigned to a clinical nurse in the role of case manager. This nurse administered and monitored prescribed medications and worked to build a therapeutic alliance with Tony. When Tony was an inpatient, as occurred frequently during the first 3 years of diagnosis, he was assigned a primary nurse on the mental health unit, who collaborated with the case manager to provide continuity of care and another avenue for Tony to develop rapport.

Over time, Tony began to engage with his two primary carers, which provided an opportunity for education about his diagnosis and treatment options. In time, Tony became more accepting of the treating team as a whole, and would discuss medication issues freely with his treating psychiatrist.

As Tony's acceptance improved, medication options were no longer restricted to depot injections, and oral medications were trialled. Tony was very sensitive to typical antipsychotics and developed extrapyramidal side effects at subtherapeutic doses. Trials of other atypical antipsychotic medications also had problems—poor symptom control and marked weight gain. Twelve months ago a trial of clozapine commenced. It took 4 months to stabilise the dose at 450 mg nocte (at

CASE STUDY 25.2 Nonadherence To Psychotropic Medications (Part B)—Cont'd

night). In doing so, Tony's mental state also stabilised. He developed considerable insight into his condition and treatment, and has developed a good degree of acceptance.

Nine months later, with encouragement from the treating team, Tony undertook a trial of abstinence from cannabis. Tony says he has used cannabis only twice since. This hasn't been objectively checked through urine samples, but his case manager has noted further improvement in symptom control and motivation to undertake activities of daily living and social interaction.

Tony has not required admission to the mental health unit for over 8 months now. If he remains stable until the new year, his case manager intends to assist Tony in seeking work.

The authors acknowledge this contribution from Paul McNamara, CNC, Consultation Liaison Team, Cairns Base Hospital, Australia.

CRITICAL THINKING CHALLENGE 25.1

1. Denial is a commonly used defence mechanism when a person is faced with issues they are not yet able to cope with on a conscious level. Discuss the concept of denial as a component of grief and loss in relation to the diagnosis of a chronic mental illness. How does the concept of denial differ from that of insight? In part A of the case study (Case Study 25.1), how could the nurse manage Tony's nonadherence while recognising the importance of denial as a coping mechanism?
2. Explore relevant strategies to address the other factors contributing to Tony's nonadherence, such as his paranoia, lack of education and understanding, and unwanted medication side effects.

CRITICAL THINKING CHALLENGE 25.2

1. In part B of the case study (Case Study 25.2), Tony was trialled on atypical antipsychotics. How does this group of medications differ from typical antipsychotics? Identify the benefits and disadvantages of each of these medication groups.
2. The incidence of extrapyramidal side effects varies according to the particular antipsychotic medication used. Identify the various extrapyramidal side effects and explore the most effective management for these.
3. Tony was trialled on clozapine. What are the benefits and disadvantages of using this particular antipsychotic medication? Why is it not necessarily the first medication of choice for patients with psychosis?
4. Cannabis is commonly used by patients with a mental illness. What are the reasons for this? What does the term 'self-medicating' mean? Explore the effect(s) of cannabis when a person has a psychosis.
5. Critically analyse the strategies in the management plan used for Tony's nonadherence. In your opinion, was the plan successful? If so (or not) explain the reason(s) for this.

DEPOT OR LONG-ACTING INTRAMUSCULAR INJECTABLE ANTIPSYCHOTICS

Depot or long-acting injectable antipsychotic preparations, introduced in the 1960s, are useful when there might be problems with adherence with oral medications, when the patient is unable to take oral medications, if intestinal absorption is questioned and where accidental overdose is a possibility. Importantly, this strategy offers a more consistent treatment option (Smith & Herber 2014). There are also occasions where patients express a preference for this form of treatment (Kane & Garcia-Ribera 2009). These long-acting, injectable forms of antipsychotic medications, produced mostly in decanoate esters dissolved in an oily base, are prescribed for up to 33% of people with schizophrenia and other mental health issues (Barnes et al. 2009). Mental health nurses are most commonly responsible for the administration of injectable antipsychotic medications; these may be delivered in both inpatient and community settings (Smith & Herber 2014). When administered by deep intramuscular (IM) injection, the medication is de-esterified to release the active medication, which slowly diffuses into the circulation. The injections are usually given every 2 to 4 weeks (Psychotropic Expert Group 2013) (see Table 25.6) and generally the release of medication must last at least 1 week to be considered a depot preparation. As depot injections involve large amounts of fluid, they should be injected into a large muscle using the z-track technique (McCuistion et al. 2014).

While this strategy is one way to manage adherence issues, it is important to remember that a well-targeted nurse–patient relationship can help promote medication adherence and that the patient has a right to be involved in choosing the route of administration of prescribed medications wherever possible. A recent study explored the ethical issues experienced by mental health nurses in relation to the administration of depot or long-acting antipsychotic medications (Smith & Herber 2014). The study revealed that mental health nurses were conflicted by their desire to do what they believed to be in the best interests of the patient, even if they thought this sometimes bordered on coercion, yet remaining aware of the need to protect the therapeutic relationship. Unfortunately, a number of studies have indicated that community nurses

TABLE 25.6 Depot Antipsychotic Medications

Name	Route	Typical Maintenance Dosage
Zuclopenthixol decanoate	IM	200–400 mg every 2–4 weeks
Fluphenazine decanoate	IM	12.5–75 mg every 4 weeks
Flupenthixol decanoate	IM	20–80 mg every 2–4 weeks
Risperdal consta	IM	25–50 mg every 2 weeks
Olanzapine pamoate	IM	150–300 mg every 2–4 weeks

IM, Intramuscular.

report spending very little time with patients at the time of administration of depot injections (Patel et al. 2005).

PSYCHOTROPIC MEDICATION USE IN SPECIAL POPULATIONS

Pregnant and Breastfeeding Women

The management of women who are pregnant or breastfeeding poses a significant challenge for the mental health nurse. The prescription and administration of psychotropic medications, if required during pregnancy and breastfeeding, presents many risks to the unborn fetus or the newborn child. Antipsychotic medications, especially the atypical antipsychotics, commonly prescribed for women who experience psychoses during pregnancy or in the immediate postpartum period, have not been proved safe in pregnancy, and their use in pregnancy is not based on evidence from randomised clinical trials (Usher et al. 2009b). However, the consequences of untreated psychiatric disorders during pregnancy must be weighed against the risk of prenatal exposure to medications, as antenatal psychological distress is known to be linked to premature labour, low birth weight, smaller head circumference and inferior functional assessments in the newborn (Viguera & Cohen 1998).

The evidence of the teratogenic effects of psychotropic medications is mixed, and their use during pregnancy can expose the fetus to an increased risk of congenital malformation. Medications such as lithium, valproate and carbamazepine are known to have teratogenic effects in early pregnancy, as well as probable adverse effects on neonates late in pregnancy (Baldessarini & Tarazi 2001; Pinelli et al. 2002). Most antidepressants appear to be safe during pregnancy. However, as antidepressants and lithium are excreted in breast milk, at least in small quantities, their safety for newborns is not established (Baldessarini & Tarazi 2001). Usher et al. (2005) proposed the following guidelines for the use of psychotropic medications by women who are pregnant or breastfeeding:

- Antipsychotics, including depot injections, should be avoided in the first trimester.
- Women using atypicals should change to typical antipsychotics as soon as pregnancy is diagnosed.
- Pregnant and breastfeeding women should be prescribed the lowest possible dose.
- Depot injections should be avoided in breastfeeding women.
- Only infants born at full term should be exposed to the potential to ingest medication via breast milk.

Children and Adolescents

Although psychotropic medications have been used with children and adolescents for several decades, the use of these medications with this group should be monitored carefully. Second-generation medications are used to treat a variety of conditions in children and adolescents. While these and other psychotropic medications are used to manage numerous conditions such as autism, Asperger syndrome, Tourette syndrome and tic disorders, nonpharmacological options are the preferred treatment. However, if pharmacological agents are used, the atypical antipsychotics are usually chosen because they have less serious side effects in children and adolescents (Usher et al. 2009b). Antidepressants should be prescribed only with extreme caution in this group, as children are particularly vulnerable to the cardiotoxic and seizure-inducing effects of high doses of tricyclic compounds. Deaths have been reported in children after accidental or deliberate overdosage with as little as a few hundred milligrams of a tricyclic medication. Therefore, nurses must be particularly vigilant if working with children who are prescribed psychotropic medications.

Older People

Psychotropic medications are prescribed for older people for conditions such as mood and anxiety disorders, bipolar affective disorder, depression and dementia. Psychotropic medications have a role in managing these conditions (Usher et al. 2009b). However, particular care must be taken when psychotropic medications are considered for use with older patients. It is generally considered that older people will experience more adverse effects from psychotropic medication use, especially people over the age of 70, due to slower medication metabolism and excretion. For example, benzodiazepines are more likely to cause dizziness, which can lead to falls and serious injury. Antidepressants in older people can be problematic and are more likely to cause dizziness, postural hypotension, constipation, delayed micturition, oedema and tremor (Usher et al. 2009b). It is important for mental health nurses to be aware of the special problems these medications may pose when used with older patients and to be vigilant in supervising and monitoring side effects. Polypharmacy may have dire consequences for this group and should be avoided wherever possible. Older people are known to take more medications than younger people and often take more than one medication.

Psychotropic medication use is common in people with dementia; however, psychotropic medications have actually been reported as being of little use in managing the behavioural and psychological symptoms related to dementia (Sink et al. 2005). Despite this evidence, a recent study of people with dementia living in specialised care units in Sweden found that antipsychotic medication use was common in this population (Gustafsson et al. 2013), which is in keeping with current international trends (Lövheim et al. 2006). However, a study of patterns of psychotropic medication use in a number of Australian nursing homes between 1993 and 2009 reported that rates of hypnotic, anxiolytic and antidepressant medication use are low compared to other countries (Snowdon et al. 2011).

CONCLUSION

This chapter has presented an overview of the issues related to psychopharmacology, including the use of prn psychotropic medications, adherence with medications as prescribed and their use with special populations. To be effective practitioners, mental health nurses need to be equipped with knowledge and understanding of the distinct medication indications, interactions, side effects and precautions related to the four major psychotropic medication groups (antianxiety, antidepressant, mood stabilising and antipsychotic). The skilled mental health nurse needs to have a working knowledge of psychopharmacology, as well as related issues, because the administration of these medications is a common but important nursing intervention. The information presented here will help to prepare the mental health nurse to make well-informed treatment decisions and engage in successful patient assessment and education. It will also help the nurse to detect and manage side effects from psychotropic medications, many of which can be harmful or even life threatening.

EXERCISES FOR CLASS ENGAGEMENT

1. In a small group discuss the legal and ethical issues that a mental health nurse needs to consider when administering psychotropic medications. In particular, consider the issues related to the administration of depot injections.
2. In small groups, outline what you believe are the important issues related to medication adherence. How might your beliefs differ from those of patients? Discuss your findings with the larger group.
3. In small groups, debate and respond to the following questions:
   - Discuss how you would manage a situation where you were of the opinion that a patient was being prescribed and administered a toxic level of a medication.
   - Describe how polypharmacy can be a problem for people taking antipsychotic medications and for members of vulnerable groups, such as older people.
   - Describe the signs of a tricyclic overdose and list those who might be at high risk of such an outcome.
   - Anticonvulsant medications are used in the management of people with bipolar disorder. Describe the action of these medications and list their potential side effects.
   - Lithium is commonly used as a mood-stabilising medication. Outline why it is important to obtain regular blood tests for people taking this medication, and outline the therapeutic range and signs of lithium toxicity.
   - Discuss the physical issues of importance when working with patients taking psychotropic medications.

REFERENCES

Allison, D.B., Mentore, J.L., Heo, M., Chandler, L.P., Cappelleri, J.C., Infante, M.C., Weiden, P.J., 1999. Antipsychotic-induced weight gain: a comprehensive research synthesis. American Journal of Psychiatry 156 (11), 1686–1696.

Ascher-Svanum, H., Zhu, B., Faries, D.E., Furiak, N.M., Montgomery, W., 2009. Medication adherence levels and differential use of mental health services in the treatment of schizophrenia. BMC Research Notes 2, 6.

Baldessarini, R.J., Tarazi, F., 2001. Drugs and the treatment of psychiatric disorders: psychosis and mania. In: Hardman, J.G., Limbard, L.E., Gilman, A.G. (Eds.), Goodman and Gilman's The Pharmacological Basis of Therapeutics, tenth ed. McGraw-Hill, New York, pp. 485–543.

Barnes, T.R.E., Shingleton-Smith, A., Paton, C., 2009. Antipsychotic long-acting injections: prescribing practice in the UK. The British Journal of Psychiatry 195 (52), S37–S42. https://doi.org/10.1192/bjp.195.52.s37.

Brown, E., Gray, R., 2015. Tackling medication non-adherence in severe mental illness: where are we going wrong? Journal of Psychiatric and Mental Health Nursing 22, 192–198.

Brown, I., Stride, C., Psarou, A., et al., 2007. Management of obesity in primary care: nurses' practices, beliefs and attitudes. Journal of Advanced Nursing 59, 329–341.

Cerovecki, A., Musil, R., Klimke, A., Seemüller, F., Haen, E., Schennach, R., Kühn, K.-U., Volz, H.-P., Riedel, M., 2013. Withdrawal symptoms and rebound syndromes associated with switching and discontinuing atypical antipsychotics: theoretical background and practical recommendations. CNS Drugs 27, 545–572.

Clyne, W., Mshelia, C., Hall, S., et al., 2011. Management of patient adherence to medications: protocol for an online survey of doctors, pharmacists and nurses in Europe. BMJ Open 1, 1.

Edwards, K.-L., Rasmussen, B., Munro, I., 2010. Nursing care of clients treated with atypical antipsychotics who have a risk of developing metabolic instability and/or type 2 diabetes. Archives of Psychiatric Nursing 24 (1), 46–53.

Geffen, J., Sorensen, L., Stokes, J., et al., 2002. Pro re nata medication for psychoses: an audit of practice in two metropolitan hospitals. Australian and New Zealand Journal of Psychiatry 36 (5), 649–656.

Gustafsson, M., Karlsson, S., Lövheim, H., 2013. Inappropriate long-term use of antipsychotic drugs is common among people with dementia living in specialized care units. BMCV Pharmacology and Toxicology 14 (10). Available at: www.biomedcentral.com/2050-6511/14/10. Accessed: 20 May 2015.

Happell, B., Manias, E., Roper, C., 2004. Wanting to be heard: mental health consumers' experiences of information about medication. International Journal of Mental Health Nursing 13, 242–248.

Healy, D., 2008. Psychiatric Drugs Explained, 5th ed. Churchill Livingstone Elsevier, USA.

Howland, R.H., 2007. Medication adherence. Journal of Psychosocial Nursing 45 (9), 15–18.

Hubbard, R.E., Peel, N.M., Scott, I.A., Martin, J.H., Smith, A., Pillans, P.I., Poudel, A., Gray, L.C., 2015. Polypharmacy among inpatients aged 70 years or older in Australia. Medical Journal of Australia 202 (7), 373–378.

Hurley, S.C., 2002. Lamotrigine update and its use in mood disorders. Annals of Pharmacotherapy 36 (5), 860–873.

Hussain, M., Mehta, M.A., 2011. Cognitive enhancement by drugs in health and disease. Trends in Cognitive Science 15 (1), 28–36.

Hyde, N., Dodd, S., Venugopal, K., Purdie, C., Berk, M., O'Neil, A., 2015. Prevalence of cardiovascular and metabolic events in patients prescribed clozapine: a retrospective observational, clinical cohort study. Current Drug Safety 10 (2), 125–131.

John, A.P., Koloth, R., Dragovic, M., Lim, S.C.B., 2009. Prevalence of metabolic syndrome among Australians with severe mental illness. Medical Journal of Australia 190 (4), 176–179.

Kane, J.M., Garcia-Ribera, C., 2009. Clinical guideline recommendations for antipsychotic long-acting injections. British Journal of Psychiatry 195 (52), S63–S67.

Kemp, R., David, A., Hayward, P., 1996. Compliance therapy: an intervention targeting insight and treatment adherence in psychotic patients. Behavioural and Cognitive Psychotherapy 24 (4), 331–335.

Kurien, R., Vattakatuchery, J.J., 2013. Psychotropic discontinuation leading to an NMS-like condition. Progress in Neurology and Psychiatry 17 (5), 11–12.

Lövheim, H., Sandman, P.O., Kallin, K., Karlsson, S., Gustafson, Y., 2006. Relationship between antipsychotic drug use and behavioural and psychological symptoms of dementia in old people with cognitive impairment living in geriatric care. International Psychogeriatrics 18, 713–726.
McCann, M., Clark, E., 2004. Embodiment of severe and enduring mental illness: finding meaning in schizophrenia. Issues in Mental Health Nursing 25, 783–798.
McCuistion, L.E., Kee, J.L., Hayes, E.R. (Eds.), 2014. Pharmacology: a Patient-Centered Nursing Process Approach, eighth ed. Elsevier Health Sciences, St Louis, MO.
McDaid, T.M., Smyth, S., 2015. Metabolic abnormalities among people diagnosed with schizophrenia: a literature review and implications for mental health nurses. Journal of Psychiatric and Mental Health Nursing 22, 157–170.
Medsafe, 2007. Clozapine: fatal 'constipation' more common than fatal agranulocytosis. Ministry of Health, Wellington. Available at: www.medsafe.govt.nz/profs/puarticles/clozgi.htm. Accessed: 15 June 2015.
Morrison, P., Gaskill, D., Meehan, T., et al., 2000. The use of the Liverpool University Neuroleptic Side Effect Rating Scale (LUNSERS) in clinical practice. Australian and New Zealand Journal of Mental Health Nursing 9 (4), 166–176.
Morrison, P., Meehan, T., Stomski, J., 2014. Living with antipsychotic medication side effects: the experience of Australian mental health consumers. International Journal of Mental Health Nursing 24, 253–261.
Mullen, A., Drinkwater, V., 2011. Pro re nata use in a psychiatric intensive care unit. International Journal of Mental Health Nursing 20, 409–417.
Murashita, M., Kusumi, I., Hosoda, H., Kangawa, K., Koyama, T., 2007. Acute administration of clozapine concurrently increases blood glucose and circulating plasma ghrelin levels in rats. Psychoneuroendocrinology 32 (7), 777–784.
Nassir Ghaemi, S., Manwani, S.G., Katzow, J.J., et al., 2001. Topiramate treatment of bipolar spectrum disorders: a retrospective chart review. Annals of Clinical Psychiatry 13 (4), 185–189.
Park, T., Usher, K., Foster, K., 2011. Description of a healthy lifestyle intervention for people with schizophrenia taking second generation antipsychotics. International Journal of Mental Health Nursing 20, 428–437.
Patel, M.X., DeZoysa, N., Baker, D., et al., 2005. Antipsychotic depot medication and attitudes of community psychiatric nurses. Journal of Psychiatric and Mental Health Nursing 12, 237–244.
Piat, M., Sabetti, J., 2009. The importance of medication in consumer definitions of recovery from serious mental illness: a qualitative study. Issues in Mental Health Nursing 30, 482–490.
Pinelli, J.M., Symington, A.J., Cunningham, K.A., et al., 2002. Case report and review of the perinatal implications of maternal lithium use. American Journal of Obstetrics and Gynecology 187 (1), 245–249.
Psychotropic Expert Group, 2013. Therapeutic Guidelines: Psychotropic, Version 7. Therapeutic Guidelines Limited, Melbourne.
Read, J., 2009. Psychiatric Drugs: Key Issues and Service User Perspectives. Palgrave Macmillan, New York.
Remington, G., Agid, O., Foussias, G., Hahn, M., Rao, N., Sinyor, M., 2013. Clozapine's role in the treatment of first-episode schizophrenia. American Journal of Psychiatry 170 (2), 146–151.
Salomon, C., Hamilton, B., 2014. Antipsychotic discontinuation syndromes: a narrative review of the evidence and its integration into Australian mental health nursing textbooks. International Journal of Mental Health Nursing 23, 69–75.
Shupikai Rinomhota, A., Marshall, P., 2000. Biological aspects of mental health nursing. Churchill Livingstone, Edinburgh.
Sink, K.M., Holden, K.F., Yaffe, K., 2005. Pharmacological treatment of neuropsychiatric symptoms of dementia: a review of the evidence. Journal of the American Medical Association 293, 596–608.
Smith, J.P., Herber, O.R., 2014. Ethical issues experienced by mental health nurses in the administration of antipsychotic depot and long-acting intramuscular injections: a qualitative study. International Journal of Mental Health Nursing 24, 222–230.
Snowdon, J., Galanos, D., Vaswani, D., 2011. Patterns of psychotropic medication use in nursing homes: surveys in Sydney, allowing comparisons over time and between countries. International Psychogeriatrics 23 (9), 1520–1525.
Thanasan, S., 2010. Clozapine withdrawal catatonia or lethal catatonia in a schizoaffective patient with a family history of Parkinson's disease. African Journal of Psychiatry 13, 402–404.
Tirupati, S., Chua, L.E., 2007. Obesity and metabolic syndrome in a psychiatric rehabilitation service. Australian and New Zealand Journal of Psychiatry 42 (2), 606–610.
Tschoner, A., Engl, J., Laimer, M., Kaser, S., Rettenbacher, M., Fleischhacker, W.W., et al., 2007. Metabolic side effects of antipsychotic medication. International Journal of Clinical Practice 61 (8), 1356–1370.
Usher, K., 2001. Taking neuroleptic medications as the treatment for schizophrenia: a phenomenological study. Australian and New Zealand Journal of Mental Health Nursing 10 (3), 145–155.
Usher, K., Baker, J., Homes, C., 2010. Understanding clinical decision making for prn medication in mental health inpatient facilities. Journal of Psychiatric and Mental Health Nursing 17, 558–564.
Usher, K., Baker, J., Holmes, C., Stocks, B., 2009a. Clinical decision-making for 'as needed' medications in mental health care. Journal of Advanced Nursing 65 (5), 981–991.
Usher, K., Foster, K., Bullock, S., 2009b. Psychopharmacology for Health Professionals. Elsevier, Sydney.
Usher, K., Foster, K., McNamara, P., 2005. Antipsychotic drugs and pregnant or breastfeeding women: the issues for mental health nurses. Journal of Psychiatric and Mental Health Nursing 12 (6), 713–718.
Usher, K., Foster, K., Park, T., 2006. The metabolic syndrome and schizophrenia: the latest evidence and nursing guidelines for management. Journal of Psychiatric and Mental Health Nursing 13 (6), 730–734.
Usher, K., Holmes, C., Baker, J., et al., 2007. Enhancing The Understanding of Clinical Decision Making for Prn Medications Within Mental Health Facilities. Final report to the Queensland Nursing Council (QNC), Brisbane.
Usher, K., Park, T., Foster, K., 2013. The experience of weight gain as a result of taking second-generation antipsychotic medications: the mental health consumer perspective. Journal of Psychiatric and Mental Health Nursing 20, 801–806.
Viguera, A.C., Cohen, L.S., 1998. The course and management of bipolar disorder during pregnancy. Psychopharmacology Bulletin 34 (3), 339–353.
Wadekar, M., Syed, S., 2010. Clozapine withdrawal catatonia. Psychosomatics 51 (4), 355.

USEFUL WEBSITES

BNF, https://bnf.nice.org.uk/
LUNSERS tool, www.reach4resource.co.uk/node/104

GLOSSARY

A

acceptance and commitment therapy (ACT) Develops acceptance of unwanted private experiences that are out of the person's control, and fosters commitment and action towards living a valued life.

adjustment disorder A clinically significant emotional or behavioural response to a significant life change or stressor such as a relationship break-up, bereavement, divorce or illness.

advance directive A means by which patients can state their preferences for future healthcare.

advanced practice A level of nursing practice characterised by clinical expertise, application of research to practice, clinical leadership and postgraduate education.

affect The observable behaviours associated with changes in a person's *mood*, such as crying and looking dejected. Some terms for affect are blunted, flat, inappropriate, labile and restricted.

ageism The systematic stereotyping of and discrimination against people because of their age alone.

aggression Actions or behaviours ranging from verbal abuse, insults and nonverbal gestures to violent physical acts such as kicks or punches.

agitation (Also known as psychomotor agitation.) Excessive nonproductive, repetitious motor activity associated with a feeling of inner tension (pacing, hand-wringing, fidgeting).

agnosia A failure to recognise objects.

agoraphobia Anxiety about being in places or situations from which escape might be difficult (or embarrassing) or in which help might not be available.

agranulocytosis A blood disorder characterised by severe depletion of white blood cells, rendering the body almost defenceless against infection.

akathisia One of the side effects of antipsychotic medication; involves the person not being able to stay or remain still, being restless and suffering from leg aches.

Alzheimer disease A form of dementia that features memory impairment as well as one or more cognitive disturbances, including aphasia (impaired understanding of language in any form), apraxia (impaired motor activities), agnosia (failure to recognise objects) and disturbance in executive functioning.

ambivalence An individual's tendency to hold conflicting views and feelings such as love and hate, making decision making difficult.

amnesia An inability to remember events from a particular period. There are a number of different amnesias, including localised amnesia, selective amnesia, generalised amnesia and systematised amnesia.

anhedonia Loss of the feelings of pleasure previously associated with favoured activities.

anorexia nervosa A disorder characterised by a refusal to maintain minimal, normal body weight for age and height; an intense fear of gaining weight; disturbed perception of body shape and size.

anticholinergic Side effects of first-generation antipsychotic medication, including dry mouth, blurred vision, orthostatic hypotension, tachycardia, urinary retention and nasal congestion.

antidepressant medication Medication that elevates mood by enhancing the transmission of neurochemicals, particularly serotonin and noradrenaline, by blocking their reuptake at the synapse, inhibiting their metabolism and destroying and/or enhancing the activity of the receptors.

antiparkinsonian medication Medication used to treat the extrapyramidal side effects of antipsychotic medication, including dystonia and akathisia.

antipsychotic medication Also known as *neuroleptic medication*, these drugs were introduced in the 1950s and revolutionised the treatment of mental illness. First-generation antipsychotics are dopamine antagonists that reduce the 'positive' symptoms of schizophrenia. Second-generation antipsychotics reduce the 'positive' symptoms of schizophrenia and can also improve the 'negative' symptoms.

antisocial Exhibiting disregard for the rights of others and engaging in reckless, aggressive, deceitful and impulsive behaviour.

anxiety A common human experience that is a normal emotion felt in varying degrees by everyone; also a state in which individuals experience feelings of uneasiness, apprehension and activation of the autonomic nervous system in response to a vague, nonspecific threat.

anxiolytic medication Also known as anti-anxiety medication; medication used when anxiety becomes debilitating. Benzodiazepines are the drug of choice for short-term treatment of anxiety states.

apathy Indifference; lack of interest or feeling.

aphasia Impairment in the understanding or transmission of ideas by language in any form (writing, reading, speaking) due to impairment of the brain centres involved in language.

apraxia Impaired motor activities.

assertive outreach teams A model of community care in which clinicians, often nurses, actively follow-up on patients with high needs in order to maintain community living and prevent hospitalisation.

assertiveness A communication skill that enhances one's interpersonal effectiveness and allows one the choice of how to respond to others. The assertive person protects the rights of each party and achieves their own goals without hurting others. This results in self-confidence and the ability to express oneself appropriately in emotional and social situations.

asylum An institution intended to provide sanctuary and care for those with mental illness.

ataxia Partial or complete loss of voluntary muscular movement and coordination.

attachment The strong bond or connection one feels for particular people in one's life; usually associated with the primary bond between infant and mother, which can influence one's self-concept, relationships and life experiences.

autism An individual's tendency to retreat into an inner world, resulting in social isolation or withdrawal and inflexible, repetitive patterns of thinking and behaviour.

autonomy The right of each person to make their own decisions, provided these decisions do not violate another person's autonomy. For people to be able to make autonomous decisions, they must be free of the control of others.

avoidance behaviour Withdrawing or turning away from occupational and/or social activities because of fear of disapproval, rejection and ridicule.

B

behaviour therapy Therapy aimed at changing behaviour by changing the patterns of reinforcement that maintain behaviour. Behaviour therapy is usually highly structured with specific measurable goals, interventions to achieve goals and a timeline for goal achievement.

beneficence The deliberate bringing about of positive action or intervention. Ethical principle of beneficence: actions taken for the benefit of others.

bereavement Deprived by death of a friend or relative.

biomedical model A model based on the idea that normal behaviour occurs because of equilibrium within the body and that abnormal behaviour results from pathological bodily or brain function.

biopsychosocial model of assessment A comprehensive assessment of all aspects of information concerning the patient—biological, psychological, sociological, developmental, spiritual and cultural.

bipolar disorder A diagnosis outlined in the DSM-5 when a person has previously experienced at least one manic episode and a depressive episode.

blunted affect Observed mood is less astute and aware than would be expected.

body image assessment Assessment of components of body image, including body image distortion, body image avoidance and body image dissatisfaction.

body dysmorphia A disturbance of cognition and affect that leads to a negative evaluation of physical appearance.

body mass index (BMI) A mathematical formula, based on the height and weight of an individual, which is used to help determine the degree of starvation or obesity.

bulimia nervosa A disorder characterised by binge-eating behaviour—eating much larger amounts of food than would normally be eaten in one sitting, and inappropriate, compensatory weight-loss behaviours such as self-induced vomiting and purging.

bullying Unwanted and repeated aggressive verbal or physical behaviour towards a person, often considered less powerful, with the aim to control, harm and intimidate.

burnout A syndrome in which healthcare workers lose concern and feeling for patients under their care, becoming detached and distancing themselves from the patients; characterised by emotional exhaustion, depersonalisation and decreased personal accomplishment.

C

carer Someone who provides unpaid assistance for family members or friends with care needs. Carers are parents, children, partners, other relatives and friends who assist with a variety of personal care, healthcare, transport, household and other activities.

case management Assessing, planning, linking, monitoring and evaluating services with the patient, with caseloads shared among the multidisciplinary team.

catatonia A severe and debilitating condition with disorganisation of motor behaviour and inability to relate to external stimuli; can be a feature of mood disorder, psychotic disorder or schizophrenia.

challenging behaviour A term used to describe behaviour that disrupts relationships with others and complicates healthcare delivery—for example, aggression, manipulation and self-harm.

circumstantiality A disturbance in form of thought, in which speech is indirect and long-winded.

clang association A disturbance in form of thought, in which words are chosen for their sounds rather than their meanings; includes puns and rhymes.

classification of mental disorders Systems of categorisation that enable information to be identified concerning the patterns of behaviour, thoughts and emotions of patients. The most commonly used classification systems are the Diagnostic and Statistical Manual and the International Classification of Diseases.

clinical formulation The process of developing with the patient a summary of the various influences on the patient's current problems, and how the patient and clinician can work towards resolving those problems.

clinical supervision A positive process that involves reflection on clinical interactions and interventions between one clinician and another more experienced clinician for support, professional development, education and development of clinical practice skills.

code of ethics Guidelines for members of professional groups as to the nature of proper ethical conduct and their obligations to patients and to the public.

coexisting/comorbid disorder Having more than one disorder at the same time, most commonly a mental health disorder and a substance use disorder. Similar terms are *comorbidity* and *dual diagnosis*.

cognition Knowing or perceiving something; related to intellect, logic and reason, not emotions and feelings.

cognitive behavioural therapy (CBT) Therapy that aims to help people to develop more efficient coping mechanisms by equipping them with strategies that promote logical ways of thinking about and responding to everyday situations.

cognitive enhancers Drugs used in the treatment of cognitive impairment to improve memory, boost energy and alertness levels and increase concentration.

cognitive restructuring A collaborative nurse–patient intervention that aims to monitor and reduce distressing negative cognitions (thoughts), especially in people who are depressed.

community care Health services available from community mental health centres and emphasising the multidisciplinary team; includes services such as counselling, follow-up treatment, referrals and supported accommodation.

community treatment orders Provisions within Mental Health Acts that enable the involuntary treatment of people with mental illness while they live in the community.

comorbidity See *coexisting/comorbid disorder* and *dual diagnosis*.

compassion Sensitivity to suffering and a desire to alleviate distress; underpins concepts of acceptance, a non-judgemental attitude, awareness, being present and listening.

competence When a person can or should decide or be permitted to decide for themselves; beyond this point another or others will need to, or should, decide for the person.

competencies A specific framework that describes the expected skill base of all practitioners within a specific discipline; set by regulatory bodies and professional nursing organisations.

compulsions Repetitive behaviours (e.g. hand washing, checking) or mental acts (e.g. praying, counting), the goal of which is to prevent or reduce anxiety or distress, not to provide pleasure or gratification.

confabulation Filling in gaps in memory with imaginary experiences.

confidentiality A primary principle of the therapeutic relationship; involves maintaining confidential information about a patient within the treatment team.

containment Provision of a place of safety; the hospital can be seen as a refuge from self-destructiveness and an opportunity to reassure the patient and others that illness will not overwhelm them.

continuity of care A continuous relationship between a patient and an identified healthcare professional or agency who ensures that the patient's health needs over time are met.

coping The way one deals with change, conflict and demands in life, which can be influenced by factors such as one's feelings, thoughts, beliefs and values.

countertransference The response of the therapist to the patient. Having strong feelings for the patient, either negative or positive, might be a cue that one is experiencing countertransference.

court liaison nurse Employed in courts to advise judges, lawyers and the police on issues regarding the mental health, addiction status and needs of people presenting to court.

credentialing A core component of clinical/professional governance or self-regulation where members of a profession set standards for practice and establish a minimum requirement for entry, continuing professional development, endorsement and recognition.

crisis An event that creates a sense of one's life being out of control, feeling that one is vulnerable and that events are unpredictable; can involve a significant loss for the person involved but also an opportunity for growth.

crisis intervention Involves assessment, planning, intervention and resolution of a crisis.

cultural assessment A process of examining individuals, groups and communities regarding their cultural beliefs, values and practices as a means to determine needs and appropriate interventions.

cultural competence A model developed from transcultural nursing to describe the role of culture in nurse–patient dynamics and to attempt to understand these cultural dynamics.

cultural safety Goes beyond describing the practices of other ethnic groups to nurses learning about their own attitudes and values in their own culture, rather than just learning about the cultures of their patients.

culture A body of learned behaviours that is used to interpret individual experience and shape individual behaviour, emotion and social responses.

cyclothymia A condition characterised by mild depression alternating with mild manic symptoms.

D

defence mechanisms Unconscious processes whereby anxiety experienced by the individual's ego is reduced by behaviours such as denial, repression, projection and displacement.

deinstitutionalisation Closure of major psychiatric hospitals and expansion of community-based care for patients, including relocation of inpatient psychiatric beds into general hospitals.

delirium A syndrome that constitutes a characteristic pattern of signs and symptoms that reduce clarity of awareness and impair the patient's ability to focus, sustain or shift attention; tends to develop quickly and fluctuate during the course of the day.

delirium tremens (DTs) A withdrawal syndrome in which the patient presents with a number of complaints that may include agitation, disorientation, fever, paranoia, hallucinations, coarse tremors and seizures.

delusion A false belief, based on incorrect inference about external reality that is firmly sustained despite what almost everyone else believes and despite incontrovertible and obvious proof or evidence to the contrary. Types of delusion include bizarre, jealous, erotomanic, grandiose, control, reference, persecution, somatic, thought broadcasting and thought insertion.

dementia A progressive illness that involves progressive cognitive, emotional and behavioural impairments; presents as a gradual failure of brain function. It is not a normal part of life or ageing.

dependence (drugs or alcohol) Can be both physical and psychological. Physical dependence is the physical symptomatology of withdrawal as evidenced by sweating, perspiration and raised blood pressure. Psychological dependence is the withdrawal-driven craving for the substance when the person stops using the substance.

depersonalisation A sense of personal reality being lost or altered, of being estranged from oneself, as if in a dream, or that one's actions are mechanical or otherwise detached from the body or mind.

depot antipsychotic medication Long-acting, injectable forms of antipsychotic medication used when the patient is unable or unwilling to take oral medication, if intestinal absorption is questioned or when there might be a medication adherence or compliance problem.

depression A disorder characterised by lowered mood, with feelings of hopelessness and helplessness, lack of pleasure or interest, appetite disturbance, sleep disturbance and fatigue.

derailment A disturbance in form of thought, in which thoughts do not progress logically and ideas are unconnected, shifting between subjects; also known as loosening of association.

derealisation A phenomenon in which the person's sense of the object world is altered. The person may perceive objects to be bigger or smaller than they really are, or once-familiar objects may now seem strange.

detoxification The process by which an alcohol- or drug-dependent person recovers from intoxication in a supervised environment so that withdrawal symptoms are minimised.

developmental psychology The scientific study of how and why human beings develop over the course of their life.

developmental theories Theories that highlight the importance of the early months and years of one's life in laying a solid foundation for mental health and wellbeing in adulthood.

diagnosis A mental illness a patient is considered to be experiencing; the act of identifying a mental illness through a process of assessment.

dialectical behaviour therapy (DBT) Similar to *cognitive behavioural therapy* but actively incorporates social skills training, dealing with distress, and validation and acceptance of the person.

differential diagnosis The process of distinguishing one illness from other illnesses presenting with similar signs and symptoms by listing, in order of likelihood, the most likely diagnoses.

diminished capacity A mitigating defence used to establish the absence of malice by a defendant who committed a violent act. Not technically 'insanity', but a suspended mental state in which the defendant's thoughts and actions were dominated by passion and emotional stress, preventing them from acting rationally or being aware of the consequences of their actions. See also *competence*.

disability An individual's impairment in one or more areas of functioning.

discontinuation syndrome A withdrawal syndrome that can result from switching between or rapid withdrawal of one of the antidepressant or antipsychotic medications.

discrimination Unfavourable treatment based on prejudice, especially regarding race, colour, age or gender.

dissociation Being focussed on one's own internal thoughts and unaware of the external environment. For example, daydreaming is considered a mild form of dissociation.

distractibility A disturbance in form of thought attention, in which nearby various stimuli cause repeated changes in the topic of speech that interfere with ability to attend to activities or interactions.

distress An unpleasant subjective emotional state that causes significant impairment in functioning.

distress tolerance A patient's capacity to recognise and manage their own experiences of distress.

diversion Arrangements between mental health services and police so that patients on petty charges can be diverted from the criminal justice system to inpatient or community mental health services.

DSM-5 *Diagnostic and Statistical Manual of Mental Disorders*, 5th edition, published by the American Psychiatric Association. Sets out concise descriptions of each mental disorder organised by explicit diagnostic information about the diagnosis, risk factors and associated features of each disorder.

dual diagnosis Having more than one disorder at the same time, most commonly a mental health disorder and a substance use disorder. See also *coexisting/comorbid disorder*.

dual disability Having a comorbid intellectual or developmental disability.

duty of care The taking of reasonable care by a nurse to avoid acts or omissions that one can reasonably foresee would be likely to injure another.

dysthymia Chronic mild depression.

dystonic reaction One of the side effects of some antipsychotic medications. May include painful muscle spasms in the head, back and torso that can last minutes or hours.

E

early intervention Can be employed with people who are identified as at risk or already showing signs of emotional or behavioural problems; may also contribute to the prevention of some types of mental illness or disorder, or to reduced severity or duration of symptoms if a disorder does emerge.

eating disorders Complex and serious disorders that involve physical, psychological, social, family and individual factors characterised by serious disturbance of eating behaviours; includes anorexia nervosa, bulimia nervosa and binge eating disorder.

echolalia A disturbance in form of thought, in which other people's words or phrases are echoed, often in a 'mocking' tone; not the same as repetition of the person's own words *(perseveration)*.

echopraxia Repetition by imitation of the movements of another person. The actions are involuntary and semiautomatic.

egocentric Focussing on oneself to the degree that other people's needs are beyond one's awareness.

ego-dystonic When a patient's symptoms are experienced as distressing to the individual.

elation A feeling of exhilaration and intense pride and joy.

electroconvulsive therapy (ECT) The application of metal electrodes to the head, through which an electric current is delivered. ECT is an effective intervention in the treatment of severe depression, although it remains a controversial intervention.

emotional dysregulation Being easily overwhelmed by negative emotions and unable to regain a sense of emotional control. Often associated with maladaptive regulation strategies such as self-harm.

empathy Observing, listening, understanding and attending; 'being' with the person physically, cognitively and emotionally, understanding their story, thoughts, feelings, beliefs and emotions.

enabling environments (Also known as supportive environments.) Inherently helpful environments that in and of themselves enable people to move towards recovery.

engagement The process of establishing rapport with a patient through interactions based on acknowledging and developing a relationship based on trust.

ethical conduct Health professional behaviour that is consistent with ethical principles of *autonomy*, *beneficence*, *nonmaleficence* and *justice*.

ethics Morals in human conduct; rules of conduct appropriate to a profession or area of life.

ethnocentrism The belief that one's own cultural values constitute the human norm and that difference is deviant and wrong.

externalising problems Personal problems that are expressed as problematical behaviour, including antisocial or undercontrolled behaviour, delinquency or aggression.

extrapyramidal side effects Side effects of antipsychotic drugs on the extrapyramidal motor system; include dystonia, parkinsonism, akathisia and tardive dyskinesia.

F

family therapy An approach to treatment based on the idea that when a family member has a problem, it usually involves the whole family. Family therapists aim to effect change in the entire family system.

fear A response to a known threat; manifests in the same way as *anxiety*.

flight of ideas A disturbance in form of thought, in which the person's ideas are too rapid for them to express and so their speech is fragmented and incoherent.

forensic patient A person who has committed a crime while mentally ill and is remanded in custody in an approved mental health service, within a prison, remand centre or forensic psychiatric hospital.

form of thought The amount and rate of production of thought, continuity of ideas and language. Disturbances in form of thought include: *circumstantiality*, *clanging*, *derailment* (loosening of associations), *distractible speech*, *echolalia*, *flight of ideas*, *illogicality*, *incoherence*, *irrelevance*, *neologisms*, *perseveration*, *tangentiality*, *thought blocking*, *thought disorder* and *word approximations*.

fugue In a long-term dissociative state; the person is unable to remember the past and may also be confused about their identity, unable to remember their name or occupation.

G

generalised anxiety disorder (GAD) Excessive worry concerning events or activities occurring more days than not for a period of at least 6 months, and which the individual finds it difficult to control.

Geriatric Depression Scale (GDS) Assessment tool designed to assist in making a diagnosis of depression in older persons and referral for treatment and to provide a baseline assessment with which to measure the outcome of treatment.

Gillick competence The ability of young people to consent to medical treatment or seek medical consultation, as seen in their cognitive ability to make an informed judgement to give consent for treatment.

Glasgow Coma Scale (GCS) A standardised system for assessing the degree of impairment of consciousness and for predicting the duration and outcome of coma, primarily in patients with head injury.

grandiosity An inflated appraisal of one's worth, power, knowledge, importance or identity.

grief A natural process that can be experienced after loss; may be an emotional response of distress, pain and disorganisation.

group cohesion An important component in creating a climate of support and involvement in a group of people. Group cohesion is important in group therapy and in inpatient care settings.

group therapy The engagement of two or more people in therapy at the same time. Interactions with others in a group situation, especially people who come together with others who experience the same or similar difficulties, have been shown to have positive and beneficial effects.

H

hallucination A sensory perception that seems real but occurs without external stimulation. Types of hallucination include auditory, gustatory, olfactory, somatic, tactile and visual (see also *illusion*).

harm reduction The guiding principle used to identify a range of strategies that target the consequences of drug use rather than the drug itself.

hazardous substance use A repetitive pattern of use that poses a risk of harmful physical, psychological or social consequences.

Health of the Nation Outcome Scales (HoNOS) Instrument used to gather information concerning key areas of mental health and social functioning for service monitoring and outcome measurement.

histrionic Displaying theatrical, dramatic and exaggerated behaviour.

holism Healing of the whole person by recognising the importance of the interrelationships between biological, psychological, social and spiritual aspects of a person.

human rights Rights that are believed to belong to every individual. Human rights are protected by various domestic and international laws and conventions.

humours The humoural theory was based on the belief that the body contained within it four humours—blood, phlegm, yellow bile and black bile—and that disease developed when internal or external factors disturbed the balance of the humours and produced injurious effects such as mental illness.

hyperarousal A state of heightened psychological alertness and physiological arousal associated with anxiety and with posttraumatic stress disorder.

hypersomnia Excessive sleepiness; prolonged nocturnal sleep, difficulty in staying awake during the day and/or undesired daytime sleep episodes.

hypervigilance A state of heightened awareness in which the person constantly scans the environment for evidence of threats.

hypomania A form of elevated mood less severe than mania.

I

ICD-10-AM *International Statistical Classification of Diseases and Related Health Problems*, 10th revision, published by the World Health Organization; provides a comprehensive listing of clinical diagnoses, each with its own numerical code. A version of the ICD-11 was released in June 2018, to allow Member States to prepare for implementation, with a view to reporting using ICD-11 from 1st January 2022.

ideas of reference Belief that an insignificant or incidental object or event has special significance or meaning for that individual.

identity Part of one's self-concept; develops over time and contributes to one's overall sense of self.

illicit drugs Drugs that are classified as illegal.

illusion A misperception or misinterpretation of a real external stimulus, such as seeing a shadow on the wall as a person, or hearing rustling leaves as people speaking.

impulsivity A tendency to act in an unpremeditated fashion, suddenly and without reflection.

incidence The number of new cases of a condition, symptom, death or injury that develop during a specific time period, such as a year.

incoherence A disturbance in form of thought in which there is verbal rambling with no clear main idea.

incongruent affect A mismatch between a person's thoughts and their emotional expression.

individual psychotherapy One-on-one psychotherapy designed to effect change in the person's character; provides the patient with opportunities to examine the historical experiences that have shaped who they are and influenced their life decisions.

informed consent Consent to treatment that is (among other requirements) voluntary and specific and comes from a competent person.

insane Coming from the Latin word 'insana' meaning not of right mind; the equivalent Greek term is 'mania'.

insight The patient's ability to understand the reason for and the meaning of their behaviour, feelings and life events.

interpersonal therapy (IPT) Therapy that targets relationships as a key factor in the contribution and maintenance of psychological or emotional disorders.

intoxication A reversible state that occurs when a person's intake of a drug exceeds their tolerance and produces behavioural and/or physical changes.

involuntary admission and treatment Compulsory detention in an approved mental health facility for treatment that will alleviate the individual's symptoms of mental illness.

J

justice (ethical principle) The equal or fair treatment of all individuals.

L

la belle indifference 'Beautiful indifference', where the patient shows a marked indifference to or unconcern about their symptoms, even if the symptom is blindness or paralysis.

labile Having rapidly shifting or unstable emotions.

learned helplessness Both a behavioural state and a personality trait of a person who believes that their control over a situation has been lost. It can also relate to hopelessness and powerlessness—an inability to escape an intolerable situation, leading to the ultimate mode of adaptation: subjugation and acceptance.

learning disability A disability typified by major limitations in intellectual functioning and in conceptual, social and practical adaptive skills that originates before the age of 18.

least restrictive practice The option of least restriction for the individual (e.g. in a community-based environment rather than hospital), with consideration of the person's level of autonomy, their acceptance and cooperation and potential for harm to self and others.

limit setting Explaining to patients what behaviours are acceptable and what are unacceptable, and informing them of the consequences of breaking the rules; aims to offer the patient a degree of control over their behaviour by setting firm, fair and consistent limits or rules.

M

mad A middle-English, pre-twelfth-century word that means having lost reason and judgement.

magical thinking The erroneous belief that one's thoughts, words or actions will cause or prevent a specific outcome in some way that defies the laws of cause and effect.

major depressive disorder A condition involving seriously depressed mood and other symptoms defined by the DSM-5 that affect all aspects of a person's bodily system and interfere significantly with daily living activities.

malingering The intentional production of symptoms in order to avoid some specific duty or responsibility; the incentive to become sick is clearly identifiable.

mania A state of euphoria that results in extreme physical and mental overactivity.

manipulation Managing a person or situation unfairly or unscrupulously to one's own advantage.

medication adherence Formerly called compliance, this refers to maintaining a prescribed medication regimen.

mental disorder A diagnosable illness that significantly interferes with an individual's cognitive, emotional or social abilities; a condition in which an individual cannot cope and function as they did previously, causing considerable personal, social and financial distress.

mental health A state in which an individual has a positive sense of self, personal and social support with which to respond to life's challenges, meaningful relationships with others, access to employment and recreational activities, sufficient financial resources and suitable living arrangements.

mental health assessment and outcome measures Standardised measures in mental health for more reliable, valid and consistent measures of initial assessment and change that occurs with treatment.

mental health first aid A course designed to raise awareness and recognition of mental illness.

mental health legislation Legislation that establishes criteria for mental health detention and treatment without consent, and protects the rights of individuals.

mental health policy Local and national policies governing the provision of mental health services and promoting mental health; and international health policy based on the World Health Organization guiding principles of access, equity, effectiveness and efficiency for all people with mental health issues.

mental health problem Diminished cognitive, emotional or social abilities but not to the extent that the criteria for a diagnosable mental disorder are met.

mental health promotion A population-health approach to mental health that attends to the mental health status and needs of the whole population, emphasising a continuum of care from universal prevention to long-term individual care with early intervention and treatment.

mental illness A condition of impairment resulting in significant changes in emotional, psychological or social functioning.

Mental Status Assessment/Examination (MSA/MSE) An assessment of the person's current neurological and psychological status using several dimensions, such as perception, affect, thought content, form of thought and speech.

mental wellbeing The state in which an individual realises their own abilities, can cope with normal stresses of life, can work productively and is able to make a contribution to their community.

mentoring Process aimed at promoting growth and development in clinicians by means of partnerships with other clinicians in the workplace, involving problem solving, feedback, support and relationship building.

metabolic syndrome A group of risk factors that together predict cardiovascular disease and type 2 diabetes. Risk factors include hypertension, elevated triglycerides, elevated high-density lipoproteins and weight gain. Metabolic syndrome is common in people taking second-generation antipsychotic agents.

milieu therapy Therapy that involves the environment in the treatment process, the participation of patients and staff in decision making, the use of a multidisciplinary team, open communication and individualised goal setting with patients.

mindfulness Deliberate awareness of the present; openly interested and receptive.

Mini-Mental State Examination (MMSE) A standardised assessment of mental state; based on observable behaviour in a patient assessment interview; results in a score between 0 and 30.

mood A subjective emotion that colours the person's perception of the world (in contrast to *affect,* which is objective and observable, the visible expression of emotions).

motivational interviewing (MI) A form of interviewing aimed at maximising a patient's ability to change a problem behaviour; proceeds from the assumption that change is produced collaboratively and cannot be imposed from outside.

mourning An emotional response to the loss of a loved person or a valued part of someone's life. See also *grief.*

multidisciplinary team (MDT) A team of clinicians from multiple disciplines, such as nurses, psychologists, psychiatrists, social workers and occupational therapists, working together to provide a holistic team approach to care.

N

narcissistic Excessive love of self.

nature versus nurture debate Discussion about the effects of biological phenomena and inheritance (nature) and the individual's environment and experiences in the world (nurture) and whether both are vital, inseparable, interdependent components of personality development that influence human behaviour.

negative symptoms of schizophrenia Signs and symptoms such as blunting of *affect, avolition* and *anhedonia.*

negligence Failure to take all reasonable action to provide an appropriate standard of care and to prevent harm.

neologism Disturbance in form of thought, in which a person creates new words or expressions that have no recognised meaning.

neuroleptic malignant syndrome A rare disorder caused by antipsychotic medication and characterised by fever, muscular rigidity, altered mental status and autonomic dysfunction; risk of death is high if it is not treated.

neuropsychiatric disorders Disorders, such as Huntington disease, in which the origin of the psychological disturbance lies in the neurological structure and function of the brain.

neurosis A historical term that was used in reference to madness caused by nervous system disease. Since Freud's time, 'neurosis' has been used to refer to nonpsychotic disorder characterised mainly by anxiety.

neurotransmitter Chemical messenger necessary for communication between neurons. Neurotransmitters involved in psychological functions include acetylcholine, noradrenaline, dopamine, serotonin (5HT) and gamma-aminobutyric acid (GABA).

non-government organisations (NGOs) Services that operate outside mainstream government authority and at a community level to support patients and carers with a range of special needs, e.g. Association of Relatives and Friends of the Mentally Ill (ARAFMI).

nonmaleficence An ethical principle that means above all to do no harm and implies both a duty of care to avoid actual harm and considering the risks of any potential harm.

non-suicidal self-injury (NSSI) Intentional, self-effected, low-lethality bodily harm of a socially unacceptable nature, performed to reduce and/or communicate psychological distress.

normalisation A humanistic model of care in which people with an intellectual disability are given the same rights and opportunities as any other person and the support of appropriate services.

nurse–patient relationship The nurse and the person work together towards the person's growth and independent problem solving. The relationship exists for the benefit of the patient and at every interaction the nurse uses self therapeutically. This is achieved by maintaining the nurse's self-awareness to prevent unrecognised needs from influencing their perception of and behaviour towards the patient.

nurse practitioner An advanced practitioner with a high degree of autonomy, who has extended education within a defined scope of practice and is licensed to practise within an extended role.

O

observation A continuous watchful presence in a nonthreatening, nonintrusive manner to maintain safety and set reasonable limits on behaviour.

obsessions Recurrent, persistent thoughts, impulses and images that are intrusive and inappropriate and cause marked anxiety or distress.

obsessive-compulsive disorder Recurrent obsessions or compulsions that are severe enough to be time consuming or cause marked distress or significant impairment.

obstructive sleep apnoea The most common form of sleep-disordered breathing. Untreated, it is associated with high morbidity and mortality due to increased risks of cardio- and cerebrovascular disease, worsening of diabetes and hypertension.

P

panic attack A discrete period of intense fear or discomfort in the absence of real danger.

panic disorder The presence of recurrent, unexpected panic attacks followed by concern about having another panic attack or significant behavioural change related to the attacks.

paranoia Unfounded suspicion and distrust of others and their actions.

Parkinson syndrome One of the side effects of *antipsychotic medication*, with the person exhibiting a rigid, mask-like facial expression, shuffling gait and drooling.

passivity A state of inactivity and submissiveness/acceptance; can involve being influenced by the will of another.

patient Someone who has the lived experience of mental distress and who has received care from mental health professionals.

peer support The provision of support to people with mental health challenges by people who have also experienced challenges with their mental health.

perinatal depression Depression occurring in the antenatal (before birth) and postpartum (after birth) periods, characterised by depressed mood, excessive anxiety, insomnia and change in weight.

perseveration A disturbance in form of thought, in which the individual persistently repeats the same word or ideas; often associated with organic brain disease.

personal agency A recovery principle; discovering a more active sense of self.

personality Expression of our feelings, thoughts and patterns of behaviour that evolve over time.

personality disorder A diagnosis made when manifestations of personality in an individual start to interfere negatively with the individual's life or with the lives of those close to them. Personality disorders include paranoid, schizoid, schizotypal, antisocial, borderline, histrionic, narcissistic, avoidant, dependent and obsessive-compulsive.

personality traits Aspects of our personality that make us unique and differentiate us from each other.

person-centred planning A process of shared responsibility whereby a person is provided with the opportunity to take full control of setting lifestyle goals and negotiating with others how those goals will be achieved.

pet therapy Use of pets and even companion robots such as animal robots to reduce agitation and improve quality of life.

pharmacodynamics The processes by which drugs and their metabolites influence biological functioning.

pharmacokinetics The study of the actions of drugs within the body, including the mechanisms of absorption, distribution, metabolism and excretion.

phobia An irrational fear of something, so that the person feels compelled to avoid it.

polypharmacy Concurrent use of multiple psychotropic medications. Although polypharmacy might be useful in some instances, it is generally not advisable as it increases the chance of side effects and interactions. Polypharmacy can be extremely problematic in older people.

positive symptoms of schizophrenia Signs and symptoms such as delusions and hallucinations.

postpartum depression A condition characterised by depressed mood, excessive anxiety, insomnia and change in weight occurring in the 6 months following giving birth.

postpartum psychosis A rare psychotic disorder in women who have recently given birth, characterised by depression, delusions and thoughts of harming herself or her infant.

posttraumatic stress disorder (PTSD) A condition where the person experiences severe psychological distress as a result of a traumatic past experience or set of experiences.

preceptoring A relationship usually based in the clinical environment, occurring between a nurse who is new to an area and a preceptor (a more experienced nurse) who is allocated to support the nurse.

pressure of speech Speech that is increased in amount, accelerated and difficult or impossible to interrupt.

prevalence A measurement of all individuals affected by a disease or who had a specific characteristic at a particular time.

primary gain Results in relief from psychological pain, anxiety and conflict. For example, having physical symptoms gives legitimacy to feeling unwell.

primary mental healthcare Strategies and interventions for reducing the prevalence and impact of mental health problems in the community; includes increasing detection, promotion, prevention, early intervention and effective treatment.

prn (pro re nata) medication Medication that is given on an as-needed basis rather than at set times.

prodrome/prodromal An early or premonitory sign or symptom of a disorder.

professional boundaries Limitations that need to be agreed upon in therapeutic relationships between the patient and the nurse. These boundaries define acceptable and expected behaviour for both the nurse and the patient that ensures a 'safe' environment based on ethical practice.

progressive muscle relaxation (PMR) Involves the progressive relaxation of the major muscles of the body while making a conscious effort to distinguish muscle tension from muscle relaxation.

protective factors A number of aspects that guard a person against mental health problems or mental illness; can include, for example, positive relationships, support from peers and a sense of humour.

psychiatric liaison A role where a mental health nurse offers assessment services, advice and assistance to staff in non–mental health settings about the management of people with mental health problems.

psychoanalytic theory Developed by Freud, this theory places strong emphasis on the role of the unconscious in determining human behaviour. Mental illness is seen as a state of being fixated at a developmental stage or conflict that has not been resolved.

psychodynamic theory Rooted in the belief that we develop a sense of self during childhood and that difficulties of living can be resolved by examining childhood development of the psyche that shaped the person's subsequent decisions.

psychoeducation Education concerning a patient's mental illness and treatment, aimed at promoting wellness and providing an opportunity for the person to gain insight into their condition.

psychological first aid (PFA) Designed to identify unobtrusively and quickly who is in need of immediate intervention. Rather than focussing on pathology, the emphasis is on reducing acute distress by encouraging adaptive coping.

psychomotor retardation Marked slowing in mental and physical activity, often associated with depression.

psychopathology A term that refers to either the study of mental illness or mental distress or the manifestation of behaviours and experiences that may be indicative of mental illness or psychological impairment. It is also a synonym for mental illness.

psychopharmacology The use of medications to treat psychiatric disorders. Psychopharmacology includes medication indications, interactions, side effects and precautions, patient experience and education, and the issues of adherence and as-needed or prn administration.

psychosis/psychotic disorder A condition in which a person has impaired cognition, emotional, social and communicative responses and interpretation of reality.

psychosocial rehabilitation Working with people who are mentally ill to assist them to reintegrate into the community.

psychotherapy A form of therapy that is concerned with the nature of the human experience; it has a number of interpersonal models with individual philosophy and set techniques, such as *cognitive behavioural therapy*, *motivational interviewing* and planned short-term *psychotherapy*.

psychotropic/psychoactive medications A collection of pharmacological agents in current psychiatric use: antianxiety sedatives, antidepressants, mood-stabilising, neuroleptic and antipsychotic drugs.

R

racism An ideology of inferiority that labels some ethnic/racial groups as inferior to others. Characterised by avoidable and unfair actions that further disadvantage the disadvantaged and advantage the advantaged, expressed through beliefs, actions and prejudice.

reality testing/confrontation Reflecting an individual's behaviour back to them; a form of giving information and sharing feelings in an acceptable way.

recidivism The repetition (relapse) of criminal behaviour.

recovery Being able to create and live a meaningful and contributing life in a community of choice with or without the presence of mental health issues. Recovery begins as soon as a person develops mental health problems, emphasising hope, positive mental health and wellness.

reflection A process of critically reviewing experiences and using them to inform and change future practice in a positive way.

reflective practice Processes that allow nurses to examine both their practice (actions) and the accompanying cognitions (thoughts) and affective meanings (feelings) in relation to their values, biases and knowledge, in the context of a particular situation.

regulation System whereby authorities set and monitor standards in the interests of the public and the professions, and maintain registers of individuals licensed to practise nursing.

relapse prevention Programmes that aim to teach patients a set of cognitive and behavioural strategies to enhance their capacity to cope with high-risk situations that could otherwise precipitate relapse.

resilience An individual's innate ability to achieve good outcomes in spite of adversity, serious threats and risks.

resocialisation Reestablishing social support networks and peer support through group therapy and individual goal setting.

respite care Planned or emergency temporary care provided to carers that affords the carer an opportunity to attend to their personal everyday activities.

risk assessment/management Assessment of a patient with regard to various factors: risk of harm to self, risk of harm to others, risk of suicide, risk of absconding and vulnerability to exploitation or abuse. Identifying and estimating risk so that structured decisions can be made as to how best to manage a risk behaviour.

rumination Repetitive and increasingly intrusive negative thoughts and ideas, which can eventually interfere with other thought processes.

S

schizophrenia A disorder characterised by major disturbances in thought, perception, thinking and psychosocial functioning; a severe mental illness.

seclusion An intervention to prevent harm to the person and others; a method of managing difficult behaviour, based on the therapeutic principles of containment, isolation and decrease in sensory input; usually instigated when other methods, such as talking and medication, have failed.

secondary gain The attention and support provided by others for a physical illness; can involve any benefit other than relief from anxiety.

self-awareness The process of becoming aware of and examining one's own personal beliefs, attitudes and motivations and recognising how these may affect others.

self-disclosure Making knowledge about oneself known to others.

self-efficacy The person's expectation that they can cope with and master life events effectively, and that their efforts will achieve satisfactory outcomes.

self-harm Behaviour occurring along a continuum, from pulling one's own hair out to cutting, piercing and burning oneself, through to suicide. These behaviours may be a mode of emotional self-regulation for the patient and can be comforting and confirming in a world that is out of control from their perspective.

self-help Listening to one's own self-wisdom; can also involve seeking assistance and support from others who have had similar experiences to learn coping skills, tap into resources and find useful information.

service user An alternative term to 'patient', 'client' or 'consumer'.

sexual abuse Unwanted sexual activity with the perpetrator using force, making threats or taking advantage of victims not able to give consent.

sexual health All aspects of sexual functioning and related healthcare, including relationships, screening for sexually transmitted diseases, sexual side effects of medications and reproductive health.

sexuality Involves people's gendered sex, their sexual feelings for others, their feelings about themselves as sexual beings, their sexual orientation and their sexual behaviour.

sleep hygiene The development of personal practices that assist in gaining adequate good-quality sleep.

social determinants of health The conditions in which people are born, grow, live, work and age.

social inclusion Involves the provision of rights and opportunities to all individuals and groups in society, such as employment, adequate housing, healthcare, education and training.

social skills training Helping people to relearn the skills they need in order to engage with other people and the communities in which they live. Social skills training groups combine instruction, modelling, rehearsal and role playing, as well as coaching, feedback and reinforcement.

sociological theories Theories that examine the influence of societal factors on the behaviour of individuals.

Socratic questioning A common technique for encouraging self-understanding and motivation, which helps the patient to come to an alternative belief of their own.

solution-focussed brief therapy (SFBT) Encourages solutions rather than dwelling on problems; based on the strengths approach, SFBT works with the person's strengths and capacities and assumes that they are capable of knowing what is best for them and of achieving self-defined goals.

somatisation A psychological process whereby anxiety or psychological conflict is translated into physical complaints, although no mechanism has been found.

spirituality Inclusive of the patient's concept of God, sources of strength and hope, religious practices and meaning and purpose in the patient's life.

splitting An attempt to split a group by appealing to individual members, by sharing 'secrets' and suggesting that one person is the 'only one' who understands them or is approachable.

stage theories Theories based on measuring and monitoring a person's individual development against a set of expected 'norms' as certain age milestones are achieved.

standards of practice Professional standards that describe the expected performance of nurses providing mental healthcare; represent the commitment to accountability of mental health nurses. Mental health nursing standards of practice include a rationale and attributes for each standard.

stepped care Mental healthcare that is staged to provide an appropriate level of intervention for the seriousness of an individual's mental illness or symptoms. Stepped care begins in primary care with stages from advice and guided self-help through to psychological intervention, medication and hospitalisation.

stigma A notion that mental illness is something to be avoided, hidden away or shameful.

strengths A person's resilience, aspirations, talents and uniqueness; what a person can do and do well.

strengths-based approach The strengths model proposes that all people have goals, talents and confidence, and that all environments contain resources, people and opportunities. Focussing on strengths and personal values promotes a person's resilience, aspirations, talents and uniqueness, what the person can do and how strengths can be mobilised to overcome current difficulties.

stress A psychological response to any demand or stressor; can be experienced as negative (distress) or positive. Individuals can respond differently to the same stressor.

stress-diathesis model A model used to understand how mental illness occurs; individuals are exposed to stressful events in the course of their lives and these events may precipitate symptoms in some people who have a predisposition to mental illness.

stress management Managing the effects of the stress one is experiencing by changing the situation, increasing one's ability to deal with the situation, changing one's perception of the situation and/or changing one's behaviour.

substance abuse The use of drugs or alcohol in a way that disrupts prevailing social norms; these norms vary with culture, gender and generations.

suicide The intentional killing of oneself.

support worker A nonprofessional mental health worker who works with people with mental illness to enable them to function well and achieve personal life goals.

supportive environments See *enabling environments.*

T

tangentiality A disturbance in form of thought in which the individual gives irrelevant or oblique replies to questions; the reply might refer to the topic but not be a complete answer.

tardive dyskinesia Stereotypical involuntary movement of the tongue, lips and feet; results from prolonged use of traditional antipsychotics.

telephone counselling Method of crisis counselling that usually involves a single session and affords anonymity to the caller at a time when the person may be feeling vulnerable. The counsellor helps the person to cope with the crisis by working through feelings and problem solving.

therapeutic relationship The development of the trusting, beneficial and understanding partnership that needs to exist between the nurse and the patient for a therapeutic relationship to develop.

therapeutic community An environment in which the emphasis is on normal functioning rather than on an illness or a disability. Decision making is shared and relationships between staff and residents are intended to be nonhierarchical.

thought blocking A disturbance in form of thought in which there are abrupt gaps in the individual's flow of thoughts; not caused by anxiety, poor concentration or being distracted.

thought broadcasting The belief that one's thoughts are being broadcast from one's head to the external world.

thought disorder A disturbance of the form in which an individual expresses their thoughts (structure, grammar, syntax, logic) or sometimes the content of their thoughts.

tic An involuntary, sudden, rapid, recurrent, nonrhythmic, stereotyped motor movement or vocalisation.

tolerance With medication or substance use, needing more and more of the substance to get the effect you want. Results from the repeated effects of daily doses of drugs such as alcohol, methamphetamines, nicotine or opioids.

toxicity Nontherapeutic, harmful effects of medication usually associated with high serum levels, sensitivity to the effects of the medication or impaired ability to metabolise or excrete the medication.

transference When a person transfers beliefs, feelings, thoughts or behaviours that occurred in a past situation to a situation happening in the present. The person with unconscious feelings or beliefs about someone in their past transfers these feelings or beliefs onto another, unfamiliar person.

trauma A severe physical injury or a specific experience that triggers mental and emotional distress and results in suffering and disruption to the person's physical and/or emotional wellbeing.

trauma-informed care Core features of trauma-informed care are safety, trustworthiness, choice, collaboration and empowerment.

triage assessment A process for decision making that occurs when alternatives for acute care are being considered. A comprehensive assessment is undertaken, including the person's symptoms and current situation.

V

victim A person who has endured a form of physical and/or psychological or emotional harm at another's hand; for example, a person who has suffered sexual assault, domestic violence and/or rape.

violence Physical or psychological attack where the intent is to cause harm to an individual or object.

voluntary admission Admission of individuals, with their full consent, who require treatment in an approved mental health setting because of the severity of their mental illness, and also for individuals suffering from an acute episode of a mental illness.

vulnerable Capable of being physically or emotionally harmed, wounded or hurt.

W

withdrawal The development of a substance-specific syndrome due to the cessation of (or reduction in) substance use that has been heavy and prolonged. Most individuals going through withdrawal have a craving to readminister the substance to reduce the symptoms.

INDEX

Note: Page numbers followed by "f" indicate figures, "t" indicate tables and "b" indicate boxes.

D

E

Q

R

S